Viral Infections of Humans

Epidemiology and Control

SECOND EDITION

Viral Infections of Humans

Epidemiology and Control

SECOND EDITION
completely revised and expanded

Edited by

Alfred S. Evans

Yale University
New Haven, Connecticut

PLENUM MEDICAL BOOK COMPANY

New York and London

Library of Congress Cataloging in Publication Data

Main entry under title:

Viral infections of humans.

Includes bibliographies and index.
1. Virus diseases. 2. Epidemiology. 3. Virus diseases—Prevention. I. Evans,
Alfred S., 1917 –   . [DNLM: 1. Virus diseases—Prevention and control. 2.
Virus diseases—Occurrence. WC 500 V8155]
RA644.V55V57 1982   614.5'7   82-3684
ISBN-13: 978-1-4613-3239-8   e-ISBN-13: 978-1-4613-3237-4   AACR2
DOI: 10.1007/ 978-1-4613-3237-4

© 1982 Plenum Publishing Corporation
Softcover reprint of the hardcover 1st edition 1982
233 Spring Street, New York, N.Y. 10013

Plenum Medical Book Company is an imprint of Plenum Publishing Corporation

Dedication

This book is dedicated to Dr. John R. Paul, who introduced me to the field of epidemiology and to the concepts of clinical and serological epidemiology; to Dr. Thomas F. Francis, who arranged and supervised my Master of Public Health degree (in epidemiology) at the University of Michigan School of Public Health; to Dr. William D. Stovall, who taught me the potential contributions of the public health laboratory to epidemiology and to preventive medicine; to Dr. David Seegal and Dr. John R. Talbott, my mentors in clinical medicine; and to Dr. Ernst J. Witebsky, Dr. Paul F. Clark, and Dr. Victor C. Seastone, my teachers and associates in immunology and microbiology.

ACKNOWLEDGMENTS. This publication was supported for editorial preparation in part by NIH grant LM 03299 from the National Library of Medicine. I also wish to thank my wife Brigitte, and children John, Barbara, and Christopher, for their patience and support.

A. S. EVANS

Contributors

Abram S. Benenson, Gorgas Memorial Laboratory, Panama, Republic of Panama. Present address: School of Graduate Studies and Public Health, San Diego State University, San Diego, California

Francis L. Black, Department of Epidemiology and Public Health, Yale University School of Medicine, New Haven, Connecticut

Carl D. Brandt, Children's Hospital National Medical Center of Washington, D.C.; and George Washington University School of Medicine and Health Sciences, Department of Child Health and Development, Washington, D.C.

Jacob A. Brody, Epidemiology, Demography, Biometry, National Institute on Aging, National Institutes of Health, Bethesda, Maryland

Jordi Casals, Department of Epidemiology and Public Health, Yale University School of Medicine, New Haven, Connecticut

Robert M. Chanock, Laboratory of Infectious Diseases, National Institute of Allergy and Infectious Diseases, National Institutes of Health, Bethesda, Maryland; Children's Hospital National Medical Center of Washington, D.C.; and George Washington University School of Medicine and Health Sciences, Department of Child Health and Development, Washington, D.C.

†Fred M. Davenport, Department of Epidemiology, School of Public Health, University of Michigan, Ann Arbor, Michigan (Deceased March, 1982)

Floyd W. Denny, Department of Pediatrics, School of Medicine, University of North Carolina, Chapel Hill, North Carolina

G. de-Thé, CNRS, Faculty of Medicine A. Carrel, Lyon and Cancer Institute—CNRS, Villejuif, France

Wilbur G. Downs, Yale Arbovirus Research Unit, Department of Epidemiology and Public Health, Yale University School of Medicine, New Haven, Connecticut

Alfred S. Evans, WHO Serum Reference Bank, Section of International Epidemiology, Department of Epidemiology and Public Health, Yale University School of Medicine, New Haven, Connecticut

Harry A. Feldman, Department of Preventive Medicine, State University of New York, Upstate Medical Center, Syracuse, New York

Hjordis M. Foy, Department of Epidemiology and International Health, School of Public Health and Community Medicine, University of Washington, Seattle, Washington

Clarence Joseph Gibbs, Jr., Laboratory of Central Nervous System Studies, National Institute of Neurological and Communicative Disorders and Stroke, National Institutes of Health, Bethesda, Maryland

W. Paul Glezen, Department of Microbiology and Immunology, Baylor College of Medicine, Houston Texas

Eli Gold, Department of Pediatrics, University of California, Davis, California

J. Thomas Grayston, Department of Epidemiology and International Health, School of Public Health and Community Medicine, University of Washington, Seattle, Washington

Harry B. Greenberg, Laboratory of Infectious Diseases, National Institute of Allergy and Infectious Diseases, National Institutes of Health, Bethesda, Maryland

Jack M. Gwaltney, Jr., Department of Internal Medicine, University of Virginia School of Medicine, Charlottesville, Virginia

J. H. C. Ho, Institute of Radiology and Oncology, Queen Elizabeth Hospital, Kowloon, Hong Kong

Dorothy M. Horstmann, Department of Epidemiology and Public Health and Department of Pediatrics, Yale University School of Medicine, New Haven, Connecticut

Karl M. Johnson, Center for Disease Control, Special Pathogens Branch, Virology Division, Bureau of Laboratories, U.S. Public Health Service, U.S. Department of Health and Human Services, Atlanta, Georgia

William E. Josey, Department of Gynecology and Obstetrics, Emory University School of Medicine, Atlanta, Georgia

Anthony R. Kalica, Laboratory of Infectious Diseases, National Institute of Allergy and Infectious Diseases, National Institutes of Health, Bethesda, Maryland

Albert Z. Kapikian, Laboratory of Infectious Diseases, National Institute of Allergy and Infectious Diseases, National Institutes of Health, Bethesda, Maryland

Hyun Wha Kim, Children's Hospital National Medical Center of Washington, D.C.; and George Washington University School of Medicine and Health Sciences, Department of Child Health and Development, Washington, D.C.

Frank A. Loda, Department of Pediatrics, School of Medicine, University of North Carolina, Chapel Hill, North Carolina

Robert W. McCollum, Department of Epidemiology and Public Health, Yale University School of Medicine, New Haven, Connecticut

Joseph L. Melnick, Department of Virology and Epidemiology, Baylor College of Medicine, Houston, Texas

George Miller, Department of Pediatrics and Department of Epidemiology and Public Health, Yale University School of Medicine, New Haven, Connecticut

Arnold S. Monto, Department of Epidemiology, School of Public Health, University of Michigan, Ann Arbor, Michigan

C. S. Muir, International Agency for Research on Cancer, Lyon, France

André J. Nahmias, Department of Pediatrics, Emory University School of Medicine, Atlanta, Georgia

George A. Nankervis, Department of Pediatrics, Medical College of Ohio, Toledo, Ohio

James C. Niederman, Department of Epidemiology and Public Health, Yale University School of Medicine, New Haven, Connecticut

James M. Oleske, Department of Pediatrics, New Jersey College of Medicine, Newark, New Jersey

Robert H. Parrott, Children's Hospital National Medical Center of Washington, D.C.; and George Washington University School of Medicine and Health Sciences, Department of Child Health and Development, Washington, D.C.

William J. Rodriguez, Children's Hospital National Medical Center of Washington, D.C.; and George Washington University School of Medicine and Health Sciences, Department of Child Health and Development, Washington, D.C.

Robert E. Shope, Department of Epidemiology and Public Health, Yale University School of Medicine, New Haven, Connecticut

Thomas H. Weller, Department of Tropical Public Health, Center for Prevention of Infectious Diseases, Harvard School of Public Health, Boston, Massachusetts

Richard G. Wyatt, Laboratory of Infectious Diseases, National Institute of Allergy and Infectious Diseases, National Institutes of Health, Bethesda, Maryland

Preface to the Second Edition

Each chapter of this second edition has been updated and expanded by the authors, and two new chapters have been added. One is on viral gastroenteritis by Albert Kapikian and his associates and deals with the rotavirus and Norwalk groups of agents. The second, by Karl Johnson, is on the African hemorrhagic fevers caused by Marburg and Ebola viruses. The reader will note that some viral groups such as cat scratch fever agent, mulluscum contagiosum, human papilloma viruses, and reoviruses are not yet included. This is because sufficient information on the agent and its epidemiology is not yet available or because it was not regarded as a common cause of human illness.

As a guide to readers familiar with the first edition, some highlights of the new material in the second edition are listed below.

I. Introduction and Concepts

Chapter 1, Epidemiological Concepts and Methods: New sections on investigating an epidemic, the host, congenital infections, hospital infections, and infections in immunosuppressed and surgical patients have been added.

Chapter 2, Surveillance and Seroepidemiology: A new section on viruses, cancer, and chronic disease is included.

II. Acute Viral Infections

Chapter 3, Adenoviruses: There are now 33 distinct immunological types. Severe infections may occur in congenital immunodeficiency, among immunosuppressed patients, and following measles. Type 7 has produced prolonged outbreaks in England. Reactivation of adenovirus infections may possibly be evoked by other respiratory agents. Healthy carrier rates may reach 18% in recruits.

Chapter 4, African Hemmorhagic Fevers: This new chapter by Karl Johnson deals with Marburg and Ebola viruses whose importation poses a continual threat outside Germany and Yugoslavia, where Marburg agent has been active, and the Sudan and Zaire, where Ebola is endemic.

Chapter 5, Arboviruses: Transovarial transmission—first of California viruses and later of all four types of dengue virus, Japanese B encephalitis virus, and yellow fever virus—has now been demonstrated, providing an important contribution to the mechanism of survival of these agents in nature. Venereal transmission of California LaCrosse virus also occurs. New outbreaks of yellow fever have occurred in Colombia and Trinidad and new outbreaks of rift valley fever have occurred in Egypt.

Chapter 6, Arenaviruses: The biochemical and physical properties have now been clarified, and they show a remarkable uniformity in the various viruses constituting the group. The possibility that prenatal infection with LCM may result in hydrocephalus and chorioretinitis has been raised. Serologic surveys have suggested the existence of Lassa virus infection in Guinea, Central African Empire, Mali, Senegal, Cameroon, and Benin, in addition to earlier identification in Nigeria, Liberia, and Sierra Leone.

Chapter 7, Coronaviruses: New studies have confirmed the important role of these viruses in common respiratory illnesses of children and adults. The viruses are now known to contain a single positive strand of RNA. About 50% of corona virus infections result in clinical illness. About 5% of common colds are caused by strain DC 43 in winter.

Chapter 8, Cytomegalovirus: Sections on pathogenesis of CMV in relation to organ transplantation and mononucleosis, as well as sections on the risk and features of congenital infection and disease, have been expanded. There are encouraging preliminary results with a live CMV vaccine, but the questions of viral persistence and oncogenicity require further evaluation.

Chapter 9, Enteroviruses: Hepatitis A is now considered an enterovirus, but it is discussed in Chapter 12. An enterovirus unrelated to any known type was isolated in South Africa mainly from patients diagnosed clinically as having poliomyelitis but from whom no poliovirus could be isolated; it could be passaged only in suckling mice and is now designated as enterovirus 71. Epidemics of acute hemorrhagic conjunctivitis caused by enterovirus 70 occurred in Asia, with small outbreaks in Europe but not yet in Australia or the Americas. Enterovirus 70 has now been recognized globally with different clinical manifestations in such areas as aseptic meningitis, encephalitis, paralysis, and the hand, foot, mouth syndrome. Chronic cardiovascular diseases may follow coxsackie carditis, and coxsackie B may induce severe neonatal infection; diabetes has resulted from coxsackie B4 in one 4-year-old boy.

Chapter 10, Epstein–Barr Virus: Advances have been made in the understanding of the immune response to EBV infections and of the pathogenesis of infectious mononucleosis. Psychosocial factors play a role in the development of clinical disease among those infected. Severe and fatal complications of the EBV infection as well as the immunoblastic B-cell sarcoma, Burkitt lymphoma, and various lytic complications occur in immunodeficient persons, especially in those genetically related as in the X-linked lymphoproliferative syndrome. Typical IM in childhood and in developing countries is now recognized through more sensitive tests, as are some syndromes such as pneumonitis and hepatitis in the absence of other features of IM.

Chapter 11, Viral Gastroenteritis: This new chapter emphasizes the importance of the rotavirus and Norwalk group of viruses. The former causes about 50% of acute gastroenteritis in children under 3 throughout the world, and the latter is an important cause of outbreaks of gastroenteritis in both children and adults.

Chapter 12, Viral Hepatitis: There is increased recognition of the importance of non-A, non-B hepatitis in transfusion hepatitis as well as in sporadic cases. Antibody tests for hepatitis A have indicated its common occurence worldwide. An important link of hepatitis B to hepatocellular cancer is being vigorously pursued. Vaccines against HBV are on clinical trial.

Chapter 13, Herpes Simplex Viruses 1 and 2: The immunological responses to infection, the mechanism of latency and reactivation in nerve tissue, and the broadening spectrum of host–response constitute new advances.

Chapter 14, Influenza Viruses: The most important advance since the appearance of the first edition is the ability to characterize RNA fragments of the viral genome. This is a technical development, and whether or not it can be applied to solution of epidemiological problems has yet to be established.

Chapter 15, Measles: There is increasing recognition of natural measles under age 1 in developing countries and of focal outbreaks in unimmunized children in developed countries. Atypical measles in persons receiving killed measles vaccine or live vaccine under age 1 occurs in the United States but will disappear over time since CDC now recommends vaccination at about "15 months of age." In developing countries, early immunization at age 6–9 months is necessary to prevent measles mortality, but whether a later booster dose is desirable has not been clearly established. The elimination of measles by vaccination is the United States is a goal of the CDC.

Chapter 16, Mumps: In the 10 years since the licensing of live vaccine in the United States and its increasing utilization in immunization programs, the reported case rates have decreased from about 88 per 100,000 in 1968 to under 10 by 1978. Since, as with measles, man is the only reservoir, there is hope of eventual eradication.

Chapter 17, Parainfluenza Viruses: Direct viral diagnosis is now possible through the examination—by immunofluorescent techniques—of epithelial cells from throat washings.

Chapter 18, Rabies: A new rabies vaccine grown in human diploid cells has now been licensed in the United States. It requires only five doses and induces an excellent antibody response. A revised schedule for use of vaccine and human immunoglobulin now recommends their combined use after almost all types of rabies exposure, irrespective of the time of initiation after exposure. Soap and water is recommended for local cleaning. New diagnostic and isolation techniques are under development.

Chapter 19, Respiratory Syncytial Virus: This remains the major pathogen of the lower respiratory tract of infancy and childhood throughout the world, but the pathogenesis of serious disease in early infancy is not well understood. Virus-specific IgA antibodies have been found in nasal secretions of infected infants but do not neutralize RSV. A vaccine is not yet available, but encouraging results have been found experimentally with a *ts* mutant and with a live vaccine grown in human diploid cells and injected parenterally into seronegative infants.

Chapter 20, Rhinoviruses: While recoverable from the lower respiratory tract, rhinoviruses are probably not an important cause of viral pneumonia, croup, or bronchiolitis. Rather, they may be a precipitant of asthmatic attacks in children through unknown mechanisms. Psychological factors may play a role in susceptibility to rhinovirus infection or illness. The multiplicity of specific antigenic types of varying epidemiological behavior has thus far limited vaccine development. Administration of interferon prior to, but not during, experimental common colds appears to reduce their severity. The evidence favoring vitamin C is inadequate to recommend its use for prevention or therapy.

Chapter 21, Rubella: The RA 27/3 vaccine, grown in WI 38 cells, is now available for use in the United States. It retains ability to infect intranasally and induces a broader antibody response—including local IgA production— and higher resistance to reinfection than earlier vaccines. There is increasing emphasis on vaccine use in adolescents and young women, especially at time of entrance to high school, but with a strong contraindiction to its use in pregnant women; serological tests to identify susceptibility to rubella are desirable prior to vaccination in women of childbearing age, as are tests for pregnancy if doubt exists.

Chapter 22, Smallpox: No case of natural smallpox has occurred since October, 1977, and on December 9, 1979 the Global Commission certified that smallpox had been eradicated from the world. Thus this chapter can be regarded as a "requiem for a heavyweight." However, the presence of "whitepox" virus in monkeys, the fact that the only known difference of this virus from variola virus is its infectivity for man, and the reports of 36 cases of monkeypox virus infection in humans up to April, 1979 all stress the need for vigilance.

Chapter 23, Varicella–Herpes Zoster Virus: New developments include new diagnostic and seroepidemiologic techniques, advances in our knowledge of the role of cellular immunity in zoster infections, the proof of effectiveness of antiviral chemotherapy, and the encouraging results with a candidate varicella vaccine developed by Japanese workers.

III. Malignant and Chronic Neurological Diseases Associated with Viruses

Chapter 24, Burkitt Lymphoma: A prospective study of 42,000 children in the West Nile area of Africa revealed that 10 of 14 sera taken 7–54 months prior to detectable tumor had anti-VCA titers to EB virus 2-fold or more higher than in matched controls; a titer increase of this magnitude carried a 30-fold increased risk of BL. EBV genome was present in tumor tissue from most biopsied cases with elevated titers and absent from those with normal titers. About 90% of BL tumors contain a 14q + chromosome marker; the marker has also been found in EBV-negative tumors. Strong evidence supports a causal role of EBV in African BL.

Chapter 25, Nasopharyngeal Carcinoma: Risk factors among high-incidence-rate Chinese are related to genetics and certain cultural practices, including feeding salted fish to infants just before and after weaning. Certain chemicals are also suspect. In the United States, the risk factors include a history of ENT disease and occupational exposure to fumes, smoke, and chemical. EBV-IgA antibody is present in both serum and nasopharyngeal washings of almost all NPC cases. In China a massive serum survey to detect this antibody has been a rewarding method of case detection: of the 56,584 persons age 30 or more tested, 117 had EBV-IgA, among whom 20 NPC cases were subsequently diagnosed.

Chapter 26, Cervical Cancer: Early results of prospective studies of women with and without HSV-2 antibody have shown a 4-fold higher frequency of severe cervical dysplasia and cancer *in situ* (CIS) in those with antibody; 6 of 28 women (21%) with a primary HSV-2 genital infection developed one of these lesions, ten times that of controls. A possible relation of cervical cancer to HLA-B12 has been reported. New antigens may yield better distinction between HSV-1 and HSV-2. Multiple disciplines are needed to resolve the possible relation of HSV-2 to cervical cancer.

Chapter 27, Chronic Neurological Diseases: Kuru and Creutzfeldt-Jakob Disease (CJD) remain rare and fatal diseases caused by agents that are probably closely related but whose biological nature and lack of immune response remain an enigma. Kuru is still localized in the Fore area of New Guinea, and no new infections have occurred since the discontinuance of cannibalism; previously infected cases are still appearing with an incubation period of up to 30 years. CJD is worldwide with an incidence throughout of about one per million. A comprehensive epidemiological study has been made in France. Oral transmission of kuru and CJD to monkeys experimentally has been reported, and the host range of CJD extends to cats, guinea pigs, and mice. The natural route of infection of CJD remains unknown although transmission by corneal transplants and brain electrodes from infected persons occurs, and transmission by transfusion is a potential hazard. Procedures for medical and surgical management of such patients have been developed. SSPE is a rare, late manifestation of measles infection early in life that has declined sharply with the widespread use of measles vaccine. It is not clear whether vaccine virus itself could occasionally induce SSPE. Progressive multifocal encephalopathy is still a very rare disease with a total of 200–250 reported cases; the ubiquitous virus that causes it produces no recognizable acute primary illness. PML has occurred in immunodeficient persons, including two children ages 5 and 11. Sections of PML brain reveal common polyomavirus antigen. The JC strain induces brain tumors in hamsters and monkeys, and in a very few human brains it has been found together with gliomatous or lymphomatous tumors.

Alfred S. Evans

New Haven

Contents

Chapter 2

Surveillance and Seroepidemiology
Alfred S. Evans

II. ACUTE VIRAL INFECTIONS

Chapter 3

Adenoviruses
Hjordis M. Foy and J. Thomas Grayston

Chapter 4

African Hemorrhagic Fevers Due to Marburg and Ebola Viruses

Karl M. Johnson

Chapter 5

Arboviruses

Wilbur G. Downs

Chapter 6

Arenaviruses
Jordi Casals

Chapter 7

Coronaviruses
Arnold S. Monto

Chapter 8

Cytomegalovirus
Eli Gold and George A. Nankervis

Chapter 9

Enteroviruses

Joseph L. Melnick

Chapter 10

Epstein–Barr Virus
Alfred S. Evans and James C. Niederman

Chapter 11

Viral Gastroenteritis

Albert Z. Kapikian, Harry B. Greenberg, Richard G. Wyatt, Anthony R. Kalica, Hyun Wha Kim, Carl D. Brandt, William J. Rodriguez, Robert H. Parrott, and Robert M. Chanock

Chapter 14

Influenza Viruses

Fred M. Davenport

Chapter 15

Measles

Francis L. Black

Chapter 16

Mumps
Harry A. Feldman

Chapter 19

Respiratory Syncytial Virus
Robert M. Chanock, Hyun Wha Kim, Carl D. Brandt, and Robert H. Parrott

Chapter 20

Rhinoviruses

Jack M. Gwaltney, Jr.

Chapter 23 | **Varicella–Herpes Zoster Virus**
Thomas H. Weller

III. MALIGNANT AND CHRONIC NEUROLOGICAL DISEASES ASSOCIATED WITH VIRUSES

Chapter 24

Burkitt Lymphoma
George Miller

Chapter 25 | Nasopharyngeal Carcinoma

G. de-Thé, J. H. C. Ho, and C. S. Muir

PART I

Introduction and Concepts

CHAPTER 1

Epidemiological Concepts and Methods

Alfred S. Evans

1. Introduction

The epidemiology of infectious diseases is concerned with the circumstances under which both infection *and* disease occur in a population and the factors that influence their frequency, spread, and distribution. This concept distinguishes between infection *and* disease because the factors that govern their occurrence may be different and because infection *without* disease is common with many viruses. Infection indicates the multiplication of an agent within the host and is determined largely by factors that govern exposure to the agent and by the susceptibility of the host. Disease represents the host response to infection when it is severe enough to evoke a recognizable pattern of clinical symptoms. The factors that influence the occurrence and the severity of this response vary with the particular viruses involved and their portal of entry, but the most important determinants for many common in-

fections lie within the host itself. Of these, the *age* at the time of infection is most crucial.

This first chapter will deal in a general way with concepts, methods, and control techniques that will be explored in detail in individual chapters concerned with specific viruses or groups of viruses. For fuller presentations of the epidemiological principles, see references 17, 44, 55, 73, 80, 92, 106, and 108.

2. Definitions and Methods

Incidence is the number of *new* cases of disease occurring in a unit of time. The incidence *rate* is the number of new cases over the total population at risk. The numerator in this ratio is usually based on the number of *clinical cases* of the disease in question as recognized by physicians and reported to public health departments over the period of a year. The denominator represents the population under surveillance. This is often the total population of the geographic area encompassed by the reporting system. In more intensive studies, the numerator may be defined as the incidence of infection (with or without disease) as determined by viral excretion

Alfred S. Evans WHO Serum Reference Bank, Section of International Epidemiology, Department of Epidemiology and Public Health, Yale University School of Medicine, New Haven, Connecticut.

and/or the appearance of antibody between two points in time. The denominator may be defined as those who are both exposed and susceptible (i.e., lack antibody). These more sophisticated definitions are usually restricted to special investigations in which antibody or viral measurements, or both, are possible.

Prevalence is the number of cases existing at one time. The *prevalence rate* is the number of such cases divided by the population at risk. The time period involved may be 1 year or other fixed period (period prevalence) or a given instant of time (point prevalence). The term *period prevalence* involves both the number of new cases (incidence) and the duration of illness (number of old cases persisting from the previous reporting period). It is used most commonly for chronic diseases.

In serological surveys, *prevalence* represents the presence of an antibody, antigen, chemical marker, or other component in blood samples from a given population at the time of the collection. The *prevalence rate* is the number of sera with that component divided by the number of persons whose blood was tested. For viral infections, the presence of antibody represents the cumulative infection rate over recent and past years depending on the duration of the antibody. For neutralizing or other long-lasting antibody, it reflects the lifetime or cumulative experience with that agent. If the antibody measured is of short duration, then prevalence indicates infection acquired within a recent period.

Descriptive epidemiology deals with the characteristics of the agent, the environment, and the host, and with the distribution of the resultant disease in terms of place, season, and secular trends. It is concerned with what the late John R. Paul[92] called "the seed, the soil and the climate." The delineation of these attributes of infection and disease in a population is the "meat" of epidemiology, and this text is largely one of this descriptive nature. The sources of data on which this volume is based are mortality and morbidity reports, field and serological surveys, and special investigations that will be described in detail in Chapter 2.

Analytical epidemiology is concerned with planned epidemiological investigations designed to weigh various risk factors or to evaluate a hypothesis of causation. Two methods of analytical study are commonly employed: the prospective and the retrospective.

The prospective method is a means of measuring incidence in a population or a cohort observed over time. In virology, incidence studies permit the direct assessment of the risk of infection or disease, or both, in a defined population group over time in terms of age, sex, socioeconomic level, and other factors. Both the numerator and the denominator are known. In practice, incidence rates are often calculated retrospectively by using data on cases and populations that have been filed away; in virology, infection rates can be determined by carrying out virus isolations or serological tests, or both, on materials that have been frozen away and for which data on the population sampled are available. Since such studies are not "prospective" in terms of the observer, calling them "cohort," "longitudinal," or "incidence" studies is more appropriate in a semantic sense. In addition to the direct measurement of risk, this type of investigation avoids the need of selecting controls, because one is merely recording the occurrence of disease or of infection in persons with different characteristics. The disadvantages of incidence studies are that they are expensive because an entire population must be kept under observation and appropriate specimens collected; the lower the incidence of the disease, the larger the denominator requiring observation and the higher the expense. They are sometimes laborious to conduct and may require much technical help.

Retrospective or case/control studies compare the presence or absence of certain suspected etiological factors in patients with a certain disease to their occurrence in subjects without this disease. An example is the relationship of smoking to the occurrence of lung cancer. Since both the disease and the characteristic are already present at the time of observation, the data obtained represent prevalence rather than incidence rates. The absolute risk of the disease in persons with different characteristics cannot be measured because no denominators are available. Only the relative prevalence of the disease in persons having the characteristic as compared with that in persons not having the characteristic can be calculated. The selection and identification of appropriate controls in retrospective studies often pose difficulties because unrecognized biases may be present. In virology, an example of the case/control method would be the evaluation of the etiological role of a given virus in a certain disease by comparison of the frequency of viral excretion and/

or antibody rises in patients having this disease with their frequency in those not having the disease. In evaluating this relationship, it must be remembered that infection *without* clinical disease is common in viral infections and might be occurring in the control group. Another recent example is comparison of the frequency of elevated viral antibody titers in the sera of patients with certain malignant or chronic diseases as compared to the antibody titers in age- and sex-matched controls as a clue to causation. Examples of this are the relationship of raised antibody levels of Epstein–Barr virus to Burkitt lymphoma and nasopharyngeal cancer as compared to controls, or of measles antibody titers in cases of subacute sclerosing panencephalitis and multiple sclerosis in relation to controls. In general, retrospective or case/control analyses are cheaper, are more quickly performed, and require smaller numbers than incidence studies, but measure relative rather than absolute risk.

Traditionally, the existence of a possible causal association between a factor and a disease is usually recognized in a clinical setting and its statistical significance is determined by comparison with controls using the case/control or retrospective method. If the results indicate the presence of an important association, an incidence study is then set up to evaluate or confirm the observation. Thus, the risk of smoking in lung cancer and that of rubella infection in congenital abnormalities were discovered by case/control methods and confirmed by incidence and cohort analyses. Other retrospective case/control investigations such as those on the relationship between certain blood groups and influenza (72) have not been confirmed when tested using incidence data.[35]

Experimental epidemiology utilizes epidemiological models and is the most elegant and sophisticated approach because all the variables should be subject to control. Unfortunately, animal models may be difficult or impossible to establish in the laboratory, and even if they are established, there is sometimes the question of the applicability of the results to the human host. Theoretically, the ideal way would be the employment of volunteers. In the past, human subjects have participated in studies of yellow fever, malaria, hepatitis, infectious mononucleosis, acute respiratory infections, measles, rubella, and even syphilis. Such investigations involve important technical, medical, ethical, and moral issues. On the

technical level, there is the question of the susceptibility of the volunteer to the disease under study; i.e., volunteer adults may already be immune as a consequence of childhood infection. Second, the host response to many infections may result in *disease* in only a small percentage of those exposed, or even of those infected, thus requiring a large volunteer group. Medically, there is concern for the seriousness of the disease produced, and for the possibility, however remote, of permanent disability or even death. Finally, the moral and ethical right to use human subjects in any medical experimentation is under debate. In today's climate, experimental studies in volunteers are subject to very strict control, and work being supported by government, foundation, or institutional funds must be scrupulously reviewed by a committee of professional and sometimes of lay and religious representatives. This peer group is required to weigh the benefits of the experiment against the risks involved and to ensure that the experimental subjects are fully aware of all possible consequences before signing a statement of "informed consent."

Serological epidemiology is a term applied to the systematic testing of blood specimens from a defined sample of a healthy population for the presence or level of various components. These include antigens, antibodies, proteins, biochemical and genetic markers, and other biological characteristics (see Chapter 2 and references 26, 37, 38, 43, 49, 51, 91, 93, 107, 113, and 116).

3. Epidemics

An *epidemic* or outbreak of disease is said to exist when the number of cases is in excess of the expected number for that population based on past experience. This determination obviously requires a knowledge of the number of both current and past cases. The definition of "excess" is an arbitrary one. The occurrence of a large number of cases, compressed in time, as when a new influenza strain is introduced, is readily identified as an "epidemic." Indeed, for influenza, a more sophisticated index has been set up by the National Center for Disease Control in the United States by which an expected threshold of deaths from influenza and pneumonia in 122 cities has been established based on a 5-year average. When this threshold is exceeded, an influenza outbreak is said to exist. In contrast, even a few cases of encephalitis over a summer may constitute an "outbreak" in areas where no cases previously existed. When several continents are involved, a disease is said to be "pandemic."

Chronic diseases pose more difficult problems in definition because their scale of occurrence must be viewed over *years* rather than months or weeks. In such a perspective, we do have current "epidemics" of chronic illnesses such as coronary artery disease or lung cancer. The key words are "an unusual increase in the expected number of cases" irrespective of whether the time period involved is short or long.

Three essential requirements for an outbreak of viral disease are the presence of an infected host, an adequate number of susceptibles, and an effective method of contact and transmission between them. If the agent is not endemic within the community, then the introduction of an infected person, animal, insect, or other vector of transmission is needed to initiate an outbreak. This is particularly important in a remote island or isolated population group where a virus disappears after no more persons remain susceptible, if persistent viral excretion does not occur to permit infection of newborns. Rubella, for example, disappeared from Barbados for 10 years despite an accumulation in the number of susceptibles to a level representing about 60% of the population and despite the existence of a large tourist trade.[39] In an isolated Indian tribe in Brazil, antibodies to respiratory-transmitted viruses including measles, influenza, and parainfluenza were essentially absent from the entire tribe.[10] The introduction of more susceptibles or of more infected persons may tip this balance. However, antibodies to viruses characterized by persistent or recurrent viral excretion such as herpes viruses and adenoviruses have been present in every population thus far tested, no matter how remote or isolated.[10]

The cumulative number of persons immune to a given disease within a community has been termed the *herd immunity* level. If this level is sufficiently high, then the occurrence of an outbreak has been regarded as highly unlikely. This concept has recently been challenged, at least for rubella. For example, in an open college community, a preexisting herd immunity level to rubella of 75% failed to prevent an outbreak of this disease.[34] Indeed, the rubella infection rate of 64% among those completely

susceptible (i.e., without detectable antibody) was even higher than the 45% infection rate in the same community for a new influenza strain to which the entire population was susceptible.[34] A rubella outbreak has even occurred among military recruits in the presence of a 95% level of herd immunity: 100% of the susceptibles were infected.[57] The spread of infection is apparently so efficient under these circumstances that a high level of herd immunity does not deter its progress. Another possibility is that reinfection of partially immune persons results in pharyngeal excretion and further spread of virus.

For smallpox, the induction of herd immunity by vaccination has resulted in the apparent global eradication of the disease through the efforts of the World Health Organization. The last case occurred in Somalia on October 26, 1977.[117] No new natural cases have been reported for at least 2 years since then, although laboratory infections have occurred and remain a hazard to laboratory personnel. Continued surveillance will be needed to assure eradication, especially from sources such as the laboratory, or biological warfare, or animal reservoirs of smallpox-related viruses.

Mathematical models have been constructed to fit the epidemic spread of certain infectious diseases or as a basis for immunization programs.[1,24] For diseases in which most infections are clinically expressed, the immunity is good, and the means of transmission is clear, such models are useful. But for other conditions with a high frequency of inapparent infections, or in which the disease depends on a reactivated rather than a primary infection, or in which the agent is intermittently excreted by the human host or intermittently present in an arthropod vector, the events leading to infection and disease are so complex that a mathematical model is difficult to construct. Other poorly understood factors are the role of the genetic makeup of the host in determining susceptibility to infection and disease, the duration and amount of viral excretion, and the varying patterns of clinical illness.

4. Investigation of an Epidemic

The investigation of an epidemic involves a sequence of steps summarized in Table 1. They do not necessarily represent the appropriate order of exe-

Table 1. Epidemic Investigation

1. *Define the problem.*
   Diagnosis? Is it an epidemic?
2. *Appraise existing data.*
   Time: date (and hour) of onset; make epidemic curve
   Place: spot map of cases; home, work, and recreational places; special meetings
   Person: age, sex, occupation, ethnic groups
   Incidence rates: infection, cases, deaths
   Possible means of transmission
   Seek common denominator and unusual exceptions
3. *Formulate hypothesis.*
   Source of infection, method of spread, possible control
4. *Test the hypothesis.*
   Search for added cases; evaluation; laboratory investigation
5. *Conclusions and practical application.*
   Long-term surveillance and prevention

cution. It may not be possible to establish a definitive diagnosis early, so that a rather specific, simple working definition should be established using *key* epidemiological and clinical features as a case-finding device. This definition can be expanded and made more sensitive later when laboratory studies are possible. Control measures should be instituted as soon as the means of spread is reasonably established. Common source outbreaks of viral infections from water, food, milk, or environmental sources are not nearly as common as with bacterial infections. However, they do occur. Some examples include spread of adenoviruses by eye tonometers in eye clinics or via swimming pools, of hepatitis A by public water supplies or by seafood, of hepatitis B by viral-contaminated yellow fever vaccines, or of enteroviruses by fecally contaminated foodstuffs or milk. Most common viral epidemics are respiratory or arthropod-borne, and more recently, spread of several types of viral infections in hospital settings has been recognized. Thus, the more classic steps in epidemic investigation outlined are in Table 1 and will not be discussed further here.

5. The Agent

This section is concerned primarily with those general properties of viruses that are important to an understanding of their epidemiology and not with their basic chemistry, morphology, genetics, or multiplication. These later aspects are dealt with in various microbiology and virology textbooks.[21, 41,56,59,]

The chief characteristics of viruses that are of importance in the production of infection in man are (1) factors that promote efficient transmission within the environment; (2) the ability to enter one or more portals in man; (3) the capacity for attachment to, entry into, and multiplication within a wide variety of host cells; (4) the excretion of infectious particles into the environment; (5) a means of developing alternate mechanisms of survival in the face of antibody, cell-mediated immunity, chemotherapeutic agents, interferon, or other hostile elements. Survival of the virus might be achieved through mutation, recombination, basic properties of resistance, or the availability of alternate biochemical pathways.

The *spread* of viruses depends on (1) the stability of the virus within the physical environment required for its transmission, including resistance to high or low temperatures, desiccation, or ultraviolet; (2) the amount of virus expelled into the proper vehicle of transmission; and (3) the availability of the proper vector or medium for its spread.

After entry through an appropriate portal, the virus must escape from ciliary activities, macrophages, and other primary defense mechanisms during its sojourn to the target cell, find appropriate receptors on the cell surface for its attachment, and be able to penetrate and multiply within the cell. The steps then include initiation of transcription of messenger ribonucleic acid (mRNA), translation of early proteins, replication of viral nucleic acids, transcription of mRNA, translation of late proteins, assembly of virions, and then viral release.[41] These aspects fall into the province of basic virology and will not be discussed in detail here. What is important in pathogenesis is the efficiency of spread from cell to cell, either by direct involvement of contiguous cells or by transport via body fluids to other susceptible cells; the number of cells infected; and the consequences of viral multiplication on the cell itself and on the organism as a whole. The long-term survival of a virus in human populations depends on its ability to establish a chronic infection without cell death, or on an effective method of viral release into the environment in a manner ensuring its transport to a susceptible host, or on a highly adaptive system for biological adversity. The prime example of adaptability among animal viruses is influenza A. Without its property for antigenic variation, it would probably behave like measles or rubella viruses and be dependent for survival on the temporal accumulation of new susceptibles.

6. The Environment

The external environment exerts its influences on the agent itself, on the manner of its spread, and on the nature of the host response to infection. While viruses survive or die within defined ranges of certain physical factors such as temperature and humidity, there is much variability from one viral group to another. A simple environmental factor such as cold may have different effects on the survival of different viruses and on their ability to multiply within cells. While environmental characteristics play an important role in the survival of a virus, they are probably of much greater significance in their influence on the routes of transmission and on the behavior patterns of the host.

For infections that require an insect vector, such as the arboviruses, the environment exerts an obvious role in restricting the occurrence of infection and disease to those areas that have the proper temperature, humidity, vegetation, amplifying animal hosts, and other features necessary for the insect involved. For viral diseases readily transmitted by water, such as hepatitis A virus, a warm environment attended by poor sanitation and fecal contamination clearly enhances the degree of exposure and the efficiency of transmission.

Perhaps the most crucial effect of climate on common viral diseases is exerted on the social behavior of the host. In tropical settings and in the summer season in temperature climates, the opportunity for transmission of gastrointestinal diseases is increased through contact with water, as in swimming in and drinking from the polluted areas. Warm weather also brings closer contact with dogs and other animal sources of rabies and with insect vectors of arboviruses. In winter, people huddle together inside, promoting the transmission of airborne and droplet infections. This spread is amplified by the opening of schools and colleges. In addition, the environ-

ment within most houses and buildings tends to be hot and dry, which impairs the protective mechanisms of human mucous surfaces and may permit easier entry and attachment of certain respiratory viruses.

While winter clearly brings with it an increase in viral respiratory illnesses, heavy rains and the monsoon similarly influence these same diseases in tropical settings. Indeed, the incidence of common upper respiratory diseases in college students was as high in the warm climate at the University of the Philippines as in the intemperate winters at the University of Wisconsin.[31,32] Viruses that cause respiratory infections in children have also been found to be active in all climates around the world.[15] Community studies in India,[87] Trinidad,[9] and Panama[79] have indicated a high morbidity from influenza and other respiratory diseases in tropical settings. As in temperate climates, factors that tend to aggregate people inside, such as heavy rainfall or schooling, also coincide with the highest incidence of respiratory-transmitted infections in the tropics.[31,79]

7. The Host

The factors that influence *infection* involve primarily exposure to the infectious agent and the susceptibility of the host. The opportunity for a susceptible host to come in contact with a source of infection depends on the means of transmission. Respiratory-transmitted agents are usually general in their exposure; those transmitted by gastrointestinal routes are related to exposure to food or water and the hygienic and socioeconomic level of the host; those that depend on arthropod-borne transmission involve persons in special settings or special occupational exposures. Others, such as sexually transmitted agents, require specific behavioral acts of the host; still others require specialized exposures such as transfusions, rabid animals, or specialized environments. The factors that influence infection are therefore mostly extrinsic to the host.

Those factors that determine whether *clinical illness* will develop in a person already infected depend in part on the dosage, virulence, and portal of entry of the agent, but more important, they depend on certain intrinsic properties of the host.

Some of these characteristics are listed in Table 2. Age at the time of infection is a critical host factor and influences whether clinical illness develops following infection with such agents as Epstein–Barr virus, hepatitis viruses, and poliomyelitis viruses. In general, the probability that clinical illness will develop increases as the age at the time of infection increases; in a similar fashion, the *severity* of the clinical response also increases with age at the time of illness. The nature of the immune response to a virus can be either beneficial to the host in limiting the infection or detrimental if the clinical disease is due to certain immunopathological consequences of infection such as immune complexes or autoimmune mechanisms. The vigor of the humoral and cell-mediated immune responses may also determine when a virus becomes persistent or is eradicated from the body. Certain host attributes also affect specific diseases: smoking enhances the severity of respiratory infections; alcohol, that of liver infections; and exercise, the development of paralytic poliomyelitis in a particular limb. We know little of the importance of nutritional or psychological factors in tipping the scale toward the clinical expression of illness, but both probably play an important role. Our knowledge of the actual cellular or molecular basis for the clinical pattern following infection is also meager, but it is clear that the immune response and the genetic controls of that response both exert profound influences.

8. Routes of Transmission

The major routes of transmission of viral infections are listed in Table 3. Many viruses have several alternate routes, thus enhancing the chance of survival. The sequence of events in transmission involves release of the virus from the cell, exit from the body, transport through the environment in a viable form, and appropriate entry into a susceptible host.

Some viruses are released from cells at the end of the cycle of multiplication. Others do not complete this cycle (incomplete viruses), and some do not effect efficient escape (cell-bound viruses). Many viruses are released from cells by budding, acquiring a lipoprotein coat or envelope as they go through the cell membrane; these include herpesviruses, to-

Table 2. Factors That Influence the Clinical Host Response

1. Dosage, virulence, and portal of entry of the agent
2. Age at the time of infection
3. Preexisting level of immunity
4. Nature and vigor of the immune response
5. Genetic factors controlling the immune response, the presence of receptor sites, and cell-to-cell spread
6. Nutritional status of the host
7. Preexisting disease
8. Personal habits: smoking, alcohol, exercise, drugs
9. Double infection or bacterial complications
10. Psychological factors (e.g., motivation, emotional crises, attitudes toward illness)

gaviruses, myxoviruses, paramyxoviruses, and coronaviruses. Nonenveloped viruses not released by budding are the adenoviruses, parvoviruses, poxviruses, picornaviruses, and reoviruses. Some of these latter are released by cell lysis. Once released, viruses find their way to new hosts via one or more portals such as the respiratory tract (e.g., influenza), skin (varicella, smallpox), blood (hepatitis viruses via blood transfusion, arboviruses via mosquitos), gastrointestinal tract (enteroviruses), genital tract (herpes simplex type 2), urine [cytomegalovirus (CMV)], and placenta (rubella, CMV). A more detailed presentation of these major routes of spread will now be given.

8.1. Respiratory

The respiratory route is probably the most important method of spread for most common viral diseases of man and is the least subject to effective environmental control. For influenza virus, the degree of transmissibility varies from one strain to another and seems to be independent of other attributes of the virus. Schulman[99] has compared the features of a strain with high transmissibility (Jap 305) and one with low transmissibility (Ao/NWS) in an experimental mouse model. The virus titer in the lung was similar for both strains, but the virus content in the bronchial secretion was low for the Ao/NWS strain compared to the Jap 305 strain. This higher degree of release into the respiratory portal of exit resulted in detectable virus in the air surrounding mice infected by the Jap 305 but not by the Ao/NWS strain. Once an aerosol was created,

Table 3. Transmission of Viral Infections

Route of exit	Routes of transmission	Examples[a]	Factors[a]	Routes of entry
Respiratory	Bite	Rabies	Animal	Skin
	Salivary transfer	EBV in adults	Kissing	Mouth
		Hepatitis B	Dental work	?Mouth
	Aerosol	Influenza and other respiratory viruses, Lassa virus	Sneeze, cough, <2-nm particles to lung	Respiratory
	Mouth → hand or object	Herpes simplex, EBV in children, rhinovirus, enterovirus, Lassa virus	Salivary contamination of hands and objects	Oropharyngeal
Gastrointestinal tract	Stool → hand	Enteroviruses, hepatitis A, rotaviruses	Poor hygiene	Mouth
	Stool → water (or milk)	Hepatitis A	Seafood	Mouth
	Thermometer	Hepatitis A	Nurse	Rectal
Skin	Air	Poxviruses	Also via objects	Respiratory
	Skin to skin	Molluscum contagiosum, warts	Abrasions	Abraded skin
Blood	Mosquitos	Arboviruses	Extrinsic I.P.	Skin
	Ticks	Group B togaviruses	Transovarial transmission	Skin
	Transfusion of blood and blood products	Hepatitis B, non-A, non-B hepatitis, CMV, EBV	Carrier state, free or with lymphs	Skin
	Needles for injection	Hepatitis B, non-A, non-B hepatitis	Addicts	Skin
Urine	Rarely transmitted	CMV, measles, mumps, congenital rubella	Unknown	Unknown
Genital	Cervix	Herpes simplex, CMV, ?rubella, ?hepatitis	?Venereal	Genital
	Semen	CMV	?Venereal	Genital
Placental	Vertical to embryo	CMV, rubella, smallpox, hepatitis B	Congenital abnormalities, abortion	Blood
Eye	Tonometer	Adenovirus	Exam for glaucoma	Eye

[a] (EBV) Epstein–Barr virus; (CMV) cytomegalovirus; (I.P.) incubation period.

the stability of both strains was similar. Protein analysis also revealed differences in the neuraminidase of the two strains; this component is associated with dissociation of viruses from the cell and thus perhaps with its transmissibility. However, high transmissibility did not go along with transfer of the gene for neuraminidase, so it was concluded that other factors were also involved in the efficacy of spread.

Other aspects that affect the transmission of respiratory viruses are the intensity and method of propulsion of discharges from the mouth and nose, the size of the aerosol droplets created, and the re-

sistance of the airborne virus to desiccation. Much work has been done by Knight[63] and his group on the transmission of respiratory viruses. At one extreme is the direct transmission of infection via personal contact such as kissing, touching of contaminated objects (hands, handkerchiefs, soft drink bottles), and direct impingement of large droplets produced by coughing or sneezing. This last method is regarded as a form of personal contact because of the short range of the heavy droplets formed. Sneezing and coughing also create aerosols varying in size from about 1 to more than 20 μm that permit transmission of infection at a distance. The dispersion of an aerosol depends on wind currents and on particle size. In still air, a spherical particle of unit density of 100-μm diameter requires 10 sec to fall the height of the average room (3 m), 40-μm particles require 1 min, 20-μm particles 4 min, and 10-μm particles 17 min. This means that particles of under 10 μm have a relatively long circulation time in the ordinary room. Once initiated, particles 6 μm or more in diameter are usually trapped in the nose while those 0.6–6.0 μm in diameter are deposited on sites along the upper and lower respiratory tract.

Hygroscopic particles of 1.5-μm diameter discharged in large numbers by coughing or sneezing lose moisture and shrink in ambient air but regain their original dimensions from the saturated air in the respiratory tract. The site of disposition of an aerosol containing virus particles does not necessarily represent the level in the respiratory tree where the greatest number of susceptible cells exist for that agent. Quantitative studies have indicated that with four different respiratory viruses, the number of viral particles necessary to produce infection in the respiratory tract is relatively small. With adenoviruses, for example, it is on the order of seven virions. The lower infective dose required for nasal implantation of rhinoviruses and coxsackievirus indicates that this route, perhaps by personal contact, leads to their effective transmission.[63] The high concentrations of rhinovirus particles on fingers, hands, and hard surfaces as opposed to the lower concentrations found in aerosols suggest that infection via hands may be an important route of spread. This is supported by the frequent inadvertent contact of hands with the nose or eyes.[52] If the importance of this mechanism is confirmed, frequent hand-washing may help control the spread of the common cold.

The size and number of viral particles in sneezes and coughs have varied from study to study depending on the methodology employed. In one study, 1,940,000 particles were present in sneezes and 90,765 in coughing, a ratio of 2.14:1.[48] Despite the high level of particles, the recovery of Coxsackie A21 virus itself was more frequent from coughs than from sneezes.[63] Many questions on the mechanics of transmission of respiratory viruses remain unanswered and any generalizations are premature, but the methodology to answer some of these is becoming available.

Aerosolization of certain viral agents may occur from suction devices and from catheters in intensive care units and from blood products in dialysis units. These include not only respiratory and intestinal agents but also blood-associated agents such as hepatitis viruses and herpes viruses (CMV, Epstein–Barr virus).

8.2. Gastrointestinal

Transmission by the oral–fecal route is probably the second most frequent means of spread of common viral infections, and the gastrointestinal tract is the second great portal of entry of infection. Viruses can directly infect susceptible cells of the oropharynx, but to induce intestinal infection, virus-containing material must be swallowed, successfully resist the hydrochloric acid in the stomach and the bile acids in the duodenum, and progress to susceptible cells in the intestine. These cells may be the epithelial cells in the intestinal mucosa or in the intestinal lymphatics, as with adenoviruses. Viruses with envelopes do not normally survive exposure to these acids, salts, and enzymes in the gut. The major enteric viruses are poliomyelitis, echo, coxsackie, and infectious hepatitis (hepatitis A) viruses. It is known that under conditions of close and prolonged contact, hepatitis B virus and non-A, non-B hepatitis may also be transmitted in this way. Multiplication and excretion in the intestinal tract also occur with adenoviruses and reoviruses, but this route of transmission is not usually of epidemiological importance. The rhinoviruses are acid-labile and do not survive passage through the stomach. Unlike the respiratory viruses, the enteriviruses rarely produce evidence of local disease as a consequence of their multiplication in cells lining that area. Thus, diarrhea, vomiting, and abdominal pain are highly unusual features of infection with these agents. Instead, their major target organs and the site of major symptomatology are at a distance: hepatitis viruses in the liver and enteroviruses in the central nervous system and skin.

Viruses excreted via the gastrointestinal tract must successfully infect other susceptible persons via the oral–intestinal route through fecally contaminated hands, food, water, milk, flies, thermometers, or other vehicles. Viruses spread via these routes are subject to much greater environmental control than are agents transmitted by the respiratory route. Thus, good personal hygiene, especially washing of hands after defecation, proper cleanliness and cooking of food, pasteurization of milk, good waste disposal, and purification of drinking water supplies are effective preventive measures. Hepatitis A virus is remarkably heat-stable and may not be inactivated by ordinary levels of chlorination in drinking water if the viral content is great and has a high infectivity. Furthermore, it can survive in oysters and clams over long periods. This is especially hazardous because these foods are so often eaten without cooking. Hepatitis viruses and the enteroviruses also flourish in certain institutional settings (mental hospitals, institutions for retarded children, some prisons) and in countries where personal hygiene is lacking or difficult to practice or where poor environmental control is present. Since some enteroviruses may also multiply in the respiratory tract and be transmitted by the respiratory route, this alternate pathway is of epidemiological importance even in the face of good personal and environmental hygiene.

8.3. Skin

Skin is the third important area for the entry and exit of viral infections. While penetration of the intact skin is an unlikely mechanism of infection, the introduction of virus particles via a bite as with rabies, or via a mosquito as with the arboviruses, or via a needle or blood transfusion as with both types of hepatitis viruses makes this route an important one. CMV and Epstein–Barr virus may also be transmitted through blood transfusions. The abraded skin may serve as the entry point of human papovavirus, which causes warts. In patients with skin lesions such as eczema, the accidental transfer of smallpox virus from the site of inoculation to other skin areas might occur.

The skin serves as a portal of *exit* only for those viruses that produce skin vesicles or pox lesions that release infectious particles on rupture. These include herpes simplex, smallpox, varicella-zoster, and vaccinia viruses. The viruses of certain maculopapular exanthems may also be present in the skin, as in rubella, but this does not seem to be an important avenue of escape, since vesicles are not formed and skin involvement occurs late in the disease at a time when the virus may be bound by antibody; indeed, the antigen–antibody complex may be responsible for the rash itself.

8.4. Genital

The genital tract serves as a portal of infection for both partners during sexual activity and as a source of infection for the fetus as it passes down the birth canal. Herpes simplex type I and II viruses, CMV, and rubella virus have all been isolated from cervical secretions.[61] CMV has also been isolated from male semen.[66] Cervical or penile lesions may result from herpes infections. There is increasing epidemiological, virological, and serological evidence establishing an association between herpes type 2 (II) infections and cancer of the cervix. This is discussed in Chapter 25. Infections of the newborn at the time of delivery can occur with herpesviruses, CMV, and rubella virus. The capacity of herpesviruses for latency emphasizes that long-term carrier states exist. Sexual practices involving oral, genital, or anal contact may result in infections in these sites with herpesviruses and CMV, and possibly hepatitis B virus.

8.5. Intrauterine or Transplacental

Viruses may infect the fetus either by direct contact via the birth canal as discussed in Section 8.4 or by hematogenous spread via the placenta to the fetus within the uterus. The term *congenital* infections is now used for both mechanisms of transmission. Viruses that produce intrauterine infection include CMV, hepatitis B, herpes simplex, rubella, and varicella viruses. CMV and rubella viruses are the most common congenital infections, and infection of the fetus may result in no symptoms, in abortion and stillbirth, in developmental abnormalities, or in persistent postnatal infection. A fine book now deals with infectious diseases of the fetus and newborn infant.[95b]

8.6. Genitourinary

While excretion of viruses such as CMV and measles occurs in the urine, this portal of exit has not been established as being of epidemiological or clinical importance. Considering the wide variety of viruses that can multiply in human kidney tissue cultures *in vitro*, it is surprising that renal infections in man from these viruses are virtually nonexistent, or at least are nonrecognized. It seems possible that viruses may play a role in immune complex nephritis in man as they do in experimental animal models, but to date this has not been clearly demonstrated, nor has it been reflected in abnormally high viral antibody levels in such patients.[114] Recently, adenovirus types 11 and 21 have been implicated as the cause of hemorrhagic cystitis in children (see Chapter 3).

8.7. Personal Contact

Direct transfer of infected discharges from the respiratory or gastrointestinal tract to a susceptible person is often included under "transmission by personal contact." Many viruses regarded as "respiratory or airborne" in spread may in fact be more direct in their transmission mechanism, as has been previously mentioned for the rhinoviruses.[52,55a]

8.8. Water and Food

Outbreaks of viral hepatitis have occurred from sewage-contaminated water, as in the large outbreak in New Delhi, India, in 1956,[75] or from seafood obtained from fecally contaminated waters, as shown in outbreaks associated with oysters in the United States[71] and in Sweden[47] and with clams in New Jersey.[23] Milk and water have also served as vehicles of transmission of hepatitis and poliomyelitis viruses. Summer outbreaks of adenovirus type 3 infections have occurred in associated with swimming pools.[6]

8.9. Arthropod-Borne

Mosquitos, flies, ticks, and other insects may transmit viral infections. One kind of transmission is a passive type, simply involving survival of the virus in or on the insect that has picked it up from skin lesions or the blood. This type requires neither incubation time in the insect vector nor any specificity for either the arthropod host or the virus. Poliomyelitis and possibly hepatitis viruses may be carried in this way. On the other hand, some viruses require multiplication in the insect vector. In this instance, virus acquired from the blood of the human or animal host during viremia requires a period of multiplication within the arthropod vector before it is infectious, and there is a high degree of vector–virus–host specificity. An example of this is the transmission of yellow fever virus by *Aedes ae-*

gypti mosquitos. The details of arthropod transmission are described in more detail in Chapter 5.

9. Pathogenesis

Since each chapter on specific viruses will deal with the subject of pathogenesis, this discussion will be limited to a general consideration of infections involving certain local or systemic features. Good general presentations will be found in other books.[41,56,78]

9.1. Respiratory

Infectious particles may be implanted directly on nasal surfaces from contaminated hands or from large droplets or may reach the lower respiratory passages from aerosols. Since man continually samples the environmental air about 20 times a minute in breathing, it is no wonder that exposure to and infection with respiratory viruses are common indeed. Furthermore, only a small number of infectious particles need to be implanted in appropriate areas to induce infection. This is on the order of three particles for influenza A by aerosol, six for Coxsackie A21 by intranasal implantation, and seven for adenovirus 4 by aerosol.[63] In general, aerosol particles of 3 μm in size reach the alveolus and those of 6 μm or greater are retained in the upper respiratory tract. The mucociliary epithelium transports particles up from the lung or down from the nasal mucosa.[78] To reach susceptible cells, viruses must pass through the mucus film and make physical contact with the cell receptors. The mucus contains mucopolysaccharide and other inhibitors, such as specific immunoglobulin A (IgA) antibody in previously exposed persons. Influenza virus is assisted in its spread by its own neuraminidase, which hydrolyzes the polysaccharides of the inhibitors; the virus attaches to cell receptors by means of surface hemagglutinin spikes. In the alveolus, small aerosol particles are ingested by macrophages, and some viruses are digested and degraded by these cells; other viruses are even capable of multiplication within macrophages themselves.

Most respiratory viruses produce illness through the direct consequences of local multiplication. Necrosis and lysis occur with desquamation of the respiratory epithelium.[21] Constitutional symptoms may then result from breakdown products of dying cells that are absorbed into the bloodstream; fever is produced by the liberation of endogenous pyrogen resulting from viral action on polymorphonuclear leukocytes. This sequence of events may be modified or altered by interferon production in infected cells, by the appearance or preexistence of secretory or local antibody, or by the presence of preexisting or produced humoral antibody. If humoral antibody is present in the absence of local antibody, then a more severe reaction may occur, possibly through antigen–antibody deposition on the cell membrane. The mechanism of this is not clear, but the phenomenon has been observed in infants with passively acquired maternal respiratory syncytial antibody who subsequently develop an infection with this virus. It has also been seen following parenteral administration of an inactivated vaccine that produces humoral antibody but little or no local antibody, such as experimental respiratory syncytial and early measles vaccines when followed by natural or purposeful exposure to live virus.[16]

The multiplication and effect of respiratory viruses such as influenza virus, parainfluenza virus, rhinoviruses, and respiratory syncytial virus are generally limited to the respiratory tract. Influenza virus has been detected in the blood only rarely,[22a,103] but has been isolated from the spleen, lymph nodes, tonsils, liver, kidney, and heart in fatal cases of Asian influenza pneumonia.[88] Systemic spread of this type appears to be unusual and associated with overwhelming viral infection.[111] More examples may come to light with more widespread use of immunosuppressive drugs. Adenoviruses and the enteroviruses multiply both in the respiratory tract and in the gut; viremia and secondary multiplication in the central nervous system are common in the latter group. Among the enteroviruses, however, only Coxsackie A21 acts primarily as a respiratory virus, and its importance is limited mainly to military recruits. Enterovirus 70 causes acute hemorrhagic conjunctivitis, and the virus is present in the conjunctiva and throat (see Chapter 9).

9.2. Gastrointestinal

Hepatitis viruses, enteroviruses, adenoviruses, reoviruses, and rotaviruses multiply within the gut. Many of the same barriers that prevent cell attachment and penetration may exist there as in the respiratory tract, including local IgA antibody. Local, humoral, and cell-mediated immunity follows natural viral infections of the intestinal tract and is the basis for immunity following oral administration of live vaccines such as poliomyelitis and adenoviruses 4 and 7. Unlike the case with respiratory viruses, local multiplication does not produce local symptoms; these occur only after implantation has occurred in secondary sites of multiplication such as the liver for hepatitis virus and the central nervous system for enteroviral infections. Exceptions are the rotavirus and parvovirus (Norwalk agent) infections of children[20a] and adults (see Chapter 11 and references 23a, 42, and 62).

9.3. Systemic Infections

Systemic infections involve viremia, with or without additional spread along other routes. Spread via the bloodstream is the major route by which many viruses locate in secondary habitats where their principal effects are produced. Some viruses become closely associated with lymphocytes in the blood during the viremia phase [measles, cytomegalovirus (CMV), poxviruses, Epstein–Barr virus (EBV)]. Some produce a chronic nonproductive infection of lymphocytes, such as EBV; some are free in the plasma, as are the arboviruses, enteroviruses, and hepatitis B virus, or circulate as immune complexes; some have a special affinity for red cells, such as the viruses of Colorado tick fever and Rift Valley fever. Viremia may be maintained by continual seeding from the liver, spleen, bone marrow, and other organs. The persistence of hepatitis B virus, CMV, and EBV in the blood for months or years poses a hazard in their transmission via blood transfusions. It also seems evident that the viruses associated with viremia may join with antibody and that such complexes may circulate with occasional deposition, fixation of complement, and local tissue injury, especially in small blood vessels. This has been shown for hepatitis B antigen in relation to periarteritis. Other viral immune complexes may involve the kidney.

9.4. The Exanthem

Our understanding of the pathogenesis of systemic infections associated with a rash such as the pox group, measles, and rubella has been enhanced by the fine studies of Fenner with mouse pox.[40,41] In each such exanthem, there is an incubation period of 10–12 days before symptoms of illness appear. After multiplication of the virus at the site of implantation and in the regional lymph nodes, a primary viremia occurs within the first few days, resulting in seeding of organs such as the liver and spleen. A secondary viremia then follows, with focal involvement of the skin and mucous membranes, the appearance of a rash, and the onset of symptoms. In mouse pox, a primary lesion then develops at the site of inoculation. While the destruction of cells involved in viral multiplication and the release of pyrogens from leukocytes may be responsible for symptoms such as fever, the appearance of antibody at this time suggests that antigen–antibody complexes may play an important role in the pathogenesis of the rash. The viruses of smallpox, herpes simplex, and varicella-zoster are present in the skin vesicles of each of these diseases.

9.5. Infections of the Central Nervous System

In a comprehensive review of the pathogenesis of viral infections of the CNS, Johnson and Mims[60] emphasize that one or more routes of infection may be involved and that the pathways differ with the particular viruses, the host, and the portal of entry. In man, the hematogenous routes to the CNS from the portal of entry and from primary multiplication sites in the gut, respiratory tract, parotid, or lymph nodes are clearly of importance in enteroviral infections, mumps, lymphocytic choriomeningitis, primary herpes simplex infections, and fetal infections with rubella virus and CMV. Secondary multiplication sites in the liver, spleen, muscle, or vascular tissue may augment or maintain the viremia; the brown fat has also received attention in this regard for a variety of viruses. Several mechanisms have been suggested as to how viruses enter the brain from the bloodstream. This may be a passive process, or the viruses may actually grow their way through the choroid plexus. Viral multiplication at this site or leakage into the cerebrospinal fluid following growth in the meningeal cells may explain the presence of echovirus and coxsackievirus in the spinal fluid during CNS infections.[60] What has been termed a "blood–brain barrier" for entry of the blood-borne viruses into the CNS appears to have no strict anatomical basis; rather,

it appears to represent a composite of those factors that influence spread to the CNS.

Neural spread along nerves can occur in rabies, poliomyelitis, and B virus infections of man. In rabies, it appears to be the predominant if not the sole method of spread to the CNS, whereas it seems to be relatively unimportant in poliomyelitis. The axons, lymphatics, and tissue spaces between nerve fibers represent three possible conduits for spread along the neural route. Transmission via the tissue spaces plus direct infection and involvement of endoneural cells seems the most likely mechanism. Spread along the olfactory pathway has also been experimentally demonstrated for poliomyelitis, herpes simplex, and certain arthropod-borne viruses. The role of this route in natural infections is uncertain. As with respiratory viruses, those that infect the CNS have different cell preferences: poliomyelitis has a predilection for anterior horn cells of the spinal cord and the motor cortex of the brain, and arboviruses have a predilection for cells of the encephalon. Herpes simplex appears to have more catholic tastes and multiplies in a wide variety of cell types. As is also true of respiratory cells, the existence of specific cell receptors for individual viruses may play a crucial role in susceptibility.

9.6. Persistent Viral Infections

The pathogenetic mechanisms discussed thus far have dealt with infections in which an acute illness results, usually after a relatively short incubation period (except for rabies) and in which recovery ensues. The virus disappears and is often eliminated from the body. Another pathogenetic mechanism under increasing study is one in which the virus persists for months or years and may result in delayed host responses. Some of these persistent viruses are also capable of evoking an acute response such as the herpesviruses, rubella virus, the adenoviruses, measles virus, and other paramyxoviruses. Other persistent viruses such as papovaviruses and polyoma viruses rarely produce any acute illness. Still other agents called "slow viruses" produce chronic degenerative disease years after exposure. This group includes kuru and Creutzfeldt–Jakob disease of man, scrapie infection of sheep, and transmissible mink encephalopathy (see Chapter 27).

Six factors that favor persistence of certain viruses have been summarized by Mims[78a]: (1) persistent viruses tend to have low or no pathogenicity for the cells they infect, in contrast to viruses with severe, destructive effects induce acute disease terminated by death or by recovery and the elimination of the virus; (2) there may be an ineffective antibody response possibly due to tolerance, autoimmunosuppression, production of nonneutralizing or blocking antibodies, not enough antigen on the surface of the infected (target) cell to induce adequate antibody formation, or spread of the virus directly from cell to cell where antibody does not reach it; (3) there may be an ineffective cell-mediated immune response for reasons similar to those involved in the poor antibody response [tolerance, autoimmunosuppression, blocking antibodies, too little antigen expressed on surface to infected cell, failure of immune cells to reach infected (target) cells]; (4) there may be a defective interferon response, such as in lymphocytic choriomeningitis in mice; other viruses may be relatively insensitive to interferon action even though it may be produced; (5) certain persistent viral infections induce neither an immune nor an interferon response; these include the "slow virus" infections such as kuru and Creutzfeldt–Jakob disease; (6) lymphocytes and macrophages are often infected in persistent viral infections, such as with adenoviruses, EBV, CMV, and measles virus, thus altering the host's immune response. Interferon produced by infected macrophages may have no protective effect on other macrophages, although there is normal activity on normal cell types; certain virus–antibody complexes still remain infectious after phagocytosis by macrophages; infected macrophages may be less active in releasing the same virus from the blood, thus favoring persistent viremia.

Such persistent and latent viral infections may reactivate, producing the acute disease again, or may result in a chronic viral infection manifested by immune complex disease, degenerative diseases of the CNS, or certain malignancies. These infections will acquire greater visibility and importance as immunosuppressive drugs are used more widely in medical therapy and in organ-transplant recipients.

10. Incubation Period

The period from the time of exposure to the appearance of the first symptoms is called the *incu-*

bation period. Viruses that do not require distant spread but are able to produce disease through multiplication at the site of implantation, such as the respiratory tract, have short incubation periods on the order of 2–5 days. Those that require hematogenous spread and involvement of distant target organs such as the skin or CNS have incubation periods of 2–3 weeks. Viruses such as rabies, dependent on spread along nerves, have very long and variable incubation periods ranging from 8 days to a year or more. The variation in incubation periods in different diseases is indicated in Fig. 1. In some diseases, early symptoms or even a rash may accompany the period of initial invasion or viremia. This has been seen in poliomyelitis, dengue, hepatitis, and infectious mononucleosis. In such instances, the apparent incubation period to the appearance of these early features is much shorter than the usually accepted period; more often, this early phase is not clinically recognized or occurs before the patient visits the physician.

Knowledge of the incubation period has many practical uses. Epidemiologically, it helps define the period of infectiousness: a patient is not usually infestious until close to the time of the appearance of clinical symptoms. The duration of infectivity depends on the persistence of the virus and its exit into the environment. Clinically, the duration of the incubation period helps to identify the likelihood of a viral exanthem after a known exposure or to differentiate hepatitis A from hepatitis B infections. Prophylactically, it determines the feasibility of prevention of the clinical illness by immune serum as in hepatitis A, varicella-zoster infections, rubella, and rabies, as well as the potential success of rabies vaccination.

In addition to the viruses that produce acute infections, there are delayed effects of certain common viruses in which the "incubation period" may be several years. An example is the relationship of measles virus to subacute sclerosing panencephalitis, in which infection in infancy may be associated with involvement of the CNS some 5–10 years later.[12]

Certain papovaviruses cause widespread inapparent infections in childhood. Rarely, reactivation occurs later in life in the form of progressive multifocal leukoencephalopathy. This is seen in patients with Hodgkin's disease in association with depression of cell-mediated immunity (see Chapter 27).

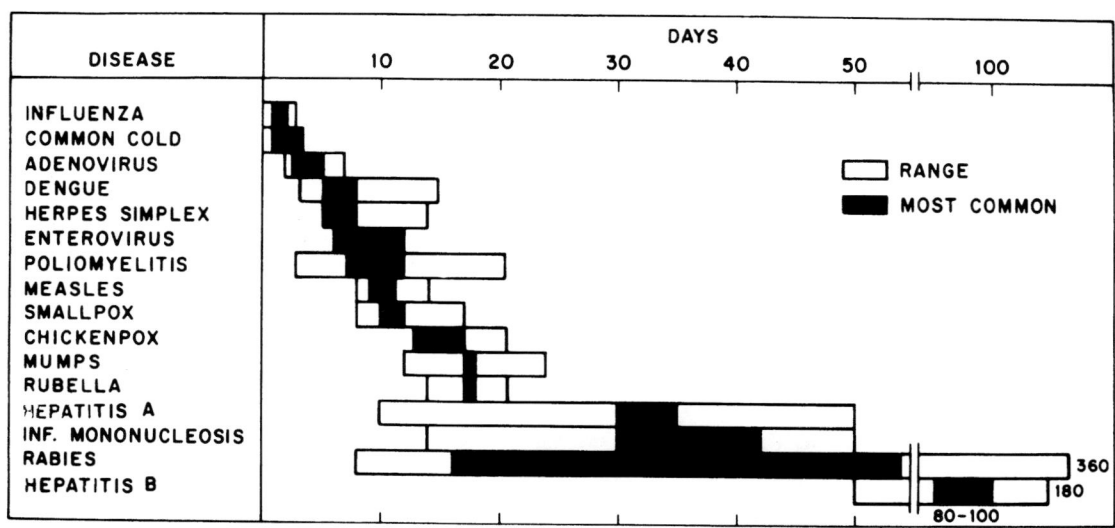

Fig. 1. Incubation periods in viral diseases. Based mostly on data from Benenson, A. S. (ed.), *Control of Communicable Diseases in Man,* 12th ed., American Public Health Association, Washington, D.C., 1975.

The term "incubation period" may be inappropriate in this setting because viral reactivation appears to be involved, and not a period of primary multiplication of the virus.

A prolonged incubation period lasting up to a year or so is involved in natural and experimental infections with kuru, an unusual disease of the CNS that occurs in New Guinea[46]; similar long incubation periods are seen in other "slow viral infections" of animals such as scrapie in sheep (see Chapter 27).

The concept of an incubation period has also been applied to putative oncogenic viruses and to chemical carcinogens in relation to the subsequent development of cancer. In various neoplastic diseases, the estimated incubation period from a defined point of exposure to a suspected carcinogen to the development of disease has ranged from 0.27 year for the development of pancytopenia after chloramphenicol to 36 years for the appearance of lung cancer after exposure to asbestos.[4]

11. The Immune Response

The immunological response of the host to a virus infection plays a role not only in the development of specific resistance but also in the pathogenesis of the signs and symptoms of the disease itself.[85] Specific immunity to viral disease is based on humoral antibody, local antibody, and cell-mediated immunity. It is evoked either by natural infection or by immunization with live or killed antigens. The immune responses are dependent on B-type lymphocytes derived from the bone marrow and on T lymphocytes derived from the thymus in cooperation with macrophages.

11.1. Humoral Immunity

Humoral immunity is dependent on antibody found in the blood and other body fluids. Of the five classes of immunoglobulins, IgG-, IgM-, and IgA-type antibodies are important in this type of protection. Viral-specific IgG antibodies usually persist for life; those of the IgM type are short-lived and characterize the primary infection. It is possible that persistence or reactivation of virus in an active antigenic form may also be accompanied by a prolonged or recrudescent IgM antibody response. Infections characterized by viremia produce the most marked humoral antibody response, and the resulting immunity is usually of long duration. Type-B lymphocytes are primarily responsible for antibody production, but T lymphocytes appear to play a helper role.

Passive transfer of convalescent sera or immune

globulins may also produce protection against those infections that are dependent on a viremia to reach target organs for their clinical expression; it does not protect against multiplication of virus at the site of initial implantation in the respiratory or gastrointestinal tract.

11.2. Local Immunity (Secretory IgA System)

Local antibody production is mediated through viral-specific immunoglobulins of the IgA class. Their presence in glandular secretions and on mucous surfaces of the respiratory tract and the gut is an effective deterrent to viral infection at these sites. The production of local antibody is elicited by natural infection or by a live vaccine given by the natural portal of entry. Less efficient production occurs with killed vaccines given by the natural route of infection or by live or killed vaccines given parenterally. Indeed, an important limitation to the effective prevention of infection with the parenteral administration of inactivated vaccines such as influenza and poliomyelitis is their failure to evoke a satisfactory local antibody response. Similarly, passive immunization as in the use of γ-globulin may prevent systemic spread and clinical disease, but does not prevent primary *infection*. Epidemiologically, it is important to recognize that passively immunized persons may continue to be a source of spread of infection to others.

11.3. Cell-Mediated Immunity

Delayed hypersensitivity is a classic manifestation of cell-mediated immunity as exemplified by positive skin-test reactions. In viral infections, lymphocytes and the lymphokines that they produce attract macrophages and with their products are participants in the destruction of antigen and antigen-infected cells. The T lymphocyte is of key importance in the recognition and management of viral and fungal infections.[2,3,50,115] When T cells are absent, depleted, or functionally impaired, severe and widespread viral or fungal infections may develop and latent viruses may reactivate. Specific receptors on T cells appear to be programmed, probably by genetic inheritance, to recognize and respond to different antigens.

There are different subclasses of T lymphocytes that play different, and sometimes opposite, roles in the immune response. These include suppressor T cells, helper T cells, and cytotoxic (killer) T lymphocytes. These functions are usually highly antigen-specific, but some killer T cells have nonspecific cytotoxic activity. Macrophages are involved in the immune response and are activated by lymphokines, by immune complexes, or by the third component of complement; these activated cells act nonspecifically to limit viral multiplication, effect complement cleavage, and carry out phagocytosis. In addition to monophages, there is another cell capable of killing, the so-called K cell, which is lymphoidlike but the lineage of which is unclear. It has a receptor for the Fc portion of IgG and can kill target cells covered by antibody. Increasing attention is being focused on the T suppressor or immunoregulatory cells. Effector responses of both B and T cells are controlled by these regulator cells; the appropriateness of their activities is under genetic control, probably from loci on the sixth chromosome. Subtle alterations in their effectiveness may lead to disease states, possibly to malignancy.

While the prevention of spread of viruses through extracellular fluids and the blood seems to be largely dependent on neutralization by humoral antibody, control of viral spread from cell to cell is probably dependent on cellular immunity. The latter form of contiguous infection might be interrupted by destroying infected cells, by severing connections between infected and uninfected cells so that the virus cannot be transferred to uninfected cells without being exposed extracellularly to neutralizing antibody, or by destroying contiguous uninfected cells so that virus must proceed extracellularly to reach target cells for further multiplication.[83,84] An important element in the destruction of infected cells is the induction of virus-induced antigens on the cell surface, which makes them appear foreign to other host cells; they are then destroyed by T-type lymphocytes as in graft-vs.-host rejection.

A two-phase response for stopping the cell-to-cell spread of herpesvirus has been postulated in which both specific and nonspecific defenses are involved[68]: The immunologically specific recognition phase consists of the interaction of antiviral antibody, complement, and virus (or virus-infected cells), as well as the stimulation of immune lymphocytes. This results in the generation of a variety of biological mediators, some of which are chemotactic for inflammatory cells. The nonspecific phase consists of the attraction of inflammatory cells to the site where they exert a toxic effect on both infected and noninfected cells and, with lymphocyte mediators, inhibit viral multiplication and/or break connections between cells, forcing extracellular passage of virus. A third form of vertical spread from parent to progeny cells may also occur if the viral genome becomes integrated into the genome of the host cell.

11.4. Immune Responses in the Pathogenesis of Viral Diseases

Viral infections may produce the symptoms of disease through a variety of mechanisms, some of which are immunological in nature.[22,85] Antibody produced by the virus may circulate until it reaches the virus and in combining with it initiate an attack on the tissue to which the virus is attached. Viruses may circulate in the blood, forming circulating immune complexes with the antibody they have induced. The consequences of this depend on the antigen–antibody balance and the size of the complex formed.[22] With large antigen excess, the complexes are small, are excreted readily, and do not activate complement. With antibody excess, large complexes are formed that are phagocytosed and removed. The pathogenic complexes are those in balance or with slight antigen excess that combine with complement and deposit in blood vessels, especially in the glomeruli of the kidney. Together with polymorphonuclear cells, they may evoke an inflammatory response and tissue injury. Immune complex nephritis is the best-studied example of this. A third mechanism of injury, referred to previously, is based on the induction by viruses of new antigens on the surface of the cell. These neoantigens are regarded as foreign by host cells and may evoke antibody formation and a cell-mediated response that results in host cell injury or in immune complex formation. If the virus-infected cell is a lymphocyte, as in the Epstein–Barr virus infection causing infectious mononucleosis, then the neoantigen induced on the B cell may result in a mixed-lymphocyte response with T-cell transformation and proliferation.[5,70,112] In this situation, the atypical lymphocytosis characteristic of the disease may result both from viral-transformed B cells and from T cells entering blast formation as an immune response to altered B cells. A fourth mechanism of immune viral injury might occur when the virus or the virus-induced antigen shares a common component with normal tissue and an autoimmune response results.

Our knowledge of cell-mediated immunity and of cell-mediated tissue injury is incomplete. An increasing understanding of the mechanisms involved, of the relationship of cellular to humoral immunity, and of the consequences of depressed cellular immunity may explain why certain viruses persist and how such persistence may relate to cancer, immune complex diseases, and chronic infections of the CNS.

12. Patterns of Host Responses

The host responses to viral infections vary along a biological gradient in terms of both the *severity* and the *nature* of the clinical syndrome produced.

12.1. The Biological Gradient

The host response to a virus may range from a completely *inapparent* infection without any clinical signs or symptoms at all to one of great clinical severity, even of death. The ratio of these inapparent (or subclinical) to apparent (or clinical) responses varies from one virus to another; representative examples are shown in Table 4. At one end of the spectrum are certain infections that are almost completely asymptomatic or unrecognizable in their pattern until some special event provokes a clinical response. The response may appear long after the initial infection and be due to viral persistence or reactivation or both. The BK and JC strains of papovavirus fall in this category: no known clinical disease has been associated with the high antibody prevalence found for this virus in various population groups.[89,101] However, in patients with Hodgkin's disease and other conditions associated with depression of cell-mediated immunity, a fatal disease of the CNS known as progressive multifocal leukoencephalopathy may develop. The virus can be isolated from the brain.[90] Antibody titers to papovavirus may reach a high level if the patient survives long enough.

A second group of viral infections are those that are predominantly mild or asymptomatic when exposure and infection occur in early childhood, but that frequently result in symptomatic and some-

Table 4. Subclinical/Clinical Ratio in Viral Infections (Inapparent/Apparent Ratio)

Virus	Clinical feature	Age at infection	Estimated subclinical/ clinical ratio	Percentage of infection with clinical features
Poliomyelitis	Paralysis	Child	±1000:1	0.1–1
Epstein–Barr	Heterophil-positive infectious mononucleosis	1–5	>100:1	1
		6–15	10–100:1	1–10
		16–25	2–3:1	50–75
Hepatitis A	Jaundice	<5	20:1	5
		5–9	11:1	10
		10–15	7:1	14
		Adult	2–3:1	50–75
Rubella	Rash	5–20	2:1	50
Influenza	Fever, cough	Young adult	1.5:1	60
Measles	Rash, fever	5–20	1:99	99+
Rabies	CNS symptoms	Any age	0:100	100

times severe clinical disease when infection is delayed until late childhood and young adult life. Examples of this are viral hepatitis, poliomyelitis, and Epstein–Barr virus (EBV) infections.

At the other end of the spectrum are infections due to measles, rabies, and Lassa fever viruses, in which clinically recognized illness usually accompanies the infection. Indeed, in rabies infection of man, death is almost inevitable after characteristic symptoms develop.

This biological gradient of host response is often pictured as an iceberg in which clinically apparent illness—i.e., above the water line—represents only a small proportion of the response pattern and the larger amount represents unrecognized and inapparent infections; a similar analogy may exist at the

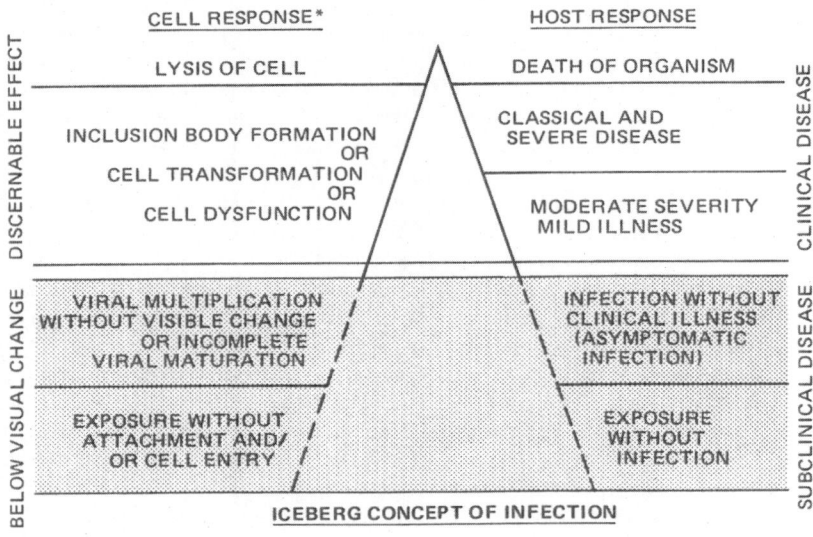

Fig. 2. "Iceberg" concept of infectious diseases at level of the cell and at level of the host. Within any cell population, varying patterns of cell response also occur. * Hypothetical.

cellular level. Figure 2 portrays these concepts. The cellular responses shown might be better considered as differences in the *nature* of the response rather than the *severity* of the response.

12.2. Clinical Syndromes

The *nature* as well as the *severity* of the host response vary widely in viral infections even with the same virus. These various clinical patterns may be due to different organ tropisms of the virus, different portals of entry, different ages at the time of infection, variations in the immune response, and differences in genetically controlled host responses. The clinician faced with the diagnosis of a patient presenting certain respiratory or CNS symptomatology, or with a rash, may be unable to identify the etiological agent on the basis of the clinical findings alone. This is because these target organs have only a limited number of ways to respond to infection and any one of several viruses or other causative agents may trigger an identical or nearly identical response. The results of specific viral tests, even if they yield a viral isolate or show a serological rise, are often available too late to make the diagnosis during the course of the acute illness. The physician must therefore rely on epidemiological and clinical *probabilities* in making a tentative etiological diagnosis. This diagnostic reasoning is based on the known frequency of a certain virus in a given clinical picture and on epidemiological features, which include age, season, year, and epidemic occurrence. Certain infections such as adenovirus pneumonia are more common in military recruits than in other young adults of the same age. A brief presentation of certain common syndromes will be made.

12.2.1. Common Respiratory Syndromes. A great many viruses and viral groups can evoke respiratory symptoms, as can bacteria, rickettsiae, and certain fungi. In children and young adults, over 90% of respiratory infections appear to be viral in nature, although only about half of these can be identified etiologically in the laboratory. In older adults, especially those over 50 years of age, bacterial infections are more common than viral infections and predominate in the severe respiratory-tract infections that require hospitalization.

A number of investigators have sorted out the relative importance of different infectious agents in the etiology of childhood and adult respiratory in-

fections.[14,20,25,29,69,81,104] "Etiological pies" based on these data for four common respiratory syndromes of young adults are depicted in Fig. 3. Some 40–50% are of unknown cause. The importance of the agents involved will vary from year to year, especially as influenza epidemics wax and wane.

In infants, respiratory syncytial virus is by far the most important viral respiratory agent, producing the syndromes of bronchitis and bronchiolitis. Recently, *Chlamydia trachomatis* has also been recognized as an important cause of pneumonia in infants, accounting for perhaps 20–30% of patients hospitalized with penumonia in the first 6 months of life.[51b] In young children, parainfluenza viruses are also an important cause of these two syndromes. The causes of pneumonia syndromes in infancy and young children and in hospitalized adults are shown in Fig. 4. It is not known whether the presence of *Streptococcus pneumoniae* alone in throat cultures from infants and children indicates a true pathogen or only a carrier state.

These etiological pies emphasize the importance of viruses in respiratory disease and explain the failure of chemotherapy. Antibiotic therapy is thus useful only in group A streptococcal pharyngitis and tonsillitis, *Mycoplasma pneumoniae* pneumonia as in young adults, and bacterial pneumonia as in adults over age 50. It is not useful therapeutically or prophylactically in any viral disease.

12.2.2. Common Infections of the Central Nervous System. Multiple agents are also involved in the causation of acute infections of the CNS. An analysis of the causes of the syndromes of infectious encephalitis in 1977 as reported to the Center for Disease Control (CDC) in the United States[13a] is given in Fig. 5 for 938 cases. In only 27.1% could a cause be identified; 72.9% were of indeterminate cause. The distribution of agents will vary from year to year. For example, in 1976, there were 1826 reported cases, of which 38.6% were identified. This included 23.4% due to arboviruses, in which St. Louis encephalitis predominated, accounting for 88.7% of the 427 cases of arboviral etiology. In contrast, in 1978, there were only 53 cases due to arboviruses in the continental United States, of which 43 were due to California virus. In addition, some 10,000 cases of dengue occurred in Puerto Rico.

In 1979, there were 8201 reported cases of aseptic meningitis reported to the CDC as of December 22. The analysis of the causes is not yet completed, but

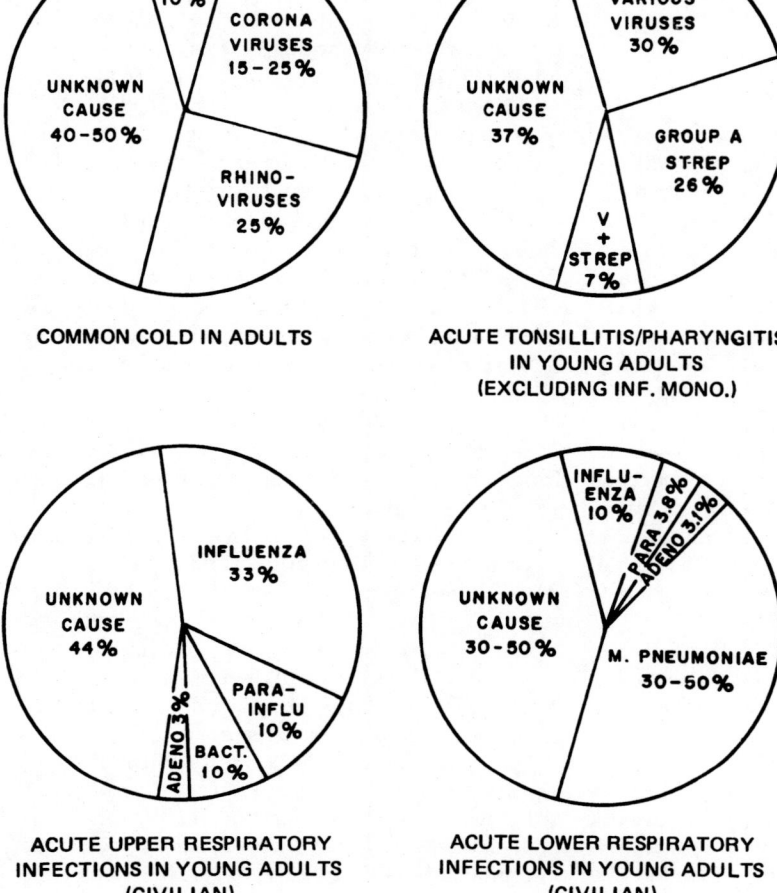

COMMON COLD IN ADULTS

ACUTE TONSILLITIS/PHARYNGITIS
IN YOUNG ADULTS
(EXCLUDING INF. MONO.)

Fig. 3. The causes of acute respiratory syndromes in young adults.

ACUTE UPPER RESPIRATORY
INFECTIONS IN YOUNG ADULTS
(CIVILIAN)

ACUTE LOWER RESPIRATORY
INFECTIONS IN YOUNG ADULTS
(CIVILIAN)

based on past experience will include about 80% of unknown cause, about 15% due to enteroviruses (depending on epidemic activity), and a small percentage due to mumps. The small number of cases of established etiology is in part related to the diagnostic need for both isolation of the agent from the stool and the demonstration of an antibody rise to that particular enterovirus, whereas identification of the causes of infectious encephalitis can be made primarily on serological grounds using a battery of about 10 known standard antigens.

Certain state laboratories have made more intensive investigations of the etiology of infections of the CNS. In California, an intensive investigation of the syndrome of aseptic meningitis in the 1950s and 1960s permitted identification of a suspected causal agent in about 65% of the cases.[67a] In more recent years, such as 1975–1976 and 1976–1977, fewer systematic and intensive studies were made, so that only about 20% were identified although essentially the same range of etiological agents was involved.[67b]

12.2.3. Common Exanthems. Acute viral syndromes involving the skin are represented by the exanthems of childhood (measles, rubella, varicella); by various strains of coxsackievirus and echo-

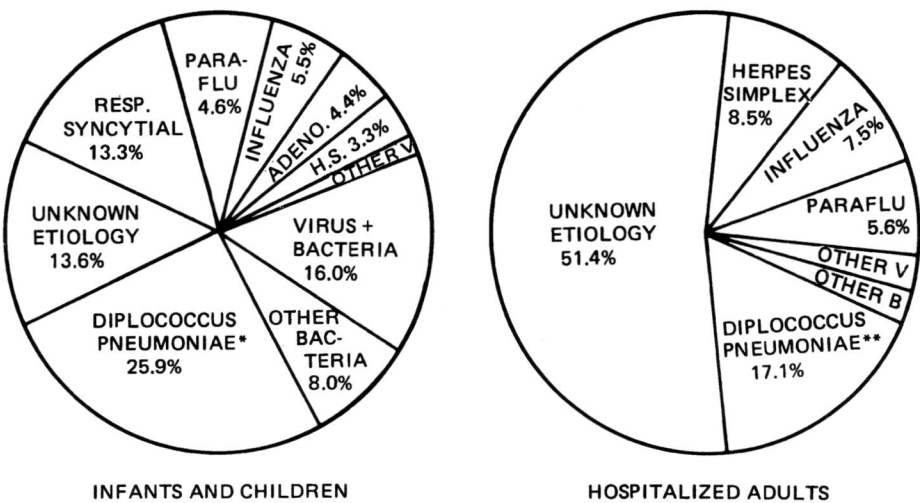

Fig. 4. Causes of pneumonia syndromes in infants and children and in hospitalized adults. * Based on pure throat culture. ** Based on pure blood culture and now called *Streptococcus pneumoniae*.

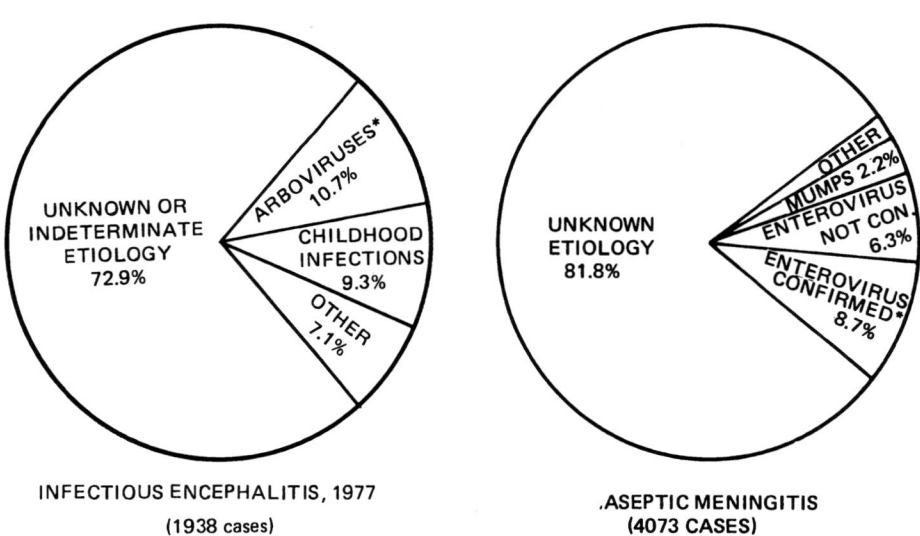

Fig. 5. Causes of syndromes involving the central nervous system in the United States. * Confirmed by virus isolation from cerebrospinal fluid and/or serological rise; not confirmed if virus isolated from stool or throat only. Arboviruses: WEE, 4.4%; SLE, 2.5%; EEE, 0.1%; CE, 3.7%. Childhood infections: Mumps, 3.3%; measles, 1.8%; varicella, 4.1%. Other: Enteroviruses, 2.3%; HSV, 3.4%; other known viruses, 1.4%. From CDC Surveillance Reports, Encephalitis, July 19, Aseptic Meningitis, May 1973.

virus; by adenoviruses, especially type 7; by EBV in infectious mononucleosis; and by the presumed viral causes of roseola infantum (exanthem subitum) and erythema infectiosum. A listing of the clinical exanthems associated with the viruses is given in Table 5.

Enteroviral exanthems are not reportable, so an overall "etiological pie" cannot be reliably constructed. Epidemics of Echo 9 such as the 1978 outbreak on Long Island[13b] occur periodically and may involve large communities. Variable expressions of rash, pharyngitis, and CNS involvement occur in different outbreaks.[4a] Of 266,136 cases of reported viral exanthems in the United States in 1977,[13a] 70.8% were chicken pox, 21.5% were measles, and 7.7% were rubella.

12.2.4. Viral Hepatitis. The wide use of laboratory tests for hepatitis B virus (HBV) now permits accurate identification of this antigen, but the very limited amounts of hepatitis A antigen (HAV) and of the "non-A, non-B" antigens available have restricted testing for these causes to a few research centers. Of over 54,132 cases of viral hepatitis reported to the CDC in 1979, 53.4% were classified as HAV, 27.0% as HBV, and 19.6% as unspecified. The diagnostic restrictions of this data should be kept in mind. It is clear that most transfusion hepatitis in the United States currently is non-A, non-B (see Chapter 12). Other viral causes of hepatitis include EBV (infectious mononucleosis) and cytomegalovirus, but neither of these is a reportable disease. Based on an estimated 100,000 cases of infectious

mononucleosis annually, of which about 5% have clinical jaundice, there may be roughly 5000 cases in the United States from this cause.

12.2.5. Viral Gastroenteritis. Rapid advances in our knowledge of the causes of acute viral gastroenteritis have occurred in the past 5 years, and these are presented in Chapter 11. The importance of rotaviruses (duoviruses, reolike viruses) as a cause of acute gastroenteritis in infants and young children throughout the world has now been established through use of immune electron-microscopy studies of stool samples[7,8,42,64a,76] and, more recently, with the enzyme-linked immunosorbent assay (ELISA) and with serological techniques.[112a] The causes of acute gastroenteritis in 378 children in Melbourne, Australia, are shown in Fig. 6: 52% were associated with rotavirus (duoviruses) in the stool in contrast to their absence in the stool of 116 control children.[20a] The contribution of rotavirus infection to acute gastroenteritis of infants and children has varied in different geographic areas. Some examples are: Canada, 11.0%[50a]; Venezuela, 41.3%[108a]; United States, 42.0%[62a]; Japan, 89%.[64a] The evidence clearly indicates that this virus is the major cause of acute childhood gastroenteritis in winter months. It may also cause diarrhea in adults.[10a] Two types of rotavirus infections have been identified using the ELISA test[112a]: of 414 isolates tested, 77% were identified as Type 2, and the rest were Type 1. Infection with Type 1 was asymptomatic in 45% of the infections, whereas every Type 2 infection was associated with gastroenteritis. The two types show no evidence of cross-immunity.

Another viral cause of acute gastroenteritis is called the "Norwalk agent" from the town in Ohio where the first isolates were obtained during an outbreak involving older children and adults. It is a parvovirus, about 27 nm in size, and is also identified by immune electron microscopy. The agent has been associated with at least six outbreaks of gastroenteritis in older children and adults in several geographic areas. There appear to be at least three different types. Its contribution to acute gastroenteritis in general is not known (see Chapter 11 for more details).

12.2.6. Congenital Infections. The acronym TORCH (toxoplasma, other viruses, rubella, cytomegalovirus, and herpes simplex) designates the most common causes.[81b,95b] Infection rates in pregnant women and their infants are given in Table 6. Cytomegalovirus (CMV) is the most frequent, pro-

Table 5. Viral Causes of Common Exanthems

Type of rash	Examples
Macular/papular	Measles and measles vaccine
	Rubella
	Echo 4, 9, 16
	Coxsackie A9, 16, B5
	Adeno
Vesicular	Varicella
	Smallpox
	Eczema hepaticum
	Eczema vaccinatum
	Herpes zoster
	Coxsackie A16
Petechial or purpuric	Coxsackie A9
	Echo 9

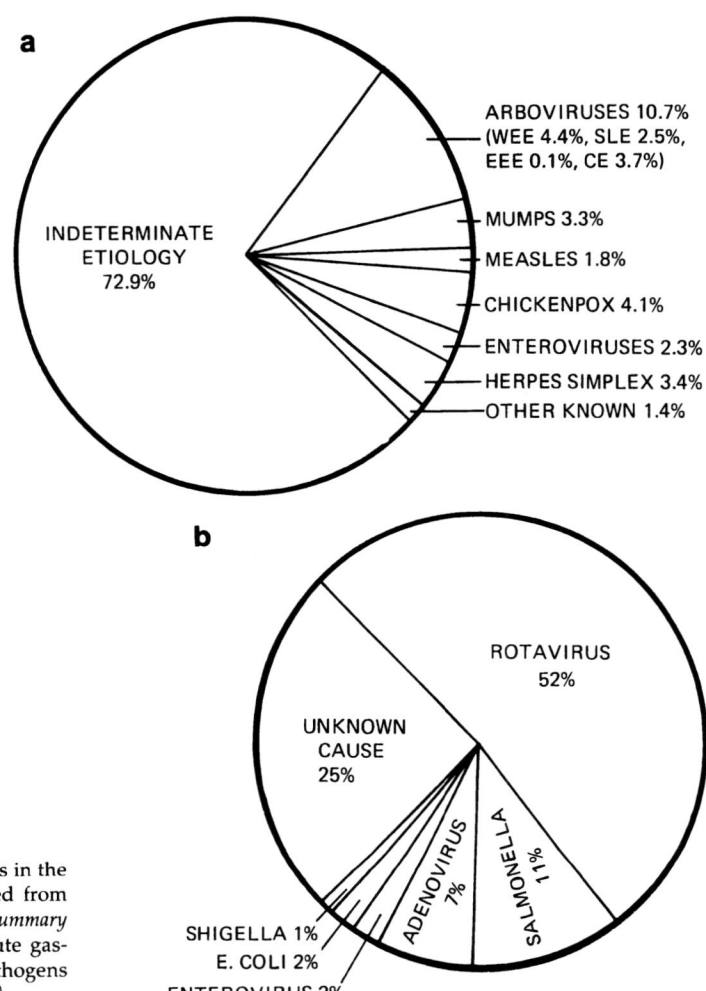

Fig. 6. (a) Causes of infectious encephalitis in the United States in 1977 (936 cases). Derived from *Morbidity Mortality Weekly Report, Annual Summary for 1977* **26**:1–80 (1978). (b) Causes of acute gastroenteritis in 378 children with enteric pathogens in feces. Adapted from Davidson *et al.*[20a]

ducing congenital anomalies manifested as microcephaly, chorioretinitis, deafness, and mental retardation; these usually result from primary infection in an antibody-negative mother, but reactivated infections of the mother may occasionally lead to congenital infection and disease. The antibody prevalence in women of child-bearing age varies in different socioeconomic and geographic settings—about 60% have antibody in the United States (see Chapter 8, Section 5.1). In prospective tests on antibody-negative women, 1.4% had a primary CMV infection during pregnancy leading to 77% infection and 11% stigma rates in their offspring. In the United States and England, about 1 in 100 live births will be CMV-infected and about 1 in 1000 have a

congenital defect. Rubella is the next most common, resulting in abortion and stillbirth and in congenital abnormalities such as cataracts, deafness, heart lesions, psychomotor retardation, and others (see Chapter 21, Section 8.1.2). Congenital abnormalities occur in 15–20% of infants from mothers infected during the first trimester; late manifestations may increase this to 30–35%. Herpes simplex (HSV) from infections of the pregnant mother due to either type 1 or type 2 can result in disseminated disease of the infant with involvement of the liver and other visceral organs, as well as localized lesions, but the importance of HSV in congenital malformation is not known (see Chapter 13, Section 9.1). Other viruses may occasionally result in congenital infection

Table 6. Estimated Rate of Infection in Pregnant Women and Their Infants in the United States[a]

Cause	Mother (per 1000 pregnancies)	Fetus (per 1000 live births)
Rubella		
Epidemic	20–40	4–30
Interepidemic	1	0.5
CMV	40–150	5–20
HSV	10–15	?
T. gondii	1.5–6.4	0.75–1.3
T. pallidum	0.2	0.1

[a] Derived from Alford *et al.*,[1a] and based on prospective serologic and virologic evidence.

with a risk per 10,000 mothers estimated as 10 for mumps, 5 for varicella zoster, and 0.6 for measles. Mumps and measles infections of the pregnant mother may result in increased fetal death, varicella-zoster, smallpox, and vaccinias with widespread infections of the infant. Maternal Coxsackie B infection may lead to neonatal encephalomyocarditis; maternal hepatitis may be more severe in pregnancy and hepatitis may appear in the infant.

12.2.7. Immunosuppressed and Surgical Patients. Reactivation of viral infections, especially the herpes group, is common in immunosuppressed, transplanted, or transfused patients. Most of these are inapparent infections, but diseases occasionally result, especially with CMV. Armstrong *et al.*[4a] found the infection rates in 26 prospectively followed renal-transplant recipients to be: CMV, 43%; HSV, 38%; EBV, 32%. With the exception of 3 primary CMV infections, all others were due to reactivation. No unusual incidence of primary or secondary infections to nonherpes viruses (parainfluenza 1, 2, 3, HBV, measles, rubella) occurred. Clinically, 5 patients developed herpetic-type sores, three of whom showed HSV antibody rises; 5 had fever of unknown origin with rises in CMV antibody titer. Hematologically, 7 patients showed atypical lymphocytosis associated with serological evidence of CMV in 6. Of 13 episodes of rejection, 5 occurred in patients with CMV antibody rises. Fever and lymphocytosis due to CMV also occur after cardiac surgery, and the mononucleosis syndrome occurs in about one third of patients after heart surgery with an extracorporeal pump (see Chapter 8, Section 8.2.3). The source of CMV in transplant and surgery patients is unclear and might be exogenous in origin, be introduced with the blood, result from reactivation in the blood of the recipient, or be present in the transplanted organ. Immunodeficiency also enhances the severity of primary viral infections, especially herpes infections, from natural exogenous sources as well as induced infections in persons receiving live polio, measles, rubella, smallpox, or yellow fever vaccines.

12.2.8. Sexually Transmitted Infections. These now include herpes simplex as an important cause.[13d] While HSV-2 is primarily involved, oral–genital and oral–rectal practices are now involving HSV-1 as well. Since HSV infections are not reportable, the contribution of HSV to the total syndrome cannot be determined on a national basis. It has been estimated that 1 case of genital herpes occurs for every 5–10 of gonorrhea[81a]; in a group of Boston clinics, genital herpes was seen 7 times more frequently than primary syphilis.[13c] In a recent survey of six clinics in the United States, 3.4% of the visits in men and 1.5% of the visits in women were diagnosed as genital herpes (Fig. 7). (See Chapter 13 for more information on HSV infections.) While hepatitis B and CMV may also be venereally transmitted, there is no known clinical expression of this infection.

12.2.9. Hospital Infections. Viruses are not widely recognized as important causative agents in nosocomial infections.[66a] However, they have been inadequately studied and clearly play a role in special settings. One is the nursery, where infections, diseases, and sometimes outbreaks of illness have occurred from herpes simplex, varicella-zoster, CMVs, enteroviruses, myxoviruses, and parainfluenza 3 virus.[62b,64a,95a] Rubella may spread to other infants or to susceptible nursery staff. A second setting is the hemodialysis unit and the laboratory, where hospital personnel are at risk to viral hepatitis, especially HBV. A third is on crowded wards, where both susceptible patients and staff are at risk to influenza and other respiratory-borne viruses. For this reason, routine influenza immunization should be carried on in hospital personnel. Fourth, patients receiving multiple transfusions or transplant organs may be infected with hepatitis B, hepatitis non-A, non-B, CMV, and sometimes EBV. Immunosuppressed patients are susceptible to primary and reactivated viral infections, especially the herpes group. Hospital personnel, especially on the obstetrics staff, may be at high risk to Lassa fever virus in endemic areas. Even smallpox has found its way

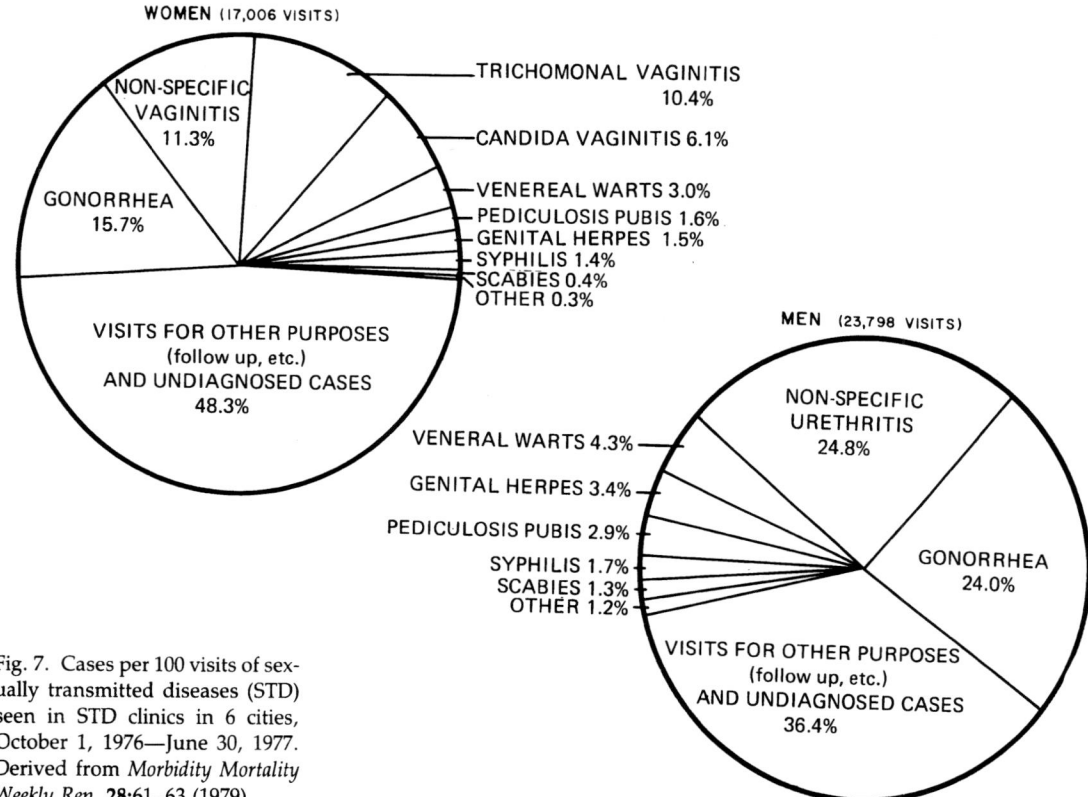

Fig. 7. Cases per 100 visits of sexually transmitted diseases (STD) seen in STD clinics in 6 cities, October 1, 1976—June 30, 1977. Derived from *Morbidity Mortality Weekly Rep.* **28**:61–63 (1979).

from the laboratory into the air vents to infect distant personnel. The transmission of Jakob–Creutzfeldt disease and of rabies constitutes an unusual hazard in corneal-transplant recipients and sometimes in neurosurgeons.

12.2.10. Renal Syndromes. In renal diseases, evidence of viral causation has not been firmly established in man, except for hemorrhagic cystitis due to adeno 11. This is despite the occasional presence of viruses in the urine and the ability of many viruses to multiply in *in vitro* tissue cultures prepared from human kidneys. The role of immune complex formation of viruses and antibody in the causation of human glomerulonephritis is unknown, although there is ample precedent in animal models[86]; except for elevated antibody titers to rubella virus in the nephritis of systemic lupus erythematosus, no other leads were found in a serological study of 106 cases of immune complex glomerulonephritis of unknown cause employing 13 different viral antigens.[114] It is likely that improved techniques of

identifying viruses and immune complexes will lead to the discovery of a role for viruses in both acute and chronic nephritis.

13. Diagnosis of Viral Diseases

The etiological diagnosis of a viral disease usually requires laboratory tests. There are four circumstances in which a probable diagnosis of the causative agent is suggested on clinical or epidemiological grounds or both. First, some viral infections have distinctive enough *clinical* features that typical cases can be recognized *if they occur* in the right geographic area, season, and/or age group. This includes chickenpox and herpes zoster, herpes simplex infection of lips or genitalia, infectious mononucleosis in a young adult, measles, mumps parotitis, paralytic poliomyelitis, rabies, rubella, smallpox, and viral hepatitis. Second, if there is an *epidemic* in which an etiological agent has been isolated, then most clinical syndromes of the same type are probably due to the same virus. Examples of this are outbreaks of influenza, arbovirus infections, enteroviral exanthems, epidemic pleurodynia, and pharyngeal–conjunctival fever. Third, special or unique epidemiological circumstances may indicate the probable diagnosis; croup or bronchiolitis in an infant is most likely due to respiratory syncytial virus, jaundice in drug users is usually hepatitis B or following a blood transfusion is often non-A, non-B hepatitis, and mononucleosis following blood transfusion and/or immunosuppression is probably due to cytomegalovirus (CMV). Fourth, the type of *organ* involvement may be a lead—i.e., 80–90% of common respiratory infections are viral in origin, nonpurulent infections of the CNS are likely to be viral, with the most likely candidates being mumps virus, enteroviruses, and arboviruses, in that order.

There are some common but not pathognomonic features of viral diseases: they are usually nonpurulent and associated with mononuclear rather than polymorphonuclear infiltrates; the onset is more likely to be insidious than with a bacterial infection; often there are prodromal symptoms; and retrobulbar headache is common. In the clinical laboratory, the presence of a normal or low white count suggests a viral infection, but typhoid, tuberculosis, brucellosis, malaria, histoplasmosis, and overwhelming bacterial infections can also produce leukopenia. The presence of lymphocytosis and of atypical lymphocytes also suggests a viral infection. Lymphocytosis of 50% or more and atypical lymphocytosis of 20% or more occur in infectious (Epstein–Barr virus) mononucleosis, cytomegalovirus mononucleosis, and rarely in *T. gondii* infections, but drugs such as *p*-aminosalicylate (PAS), Dilantin, and tetrachlorethylene may also evoke lymphocytosis. Less intense lymphocyte responses are seen in a variety of viral infections such as rubella, hepatitis A, adenovirus, mumps, herpes, and varicella infections. They may occasionally occur in tuberculosis, histoplasmosis, and other nonviral infections.

The diagnostic procedures used for viral infections are presented in individual chapters of this book. However, there are certain common aspects of collection, requests for testing, and interpretation that merit comment here. A detailed description can be found in the APHA diagnostic handbook[67] and in a fine book by Hsiung.[57a]

13.1. Collection

Materials for viral isolation should be obtained from the site of the lesion, if feasible. Usually, a swab or gargles from the throat and a rectal swab or a stool sample are useful for all suspected respiratory and CNS infections and for the viral exanthems. Nasopharyngeal washings using an infant-sized catheter and suction apparatus should be taken for direct fluorescent-antibody identification of respiratory viruses.[47a] In suspected arboviruses infections, a sample of whole blood should be collected, and in vesicular exanthem, an aspiration or scraping of the lesion. Direct viral fluorescent-antibody identification of rabies and certain other infections may be possible with small skin biopsies; brain biopsies are needed to identify herpes simplex virus meningoencephalitis. All such materials should be frozen immediately at $-70°C$ and shipped in dry ice or liquid nitrogen to the nearest viral diagnostic laboratory—usually a governmental (state, Federal) or university laboratory. Collection and shipping kits are often available. For some more stable viruses, freezing may not be necessary if transportation time is short. Certain laboratories now provide tubes with a transport medium. These include tissue-culture tubes with one or even two tissue-culture cell types already grown and ready for bedside inoculation of the specimen and shipment to the laboratory for further study.[77]

Serological tests are carried out on serum from a sample of blood, usually 10 ml collected in the acute illness, and on a convalescent sample obtained 2–3 weeks later; a third sample drawn about a month after the second may be useful in some infections. The sera should be sterilely separated immediately after clotting and either frozen ($-20°$ or $-70°C$) or kept at 4°C. Serum may be stored in a freezer in the hospital or clinic where it has been collected or in the laboratory where the test is performed. In infectious-disease hospitals or units, *routine* collection and storage of acute and convalescent sera from all febrile patients should be carried out to permit retrospective testing.

13.2. Requests for Testing

Most common clinical syndromes have more than one cause, so that a request for a battery of serological tests should be made for most individual cases. The laboratory needs clinical and epidemiological information as a guide for these determinations. At a minimum, the age of the patient, date of onset, and the major organ system involved should be indicated on the request slip. The term "viral disease" or "FUO" leaves the laboratory at a loss as to the best way to proceed.

13.3. Tests Employed

Isolation or identification of the virus, preferably from the lesion itself, and demonstration of a serological response to it are the common criteria for viral diagnosis. Unfortunately, the isolation of a virus in tissue culture, embryonated eggs, or suckling mice may require at least a week and often longer if identification of the virus is involved, and serological diagnosis is usually dependent on tests of a convalescent serum sample. Such viral diagnosis is therefore of little help to the clinician in recognition and management of the acute viral disease. Progress is being made in rapid diagnostic techniques.[74,117a,105] These include the identification of respiratory syncytial and influenza viral infections by fluorescent identification of antigen in nasopharyngeal cells[47a]; the demonstration of rotaviruses, parvoviruses, and hepatitis A virus particles in stool samples by immune electron microscopy or by the enzyme-linked immunosorbent assay (ELISA)[112a,117a]; and the recognition of several viruses in clinical material by radioimmunoassay. The electron microscope has also been used to identify herpes and pox viruses in vesicle fluid and CMV in urine.

13.4. Interpretation of Tests

Isolation of the virus and a 4-fold or greater rise in antibody titer between the acute and convalescent sera are classic criteria for viral diagnosis. For some viral infections, isolation of the virus first and then tests for a serological rise against that isolate are required. This is true of virus groups in which there are too many antigenically distinct strains to carry out a battery of serological tests such as the echovirus, coxsackievirus, and rhinovirus groups. The adenoviruses, group B arboviruses, and influenza A and B groups have common intragroup antigens, particularly in the complement-fixation test. These permit one test to be used to reflect infection for all members of that viral group.

If it has been possible to obtain only a single convalescent serum sample and a high antibody titer is found, or if high titers are present in both acute and convalescent sera without a 4-fold difference, then the question is whether these results reflect current infection or persistently high titers from a previous infection. Significance may be attached to these findings if the disease is a rare one in which the presence of this antibody is unique, if the test reflects a short-lasting antibody, or if IgM-type antibody can be demonstrated. A rapid drop in antibody titer in a subsequent specimen is also suggestive of a recent infection. Sequential testing of other family members may also be useful, since they may be in different stages of apparent or inapparent infection with the same virus. In an epidemic setting, comparison of the geometric mean antibody titer of sera collected early in illness from one group of patients with the titer in sera from another group of patients convalescing from the same illness may permit rapid identification of the outbreak.

Sometimes a virus may be isolated or an antibody rise may be demonstrated that is not, in fact, causally related to the illness. Sometimes two viruses, or a virus and a bacteria, are implicated in the infection, and the interpretation of their causal role may be very difficult. On other occasions, no virus can be isolated or a serological rise is not demonstrable when a specific virus is the real cause of the illness. A list of some common causes for these false-positive and false-negative results is given in Table 7.

14. Proof of Causation

The classic concepts of causation in infectious diseases are those elaborated by Jakob Henle (1809–1885) in 1840 and by his student Robert Koch (1843–1910) in 1884 and 1890. These are termed the Henle–Koch postulates. The basic criteria (Table 8, column 1) included the consistent presence of the parasite in the disease in question under circumstances that can account for the pathological changes and clinical course, the absence of the parasite in other diseases as a fortuitous or nonpathogenic parasite, and the experimental reproduction of the dis-

Table 7. Viral Diagnosis: Some Causes of False-Positive and False-Negative Tests

False positive
Viral isolation
1. Persistent or reactivated virus from prior and unrelated infection has been isolated.
2. A viral contaminant is present in the tissue culture or other isolation system.
3. Nonspecific cytopathic effects occur due to toxicity of specimen or presence of bacteria, or to other causes, and are mistaken for a virus.
4. Two microbial agents are present and the one isolated is not the cause of the disease.

Serological rise
1. Cross-reacting antigens.
2. Nonspecific inhibitors.
3. Double infection, with only one agent producing the illness.
4. Rise to vaccination rather than natural infection.

False negative
Viral isolation
1. Viral specimen taken too late or too early in illness.
2. Wrong site of multiplication sampled (e.g., throat rather than rectal swab).
3. Improper transport or storage of specimen—not kept frozen.
4. Wrong laboratory animal or tissue-culture system selected for isolation.
5. Toxicity of specimen kills the tissue culture, obscuring the presence of virus.

Serological rise
1. Specimens not taken at proper time—i.e., too late in illness or too close together to show antibody rise.
2. Poor antibody response—low antigenicity of the virus or removal of antibody by immune-complex formation.
3. Wrong virus or wrong virus strain used in the test.
4. Nonspecific inhibitor obscures true antibody rise.
5. Wrong test used for the timing of the serum specimens.

---

ease by the organism after having been grown repeatedly in pure culture. The rigidity of these criteria and the inability of many clear-cut causes of certain diseases to fulfill them was recognized by Koch himself. He recognized that while the bacteria of anthrax, tuberculosis, tetanus, and many animal diseases fulfilled the proof, those of many other diseases did not. These latter included typhoid fever, diphtheria, leprosy, relapsing fever, and Asiatic cholera. He felt particularly strongly about cholera because he himself had discovered the causative organism. For these diseases, he felt that fulfillment of only the first two criteria was needed and that experimental reproduction of the disease was not essential to proof of causation. Rivers[96] reviewed the Koch postulates in terms of viral infections in his presidential address to the American Immunological Society in 1937 and found them lacking. Included in his objections were (1) the idea that a disease is necessarily caused by only one agent, citing the work of Shope[102] with swine influenza, in which both a virus and a bacteria are required; (2) the necessity of demonstrating the presence of

viruses in *every* case of the disease produced by it; and (3) the fact that the existence of virus carriers must be recognized. He set forth two conditions for establishing the specific relationship of a virus to a disease (Table 8, column 2): (1) a specific virus must be present with a degree of regularity in association with the disease and (2) the virus must occur in the sick individual not as an incidental or accidental finding but as a cause of the disease. In support of the latter, he stressed the importance of the experimental reproduction of the disease in susceptible experimental hosts with the inclusion of suitable controls to eliminate the fortuitous presence of other viral agents either in the patient or in the experimental host. The absence of antibody to a virus in the patient's sera at the onset of illness and its appearance during recovery were recognized as an important but not absolute link in causation; Rivers was cautious in this statement because of the possible presence of passenger viruses to which antibody appeared but which were not of etiological significance. He also noted that recovery from viral infection sometimes takes place without the devel-

Table 8. Postulates of Causation

Bacteria[a] Henle (1840); Koch (1890)	Viruses[b] Rivers (1937)	Viruses[c] Immunological proof (1973)
1. Parasite occurs in every case of the disease in question and under circumstances that can account for the pathological changes and clinical course of the disease.	1. A specific virus must be found associated with a disease with a degree of regularity.	1. Viral-specific antibody is regularly absent prior to illness.
2. Occurs in no other disease as fortuitous and nonpathogenic parasite.	2. Virus occurs in the sick individual not as incidental or accidental finding but as cause of the disease.	2. Antibody regularly appears during illness, including: a. Transient viral-specific IgM antibody b. Persistent IgG antibody c. Local antibody (IgA)—at site of primary multiplication.
3. After being fully isolated from the body and repeatedly grown in pure culture, can induce the disease anew.	3. Transmissible infection is produced with a degree of regularity in susceptible experimental hosts by means of inoculation of material, free from ordinary microbes or rickettsiae, obtained from patients with the disease, and proper control and immunological studies demonstrate that the virus was neither fortuitously present in the patient nor accidentally picked up in the experimental animals.	3. Antibody production is accompanied by presence of viruses in appropriate tissues.
Only 1 and 2 were regarded as essential by Koch.		4. Absence of IgG antibody indicates susceptibility to the disease. 5. Presence of IgG antibody indicates immunity to the disease. 6. No other virus or antibody is similarly associated. 7. Production of the antibody (immunization) prevents the disease.

[a] Koch[64] (see Rivers[96]). [b] Rivers.[96] [c] Derived from Rivers[96] and Evans.[29a]

opment of antibodies and that occasionally an individual already possessing antibodies against a virus succumbs to a disease caused by it (i.e., reinfection or reactivation).

The "virologists' dilemma" was further discussed in 1957 by Huebner,[58] who revised the Koch and Rivers postulates into the following criteria: (1) the virus must be a "real entity," i.e., well-established on animal or tissue culture passage in the laboratory; (2) the virus must originate in human tissues and be repeatedly present therein and not in the experimental animals, cells, or the media used to grow it; (3) the agent should be characterized early to permit differentiation from other agents, including immunological comparisons; (4) the virus should have a constant association with the clinical entity in question; (5) the clinical syndrome should be experimentally reproducible in volunteers inoculated with the agent in a "double-blind" study; (6) carefully conceived epidemiological cross-sectional and longitudinal studies are indispensable in establishing the role of highly prevalent viruses in human diseases; (7) the disease should be prevented by a specific vaccine. He also added an eighth consideration—financial support—which is so needed to carry out the virological and epidemiological analyses required in establishing proof of causation.

The problem of establishing causality for viral infections has been exemplified by the relationship of Epstein–Barr virus (EBV) to infectious mononucleosis. In the beginning, no method of virus isolation existed, no susceptible laboratory animal was known, and EBV antibody was already present at the time the patient with infectious mononucleosis was first seen by the physician. The proof of causation had to rest on prospective serological investigations that fulfilled certain immunological criteria.[29a,54,82,98,109] The most important of these were the regular absence of antibody prior to disease, its regular appearance during illness, and the relationship of antibody to susceptibility and immunity[33,82] (see Table 8, column 3). To date, a vaccine has not been developed to prevent the disease. Advances in viral technology later permitted the identification of the presence and persistence of EBV in the pharynx of patients having acute infectious mononucleosis. Human and monkey transmission experiments with EBV have resulted in the reproduction of some but not all of the features of the disease (see Chapter 10). The web of causation is now firm that EBV causes all heterophil-antibody-positive infectious mononucleosis and most heterophile negative cases.[30]

Similar seroepidemiological techniques have been needed in studying the spectrum of infections produced by hepatitis B antigen (HBAg) because of the difficulty of isolating the virus in the laboratory and the lack of a good experimental animal (see Chapter 12).

The most difficult and challenging problems of causation are arising in the possible relationship between certain viruses and the development of various malignant and chronic diseases. These include EBV in relation to Burkitt lymphoma and nasopharyngeal cancer,[28,29,36] herpesvirus type 2 in relation to cervical cancer,[19] measles virus in relation to subacute sclerosing panencephalopathy and to multiple sclerosis,[18,99,110] and papovaviruses in

relation to progressive multifocal leukoencephalopathy. High antibody titers to the viruses in question are common in many of these conditions, as well as sarcoidosis[13] and systemic lupus erythematosis.[94,97] But it is not known whether they precede the illness, accompany it, or occur in its wake. The persistence and/or reactivation of these viruses under circumstances of impaired cell-mediated immunity (CMI) have been postulated as a possible common mechanism.[27,110] Such an impairment in CMI could arise when the viral infection occurs very early in infancy or during pregnancy; it might also result from the presence of a concomitant infection (malaria) that depresses the immune response, from the use of immunosuppressive drugs, from genetic defects in the ability of T-type lymphocytes to recognize or respond to certain viruses, from serum inhibitors of cellular immunity, or from disease-induced immunosuppression.

Current evidence suggests that certain cancers and certain chronic diseases of man are due to the persistence and/or reactivation of common, ubiquitous viruses in an immunologically compromised host. Those viruses with a capacity for latency such as the herpes, papova, measles, rubella, and adenoviruses appear to be the most likely candidates for the causation of these conditions. Present and future work to determine the elements of causation include (1) large-scale multipurpose prospective studies of populations, seeking evidence of viral persistence, high viral antibody levels, and/or impaired lymphocyte response to viral agents as a possible prelude to malignancy and chronic disease, and then the appearance of the disease itself as more definitive proof of causation; (2) the demonstration of the virus or viral genome in afflicted tissues but not in normal tissues; (3) the occurrence or reproduction of the condition in man and/or experimental hosts, or both, under natural or induced viral infection. It must be stressed that cancer or a chronic disease will not always result even under propitious circumstances. The host response will probably fall along a biological gradient from very mild to severe. It also seems likely that any given malignant or chronic condition may be produced by more than one cause or group of causes. The current evidence on viruses, cancer, and their relationship to chronic neurological diseases is discussed in later chapters of this book. The developments in our concepts of causation and the limitations of the Henle–Koch postulates have been recently reviewed.[30a–c]

15. Control and Prevention

The basic concept in controlling a viral disease is to break a link in the chain of causation. Interruption of a single known essential link may effectively control a disease even if knowledge of other links, or of the etiology itself, is incomplete. Despite this, very little has been accomplished in most viral diseases by environmental changes, except for the arboviruses, in which the appropriate insect vector can be controlled. Improved water supplies, proper sewage disposal, and improved personal hygiene could potentially decrease the incidence of poliomyelitis and other enterovirus and hepatitis A infections, but in general the results have been disappointing because so many pathways of infection exist. Furthermore, improved sanitation may delay the age of exposure to later childhood and young adult life, when infections are more often clinically apparent and more severe.

15.1. Immunization

The difficulty in the environmental control of viral infections spread by close personal contact, by the respiratory route, or even by oral–intestinal spread has directed the main thrust of prevention to immunization of the host. The requirements of a good vaccine are listed in Table 9. The overall objective is to create the same degree and duration of protection as with natural infection but without the ac-

Table 9. Objectives of Immunization

1. Produce a good humoral, cellular, and local immune response similar to natural infection.
2. Produce protection against clinical disease and reinfection.
3. Give protection over several years, preferably a lifetime.
4. Result in minimal immediate side reactions or mild disease and with no delayed effects such as late reactivation, CNS involvement, or cancer.
5. Can be administered simply in a form acceptable to the public.
6. Cost and benefits of administration should clearly outweigh the cost and risk of natural disease.

companying clinical illness. Both live and killed vaccines have been used. In general, live viral vaccines are more desirable and induce a longer and broader immune response, especially if given by a natural route. Some of the problems include successful attenuation without reversion to virulence, avoidance of viral persistence and of the risk of reactivation, and the elimination of possible oncogenicity. These are major hurdles for vaccines against herpes viruses, and it is difficult to measure some of these attributes in the laboratory. There are efforts to produce live vaccines with temperature-sensitive mutants for respiratory syncytial and influenza viruses that would multiply only in the colder temperature of the upper respiratory host but not in the lung where clinical disease might result. Table 10 summarizes current information on the use of viral vaccines (see individual chapters for more details).

The most successful of these efforts toward vaccine development have used an attenuated live virus as the antigen (adenovirus, measles, mumps, poliovirus, rubella, and smallpox). Administration by the natural portal of entry to produce local immunity has also been important (poliovirus, adenovirus). Inactivated viral vaccines such as influenza vaccine have met with limited success, although highly purified and concentrated preparations are giving more promising results[45]; a successful inactivated polio vaccine has also provided good protection in Scandinavian countries. Passive immunization is a short-term expedient useful only when the γ-globulin can be administered early after exposure and when it contains a sufficiently high titer of specific antibody. Today, well-defined exposures to hepatitis A, vaccinia virus, and rabies virus under circumstances of high risk constitute the major indications for passive antibody. In rabies, this approach is probably the most important one in preventing the disease following severe exposures; it is successful because early administration may interrupt the virus before it reaches the CNS. In the past, immunoglobulin was also used after exposure to measles, mumps, or rubella viruses, but such preparations are not commonly employed today because of the availability of effective live vaccines and the difficulty in administering the immune globulin early enough.

Our greatest needs today for the prevention of viral diseases are the development of effective vaccines against hepatitis viruses, syncytial virus, parainfluenza viruses, and the human herpesvi-

Table 10. Viral Prophylaxis[a]

Vaccine	Type[b]	Persons to be immunized	Age	Product[c]	Dosage (ml)	Route	Number of doses or repeats
Adenovirus	L	Military recruits	Young adults	Type 4 and 7	0.5	Oral (enteric capsule)	1
Hepatitis A	P	1. Household and institutional contacts in 1st 2 wk after exposure	All	ISG	0.02 ml kg	i.m.	1
B	P	1. Accidental needle-stick or mucosal exposure in 7 days	All	HBIG (or use ISG in same dose)	0.05–0.07 ml/kg	i.m.	2 (25–30 day later)
		2. Infants with mothers with acute hepatitis in 3rd trimester and HBsAG in 7 days of birth.	Infant	HBIG or ISG	0.13 ml/kg 0.5 ml/kg	i.m. i.m.	1 1
		3. High-risk hemodialysis units (sanitation poor)		ISG	0.05–0.07 ml/kg	i.m.	Every 4 mo
		4. Possible use in custodial institution for mentally retarded		ISG	0.05–0.07 ml/kg	i.m.	Every 4 mo
Influenza	I	1. High risk[d]	6–35 mo 3–12 yr 13–25 yr	Split virus Split virus Whole or split	0.15 0.25 0.5	s.c. or i.m. s.c. or i.m. s.c.	2 (1 mo later) 2 (1 mo later) 2 (1 mo later) 2 (1 mo later)
		2. Over 65	≥26 yr	Whole or split	0.5	s.c.	1
Measles	P	1. Susceptible, exposed under 6 days before	Especially < 1 yr	ISG	0.25 ml/kg	i.m.	1
	L	2. Infants and other susceptibles	≥15 mo (earlier if exposure likely)	Live (MMR in infants)		s.c.	Repeat if given <12 mo
Mumps	L	Children— especially near puberty and males with no history	Children over 12 mo	Live virus (MMR in infants)	As indicated by manufacturer	s.c.	1
Polio	L	1. Infants and children through 18 yr	6–12 wk thru age 18	TOPV		Oral	3 initial and at school entry and possibly ± 11–12 yr

Continued

Table 10. Viral Prophylaxis[a] (*Continued*)

Vaccine	Type[b]	Persons to be immunized	Age	Product[c]	Dosage (ml)	Route	Number of doses or repeats
Polio	L or I	2. Susceptible adults in high-risk area	Adult	TOPV IVP		Oral s.c.	3 4
Rabies	P	1. Bite by wild skunk, fox, raccoon, coyote, bat, or rabid or suspected rabid dog, cat, or escaped animal	Any	RIG and vaccine (sec below)	20 IU/kg	i.m. and local	1
				ARS, if RIG not available	40 IU/kg	i.m. +	1
	I	Same as above		HDCV	1.0	i.m.	5
Rubella	L	All children, many adolescents, some adults (*not in pregnant women*) and women in hospitals and clinics, possibly in colleges, work	≥12 mo	Human or diploid live virus (MMR in infants) or DEV (second choice)	As per manufacturer	s.c.	1
Smallpox	L	1. Travelers to areas *requiring* vaccination 2. Laboratory workers with virus 3. None for entry into U.S.	Any	Glycerinated or lyophilized		Drop i.c.	1
Yellow fever		1. Travelers to infected areas 2. Laboratory workers with virus	>6 mo	Live, attenuated	0.5	s.c.	1

[a] Derived from the *Morbidity Mortality Weekly Rep.* hepatitis **26**:425 (1978); influenza **27**:285 (1978); measles **27**:427 (1978); mumps **26**:393 (1977); polio **26**:329 (1977); rabies **29**:265 (1980); rubella **27**:451 (1978); smallpox **27**:156 (1978); **27**:295 (1978); yellow fever **27**:268 (1978).
[b] (I) Inactivated vaccine; (L) live vaccine; (P) passive (immune globulin).
[c] (ISG) Immune serum globulin; (HBIG) anti-hepatitis B serum; (MMR) measles–mumps–rubella vaccine for infants; (TOPV) trivalent oral polio vaccine; (IVP) inactivated polio vaccine; (RIG) rabies immune globular, human; (ARS) anti-rabies, equine; (DEV) duck embryo vaccine; (HDCV) human diploid cell rabies vaccine.
[d] (1) Acquired or congenital heart disease; (2) chronic pulmonary disease; (3) chronic renal disease with azotemia or nephrotic syndrome; (4) diabetes mellitus and other metabolic diseases; (5) chronic severe anemia; (6) conditions that compromise the immune system.

ruses. An effective rhinovirus vaccine would reduce morbidity from the common cold about 25%, but the existence of over 100 antigenic strains makes this impossible; a multiplicity of antigenic strains also deters immunization against coxsackieviruses and echoviruses. The available vaccines and recommended applications are listed in Table 10 (see also individual chapters).

15.2. Chemoprophylaxis and Therapy

The uses of amantadine and vidarabine are summarized in Table 11.[54a] Chemoprohylaxis against viral infections has met with limited success for influenza and smallpox, but has not been useful for most other infections. Amantadine hydrochloride is effective against infection with most strains of influenza A. Amantadine is recommended for non-vaccinated persons at high risk to severe disease or essential to the community in the presence of an established A outbreak. It also appears to have some therapeutic value when given early in illness and should be considered in high-risk groups and influenza pneumonia. A semicarbazone preparation used in India in the prevention of smallpox among exposed contacts would now seem outdated by the success of the eradication program. Effective therapeutic results against fatal herpes encephalitis have been obtained with vidarabine (ara-A adenine arabinoside) and its analogues if given early in biopsy-diagnosed illness. It is useful locally for herpetic eye infections; other used are in herpes zoster immunocompromised patients.

Interferons show much promise for antiviral therapy of selected infections.[54a] They consist of viral-induced interferon (Type 1) and lymphocyte-produced (Type II), which differ in host range, pH, and heat stability. Most clinical trials have used human leukocyte interferon produced in Finland. The sup-

Table 11. Antiviral Agents Useful in Prophylaxis or Therapy

Agent	Viral infection	Use	Application	Toxicity	Effectiveness
Amantadine	Only influenza A	Prophylaxis	During proved influenza A outbreak for persons not vaccinated against current strain who: a) Have underlying disease (e.g., cardiac respiratory) that puts them at risk to serious illness b) Are older persons in institutional settings c) Are adults essential for medical care and other inpatient community services d) Are possibly certain hospitalized patients	3–7% develop CNS symptoms: confusion, hallucinations, anxiety, insomnia; reversible	60% vs. clinical illness 50% vs. influenza infection
		Therapy	Consider use in 1st 24–48 hr after onset in persons (a) and (c) above plus those with influenza pneumonia.		50% reduction in fever; duration shortened 1–2 days
Vidarabine (Ara A, Vira-A adenine arabinoside)	Herpes simplex, herpes zoster	Therapy	Proved herpes simplex encephalitis (HSV) Infants with proved disseminated HSV infections or CNS Topically for HSV acute keratoconjunctivitis or recurrent epithelial hepatitis Possibly herpes zoster in immunocomposed patients	Low: occasional nausea, vomiting, disorientation, or skin rash; rare CNS symptoms	Reduced HSV encephalitis mortality from 70 to 28%

plies are very limited and preparations vary in purity. New methods of production such as by Epstein–Barr-virus-infected lymphoblastoid lines and through genetic recombinant techniques may answer this problem. Exogenous interferon inducers have at present greater availability and lower cost, but have not yet been shown to be safe and effective in humans. When sufficient interferon is available, the promising areas for clinical evaluation on the basis of experimental trials include varicella-zoster infections in cancer patients, cytomegaloviral infections in renal-transplant recipients, patients with recurrent hepatitis, chronic active hepatitis B and viral respiratory tract infections, and infections in bone-marrow transplants.[54a]

Acyclovir [acycloguanosine, 9-(2-hydroxyethoxymethyl) guanine] is a new experimental drug with a high level of activity against herpesviruses in tissue culture and in experimental herpes infections in laboratory animals. It has limited toxicity and merits controlled clinical trials in humans.

Additional information on the control and prevention of specific viral infections is included in the appropriate sections of subsequent chapters of this book.

ACKNOWLEDGMENTS

I wish to thank the following persons for their review of part or all of this chapter and their many helpful suggestions and corrections: Dr. Philip Brachman; Dr. Roger Feldman and others at the Bureau of Epidemiology, Center for Disease Control, Atlanta, Georgia; Drs. Harry A. Feldman and Paul Sheehe, Department of Preventive Medicine, State University of New York at Syracuse, New York; and Drs. John Dwyer, Fred Kantor, and Elisha Atkins, Department of Medicine, Yale University School of Medicine, New Haven, Connecticut.

16. References

1. ABBEY, H., An examination of the Reed–Frost theory of epidemics, *Hum. Biol.* **24**:201–233 (1952).

1a. ALFORD, C. A., STAGNO, S., AND REYNOLDS, D. W., Perinatal infections caused by viruses, toxoplasma and *Treponema pallidum*, in: *Clinical Perinatology* (S. ALADJEM AND A. K. BROWN, eds.), pp. 183–204, C. V. Mosby Co., St. Louis, 1974.

2. ALLISON, A. C., *The Scientific Basis of Medicine*, p. 49, Annual Reviews, London (1972).

3. ALLISON, A. C., Immune responses in persistent viral infections, *J. Clin. Pathol. Suppl.* **6**:121 (1972).

4. ARMENIAN, H. K., AND LILIENFELD, A. M., The distribution of incubation periods of neoplastic diseases, *Am. J. Epidemiol.* **99**:92–100 (1974).

4a. ARMSTRONG, J. A., EVANS, A. S., RAO, N., AND HO, M., Viral infections in renal transplant recipients, *Infect. Immunol.* **14**:970–975 (1976).

5. BAUSCHER, J. C., AND SMITH, R. T., Studies of the Epstein–Barr virus–host relationship: Autochthonous and allogeneic lymphocyte stimulation by lymphoblast cell lines in mixed cell culture, *Clin. Immunol. Immunopathol.* **1**:270–281 (1973).

6. BELL, J. A., ROWE, W. P., ENGLER, J. I., PARROT, R. H., AND HUEBNER, R. J., Pharyngeal conjunctival fever: Epidemiological studies of a recent recognized disease entity, *J. Am. Med. Assoc.* **175**:1083–1092 (1955).

7. BISHOP, R. F., DAVIDSON, G. P., HOLMES, I. H., AND RUCK, B. J., Virus particles in epithelial cells of duodenal mucosa from children with acute nonbacterial gastroenteritis, *Lancet* **2**:1281–1283 (1973).

8. BISHOP, R. F., DAVIDSON, G. P., HOLMES, I. H., AND RUCK, B. J., Detection of a new virus by electron microscopy of fecal extracts of children with acute gastroenteritis, *Lancet* **1**:149–151 (1974).

9. BISNO, A. L., BARRATT, N. P., SEVANSTON, W. H., AND SPENSE, L. P., An outbreak of acute respiratory disease in Trinidad associated with para-influenza virus, *Am. J. Epidemiol.* **91**:68–77 (1970).

10. BLACK, F. L., HIERHOLZER, W. J., PINHEIRO, F. DE P., EVANS, A. S., WOODHALL, J. P., OPTON, E. M., EMMONS, J. E., WEST, B. S., EDSALL, G., DOWNS, W. G., AND WALLACE, G. D., Evidence for persistence of infections agents in isolated human populations, *Am. J. Epidemiol.* **100**:230–250 (1974).

10a. BONSDORFF, C. H., HOVI, T., MAKELA, P., HOVI, L., AND TEVALVOTO-AARMO, M., Rotavirus associated with acute gastroenteritis in adults, *Lancet* **2**:423 (1976).

11. BLUMBERG, B. S., ALTER, H. J., AND VISNICK, S., A "new" antigen in leukemia sera, *J. Am. Med. Assoc.* **191**:541–546 (1965).

12. BRODY, J. A., AND DETELS, R., Subacute sclerosing panencephalitis: A zoonosis following aberrant measles, *Lancet* **2**:500–501 (1970).

13. BYRNE, E. B., EVANS, A. S., FONTS, D. W., AND ISRAEL, H. L., A seroepidemiological study of Epstein–Barr virus and other viral antigens in sarcoidosis, *Am. J. Epidemiol.* **97**:355–363 (1973).

13a. CENTER FOR DISEASE CONTROL, Reported Morbidity and Mortality in the United States, Annual Summary 1978, *Morbidity Mortality Weekly Rep.* **27**:1–94 (1979).

13b. CENTER FOR DISEASE CONTROL, ECHO virus 9 outbreak—New York, *Morbidity Mortality Weekly Rep.* **27**:392–394 (1978).

13c. CENTER FOR DISEASE CONTROL, Nonreported sexually transmissible diseases—United States, *Morbidity Mortality Weekly Rep.* **28**:61–63 (1979).

13d. CHANG, T., FIUMARA, N. J., AND WEINSTEIN, L., Genital herpes: Some clinical and laboratory observations, *J. Am. Med. Assoc.* **229**:544–545 (1974).

14. CHANOCK, R. M., AND PARROT, R. H., Acute respiratory disease in infancy and childhood, present understanding and prospects for prevention, *Pediatrics* **36**:21–40 (1965).

15. CHANOCK, R., CHAMBON, L., CHANG, W., FERREIRA, F. G., GHARPURE, P., GRANT, L., HATEM, J., IMAN, I., KALRA, S., LIM, K., MADALENGOITIA, J., SPENSE, L., TENG, P., AND FERREIRA, W., WHO respiratory survey in children: A serological study, *Bull. WHO* **37**:363–369 (1967).

16. CHANOCK, R. M., PARROTT, R. H., KAPIKIAN, A. Z., KIM H. W., AND BRANDT, C. D., Possible role of immunological factors in pathogenesis of RS virus lower respiratory tract disease, *Perspect. Virol.* **6**:125–135 (1968).

17. CHRISTIE, A. B., *Infectious Diseases: Epidemiology and Clinical Practice*, E. and S. Livingston, Edinburgh, 1969.

18. CIONGOLI, A. K., PLATZ, P., DUPONT, B., SVEJGAAD, A., FOG, T., AND JERSILD, C., Lack of antigenic response to myxoviruses in multiple sclerosis, *Lancet* **2**:1147 (1973).

19. CONNOLLY, J. H., ALLEN, I. V., HURWITZ, L. J., AND MILLAR, J. H. D., Measles-virus antibody and antigen in subacute sclerosing panencephalitis, *Lancet* **1**:542–544 (1967).

20. CORRIEL, L. L., Clinical syndromes in children caused by respiratory infection, *Med. Clin. North Am.* **51**:819–830 (1967).

20a. DAVIDSON, G. P., BISHOP, R. F., TOWNLEY, R. R. W., HOLMES, I. H., AND RUCK, B. J., Importance of a new virus in acute sporadic enteritis in children, *Lancet* **1**:242–245 (1975).

21. DAVIS, B. D., DULBECOO, R., EISEN, H. N., GINSBERG, H. S., AND WOOD, W. B., *Microbiology*, Harper and Row, New York, 1968.

22. DIXON, F. J., Mechanisms of immunologic injury, in: *Immunobiology* (R. A. GOOD AND D. W. FISCHER, eds.), pp. 161–166, Sinauer, Stamford, Connecticut, 1971.

22a. DOUGLAS, R. G., JR., Influenza in Man, in: *The Influenza Viruses and Influenza* (E. D. KILBOURNE, ed.), pp. 395–447, Academic Press, New York, 1975.

23. DOUGHERTY, W. J., AND ALTMAN, R., Viral hepatitis in New Jersey 1960–1961, *Am. J. Med.* **32**:704–716 (1962).

23a. Editorial, Rotaviruses of man and animals, *Lancet* **1**:257–259 (1975).

24. ELVEBACK, L. R., ACKERMAN, E., YOUNG, G., AND FOX, J. P., A stochastic model for competition between viral agents in the presence of interference. 1. Live virus vaccine in randomly mixing population, model III, *Am. J. Epidemiol.* **87**:373–384 (1968).

25. EVANS, A. S., Clinical syndromes in adults caused by respiratory infection, *Med. Clin. North Am.* **5**:803–818 (1967).

26. EVANS, A. S., Serological surveys: The role of the WHO Reference Serum Bank, *WHO Chron.* **21**:185–190 (1967).

27. EVANS, A. S., The spectrum of infections with Epstein–Barr virus: A hypothesis, *J. Infect. Dis.* **124**:330–337 (1971).

28. EVANS, A. S., Clinical syndromes associated with EB virus infection. *Adv. Intern. Med.* **18**:77–93 (1972).

29. EVANS, A. S., Diagnosis and prevention of common respiratory infection, *Hosp. Pract.* **10**:31–41 (1974).

29a. EVANS, A. S., New discoveries in infectious mononucleosis, *Mod. Med.* **42**:18–24 (1974).

30. EVANS, A. S., EB virus, infectious mononucleosis and cancer: The closing of the web, *Yale J. Biol. Med.* **47**:113–122 (1974).

30a. EVANS, A. S., Causation and disease: The Henle–Koch postulates revisited, *Yale J. Biol. Med.* **49**:175–195 (1976).

30b. EVANS, A. S., Causation and disease: A chronological journey, *Am. J. Epidemiol.* **108**:249–258 (1978).

30c. EVANS, A. S., Limitations of Koch's postulates, *Lancet* **2**:1277–1278 (1977).

31. EVANS, A. S., CAMPOS, L. E., D'ALLESSIO, D. A., AND DICK, E. C., Acute respiratory disease in University of the Philippines and University of Wisconsin students: A comparative study, *Bull. WHO* **36**:397–407 (1967).

32. EVANS, A. S., AND CAMPOS, L. E., Acute respiratory disease in students at the University of the Philippines, *Bull. WHO* **45**:103–112 (1971).

33. EVANS, A. S., NIEDERMAN, J. C., AND MCCOLLUM, R. W., Seroepidemiologic studies of infectious mononucleosis with EB virus, *N. Engl. J. Med.* **279**:1123–1127 (1968).

34. EVANS, A. S., NIEDERMAN, J. C., AND SAWYER, R. N., Prospective studies of a group of Yale University freshman. II. Occurrence of acute respiratory infections and rubella, *J. Infect. Dis.* **123**:271–278 (1971).

35. EVANS, A. S., SHEPARD, K. A., AND RICHARDS, V. A., ABO blood groups and viral diseases, *Yale J. Biol. Med.* **45**:81–92 (1972).

36. EVANS, A. S., KLEIN, G., NIEDERMAN, J. C., RICHARDS, V., AND WANAT, J., Viral antibody levels in nasopharyngeal carcinoma (1974), Unpublished.

37. EVANS, A. S., CASALS, J., OPTON, E. M., BORMAN, E. K., LEVINE, L., AND CUADRADO, R. R., A nationwide serum survey of Colombian military recruits, 1966.

I. Description of sample and antibody patterns with arboviruses, polioviruses, respiratory viruses, tetanus and treponematosis, *Am. J. Epidemiol.* **90**:292–303 (1969).

38. EVANS, A. S., CASALS, J., OPTON, E. M., BORMAN, E. E., LEVINE, L., AND CUADRADO, R. R., A nationwide serum survey of Argentinian military recruits, 1965–1966. I. Description of sample and antibody patterns with arboviruses, polioviruses, respiratory viruses, tetanus and treponematosis, *Am. J. Epidemiol.* **93**:111–121 (1971).

39. EVANS, A. S., COX, F., NANKERVIS, G., OPTON, E., SHOPE, R., WELLS, A. V., AND WEST, B., A health and seroepidemiological survey of a community in Barbados, *Int. J. Epidemiol.* **3**:167–175 (1974).

40. FENNER, F., The pathogenesis of the acute exanthems; an interpretation based on experimental investigations with mousepox (infectious ectromelia of mice), *Lancet* **2**:915–920 (1948).

41. FENNER, F. J., AND WHITE, D. O., *Medical Virology,* Academic Press, New York, 1970.

42. FLEWETT, T. H., BRYDEN, A. S., WOODE, G. N., BRIDGER, J. C., AND DERRICK, J. M., Relation between viruses from acute gastroenteritis of children and newborn calves, *Lancet* **2**:61–63 (1974).

43. FLOREY, C. DU V., CUADRADO, R. R., HENDERSON, J. R., AND DE GOES, P., A nationwide serum survey of Brazilian military recruits, 1964. I. Method and sampling results, *Am. J. Epidemiol.* **86**:314–318 (1967).

44. FOX, J. P., HALL, C. E., AND ELVEBACK, L. R., *Epidemiology: Man and Disease,* Collier-Macmillan, Ltd., London, 1970.

45. FOY, H. M., COONEY, M. I. C., AND McMAHAN, R. A., A/Hong Kong influenza immunity three years after immunization, *J. Am. Med. Assoc.* **226**:758–761 (1973).

46. GAJDUSEK, D. C., AND GIBBS, C. J., JR., Slow, Latent and Temperate Infections of the Central Nervous System, in: *Infections of the Nervous System,* Vol. XLIV, The Association for Research in Nervous and Mental Disease, Williams and Wilkins, Baltimore, 1968.

47. GARD, S., AND ALLIN, K., Studies on the hepatitis virus, in: *Hepatitis Frontiers* (F. W., HARTMAN *et al.,* eds.), pp. 169–172, Little, Boston, 1957.

47a. GARDNER, P. S., AND McQUILLAN, J., *Rapid Viral Diagnosis: Application of Immunofluorescence,* Butterworths, London, 1974.

48. GERONE, P. J., COUCH, R. B., KEEFER, G. V., DOUGLAS, R. G., DERRENBACHER, E. B., AND KNIGHT, V., Assessment of experimental and natural viral aerosols, *Bacteriol. Rev.* **30**:576–584 (discussion 584–588) (1966).

49. GESER, A., CHRISTENSEN, S., AND THORUP, I. B., A multipurpose serological survey in Kenya. I. Survey methods and progress of field work, *Bull. WHO* **43**:521–537 (1970).

50. GREAVES, M. F., OWENS, J. J. T., AND RAFF, M. C., *T and B Lymphocytes, Origins, Properties and Roles in Immune Responses,* Exerpta Medica, Amsterdam, American Elsevier, New York, 1973.

50a. GURWITH, M. J., AND WILLIAMS, T. W., Gastroenteritis in children: A two-year review in Manitoba. I. Etiology, *J. Infect. Dis.* **136**:239–247 (1977).

51. GUTHE, T., RIDET, J., VORST, F., D'COSTA, J., AND GRAB, B., Methods for surveillance of endemic treponematosis and sero-immunological investigations of "disappearing" disease, *Bull. WHO* **46**:1–14 (1972).

51a. GWALTNEY, J. M., JR., AND HENDLEY, J. O., Rhinovirus transmission: One if by air, two if by hand, *Am. J. Epidemiol.* **107**:357–361 (1978).

51b. HARRISON, H. R., ENGLISH, N. G., LEE, C. K., AND ALEXANDER, E. R., *Chlamydia Trachomatis* infant pneumonitis: Comparison with matched controls and other infant pneumonitis, *N. Engl. J. Med.* **298**:702–708 (1978).

52. HENDLEY, J. O., WENZEL, R. P., AND GWALTNEY, J. M., JR., Transmission of rhinovirus colds by self-induction, *N. Engl. J. Med.* **288**:1361–1364 (1973).

53. HENLE, G., AND HENLE, W., Immunofluorescence in cells derived from Burkitt lymphoma, *J. Bacteriol.* **91**:1248–1258 (1966).

54. HENLE, G., HENLE, W., AND DIEHI, V., Relation of Burkitt's tumor-associated herpes-type virus to infectious mononucleosis, *Proc. Natl. Acad. Sci. U.S.A.* **59**:94–101 (1968).

54a. HIRSCH, M. S., AND SWARTZ, M. N., Antiviral agents, *N. Engl. J. Med.* **302**:949–953 (1980).

55. HOEPRICH, P. D. (ed.), *Infectious Diseases,* Harper and Row, Hagerstown, Maryland, 1972.

56. HORSFALL, F. L., AND TAMM, I., (eds.), *Viral and Rickettsial Infections of Man,* Lippincott, Philadelphia, 1965.

57. HORSTMANN, D. M., LIEBHABER, H., LeBOUVEIR, G. L., ROSENBERG, D. A., AND HALSTEAD, S. B., Rubella: Reinfection of vaccinated and naturally immune persons exposed in an epidemic, *N. Engl. J. Med.* **283**:771–778 (1970).

57a. HSIUNG, G. D., *Diagnostic Virology: An Illustrated Handbook,* Yale University Press, New Haven and London, 1973.

58. HUEBNER, R. J., The virologist's dilemma, *Ann. N.Y. Acad. Sci.* **67**:430–442 (1957).

59. JAWETZ, E., ADELBERG, E. A., AND MELNICK, J. L., *Review of Medical Microbiology,* 13th ed., Lange Medical Press, Los Altos, 1978.

60. JOHNSON, R. T., AND MIMS, C. A., Pathogenesis of viral infections of the nervous system, *N. Eng. J. Med.* **278**:23–30, 84–92 (1968).

61. JORDON, M. C., ROUSSEAU, W. E., NOBLE, G. R.,

STEWART, J. A., AND CHIN, T. D. Y., Association of cervical cytomegaloviruses with venereal disease, *N. Engl. J. Med.* **288**:932–934 (1973).

62. KAPIKIAN, A. Z., WYATT, R. G., DOLIN, R., THORN-HILL, T. S., KALICA, A. R., AND CHANOCK, R. M., Visualization by immune electron microscopy of a 27-nm particle associated with acute infectious non-bacterial gastroenteritis, *J. Virol.* **10**:1075–1081 (1972).

62a. KAPIKIAN, A. Z., KIM, H. W., WYATT, R. G., *et al.*, Human reovirus-like agent as the major pathogen associated with "winter gastroenteritis" in hospital-ized infants and young children, *N. Engl. J. Med.* **294**:965–972 (1976).

62b. KLOENE, W., BANG, F. B., CHAKRABORTY, S. M., COOPER, M. R., KULEMANN, H., OTA, M., AND SHAW, K. V. A two-year respiratory virus survey in four villages in West Bengal, India, *Am. J. Epidemiol.* **92**:307–320 (1970).

63. KNIGHT, V. (ed.), *Viral and Mycoplasma Infections of the Respiratory Tract*, Lea and Febiger, Philadelphia, 1973.

64. KOCH, R., Über bacteriologische Forsching, *Verhandl, X. Int. Med. Cong. Berlin* **1**:35 (1891).

64a. KONNO, T., SUZUKI, H., IMAI, A., AND IHIDA, N., Reovirus-like agent in acute epidemic gastroenteritis in Japanese infants: Fecal shedding and serologic response, *J. Infect. Dis.* **135**:259–266, 1977.

65. KRUGMAN, S., GILES, J. P., AND HAMMOND, J., Infectious hepatitis: Evidence for two distinctive clinical, epidemiological and immunological types of infections, *J. Am. Med. Assoc.* **200**:365–373 (1967).

66. LANG, D. J., AND KUMMER, J. F., Demonstration of cytomegalovirus in semen, *N. Engl. J. Med.* **287**:756–758 (1972).

66a. LE FROCK, J. L., AND KLAINER, A. S., Nosocomial infections, Current Concepts, Scope Publications, Upjohn Co., Kalamazoo, Michigan (1976).

67. LENNETTE, E. H., AND SCHMIDT, N. J. (eds.), *Diagnostic Procedures from Viral and Rickettsial Infections*, APHA Inc., New York, 1969.

67a. LENNETTE, E. H., MAGOFFIN, R. L., AND KNAUF, E. G., Viral central nervous system disease: An etiologic study conducted at the Los Angeles General Hospital, *J. Am. Med. Assoc.* **179**:687–695 (1962).

67b. LENNETTE, E. H., AND EMMONS, R. W., Viral and Rickettsial Disease Laboratory, *California Department of Health Services*, Unpublished laboratory records.

68. LODMELL, D. L., NIWA, A., HAYASHI, K., AND NOTKINS, A. L., Prevention of cell-to-cell spread of herpes simplex virus by leukocytes, *J. Exp. Med.* **137**:706–720 (1973).

69. MACASAET, F. F., KIDD, P. A., BOLANO, C. R., AND WENNER, H. A., The etiology of acute respiratory infections. III. The role of viruses and bacteria, *J. Pediatr.* **72**:829–839 (1968).

70. MANGI, R. J., NIEDERMAN, J. C., KELLEHER, J. E., DWYER, J. M., EVANS, A. S., AND KANTOR, F. S., Depression of cell-mediated immunity during infectious mononucleosis, *N. Engl. J. Med.* **291**:1149–1153 (1974).

71. MASON, J. O., AND MCLEAN, W. R., Infectious hepatitis traced to consumption of raw oysters: An epidemiologic study, *Am. J. Hyg.* **75**:90–111 (1962).

72. MCDONALD, J. D., AND ZUCKERMAN, A. J., ABO blood groups and acute respiratory disease, *Br. Med. J.* **1**:89–90 (1962).

73. MCMAHON, B., PUGH, T. F., AND IPSEN, J., *Epidemiologic Methods*, Little, Brown, Boston, 1960.

74. MCQUILLIN, J., GARDNER, P. S., AND MCGUCKIN, R., Rapid diagnosis of influenza by immunofluorescent techniques, *Lancet* **2**:690–695 (1970).

75. MELNICK, J. L., A water-borne urban epidemic of hepatitis, in: *Hepatitis Frontiers* (F. W. Hartman *et al.*, eds.), Churchill, London, 1957.

76. MIDDLETON, P. J., SZYMANSKI, M. T., ABBOTT, G. D., BORTOLUSSI, R., AND HAMILTON, J. R., Orbivirus acute gastroenteritis of infancy, *Lancet* **1**:1241–1243 (1974).

77. MILLER, D. G., GABRIELSON, M. O., AND HORSTMANN, D. M., Clinical virology and viral surveillance in a pediatric group practice: The use of double-seeded cultures for primary virus isolation, *Am. J. Epidemiol.* **88**:245–256 (1968).

78. MIMS, C. A., *Pathogenesis of Infectious Diseases*, Academic Press, London, Grune and Stratton, New York, 1976.

78a. MIMS, C. A., Factors in the mechanisms of persistence of viral infections, *Prog. Med. Virol.* **18**:1–14 (1974).

79. MONTO, A. S., AND JOHNSON, K. M., A community study of respiratory infections in the tropics. I. Description of the community and observation on the activity of certain respiratory agents. *Am. J. Epidemiol.* **86**:78–92 (1967).

80. MORRIS, J. N., *The Uses of Epidemiology*, E. and S. Livingstone, Edinburgh, 1957.

81. MUFSON, M. A., CHANG, V., GILL, V., WOOD, S. C., ROMANSKY, M. J., AND CHANOCK, R. M., The role of viruses, mycoplasmas and bacteria in acute pneumonia in civilian adults, *Am. J. Epidemiol.* **86**:526–544 (1967).

81a. NAHMIAS, A. J., VON REYN, C. F., JOSEY, W. E., NAIB, Z. M., AND HUTTON, R., Genital herpes simplex virus infection and gonorrhea—association and analogues, *Br. J. Vener. Dis.* **49**:306–309 (1973).

81b. NAHMIAS, A. J., The Torch Complex, *Hosp. Pract.* **9**:65–72 (1974).

82. NIEDERMAN, J. C., MCCOLLUM, R. W., HENLE, G., AND HENLE, W., Infectious mononucleosis: Clinical manifestations in relation to EB virus antibodies, *J. Am. Med. Assoc.* **203**:205–209 (1968).

83. NOTKINS, A. L., Commentary: Immune mechanisms by which the spread of viral infections is stopped, *Cell. Immunol.* **11**:478–483 (1974).

84. NOTKINS, A. L., AND KOPROWSKI, H., How the immune response to a virus can cause disease, *Sci. Am.* **228**:22–31 (1973).

85. NOTKINS, A. L., MERGENHAGEN, S. E., AND HOWARD, R. J., Effect of virus infections on the function of the immune system, *Annu. Rev. Microbiol.* **24**:525–538 (1970).

86. OLDSTONE, M. B. A., AND DIXON, F. J., Pathogenesis of chronic disease associated with persistent lymphocytic choriomeningitis viral infection. I. Relationship of antibody production to disease in neonatally infected mice, *J. Exp. Med.* **129**:483–505 (1969).

87. OLSON, L. C., LEXOMBOON, U., SITHISARN, P., AND NOYES, H. E., The etiology of respiratory tract infections in a tropical country, *Am. J. Epidemiol.* **97**:34–43 (1973).

88. OSEASOHN, R., ADELSON, L., AND KAJI, M., Clinical pathological study of 33 fetal cases of Asian influenza, *N. Engl. J. Med.* **260**:509–518 (1959).

89. PADGETT, B. L., AND WALKER, D. L., Prevalence of antibodies in human sera against J. C. virus, an isolate from a case of progressive multifocal leukoencephalopathy, *J. Infect. Dis.* **127**:467–470 (1973).

90. PADGETT, B. L., WALKER, D. J., ZURHEIN, G. M., ECKROADE, R. J., AND DESSEL, B. H., Cultivation of papova-like virus from human brain with progressive multifocal leucoencephalopathy, *Lancet* **1**:1257–1260 (1971).

91. PAUL, J. R., The story to be learned from blood samples: Its value to the epidemiologist, *J. Am. Med. Assoc.* **175**:601–605 (1961).

92. PAUL, J. R., *Clinical Epidemiology*, rev. ed., University of Chicago Press, Chicago, 1966.

93. PAUL, J. R., AND WHITE, C. (eds), *Serological Epidemiology*, Academic Press, New York (1973).

94. PAUL, J. R., NIEDERMAN, J. C., PEARSON, R. J. C., AND FLOREY, DuV., A nationwide serum survey of United States military recruits, 1962: General considerations, *Am. J. Hyg.* **80**:286–292 (1964).

95. PHILIPS, P. E., AND CHRISTIAN, C. L., Myxovirus antibody increases in human connective tissue disease, *Science* **168**:982–984 (1970).

95a. PUGH, R. C. B., DUDGEON, J. A., AND BODIAN, M., Kapsoi's varicella form eruption (eczema hepeticum) with typical and atypical visceral necroses, *J. Pathol. Bacteriol.* **69**:67–80 (1955).

95b. REMINGTON, J. S., AND KLEIN, J. O. (eds.), *Infectious Diseases of the Fetus and Newborn Infant*, W. B. Saunders, Philadelphia, 1976.

96. RIVERS, T., Viruses and Koch's postulates, *J. Bacteriol.* **33**:1–12 (1937).

97. ROTHFELD, N. F., EVANS, A. S., AND NIEDERMAN, J.

C., Clinical and laboratory aspects of raised virus antibody titers in systemic lupus erythematosis, *Ann. Rheum. Dis.* **32**:238–246 (1973).

98. SAWYER, R. N., EVANS, A. S., NIEDERMAN, J. C., AND McCOLLUM, R. W., Prospective studies of a group of Yale University freshmen. I. Occurrence of infectious mononucleosis, *J. Infect. Dis.* **123**:263–270 (1971).

99. SCHULMAN, J., Transmissibility as a separate genetic attribute of influenza viruses, in: *Aerobiology* (I. H. SILVER, ed.), Proceedings of the Third International Symposium, Academic Press, New York, 1970.

100. SEVER, J. L., KURTZKE, J. F., ALTER, M., SCHUMACHER, G. A., GILKESON, M. P., ELLENBERG, J. H., AND BRODY, J. A., Virus antibodies and multiple sclerosis, *Arch. Neurol.* **24**:489–494 (1971).

101. SHAW, K. V., DANIEL, R. W., AND WARZAWSKI, R. M., High prevalence of antibodies to BK virus, and SV40-related papovavirus, in residents of Maryland, *J. Infect. Dis.* **128**:784–787 (1973).

102. SHOPE, R. E., Swine influenza. I. Experimental transmission and pathology, *J. Exp. Med.* **54**:349–359 (1931).

103. STANLEY, E. D., AND JACKSON, G. G., Viremia in Asian influenza, *Trans. Assoc. Am. Physicians* **79**:376–387 (1966).

104. STUART-HARRIS, C. H., *Influenza and Other Virus Infections of the Respiratory Tract*, 2nd ed., Edward Arnold, London, 1975.

105. TABER, L. H., ADAM, V., ELLIS, S. S., MELNICK, J. L., MIRKOVIC, R. R., AND YOW, M. D., Rapid diagnosis of enterovirus meningitis by immunofluorescent staining of CSF leukocytes, *Intervirology* **1**:127–134 (1973).

106. TAYLOR, I., AND KNOWLDEN, J., *Principles of Epidemiology*, Little, Brown, Boston, 1957.

107. THOMPSON, W. H., AND EVANS, A. S., California virus studies in Wisconsin, *Am. J. Epidemiol.* **81**:230–234 (1965).

108. TOP, F. H., AND WEHRLE, P. F. (eds.), *Communicable and Infectious Diseases*, 7th ed., C. V. Mosby, St. Louis, 1972.

108a. TORRES, B. V., ILJA, R. M., AND ESPARZA, J., Epidemiological aspects of rotavirus infection in hospitalized Venezuelan children with gastroenteritis, *Am. J. Trop. Med. Hyg.* **27**:567–572 (1978).

109. UNIVERSITY HEALTH PHYSICIANS AND PHLS LABORATORIES, A joint investigation: Infectious mononucleosis and its relationship to EB virus antibody, *Br. Med. J.* **4**:643–646 (1971).

110. UNTERMOHLEN, V., AND ZABRISKIE, J. F., Suppressed cellular immunity to measles antigen in multiple-sclerosis patients, *Lancet* **2**:1147–1148 (1973).

111. URQUHARDT, G. E. D., AND STOTT, E. J., Rhinoviremia, *Br. Med. J.* **4**:28 (1970).

112. VIROLAINER, M., ANDERSSON, L. C., LALLA, M., AND VON ESSEN R., T lymphocyte proliferation in mononucleosis, *Clin. Immunol. Immunopathol.* **2:**114–120 (1973).

112a. YOLKEN, R. H., WYATT, R. G., ZISAIS, G., BRANDT, C. D., *et al.*, Epidemiology of human rotavirus types 1 and 2 as studied by enzyme-linked immunosorbent assay, *N. Engl. J. Med.* **299:**1156–1161 (1978).

113. WIDELOCK, D., SCHAEFFER, M., AND MILLIAN, J., Surveillance of infectious disease by serologic methods, *Am. J. Public Health* **55:**578–586 (1965).

114. WILSON, C. B., DIXON, F. J., EVANS, A. S., AND GLASSOCK, R. J., Anti-viral antibody responses in patients with renal disease, *Clin. Immunol. Immunopathol.* **2:**114–120 (1973).

115. WHO TECHNICAL REPORT SERIES, Cell-Mediated Immunity and Resistance to Infection, No. 519, Geneva (1973).

116. WHO TECHNICAL REPORT SERIES, Immunological and Hematological Surveys, No. 181, Geneva (1973).

117. WHO WEEKLY EPIDEMIOLOGICAL RECORD, Smallpox Surveillance **54:**1–6 (1979).

117a. WHO, Progress in the rapid diagnosis of viral infections: A memorandum, *Bull WHO* **2:**241–244 (1978).

17. Suggested Reading

BENENSON, A. S. (ed.), *Control of Communicable Diseases in Man*, 13th ed., American Public Health Association, Washington, D.C., 1981.

FENNER, F. J., AND WHITE, D. O., *Medical Virology*, Academic Press, New York, 1970.

FOX, J. P., HALL, C. E., AND ELVEBACK, L. R., *Epidemiology: Man and Disease*, Collier-Macmillan, Ltd., London, 1970.

HIRSCH, M. S., AND SWARTZ, M. N., Antiviral agents, *N. Engl. J. Med.* **302:**949–953, 1980.

HOEPRICH, P. D. (ed.), *Infectious Diseases*, Harper and Row, Hagerstown, Maryland, 1972.

LILIENFELD, A. M., AND LILIENFELD, D., *Foundations of Epidemiology*, 2nd ed., Oxford University Press, New York, 1980.

MANDELL, G. L., DOUGLAS, R. G., JR., AND BENNETT, J. E. (eds.), *Principles and Practice of Infectious Diseases*, 2 vols., Wiley, New York, 1970.

PAUL, J. R., *Clinical Epidemiology*, rev. ed., University of Chicago Press, Chicago, 1966.

CHAPTER 2

Surveillance and Seroepidemiology

Alfred S. Evans

1. Introduction

Surveillance has been described as the systematic collection of data pertaining to the occurrence of specific diseases, the analysis and interpretation of these data, and the dissemination of consolidated and processed information to contributors to the program and other interested persons.[57] The principles have been well set forth by Langmuir[41] for the United States Center for Disease Control (CDC) and by Raška[57] for the World Health Organization (WHO), and were a major focus of discussion of the Twenty-first World Health Assembly in 1968.[70] The techniques of surveillance have become a part of national and international programs of disease control. This chapter will discuss the background and elements of traditional surveillance, the concept and uses of serological epidemiology, and their application to the control of infectious diseases.

2. Surveillance

The traditional methods of reporting and surveillance are based on the occurrence of a case of

Alfred S. Evans   WHO Serum Reference Bank, Section of International Epidemiology, Department of Epidemiology and Public Health, Yale University School of Medicine, New Haven, Connecticut.

clinical disease or of a death from clinical disease. They form the basis of public health control and immunization programs throughout the world.

2.1. Historical Background

The use of mortality and morbidity data as a basis for public-health action goes back for centuries. The occurrence of the "Black Death" or pneumonic plague in Europe about 1348 resulted in the appointment of three guardians of public health by the Venetian Republic to exclude ships with affected persons aboard. The detention of travelers from plague-infected areas for 40 days in Marseilles (1377) and in Venice (1403) led to our current concept of quarantine.

The term *surveillance* has been employed for years in the restrictive sense of follow-up of persons who have had contact with plague or of infectious syphilis patients to determine whether disease developed within the limits of the incubation period. The dictionary defines the word in terms of police surveillance as meaning to "watch or guard over a person, especially a suspected person, a prisoner, or the like."[49] In public health practice, the suspect is the disease.

The principles of surveillance were first exemplified by William Farr, Superintendent of the Statistical Department of the General Registry in London, in a series of classic letters on the causes of death in England appearing from 1839 to 1870 and through a collection of papers on "Vital Statistics" published in 1885. The WHO Influenza Centers for recognition of influenza outbreaks and new viral strains were established in 1948 prior to the introduction and general use of the term. Formal development of the concept of surveillance is of more recent origin and was in response to national needs for disease surveillance or to major new epidemic problems. These needs involved the requirement for a nationally centralized clearinghouse of essential information in order to define the magnitude of the problem, to inform the appropriate authorities on whom responsibility fell for public-health control measures, and as a means of evaluating the effectiveness of such measures. Use of the term in the United States began in 1949 with the development of a modified program at the CDC called "Surveillance and Appraisal of Malaria." In 1951, the concept was applied to the residual smallpox cases in the United States.

Surveillance really became an established concept and public-health practice on April 28, 1955, when the Surgeon General directed the establishment of a "National Poliomyelitis Surveillance Program" in response to paralytic polio cases following the use of Salk vaccine (the "Cutter incident"). This program was set up at the CDC. The technique became an effective tool in following trends in the disease, in measuring the effectiveness of polio immunization programs, and in detecting suspected vaccine-associated cases.

On July 5, 1957, the Asian influenza surveillance program was initiated and consisted of bimonthly reports from the CDC to keep everyone informed of the progress of the outbreak, including the public press. It served as an essential system tying together the massive national program to control the pandemic. Influenza surveillance has continued at the CDC in conjunction with the WHO ever since and has provided critical data on the occurrence of influenza outbreaks throughout the world.

The surveillance of hepatitis similarly followed an epidemic in 1961 in which shellfish from contaminated waters were identified as the source of an outbreak. Salmonella surveillance was initiated in 1962 following 18 hospital outbreaks. Many other diseases were added to this list over time, and now the CDC publishes special surveillance reports on about 20 categories of infectious disease. In Europe,

Dr. Kǎrél Raška was an enthusiastic supporter of the surveillance concept, initiated both traditional and serological surveillance in his own country, Czechoslovakia, and promoted the principles as Director, Division of Communicable Disease, WHO. A special unit called "Epidemiological Surveillance of Communicable Diseases" was established in the WHO by Dr. A. M.-M. Payne to coordinate and extend this program; three WHO Serum Reference Banks that are currently concerned with serological surveys and serological surveillance are under the jurisdiction of this unit.* Currently, only three diseases are under International Sanitary Regulation: plague, yellow fever, and smallpox; other important communicable diseases are kept under surveillance.[58]

2.2. Elements of Surveillance

As applied to communicable diseases, *surveillance* has been defined as "the exercise of continuous scrutiny of, and watchfulness over, the distribution and spread of infections and factors related thereto, of sufficient accuracy and completeness to be pertinent to effective control."[70] A wide variety of sources of data on disease occurrence and on the characteristics of the populations at risk contribute to surveillance. These sources vary from country to country depending on the stage of development and sophistication of the public health services, the quality and extent of laboratory facilities, the available funds, and the characteristics of the indigenous diseases. The major features have been summarized in ten "elements of surveillance" by the WHO (1968) and are listed in Table 1.

2.2.1. Mortality Registration. Mortality registration is the oldest form of disease reporting and has the advantage of being legally required and of a high order of completeness in most countries. Since a physician or other health practitioner is usually in attendance, there is a reasonable expectation that

---

* The WHO Serum Reference Banks are located at the Institute of Epidemiology and Microbiology, Prague, Czechoslovakia; Department of Epidemiology and Public Health, Yale University School of Medicine, New Haven, Connecticut; and the National Institutes of Health, Tokyo, Japan. A fourth established at the South African Institute of Medical Research, Johannesburg, South Africa, is no longer an official WHO unit.

Table 1. Elements of Surveillance

1. Mortality registration
2. Morbidity reporting
3. Epidemic reporting
4. Laboratory investigations
5. Individual case investigations
6. Epidemic field investigations
7. Surveys
8. Animal-reservoir and vector-distribution studies
9. Biologics and drug utilization
10. Knowledge of the population and environment

most infectious diseases of sufficient severity to cause death *may* exhibit enough clinical characteristics to permit diagnosis. The possibility of an autopsy may also contribute to the accuracy of identification of the disease process. On the other hand, some deaths such as those from coronary artery disease may be sudden and unattended by a physician; multiple causes of death may be involved, and the one of most public-health significance may be lost in the order of causation recorded on the death certificate. There is often a long delay in the tabulation and publication of mortality data; autopsy information may not be added to amend information on the original death certificate. In general, mortality data reflect incidence only when there is some relatively constant ratio between deaths and cases. With the exception of rabies, Lassa fever, and certain hemorrhagic fevers, most viral diseases are not fatal, so that mortality data have limited usefulness as a barometer of disease occurrence. However, the occurrence of an excess of deaths from influenza and pneumonia above the expected level has been a sensitive index of influenza. It was first used by William Farr in 1847 and has been consistently reported in the United States since 1918. At present, weekly data on deaths from influenza and pneumonia in 122 cities are compared to the average number of deaths in the same week in the previous 5 years. Current deaths that exceed this "epidemic threshold" can usually be attributed to epidemic influenza. Heat exhaustion and smog may also increase deaths above this level, but such events are geographically localized and can be readily identified from environmental data. Unfortunately, the time required for reporting and analyzing these mortality data results in a delay of a month or so in recognition of an outbreak; this period is

longer during Christmas or holiday periods for public-health workers.

2.2.2. Morbidity Reporting. The reporting of cases of specified communicable diseases is legally required in most countries, and as many as 40 conditions may be involved. A simple and effective reporting system is the backbone of surveillance for most health departments. The advantages are that (1) such reports are usually made by physicians who are best qualified to identify the diseases; (2) laboratory confirmation may be available; and (3) there is usually an organized system of regional or national tabulation and reporting. The disadvantages are (1) the absence of many viral diseases from the required list; (2) the notorious underreporting of the occurrence of *required* diseases because of failure of physicians to notify the public health authority due to lack of motivation, of secretarial help, or of time; (3) the uncertainty of diagnosis (especially without laboratory confirmation)—a major issue for many viral infections; (4) the variability of reporting efficiency from one time period to another, being in general highest during epidemics. A recent analysis of the efficacy of reporting of 570 cases of notifiable communicable diseases from 11 hospitals in Washington, D.C., revealed an overall reporting rate of 35%.[42a] For individual diseases, the rates were as follows: viral hepatitis, 11%; *H. influenza* meningitis, 32%; meningococcal meningitis, 50%; shigellosis, 62%; and tuberculosis, 11%.

2.2.3. Epidemic Reporting. The recognition and identification of epidemic viral diseases are commonly more accurate than individual reports because public-health officials and laboratory facilities are usually involved. This is true of outbreaks of yellow fever, influenza, rubella, hepatitis, viral exanthems, and certain arbovirus infections. Unfortunately, this may not always be the case, particularly if the viral agent produces primarily mild or inapparent infections or if the outbreak occurs in areas with poor medical care or inadequate public-health and laboratory facilities. Unrecognized epidemics of dengue involving thousands of people have taken place under such circumstances. Sometimes outbreaks of diseases such as poliomyelitis, hemorrhagic fevers, and influenza may be recognized by local health authorities but not reported to the WHO because of fear of the economic impact of this knowledge on tourist or export trade. However, local outbreaks of diseases that have a high mortality or that involve tourists or other persons from outside the country are now being recognized through better surveillance, even in more remote areas. Examples are Lassa, Ebola, and Marburg fevers and certain animal pox viruses, such as camel, gerbil, and monkeypox, that may occasionally involve humans.

2.2.4. Laboratory Investigations. Laboratory identification of the causative agent is an almost absolute requirement for the etiological diagnosis of individual cases and for most epidemics of viral diseases; the exceptions are poliomyelitis and certain viral exanthems in which the clinical features are characteristic enough to permit diagnosis. Sophisticated laboratory facilities and experienced personnel are therefore needed for the isolation and/or serological identification of the majority of viral infections. These may exist in the national or regional public-health laboratories, in specialized virus diagnostic institutes, or in university settings. The WHO has established a broad network of regional, national, and international reference laboratories for specific viral infections to assist in this task. These include laboratories for influenza, other viral respiratory infections, arboviruses, and enteroviruses, as well as a group of about 15 other collaborating virus-diagnostic laboratories around the world. A few WHO-supported multipurpose viral-diagnostic facilities in key areas of the world that are otherwise devoid of such laboratories are also being established. The need for trained personnel, special equipment, standardized antigens and antisera, protection against laboratory infections, good water, reliable refrigeration, and proper sterilizing equipment makes viral laboratories expensive and difficult to maintain without this type of support.

2.2.5. Individual Case Investigations. The occurrence of a disease of public-health importance in an area previously free of the disease or where control measures have been established demands rapid and intensive investigation. This includes viral infections such as smallpox, yellow fever, certain types of viral encephalitis, the hemorrhagic fevers, rabies (either in humans or in a new animal species), and paralytic poliomyelitis. Of special importance is the follow-up of persons returning to their own country from areas where these infections are known to occur. This is done in the United States through an alert card issued to incoming travelers from foreign countries; the card requires notification and investigation of any illness developing within a defined period after arrival (currently 6 weeks). Since the discontinuance of the requirement for routine smallpox vaccination for returning American travelers and the presumed global eradication of the natural disease as of October 1977, the possibility of imported cases of smallpox seems remote. However, surveillance and accurate diagnosis of persons developing poxlike illness on return from potential geographic foci, such as Ethiopia, Somalia, and Bangladesh, should be continued for several years. Political upheaval, enemy action, or lack of funds or interest may disrupt the present high order of surveillance, immunization, and control in these "high-risk" areas.

2.2.6. Epidemic Field Investigations. When there is an increase in the number of cases or deaths from a viral disease of public-health significance, an epidemic team must be dispatched to make further study. The team should include an epidemiologist and a virologist, with appropriate equipment for the collection and transportation of specimens. New rapid diagnostic techniques, such as fluorescent antibody or enzyme-linked immunosorbent assay (ELISA) tests on throat or skin specimens or on infected insects, may permit direct identification of the causative agent in the field. These teams are usually composed of experts from regional or national health services that operate in support of local health officials. In the United States, the Epidemic Intelligence Service and the Laboratory Division of the CDC in Atlanta, Georgia, fulfill this role on the request of state health departments. On a worldwide basis, the WHO in Geneva, its regional branches, or WHO-designated laboratories may be able to render assistance. More routine outbreaks are handled by state or municipal health departments, often assisted by laboratory personnel. There is increasing need for better integration and cooperation between epidemiologists and public-health laboratory personnel in this task.[14] The establishment of an Epidemiological Investigation Unit in affiliation with each public-health laboratory should be promoted not only for epidemic analysis but also for the evaluation of the need for and effectiveness of immunization programs as well as day-to-day surveillance work involving both epidemiological and laboratory data. The public-health service in England has created such a unit,[10] and it has been proposed for developing countries as well.[12,15,17]

2.2.7. Surveys. Many types of surveys of infectious disease are used in public-health work. These may use epidemiological markers to identify certain diseases; such markers include splenomegaly or positive blood smears for malaria, scars for smallpox vaccination, and positive skin tests for tuberculosis. Immunization histories, personal interviews, or clinic records may also be used to assess the vaccination status of the population. For many viral diseases, major reliance must be placed on antibody surveys or, in the case of hepatitis, tests for hepatitis B antigen in blood specimens. The use and application of serological surveys to these ends are discussed in detail in Section 3.

2.2.8. Animal-Reservoir and Vector-Distribution Studies. Surveillance of human diseases acquired from animals or of diseases in which the vector is arthropod-borne requires the collection of data on the zoonoses and the presence of appropriate vectors in the area. Examples for which such data are needed are yellow fever and other arthropod-borne diseases, especially dengue and the hemorrhagic fevers, rabies, and perhaps monkey pox as a potential source of human smallpox. The emergence of a group of unusual but frequently lethal diseases such as Lassa fever and the Argentinian and Bolivian hemorrhagic fevers involves study of the rodents that are suspected as the reservoirs. The surveillance of these infections requires a special investigation team and/or close cooperation among existing epidemiological, veterinary, and entomological services.

2.2.9. Biologics and Drug Utilization. The establishment of an effective system of determining the scale and utilization of viral vaccines and immune globulins may not only provide a lead to the immunization status of an area but might also give supplementary information to permit the recognition of an outbreak or of other special problems.

2.2.10. Knowledge of the Population and Environment. The denominator used in determining incidence and prevalence rates is the population at risk to the disease in the area from which the cases are reported. Necessary information includes age, sex, ethnic, economic, and other demographic data in order to interpret disease trends. Other background information often needed relates to sanitary conditions, food and water supplies, housing, insects, nutrition, and cultural habits. The accessibility, utilization, and quality of medical care must be known in order to evaluate the potential efficacy of case-reporting, mortality data, and other indices of the health of the population.

2.3. Other Surveillance Methods

Additional sources of data may be utilized in supplementing routine surveillance techniques or in evaluating special disease situations. Some of these are listed in Table 2.

2.3.1. Hospital and Medical Care. The existence of national health plans in many countries and the extension of prepaid health-insurance schemes in other areas make computerized accounting necessary. This provides the opportunity for including morbidity and mortality information in the data system. Large-scale health plans such as the Kaiser-Permanente Plan in California, the Cooperative Group Health Insurance Plan in Seattle, and the Health Insurance Plan (HIP) of greater New York City are now being utilized for these purposes. Centralized data-processing centers for hospitals such as the Professional Activities Services (PAS) operating out of Ann Arbor, Michigan, provide another opportunity; this system, which covers some 200 hospitals and a hospital population of over 2 million persons, is based on a hospital discharge sheet that incorporates much useful information on diagnosis, surgical procedures, complication, length of stay, laboratory data, and other factors. Surveillance of the number of patients with acute respiratory infections in emergency rooms, outpatient clinics, and pediatric clinics in large community hospitals[58a] combined with prospective virological surveillance of such patients[32a] provides sensitive and specific indicators of an influenza outbreak.

2.3.2. Panels of Cooperating Physicians. In some areas, data networks have been established by groups of cooperating physicians to record morbid-

Table 2. Other Sources of Surveillance Data

1. Hospital and medical care statistics
2. Panels of cooperating physicians
3. Public-health-laboratory reports
4. Absenteeism from work or school
5. Telephone and household surveys
6. Newspaper and newsbroadcasting reports

ity data and analyses of their medical care programs. For example, the *National Disease and Therapeutic Index*[47] is an outcome of one such operation that provides analyses of the frequency of different diagnoses in over 1500 private physicians' offices in randomly selected parts of the United States.

2.3.3. Public-Health-Laboratory Reports. The state and municipal public-health laboratories provide a wide range of diagnostic facilities for communicable diseases. Backed by the fine laboratories of the USPHS CDC in Atlanta, Georgia, these represent the predominant diagnostic services in viral infections in the country. They are supplemented by virus research and diagnostic laboratories in universities and a few large hospitals. These usually operate in close communication with the public-health laboratories of the area. The consolidation and utilization of information from these various sources represent the best ongoing method for surveillance of viral infections. This is especially true for viral diseases, since many are not reportable and because accurate diagnoses are often dependent on laboratory identification of the viral agent. The use of sera sent to such laboratories for multipurpose viral testing is discussed in Section 3.5.3.

2.3.4. Absenteeism from Work or School. A sensitive barometer of any major epidemic in children is an increase in school absentee rates; in adults, it is a jump in absenteeism in industry. Since an absence of any duration in schools may be investigated by the school or public-health nurse and any significant loss of time from work may require a physician's certificate of illness, additional data on the nature and duration of the condition may be obtained. The active cooperation of a few geographically representative schools and key industries may provide public-health officials with valuable leads on epidemic illness.

2.3.5. Telephone and Household Surveys. The CDC has utilized telephone surveys to verify the presence and the extent of an epidemic such as influenza. A defined subsample selected from the local telephone book is sequentially called to determine whether illness exists in the household. Research studies of the occurrence of minor illnesses such as acute respiratory infections in Tecumseh, Michigan, have used telephone interviews as the basis of data collection.[46] The limitations of this method are obvious: (1) the family must have a phone; (2) someone must be at home to answer it; (3) the person answering must be aware of illnesses in other members of the family; (4) the disease involved must be characteristic enough to permit recognition by a layman; (5) the presence of illness can be inquired about over only short periods because of imperfect memory; and (6) the person answering must be willing to cooperate in the survey.

Household surveys by skilled interviewers form the basis of the U.S. National Health Survey, in which a carefully selected random sample consisting of about 55,000 families is the source of data. An extensive series of morbidity and health analyses and much useful surveillance information have resulted from these repeated surveys. They are not helpful in providing *immediate* surveillance of common diseases, but reveal long-term trends of importance.

2.3.6. Newspaper and Newsbroadcasting Reports. The news media often report outbreaks of disease before they have been announced by the slower process of most health-reporting mechanisms. Furthermore, there may be epidemics of nonreportable diseases picked up by an active news-surveillance system that may be missed or never officially reported to public-health authorities. A systematic clipping and recording service from local news services may thus provide important leads to an alert epidemiological surveillance program. The earliest reports of influenza outbreaks in Hong Kong, or of Lassa fever in Africa, or of an outbreak of hemorrhagic fever in South America may be found on the pages of newspapers with extensive coverage such as the *New York Times*.

2.4. Surveillance in Research Studies

The methods thus far discussed contribute directly to official public-health agencies. In research, specialized surveillance systems have been established for various viruses or groups of viruses. The Virus Watch Programs established by Fox and his associates[11,30] in New York City and then in Seattle, Washington, are excellent examples of this method, which involves systematic sampling of a population of families for enteric and respiratory viruses, antibody testing, and analyses of coincident illness patterns. An earlier effort of special surveillance of this type was the extensive analyses of common illnesses in a group of Cleveland families carried out by Dingle *et al.*[13] Special population groups such as Tecumseh, Michigan, used for analyses of chronic disease are also being utilized for studies of viral infections, especially acute respiratory disease.[46] In children, the massive long-term study of viral infections in Junior Village carried out by Bell *et al.*[5] at the National Institutes of Health has yielded sequential data on the behavior of common viruses in such a closed setting.

2.5. Publications on Surveillance

The dissemination of data derived from surveillance programs is an essential requirement for public-health action. Table 3 lists the common publications reporting current and long-term trends in infectious diseases. The most current and useful are the *WHO Weekly Epidemiological Record* and the *Morbidity and Mortality Weekly Report* from the U.S. Public Health Service.

The *WHO Technical Report Series* provides up-to-date information on various viral infections as well as other diseases, prepared by expert committees.

2.6. Predictive Surveillance

The ability to predict the occurrence of infection or of an outbreak is theoretically possible if there are adequate epidemiological data on hand. This has been tried with varying success for influenza epidemics; here the problem is confounded by our sparse knowledge of the factors governing the emergence of new antigenic variants of influenza virus. For infections in which quite precise requirements exist, such as an insect vector, intermediate hosts, animal reservoirs, or special terrain, the *potential* existence of the infection in certain geographic areas can be presumed and its probable *absence* in other areas can be predicted. This approach has special interest to the armed forces because the introduction of susceptible military units into areas in which few health data are available poses hazardous conditions for the men and for the success of the mission. In this connection, three infections have been analyzed in detail by Baker[3] employing computer analysis of existing epidemiological and ecological information: schistosomiases, malaria, and leptospirosis. The name "infectious disease

Table 3. Publications Dealing with Surveillance Data[a]

1. Worldwide
   WHO Weekly Epidemiological Record
   WHO Epidemiological and Vital Statistics Report (monthly)
   WHO Annual, Vol. II: *Infectious Diseases; Cases, Deaths, Vaccinations*
2. North America
   PAHO—*Weekly Epidemiological Report*
   PAHO—*Quarterly Information Bulletin*, Pan American Zoonoses Center
   PAHO—*Annual Report of the Director*
   CAREC—*Carribbean Epidemiology Center Surveillence Report* (monthly)
3. United States (USPHS)
   Morbidity and Mortality Weekly Report, CDC, U.S. Department of Health and Human Services
   Annual Supplement, Reported Incidence of Notifiable Diseases in the United States, CDC, U.S. Department of Health and Human Services
   Special Surveillance Reports (including the following viral diseases) from CDC, U.S. Department of Health, Education, and Welfare
      Hepatitis
      Infectious mononucleosis
      Measles
      Neurological viral diseases (aseptic meningitis, encephalitis, enteroviruses, poliomyelitis)
      Rabies
      Rubella
      Smallpox-vaccinia

[a] From National Health Survey: Health Statistics Publications, National Center for Vital Statistics.

prognostication" has been applied to this methodology. Similar predictions might be made for viral infections such as the arboviruses, which require insect vectors with well-defined ecological features. Serological surveys can also provide valuable data on the potential danger of certain infections; these may be especially useful in areas in which health reporting is poor, or in the case of a virus that produces largely subclinical infections. For example, the presence in persons of all ages and especially young children of antibody to viruses such as poliomyelitis, hepatitis B, Epstein–Barr virus (EBV), or dengue indicates the continuing activity of that agent in that environment, irrespective of the apparent absence of clinical illness or of reported cases due to these viruses. If soldiers, tourists, Peace Corps volunteers, or other visitors who lack antibody to the agent intermix with the local population and/or are exposed to the local environment and population, infection may result. Such infection is often accompanied by a higher risk of clinical disease than in the indigenous population because infection of older children and adults results in more severe host response than infection very early in life.

3. Seroepidemiology

3.1. Introduction

Seroepidemiology is the systematic collection and testing of blood samples from a target population, or a representative sample thereof, to identify current and past experiences with infectious diseases by means of antibody and antigen tests and by measurement of cell-mediated immunity (CMI). Additional uses are to seek biochemical markers for various chronic diseases, to measure certain nutritional components, and to characterize the genetic aspects of red cells, leukocytes, and serum proteins. In infectious diseases, serological epidemiology contributes to two broad and overlapping areas:

1. Serological surveillance to provide supplementary data as the basis for public-health planning and immunization programs.
2. In research, as an epidemiological tool to investigate the risk and occurrence of infectious diseases and to study the behavior of old and

newly recognized microbiological agents in different population groups.

Serological surveys may be carried out to determine the patterns of a single agent such as poliomyelitis but are more commonly "multipurpose" in nature. This section will consider the history, methods, and uses of seroepidemiology with particular reference to its application as an important adjunct to traditional methods of surveillance of infectious diseases. The WHO has sponsored two expert committee reports on the subject,[71,72] and a book[56] has been published.

Just as epidemiology is concerned with the occurrence and distribution of *clinical cases* in different populations, so serological epidemiology, as noted above, is concerned with the occurrence and distribution of various *components* of the blood that indicate past or current infection, that are biochemical markers for certain chronic diseases, or that reveal the genetic attributes of various population groups. The epidemiological characteristics are detected in the laboratory rather than at the bedside. The name "serological surveys" has been used interchangeably with "immunological surveys." No satisfactory expression has been found to indicate the whole spectrum of components in the red cells, white cells, plasma, and serum that may be measured in population surveys; perhaps the term "immunoserological surveys" comes closest to include the measurements of immunity, genetic attributes, and chemical components in the blood. Of current interest are the lymphocyte responses to different antigens and the genetic control of that response as reflected by the human leukocyte antigen (HLA) systems.

3.2. Historical Background

The introduction of serological tests for the diagnosis of disease provided the basis for later serological surveys. As early as 1916, the Wassermann test was applied routinely to patients attending a prenatal clinic at John Hopkins Hospital by Williams,[74] but this was more of a case-finding procedure than an attempt to delineate disease patterns. In 1930, the development of a neutralization test for poliomyelitis led Aycock and Kramer[2] to use the procedure to define the immunity pattern of a given population; this is a landmark in the history of serum surveys. In 1932, Soper *et al.*[65] mapped out the occurrence of yellow fever in Brazil by antibody surveys under the auspices of the Rockefeller Foundation, and this technique has been widely used subsequently in studying arbovirus infections. Antibody surveys for influenza also date back to the mid-1930s. The discovery of swine influenza virus by Shope[63] in 1931 and of human influenza virus by Smith *et al.*[66] in 1933 was rapidly followed by population studies to measure antibody to these viruses in persons of different age groups.[1,8,31]

The Yale Poliomyelitis Study Unit under Dr. John R. Paul employed serological survey techniques as long ago as 1935,[55] and his analysis with Riordan of the poliomyelitis pattern in Alaskan Eskimos is a classic study.[54] He became one of the foremost users and promoters of the concept of serological epidemiology, and through his work and writing,[50,56] the utilization of this technique in public-health practice and research studies has become a reality. The World Health Organization also took note of this development in 1960 and established three WHO Serum Reference Banks to practice and promote seroepidemiology. These were located in the Department of Epidemiology and Public Health at Yale University, New Haven, Connecticut; at the Institute of Epidemiology and Microbiology, Prague, Czechoslovakia; and the South African Institute for Medical Research, Johannesburg, South Africa.* An additional bank was established in 1971 at the National Institutes of Health in Tokyo, Japan. The activities and principles of these banks have been reviewed in two *WHO Technical Reports*,[71,72] in a book,[56] and in several other publications.[15,51,52]

3.3. Methodology

3.3.1. Sources of Sera. A list of several sources of sera for survey analysis is given in Table 4. By far the most important method is the collection of blood specimens and of health data from a carefully selected sample from the target population at risk. To achieve the highest yield from this type of study, serological surveys should be multipurpose in nature and include measurement of antibodies to all prevalent infections. The sera collected in household surveys in rural areas by the WHO for the

* This one is no longer an official WHO Bank.

Table 4. Sources of Sera for Serological Surveillance

1. Planned serum surveys from target populations
2. Entrance and periodic examinations of different groups:
   a. Military
   b. Industry
   c. Health clinics
3. Blood donors in Red Cross and similar programs
4. Public-health laboratories:
   a. Serological tests for syphilis (e.g., premarital)
   b. Other immunological and diagnostic tests
5. Hospitals:
   a. Entry tests for blood chemistries or syphilis
   b. Diagnostic tests for infectious diseases
   c. Blood banks
   d. Prenatal clinics

evaluation of the effectiveness of penicillin in mass eradication programs for yaws have also been an important source for multipurpose testing.[35]

Because of the cost of collecting sera from a properly selected sample of a population, other sources of sera have been utilized. These have included utilization of blood specimens collected for other purposes, especially for routine tests during physical examinations for the armed forces or industry, or during an outpatient visit or admission to a hospital. Sera sent to a public-health laboratory for serological tests for syphilis, viral diagnosis, or other diagnostic tests have also been employed. These collections of sera may not be representative of the age, sex, and geographic distribution of the entire population; the nature of the biases introduced must be recognized and evaluated. However, they are economical to obtain and sometimes may reveal important information on the presence or absence of a certain virus in the community or of the occurrence of a recent outbreak. For most multipurpose surveys, a representative sample carefully selected from the community at risk is important. A broad representation of all younger age groups is essential if the sera are to be used in evaluating the immunization needs of the population or in measuring the impact of a vaccination program. As a rough guide for multipurpose surveys, the reports of the WHO have suggested a sample of 300–600 persons divided into 25 sera per age group (e.g., single-year groups under 5 years, 5-year groups up to 19 years, and broader groups thereafter).[71,72]

The blood must be collected and separated under sterile conditions. Aliquots of 0.5 ml each are used by the WHO and CDC serum banks and are very useful for microtiter tests; several replicates of the entire collection may be prepared at the time of aliquoting so they can be shipped to other laboratories for testing. Sera are usually stored at −20°C, often in a commercial warehouse. Temperatures of −70°C are best, but are expensive to maintain. Lymphocytes can also be separated from anticoagulated blood, frozen at low temperatures in fetal calf serum and dimethylsulfoxide (DMSO), and later thawed for measurement of CMI and HLA characteristics.[48a]

3.3.2. Laboratory Tests. The antibody tests most suitable to serological surveys of specific viruses are detailed in each chapter of this book. The criteria for a satisfactory test include simplicity, sensitivity, specificity, reliability, ability to detect long-lasting antibody, minimal interference from nonspecific inhibitors, the availability of satisfactory reagents, and the safety of the test for the laboratory technician.[16,72] The microtiter procedure developed by Takatsy in 1950 in Hungary and popularized in this country by Sever[62] in 1962 has become the standard method in serological survey laboratories. It is adaptable to a wide variety of antibody determinations, it requires a minimal amount of sera (usually 0.1 ml) and other ingredients, and large numbers of sera can be efficiently tested. Several automated methods of dilution and of adding various reagents have been introduced to speed the testing even more.[72]

3.4. Advantages and Limitations

The traditional methods of surveillance are based on *cases* of clinical disease reported by physicians or identified by some survey technique. The sequence usually involved includes the requirements listed in Table 5. In underdeveloped and developing countries, many of these requirements for surveillance may be missing or inadequate, and even in highly developed countries the reporting of communicable diseases is less than satisfactory and involves much variability.[42a] The use of serological surveys is an important means of supplementing morbidity information. Because many viral infections may be clinically mild or inapparent, may require laboratory confirmation for accurate diagnosis of even overt cases, and may not be on the list of reportable diseases, the serological survey technique is an important tool: it reveals *total* infection rates (apparent and inapparent), both currently and in the past. Selection of tests that reflect antibody of long duration permits measurement of the cumulative experience of the population tested with the disease in question; selection of a test based on short-lived antibody allows identification of a recent epidemic or infection. Testing of two sera spaced in time permits measurement of the incidence of infection.

The disadvantages of seroepidemiology are the cost and effort involved in the selection and bleeding of the target population and in the collection and analysis of data, and the need for and cost of laboratory facilities equipped to carry out the tests. There must also be a satisfactory means of measuring antibody for the particular virus to be studied, and the method of carrying it out must be simple enough to allow performance on a large-scale basis. Because aliquots of sera from a collection can be shipped long distances in the frozen state to a number of specialized reference laboratories for testing, the work can be divided among participating laboratories. The establishment and funding of more WHO, national, or regional laboratories for multipurpose testing may come in the future. Currently, the funds for seroepidemiological surveys are grossly inadequate.

3.5. Uses of Seroepidemiology

The uses discussed below encompass both public-health and research applications, and there is some overlapping in the various categories. The utilization of serological techniques in the surveillance of disease (serological surveillance) is clear in many of the "uses" described.

3.5.1. Prevalence. The presence in the serum of one or more antibodies to specific infectious agents at the time of collection is called *antibody prevalence.*

Table 5. Requirements for Surveillance Based on Clinical Cases

1. Occurrence of clinical illness
2. Sufficient severity to seek medical care
3. Availability of medical care
4. Capability of physicians to diagnose illness
5. Laboratory support of diagnosis
6. Reporting of disease to health department
7. Collection and analysis of data by health department

The antibody prevalence *rate* is the number of persons whose sera contain a particular antibody in the lowest dilution tested divided by the total number of persons examined. Unlike "case prevalence," which indicates the existence of disease at the time of the survey, antibody prevalence reflects the cumulative experience, past and present, with an infectious agent. The prevalence rate is a function both of prior and current infection and of the durability of the antibody produced.

Many antibodies such as the neutralization antibody for poliomyelitis or yellow fever virus and the hemagglutination-inhibition antibody for influenza, parainfluenza, rubella, measles, or arboviruses last for years, perhaps a lifetime. Thus, the cumulative experience of a population can be measured and infection acquired in childhood can be detected in persons of middle or perhaps even old age. Some dropoff in antibody titer (sometimes below the lowest detectable levels) may occur in older age groups after a childhood infection. Similarly, the antibody to EBV measured by the indirect immunofluorescence test has been found to be of long duration; even complement-fixing antibodies to cytomegalovirus (CMV), herpesviruses, or dengue virus have been found to persist for years following infection. It should also be emphasized that unlike prevalence data for *clinical* infectious disease, serological prevalence data reflect *total infection* rates, representing both clinical and subclinical (or asymptomatic) infections.

Multipurpose antibody surveys have been carried out in a number of countries under WHO auspices as an extension of evaluation surveys for penicillin campaigns to eradicate yaws, as noted above. They have been largely in rural areas of Nigeria, Toga, Afghanistan, the Philippines, Samoa, Thailand, and Yugoslavia.[35] Unfortunately, the results of most of these surveys have not been published. Published multipurpose surveys include those of military recruits in the United States,[53] Brazil,[20,27] Colombia,[20a] and Argentina.[21] There is an initial report of a survey of Kenya[32] and recent health and serological surveys of Barbados[22,25a] and of St. Lucia.[21a] In the Barbados study, a 10% household sample was randomly selected from a middle- and lower-socioeconomic-level community of 10,000 persons in Bridgetown. The results will be discussed to indicate the type of information that can be derived from this type of study. Of 100 sera from children under

age 10 tested, 30% lacked protective levels of antitoxin against both diphtheria and tetanus, indicating the need for intensifying the immunization program against these diseases. The prevalence of protective levels against tetanus is a good indicator of the level of public-health practice, since this antitoxin is acquired almost exclusively by immunization procedures and not through natural infection. The age distribution of antibodies to various viruses may provide useful information on the behavior of these infections in the community and of the need for immunization programs. Antibodies to EBV were acquired very early in life, reaching a plateau of about 95% positive by age 5. Antibodies to CMV were present in 60% by age 5, rose to 78% by age 15, and reached a plateau of about 85% by age 30 (Fig. 1A). This means that clinical illness due to these viruses would be rare because they usually cause mild and inapparent infection when acquired by young age groups. In contrast, rubella antibody, while present in 41.4% of the females, was essentially absent from children under 11 years old (Fig. 1A). This indicates that there had been no rubella infection for the previous 10 years and that a female population was entering childbearing age without any protection against rubella. On this basis, an active rubella immunization program of girls of 12 and under has been initiated. In subsequent years through 1978, a few sporadic cases have been reported yearly, but no epidemic has occurred. A similar age pattern was seen for all three types of dengue antibody: it was absent in persons under age 25, but antibody prevalence rose rapidly after this to reach levels of 50–60% (Fig. 1B). This suggested that dengue virus had not been introduced in the past 25 years, or that mosquito and other control measures had been effective, or both. However, in 1978, Barbados experienced a small outbreak of dengue as part of the Caribbean-wide outbreak that had severely affected Puerto Rico in late 1977. The information obtained on the patterns of susceptibility and immunity to these viral infections could not have been obtained by ordinary surveillance methods based on the reporting of clinical cases.

Initial tests for poliomyelitis antibody employing conventional microtiter neutralization procedures indicated that 27, 42, and 53.8% of those tested at 1:5 or 1:8 serum dilution lacked antibody to poliomyelitis types 1, 2, and 3, respectively.[22] Subsequent tests on 304 sera using a 1:2 serum dilution

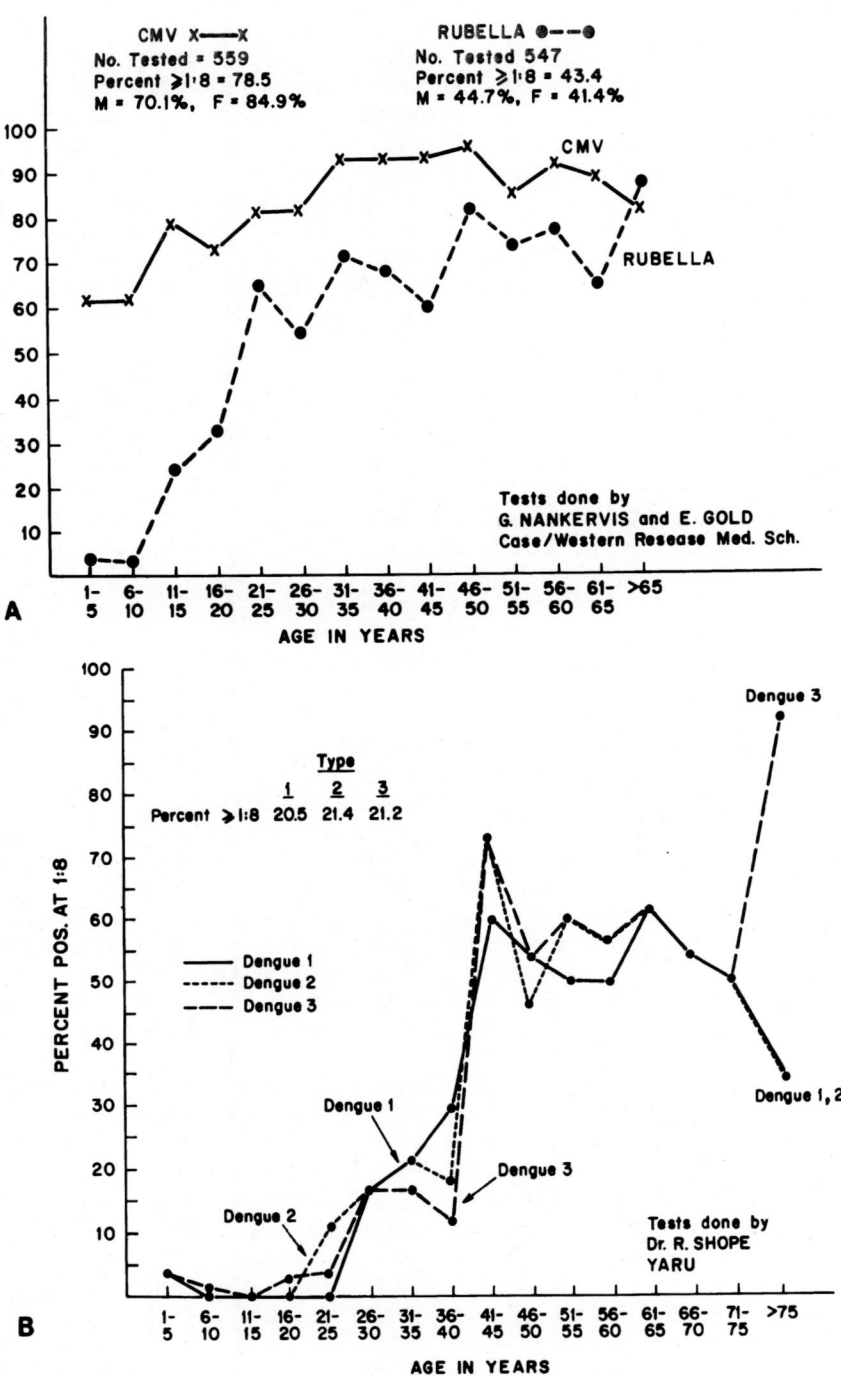

Fig. 1. Results of serologic tests in Barbados, West Indies. CF, Complement fixation; HI, indirect hemagglutination. (A) Age distribution of antibody to cytomegalo and Rubella (HI) viruses. (B) Survey of Dengue (CF) titer in 336 persons.

and longer serum–virus incubation periods indicated that only 13.1% lacked type 1 antibody, 6.5% type 2 antibody, and 14.3% type 3 antibody.[25a] This emphasizes the need for sensitive methods for detecting low levels of antibody. Two mass poliomyelitis programs have been carried out since the 1972 survey, one in 1974–1975 and one in 1977–1978. There have been no reported cases of poliomyelitis since 1972.

3.5.2. Incidence. The *appearance* of antibody to a virus in the second of two sequentially collected specimens indicates infection with that agent somewhere between the two times of collection. A 4-fold or greater *rise* in antibody titer over a preexisting level indicates *reinfection* with that agent. If surveillance of clinical illness can also be maintained between serum collections, then the ratio of apparent (i.e., clinical) to inapparent (i.e., subclinical) infections can be ascertained. An example of this is a study in which a group of Yale college students were followed clinically and serologically during their freshman year for acute respiratory infections, rubella, and infectious mononucleosis[24,60] (Table 6). During the year, epidemics of influenza and rubella occurred. The serological infection rate for influenza was 43.6% in susceptible students, with 59% of infected persons exhibiting clinical illness. For rubella, 25% lacked antibody on entry; of these, 61.4% became infected, of whom 39% had a clinical illness with rash. No clinical rubella cases occurred in persons with titers 1:64 or higher. With EBV an infection rate of 13.1% occurred among the 49% lacking antibody; this was clinically manifested as definite infectious mononucleosis in 74% of those infected.[60]

Other prospective serological studies have been made of respiratory infections, rubella, EBV, CMV, and other viral infections in a variety of settings. They offer the advantages of (1) defining total infection rates, (2) identifying risk factors, and (3) relating infection rates to prior antibody levels. They are especially useful in defining the risk in pregnant women of CMV and rubella infections and the risk in the infected fetus of subsequent congenital malformations. They have been used to portray the infection pattern in military recruits during training[19b] or in college students during various years.[24,60] The level of antibody in the first serum sample that protects against reinfection or clinical illness or both over the period until the next serum specimen is drawn has been used to evaluate the quality and duration of both natural and vaccine-induced antibody to influenza and rubella.[19b,24,29,37,38]

3.5.3. Diagnostic Serology. Sera sent to large hospitals or public-health laboratories for various tests can be frozen and stored for later antibody testing against other antigens. The specimens must be adequate in amount and free of bacterial contamination. Specimens sent for viral antibody tests usually fulfill these criteria and are accompanied by age, sex, address, and clinical data concerning the patient. There are many uses for this type of collection. All sera coming from patients with central nervous system, gastrointestinal, or respiratory infections, or the exanthems can be tested at the time of receipt, or later, against a battery of viral antigens in order to reveal the "etiological pie" involved in the causation of the syndromes. The later discovery of a new agent involved in one of these conditions permits a retrospective assessment of its importance using sera previously collected and stored. An example of this was the evaluation of the importance of California virus in the causation of infections of

Table 6. Infection and Illness Rates for Influenza, Rubella, and Epstein–Barr Viruses in a Group of Yale University Students during Their Freshman Year[a]

Virus	Number studied	Susceptible on entry to Yale (%)[b]	Susceptibles infected over year (%)[c]	Infected developing clinical illness (%)[c]
Influenza (A₂/HK)	281	91.1	43.6	59.0
Rubella	256	25.0	64.1	39.0
EBV	355	49.0	13.1	74.0

[a] Derived from Evans *et al.*[24] and Sawyer *et al.*[60]
[b] Lacking antibody in lowest dilution tested.
[c] Seroconversion during year.

the central nervous system by testing of all sera received in a state public-health laboratory for this syndrome. In Wisconsin, 5.7% of 351 sera received in the state laboratory over the period 1961–1964 revealed evidence of this infection[68]; in Minnesota, 4.1% of 1617 retrospectively tested sera contained this antibody.[4] A second and related application is the determination of the clinical spectrum associated with a newly discovered virus; this is accomplished by testing stored sera from patients with a variety of clinical syndromes and looking for evidence of infection with the new agent.

A third application for sera stored over time is the measurement of *secular trends* or antigenic shifts in viruses over time. This is especially useful in relation to influenza viruses. A fourth use, employing freshly received sera for VDRL or other tests, is the search for influenza antibody patterns that may reveal the beginning of an outbreak or a change in the antigen composition of currently circulating strains; this has been used by Widelock *et al.*[73] at the public health laboratories of New York City. Comparison of the geometric mean antibody titer to influenza sera from persons in the acute phase of an unidentified respiratory illness with the titer in others convalescing from a similar illness may permit early identification of an outbreak without the wait for serial samples from the same persons.

3.5.4. Evaluation of Immunization Programs. Serological surveys should play an increasing role in immunization programs because of the inadequacy and imprecision of traditional surveillance techniques in determining the need for and the effectiveness of a given vaccine. Currently, our knowledge of the utilization of a vaccine depends on sales records of pharmaceutical houses, clinic and physicians' data, and special interview surveys. In the United States, a household interview on immunization utilization is conducted by the Bureau of the Census in the fall; it is based on about 35,000 households. Problems of poor memory, and of the difficulty in identification of the actual immunizations given, and questions relating to absentee members at the time of the interview pose limitations to this approach.

The effectiveness of an immunization program is traditionally judged on the basis of clinical cases or epidemic behavior. A program is regarded as effective when cases decrease or epidemics do not occur. This is a negative type of information in the sense that while true protection may have resulted, it is also possible that the decrease in clinical cases is due to poor reporting or that insufficient time has elapsed for another epidemic to have occurred.

The uses of serological epidemiology in immunization programs are summarized in Table 7. Much of this information could be obtained in no other way. Immunoserological surveillance is of particular importance for the new epidemiological settings created by substituting vaccine immunity for natural immunity as a poliomyelitis, measles, and rubella,[19e] and to a lesser extent in mumps and influenza. Patterns of susceptibility and immunity will now vary from place to place, from age group to age group, and in various socioeconomic settings, depending on the immunization program instituted by the health department and the activities of physicians and clinics, rather than on the inherent epidemiological characteristics of the natural disease. The methods of immunization practice, the fre-

---

Table 7. Uses of Seroepidemiology in Immunization Programs

---

1. Cross-sectional surveys to determine the need for immunization programs in:
    a. Different age groups
    b. Different geographic areas
    c. Different socioeconomic classes
2. Follow-up measurements of immunized persons to determine the:
    a. Percentage developing local, humoral, and cell-mediated immune responses
    b. Quality and extent of the immune response
    c. Duration of the immune response
    d. Level of protection afforded against clinical disease and asymptomatic reinfection
    e. Degree of spread of live vaccines to exposed and susceptible contacts
3. Periodic serological surveillance to identify groups who are not receiving vaccines or who have inadequate antibody responses

---

**Table 8. Protocol for Serological Approach to Agents
in Search of Disease**

1. Develop serological test for mass screening.
2. Test representative population groups.
3. Test paired sera from infectious diseases.
4. If associated syndrome is identified:
   a. Test for frequency of association with the agent.
   b. Exclude presence of agent in other infections.
   c. Determine frequency in close contacts.
5. Carry out prospective study of susceptible persons at high risk to infection, for:
   a. Incidence of infection.
   b. Clinical/subclinical ratio.
   c. Determination of clinical spectrum.
   d. Pattern of incidence related to antibody level.

quency of repeated immunization programs, and the quality and duration of vaccine immunity now constitute the major determinants of the behavior of these diseases.

Serological surveys in several American cities such as Syracuse, New York,[40] Cleveland, Ohio,[33] and Houston, Texas,[44] have uncovered serious deficiencies in the antibody patterns for viral diseases for which vaccines are available. Part of the problem lies in the failure of immunization programs to reach certain segments of the community, and part lies in the loss of interest on the part of the public in seeking and of the physician in giving the available vaccines. There are also inherent difficulties in the preservation of the viability of certain live virus vaccines and inherent inadequacies in the quantity and quality of the antibody response produced by some vaccine preparations. The need for surveillance programs and serological surveys to evaluate immunization programs has been stressed by several authors.[17,19e,37]

3.5.5. Agents in Search of Disease. The application of new immunological and microbiological techniques has sometimes led to the discovery of a new antigen or a new antibody before anything is known of the disease, if any, with which it is associated. The use of seroepidemiological techniques to identify possible associations is one important research application of the method. The discovery of EBV and that of hepatitis B antigen are examples. The sequence in developing an association with illness is outlined in Table 8. In the case of EBV, a fluorescent antibody method developed by Henle and Henle[36] in 1966 provided the key tool. The

virus had been found in cultured cells derived from Burkitt lymphoma, but it could not be isolated in the usual tissue-culture systems. By application of serological techniques, the presence of antibody to the virus was found commonly not only in sera from Burkitt lymphoma patients but also in sera from healthy African and American children. The fortuitous development of infectious mononucleosis in the Henles' technician provided the clue to a disease association,[36a] which was confirmed by prospective studies carried out at Yale University.[23,48,60] The sequence of events is presented in detail in Chapter 24 and has been reviewed.[18] Through this approach, EBV has been firmly established as the sole cause of heterophil-positive infectious mononucleosis.[19]

A second example of the use of seroepidemiological techniques is the discovery by Blumberg *et al.*[6] in 1965 of a particular antigen in the sera of an Australian aborigine; it was uncovered in the course of genetic studies of β-lipoprotein. Since the antigen could not be isolated or cultivated in the laboratory, serological surveys using immunodiffusion tests were carried out to detect its presence in the sera of different population groups and different disease entities. The results provided the sole initial evidence that this "Australia antigen" was associated causally with hepatitis B or "long-incubation hepatitis."[7] Many other investigators contributed to and expanded these studies; their contributions are reviewed in Chapter 12.

3.5.6. Evaluation of Immunological Function in Healthy Populations. Two important developments in immunology bear on future serological surveys. First, standardization and simplification of the means of measuring the various serum immunoglobulins (Ig's) permit assessment of large population groups to establish normal levels for these proteins in different geographic areas and to detect abnormal levels and abnormal Ig's in relation to various infectious diseases. The identification of illnesses associated with primary or secondary Ig deficiencies or with Ig dysfunction may become possible on a large scale. Second, there are exciting advances in our understanding of CMI and advances in the methods available for measuring altered functions. Some of the applications in these two areas are summarized in Table 9. The response of lymphocytes to nonspecific stimuli such as phytohemagglutinin and pokeweed mitogen and the mixed-lymphocyte reaction reflects the functional integrity of the cell-mediated immune system. The response of lymphocytes to *specific* antigens to which the individual has been previously exposed provides an additional epidemiological marker of past infection for those agents; it is especially useful for detecting prior exposure to microbiol agents for which antibody measurement is difficult or not available, such as tuberculosis, leprosy, fungi, and certain viruses. The sensitization of lymphocytes to tumor antigens, par-

ticularly viral-associated tumors, has been demonstrated not only in the tumor patients themselves but also in lymphocytes from household contacts. These observations are of potentially great epidemiological importance because they suggest a common environmental antigen at work, with cancer occurring in only a small proportion of those so exposed.

Just as the lymphocyte response to a virus indicates prior exposure to that agent, the *failure* to respond to an antigen for which there is *known* or *probable* exposure may indicate a high susceptibility to certain chronic viral diseases. For example, the recent demonstration that lymphocytes from some patients with multiple sclerosis fail to produce migratory-inhibiting factor on exposure to measles virus[9,69] is an important lead to viral persistence and to possible disease causation. The adaptation of measurements of lymphocyte function to microtechniques may soon permit large-scale population and prospective studies to be made. Through these surveys, individuals may be identified who have high viral antibody levels but no lymphocyte response to a particular antigen. Such a setting may reflect viral persistence and place the individual at high risk to certain cancers, viral infections of the

Table 9. Measurement of Different Aspects of the Immune System in Seroepidemiological Studies

1. Immunoglobulin measurements of:
   a. Normal levels of different immunoglobulin classes
   b. Deficiency states
   c. High levels as reflection of chronic infections
2. Test for humoral antibody:
   a. Viral-specific IgG antibody in relation to current and past infections
   b. Viral-specific IgM antibody as reflection of recent or recurrent infections
   c. Abnormally high levels of certain viral antibodies as marker of persistent viral infections
3. Cell-mediated immunity assays of:
   a. Lymphocyte function:
      (1) Absolute number of B and T cells
      (2) Response to nonspecific mitogens (phytohemagglutinin, pokeweed, mixed lymphocytes)
      (3) Response to specific viral antigens
      (4) HLA and LD antigens as genetic markers
      (5) Chronic carrier status of EBV, CMV, and other viruses
   b. Skin-test responses to viral antigens
4. Search for circulating immune complexes in:
   a. Immune complex glomerulonephritis
   b. Systemic lupus erythematosus
   c. Hepatitis B infections
   d. Viral exanthems

Table 10. Association of Certain Viruses with Cancer and Chronic Disease

Virus	Disease[a]	Strength of association	High viral antibody titers	Virus or genome in tissues
EBV	Burkitt lymphoma	Strong	+ + +	+ + +
	Nasopharyngeal cancer	Strong	+ + +	+ + +
	Hodgkin's disease	Weak	+ +	0
Hep. B	Heptacellular cancer	Strong	(Persistent antigenemia)	
	Periarteritis nodosa	Moderate	(Immune-complex deposition)	
HSV-Type 2	Cervical cancer	Moderate	+	±
Measles	SSPE	Strong	+ + +	+ + +
Papova	PML	Strong	+	+ + +

[a] (SSPE) Subacute sclerosing panencephalitis; (PML) progressive multifocal leukoencephalopathy.

central nervous system, immune-complex diseases, and other diseases. The observation that transfer factor prepared from persons who have a normal lymphocyte response to a specific antigen can restore function when administered to a deficient individual offers an exciting lead to therapy.

3.5.7. Interrelationship of Disciplines. Seroepidemiological techniques can contribute to our understanding of the possible links among infectious diseases, chronic diseases, cancer, nutrition, and genetics. The general problems relating a possible cause to a disease have been recently reviewed.[19c,19d] Some examples related to viral disease can be cited.

a. Viruses, Cancer, and Chronic Diseases. Evidence of the persistence of viruses as reflected by persistent antigenemia (hepatitis B), by immune complexes (hepatitis B), or by higher antibody titers than in matched controls (EBV, measles, papovaviruses) has suggested a causal relationship to certain cancers and chronic diseases. The presence of one of these immunological markers may be a risk factor in the development of these diseases. The major associations among viruses, cancer, and chronic diseases of the central nervous system are listed in Table 10 and discussed in detail in the appropriate chapters of this volume and in recent papers.[19a,66a] Some will be briefly summarized here. High viral antibody titers might precede the development of a cancer or chronic disease and play a role in its pathogenesis, accompany the onset of disease due to a common immunological mechanism, or arise after the onset of the disease due to the disease process itself or to immunosuppressive drugs used in therapy. The mechanism may vary from one dis-

ease to another. In Burkitt lymphoma, a massive prospective study of some 45,000 children in the West Nile district of Africa[12a] has demonstrated that (1) EBV infection precedes the development of the tumor by 7–54 months; (2) high EBV antibody titers often precede the disease; and (3) antibody titers to other viruses are not elevated. In other studies, EBV genome has been demonstrated in the tumor cells, and a malignant lymphoma can be induced in cotton-top marmosets and owl monkeys with the virus or with EBV-infected lymphocytes. Thus, EBV, in conjunction with malaria, has a very strong causal association with African Burkitt lymphoma, a tumor of childhood. However, these cannot be unique associations, since most cases of Burkitt lymphoma occurring in the United States are not related to either EBV or malaria. In nasopharyngeal cancer, high EBV antibody titers also occur, and EBV genome is demonstrable in the cancer cells. The tumor occurs in adults, and no prospective study has been done to determine whether EBV infections precede the tumor or not, nor has the tumor been reproduced in experimental animals. However, there is increased risk in Chinese with HLA-2 and SIN-2 antigens. In Hodgkin's disease, modestly elevated EBV antibody titers occur in 30–40% of patients, but EBV genome has not been found in the tumor tissue. The antibody elevations have been consistently found in different geographic areas,[20] but it is not known whether they precede or follow the disease. Genetic susceptibility may play a role.[26]

There is also serological and virological evidence relating herpes type 2 to cervical cancer (see Chapter 26) and stronger virological evidence relating hepatitis B to hepatocellular cancer (see Chapter 12). In several chronic diseases, such as sarcoidosis, systemic lupus erythematosus, and chronic liver disease, there may occur elevated antibody titers to EBV, and to other herpes viruses, as well as to measles, rubella, and parainfluenza viruses. These elevated titers are probably the consequence of immunological factors related to the disease itself, especially polyclonal activation of B cells. In subacute sclerosing panencephalitis (SSPE), measles infection, especially in the first two years of life, precedes the development of the disease, and high antibody titers also probably precede the appearance of symptoms of SSPE. In progressive multifocal leukoencephalopathy (PML), the disease appears to be the consequence of the reactivation of a prior infection with a papovirus in the presence of immunosuppression. These relationships of viruses to cancer and chronic disease are emphasized here because it may be possible to identify persons at risk to or developing these conditions through demonstration of high viral antibody titers or hepatitis B antigenemia during seroepidemiological surveys of presumably healthy populations. Once identified by these risk markers, such persons can be followed over time in search of clues to pathogenesis, early detection, or perhaps even the prevention of the disease.

b. Genetics and Viral Disease. Controversy has long existed as to whether the blood group of an individual is associated with a higher risk of certain diseases, including viral infections. For example, retrospective studies suggested a relationship between blood group O and influenza.[43] The validity of this association was tested in prospective serological surveys that permit determination of the actual risk of infection and of disease for each blood group. An extensive prospective analysis carried out in military recruits, college students, and Peace Corps volunteers failed to identify any clear-cut differential risk of persons of different blood types to influenza, parainfluenza, rubella, EBV, and certain other viral infections.[25] In addition, no relationship between serologically proved clinical influenza and any blood groups was found.

The possible relationship between human leukocyte antigens (HLA) and certain diseases is under current vigorous investigation. Differences between the frequency of certain HLA antigens in persons with certain diseases as compared with healthy controls have been found. They have been demonstrated in ankylosing spondylitis,[61] coeliac disease,[67] psoriasis,[59] chronic active hepatitis,[42] Hodgkin's disease,[28] systemic lupus erythematosus,[34] and others. Of particular interest to the virologist are recent reports on multiple sclerosis and nasopharyngeal cancer. In multiple sclerosis, several retrospective analyses have indicated an increased frequency of HLA-3 and HLA-7 antigens as well as a specific lymphocyte determinant, LD-7a.[39] Patients with these antigen patterns have a more rapid course and may also have high measles antibody titers; their lymphocytes may not respond to measles antigen.[9,69] An increased risk for nasopharyngeal carcinoma has been shown in Chinese with an increase in frequency of HLA-A2 antigen[64,64a] and an antigen at the second locus, now termed SIN-2.[64b] One implication of these observations is that there may be genetic control of the immune response; lymphocyte receptors may be absent or may not respond to specific viral antigens, leading to persistence of the virus and perhaps to the development of disease. Much evidence is accumulating bearing on the genetic control of the immune response and the dual specificity of T lymphocytes dependent both on viral antigens, or those expressed on target-cell surfaces, and on a self-component expressed in the major histocompatibility complex.[75] Study of viral infections in humans with certain inherited cell-mediated deficiencies is leading in the same direction; the relationship of EBV to an X-linked lymphoproliferative syndrome may be an example of an inherited T-cell deficiency.[56a]

As with earlier work with ABO blood groups, the association of HLA antigens and disease is currently based on retrospective analyses. As techniques are improved and simplified, the distribution of HLA types may become part of prospective surveys in which the *risk* of infection and disease in persons of certain HLA patterns can be directly measured. A pool of data of this type is now accumulating in organ-transplant centers and includes information on relatives and other tissue donors. Long-term clinical follow-up of these individuals with known HLA configurations might give early clues to risk factors for various chronic diseases.

ACKNOWLEDGMENTS

I wish to express my appreciation to Dr. Alexander D. Langmuir, formerly Chief, Epidemiology Section, U.S. Center for Disease Control, and Dr. Dorothy Horstmann, Professor of Epidemiology and Pediatrics, Yale University School of Public Health, for many helpful comments and careful review of this chapter.

4. References

1. ANDREWS, C. H., LAIDLAW, P. P., AND SMITH, W., Influenza: Observations on the recovery of virus from man and on the antibody content of human sera, *Br. J. Pathol.* **16**:566–582 (1935).
2. AYCOCK, W. L., AND KRAMER, S. D., Immunity to poliomyelitis in normal individuals in urban and rural communities as indicated by the neutralization test, *J. Prev. Med.* **4**:189–200 (1930).
3. BAKER, H., Infectious disease information and preparedness, Presented at meeting of the Society of Medical Consultants to the Armed Forces, U.S.A., Washington, D.C., 1973.
4. BALFOUR, H. H., JR., SIEM, R. A., BAUER, H., AND QUIE, P. G., California arbovirus (LaCrosse) infections. 1. Clinical and laboratory findings in 66 children with meningoencephalitis, *Pediatrics* **52**:680–691 (1973).
5. BELL, J. A., HUEBNER, R. J., ROSEN, L., ROWE, W. P., COLE, R. M., MASTROT, F. M., FLOYD, T. M., CHANOCK, R. M., AND SHOEDOFF, R. A., Illness and microbial experiences of nursery children at Junior Village, *Am. J. Hyg.* **74**:267–292 (1961).
6. BLUMBERG, B. S., ALTER, H. J., AND VISNICH, S., A "new" antigen in leukemia sera, *J. Am. Med. Assoc.* **191**:541–546 (1965).
7. BLUMBERG, B. S., GERSTEY, B. J. S., HUNGERFORD, D. A., LONDON, W. T., AND SUTNIK, A. I., A serum antigen (Australia antigen) in Down's syndrome, leukemia, and hepatitis, *Ann. Intern. Med.* **66**:924–931 (1967).
8. BROWN, H. W., The occurrence of neutralizing antibodies for human influenza virus in the sera of persons with various histories of influenza, *Am. J. Hyg.* **24**:361–380 (1936).
9. CIONGOLI, A. K., PLATZ, P., DUPONT, B., SVEJGAARD, A., FOG, T., AND JERSILD, C., Lack of antigen response to myxoviruses in multiple sclerosis, *Lancet* **2**:1147 (1973).
10. COOK, G. T., AND PAYNE, A. M., Epidemiological control of infectious diseases, *Br. Med. Bull.* **7**:185–187 (1951).
11. COONEY, M. K., HALL, C. E., AND FOX, J. P., The Seattle Virus Watch Program. I. Infection and illness experience of Virus Watch Families during a community-wide epidemic of echovirus 30 aseptic meningitis, *Am. J. Public Health* **60**:1456–1465 (1970).
12. CRUICKSHANK, R., Epidemiological surveillance of communicable diseases and development of public health laboratory facilities in the developing countries, in: *Fourth International Congress on Global Impacts of Applied Microbiology*, São Paulo, Brazil, abstracts (1973).
12a. DE-THÉ, G., GESER, A., DAY, N., INKEI, P. M., WILLIAMS, E. H., BERI, D. P., SMITH, P. G., DEAN, A. G., BORNKAMM, G. W., FEORINO, P., AND HENLE, W., Epidemiological evidence for causal relationship between Epstein–Barr virus and Burkitt's lymphoma from Ugandan prospective study, *Nature (London)* **274**:756–766 (1978).
13. DINGLE, J. H., BADGER, G. F., AND JORDAN, W. S., JR., *Illness in the Home: A Study of 25,000 Illnesses in Group of Cleveland Families*, Press of Western Reserve University, Cleveland, 1964.
14. EVANS, A. S., Epidemiology and the public health laboratory, *Am. J. Public Health* **57**:1041–1052 (1967).
15. EVANS, A. S., Serological surveys: The role of the WHO Serum Reference Bank, *WHO Chron.* **21**:185–190 (1967).
16. EVANS, A. S., Serological Techniques, in: *Serological Epidemiology* (J. R. PAUL AND C. WHITE, eds.), pp. 42–54, Academic Press, New York, 1973.
17. EVANS, A. S., Surveillance of mass vaccination program, in: *Proceedings of the Fourth International Conference on Global Impacts of Applied Microbiology*, São Paulo, Brazil (1973).
18. EVANS, A. S., The history of infectious mononucleosis, *Am. J. Med. Sci.* **267**:189–195 (1974).
19. EVANS, A. S., New discoveries in infectious mononucleosis, *Mod. Med.* **42**:18–24 (1974).
19a. EVANS, A. S., EB virus, infectious mononucleosis and cancer: The closing of the web, *Yale J. Biol. Med.* **47**:113–122 (1974).
19b. EVANS, A. S., Serologic studies of acute respiratory infections in military personnel, *Yale J. Biol. Med.* **48**:201–209 (1975).
19c. EVANS, A. S., Causation and disease: The Henle Koch postulates revisited, *Yale J. Biol. Med.* **49**:175–195 (1976).
19d. EVANS, A. S., Causation and disease: A chronological journey, *Am. J. Epidemiol.* **108**:249–258 (1978).
19e. EVANS, A. S., The need for serologic evaluation of immunization programs, *Am. J. Epidemiol.* **112**:725–731 (1980).
20. EVANS, A. S., CARVALHO, R. P. S., FROST, P., JAMRA, M., AND POZZI, D. H. B., Epstein–Barr virus infections in Brazil. II. Hodgkin's disease, *J. Natl. Cancer Inst.* **61**:19–26 (1978).
20a. EVANS, A. S., CASALS, J., OPTON, E. M., BORMAN, E. K., LEVINE, L., AND CUADRADO, R., A nationwide survey of Colombian military recruits, 1966. 1. Description of sample and antibody patterns with arbovi-

ruses, polioviruses, respiratory viruses, tetanus, and treponematosis, *Am. J. Epidemiol.* **90**:92–303 (1969).

21. Evans, A. S., Casals, J., Opton, E. M., Borman, E. K., Levine, L., and Cuadrado, R., A nationwide survey of Argentine military recruits, 1965–1966. I. Description of sample and antibody patterns with arboviruses, polioviruses, respiratory viruses, tetanus, and treponematosis, *Am. J. Epidemiol.* **93**:111–121 (1971).

21a. Evans, A. S., Cook, J. A., Kapikian, A. Z., Nankervis, G., Smith, A. L., and West, B., Serological Survey of St. Lucia, *Int. J. Epidemiol.* **8**:327–332, (1979).

22. Evans, A. S., Cox, F., Nankervis, G., Opton, E., Shope, R., Wells, A. V., and West, B., A health and seroepidemiological survey of a community in Barbados, *Int. J. Epidemiol.* **3**:167–175 (1974).

23. Evans, A. S., Niederman, J. C., and McCollum, R. W., Seroepidemiologic studies of infectious mononucleosis with EB virus, *N. Engl. J. Med.* **279**:1121–1127 (1968).

24. Evans, A. S., Niederman, J. C., and Sawyer, R. N., Prospective studies of a group of Yale University freshman. II. Occurrence of acute respiratory infections and rubella, *J. Infect. Dis.* **123**:271–278 (1971).

25. Evans, A. S., Shepard, K. A., and Richards, V., ABO blood groups and viral diseases, *Yale J. Biol. Med.* **45**:81–92 (1972).

25a. Evans, A. S., Wells, A. V., Ramsey, F., Drabkin, P., and Plamer, K., Poliomyelitis, rubella, and dengue antibody survey in Barbados: A follow-up study, *Int. J. Epidemiol.* **8**:235–241 (1979).

26. Falk, J., and Osoba, D., HL-A antigens and survival in Hodgkin's disease, *Lancet* **2**:1118–1121 (1971).

27. Florey, C., DuV., Cuadrado, R. R., Henderson, J. R., and De Goes, P., A nationwide serum survey of Brazilian military recruits, 1964: Method and sampling results, *Am. J. Epidemiol.* **86**:314–318 (1967).

28. Forbes, J. F., and Morris, P. J., Leucocyte antigens in Hodgkin's disease, *Lancet* **2**:849–851 (1970).

29. Foy, A. M., Cooney, M. K., McMahan, R., Bor, R., and Grayston, J. T., Single-dose monovalent A₂/ Hong Kong influenza vaccine—Efficacy 14 months after immunization, *J. Am. Med. Assoc.* **217**:1067–1071 (1971).

30. Fox, J., Elveback, L. R., Spigland, I., Frothingham, T. E., Stevens, D. A., and Huger, M., The Virus Watch Program: A continuing surveillance of viral infections in metropolitan New York families. 1. Overall plan, methods of collecting and handling information and a summary report of specimens collected and illnesses observed, *Am. J. Epidemiol.* **83**:389–412 (1966).

31. Francis, T. F., and Magill, T. P., The incidence of neutralizing antibody for human influenza virus in the serum of human individuals of different ages, *J. Exp. Med.* **63**:655–668 (1936).

32. Gezer, A., Christensen, S., and Thorup, B., A multipurpose serological survey in Kenya. 1. Survey methods and progress of field work, *Bull. WHO* **43**:521–537 (1970).

32a. Glezon, W. P., and Couch, R. B., Interpandemic influenza in the Houston area, 1974–1976, *N. Engl. J. Med.* **298**:587–592 (1978).

33. Gold, E., Fevrier, A., Hatch, M. H., Hermann, K. L., Jones, W. L., Krugman, R. D., and Parkman, P. D., Immune status of urban children determined by antibody measurement, *N. Engl. J. Med.* **289**:231–234 (1973).

34. Grumet, F. C., Coukell, A., Bodmer, J. G., Bodmer, W. F., and McDevitt, H. O., Histocompatibility (HL-A) antigens associated with systemic lupus erythematosus: A possible genetic predisposition to disease, *N. Engl. J. Med.* **285**:193–196 (1971).

35. Guthe, T., Ridet, J., Vorst, F., D'Costa, J., and Grab, B., Methods for the surveillance of endemic treponematosis and seroimmunological investigations of "disappearing" disease, *Bull. WHO* **46**:1–14 (1972).

36. Henle, G., and Henle, W., Immunofluorescence in cells derived from Burkitt's lymphoma, *J. Bacteriol.* **91**:1248–1256 (1966).

36a. Henle, G., Henle, W., and Diehl, V., Relationship of Burkitt's tumor-associated herpes-type virus to infectious mononucleosis, *Proc. Natl. Acad. Sci. U.S.A.* **59**:94–101 (1968).

37. Horstmann, D. M., Need for monitoring vaccinated populations for immunity levels, *Prog. Med. Virol.* **16**:215–240 (1973).

38. Horstmann, D. M., Liebhaber, H., LeBouvier, G. L., Rosenberg, D. A., and Halstead, S. G., Rubella: Reinfection of vaccinated and naturally immune persons exposed in an epidemic, *N. Engl. J. Med.* **283**:771–778 (1970).

39. Jersild, C., Fog, T., Hansen, G. S., Thomsen, M., Svejgaard, A., and Dupont, B., Histocompatibility determinants in multiple sclerosis, with special reference to clinical course, *Lancet* **2**:1221–1225 (1973).

40. Lamb, G. A., and Feldman, H. A., Rubella vaccine response and other viral antibodies in Syracuse children, *Am. J. Dis. Child.* **122**:117–121 (1971).

41. Langmuir, A. D., The surveillance of communicable diseases of national importance, *N. Engl. J. Med.* **268**:182–192 (1963).

42. Mackay, I. R., and Morris, P. J., Association of autoimmune active chronic hepatitis with HL-A1,8, *Lancet* **2**:793–795 (1972).

42a. Marier, R., The reporting of communicable diseases, *Am. J. Epidemiol.* **105**:587–590 (1977).

43. McDonald, J. D., and Zuckerman, A. J., ABO blood

groups and acute respiratory disease, *Br. Med. J.* **1**:89–90 (1962).

44. MELNICK, J. L., BURKHARDT, M., TABER, L. T., AND ERCKMAN, P. N., Developing gap in immunity to poliomyelitis in an urban area, *J. Am. Med. Assoc.* **209**:1181–1185 (1969).

45. MILLER, D., GABRIELSON, M. O., AND HORSTMANN, D. M., Clinical virology and viral surveillance in a pediatric group practice: The use of double-seeded tissue culture tubes from primary virus isolation, *Am. J. Epidemiol.* **88**:245–256 (1968).

46. MONTO, A. S., AND ULLMAN, B. M., Acute respiratory illness in an American community, *J. Am. Med. Assoc.* **227**:164–169 (1974).

47. *National Disease and Therapeutic Index*, Lea Associates, Ambler, Pennsylvania, 1969.

48. NIEDERMAN, J. C., MCCOLLUM, R. W., HENLE, G., AND HENLE, W., Infectious mononucleosis in relation to EB virus antibodies, *J. Am. Med. Assoc.* **203**:205–209 (1968).

48a. OLDHAM, R. K., DEAN, J. H., CANNON, G. B., ORTALDO, J. R., DUNSTON, G., APPLEBAUM, F., MCCOY, J. L., DJEN, J., AND HERBERMAN, R. B., Cryopreservation of human lymphocytes function as measured by *in vitro* assays, *Int. J. Cancer* **18**:145–155 (1976).

49. *Oxford Universal Dictionary*, Clarendon Press, Oxford, 1955.

50. PAUL, J. R., Aims, purposes, and method of the World Health Organization Serum Banks, *Yale J. Biol. Med.* **36**:2–4 (1963).

51. PAUL, J. R., The story to be learned from blood samples: Its value to the epidemiologist, *J. Am. Med. Assoc.* **175**:601–605 (1961).

52. PAUL, J. R., *Serological Epidemiology in Clinical Epidemiology*, rev. ed., University of Chicago Press, Chicago, 1966.

53. PAUL, J. R., NIEDERMAN, J. C., PEARSON, R. J. C., AND FLOREY, C. DU V., A nationwide serum survey of United States military recruits. 1. General considerations, *Am. J. Hyg.* **80**:286–292 (1964).

54. PAUL, J. R., AND RIORDAN, J. T., Observations on serological epidemiology: Antibodies to the Lansing strain of poliomyelitis virus in sera from Alaskan Eskimos, *Am. J. Hyg.* **52**:202–212 (1950).

55. PAUL, J. R., AND TRASK, J. E., Neutralization test in poliomyelitis, comparative results with four strains of the virus, *J. Exp. Med.* **61**:447–464 (1935).

56. PAUL, J. R., AND WHITE, C. (eds.), *Serological Epidemiology*, Academic Press, New York, 1973.

56a. PURTILO, D. T., BHAWAN, J., HUTT, L. M., DENIKOLA, L., SZYMANSKI, I., YANG, J. P. S., BOTO, W., MAIER, R., AND THORLEY-LAWSON, D., Epstein–Barr virus infections in the X-linked recessive lymphoproliferative syndrome, *Lancet* **1**:798–801 (1978).

57. RAŠKA, K., National and international surveillance of communicable diseases, *WHO Chron.* **20**:313–321 (1966).

58. ROLESGAARD, E., Health regulations and international travel, *WHO Chron.* **28**:265–268 (1974).

58a. RUBIN, R. J., AND GREGG, M. B., A national influenza surveillance system: Methods and results, 1972–1974, *Am. J. Epidemiol.* **100**:516–517 (1974).

59. RUSSELL, T. J., SCHULTES, L. M., AND KUBAN, D. J., Histocompatibility (HL-A) antigens associated with psoriasis, *N. Engl. J. Med.* **287**:738–740 (1972).

60. SAWYER, R. N., EVANS, A. S., NIEDERMAN, J. C., AND MCCOLLUM, R. W., Prospective studies of a group of Yale University freshman. 1. Occurrence of infectious mononucleosis, *J. Infect. Dis.* **123**:263–270 (1971).

61. SCHFOSSTEIN, L., TERASAKI, P. I., BLUESTONE, R., AND PEARSON, C. M., High association of an HL-A antigen, W27, with anklylosing spondylitis, *N. Engl. J. Med.* **288**:704–706 (1973).

62. SEVER, J. L., Applications of a microtechnique to viral serologic investigations, *J. Immunol.* **88**:320–329 (1962).

63. SHOPE, R. E., Swine influenza. 1. Experimental transmission and pathology, *J. Exp. Med.* **54**:349–359 (1931).

64. SIMONS, M. J., WEE, G. B., DAY, N. E., MORRIS, P. J., SHANMUGARATNAM, K., AND DE THE, G. B., Immunogenetic aspects of nasopharyngeal carcinoma. 1. Differences in Hl-A antigen profiles between patients and control groups, *Int. J. Cancer* **13**:122–134 (1974).

64a. SIMONS, M. J., WEE, G. B., CHAN, S. H., SHANMUGARATNAM, K., DAY, N. E., AND DE THE, G. B., Immunogenetic aspects of nasopharyngeal carcinoma (NPC). III. HL-A type as a genetic marker of NPC predisposition to test the hypothesis that EBV is an etiologic agent in NPC, in: *Second International Conference on Oncogenesis and Herpesviruses*, Nuremberg, Germany, October 14–16, 1974.

64b. SIMONS, M. J., CHAN, S. H., WEE, G. B., SHANMUGARATNAM, K., DAY, N. E., AND DE-THE, G. B., Probable identification of HL-A second-locus antigen associated with a high risk of nasopharyngeal carcinoma, *Lancet* **1**:142–143 (1975).

65. SOPER, F. L., PENNA, H., CARDOSA, E., SERAFIM, J., JR., FROSBISHER, M., JR., AND PINHIERO, J., Yellow fever without *Aedes aegypti*: Study of a rural epidemic in the Valle do Chanaan, Espirito Santo, Brazil, *Am. J. Hyg.* **18**:555–587 (1932).

66. SMITH, W., ANDREWES, C. H., AND LAIDLAW, P. O., A virus obtained from influenza patients, *Lancet* **2**:66–68 (1933).

66a. SZMUNESS, W., Hepatocellular carcinoma and the hepatitis B virus: Evidence for a causal association, *Prog. Med. Virol.* **24**:40–69 (1978).

67. STOKES, P. L., ASQUITH, P., HOLMES, G. K. T., MACK-

INTOSH, P., AND COOKE, W. T., Histocompatibility antigens associated with adult coeliac disease, *Lancet* **2**:162–164 (1974).

68. THOMPSON, W. H., AND EVANS, A. S., California virus encephalitis studies in Wisconsin, *Am. J. Epidemiol.* **81**:230–244 (1965).

69. UNTERHOLER, V., AND ZABRISKIE, J. B., Suppressed cellular immunity to measles antigen in multiple sclerosis patients, *Lancet* **2**:1147 (1973).

70. WHO, Proceedings of the Twenty-first World Health Assembly (1968).

71. *WHO Tech. Rep. Ser.*, Immunological and Hematological Surveys, No. 181, Geneva (1959).

72. *WHO Tech. Rep. Ser.*, Multipurpose Serological Survey and WHO Serum Reference Banks, No. 454, Geneva (1970).

73. WIDELOCK, D., KLEIN, S., PEIZER, L. R., AND SIMONOVIC, O., Laboratory analyses of 1957–1958 influenza outbreak (A/Japan) in New York City. I., Preliminary report on seroepidemiologic investigation and variant A/Japan isolate, *J. Am. Med. Assoc.* **167**:541–543 (1958).

74. WILLIAMS, J. W., The value of the Wassermann reaction in obstetrics, based upon the study of 4547 consecutive cases, *Johns Hopkins Hosp. Bull.* **31**:335–342 (1920).

75. ZINKERNAGEL, R. M., Major transplantation antigens in host responses to infection, *Hosp. Pract.* **13**:83–92 (1978).

PART II

Acute Viral Infections

CHAPTER 3

Adenoviruses

Hjordis M. Foy and J. Thomas Grayston

1. Introduction

Adenoviruses derived their name from the fact that they were first isolated from adenoid tissues (tonsils) and have a certain affinity for lymph glands, where they may remain latent for years. They also invade the respiratory tract, the gastrointestinal tract, and the conjunctiva. In the respiratory tract, they may cause a variety of clinical manifestations ranging from pharyngitis to bronchitis, croup, and pneumonia. Adenovirus infections are widely distributed and common. Most infections occur in childhood.

A recognized syndrome seen especially among military recruits is febrile acute respiratory disease (ARD). Other disease syndromes caused by certain specific serotypes of adenovirus are pharyngoconjunctival fever (PCF) and epidemic keratoconjunctivitis (EKC). Several other disease syndromes that usually occur in children (hemorrhagic cystitis, pertussislike disease, skin rashes, intussusception) have been associated with adenoviruses.

Although some serotypes have been found to be oncogenic in animals, oncogenicity has not been observed in humans. Viral hybridization and cell transformation with adenovirus have been observed.[43,67a] Because of the latency of the infections, late sequelae are at least a theoretical possibility.

Hjordis M. Foy and J. Thomas Grayston · Department of Epidemiology and International Health, School of Public Health and Community Medicine, University of Washington, Seattle, Washington.

The viruses are unusually resistant to inactivation and degradation, allowing purification and molecular investigation. As much detailed structure and biochemistry of adenovirus are known as for any microorganism.[67a] Although many problems remain concerning production and use of adenovirus vaccines, both inactivated and live vaccines have been developed and found effective. Subunit vaccines are possible.

2. Historical Background

In 1953, a few years after cell culture became practical for isolation of viruses, Rowe et al.[70] described an agent that caused spontaneous degeneration of tissue culture originating from surgically removed human tonsils and adenoids. In 1954, Hilleman and Werner[41] reported isolation of similar agents from military personnel ill with febrile respiratory disease. Epidemics of such had been a serious problem in recruit training, and the Commission on Acute Respiratory Diseases of the U.S. Armed Forces Epidemiological Board initiated a series of studies revealing that the newly discovered agents were the cause of a large proportion of febrile acute respiratory disease among military recruit populations.[16,21] Several names were used for the new viruses, but in 1956 the term *adenoviruses* was adopted.[25]

Although the laboratory techniques for diagnosing adenovirus infections were not available until the 1950s, human adenoviruses have probably been present for a long time. Most illnesses caused by adenoviruses cannot be diagnosed by clinical observation alone. However, epidemics of acute respiratory diseases were recognized as causing disruption in military-recruit training as far back as the Civil War. During World War II, the Commission on Acute Respiratory Diseases defined the entity termed "ARD" through epidemiological and human-volunteer investigations.[21] This syndrome was an entity often distinguishable from other definable acute respiratory tract diseases, had an incubation period of 5–6 days, and was caused by a filtrable agent. The finding that this syndrome was caused by adenovirus suggests that this agent was responsible for the similar disease at the times of previous military mobilization.

There is also evidence that other adenovirus infections were present long before the 1950s. The disease syndrome now classified as EKC, caused primarily by adenovirus type 8, was clinically described by German workers at the end of the 19th century.[42,44] Several epidemics of conjunctivitis with fever, pharyngitis, and systemic symptoms centering around swimming baths were reported by German workers in the 1920s,[64] a disease that fits the description of PCF (see Section 5.2.3).

3. Methodology Involved in Epidemiological Analysis

3.1. Sources of Data

A good deal of the basic information on adenoviral disease comes from investigations of epidemics of ARD, PCF, and EKC. Because the disease syndromes caused by adenoviruses are not easily distinguished purely on clinical criteria in the absence of epidemics, general epidemiological studies require virus isolation and serological evidence. Adenovirus disease is not reportable, and there are no national or other general-population mortality and morbidity data. Many epidemiological data come from selected representative population samples under appropriate surveillance. Important studies have included military populations (especially recruits),[1a,16,21,22,29a,57,84] children's institutions,[3,39,78,87] groups of families,[18,30,38,45,88,90] and even an entire city.[58]

Adenovirus infections (types 4 and 7) were first recognized to cause significant illness in military-recruit populations. They have been extensively studied in the military. Not only were illnesses diagnosed with the appropriate laboratory tests, but also serological specimens collected at the beginning and end of training provided data on susceptibility and infection rates (whether symptomatic or asymptomatic). The epidemiological pattern of the disease in the four military services, including the serotypes involved under various training conditions and at different geographic locations, including international differences, has been studied.[1a,16,21,28,29,29a,81,82,84]

The epidemiological pattern of adenovirus infection in civilian populations comparable to military recruits was found to be very different.[34] Adenovirus disease was uncommon among college students.[27] On the other hand, longitudinal studies in orphanages and children's homes revealed that high rates of infection with several low-numbered serotypes occurred in infancy.[3,87] In such settings, certain viruses (types 1, 2, and 5) were often found to be endemic, whereas other serotypes (3 and 7) occurred in epidemics. The incubation period, communicability, rate of symptomatic vs. asymptomatic infection, spectrum of clinical manifestations, and cross-immunity have been investigated.

When asymptomatic children were studied as controls of clinic or hospitalized patients, adenoviruses were frequently isolated. It was quickly recognized that isolation of the virus from a sick patient did not establish a causal relationship. Much of our understanding of the epidemiology of adenovirus infection in children comes from continuous observations of panels of families conducted in Cleveland,[45] Kansas,[90] New Orleans,[38] New York,[30] Seattle,[18,30a] and also India.[50] In the first studies, respiratory and serological specimens were utilized. The broadest approach in family studies is exemplified by the Virus Watch studies, conducted in New York and Seattle, in which biweekly collections of both fecal and respiratory specimens for virus isolation were included in the routine observations. The latter type of studies uncovered a large number of asymptomatic infections, particularly with the lower-numbered serotypes, and demonstrated the high frequency of recrudescent shedding of virus.

3.2. Interpretation of Laboratory Tests

Antibody tests and virus isolation with serotyping have been used to provide epidemiological information on adenovirus infection. Properly interpreted, virus isolation provides the most conclusive evidence of infection and offers the opportunity to determine the serotype. To prevent excessive expense in population studies, isolation attempts are restricted by sampling techniques. Recovery of the virus is not difficult in the acute phase of illness in the majority of cases with upper respiratory tract and eye infections. Adenoviruses are isolated easily in cell cultures of human origin, especially HEK, Hep-2, and HeLa cells.[18,43] Monkey-kidney cells are less suitable. The optimal temperature is 37°C (rather than the frequently used 33°C).[32a] Typical cytopathogenic effect (CPE)—rounding of cells, often to grapelike clusters—may take 1–2 weeks, and sometimes cultures must be observed as long as 4 weeks before CPE is seen. Blind passage is recommended to recover the higher-numbered serotypes (above 7) and when the virus concentration in the specimen is low.[26,35,91] Demonstration of group-specific complement-fixing antigen identifies the isolate as a member of the adenovirus group. Serotyping is usually performed in a neutralization test using type-specific rabbit antisera. Counter immunoelectrophoresis has been introduced for rapid typing.[39a] Immunofluorescent antibody tests will detect group antigen and may be useful as rapid diagnostic tests, but they are not specific enough for epidemiological studies.

Since the adenovirus is often present for a prolonged period in the gastrointestinal tract, it may be recovered from fecal or rectal swab specimens after it has disappeared from the upper respiratory tract. Fecal excretion may continue intermittently for months or even years after acquisition,[30] and the diagnostic significance of recovery from this site in illness is often in doubt. Isolation from the respiratory tract has a greater probability to be associated with illness (carriage rate can be as high as 7% in healthy children[9,30,30a]). The virus usually disappears from the eye and pharynx as acute symptoms abate, but recrudescent infection may also occur in the throat. A serological antibody titer rise suggests recent infection, or possibly reactivation.

The three commonly applied serological tests in adenovirus epidemiology are the complement-fixation (CF), neutralization (N), and hemagglutination-inhibition (HI) antibody tests.[43] The CF test measures group-specific antibody. It is the easiest to perform and the most useful in diagnosis of acute infections, since CF antibodies tend to disappear rather rapidly. The production of CF antibodies in

infants may be poor, and the test can be erroneously negative. In older persons, CF antibodies from previous infections can cause difficulty in demonstrating a new infection. N and HI tests are more laborious to carry out, but they are type-specific and the antibody is long-lasting.

The HI and N tests are useful for serological epidemiology. A variety of such studies are available, comparing age of acquisition of antibody by type in different population groups including international comparisons.[80] Caution must be employed in comparing different studies, both of isolation and of antibody titers, because of variation in laboratory techniques.

4. Characteristics of the Virus

Adenoviruses are double-stranded DNA viruses lacking an envelope.[43,67a] The capsid contains 252 capsomeres and shows icosahedral symmetry. The capsomeres consist of hexons, pentons, and fibers, so named after their configuration. Hexons are similar for all types of adenoviruses and induce primarily group-specific CF antibodies; the fibers are largely responsible for type-specific antibodies. The pentons have mixed functions, and are especially active in hemagglutination.[67a] The size is 60–90 nm and the number of genes approximately 50. Thirty-three immunologically distinct types are recognized to cause human infection.

Adenoviruses are recognized by a common group antigen in a CF test. The common antigen consists primarily of hexons of the capsid.

By hemagglutination, the human adenoviruses can be divided into three groups[43,62]: Group I includes types 3, 7, 11, 14, 16, 20, 21, 25, 28, 32, and 33. They agglutinate rhesus erthrocytes. Group II includes types 8, 9, 10, 13, 15, 17, 19, 22, 23, 24, 26, 27, 29, and 30. This group agglutinates rat erythrocyte cells. Group III includes types 1, 2, 4, 5, 6, 12, 18, and 31, which agglutinate rat cells partially and not rhesus cells. Group III includes the viruses most commonly found in humans. Several viruses of group I cause severe respiratory infections. With the exception of types 8 and 19, the major causes of EKC, the group II viruses have been infrequently isolated and then usually in tropical countries.

Adenoviruses have also been grouped according to their degree of oncogenicity. Group A contains viruses of the highest oncogenic potential, types 12,

18, and 31, which are in Group III above. Group B has viruses of low oncogenicity and overlaps with group I above; viruses of groups C and D are without known oncongenicity, and most belong to groups II and III.

Adenoviruses are unusually stable to physical and chemical agents and adverse pH conditions, resulting in prolonged survival outside the host cells and great potential for spread. They are ether-resistant, but are destroyed by heat at 56°C for 30 min. Type 4 is especially heat-resistant. The viruses endure a pH range of 5.0–9.0 and temperatures ranging between 4 and 36°C. They survive freezing with minimal loss of infectivity.

The content of guanidine-cytosine in their DNA varies between 48 and 60%, and viruses with low contents (types 12, 18, and 31) are known to be oncogenic in laboratory animals, possibly reflecting a percentage of guanidine-cytosine content similar to that in the host cells. Hybridization has been observed between closely related adenovirus types. Adenoviruses can hybridize with simian virus 40 (SV40), a simian papovavirus known for its oncogenic potential.[67a]

Adenovirus-associated viruses (AAVs) are small (20–25 nm), contain DNA particles, and are found only in association with adenoviruses, which act as "helpers." AAVs were originally discovered with special staining techniques in electron microscopy. Now their presence is more easily indicated by serological techniques. These viruses do not cause cytopathogenicity. They are resistant to heating, ether, and chloroform, and can be stored at 1–4°C for many months. They are antigenically distinct from the adenoviruses. At least four immunotypes are known. So far, no disease syndrome has been associated with these viruses. They may become useful as epidemiological markers, since in an outbreak of PCF in Seattle, almost all those infected with adenovirus type 3 also had evidence of infection with AAV type 3.[71]

5. Descriptive Epidemiology

The following synopsis outlines the major epidemiological features of adenovirus infections. More detailed epidemiological characteristics are presented under the various clinical syndromes constituting the host response.

5.1. Synopsis of Descriptive Epidemiology

5.1.1. Incidence and Prevalence. See Section 5.2.1.

5.1.2. Epidemic Behavior. Types 1, 2, 5, and 6 are endemic in most areas of the world; types 4, 7, 14, and 21, which cause ARD (see Section 5.2.2), occur mostly in epidemics; type 3 is sometimes endemic, sometimes epidemic (see Section 5.2.3). Type 8 is endemic in the Far East, but occurs only in epidemics (and usually iatrogenic) in Western countries (see Section 5.2.4).

5.1.3. Geographic Distribution. Most types have been recovered from all areas of the world where they have been sought. Some of the higher-numbered types (8 and above) have been isolated more frequently in underdeveloped countries such as Saudi Arabia and Africa.

5.1.4. Temporal Distribution. The incidence of adenovirus-associated respiratory disease is higher in the late winter, spring, and early summer than in the remaining seasons of the year. This holds true for endemic childhood diseases as well as for military-recruit epidemics (see Section 5.2.2). Type 3 epidemics (PCF), associated with swimming, have been described most frequently in the summer.

5.1.5. Age. Most children have been exposed to several types of the endemic viruses by the time they enter school (see Fig. 1). Types 4, 7, 8, 14, and 21 infections may occur later in life.

5.1.6. Sex. There is no significant difference between the sexes except for ARD, a disease to which primarily males are exposed.

5.1.7. Occurrence in Different Settings. The family constitutes the most important unit for transmission of the endemic types (1, 2, 5, and 6). Rates of adenovirus infections (all types) are higher in children's institutions and daycare homes than in families. The incidence is higher in lower socioeconomic groups. Types 4 and 7 (and to some extent types 14, 21, and 11) occur as a recruit disease. Type 3 epidemics have been associated with swimming (see Section 5.2.3).

5.1.8. Occupation. ARD caused by types 4 and 7 (and to some extent 14, 21, and 11) occurs primarily in military recruits. Type 8 epidemics (EKC) have been associated with shipyards and physicians' offices.

5.1.9. Other Factors. Persons with deficient cell-mediated immunity appear at higher risk of severe adenovirus infection. This has been observed in congenital immunodeficiency, among immunosuppressed transplant patients,[76a] and following measles.[13,71a,89]

5.2. Epidemiological and Clinical Aspects of Specific Syndromes

5.2.1. Endemic Adenovirus Infections.

Most children become infected with some of the common types of adenoviruses early in life. Types 1, 2, and 5 are endemic in those parts of the world where studies have been conducted. By the age of 1 year, 80% of children in the New Orleans area had acquired antibodies to the virus, whereas the proportion with such antibodies was lower in New York and Seattle,[18,38] and slightly lower still in Stockholm, Sweden.[78] In studies including isolation of the adenovirus, the most frequently occurring types were 1 and 2. Other frequent adenovirus types occurring in childhood are types 5, 3, and 6, in that order. Neutralizing antibody studies in children and adults in four areas of the world are summarized in Fig. 1. The highest prevalence of adenovirus antibody is observed among crowded populations in tropical areas.

Overall, only about 50% of childhood adenovirus infections result in disease.[9,30] However, this proportion approaches two thirds when infection is associated with pharyngeal location of the virus. A lower percentage of symptomatic infection has been reported in some studies for type 2 than for any other adenovirus type.[3,5,10] The most significant contribution of adenoviruses to illness is in childhood, particularly under age 5, when about 5% of all acute respiratory illnesses can be associated with these viruses. The symptoms are usually nonspecific, described as stuffy nose and cough. Older children acquiring adenovirus infection often have symptoms of pharyngitis, which may mimic and be clinically indistinguishable from streptococcal pharyngitis.[39]

Studies of ill children in several hospitals and clinics suggest that 2–7% of all lower-respiratory-tract illnesses in young children seeking medical care can be attributed to adenoviruses.[10,32] Such illnesses are rare under the age of 6 months, when the child is protected by maternal antibody. The disease syndromes attributed to adenoviruses include pharyngitis, bronchitis, bronchiolitis, croup, and pneumonia. Adenovirus pneumonia in children has been particularly associated with type 7, and occasionally the disease is fatal.[8,11,13,14,74] It sometimes occurs as a complication to measles, especially in developing countries.[44a,71a,89] Adenovirus infections occur all year round, but the incidence of disease is higher in late winter, spring, and early summer.[9] When exposure is equal, both sexes are equally affected.

Public-health laboratories in England have reported a prolonged epidemic of adenovirus type 7 virus moving slowly through the country from 1971 to 1974; children manifested sore throats, conjunc-

Fig. 1. Comparison of adenovirus-neutralizing antibodies (types 1–8) in populations of four countries. The bar graphs indicate the percentage of antibody in children. If adults had a higher percentage of antibody, it is shown by a dashed-line extension. Reproduced with permission from Tai and Grayston[80] and the *Proceedings of the Society for Experimental Biology and Medicine*, with data added from Sterner.[78]

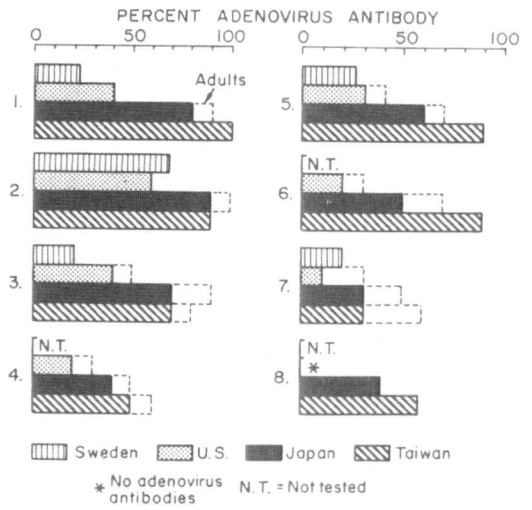

tivitis, and abdominal pain.[78a] Localized outbreaks of adenovirus pneumonia (types 7 and 21) have been reported in native Canadian,[11] New Zealand,[51] and northern Finnish infants and children.[74] It is not known whether this severe form of infection in these mostly nonwhite population groups is due to racial differences or to low socioeconomic status with crowding in a cold climate. There are no reports suggesting that American black children are more severely affected by adenovirus infection. Sequelae in the form of bronchiectasis and radiolucent lung have been frequently reported in these special groups.[11,51]

The mode of transmission in early life is thought to be primarily fecal–oral.[30] A child born into a family where other members harbor the virus in the intestinal tract will eventually become an excretor, but it may take several months before intrafamilial transmission occurs.[30,90] In family spread, the duration of shedding of the introducer seemed important: if shedding was brief, 42% of susceptibles and 6% of immunes were infected; if persistent, the rates were 65 and 21%, respectively.[30a] Figure

2 shows examples of typical fecal–oral spread of type 2 in families with newborn infants. Transmission shown in Fig. 2 contrasts with a family transmission of PCF in Fig. 3, where all became infected with type 3 shortly after the onsets of the index cases, and all but the father were symptomatic. An infected child may first excrete the virus from the respiratory tract, but the virus usually disappears from this location and may instead be found intermittently in fecal specimens for extended time periods.[30] Many apparently purely enteric infections occur that are usually asymptomatic. Intermittent excretion for up to 906 days has been reported.[30] The fact that the adenoviruses can be found in more than 50% of surgically removed tonsils suggests that the infection may lie dormant for many years.[26] The long-term effect of chronic adenovirus infections is unknown.

Children brought up in institutions acquire adenoviruses sooner than children living at home. Epidemics of infection with adenovirus types 5 and 7 have been described in orphanages and daycare facilities.[3,78,87] Whereas studies in free-living families

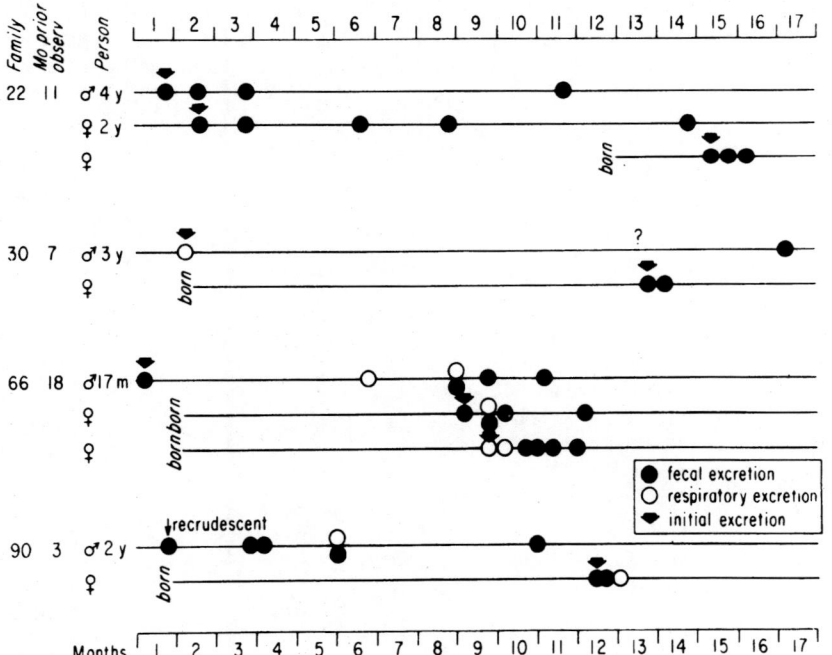

Fig. 2. Spread of type 2 adenovirus to infants born into families with siblings excreting the virus. Reproduced with permission from Fox et al.[30]

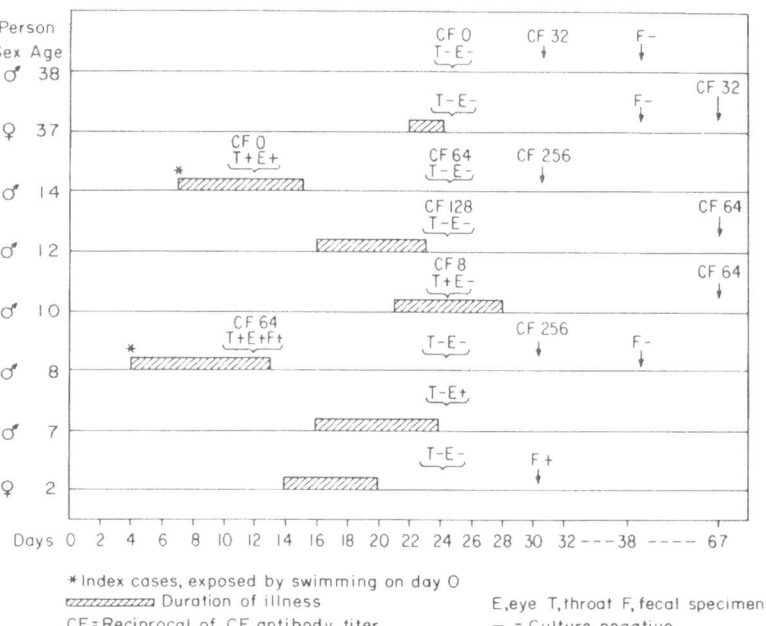

Fig. 3. Sequence of illnesses in a family where the two index cases, boys of 8 and 14 years, contracted PCF through exposure in a swimming pool. The first secondary family case occurred 10 days after onset of the first index case; within 17 days, all family members became infected. Only the father was asymptomatic; the mother's illness lasted only 2 days and was mild. Isolates from throat and eye were obtained only during acute illness (or at the latest 1 day after), whereas fecal excretion lasted longer. Isolates from the eyes were obtained only from those with conjunctivitis. Not shown in the illustration is the fact that all members developed antibodies to AAV 3. Reproduced (modified) from Foy et al.[31]

have rarely revealed the presence of other than types 1, 2, 3, 5, and 6, the studies in Junior Village,[3] an institution for homeless children in Washington, D.C., revealed spread of higher-numbered types, and studies among African children showed fecal excretion of types 8, 12, and 16.[84] The higher-numbered serological types (from type 9) are usually recovered only from fecal specimens,[3] and with the exceptions of types 11, 12, 19, 21, and 29, they have not been associated with respiratory, eye, or other illnesses. In 1975, an epidemic of type 31 was observed in New York families under continuous observation; the virus may have caused some mild respiratory disease.[88]

5.2.2. Acute Respiratory Disease of Military Recruits. Soon after adenoviruses were first isolated from cases of ARD among military personnel, it became clear that these viruses were the primary cause of morbidity among recruits, especially among North American and northern European forces.[16,21] Morbidity rates have been reported as high as 6–17/100 per week. Epidemics usually peak at about 3–6 weeks after onset of training, although sometimes the epidemic occurrence has been delayed. The sea-

sons for highest rates of adenovirus infections are winter and spring, independent of geographic locations and climatic conditions of training posts within the United States.[22] In one study, it was shown that recruits from the southern United States were less susceptible than those from the North, probably reflecting a more intensive exposure to adenoviruses during childhood and subsequent immunity for those brought up in the South.[57] In contrast to recruits, seasoned troops have low incidence of adenovirus infections, suggesting that lasting immunity is acquired early in military life[21] (Fig. 4).

The spectrum of clinical manifestations caused by adenoviruses in military recruits spans mild respiratory disease, usually with fever; febrile pharyngitis, often including adenitis; and pneumonia. Typical ARD is a febrile respiratory disease with symptoms of sore throat and cough, sometimes coryza, headache, and chest pain. Malaise is characteristic, and the illness lasts for approximately 10 days. White blood cell counts are normal or slightly elevated. It is estimated that 10% of recruits reporting to sick bay with ARD have pneumonitis on

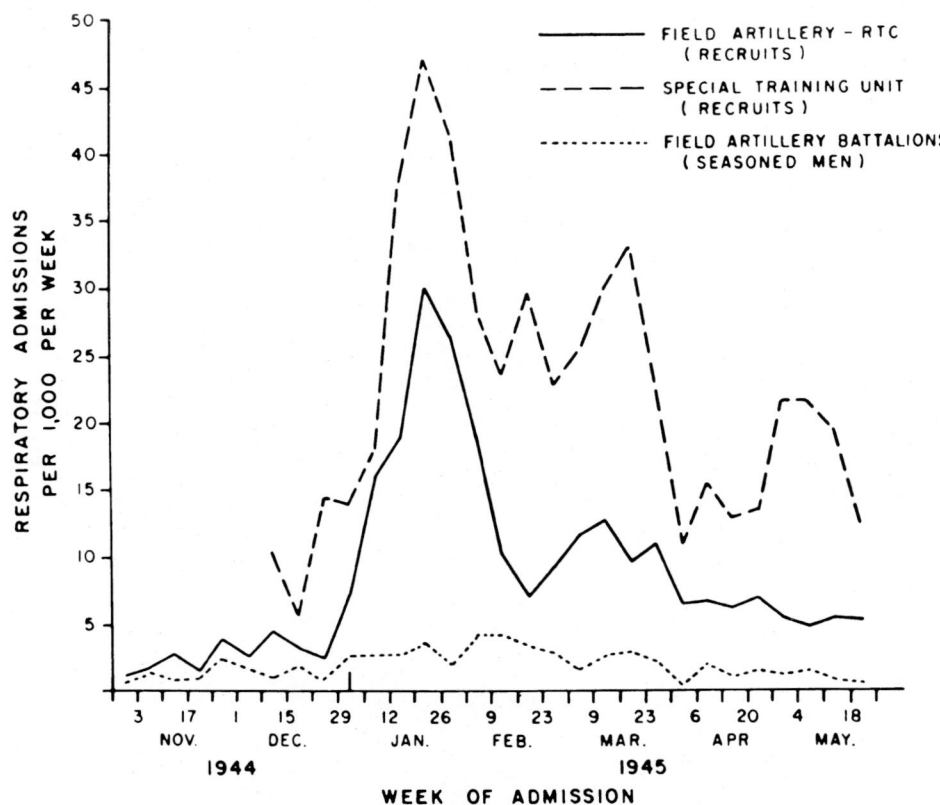

Fig. 4. Respiratory admission rates for two recruit groups and one seasoned army group at Fort Bragg, North Carolina, November 1944 to May 1945. Reproduced with permission from Dingle and Langmuir.[21]

X-ray examination. Chest films characteristically have feathery or mottled infiltrates. Deaths due to adenovirus pneumonia in the military are rare, but do occur.[23]

Epidemics of ARD are usually caused by adenovirus type 4 and less frequently by type 7. Occasionally, types 3, 11, 14, and 21 have caused epidemic ARD.[22,57,68,84]

The epidemiology of adenovirus infection among military populations has been studied extensively in the United States. Epidemics have been sharper and occurred sooner in Navy base camps, where extensive mingling of new and old recruits took place, than in Marine training camps, where new recruits were segregated in separate living quarters. The situation is similar in most European countries from which reports are available.[55,84] The incidence

in the British Army and Navy was less than in the Air Force, reflecting different management of recruit populations, with less contact between previously and recently inducted recruits.

Incidence has been reported to be low in Argentina[28] and Colombia[29] among Chinese recruits on Taiwan.[81] The types of adenoviruses prevalent in military forces of various countries have varied. Adenovirus type 4 was rarely observed among South American forces. Types 4 and 3 were epidemic in two different garrisons in Finland,[55] whereas type 7 was not. In the Netherlands, type 21 became epidemic in 1960–1961 among military recruits.[84] On Taiwan, type 5 was found in one outbreak.[81]

Despite the epidemic occurrence of adenoviruses in military populations, little spread has been noticed from the military bases to the civilian populations, including military dependents. An exception was Holland, where epidemics due to type 21 were observed among the military and children in civilian communities simultaneously.[84] Type 4 has been uncommonly associated with disease in civilians.

The sharp contrast between the epidemiology of adenovirus infections among civilian and military groups remains unexplained. Studies in adult civilian populations, including college students, have shown that adenoviruses can be associated with only a very small portion (0.5–3%) of respiratory disease.[27,34] In recruit training, a number of factors known to encourage epidemics exist. Persons are brought together from different geographic areas and backgrounds and subjected to crowding and stress. This situation is known to encourage spread in the military of many other infections often classified as childhood diseases such as mumps, rubella, chickenpox, and meningococcal disease. Methods of processing recruits may potentiate an epidemic; thus, it has been found that when new recruits are allowed to mix with those already present and presumably infected, epidemics readily occur.[1a] In the Marine Corps, when each training unit was kept separate, the overall incidence was lower. The prevalence of neutralizing antibodies in the incoming recruits to the virus types causing epidemics has generally been low.

5.2.3. Pharyngoconjunctival Fever. PCF is a syndrome characterized by pharyngitis, conjunctivitis, and fever. The fever is often spiking in character. Either one or both eyes may be involved, and only rarely is the cornea affected. Diarrhea, coryza, and occasionally otitis may be present. The tonsils may show an exudate, and lymphadenopathy is often observed.

In the 1920s, epidemics of a febrile disease with conjunctivitis centering around swimming activities were first described from Germany[64] and later from the United States.[2] The clinical epidemiological characteristics of these epidemics are highly suggestive of adenovirus infection, and the epidemics were thought to be caused by inadequate chlorination. However, the only nonbacterial agent known to cause conjunctivitis at that time was trachoma-inclusion conjunctivitis agent (*Chlamydia trachomatis*), and it was believed that these epidemics were caused by such agents, since inclusions were seen

in a few patients. After the 1950s, when adequate diagnostic tools for isolation of both inclusion conjunctivitis and adenovirus were developed, all swimming-pool-centered epidemics have been traced to adenovirus infections.[31,46,65] Thus, the name "swimming pool conjunctivitis" for inclusion conjunctivitis infections is probably a misnomer.

The association of PCF with adenovirus type 3 was first described by Bell *et al.*[4] in 1955. The syndrome is caused most frequently by adenovirus type 3 or 7, but has also been associated with other adenovirus types, such as types 1, 4, and 14. The disease may be seen sporadically and cause epidemics in families and other closed population groups,[4,31,78] but is best known as an epidemic disease centering around summer camps and especially swimming pools and small lakes.[31,46,48,65] It usually affects children and young adults. The fact that the youngest age groups (under age 4), who waded rather than swam, had the lowest attack rate in the original outbreak described by Parrott *et al.*[65] suggests that direct contact with the water, possibly allowing introduction of the virus into the eye or upper respiratory tract, is the important mode of spread. However, once the virus is introduced into a family, secondary spread to other family members frequently occurs. This secondary spread may be by direct contact or possibly droplet transmission. In a study conducted in Seattle, it was found that parents secondarily infected from children usually had milder symptoms, often only conjunctivitis.[31] This suggests that they possessed some immunity, most likely humoral, but that the conjunctiva lacked sufficient defense mechanism.

The incubation period is estimated at 6–9 days. In a common-source epidemic originating from a swimming pool open only for 1 day, the incubation period was estimated at an average of 6 days.[46] An incubation period of 6 days was also observed by Bell *et al.*[4] when a patient exposed his physician by coughing in his face. On the other hand, the incubation period observed in experimental inoculation of volunteers has been as short as 2 days.[6] This shortening of the incubation period may be dose-related.

Although several epidemic outbreaks have been traced to common exposure at a swimming pool or a small lake, the virus has never been isolated from the water of a swimming pool. However, most attempts at such isolation have taken place after the epidemic was identified, when measures to remedy the unsatisfactory conditions had already been taken. Several outbreaks have clearly been associated with unsatisfactory chlorination of swimming-pool water. The virus has been isolated from a water sample near a sewage outlet in a lake where swimmers had experienced PCF.[48] In the laboratory, adenovirus type 3 appears as susceptible to chlorination as *Escherichia coli* bacteria.

5.2.4. Epidemic Keratoconjunctivitis. EKC is a disease entity that was first described by German workers in the latter part of the 19th century.[42,44] During World War II when ship-building flourished, it was observed in industrial outbreaks first on Hawaii, then on the United States West Coast, and finally on the East Coast.[44] Transmission probably took place in the medical facilities, where the workers sought treatment for foreign bodies and chemical irritation of the eye.

It was during this period that the disease was named "epidemic keratoconjunctivitis" because of its clinical characteristics, but it was often popularly called "shipyard eye." The illness characteristically has an incubation period of 8–10 days and starts with conjunctivitis that may be follicular, followed by edema of the eyelids, pain, photophobia, and lacrimation. After a couple of days, superficial erosions of the cornea may develop, followed in a full-blown case by deeper subepithelial corneal infiltrates with characteristic round shape, located in the center of the cornea. These may interfere with vision and cause lasting visual impairment. Preauricular lymph-gland swelling is common, and occasionally cervical and submaxillary lymph glands are involved. Frequently, only one eye is infected. Constitutional symptoms may occur among children, but are usually mild.

Adenovirus type 8 was the almost exclusive cause of the typical disease in Western countries until 1973, when type 19 appeared almost simultaneously in several European countries and North America.[11a,20a,37a,86] Rarely have other types such as 4, 10, 11, and 14 been implicated.[11a,36] The virus can be isolated during the acute disease from the eye, occasionally from the throat, and for a longer period from the feces.

During recent decades, outbreaks have been reported centering around the offices of ophthalmologists.[11a,44,76,79] Since the virus is unusually hardy, ether and alcohol treatment of ophthalmological in-

struments (in particular tonometers) is insufficient as a means of sterilizing equipment, and heat sterilization (240°C or 465°F) is necessary. Spread may also occur directly by fingers during manipulation of the lids or by use of eye solutions and ointments. Patients acquiring the infection by a visit to the ophthalmologist's office only occasionally transmit the infection to family members. Direct inoculation into the eye appears necessary to cause disease.

In areas of Japan and Taiwan, a yearly epidemic of EKC has been observed in the late summer and fall.[36] The spread presumably occurs by direct contact between children and between family members. In camps for recently arrived Vietnamese refugees, adenovirus keratoconjunctivitis has been rampant, spreading also to the indigenous Americans.[92] Thus, the more crowded and less hygienic living conditions promote the spread of the virus. It is also noteworthy that many of the higher-numbered serological adenovirus types were first isolated from eyes in Saudi Arabia, where trachoma is highly endemic, suggesting environmental and hygienic requirement for spread of both these eye diseases.[7] Serological studies in the late 1950s revealed that 40–60% of Japanese and Taiwanese school children have acquired neutralizing antibody to type 8, whereas virtually no American children have antibodies to adenovirus type 8[80] (see Fig. 1).

5.2.5. More Unusual Syndromes Associated with Adenovirus Infections. *Acute hemorrhagic cystitis* is a rare self-limited disease primarily of childhood, characterized by polyuria, dysuria, and hematuria. Isolation of adenovirus type 11 from this disease by use of special techniques was first accomplished in Sendai, Japan, in 1968.[63] The patients showed significant increase in antibody titers by N and CF but not by HI test. Subsequently, isolation of adenovirus type 11 and also type 21 from the urine of children with this disease was reported from Chicago.[60] Other and previously unrecognized adenovirus types (candidate types 34 and 35) have been recovered from urine sporadically, especially from immunosuppressed recipients of kidney transplants.[76a] Such infections have led to dissemination with a fatal outcome.

Intussusception, an acute illness of infancy, is characterized by "telescoping" one part of the intestine into the next distal portion. The disease usually requires prompt surgical intervention because of risk of necrosis as the blood supply of the involved bowel segment becomes obstructed. Lymph-tissue enlargement from adenovirus infection may initiate such telescoping, and based on reports of high isolation rate of adenoviruses from such patients, an etiological role for adenoviruses has been suggested.[15,33,69] However, although the rate of isolation of adenovirus from children with intussusception is higher than in children serving as controls, not all patients with intussusception have evidence of adenovirus infection, and the etiology of this syndrome may be complex.

Pertussislike syndrome in association with various serological types of adenovirus infection has been described.[17,49] Patients selected to serve as controls have generally had less evidence of virus infection. On the other hand, in a recent in-depth study of pertussis, *Bordatella pertussis* was isolated from 45 of 65 patients, and adenovirus was shed in 8 cases. In convalescence, adenovirus was isolated in only 1 of 33 cases. The course was no worse in patients shedding adenovirus. It has been postulated that pertussis merely reactivates adenovirus infection.[2a,62]

Skin rashes have been associated with adenovirus infection, but in most such incidences, the rash could be attributed to preceding or concurrent measles or rubella.[13,37,61,71a,74]

6. Mechanisms and Route of Transmission

Adenovirus infections in man are spread from person to person by various routes. Although many lower animals have adenoviruses, there is no evidence that these are human in origin or that animal adenoviruses infect humans. There is no known spread by vectors. In childhood and in family transmission, the fecal–oral route undoubtedly plays the major role. This route is the most important for transmission of adenovirus types 1, 2, 5, and 6. Respiratory transmission of these and other types is possible at all ages in association with ARD. The respiratory route is of prime importance when ARD becomes epidemic in military-recruit camps. Pharyngeal carriage rates as high as 18% have been reported among healthy recruits.[29a] In volunteer studies, inhalation of small doses of adenoviruses in aerosols usually resulted in infection accompanied by febrile ARD, sometimes with pneumonia.[19] In contrast, nasopharyngeal administration was

much less effective in producing disease[6]; even inoculation of the conjunctiva was more successful. The eye is an important portal of entry for virus types 3 and 7, particularly when PCF is transmitted in swimming pools or lakes. EKC is often an iatrogenic disease spread by ophthalmological instruments, ointments, or fingers in physicians' offices. Adenoviruses occasionally cause nosocomial infections in hospitals.[4,13,87]

7. Pathogenesis and Immunity

Most disease caused by adenoviruses is acute and self-limited. Type-specific neutralizing antibody has been associated with prevention of symptomatic reinfection. While adenovirus disease is short-lasting, infection may be prolonged and asymptomatic infections are common. Viral shedding in the gastrointestinal tract may recur for years. Adenoviruses can be isolated from at least 50% of surgically removed tonsils,[26] occasionally from the kidney,[76a] and also from the lymphocytes,[1] suggesting that infection may remain latent for a very long time, possibly for life.

The virus may invade the bloodstream in the early stages of the disease, and viremia has been associated with a maculopapular skin rash.[8,13,37,74] However, these rashes may have been due to measles and rubella, and the adenovirus merely reactivated. Adenovirus has been isolated from cerebrospinal fluid in patients with meningoencephalitis.[47a]

In the rare fatal illness, the virus has been recovered from most body organs.[8] In such cases, extensive pathology is found in the lungs with microscopic necrosis of tracheal and bronchial epithelium characterized as necrotizing bronchiolitis. In bronchial epithelial cells, acidophilic intranuclear inclusions have been described, as well as basophilic masses of cells surrounded by characteristic clear halos. The latter may represent aggregation of a larger amount of viral material.[8,11,61,71a] Rosette formation, a mononuclear cell infiltrate, and focal necrosis of mucous glands appear to be characteristic. Typical intranuclear virus particles have been observed in alveolar lining and bronchiolar cells by electron microscopy.[61] In infants who recover from adenovirus pneumonia, severe sequelae may follow, including radiolucent lung syndrome, bronchiectasis, and persistent lobar collapse.[11,51,74]

Neurotropism of the virus, especially type 7, has been suggested by isolation from the central nervous system.[8,73]

Rates of adenovirus pneumonia in children are lower under the age of 6 months than in older infants, suggesting that maternally derived humoral antibodies are protective and that humoral antibody plays a major part in the defense mechanism. Studies of volunteers have shown that even artificial challenge with virus in persons already having neutralizing antibody for that type rarely results in symptomatic infection. Intracellular location probably protects the virus from the effect of humoral antibody and permits persistent latent infection.

The incubation period in volunteers challenged artificially can be as short as 2 days, which may be a dose-related response.[4] Under the natural challenge, the incubation period averages 6–9 days, sometimes longer, particularly in EKC.

8. Patterns of Host Response

The host response to adenovirus infection is dependent on the route of transmission and primary site of viral localization and on serological type and dose. Disease syndromes (ARD, PCF, EKC) occurring in special situations have been described above. In persons with normal immune systems, the presence of humoral antibodies plays a major role in determining the outcome of infection. Persons with poor IgA antibody response to infection have been shown to have increased severity of symptoms.[56] Immunodeficient and immunosuppressed patients appear to be at risk of disseminated infection.[76a,85] Postponement and spacing of the several routine immunizations given military recruits have been associated with reduction of ARD, pointing out an interesting type of host stress immunologically associated with adenovirus disease.[57,67]

Primary localization of adenoviruses in the respiratory tract or conjunctiva results in a higher rate of symptomatic infection than gastrointestinal localization.

The relationship of immunotype to disease severity is difficult to separate from host and environmental factors. Types 8 and 19 cause more severe eye disease than other types. Types 4, 7, and 21 have been associated with severe respiratory disease.

Why some infections cause pneumonia and even

death is not well understood. Host age of 6 months to 2 years is clearly associated with adenoviral pneumonia, as is general host deprivation associated with lower socioeconomic status. A poor nutritional state and measles both lead to suppressed cell-mediated immunity and may explain why severe adenovirus pneumonia occurs in certain situations.[44a,71a] Type 7 and to some extent type 21 have been particularly associated with fatal infant pneumonia.[8,13,14,51,74]

Reactivation of adenovirus infection may possibly be evoked by other respiratory agents.[2a,14,33a,41,62] It has been reported that during mumps infection, adenovirus excretion reappeared.[30] In studies of pneumonia etiology, an unexpectedly high rate of serological titer rises to adenoviruses was found to occur at the same time as antibody rises to influenza, parainfluenza, and *Mycoplasma pneumoniae*, which were implicated as etiological agents of the pneumonia.[32,40]

9. Control and Prevention

Of the various approaches to the prevention or control of adenovirus infections, bolstering the host's resistance through immunization has shown the most promise. In certain situations, environmental control has been effective.[52,54] Control or treatment with antiviral compounds, interferon, or interferon inducers has shown no practical value.[43]

Because of the major disruption and economic impact of ARD epidemics in military recruits, most of the efforts in the development of human adenoviral vaccines have been directed at this population. The first widely used vaccines were inactivated adenoviruses grown in monkey-kidney tissue culture.[12,66] They were shown to be effective against adenoviral infection with types 3, 4, and 7. However, potency varied among lots of vaccine because of poor growth in the monkey-cell culture. Efforts to meet minimal standards for military use were often unsuccessful. A major production difficulty was contamination of the cell culture with SV40. This virus is recognized as oncogenic in animals, and in addition it was found that adenoviruses were able to incorporate part of the SV40 genome (hybridization) when the viruses grew in the same culture.

The extensive molecular studies of adenoviruses

had shown the possibility of developing a highly purified subunit vaccine.[47] However, production problems for such a vaccine have not been solved.

In recent years, major vaccine efforts have been made with live attenuated virus given orally.[12,24,66, 68,75,83] This approach has been based on the theory that by bypassing the respiratory tract and introducing a live virus into the gastrointestinal tract, where the virus was known to multiply, respiratory disease could be avoided while the subject acquired solid immunity. For this purpose, live adenoviruses grown in human cells were placed in enteric-coated gelatin capsules. Following experimental studies, this approach to immunization has been shown to be highly effective in military-recruit populations. However, when type 4 military epidemics were controlled by live, oral immunization, type 7 epidemics occurred. Bivalent immunization has successfully controlled these two types.[82] The fear that another type of adenovirus, for example, type 21, would take over and fill the "ecological niche" has not yet been substantiated.[68]

The experimental studies with these vaccines have shown a number of interesting facts about adenoviral spread.[20,66,83] Neither type 4 nor 7 spread from adults infected by enteric capsules to susceptible adults housed together for a prolonged period.[20,66] On the other hand, when enteric live adenovirus type 4 vaccine was introduced to one partner of each of 39 married couples and a placebo was given to the other, viral isolates were obtained from 70% of the placebo recipients, suggesting that intimate physical contact facilitated transmission of the virus.[77] No serious symptoms were encountered in the placebo group. In another study, conjunctivitis occurred in two of six volunteers infected in the gastrointestinal tract, probably by fecal–conjunctival contamination.[20] When children in a household were immunized by this route, transmission of the virus (type 4) to other members of the household was demonstrated with occasional illness.[59]

There have been no efforts to protect children or other civilian populations from adenovirus infections by immunization with oral vaccine. Successful immunization by the gastrointestinal route has been demonstrated with types 1, 2, and 5 in adult volunteers.[72] Since none of the virus in these vaccines has been demonstrated to be significantly attenuated, there is the risk that administration of live

vaccines to infants may cause spread of adenoviral disease. The practical problems of spread of infection and the hypothetical concerns that remain concerning oncogenicity would make an effort to immunize infants and children with live adenoviruses a dubious undertaking.

Environmental control is effective in certain situations. Thus, the evidence suggests that adequate chlorination of swimming pools prevents the spread of PCF. The spread of keratoconjunctivitis through contaminated ophthalmological instruments, ointments, and solutions can be prevented by heat sterilization and appropriate hygienic measures.

Since adenovirus infections in military-recruit populations appear to be associated with crowding and airborne transmission, various environmental control attempts have been tried. Modification of the sleeping arrangements in barracks has met with, at best, limited success.[53] Attempts at dust suppression have been more successful,[54] whereas air purification with ultraviolet light and germicidal sprays has failed.[52,53] More extensive changes in the patterns of recruit housing and training can modify ARD occurrence, but may be impractical in times of mobilization.[1a]

10. Unresolved Problems

Great strides have been made during the last decade in describing and understanding the molecular biology of adenoviruses, yet no effective antiviral agent has been found. Although several types of vaccines have been developed, none is ideal, and the possibility of using a purified subunit of the virus for vaccine is an attractive prospect. Such a vaccine should be highly immunogenic but not pathogenic.

The exact mechanism whereby adenoviruses cause tissue damage and systemic disease, including the role of cell-mediated and humoral immunity, is not fully understood. The role of the high-numbered serological types, best known for their presence in some underdeveloped and tropical countries and incompletely studied in the United States, is yet to be determined. The role of concomitant or subsequent viral or bacterial infection in precipitating more severe adenoviral disease remains to be worked out. Why some types, especially 4, 7, and 21, are highly epidemic in the military, but rarely seen in the community, is unknown.

The long-term effect of latent adenovirus infection or reactivation later in life is open to speculation. What is the mechanism for latency: chronic low-grade infection, lysogenicity, or incorporation of the virus genome in the host cell? How long does latency last? Oncogenicity has been shown only when human adenoviruses have been introduced into animal models. Although the search for oncogenic potentiality in humans by investigation for T (tumor) antigens has so far been negative, an oncogenic effect in humans cannot be totally ruled out. To conduct long-term studies of human populations to resolve this dilemma would be a formidable task. One approach is to study the prevalence of adenovirus genome in patients with and without neoplasm using a DNA hybridization technique.

11. References

1. ANDIMAN, W. A., JACOBSON, R. I., AND TUCKER, G., Leukocyte-associated viremia with adenovirus type 2 in an infant with lower respiratory tract disease, *N. Engl. J. Med.* **297**:100–101 (1977).
1a. ARLANDER, T. R., PIERCE, W. E., EDWARDS, E. A., PECKINPAUGH, R. O., AND MILLER, L. F., IV. An epidemiologic study of respiratory illness patterns in Navy and Marine Corps recruits, *Am. J. Public Health* **55**:67–80 (1965).
2. BAHN, C., Swimming bath conjunctivitis, *New Orleans Med. Sci. J.* **79**:586–590 (1927).
2a. BARAFF, L. J., WILKINS, J., AND WEHRLE, P. F., The role of antibiotics, immunizations, and adenoviruses in pertussis, *Pediatrics* **61**:224–230 (1978).
3. BELL, J. A., HUEBNER, R. J., ROSEN, L., ROWE, W. P., COLE, R. M., MASTROTA, F. M., FLOYD, T. M., CHANOCK, R. M., AND SHVEDOFF, R. A., Illness and microbial experiences of nursery children at Junior Village, *Am. J. Hyg.* **74**:267–292 (1961).
4. BELL, J. A., ROWE, W. P., ENGLER, J. I., PARROTT, R. H., AND HUEBNER, R. J., Pharyngoconjunctival fever: Epidemiological studies of a recently recognized disease entity, *J. Am. Med. Assoc.* **175**:1083–1092 (1955).
5. BELL, J. A., ROWE, W. P., AND ROSEN, L., II. Adenoviruses, *Am. J. Public Health* **52**:902–907 (1962).
6. BELL, J. A., WARD, T. G., HUEBNER, R. J., ROWE, W. P., SUSKIND, R. G., AND PAFFENBARGER, R. S., JR., Studies of adenoviruses (APC) in volunteers, *Am. J. Public Health* **46**:1130–1146 (1956).
7. BELL, S. D., JR., ROTA, T. R., AND MCCOMB, D. E., Adenoviruses isolated in Saudi Arabia. III. Six new serotypes, *Am. J. Trop. Med.* **9**:523–526 (1960).
8. BENYESH-MELNICK, M., AND ROSENBERG, H. S., The isolation of adenovirus type 7 from a fatal case of pneumonia and disseminated disease, *J. Pediatr.* **64**:83–87 (1964).
9. BRANDT, C. D., KIM, H. W., JEFFRIES, B. C., PYLES, G., CHRISTMAS, E. E., REID, J. L., CHANOCK, R. M., AND PARROTT, R. H., Infections in 18,000 infants and children in a controlled study of respiratory tract disease. II. Variation in adenovirus infections by year and season, *Am. J. Epidemiol.* **95**:218–227 (1972).
10. BRANDT, C. D., KIM, H. W., VARGOSKO, A. J., JEFFRIES, B. C., ARROBIO, J. O., RINDGE, B., PARROTT, R. H., AND CHANOCK, R. M., Infections in 18,000 infants and children in a controlled study of respiratory tract disease. I. Adenovirus pathogenicity in relation to serologic type and illness syndrome, *Am. J. Epidemiol.* **90**:484–500 (1969).
11. BROWN, R. S., NOGRADY, M. B., SPENCE, L., AND WIGLESWORTH, F. W., An outbreak of adenovirus type 7 infection in children in Montreal, *Can. Med. Assoc. J.* **108**:434–439 (1973).
11a. CENTER FOR DISEASE CONTROL, International notes: Keratoconjunctivitis due to adenovirus type 19—Canada, *Morbidity Mortality Weekly Rep.* **23**:185–186 (1974).
12. CHANOCK, R. M., LUDWIG, W., HUEBNER, R. J., CATE, T. R., AND CHU, L. W., Immunization by selective infection with type 4 adenovirus grown in human diploid tissue culture. I. Safety and lack of oncogenicity and tests for potency in volunteers, *J. Am. Med. Assoc.* **195**:151–158 (1966).
13. CHANY, C., LEPINE, P., LELONG, M., VINH, L. T., SATGE, P., AND VIRAT, J., Severe and fatal pneumonia in infants and young children associated with adenovirus infections, *Am. J. Hyg.* **67**:367–378 (1958).
14. CHIN-HSIEN, T., Adenovirus pneumonia epidemic among Peking infants and pre-school children in 1958, *Chin. Med. J.* **80**:331–339 (1960).
15. CLARKE, E. J., PHILLIPS, I. A., AND ALEXANDER, E. R., Adenovirus infection in intussusception in children in Taiwan, *J. Am. Med. Assoc.* **208**:1671–1674 (1969).
16. COMMISSION ON ACUTE RESPIRATORY DISEASES, Experimental transmission of minor respiratory illness to human volunteers by filter-passing agents. I. Demonstration of two types of illness characterized by long and short incubation periods and different clinical features, *J. Clin. Invest.* **26**:957–973 (1947).
17. CONNOR, J. D., Evidence for an etiologic role of adenoviral infection in pertussis syndrome, *N. Engl. J. Med.* **283**:390–394 (1970).
18. COONEY, M. K., HALL, C. E., AND FOX, J. P., The Seattle Virus Watch. III. Evaluation of isolation methods and summary of infections detected by virus isolations, *Am. J. Epidemiol.* **96**:286–305 (1972).
19. COUCH, R. B., CATE, T. R., FLEET, W. F., GERONE, P.

J., AND KNIGHT, V., Aerosol-induced adenoviral illness resembling the naturally occurring illness in military recruits, *Am. Rev. Resp. Dis.* **93**:529–535 (1966).

20. COUCH, R. B., CHANOCK, R. M., CATE, T. R., LANG, D. J., KNIGHT, V., AND HUEBNER, R. J., Immunization with types 4 and 7 adenovirus by selective infection of the intestinal tract. *Am. Rev. Respir. Dis.* **88**:394–403 (1963).

20a. DAROUGAR, S., QUINLAN, M. P., GIBSON, J. A., JONES, B. R., AND McSWIGGAN, D. A., Epidemic keratoconjunctivitis and chronic papillary conjunctivitis in London due to adenovirus type 19, *Br. J. Ophthalmol.* **61**:76–85 (1977).

21. DINGLE, J., AND LANGMUIR, A. D., Epidemiology of acute respiratory disease in military recruits, *Am. Rev. Respir. Dis.* **97**:1–65 (1968).

22. DUDDING, B. A., TOP, F. H., JR., WINTER, P. E., BUESCHER, E. L., LAMSON, T. H., AND LEIBOVITZ, A., Acute respiratory disease in military trainees: The adenovirus surveillance program, 1966–1971, *Am. J. Epidemiol.* **97**:187–198 (1973).

23. DUDDING, B. A., WAGNER, S. C., ZELLER, J. A., GMELICH, J. T., FRENCH, G. R., AND TOP, F. H., JR., Fatal pneumonia associated with adenovirus type 7 in three military trainees, *N. Engl. J. Med.* **286**:1289–1292 (1972).

24. EDMONDSON, W. P., PURCELL, R. H., GUNDERFINGER, B. F., LOVE, J. W. P., LUDWIG, W., AND CHANOCK, R. M., Immunization by selective infection with type 4 adenovirus grown in human diploid tissue culture. II. Specific protective effect against epidemic disease, *J. Am. Med. Assoc.* **195**:159–165 (1966).

25. ENDERS, J. F., BELL, J. A., DINGLE, J. H., FRANCIS, T., JR., HILLEMAN, M. R., HUEBNER, R. J., AND PAYNE, A. M. M., "Adenoviruses": Group name proposed for new respiratory-tract viruses, *Science* **124**:119–120 (1956).

26. EVANS, A. S., Latent adenovirus infections of the human respiratory tract, *Am. J. Hyg.* **67**:256–266 (1958).

27. EVANS, A. S., Clinical syndromes in adults caused by respiratory infections, *Med. Clin. North Am.* **51**:803–818 (1967).

28. EVANS, A. S., CENABRE, L., WANAT, J., RICHARDS, V., NEIDERMAN, J. C., AND ACTIS, A., Acute respiratory infections in different ecologic settings. I. Argentine military recruits, *Am. Rev. Respir. Dis.* **108**:1311–1319 (1973).

29. EVANS, A. S., JEFFREY, C., AND NIEDERMAN, J. C., The risk of acute respiratory infections in two groups of young adults in Colombia, South America: A prospective seroepidemiologic study, *Am. J. Epidemiol.* **93**:463–471 (1971).

29a. FORSYTH, B. R., BLOOME, H. H., JOHNSON, K. M., AND

CHANOCK, R. M., Etiology of primary atypical pneumonia in a military population, *J. Am. Med. Assoc.* **191**:364–369 (1965).

30. FOX, J. P., BRANDT, C. D., WASSERMANN, F. E., HALL, C. E., SPIGLAND, I., KOGON, A., AND ELVEBACK, L. R., The Virus Watch Program: A continuing surveillance of viral infections in metropolitan New York families. VI. Observations of adenovirus infections: Virus excretion patterns, antibody response, efficiency of surveillance, patterns of infection, and relation to illness, *Am. J. Epidemiol.* **89**:25–50 (1969).

30a. FOX, J. P., HALL, C. E., AND COONEY, M. K., The Seattle Virus Watch. VII. Observations of adenovirus infections, *Am. J. Epidemiol.* **105**:362–386 (1977).

31. FOY, H. M., COONEY, M. K., AND HATLEN, J. B., Adenovirus type 3 epidemic associated with intermittent chlorination of a swimming pool, *Arch. Environ. Health* **17**:795–802 (1968).

32. FOY, H. M., COONEY, M. K., McMAHAN, R., AND GRAYSTON, J. T., Viral and mycoplasmal pneumonia in a prepaid medical care group during an eight-year period, *Am. J. Epidemiol.* **97**:93–102 (1973)

32a. FUCHS, N., AND WIGAND, R., Virus isolation and titration at 33° and 37°C., *Med. Microbiol. Immunol.* **161**:123–126 (1975).

33. GARDNER, P. S., KNOX, E. G., COURT, S. D. M., AND GREEN, C. A., Virus infection and intussusception in childhood, *Br. Med. J.* **2**:697–700 (1962).

33a. GLEZEN, W. P., WULFF, H., LAMB, G. A., RAY, C. G., CHIN, T. D. Y., AND WENNER, H. A., Patterns of virus infections in families with acute respiratory illnesses, *Am. J. Epidemiol.* **86**:350–361 (1966).

34. GRAYSTON, J. T., LASHOF, J. C., LOOSLI, C. G., AND JOHNSTON, P. B., Adenoviruses. III. Their etiological role in acute respiratory disease in civilian adults, *J. Infect. Dis.* **103**:93–101 (1958).

35. GRAYSTON, J. T., LOOSLI, C. G., SMITH, M., McCARTHY, M. A., AND JOHNSTON, P. B., Adenoviruses. I. The effect of total incubation time in HeLa cell cultures on the isolation rate, *J. Infect. Dis.* **103**:75–101 (1958).

36. GRAYSTON, J. T., YANG, Y. F., JOHNSTON, P. B., AND KO, L. S., Epidemic keratoconjunctivitis on Taiwan: Etiological and clinical studies, *Am. J. Trop. Med.* **13**:492–498 (1964).

37. GUTEKUNST, R. R., AND HEGGIE, A. D., Viremia and viruria in adenovirus infections: Detection in patients with rubella or rubelliform illness, *N. Engl. J. Med.* **264**:374–378 (1961).

37a. GUYER, B., O'DAY, D. M., HIERHOLZER, J. C., AND SCHAFFNER, W., Epidemic keratoconjunctivitis: A community outbreak of mixed adenovirus type 8 and type 19 infection, *J. Infect. Dis.* **132**:142–150 (1975).

38. HALL, C. E., BRANDT, C. D., FROTHINGHAM, T. E., SPIGLAND, I., COONEY, M. K., AND FOX, J. P., The Virus Watch Program: A continuing surveillance of viral

infections in metropolitan New York families. IX. A comparison of infections with several respiratory pathogens in New York and New Orleans families, *Am. J. Epidemiol.* **94:**367–385 (1971).

39. HARRIS, D. J., WULFF, H., RAY, C. G., POLAND, J. D., CHIN, T. D. Y., AND WENNER, H. A., Viruses and disease. III. An outbreak of adenovirus type 7A in a children's home, *Am. J. Epidemiol.* **93:**399–402 (1971).

39a. HIERHOLZER, J. C., AND BARME, M., Counterimmunoelectrophoresis with adenovirus type-specific antihemagglutinin sera as a rapid diagnostic method, *J. Immunol.* **112:**987–995 (1974).

40. HILLEMAN, M. R., HAMPARIAN, V. V., KETLER, A., REILLY, C. M., MCCLELLAND, L., CORNFIELD, D., AND STOKES, J., JR., Acute respiratory illness among children and adults: Field study of contemporary importance of several viruses and appraisal of the literature, *J. Am. Med. Assoc.* **180:**445–453 (1962).

41. HILLEMAN, M. R., AND WERNER, J. H., Recovery of new agents from patients with acute respiratory illness, *Proc. Soc. Exp. Biol. Med.* **85:**183–188 (1954).

42. HOGAN, M. J., AND CRAWFORD, J. W., Epidemic keratoconjunctivitis (superficial punctate keratitis, keratitis subepithelialis, keratitis maculosa, keratitis nummularis), *Am. J. Ophthalmol.* **25:**1059–1078 (1942).

43. JACKSON, G. G., AND MULDOON, R. L., Viruses causing common respiratory infection in man. IV. Reoviruses and adenoviruses, *J. Infect. Dis.* **128:**834–866 (1973).

44. JAWETZ, E., The story of shipyard eye, *Br. Med. J.* **1:**873–878 (1959).

44a. JEN, K. F., TAI, Y., LIN, Y. C., AND WANG, H. Y., The role of adenovirus in the etiology of infantile pneumonia and pneumonia complicating measles, *Chin. Med. J.* **81:**141–148 (1962).

45. JORDON, W. S., JR., The frequency of infection with adenoviruses in a family study population, *Ann. N. Y. Acad. Sci.* **67:**273–278 (1957).

46. KAJI, M., KIMURA, M., KAMIYA, S., TATEWAKI, E., TAKAHASHI, T., NAKAJIMA, O., KOGA, T., ISHIDA, S., AND MAJIMA, Y., An epidemic of pharyngoconjunctival fever among school children in an elementary school in Fukuoka Prefecture, *Kyushu J. Med. Sci.* **12:**1–8 (1961).

47. KASEL, J. A., ALFORD, R. H., LEHRICH, J. R., BANKS, P. A., HUBER, M., AND KNIGHT, V., Adenovirus soluble antigens for human immunization, *Am. Rev. Respir. Dis.* **94:**170–174 (1966).

47a. KELSEY, D. S., Adenovirus meningoencephalitis, *Pediatrics* **61:**291–293 (1978).

48. KJELLEN, L., ZETTERBERG, B., AND SVEDMYR, A., An epidemic among Swedish children caused by adenovirus type 3, *Acta Paediatr. Scand.* **46:**561–568 (1957).

49. KLENK, E. L., GWALTNEY, J. M., AND BASS, J. W., Bacteriologically proved pertussis and adenovirus infection, *Am. J. Dis. Child.* **124:**203–207 (1972).

50. KLOENE, W., BANG, F. B., CHAKRABORTY, S. M., COOPER, M. R., KULEMANN, H., OTA, M., AND SHAH, K. V., A two-year respiratory virus survey in four villages in West Bengal, India, *Am. J. Epidemiol.* **92:**307–320 (1970).

51. LANG, W. R., HOWDEN, C. W., LAWS, J., AND BURTON, J. F., Bronchopneumonia with serious sequelae in children with evidence of adenovirus type 21 infection, *Br. Med. J.* **1:**73–79 (1969).

52. LANGMUIR, A. D., JARRETT, E. T., AND HOLLAENDER, A., Studies of the control of acute respiratory disease among Navy recruits, *Am. J. Hyg.* **48:**240–251 (1948).

53. LEHANE, D. E., NEWBERG, N. R., AND BEAM, W. E., Environmental modifications for controlling acute respiratory disease, *Am. J. Epidemiol.* **99:**139–144 (1974).

54. LOOSLI, C. G., LEMON, H. M., ROBERTSON, O. H., AND HAMBURGER, M., Transmission and control of respiratory disease in Army barracks, *J. Infect. Dis.* **90:**153–164 (1952).

55. MANTYJARVI, R., Adenovirus infections in servicemen in Finland, *Ann. Med. Exp. Fenn.* **44:**1–43 (1966).

56. MCCORMICK, D. P., WENZEL, R. P., DAVIES, J. A., AND BEAM, W. E., Nasal secretion protein responses in patients with wild-type adenovirus disease, *Infect. Immun.* **6:**282–288 (1972).

57. MILLER, L. F., RYTEL, M., PIERCE, W. E., AND ROSENBAUM, M. J., Epidemiology of nonbacterial pneumonia among Naval recruits, *J. Am. Med. Assoc.* **185:**92–99 (1963).

58. MONTO, A. S., NAPIER, J. A., AND METZNER, H. L., The Tecumseh study of respiratory illnesses. I. Plan of study and observations on syndromes of acute respiratory disease, *Am. J. Epidemiol.* **94:**269–279 (1971).

59. MUELLER, R. E., MULDOON, R. L., AND JACKSON, G. C., Communicability of enteric live adenovirus type 4 vaccine in families, *J. Infect. Dis.* **119:**60–66 (1969).

60. MUFSON, M. A., BELSHE, R. B., HORRIGAN, T. J., AND ZOLLAR, L. M., Cause of acute hemorrhagic cystitis in children, *Am. J. Dis. Child.* **126:**605–609 (1973).

61. NAHMIAS, A. J., GRIFFITH, D., AND SNITZER, J., Fatal pneumonia associated with adenovirus type 7, *Am. J. Dis. Child.* **114:**36–41 (1967).

62. NELSON, K. E., GAVITT, F., BATT, M. D., KALLICK, C. A., REDDI, K. T., AND LEVIN, S., The role of adenoviruses in the pertussis syndrome, *J. Pediatr.* **86:**335–341 (1975).

63. NUMAZAKI, Y., KUMASAKA, T., YANO, N., YAMANAKA, M., MIYAZAWA, T., TAKAI, S., AND ISHIDA, N., Further study of acute hemorrhagic cystitis due to adenovirus type 11, *N. Engl. J. Med.* **289:**344–347 (1973).

64. PADERSTEIN, R., Was ist Schwimmbad-Konjunktivitis?, *Klin. Monatsbl. Augenheilkd.* **72:**634–642 (1925).

65. PARROTT, R. H., ROWE, W. P., HUEBNER, R. J., BERNTON, H. W., AND MCCULLOUGH, N. B., Outbreak of

febrile pharyngitis and conjunctivitis associated with type 3 adenoidal–pharyngeal–conjunctival virus infection, *N. Engl. J. Med.* **251**:1087–1090 (1954).

66. PIERCE, W. E., ROSENBAUM, M. J., EDWARDS, E. A., PECKINPAUGH, R. O., AND JACKSON, G. G., Live and inactivated adenovirus vaccines for the prevention of acute respiratory illness in Naval recruits, *Am. J. Epidemiol.* **87**:237–246 (1968).

67. PIERCE, W. E., STILLE, W. T., AND MILLER, L. F., A preliminary report on effects of routine military inoculations on respiratory illness, *Proc. Soc. Exp. Biol. Med.* **114**:369–372 (1963).

67a. PHILIPSON, L., PETERSON, U., LINDBERG, U., Molecular biology of adenoviruses, *Virol. Monogr.* **14**:1–115 (1975).

68. ROSE, H. M., LAMSON, T. H., AND BUESCHER, E. L., Adenoviral infection in military recruits: Emergence of type 7 and type 21 infections in recruits immunized with type 4 oral vaccine, *Arch. Environ. Health* **21**:356–361 (1970).

69. ROSS, J. G., POTTER, C. W., AND ZACHARY, R. B., Adenovirus infection in association with intussusception in infancy, *Lancet* **2**:221–223 (1962).

70. ROWE, W. P., HUEBNER, R. J., GILMORE, L. K., PARROTT, R. H., AND WARD, T. G., Isolation of a cytopathogenic agent from human adenoids undergoing spontaneous degeneration in tissue culture, *Proc. Soc. Exp. Biol. Med.* **84**:570–573 (1953).

71. SCHMIDT, O. W., COONEY, M. K., AND FOY, H. M., Adenovirus-associated virus in adenovirus type 3 conjunctivitis, *Infect. Immun.* **11**:1362–1370 (1975).

71a. SCHONLAND, M., STRONG, M. L., AND WESLEY, A., Fatal adenovirus pneumonia: Clinical and pathological features, *S. Afr. Med. J.* **50**:1748–1751 (1976).

72. SCHWARTZ, A. R., TOGO, Y., AND HORNICK, R. B., Clinical evaluation of live, oral types 1, 2, and 5 adenovirus vaccines, *Am. Rev. Respir. Dis.* **109**:233–238 (1974).

73. SIMILA, S., JOUPPLIA, R., SALMI, A., AND POHJONEN, R., Encephalomeningitis in children associated with an adenovirus type 7 epidemic, *Acta. Paediatr. Scand.* **59**:310–316 (1970).

74. SIMILA, S., YLIKORKALA, O., AND WASZ-HOCKERT, O., Type 7 adenovirus pneumonia, *J. Pediatr.* **79**:605–611 (1971).

75. SMITH, T. J., BUESCHER, E. L., TOP, F. H., JR., ALTEMEIER, W. A., AND McCOWN, J. M., Experimental respiratory infection with type 4 adenovirus vaccine in volunteers: Clinical and immunological responses, *J. Infect. Dis.* **122**:239–248 (1970).

76. SPRAGUE, J. B., HIERHOLZER, J. C., CURRIER, R. W., II, HATTWICH, M. A. W., AND SMITH, M. D., Epidemic keratoconjunctivitis: A severe industrial outbreak due to adenovirus type 8, *N. Engl. J. Med.* **289**:1341–1346 (1973).

76a. STALDER, H., HIERHOLZER, J. C., AND OXMAN, M. N., New human adenovirus (candidate adenovirus type 35) causing fatal disseminated infection in a renal transplant recipient, *J. Clin. Microbiol.* **6**:257–265 (1977).

77. STANLEY, E. D., AND JACKSON, G. G., Spread of enteric live adenovirus type 4 vaccine in married couples, *J. Infect. Dis.* **119**:51–59 (1969).

78. STERNER, G., Adenovirus infection in childhood: An epidemiological and clinical survey among Swedish children, *Acta Paediatr. Scand. Suppl.* **142**:1–30 (1962).

78a. SUTTON, R. N. P., PULLEN, H. J. M., BLACKLEDGE, P., BROWN, E. H., SINCLAIR, L., AND SWIFT, P. N., Adenovirus type 7: 1971–74, *Lancet* **2**:987–991 (1976).

79. SVARTZ-MALMBERG, G., AND GERMANIS, M., Adenovirus type 8-associated keratonconjunctivitis: Hospital infections and secondary spread in Stockholm, 1967, *Scand. J. Infect. Dis.* **1**:161–168 (1969).

80. TAI, F. H., AND GRAYSTON, J. T., Adenovirus neutralizing antibodies in persons on Taiwan, *Proc. Soc. Exp. Biol. Med.* **109**:881–884 (1962).

81. TAI, F. H., GRAYSTON, J. T., JOHNSON, P. B., AND WOOLDRIDGE, R. L., Adenovirus infections in Chinese Army recruits on Taiwan, *J. Infect. Dis.* **107**:160–164 (1960).

82. TOP, F. H., JR., Control of adenovirus acute respiratory disease in U.S. Army trainees, *Yale J. Biol. Med.* **48**:185–195 (1975).

83. TOP, F. H., JR., GROSSMAN, R. A., BARTELLONI, P. J., SEGAL, H. E., DUDDING, B. A., RUSSELL, P. K., AND BUESCHER, E. L., Immunization with live types 7 and 4 adenovirus vaccines. I. Safety, infectivity, and potency of adenovirus type 7 vaccine in humans, *J. Infect. Dis.* **124**:148–154 (1971).

84. VANDERVEEN, J., The role of adenoviruses in respiratory disease, *Am. Rev. Respir. Dis.* **88**:167–180 (1963).

85. VARSANO, I., SCHONFELD, T. M., MATOTH, Y., SHOHAT, B., ENGLANDER, T., ROTTER, V., AND TRAININ, N., Severe disseminated adenovirus infection successfully treated with a thymic humoral factor, THF, *Acta Paediatr. Scand.* **66**:329–331 (1977).

86. VASTINE, D. W., WEST, C. E., YAMASHIROYA, H., SMITH, R., SAXTAN, D. D., GIESER, D. I., AND MUFSON, M. A., Simultaneous nosocomial and community outbreak of epidemic keratoconjunctivitis with types 8 and 19 adenovirus, *Trans. Am. Acad. Ophthalmol. Otolaryngol.* **81**:OP826–OP840 (1976).

87. VIHMA, L., Surveillance of acute viral respiratory disease in children, *Acta Paediatr. Scand. Suppl.* **192**:8–52 (1969).

88. WANG, S. S., AND FELDMAN, H. A., Pharyngeal isolations of adenovirus 31 from a family population, *Am. J. Epidemiol.* **104**:272–277 (1976).

89. WARNER, J. O., AND MARSHALL, W. C., Crippling lung

disease after measles and adenovirus infection, *Br. J. Dis. Chest* **70**:89–94 (1976).

90. WENNER, H. A., BERAN, G. W., WESTON, J., AND CHIN, T. D. Y., WITH COLLABORATION OF ANDERSON, N. W., AND GOLDSMITH, R., The epidemiology of acute respiratory illness I. Observations on adenovirus infections prevailing in a group of families, *J. Infect. Dis.* **101**:275–286 (1957).

91. WIGAND, R., AND SCHULZ, R., Laboratoriumspraxis be Adenoviren. II. Empfindlichkeit verschiedener Zellkulturen bie Endpunkttitration, *Zentralbl. Bakteriol. Parasitenkd. Infektionskr. Abt. 1: Orig. Reihe A* **231**:31–41 (1975).

92. ZWEIGHAFT, R. M. HIERHOLZER, J. C., AND BRYAN, J A., Epidemic keratoconjunctivitis at a Vietnamese refugee camp in Florida, *Am. J. Epidemiol.* **106**:399–407 (1977).

12. Suggested Reading

EVANS, A. S., Acute respiratory infections, in: *Communicable and Infectious Diseases* (F. H., TOP, SR., AND P. F. WEHRLE, eds.), pp. 510–532, C. V. Mosby, St. Louis, 1972.

GINSBERG, H. S., AND DINGLE, J. H., The adenovirus group, in: *Viral and Rickettsial Infections of Man* (F. L. HORSFALL AND I. TAMM, eds.), pp. 860–891, J. B. Lippincott, Philadelphia, 1965.

JACKSON, G. G., AND MULDOON, R. L., Viruses causing common respiratory infection in man. IV. Reoviruses and adenoviruses, *J. Infect. Dis.* **128**:811–866 (1973).

KNIGHT, V., AND KASEL, J. A., Adenoviruses, in: *Viral and Mycoplasmal Infections of the Respiratory Tract* (V. KNIGHT, ed.), pp. 65–86, Lea and Febiger, Philadelphia. 1973.

PHILIPSON, L., PETERSON, U., AND LINDBERG, U., Molecular biology of adenoviruses, *Virol. Monogr.* Springer-Verlag, New York, **14**:1–115 (1975).

CHAPTER 4

African Hemorrhagic Fevers Due to Marburg and Ebola Viruses

Karl M. Johnson

1. Introduction

Marburg and Ebola viruses are morphologically similar, immunologically distinct rod-shaped agents of African origin. They produce acute hemorrhagic fever in man. Although other viruses cause a rather similar disease in Africa and differential diagnosis of a sporadic case cannot be made on clinical grounds, the syndrome associated with infection by

Karl M. Johnson · Center for Disease Control, Special Pathogens Branch, Virology Division, Bureau of Laboratories, U.S. Public Health Service, U.S. Department of Health, and Human Services, Atlanta, Georgia. Use of trade names is for identification only and does not constitute endorsement by the Public Health Service or by the U.S. Department of Health and Human Services.

these two agents is sufficiently unique and unvarying to distinguish it from yellow fever, Lassa fever, and other infections whenever a cluster of cases occurs. For this reason, the term African hemorrhagic fever (AFHF), rather than Marburg or Ebola disease, is used here to refer to clinical infection caused by either virus. Recent emergence, high mortality, nosocomial secondary transmission, and ecological mystery have combined to draw worldwide attention to these infections.

2. Historical Background

These viruses have the briefest of histories. Information to be presented is derived largely from four rather dramatic epidemics. Marburg virus was first isolated during an epidemic in laboratory workers processing kidney cells from African monkeys in 1967. Cases occurred in Marburg and Frankfort an Main, Germany, and Belgrade, Yugoslavia.[38,59,60] A second focal outbreak took place in South Africa in 1975.[22] Ebola virus was discovered nearly concurrently in Zaire and Sudan,[5,31,44] in association with epidemics comprising more than 500 cases during 1976.[14,15] Because of the severe disease produced by these viruses and the high potential hazard incurred during laboratory manipulation of them, progress in understanding both viral biology and epidemiology has been limited. Few laboratories in the world possess the safety facilities necessary for making specific diagnosis of infection, much less the resources required for intensive research.

3. Methodology Used in Epidemiological Analysis

3.1. Sources of Morbidity and Mortality Data

No country where these viruses are known or presumed to be endemic has established a formal requirement for reporting cases of viral hemorrhagic disease other than yellow fever. Nevertheless, all known cases of such disease caused by Marburg and Ebola viruses have been reported to the World Health Organization (WHO), and this body has urged that this clinical syndrome be added to the list of internationally notifiable communicable diseases.[64] It is likely that sporadic human illness due to these and other viruses that produce hemorrhagic fever in Africa has been, and continues to be, unrecognizable due to the lack of specific diagnostic capability on that continent. Furthermore, despite the high mortality observed during recent outbreaks, which suggests that such events are likely to be recognized, it seems quite possible that future serological surveys will disclose that human infection with these agents is more common and geographically widespread than is now believed.

3.2. Laboratory Diagnosis

3.2.1. Recovery of Virus. Marburg and Ebola viruses can be isolated from acutely ill patients.[9,15,50,68] In a very few cases examined, viremia was present until death or for an interval of at least 1 week during acute illness. Virions have been seen by direct examination of blood with the electron microscope.[7,45]

Although not yet applied in an epidemiological fashion, it also appears likely that diagnosis can reliably be made in fatal cases by electron-microscopic visualization of virions in liver sections fixed in formalin.

3.2.2. Measurement of Virus-Specific Antibodies. Persons who survive acute infection develop low-titered complement-fixing (CF) antibodies as well as antibodies detectable by indirect immunofluorescence (IIF).[7,32,50,57] Antibodies appear sooner, reach higher levels, and persist for much longer when measured by the latter method. The IIF procedure also can be used to detect specific antibodies of the immunoglobulin M (IgM) class.[68] These rarely persist longer than 3 months and thus can serve to make valid retrospective diagnosis where specimens are not available during the acute stage of infection.

Despite much effort, no successful test for neutralizing antibodies has been developed for either Marburg or Ebola virus.[65,66] Pending further work on the serology of these agents, the IIF method has been employed as the sole source of data bearing on this fundamentally important problem.

3.2.3. Interpretation. When appropriate specimens are obtained, Marburg and Ebola virus infections are recovered from blood of nearly all patients tested. Similarly, these agents were visualized in 5 of 6 postmortem cases so far examined.[19,31] Every virus-confirmed survivor of either infection has developed specific antibodies. Thus, the tools for recognition of infection, at least in its severe clinical form, are highly sensitive and reliable.

3.3. Surveys

Although IIF antibodies in titers of at least 1:32 uniformly appear in sera of patients who survive AFHF, the interpretation of data derived from population surveys using this method is somewhat less certain. This situation derives from the fact that a few Ebola-positive sera with titers of 1:4–1:64 were found in an indigenous Indian population in Panama, a country and even a continent not thought to harbor this virus.[62]

3.4. Clinical Diagnosis of Acute Infection

The clinical features of AFHF are detailed in Section 8. The occurrence of acute fever, hemorrhagic signs, and high mortality was used to estimate incidence of disease caused by Ebola virus in both Zaire and Sudan.[14,15] Residents of the affected regions repeatedly reported that this disease pattern in epidemic form was a singular event never before seen in their villages.

Clinical diagnosis of AFHF in epidemic situations is probably quite reliable, except possibly in infants less than 1 year of age, for whom no confirmatory laboratory data are available. This judgment is based on the high rate of laboratory confirmation of suspected cases and the absence or paucity of specific antibodies among persons suffering no or mild illness after direct contact with cases or even residence in the same area.

4. Characteristics of Marburg and Ebola Viruses

4.1. Morphology and Morphogenesis

Marburg and Ebola viruses are indistinguishable large rods, about 80–90 nm in diameter but varying in length from 600 nm to several micrometers.[1,19,31,46] Brushlike spikes protrude from an outer virionic membrane. Branching forms are commonly seen, as are twisted rods and bulbous protrusions at ends of particles. These viruses contain RNA,[35,47,54] have essential lipids on their surface membranes,[4,37] and contain an internal helical core that is presumed to be the nucleocapsid. Morphogenesis occurs in the cytoplasm of infected cells, inclusions composed of a matrix containing nucleocapsids are formed, and virus maturation and release occurs by budding through the host-cell plasma membrane.[42]

4.2. Physical Properties

Marburg and Ebola viruses are moderately thermolabile, but complete inactivation requires heating to 60°C for 1 hr. They are stable indefinitely at −70°C and persist well at 4°C for several days.[4] Infectivity is preserved by lyophilization but destroyed after variable intervals of exposure to ultraviolet or gamma irradiation.[18,37] Virions have a bouyant density of about 1.14 g in potassium tartrate gradients.[34]

4.3. Chemical Properties

These viruses are inactivated by brief exposure to a variety of chemicals including phenol, peracetic acid, sodium hypochlorite, methyl alcohol, ether, and sodium deoxycholate.[4] Ebola virus contains a single, biologically negative strand of RNA with a molecular weight of 4.6×10^6.[47] Four proteins have been isolated from Ebola virions. The largest of these contains sugar and is thought to represent the surface spikes of the virus.[34] The proteins of Marburg virus are similar to, but of slightly different weight and separate from, those of Ebola virus by sedimentation.

4.4. Biological Properties

Marburg and Ebola viruses infect a wide range of cultured cells from mammals, but do not replicate in cells of birds, amphibians, reptiles, or arthropods so far tested.[30,63] Although a ragged cytopathic effect has been observed in some continuous cell lines, this property is not useful for assay of infectivity because IIF reveals infection well beyond the dilutions at which morphological cell changes are observed.[54,55,65] These viruses also infect most commonly used laboratory animals. Monkeys are highly sensitive and usually succumb to infection after an illness resembling that seen in man.[8,25,52] Serial passages are usually required to induce death in hamsters and guinea pigs, which otherwise serve as convenient hosts for preparation of immune reagents.[5,49,65,69] Marburg virus is not pathogenic for mice,[36] but a Zaire strain of Ebola virus induced lethal infection in suckling mice.[44]

4.5. Serological Relationships

Marburg virus and specific antisera to this agent were tested against reagents for all previously known viruses causing hemorrhagic fever and a large number of arthropod-transmitted viruses by CF, hemagglutination-inhibition, or neutralization methods. No immunological relationships were demonstrated.[11] Somewhat surprisingly, in view of their morphological similarity, Ebola and Marburg viruses were found not to share antigens when examined by IIF and CF techniques.[31,65]

5. Descriptive Epidemiology

5.1. Prevalence and Incidence

Current information is inadequate to indicate the prevalence and incidence of Marburg and Ebola virus infections in the general population in endemic areas. Their occurrence has thus far been recognized only through outbreaks of clinically typical cases that have occurred in localized geographic areas.

5.2. Epidemic Behavior and Contagiousness

5.2.1. Marburg Virus. In August and September 1967, 30 cases of acute hemorrhagic fever occurred in Marburg and Frankfurt an Main, Germany, and Belgrade, Yugoslavia. There were 7 deaths, and 5 of the illnesses resulted from secondary infection of persons in contact with patients. Each outbreak occurred among personnel of laboratories engaged in processing tissues from vervet monkeys (*Cercopithecus aethiops*) for production of poliovirus vaccine, and all the monkeys had come from a single source in Uganda during the month prior to the outbreak.[26] Use of gloves and gowns for handling animals and tissues, suspension of further processing of tissues from the animals, and destruction of remaining monkeys brought the outbreak to an abrupt halt. From careful histories of exposure, an incubation of 3–7 days was determined for primary infection and 5–8 days for secondary cases.[27]

During January 1975, a chain of three Marburg infections occurred in Johannesburg, South Africa.[22] The index case was a young man who had made a hitchhiking trip from Johannesburg to Victoria Falls in Rhodesia and return. Exposure to the virus was deemed to have occurred in Rhodesia. A female traveling companion fell ill within 2 days of death of the first patient but survived, and a nurse who attended this patient later acquired the disease. Incubation periods were similar to those seen in Europe, as were the clinical features of these infections. These are the only cases of Marburg infection in man so far recorded.

5.2.2. Ebola Virus. Severe outbreaks of acute hemorrhagic fever due to Ebola virus took place in southwestern Sudan from July through November 1976, and in northwestern Zaire from September to November of that year.[14,15] Both regions are within 5° of the equator, and each outbreak was centered on a rural town with a large hospital: Maridi, Sudan, and Yambuku, Zaire. There were 284 clinically recognized cases in Sudan and 318 in Zaire. Mortality rates were calculated as 53 and 88%, respectively. Attack rates were not estimated in Sudan, but most illnesses occurred among adults and many were "hospital"-associated. A similar pattern was noted in Zaire, where 13 of 17 members of a hospital staff became ill and 11 died. Cases occurred in 55 of some 250 villages in the epidemic area of Zaire, and 56% of these were in females. Few cases occurred in children less than 10 years of age, and attack rates in adults ranged from 10 to 14 per 1000. The incubation period of disease was about 1 week in both Zaire and Sudan.

Another Ebola virus outbreak occurred during August–September 1979 in the area of Nzara, near Maridi, Sudan. Of 33 confirmed cases, 22 were fatal.[16] As in 1976, transmission of virus occurred after close contact with a sporadic index case at a local hospital, and further dissemination of the virus was observed among family members caring for patients in homes.

5.3. Other Epidemiological Features

Since available information is limited to outbreaks of Marburg and Ebola viruses, it is not possible to delineate the age, sex, geographic distribution, and other features of these infections at the present time except as given above.

6. Mechanism and Route of Transmission

6.1. Spread of Virus

6.1.1. Marburg Virus. The original Marburg outbreaks in Europe were the direct result of human contact with infected green monkeys (*C. aethiops*) that originated from a single dealer in Uganda. All these animals had been captured in the district near Lake Kyoga. Twenty-five primary infections occurred among personnel of three laboratories where polio vaccines were in production. It was noteworthy that 20 of 29 persons having contact with the blood or organs of live monkeys became infected, while only 4 of 13 persons exposed exclusively to cultured kidney cells from these monkeys became ill.[28] Animal caretakers suffered no infections, and this fact, together with the observation that many monkeys apparently survived until sacrifice as part of a thorough "clean-up" of premises, strongly suggests that infectious aerosols were not important in virus transmission. A total of seven secondary human infections occurred in Europe and South Africa. Only one of these seems a possible aerosol transmission; the others resulted from continued close contact with patients and their body fluids. One notable event was sexual transmission from husband to wife some 3 months after clinical convalescence.[39] No instance of subclinical infection by Marburg virus has been recorded.

6.1.2. Ebola Virus. Transmission of Ebola virus in Sudan and Zaire was either by close contact in the course of patient care or by virus-contaminated syringe and needle. Each outbreak originated in one or a very few apparently sporadic cases, and amplification was the result of substandard hospital practice. In Zaire, none of 85 patients infected by parenteral inoculation survived.[15] Secondary attack rates calculated for several generations of cases ranged from 3 to 14%. Five generations of transmission were observed in Zaire and 13 in Sudan. When close family relatives were considered, however, these rates often exceeded 20%, and hospital personnel attending patients suffered infection and illness at even higher rates.[10,14] The excess morbidity among adult females in Zaire was largely related to infections acquired parenterally at a prenatal clinic of the hospital where the outbreak was centered. The institution of patient isolation and basic personnel precautions resulted in rapid termination of epidemics in both countries. Thus, available data point to the conclusion that aerosols were not an important vehicle of virus transmission.

6.2. Reservoir

The true origin and the natural cycle of maintenance for Marburg and Ebola viruses remain unsolved. For Marburg virus, the experimental work with green monkeys disclosed that all animals that received even tiny amounts of virus experienced fatal infection within 12 days. Furthermore, neither virus nor specific antibodies were detected subsequent to the original outbreak among monkeys captured in the area of Uganda where the implicated group originated.[56] Despite exhaustive investigation, specimen collection, and testing, no trace of Marburg virus was uncovered in southern Africa.

For Ebola virus, the story remains equally elusive. Monkeys are highly sensitive to lethal infection, and more than 200 sera from several primate species in Zaire were negative for specific antibodies.[33] In the case of Marburg infection, it is not at all clear over what area in Africa the virus may be present. But sporadic cases of Ebola virus infection were documented in the Zaire River basin in 1977, and retrospectively (autopsy accident with illness, survival, and persistent antibody) in 1972.[29] Furthermore, Ebola antibodies have been found in 5–8% of persons in several localities· in Zaire and Cameroon. These data imply that the virus resides in the tropical rain forest of Central Africa and that mild or no disease may be a common event where secondary human transmission does not occur.

7. Pathogenesis and Immunity

7.1. In Guinea Pigs and Hamsters

Inoculation of unpassaged Marburg virus produces febrile infection in guinea pigs but no overt signs of disease in this species or the Syrian hamster. Specific antiviral antibodies appear within 2–3 weeks. After serial passage of the agent in guinea pigs and monkeys, however, a uniformly fatal disease is induced in adult guinea pigs and suckling hamsters. The pathogenesis of infection is generally similar in both species.[25,51,53,69] Animals become viremic within 2–4 days and die 5–8 days after inoculation. There is widespread necrosis without inflammatory reaction in the lymphoid elements of nodes and spleen and in the liver. Interstitial pneumonia is common, and there is evidence of diffuse intravascular clotting as well as hyperplasia of fixed macrophages often containing partially destroyed erythrocytes. In addition, hamsters display vascular changes in the central nervous system typical of viral encephalitis.

7.2. In Nonhuman Primates

Rhesus, vervet, and squirrel monkeys are highly susceptible to parenteral and/or intranasal infection by Marburg and Ebola viruses. The outcome of infection is always fatal, even with unpassaged virus, and the disease is very similar to that noted in man. Infected monkeys develop high fever within 2–5 days and generally die after 6–9 days.[8,25,52] Animals become anorectic and lethargic 1–2 days before death, and some develop a maculopapular skin rash during this time. Death is preceded by a drop in temperature to subnormal levels, strongly suggesting terminal shock. Mild leukopenia and thrombocytopenia are frequently observed, and gross impairment of blood coagulation is sometimes noted prior to death. Virus is present in blood of all monkeys from 1 to 4 days after infection until death. Titers in excess of 10^6 infectious units/ml were found in Ebola virus infection.[8] Large amounts of virus are present in most organs examined, but data on brain content have not been obtained. From 10^3 to 10^6 infectious doses of Marburg virus can be recovered from saliva and urine of infected monkeys.[52] Antibodies to the viruses are not present prior to death.

Pathological changes associated with infection consist of (1) necrosis of lymphoid elements with reticuloendothelial hypertrophy in nodes and spleen; (2) focal, often severe necrosis of hepatocytes with little inflammatory response but with development of large eosinophilic inclusions reminiscent of Councilman bodies of yellow fever; (3) variable degrees of interstitial pneumonia; and (4) widespread microintravascular coagulation with extravasation of erythrocytes.[2,43] Immunofluorescent and ultrastructural examination of Marburg-infected animals reveals large amounts of viral antigen in liver, spleen, and lungs, with accumulation of virions principally in liver, only moderately in spleen, and not at all in the lung, where no evidence for virus replication is found.[40]

7.3. In Man

The clinical features of AFHF are described in Section 8. Pathologically, the disease caused in humans by both Marburg and Ebola viruses is remarkably similar to that documented for monkeys. High persistent viremia is typical, and large amounts of virus are present in many Marburg-infected viscera at autopsy.[67] Histological features are also similar.[3,13,23,41] In addition, renal tubular necrosis was observed in several patients, but this may have been nonspecifically related to terminal shock. Marburg patients also display a diffuse glial-nodule type of encephalitis together with a mononuclear vasculitis reminiscent of a pattern produced by certain arthropodborne viruses.[23] Small amounts of Marburg virus were present in the brain of a single case that was tested.[67] Pathological evidence for disseminated intravascular coagulation was regarded as definitive.[17,22]

8. Patterns of Host Response

8.1. Clinical Features

Marburg and Ebola infections are marked by the appearance of headache, progressive fever, sore throat, myalgia, and diarrhea.[15,38,58] Conjunctivitis is sometimes present, as is a papular exanthem of the palate. By the 4th or 5th day of evolution, there is chemical evidence of hepatitis, and most patients develop a centripetal maculopapular rash that rarely lasts more than 3 days. Some patients experience symptoms suggesting acute pancreatitis, and this has been documented by chemical tests in Marburg infection.[22] Most patients who survive fail to develop a hemorrhagic diathesis, although severe weight loss, asthenia, and psychological depression are common features of a convalescence requiring several weeks. In fatal cases, melena, hematemesis, and bleeding from other sites generally begin on the 5th or 6th day of disease, and such patients rarely survive beyond 9 days of evolution. There is ample evidence for disseminated intravascular coagulation. Terminal shock is an unvarying finding. Patients infected with Ebola virus in Sudan in 1976 had a high incidence of dry nonproductive cough, not seen in any other outbreak.[14]

8.2. Diagnosis

In fatal cases, electron microscopy can be expected to reveal virus particles in liver. Surviving patients generally develop specific IgM and IgG antibodies about 7–10 days after onset of symptoms.[68] CF antibodies generally appear about 1 week later. To date, no satisfactory method for measuring virus-neutralizing antibodies has been developed.

9. Prevention and Control

9.1. General Concepts

In the absence of significant knowledge concerning the ecology of Marburg and Ebola infections, there is little that can be said at this time regarding control of infection. Monitoring of monkeys to be used in biomedical research or industry for infection with either agent now appears to be pointless. But basic hygienic practices in hospitals can be relied on to prevent further major epidemics. Since both viruses multiply to high titers in cell cultures, it may be possible to develop experimental vaccines for protection of key laboratory and clinical personnel. Without data on incidence of these diseases in Africa, vaccination of human populations does not seem to warrant a high priority at present.

9.2. Management and Disposition of Patients

Patients with AFHF should be placed in strict isolation. Where air-circulating systems are employed, they should be unidirectional, nonrecirculating, and away from corridors. All materials leaving the patient's room must be disinfected chemically or, preferably, by steam under pressure. Medical personnel must use gloves, gowns, and masks, and where possible, primary isolation systems for either the patient (bed isolator) or the medical team (positive-pressure hood or suit) should be utilized. Clinical pathological procedures should be carried out under strict isolation, and if maximum primary containment of potential aerosols is feasible, it should be employed.

Clinical management of patients is largely supportive. Fluid and electrolyte balance is an important consideration, and nasogastric suction with acid neutralizion is indicated in patients with evidence of acute pancreatitis. Careful anticoagulation of two Marburg virus infections with intravenous heparin prior to the potential onset of bleeding was associated with clinical recovery.[22] Whether or not there was a cause–effect relationship is not clear.

The only known survivor of a confirmed clinical Ebola virus infection acquired by parenteral injection, a laboratory worker accidentally infected by a needle puncture, was treated with both plasma containing Ebola antibodies and large doses of interferon beginning on the third day of illness. The virus titer in this patient's blood fell from $10^{4.5}$ infectious units/ml to barely detectable levels within 24 hr after administration of plasma.[20] Subsequent experimental studies in monkeys showed that interferon was unable to prevent death following infection.[6]

Thus, it may be that passive antibodies administered before the onset of bleeding are of specific value in treatment of AFHF. Interestingly, this patient developed the typical rash at the expected time and also had virus in seminal fluid for 2 months after clinical recovery.

9.3. General Strategy for Isolation and Management of Suspect "Exotic" Infections

In view of the medical drama so far associated with "exotic" diseases, the residual uncertainty regarding their potential for transmission by aerosol, and the problems of differentiation from other hazardous viral infections such as Lassa fever, it is not at all clear what the optimum course of action should be whenever a patient presents for medical care after recent travel in rural Africa. The probability of such an event is quite low. Diagnostic services are available at present in Atlanta, Georgia; Frederick, Maryland; Porton Down, England; Antwerp, Belgium; and Johannesburg, South Africa. Containment facilities for patient care and clinical pathology also exist at or near all these centers, primarily as protection for laboratory workers.[12,21,24,61] Their utilization otherwise depends on availability of safe air transport from point of patient intake. Alternately, patients might be isolated at the hospital where they are initially seen and portable, contained, clinical pathological instrumentation be flown to the hospital.[48] Resolution of these issues can be expected to vary in different countries depending on geography, political and economic structure, and continuing expenditures of time and money on feasibility study.[70] As always, energy devoted to such problems, and the configurations reached, will depend on experience and the outcome of individual, and unusual, events.

10. Unresolved Problems: Detection of Infection and Disease

We are still without the necessary basic tools. Since even a single case of AFHF represents a true medical, and a potential public-health, emergency, it is vital that rapid specific diagnosis be made. Monkey studies are urgently needed to determine the quantitative limits of detection of virus particles or antigens in blood. The IIF method for measuring antibodies in human populations is somewhat suspect, and not really applicable to the problem of elucidation of virus reservoirs. Methods for precise measurement of antibodies to virus-specific, presumably virion surface, antigens are required. Such work in turn necessitates expensive maximum-containment laboratories, which are in very short world supply.

11. References

1. ALMEIDA, J. D., WATERSON, A. P., AND SIMPSON, D. I. H., Morphology and morphogenesis of the Marburg agent, in: *Marburg Virus Disease* (G. A. MARTINI AND R. SIEGERT, eds.), pp. 84–97, Springer-Verlag, New York, 1971.
2. BASKERVILLE, A., BOWEN, E. T. W., PLATT, G. S., McARDELL, L. B., AND SIMPSON, D. I. H., The pathology of experimental Ebola virus infection in monkeys, *J. Pathol.* **125**:131–138 (1978).
3. BECHTELSHEIMER, H., JACOB, H., AND SOLCHER, H. The neuropathology of an infectious disease transmitted by African green monkeys (*Cercopithecus aethiops*), *Ger. Med. Monthly* **141**:10–12 (1969).
4. BOWEN, E. T. W., SIMPSON, D. I. H., BRIGHT, W. F., ZLOTNIK, I., AND HOWARD, D. M. R., Vervet monkey disease: Studies on some physical and chemical properties of the causative agent, *Br. J. Exp. Pathol.* **50**:400–407 (1969).
5. BOWEN, E. T. W., PLATT, G. S., LLOYD, G., BASKERVILLE, A., HARRIS, W. J., AND VELLA, E. E., Viral haemorrhagic fever in southern Sudan and northern Zaire, *Lancet* **1**:571–573 (1977).
6. BOWEN, E. T. W., BASKERVILLE, A., CANTELL, K., MANN, G. F., SIMPSON, D. I. H., AND ZUCKERMAN, A. J., The effect of interferon on experimental Ebola virus infec-

tion in rhesus monkeys, in: *Ebola Virus Haemorrhagic Fever* (S. R. PATTYN, ed.), pp. 245–252, Elsevier/North-Holland, Amsterdam, 1978.
7. BOWEN, E. T. W., LLOYD, G., PLATT, G., McARDELL, L. B., WEBB, P. A., AND SIMPSON, D. I. H., Virological studies on a case of Ebola virus infection in man and in monkeys, in: *Ebola Virus Haemorrhagic Fever* (S. R. PATTYN, ed.), pp. 95–100, Elsevier/North-Holland, Amsterdam, 1978.
8. BOWEN, E. T. W., PLATT, G. S., SIMPSON, D. I. H., McARDELL, L. B., AND RAYMOND, R. T., Ebola haemorrhagic fever: Experimental infection of monkeys, *Trans. R. Soc. Trop. Med. Hyg.* **72**:188–191 (1978).
9. BOWEN, E. T. W., PLATT, G. S., LLOYD, G., McARDLE, L., SIMPSON, D. I. H., SMITH, D. H., FRANCIS, D. P., HIGHTON, R. B., CORNET, M., DRAPER, C. C., ELTAHIR, B., MAYOM DENG, I., LOLIK, P., AND DUKU, O., Viral haemorrhagic fever in the Sudan, 1976: Human virological and serological studies, in: *Ebola Virus Haemorrhagic Fever* (S. R. PATTYN, ed.), pp. 143–151, Elsevier/North-Holland, Amsterdam, 1978.
10. BREMAN, J. G., PIOT, P., JOHNSON, K. M., WHITE, M. K., MBUYI, M., SUREAU, P., HEYMANN, D. L., VAN NIEUWENHOVE, S., McCORMICK, J. B., RUPPOL, J. P., KINTOKI, V., ISAACSON, M., VAN DER GROEN, G., WEBB, P. A., AND NGUETE, K., The epidemiology of Ebola haemorrhagic fever in Zaire, 1976, in: *Ebola Virus Haemorrhagic Fever* (S. R. PATTYN, ed.), pp. 103–124, Elsevier/North-Holland, Amsterdam, 1978.
11. CASALS, J., Absence of serological relationship between Marburg virus and some arboviruses, in: *Marburg Virus Disease* (G. A. MARTINI, AND R. SIEGERT, eds.), pp. 98–104, Springer-Verlag, New York, 1971.
12. CLAUSEN, L., BOTHWELL, T. H., ISAACSON, M., KOORNHOF, H. J., GEAR, J. H., McMURDO, J., PAYN, E. M., MILLER, G. B., AND SHER, R., Isolation and handling of patients with dangerous infectious disease, *S. Am. Med. J.* **53**:238–242 (1978).
13. DIETRICH, M., SCHUMACHER, H. H., PETERS, D., AND KNOBLOCH, J., Human pathology of Ebola (Maridi) virus infection in the Sudan, in: *Ebola Virus Haemorrhagic Fever* (S. R. PATTYN, ed.), pp. 37–42, Elsevier/North-Holland, Amsterdam, 1978.
14. Ebola haemorrhagic fever in Sudan, 1976, *Bull. WHO* **56**:247–270 (1978).
15. Ebola haemorrhagic fever in Zaire, 1976, *Bull. WHO* **56**:271–293 (1978).
16. Ebola hemorrhagic fever—southern Sudan, Center for Disease Control, *Morbidity Mortality Weekly Rep.* **28**:557–559 (1979).
17. EGBRING, R., SLENCZKA, W., AND BALTZER, G., Clinical manifestations and mechanism of the haemorrhagic diathesis in Marburg virus disease, in: *Marburg Virus Disease* (G. A. MARTINI AND R. SIEGERT, eds.), pp. 41–49, Springer-Verlag, New York, 1971.

18. Elliott, L., Dudley, M., and Johnson, K. M., Center for Disease Control, Unpublished observations (1979).
19. Ellis, D. S., Simpson, D. I. H., Francis, D. P., Knobloch, J., Bowen, E. T. W., Lolik, P., and Mayom Deng, I., Ultrastructure of Ebola virus particles in human liver, *J. Clin. Pathol.* **31:**201–208 (1978).
20. Emond, R. T. D., Evans, B., Bowen, E. T. W., and Lloyd, G., A case of Ebola virus infection, *Br. Med. J.* **2:**541–544 (1977).
21. Emond, R. T. D., Smith, H., and Welsby, P. D., Assessment of patients with suspected viral haemorrhagic fever, *Br. Med. J.* **1:**966–967 (1978).
22. Gear, J. S. S., Cassel, G. A., Gear, A. J., Trapper, B., Clausen, L., Meyers, A. M., Kew, M. C., Bothwell, T. H., Sher, R., Miller, G. B., and Schneider, J., Outbreak of Marburg virus disease in Johannesburg, *Br. Med. J.* **4:**489–493 (1975).
23. Gedigic, P., Bechtelsheimer, H., and Korb, G., The morbid anatomy of Marburg-virus-disease, *Ger. Med. Monthly* **14:**68–77 (1969).
24. Gomperts, E. D., Isaacson, M., Koornhof, H. J., Metz, J., Gear, J. H., Schoub, B. D., McIntosh, B., and Prozesky, O. W., Handling of highly infectious material in a clinical pathology laboratory and in a viral diagnostic unit, *S. Afr. Med. J.* **53:**243–248 (1978).
25. Haas, R., and Maass, G., Experimental infection of monkeys with the Marburg virus, in: *Marburg Virus Disease* (G. A. Martini and R. Siegert, eds.), pp. 136–143, Springer-Verlag, New York, 1971.
26. Hennessen, W., A hemorrhagic disease transmitted from monkeys to man, *Natl. Cancer Inst. Monogr.* **29:**161–171 (1968).
27. Hennessen, W., Bonin, O., and Mauler, R., Zur Epidemiologie der Erkrankung von Menschen durch Affen, *Dtsch. Med. Wochenschr.* **93:**582–587 (1968).
28. Hennessen, W., Epidemiology of "Marburg Virus" disease, in: *Marburg Virus Disease* (G. A. Martini and R. Siegert, eds.), pp. 161–165, Springer-Verlag, New York, 1971.
29. Heymann, D. L., Weisfeld, J. S., Webb, P. A., Johnson, K. M., Cairns, T., and Berquist, H., Ebola hemorrhagic fever: Tandala, Zaire, 1977–1978, *J. Infect. Dis.* **142:**372–376 (1980).
30. Hofmann, H., and Kunz, C. H., Cultivation of the Marburg virus (*Rhabdovirus simiae*) in cell cultures, in: *Marburg Virus Disease* (G. A. Martini and R. Siegert, eds.), pp. 112–116, Springer-Verlag, New York, 1971.
31. Johnson, K. M., Webb, P. A., Lange, J. V., and Murphy, F. A., Isolation and partial characterization of a new virus causing acute haemorrhagic fever in Zaire, *Lancet* **1:**569–571 (1977).
32. Johnson, K. M., Webb, P. A., and Heymann, D. L., Evaluation of the plasma-pheresis program in Zaire, in: *Ebola Virus Haemorrhagic Fever* (S. R. Pattyn, ed.), pp. 219–222, Elsevier/North-Holland, New York, 1978.
33. Johnson, K. M., Van Der Groen, G., Elliott, L., and Robbins, B., Center for Disease Control, Unpublished observations (1979).
34. Kiley, M. P., Regnery, R. L., and Johnson, K. M., Ebola virus; Identification of virion structural proteins, *J. Gen. Virol.* **49:**333–341 (1980).
35. Kissling, R. E., Robinson, R. Q., Murphy, F. A., and Whitfield, S. G., Agent of disease contracted from green monkeys, *Science* **160:**888–890 (1968).
36. Kunz, C., Hofmann, H., Kovac, W., and Stockinger, L., Biologische und morphologische Charackteristica des Virus des in Deutschland aufgetretenen "Hämorrhagischen Fiebers," *Wien. Klin. Wochenschr.* **80:**161–166 (1968).
37. Malherbe, H., and Strickland-Cholmley, M., Studies on the Marburg virus, in: *Marburg Virus Disease* (G. A. Martini and R. Siegert, eds.), pp. 188–194, Springer-Verlag, New York, 1971.
38. Martini, G. A., Knauff, H. G., Schmidt, H. A., Mayer, G., and Baltzer, G., A hitherto unknown infectious disease contracted from monkeys, *Ger. Med. Monthly* **13:**457–470 (1968).
39. Martini, G. A., and Schmidt, H., Spermatogene Übertragung des Marburg virus, *Klin. Wochenschr.* **46:**391–393 (1968).
40. Murphy, F. A., Simpson, D. I. H., Whitfield, S. G., Zlotnik, I., and Carter, G. B., Marburg virus infection in monkeys: Ultrastructural studies, *Lab. Invest.* **24:**279–291 (1971).
41. Murphy, F. A., Pathology of Ebola virus infection, in: *Ebola Virus Haemorrhagic Fever* (S. R. Pattyn, ed.), pp. 43–59, Elsevier/North-Holland, Amsterdam, 1978.
42. Murphy, F. A., Van Der Groen, G., Whitfield, S. G., and Lange, J. V., Ebola and Marburg virus morphology and taxonomy, in: *Ebola Virus Haemorrhagic Fever* (S. R. Pattyn, ed.), pp. 61–82, Elsevier/North-Holland, Amsterdam, 1978.
43. Oehlert, W., The morphological picture in livers, spleens, and lymph nodes of monkeys and guinea pigs after infection with the "vervet agent," in: *Marburg Virus Disease* (G. A. Martini and R. Siegert, eds.), pp. 144–156, Springer-Verlag, New York, 1971.
44. Pattyn, S., Van Der Groen, G., Jacob, W., Piot, D., and Courteille, G., Isolation of Marburg-like virus from a case of haemorrhagic fever in Zaire, *Lancet* **1:**573–574 (1977).
45. Peters, D., and Müller, G., Elektronenmikroskopische Erkennung und Charakterisierung des Marburger Erregers, *Dtsch. Aerztebl.* **65:**1831–1834 (1968).
46. Peters, D., Müller, G., and Slenczka, W. Morphology, development and classification of the Marburg virus, in: *Marburg Virus Disease* (G. A. Martini and R. Siegert, eds.), pp. 68–83, Springer-Verlag, New York, 1971.

47. REGNERY, R. L., JOHNSON, K. M., AND KILEY, M. P., The nucleic acid of Ebola virus, *J. Virol.* **36**:465–469 (1980).

48. RUTTER, D. A., Safety cabinet for use in laboratory studies on hazardous infectious diseases, *Br. Med. J.* **2**:24 (1977).

49. SIEGERT, R., SHU, H. L., SLENCZKA, W., PETERS, D., AND MÜLLER, G., The etiology of a hitherto unknown infectious disease transmitted from monkeys to man, *Ger. Med. Monthly* **13**:1–3 (1968).

50. SIEGERT, R., SHU, H. L., AND SLENCZKA, W., Isolierung und Identifierung des "Marbury virus," *Dtsch. Med. Wochenschr.* **93**:604–612 (1968).

51. SIMPSON, D. I. H., ZLOTNIK, I., AND RUTTER, D. A., Vervet monkey disease: Experimental infection of guinea-pigs and monkeys with the causative agent, *Br. J. Exp. Pathol.* **49**:458–464 (1968).

52. SIMPSON, D. I. H., Marburg virus disease: Experimental infection of monkeys, *Lab. Anim. Handb.* **4**:149–154 (1969).

53. SIMPSON, D. I. H., Vervet monkey disease: Transmission to the hamster, *Br. J. Exp. Pathol.* **50**:389–392 (1969).

54. SLENCZKA, W., Growth of Marburg virus in Vero cells, *Lab. Anim. Handb.* **4**:143–147 (1969).

55. SLENCZKA, W., AND WOLFF, G., Biological properties of the Marburg virus, in: *Marburg Virus Disease* (G. A. MARTINI, AND R. SIEGERT, eds.), pp. 105–108, Springer-Verlag, New York, 1971.

56. SLENCZKA, W., WOLFF, G., AND SIEGERT, R., A critical study of monkey sera for the presence of antibody against the Marburg virus, *Am. J. Epidemiol.* **93**:496–505 (1971).

57. SMITH, C. E. G., SIMPSON, D. I. H., BOWEN, E. T. W., AND ZLOTNIK, I., Fatal human disease from vervet monkeys, *Lancet* **2**:1119–1121 (1967).

58. SMITH, D. H., FRANCIS, D. P., AND SIMPSON, D. I. H., African haemorrhagic fever in the southern Sudan: The clinical features, in: *Ebola Virus Haemorrhagic Fever* (S. R. PATTYN, ed.), pp. 21–26, Elsevier/North-Holland, Amsterdam, 1978.

59. STILLE, W., BÖHLE, E., HELM, E., VAN REY, W., AND SIEDE, W., Über eine durch *Cercopithecus aethiops* übertragene infektious Krankheit ("Grüne-meir-katzen-krankheit," "Green monkey disease"), *Dtsch Med. Wochenschr.* **93**:572–582 (1968).

60. STOJKOVIC, L. J., BURDJOSKI, M., GLIGIC, A., AND STEFANOVIC, Z., Two cases of *Cercopithecus*-monkeys-associated haemorrhagic fever, in: *Marburg Virus Disease* (G. A. MARTINI AND R. SIEGERT, eds.), pp. 24–33, Springer-Verlag, New York, 1971.

61. TREXLER, P. C., EMOND, R. T. D., AND EVANS, R., Negative-pressure isolator for patients with dangerous infections, *Br. Med. J.* **2**:559–561 (1977).

62. VAN DER GROEN, G., JOHNSON, K. M., WEBB, P. A., WULFF, H. T., AND LANGE, J. V., Results of Ebola antibody surveys in various population groups in: *Ebola Virus Haemorrhagic Fever* (S. R. PATTYN, ed.), pp. 203–205, Elsevier/North-Holland, Amsterdam, 1978.

63. VAN DER GROEN, G., WEBB, P. A., JOHNSON, K. M., LANGE, J. V., LINDSAY, H., AND ELLIOTT, L., Growth of Lassa and Ebola viruses in different cell lines, in: *Ebola Virus Haemorrhagic Fever* (S. R. PATTYN, ed.), pp. 255–260, Elsevier/North-Holland, Amsterdam, 1978.

64. Viral haemorrhagic fever, *Weekly Epidemiol. Rep. (WHO)* **52**:185–192 (1977).

65. WEBB, P. A., JOHNSON, K. M., WULFF, H. T., AND LANGE, J. V., Some observations on the properties of Ebola virus, in: *Ebola Virus Haemorrhagic Fever* (S. R. PATTYN, ed.), pp. 91–94, Elsevier/North-Holland, Amsterdam, 1978.

66. WULFF, H., AND CONRAD, L., Marburg virus disease, in: *Comparative Diagnosis of Viral Diseases* (E. KURSTAK AND C. Kurstak, eds.), pp. 3–33, Academic Press, New York, 1977.

67. WULFF, H., SLENCZKA, W., AND GEAR, J. H. S., Early detection of antigen and estimation of virus yield in specimens from patients with Marburg virus disease, *Bull. WHO* **56**:633–639 (1978).

68. WULFF, H., AND JOHNSON, K. M., Immunoglobulin M and G responses measured by immunofluorescence in patients with Lassa and Marburg virus infections, *Bull. WHO* **57**:631–635 (1979).

69. ZLOTNIK, I., AND SIMPSON, D. I. H., The pathology of experimental vervet monkey disease in hamsters, *Br. J. Exp. Pathol.* **50**:393–399 (1969).

70. ZWEIGHAFT, R. M., FRASER, D. W., HATTWICK, M. A. W., WINKLER, W. G., JORDAN, W. C., ALTER, M., WOLFE, M., WULFF, H., AND JOHNSON, K. M., Lassa fever: Response to an imported case, *N. Engl. J. Med.* **297**:803–807 (1977).

12. Suggested Reading

MARTINI, G. A., AND SIEGERT, R. (eds.), *Marburg Virus Disease*, Springer-Verlag, New York, 1971, 230 pp.

PATTYN, S. R. (ed.), *Ebola Virus Haemorrhagic Fever*, Elsevier/North-Holland, Amsterdam, 1978, 436 pp.

Viral haemorrhagic fever, *Weekly. Epidemiol. Rep. (WHO)* **52**:177–192 (1977).

CHAPTER 5

Arboviruses

Wilbur G. Downs

1. Introduction

Well over 400 arboviruses are distinguishable by serological procedures. Theiler and Downs[74] list 273 as of 1973. The American Committee on Arthropod-Borne Viruses published the *Catalogue of Arthropod-Borne Viruses of the World* (ACAV), compiled by R. M. Taylor, in 1967,[2] and this was supplemented by additional listings in 1970[3] and 1971.[4] A complete updated revision of the catalogue appeared in 1975[2] and an additional listing in 1978.[4a] These publications contain basic information on geographic distribution, hosts and vectors, pathogenesis and pathology, cultural characteristics, and composition and morphology, plus a bibliography for each virus.

With the 1978 updating, the ACAV lists 388 viruses. There are 48 recognized groups, many of these consisting of a pair of serologically related viruses. Table 1 gives a synopsis of the present position with the more important arbovirus groupings.

The term *arbovirus* is defined in the ecological sense to include any virus of vertebrates that is biologically transmitted by arthropods. Arthropods include mosquitoes, sandflies (*Phlebotomus* and related genera and *Culicoides* and related genera), hard (ixodid) and soft (argasid) ticks, and, of lesser importance to arbovirus epidemiology, horseflies (Tabanidae), blackflies (Simuliidae), bedbugs (Cimici-

dae), and mites. Limited explorations of fleas, lice, hippoboscids, muscids, streblids, and nycteribiids have not yielded encouraging leads. *Biological transmission* implies an obligatory phase of virus multiplication in the arthropod, before transmission to the next host. *Mechanical transmission* of an arbovirus can of course occur if an arthropod bites a viremic host and then bites an uninfected host, hours or even days later, with the arthropod mouth parts or foregut still virus-contaminated. Such a mechanism has been postulated for hepatitis B virus transmission.[53] In extraordinary arbovirus epidemic situations, mechanical transmission could be a significant adjunct to biological transmission, although this has never been demonstrated in an epidemic.

2. Historical Background

The concept of arthropod-transmitted diseases slowly evolved from a background of centuries of speculations and hypotheses concerning various major plagues of man, including malaria, yellow fever, plague, typhus, filariasis, and trypanosomiasis, and of animals, including babesiosis, trypanosomiasis, African horsesickness, bluetongue of sheep, and equine encephalomyelitis.

In 1878, Patrick Manson described mosquito infection with and transmission of the filarial worm *Wuchereria bancrofti*. Theobald Smith described tick transmission of red water fever in cattle, caused by *Babesia bigemina*, in 1893. In 1897, Ross succeeded in transmitting a malarial infection by mosquito bite.

Wilbur G. Downs · Yale Arbovirus Research Unit, Department of Epidemiology and Public Health, Yale University School of Medicine, New Haven, Connecticut.

Table 1. Some Important Arbovirus Groupings and Associated Vectors

Arboviruses	Number of viruses in grouping	Vectors				Vector not known
		Mosquitoes	Phlebotomus	Culicoides	Ticks	
Togaviruses						
Alphaviruses (group A)	20	20	—	—	—	—
Flaviviruses (group B)	60	30	—	—	14	16
Bunyamwera supergroup						
Bunyamwera group	18[a]	17	—	2	—	—
Group C	11	11	—	—	—	—
California	11	10	—	—	—	1
Bunyamwera-like						
Sandfly fever group	22	4	13	—	—	5
Congo-Crimean hemorrhagic fever group	2	—	—	—	—	2
Orbivirus groups						
African horse sickness (9 immunotypes)	1	—	—	1	—	—
Blue tongue (11 immunotypes)	1	—	—	1	—	—
Colorado tick fever	2	—	—	—	2	—
Kemerovo	16	—	—	—	—	16
Rhabdovirus group						
Vesicular stomatitis	7[a]	1	3	—	—	4

[a] Vectors in more than one anthropod category have been noted for a few viruses.

Carlos Finlay attempted transmission of yellow fever virus by mosquito bite before 1900, and Walter Reed and associates succeeded in transmitting the virus by bite of *Aedes aegypti* in 1901. Not until 1928 did Stokes, *et al.*[70] demonstrate that the agent that caused yellow fever was indeed a virus. Indeed, biological transmission of the viruses of yellow fever (1901), phlebotomus fever (1909), and dengue (1920–1924) was accomplished before the viruses themselves were known. Several of the most important arboviruses were identified in the 1930s, including the viruses of eastern equine encephalitis, western equine encephalitis, St. Louis encephalitis, Russian spring-summer encephalitis, Japanese encephalitis, Murray Valley encephalitis, and Rift Valley fever. This list was expanded in the 1940s by addition of several more viruses encountered during the course of yellow fever field studies in Africa and South America and encephalitis studies in the Americas. An intensified program directed toward determining the worldwide arbovirus picture was initiated by the Rockefeller Foundation in 1952, and this, plus efforts of many investigators in other laboratories, has led to the present recognition of over 400 serologically distinct agents. Casals in 1957[16] listed 47 viruses and in 1958[17] listed 72; by 1962,

the list had reached 161. A similar increase in numbers of recognized respiratory, enteric, and other nonarboviruses has been paralleling the arbovirus explosion. The increase in numbers of recognized arboviruses is directly referable to the introduction of the infant mouse intracerebral inoculation technique for virus isolation, with cell-culture methods playing a very minor role. The infant-mouse technique was used by Dalldorf to isolate many of the coxsackieviruses, but in other areas of respiratory and enteric virology, the explosion followed introduction of cell-culture techniques.

The systems employed for arbovirus identification and classification have been largely serological, and only recently has electron microscopy been extensively and usefully employed. The serological techniques have included complement fixation (CF), hemagglutination inhibition (HI), and neutralization (N). Modern modifications of these classic techniques rooted in the same basic principles include the use of "tagged" antibodies (ferritin, fluorescein, radioactive isotopes) and antigens. Highly purified virus and virus-component preparations have been made possible by ultracentrifugation and chromatographic techniques.

With the N test, Smithburn[68] in 1942 showed

some immunological relationship among West Nile, St. Louis, and Japanese encephalitis viruses. Casals[15] confirmed this relationship by CF test, and Sabin[60] in 1949 showed a relationship among yellow fever, Japanese encephalitis, dengue, and St. Louis viruses, also by CF test. Smithburn[69] in 1954 showed that monkeys immune to one arbovirus, when inoculated with a related virus, in proper sequence, developed antibodies capable of neutralizing the second virus and an increased capacity to neutralize the original virus.

Development of the techniques of hemagglutination and HI began with the demonstration by Hallauer[32] in 1946 of a hemagglutinating antigen from a yellow fever virus strain. Sabin and Buescher[61] in 1950 described a hemagglutinin for Japanese encephalitis, and in short order, Sabin and other collaborators extended the list to include several group B arboviruses and one group A arbovirus. Casals and Brown[20] in 1954 made further additions when they prepared and used acetone and acetone–ether extracted antigens. Clarke and Casals[22] in 1958 described techniques that have been but little modified to date, including the sucrose–acetone technique for preparation of hemagglutinins and the kaolin and acetone techniques for extraction of nonspecific inhibitors from sera to be studied in tests for HI. Ardoin et al.[5] in 1969 described sonication and trypsin treatment of virus preparations to achieve hemagglutinins in instances where commonly used procedures did not work well, if at all. Beaty et al.[7a] showed that change, mainly an increase, in tonicity could increase the hemagglutinating ability of certain antigens, but by no means of all.

Casals[16] in 1957 outlined a scheme for classifying arboviruses according to serological interreactions, intending this as a helpful device for subsorting or categorizing the numerous viruses. The concept has been an invaluable one in bringing order out of chaos, and the original schema has been greatly extended. Later actions of the Virus Subcommittee of the International Nomenclature Committee have recommended the adoption of a universal system of classification in which the properties of the virion should be the sole basis for the establishment of taxa. The various arbovirus serogroups have been distributed among various taxa such as togaviruses, including alphaviruses (group A arboviruses) and flaviviruses (group B arboviruses); bunyaviruses (including the viruses of the Bunyamwera super-

group); rhabdoviruses; and orbiviruses. This does not disturb the original arbovirus definition, which continues to insist on biological transmission as the prerequisite for inclusion in the epidemiological concept.

A landmark in virology was the development of attenuated strains of yellow fever virus for vaccines in the mid-1930s.[67] The 17D yellow fever virus vaccine strain developed by Theiler and co-workers in the Virus Laboratories of the International Health Division of the Rockefeller Foundation is in worldwide use. The French neurotropic virus vaccine strain developed at the Institut Pasteur, Dakar, is now but little used. Yellow fever virus vaccination has neutralized a major hazard to residents, immigrants, and tourists in the African and South American tropics, permitting the accelerating development of these regions.

The input of field epidemiological teams (physicians, entomologists, mammalogists, ornithologists, virologists, immunologists, and ecologists) working on all the continents except Antarctica, coupled with technical improvements, has been essential in gaining an understanding of the epidemiology of arboviruses. The basic principles that determine the mode of propagation and transmission of many arboviruses have been of fundamental importance in our understanding of the epidemiology of several important diseases of human beings. They may eventually contribute to an understanding of the origin and evolution of various virus groups. Mattingly[47] discussed this in 1960, and there is much new knowledge now at hand, but few reinterpretations.

The material from field investigators has supplied bench virologists with a number of viruses that have proven to be very useful as tools to permit exploration of fundamentals of virus composition and structure, infection of the host cell, replication, and transmission. Among such viruses are the togaviruses of yellow fever, West Nile, Sindbis, the dengues, and Semliki Forest, plus the encephalitogenic viruses (also togaviruses) of St. Louis, eastern, western, Japanese, and Venezuelan encephalitis; the rhabdoviruses, including the vesicular stomatitis viruses (Indiana and New Jersey serotypes, plus Cocal, Chandipura, and Piry); the bunyaviruses (including California encephalitis virus); and the orbiviruses (including bluetongue virus of sheep and the epidemic hemorrhagic disease virus of deer).

Transovarial passage of several tick-transmitted arboviruses has been demonstrated repeatedly, but until recently, attempts to demonstrate this with viruses in mosquitos were unsuccessful. The recent demonstration of transovarial transmission of LaCrosse virus (a California encephalitis relative) in mosquitoes in Wisconsin[80] may be of epidemiological significance in that it may provide an explanation for long-term survival of a virus in nature. Venereal transmission of virus in insect vectors has also been demonstrated.[77a] Transovarial transmission of dengue virus—four types,[72a] Japanese encephalitis virus,[58a] and yellow fever virus[1a] has also been demonstrated. Extrapolations in the realm of epidemiology from these positive demonstrations must, however, be made with caution.

Some of the less pathogenic of the arboviruses are used as models or "tools" for biochemical and biophysical studies with little realization of the origins of the tool or of the close relationship of the virus to other viruses of much greater pathogenicity. The possibility that genetic change in such a tool virus of low virulence, might induce an exaltation of virulence has not gone unremarked.

The history of the treatment of arthropod-borne virus infections can be dismissed briefly, therapy being directed toward the care and support of the patient. Specific remedial measures are lacking.

3. Methodology Involved in Epidemiological Analysis

3.1. Sources of Mortality Data

The World Health Organization (WHO) publishes the *Weekly Epidemiological Record*, the Center for Disease Control (CDC) of the USPHS publishes *Morbidity and Mortality: Weekly Report*, and the Pan American Health Organization (PAHO) publishes the *Weekly Epidemiological Report*. A surveillance report is published monthly by the Caribbean Epidemiological Center (CAREC). Various states of the United States also send out periodic reports, as do many governments. These agencies report on officially notified deaths, and often include additional epidemiological information for important diseases. As valuable as such reports may be for retrospective analysis, however, they are too many weeks behind the actual events to be of much service to the epi-

demiologist in the field. It is also widely accepted, although difficult to prove, that certain diseases such as yellow fever and hemorrhagic dengue are seriously underreported in the tropical countries. Even in temperate countries, the epidemic encephalitides are undoubtedly not fully recorded. Delay in reporting presents another problem, and such delay may be a serious matter if it results in delay in application of disease-control measures.

3.2. Sources of Morbidity Data

The sources for mortality data (WHO, USPHS-CDC, and PAHO) also serve as sources for morbidity data. The morbidity reports must be regarded even more skeptically than mortality data, for virus diseases in general and arbovirus infections in particular. Cases of encephalitis, determined or suspected, are indeed reported in most states. Even when reported and followed up by epidemiological and laboratory studies, many such cases receive no specific diagnosis—"many" meaning anywhere between 40 and 65%, depending on the completeness of the workup and on the immediate epidemiological circumstances. Table 2 illustrates this point.

In the state of Connecticut, for example, although the viruses of eastern equine, western equine, and California encephalitis are found, and the tick-borne agent Powassan virus is also probably present, no case of arbovirus encephalitis or infection in man has yet been detected. Prevalence rates of antibodies to these viruses in the population are also very low, indicating that the human population has not been affected. The demonstration of the presence of a virus in field studies of arthropod or vertebrate populations cannot be used as an indication of human morbidity from the virus, but such demonstrations do serve to heighten suspicion and to orient diagnosis.

In a 1967–1968 Connecticut study[62] carried out with the help of the State Health Department, numerous hospitals and physicians were contacted, and some 70 cases of encephalitis or suspect encephalitis were seen. Those for which no specific causative agent had been identified had early and convalescent serum specimens taken and tested. No evidence of arbovirus activity was uncovered.

In the Midwestern states, aggressive case-finding and follow-up have served to uncover 50–60 cases annually of California encephalitis, and in the irri-

Table 2. Causes of Infectious Encephalitis in the United States
in 1976 and 1977[a]

Causes	1976		1977[b]	
	Cases	%	Cases	%
Arboviruses				
Western equine encephalitis	1	—	41	4.4
St. Louis encephalitis	379	20.8	23	2.5
Eastern equine encephalitis	0	—	1	0.1
California encephalitis	47	2.6	35	3.7
	427	23.4	100	10.7
Childhood infections				
Mumps	71	3.9	31	3.3
Measles	44	2.4	17	1.8
Chickenpox	58	3.2	39	4.1
Rubella	2	—	0	—
	175	9.6	87	9.3
Other				
Enteroviruses	13	0.7	22	2.3
Herpes simplex	69	3.8	32	3.4
Other known	21	1.1	13	1.4
	103	5.6	67	7.1
Indeterminate etiology	1121	61.4	684	72.9
TOTAL:	1826	100.0	938	100.0

[a] From: Reported Morbidity and Mortality in the United States, Annual Summary, 1977, Center for Disease Control, *Morbid. Mortal. Weekly Rep.* **26**:1–80 (1978). In 1978, there were only 53 cases of arbovirus infections reported in the continental United States—43 California, 3 St. Louis, 3 western, and 4 eastern encephalitis cases. In addition, 52 imported cases of dengue were reported from a large outbreak of 10,000 cases in Puerto Rico; Tahiti and other Caribbean islands were also involved.

[b] Includes both laboratory-confirmed and presumptive cases. Data provisional.

gated regions of the Southwest and West, aggressive case-hunting provides evidence of infection with St. Louis and western equine encephalitis particularly. Nonetheless, a high proportion of the encephalitis cases remain without specific causative diagnosis. When the clinical diagnosis is on even weaker grounds—undifferentiated fever, "PUO," "FUO," "flu," or "grippe"—then one may presume that sporadic cases of arbovirus infections never do get reported or investigated. Indeed, reporting of such cases is likely only when they are seen in connection with an already recognized epidemic. This is certainly the case when epidemics of dengue or Venezuelan, St. Louis, western, or eastern encephalitis occur, and is also true with yellow fever.

A common pattern of events when epidemics of these diseases occur is for dozens, hundreds, even thousands of cases to be present weeks or even months before the first specific diagnosis is made.

Prompt diagnosis of an epidemic situation is directly dependent on a high index of suspicion. Individual clinicians, epidemiologists, and health services vary greatly in the degree of alertness maintained for possible epidemic incidents.

3.3. Serological Surveys

Serological surveys continue to be the best source of information on worldwide prevalence of the hundreds of arboviruses, and the information obtained is invaluable in extending the concepts of specific virus–arthropod vector–vertebrate host interrelationships. In contrast to the ubiquitous viruses that cause human disease, such as measles, mumps, and smallpox, which are found in practically all human societies, no single arbovirus is worldwide in distribution and only a limited number even extend to two continents. Even within the limits of a continent or country, the occurrence of a single arbovirus remains inexorably delimited by the features of geography and climate that determine the distribution of the specific arthropod vector(s) and the vertebrate host(s) of the virus in question. Such boundaries are ecologically imposed and may have no relationship to political boundaries of counties, states, or countries. In international border areas, international collaboration is imperative for epidemiological investigations. WHO and PAHO are of great help in facilitating such collaboration and also actively initiate and sponsor collaborative studies.

Serological surveys can be directed toward exploring the immunity patterns of a population with reference to a specific epidemic situation, threat, or control procedure. A survey of an Amerindian tribe in Amazonas, for example, can provide information on prevalence of yellow fever in the region and on past vaccination coverage. Again, the survey can be directed toward identifying general and specific arbovirus prevalence in regions of high and low rainfall, high and low altitude, coastal regions and inland regions, forested regions and savannah regions, and rural and urban settings, and in relation to agricultural practices of crop types, irrigation, deforestation, fertilization, and deinsectization. A 1970 report of Surtees et al.[71] on arbovirus epidemiology in a rice field development project in the Kano Plain, Kenya, is an example of a carefully planned investigation, prefaced by ecological studies of the region (including agricultural practices) and embracing arthropod-vector studies; virus-isolation studies on arthropods, wild and domesticated vertebrates, and human beings; and serological studies on man, animals, and birds.

Multipurpose serological surveys of healthy populations that include the determination of the prevalence of antibodies to arboviruses as well as to other viral, bacterial, and parasitic agents may provide useful information on their distribution in different geographic areas, ages, and occupational groups as a basis of control and immunization programs. Example of this are the collaborative studies of the WHO Serum Reference Bank and the WHO International Arbovirus Reference Centre, both at Yale University, on military recruits in Argentina,[26b] Brazil,[50a] Colombia,[26a] and the United States,[77a] and on healthy population groups in Barbados[26] and St. Lucia[26c] (see Chapter 2 for details).

The interpretation of serological surveys is complicated by cross-reactivity of antisera within a number of the groupings (alphaviruses, flaviviruses, bunyaviruses, orbiviruses, rhabdoviruses, and others). There is no magic formula to resolve the problem. A serosurvey report based only on CF or HI testing (or both) does not carry as much weight as one based on N test results, or one with N test confirmations of CF and HI positive-reacting sera.

3.4. Laboratory Methods

Positive serological findings on survey sera are greatly bolstered by virus isolations from the vector, vertebrate, and human being. Virus isolation procedures for serum specimens require inoculation of a small amount of serum into laboratory animals, or cell cultures, or both. The usual inoculum for intracerebral inoculation of a 1-day-old mouse is 0.02 ml, and for the adult mouse 0.03 ml. Mice are observed daily, or more than once a day, for evidence of illness. A subpassage may be made to attempt to enhance the virulence of the virus, and when one is assured that a virus has been isolated, a stock pool of virus is established and hyperimmune mouse serum or ascitic fluid is prepared if needed. In fatal cases, 40% suspension of tissue—brain, liver, lung, and spleen (purified by ultracentrifugation)—may be inoculated as for serum.

Cell-culture systems (vertebrate or insect cell cultures) can be used for virus isolation. For certain viruses and certain cell cultures, the cell-culture systems, employing usually a 0.1-ml inoculum, are as sensitive as laboratory animals. Arbovirus outbreaks often occur far from established cell-culture laboratories so that inoculation of more readily available laboratory animals is still more widely done than inoculation of cell-culture systems. This situation will probably change. It must be remembered, however, that intracerebral inoculation of infant mice will serve to isolate a much wider total range of arboviruses than will any single cell-culture system. This factual position is not likely to change. Conversely, in the investigation of a specific virus, a cell-culture system that has been predetermined to be suited to the virus can be easier, cheaper, and as reliable as or more reliable than techniques that require laboratory animals.

In the study of material derived from patients, it is highly desirable to have a pair of serum specimens to work with. The first should be taken early in the course of illness and can serve as material both for virus isolation and for the determination of baseline serum antibody levels before the patient has developed antibodies to the infecting virus. A second serum should be obtained at least 3 weeks after onset of illness, even as late as a month or several months after onset. A seroconversion demonstrable between the early and later specimens is strong evidence of a recent virus infection. Even should a specimen taken early in the course of illness not be available, a high antibody titer in the specimen(s) taken during convalescence may be meaningful, providing a provisional diagnosis without possibility of actual proof.

Details of the techniques of CF, HI, and virus neutralization, relating specifically to arboviruses, are available in current manuals.[64,64a] Fluorescent-antibody (FA) techniques and the enzyme-linked immunosorbent assay (ELISA) are under development for measurement of antibody and for antigen detection, including field identification in infected mosquitoes.

4. Biological Characteristics of the Virus That Affect the Epidemiological Pattern

Arboviruses by definition share one common feature, the requirement of propagating in some intact arthropod. Transmission by the arthropod is a necessary postlude. For some years, it was considered that all arboviruses were RNA viruses, although any explanation as to why only RNA viruses (and indeed only *certain* RNA viruses) would multiply in the arthropod is lacking. This position was challenged by the demonstration[1,51] that African swine fever virus, which has been shown to multiply in and be transmitted through the bite of certain ticks,[52] is a DNA virus.

The property of sensitivity to deoxycholic acid (DCA) and to other lipid solvents and detergents has been useful as a screening procedure for candidate arboviruses. However, various nonarboviruses, such as influenza virus and smallpox and ectromelia viruses, are also inactivated by such reagents. Theiler[73] and others also noted that several viruses, unquestionably able to multiply in arthropods and to be transmitted by arthropods, were

partially resistant to the action of DCA and the lipid solvents. From this beginning, Borden, Murphy, Shope, and Harrison have proposed the group of orbiviruses,[10,50] which includes several important viruses such as African horsesickness, bluetongue of sheep, and epidemic hemorrhagic disease of deer. The orbiviruses share morphological and physicochemical features, but serological relationships between or among them may be marginal or lacking.

Another challenging circumstance relates to the specificity of various arboviruses for particular arthropod species. Many workers have attempted to infect arthropods with many of the arboviruses. Group B arboviruses can be conveniently divided into two sections: mosquito-transmitted and tick-transmitted. Attempts to infect ticks with certain mosquito-transmitted group B viruses such as yellow fever virus have consistently failed. Attempts to infect mosquitos with the group B virus of tick-borne encephalitis have likewise failed. However, Whitman and Aitken[83] have shown that an argasid tick can be infected by feeding on a viremic host and can transmit West Nile virus, a group B mosquito-transmitted virus. Also, L'Vov et al.[44] have shown that Tyuleniy virus, a tick-transmitted group B virus, can multiply in and can be transmitted by a mosquito. Attempts to infect mosquitoes with *Phlebotomus*-transmitted viruses have yielded conflicting results. The reverse of this has not been tried, it being difficult to manipulate *Phlebotomus* flies in the laboratory.

When Grace succeeded in cultivating insect cells in culture systems and in 1966 reported establishment of a line of mosquito (*Aedes aegypti*) cells in continuous culture,[31] the susceptibility of such cell lines to arboviruses was tested. It was early established that the cells were susceptible to infection with mosquito-transmitted viruses. Singh, working with clones of mosquito cells,[65] showed that tick-borne group B viruses did not multiply in mosquito-cell culture.[66] Buckley[12] extended these observations and showed that even *Phlebotomus*-transmitted viruses did not multiply in mosquito-cell cultures. Further observations on tick-transmitted viruses indicated that only Colorado tick fever virus, a tick-transmitted orbivirus, gave evidence of growth in mosquito-cell cultures. Libíková and Buckley[40] later reported limited growth of Kemerovo virus, a tick-transmitted virus, in a mosquito cell line. Řeháček and Pesek[57] have noted limited growth of eastern equine encephalitis in tick-tissue explants. If efforts to cultivate tick tissues, *Phlebotomus* tissues, and tissues of other arthropods succeed, the problem of specificity can be explored from new angles.

A prerequisite for the survival of an arbovirus in nature is a period of viremia in a vertebrate host at a level sufficient to infect the arthropod vector. Even with a very virulent virus and a very receptive vector, a virus titer in excess of 100,000 infectious doses of virus per milliliter of blood is usually necessary. Such high levels of viremia are presumed to occur in the natural host system, and often are attained in the more commonly used laboratory animals such as mice, hamsters, guinea pigs, chicks, and monkeys. For many of the more esoteric arboviruses, however, the natural hosts or natural vectors, or both, are either unavailable or not known, so that the postulate of a level of viremia in the vertebrate adequate to infect a susceptible vector remains undemonstrated.

5. Epidemiology

The epidemiology of arbovirus infections in man is influenced by three major determinants: (1) the behavior of the arthropod vector, including the ecological setting in which its breeding occurs, its pattern and range of mobility, its biting habits and species preferences for feeding, its longevity, and the factors affecting the entry, multiplication, and excretion of virus within the arthropod host; (2) the frequency, nature, and duration of exposure of human beings to the infected arthropod vectors, as influenced by the presence, level, and specificity of humoral antibody, and by use in the population of insecticides, insect repellents, and protective clothing; and (3) the requirements for the presence of a necessary and/or amplifying vertebrate host for the virus, such as horses, birds, or rodents, and of the availability of man as a diversion in the arthropod–vertebrate cycle.

The great variability in these three determinants does not permit broad generalization on the epidemiology of over 400 arboviruses. Instead, this section and the sections on transmission, pathogenesis, host response, and control will focus on the most common and important arbovirus infections of man in the United States and on certain common features. Subsequent sections will present these in

more detail and deal briefly in descriptive and tabular form with arboviruses important outside the United States.

5.1. Incidence and Prevalence

No general statement can be made about incidence, which varies greatly from area to area depending on the presence of an appropriate vector and the presence or absence of an outbreak. The occurence of a fresh outbreak in a region with susceptible and exposed humans may result in very high infection rates. In epidemics of St. Louis encephalitis, for example, a high proportion of susceptibles in a region where an epidemic is in progress may be infected, even though comparatively few clinical cases may be detected.[11]

The presence of antibody to most arboviruses reflects the cumulative and lifelong prevalence of infection. A classic arbovirus study was the mapping of the worldwide distribution of yellow fever by Sawyer et al.[63] in 1937. The virus neutralization test was performed using adult white mice as test animals. Yellow fever virus was found to be more widely distributed in South America and Africa than had been earlier suspected and was absent from Europe, Asia, and Australia. Much has been learned about group relationships of arboviruses since the 1937 report, and many serological cross-relationships have been demonstrated, particularly among the flaviviruses (group B arboviruses), of which group yellow fever virus is a member. Such cross-reactivity has been demonstrated not only by CF and HI tests, but also by virus neutralization procedures. Theiler and Downs[74] show, in Tables 24, 25, and 26 of their book, development of cross-immune reactions in proven primary and secondary cases of yellow fever. *Secondary* means an infection in a person who had had prior experience with another group B arbovirus. However, the serological response to the current incitant agent is usually more pronounced than the reaction to other members of the serogroup, enabling specific diagnosis (if the current agent is included in the test). The whole area of cross-immune responses is regarded with something akin to awe. It would be a courageous worker today who would attempt a project such as the 1937 yellow fever serosurvey, with just a single virus and a single test. The 1937 study relied on a relatively insensitive testing procedure, not very responsive to the nuances of cross-reacting antibodies, yet the mapping of yellow fever that resulted has required but little alteration.

Neutralization tests measure durable antibody that persists for years. High rates of antibody prevalence could result from continued, widespread virus activity and/or from a large outbreak with a high attack rate. For example, yellow fever neutralization tests performed on sera collected from residents of Trinidad, West Indies, in 1953 revealed no immunes under the age of 15 years, and therefore no apparent virus activity later than 1938. This situation changed dramatically with the reappearance of yellow fever on the island in epidemic form in 1954.[23]

Antibody patterns to California virus infection in Wisconsin[49] revealed varying prevalence rates depending on the frequency and duration of exposure: it was 48% of Indian forest workers, 34% of wildlife conservation workers, 23% of veterinarians, and 11% of short-term summer workers in forestry camps. Interpretation is difficult, since it is known that those antibodies included not only one La-Crosse strain but also several nonpathogenic members of the California-virus complex.

5.2. Epidemic Behavior

Outbreaks of arbovirus infections in the United States involving human beings occur periodically and unpredictably. Table 3 summarizes the experience from 1965 through 1978. Only 46 cases of eastern equine encephalitis (EEE) were reported during this time, of which 12 cases and 6 deaths were in 1968; during the same period, 486 cases of western equine encephalitis (WEE) were reported, of which 172 occurred in 1965, with 4 deaths, and 133 in 1975, with 6 deaths. Outbreaks of St. Louis encephalitis (SLE) were first recognized in St. Louis in 1932; recent outbreaks occurred in 1966, in 1974 in Memphis, Tennessee,[78] and the largest in 1975 mostly in Mississippi with 1815 cases and 142 deaths. Venezuelan equine encephalitis (VEE) produced its first outbreak in the United States in Texas in 1971, with no epidemic activity since that date.

5.3. Geographic Distribution

Arbovirus infections are worldwide in distribution and may occur whenever the appropriate mosquito or other arthropod vectors abound in prox-

Table 3. Human Cases and Deaths: Arthropod-Borne Encephalitis (including Colorado Tick Fever) 1965–1975[a]

Year	EEE	WEE	SLE	CE	Totals	CTF[b]
1965	8 (4)	172 (4)	58 (0)	59 (0)	297 (8)	188 (0)
1966	4 (2)	47 (2)	323 (28)	64 (0)	438 (32)	156 (0)
1967	1 (1)	18 (0)	11 (0)	53 (1)	83 (2)	137 (0)
1968	12 (6)	17 (1)	35 (3)	66 (0)	130 (9)	88 (0)
1969	3 (2)	21 (0)	16 (0)	67 (0)	107 (3)	114 (0)
1970	2 (0)	4 (0)	15 (2)	89 (1)	110 (3)	92 (0)
1971	4 (2)	11 (1)	57 (3)	58 (0)	130 (6)	116 (0)
1972	0 (0)	8 (0)	13 (0)	46 (0)	70 (0)	162 (0)
1973	0 (0)	8 (0)	13 (0)	45 (0)	66 (0)	321 (0)
1974	4 (2)	2 (0)	72 (5)	30 (0)	108 (7)	237 (0)
1975	3 (1)	133 (6)	1815 (142)	160 (1)	2113 (150)	357 (0)
1976[c]	0	1	379	47	427	NA
1977[c]	1	41	23	35	100	79
1978[c]	4	3	3	43	53	NA
	46 (20)	486 (14)	2833 (183)	202 (3)	4232 (220)	—

[a] From USPHS—Center for Disease Control, *Neurotropic Viral Diseases: Encephalitis: Annual Encephalitis Summary 1972* (July 1974) and from USPHS—Center for Disease Control, *Morbidity and Mortality Weekly Report: Reported Morbidity and Mortality in the United States 1973*, **22**(53) (1973). Also *Morbidity Mortality Weekly Rep.* **26**:1–80 (1978). (EEE) Eastern equine encephalitis; (WEE) western equine encephalitis; (SLE) St. Louis encephalitis; (CE) California encephalitis; (CTF) Colorado tick fever. The number of deaths is given in parentheses.
[b] (NA) Not available.
[c] Mortality data not available 1976–1978.

imity to man and a suitable amplifying host. Table 4 includes the geographic distribution of arboviruses in the United States and Table 5 that in South America, Europe, Asia, Africa, and Australia.

5.4. Temporal Distribution

In the United States, mosquito-borne arbovirus infections produce human infections primarily in late summer and fall; Colorado tick fever (CTF) has involved hunters, fishermen, and campers from spring through fall (see Table 4).

5.5. Age and Sex

Infections with arboviruses can occur at any age. The age distribution depends on the degree of exposure to the particular transmitting arthropod relating to age, sex, and occupational, vocational, and recreational habits of the individual or group of individuals. For example, California encephalitis (CE) virus infections primarily involve children, especially boys who climb in trees, because the mosquito vector breeds in small accumulations of water sometimes found where tree branches join the main trunk of a tree—an ideal spot for a child to sit or build a treehouse. On the other hand, adult males are more commonly infected with CTF virus, since they dominate the hunter and fisherman population who become exposed to the ticks in forested areas.

Once humans have been exposed and infected, the severity of the host response may also be influenced by age. WEE tends to produce the most severe clinical infections in young persons, and SLE in older persons.

5.6. Other Factors

Nutritional and genetic factors are not known to directly influence the epidemiology of arbovirus infections. Socioeconomic factors may play a part insofar as they relate to life patterns in seedy suburbs, barrios, or rural regions, where insect-vector populations may flourish under conditions of poor sanitation. It may emerge that cell-mediated immunity under genetic control plays a part in the nature and severity of the host response, the persistence of virus, and the formation of immune complexes, but no data are on hand to support these conjectures.

6. Mechanism and Route of Transmission

By definition, arboviruses must be transmitted by arthropod vectors within which multiplication of the virus is a necessary requirement. This biological transmission may be supplemented by mechanical transmission in which the virus is passively carried externally on the vector or even passively excreted. The primary vectors are mosquitos, sandflies (*Phlebotomus* and *Culicoides*), and ticks. Of far less importance are horseflies, mites, and blackflies. There is often a high-level virus–vector specificity.

The duration of the necessary period of virus multiplcation within the arthropod host before it becomes infectious varies from virus to virus and vector to vector, and is also directly temperature-dependent.[82] For most viruses under average summer temperature conditions, the extrinsic incubation period falls in the 7- to 14-day range. Once infected, vectors may remain infected and able to transmit for many weeks or months.

Transmission of virus transovarially in arthropods, often referred to as "vertical transmission," has been demonstrated (specific examples: tick-borne encephalitis in ticks, LaCrosse strain of California encephalitis in mosquitos, and Sicilian sandfly fever virus in phlebotomine sandflies). Venereal transmission of LaCrosse virus in vector mosquitoes has been described.[77a] These mechanisms may be important for survival of some arboviruses in nature, permitting overwintering or survival over a protracted dry spell. Birds are important reservoir vertebrates for the viruses of EEE, WEE, and SLE, and small mammals for CE and CTF viruses.

Table 6 summarizes some features of arbovirus infections important in the United States.

7. Pathogenesis and Immunity

Arbovirus infections are transmitted by the bite of the appropriate vector, so that the skin represents the sole portal of entry. With penetration of the skin by the biting mouth parts of the arthropod, the virus is deposited directly into lymph or the bloodstream, in addition to forming a local pool. With early wide dissemination throughout the host, multiplication follows in as yet inadequately identified target cells and tissues. Viremia in the host then provides the

Table 4. Descriptive Epidemiology of Arboviruses Important as Causative Agents of Disease in Human Beings in the 48 Contiguous United States

Virus[a]	Arbovirus grouping	Incidence and prevalence data	Geographic distribution	Temporal distribution of cases	Age	Sex	Race	Occupation	Occurrence in different settings
EEE	Group A togavirus	Encephalitis rare; immunity rates low	Eastern Seaboard from Massachusetts to Florida and Louisiana	Late summer and fall; sporadic cases or restricted sharp epidemics	Any age	—	—	—	Rural and suburban
WEE	Group A togavirus	Encephalitis uncommon; immunity rates may be high locally	Virus widespread; human disease restricted to West and Southwest	Summer and fall; broadly endemic and occasional epidemic peaks	Cases more severe in young	—	—	—	Rural and suburban
SLE	Group B togavirus	Encephalitis uncommon; immunity rates may be high locally	Widespread in southern, central, and western states	Summer and fall; broadly endemic and occasional epidemic peaks	Cases more severe in older people	—	—	—	Rural and suburban
CE	Bunyamwera supergroup, California group togavirus	Encephalitis uncommon; immunity rates low; infections sporadic	North central states; virus occurrence in some eastern and western states, but cases rare or absent	Summer; broadly endemic; sporadic cases	Any age	—	—	Sylvan picnic settings; woodland workers	Forested regions; campsites
CTF	—	Immunity rates low; infections sporadic	Rocky Mountain states	Spring through fall; broadly endemic; sporadic cases	Adults more likely to be exposed	Males more likely to be exposed	—	Hunters, fisherman, outdoor people	Mountain foothills and medium altitude slopes

[a] For definitions of abbreviations, see Table 3, footnote a.

Table 5. Important Arbovirus Infections of Human Beings in South America, Europe, Asia, Africa, and Australia

Disease	Geographic region(s)	Vector(s)	Vertebrate host(s)	Features of disease in human beings		Diagnosis	Control measures
				Disease pattern	Description of disease		
Yellow fever Urban	New World and African cities (seaports usually)	Aedes aegypti	Man	Epidemic	Acute onset, high fever, prostration, later jaundice, proteinuria; fatalities common, although ratio of inapparent/apparent infections is high	Virus isolation, CF, HI, N tests	Vaccination with 17D vaccine; Aedes aegypti control
Jungle	New World and African tropics	Mosquitos: Haemagogus and aedines	Forest primates	Endemic	As above; cases occur sporadically in people exposed in forested regions in Africa and New World	Virus isolation, CF, HI, N tests	Vaccination with 17D vaccine; mosquito control not practicable
Dengue(s)	New World and Old World tropics and subtropics	Aedes aegypti and other aedines	Man; possibly a "jungle" cycle in primates	Endemic and epidemic	Acute onset with rash in many cases and joint pains; simulates an influenzalike syndrome	Virus isolation, CF, HI, N tests	Mosquito control and protection against mosquito bites; no vaccines yet
Dengue hemorrhagic fever	Southeast Asia	Aedes aegypti	Man	Endemic and epidemic	Serious illness with hemorrhagic complications, shock syndrome, and high mortality—almost exclusively in children, and following a second infection with a different dengue virus	CF, HI, N tests in animals or cell-culture system	Mosquito control
Japanese encephalitis	Orient, Korea to India, and East Indies	Culex tritaeniorhynchus and other culicines	Wild birds; pigs can serve as amplifying hosts	Endemic and epidemic	Infection usually mild, but encephalitic complications can be serious in young and in elderly; very important disease in the Orient	CF, HI, N tests	Mosquito control; vaccination with an inactivated vaccine

Disease	Geographic distribution	Vector	Reservoir host	Epidemiology	Clinical features	Diagnosis	Prevention and control
Murray Valley encephalitis	Australia	*Culex annulirostris* and other mosquitos	Birds	Epidemic, sporadic, over wide areas	Infection usually mild, but encephalitis may occur, with greatest probability in children, and high fatality rates in the young	CF, HI, N tests	Mosquito control measures and protection against mosquito bite
Chikungunya	Africa, and Asia, tropics and subtropics	*Aedes aegypti*	Possibly primates	Epidemic	Acute onset, often with rash; rarely with hemorrhagic manifestations; joint aching and swelling are prominent features	CF, HI, N tests and virus isolation	Mosquito control
Tick-borne encephalitis	USSR and Northern Europe	Ticks—*Ixodes ricinus* and others	Small wild mammals and birds	Endemic in forested regions	Acute onset, violent headache, fever, nausea, vomiting, hyperesthesia, photophobia, drowsiness, delirium, coma may follow; mortality rate about 20%	Virus isolation, CF, HI, N tests	Tick control where possible; an inactivated vaccine has been tried
Kyasanur Forest disease	India (Mysore State)	Ticks—mainly *Haemaphysalis*	Monkeys; possibly also small mammals	Endemic and epidemic	Sudden onset, fever, headache, severe myalgia; there may be a disphasic course with second phase after an afebrile period of 7–15 days; mortality rates under 5%	Virus isolation, CF, HI, N tests	Protection against tick bite
Crimean hemorrhagic fever (Congo)	Southern USSR, Bulgaria	Ticks—*Hyalomma marginatum*	Probably small mammals	Endemic	Sudden onset, chills, fever, headache, nausea, vomiting, hemorrhagic manifestations common; mortality rate 5–10%	Virus isolation, CF test	Protection against tick bite
Venezuelan equine encephalitis	Central and South America and Southern United States	Mosquitos of several species	Horses; possibly small mammals	Probably endemic; sharply epidemic	Fever, encephalitic signs, usually mild, fatalities rare	Virus isolation, CF, HI, N tests	Mosquito control and protection against mosquito bites; attenuated vaccine exists for equines

Table 6. Mechanisms and Route of Transmission, Pathogenesis, and Immunity Features of Arboviruses Important as Causative Agents of Disease in Human Beings in the 48 Contiguous United States

Virus[a]	Transmission mechanism	Vector(s)	Animal reservoirs	Pathogenesis in man	Immunity	Patterns of host response		
						Key clinical features	Biological spectrum	Ratio of inapparent to apparent infections
EEE	Mosquito bite	*Culiseta melanura* and various *Aedes*	Wild birds; penned pheasants; equines affected but not reservoirs	Encephalitis, frequently fatal; nerve-cell damage often focal	Long-lasting, probably lifetime	Abrupt onset, high fever, signs of encephalitis, often becoming severe or fatal in 3–5 days	Severe cases mostly in small children; sequelae common; adults who recover usually have few or no sequelae	Few mild or clinically inapparent infections; immunity rates in populations low
WEE	Mosquito bite	*Culex tarsalis* in the West; *Culiseta melanura* in the East; other mosquitos	Wild birds; equines affected but not reservoirs	Encephalitis with mortality rates 2–18%; nerve-cell damage often focal	Long-lasting, probably lifetime	Fever, drowsiness, and other signs of encephalitis, remission is sudden, with recovery in 5–10 days	Children have sequelae, more severe in younger children; adults rarely have sequelae	Many mild or inapparent infections occur (ratio 58:1 in children, 1150:1 in adults)

SLE	Mosquito bite	Culex pipiens and C. quinquefasciatus, C. nigripalpus and other culicines	Wild birds	Encephalitis, with diffuse nerve-cell damage	Long-lasting, probably lifetime	Brief febrile illness with severe encephalitis in small proportion of cases	Cases of greater severity more frequently in elderly patients; sequelae rare	Ratio high, 64:1; attack rate of clinically apparent infections 280/100,000
CE	Mosquito bite	Aedes triseriatus and other Aedes and Culex; transovarial transmission demonstrated	Small mammals	Mild encephalitis	Probably long-lasting	Brief febrile illness and sometimes mild encephalitis	Encephalitis of mild to moderate severity in children and adults	Probably high
CTF	Tick bite	Dermacentor andersoni	Small mammals	Febrile illness of several days' duration; leukopenia	Probably long-lasting	Diphasic fever leukopenia; CNS or hemorrhagic complications occasionally in young children	Affects all ages; cases in children more severe	Mild and inapparent infections occur; frequency undetermined

[a] For definitions of abbreviations, see Table 3, footnote a.

seedbed for infection of succeeding cohorts of biting arthropods.

The site of multiplication of most arboviruses remains undetermined, but is presumed to be in the vascular epithelium and the reticuloendothelial cells on the lymph nodes, liver, spleen, and elsewhere. Liberation of virus from these organs constitutes the "systemic phase of viremia," resulting after 4–7 days in fever, chills, and aching. A number of arbovirus infections have two phases—this early phase and then a second phase with or without a few days of freedom from illness. The second phase may be attended by encephalitis, joint involvement, rash (sometimes hemorrhagic), and involvement of liver and kidneys. In most arbovirus infections, only the first phase occurs, and the disease is mild and "nonspecific." In other instances, the early phase may be missed and only the severe manifestations occur. The early phase is accompanied by leukopenia and the second phase often by leukocytosis. Tissue injury may be the direct effect of viral multiplication in susceptible cells, as is the case with liver involvement in yellow fever. The role of immunological injury is not clear, although antigen–antibody complexes are suspected of playing an important part in the pathogenesis of the dengue shock syndrome.[33]

Humoral antibodies regularly appear early in the course of arbovirus infection and constitute the major basis of immunity. Such immunity may be lifelong. No infection with yellow fever virus has been recorded in an individual who either had antibodies from an earlier infection or had a history of yellow fever vaccination with development of postvaccination antibody. The presence of antibodies in the blood at the time of exposure to an infected arthropod vector provides a primary deterrent to reinfection with the homologous virus. Later infection may occur with a virus strain related to but not identical with the original infecting virus. This has been reported for dengue (which has four "types"). Such an event has been demonstrated to produce an exaggerated antibody response, and such a response with the resulting antigen–antibody complexes is suspected of precipitating the host responses seen clinically as dengue hemorrhagic fever or dengue shock syndrome.[33]

The long persistence of CF antibody to dengue in the absence of reexposure and of reinfection[26] raises the possibility of persistence of the virus, per-haps in association with circulating macrophages. Marchete et al.[46] have shown that dengue virus multiplies in lymphocytes from individuals previously sensitized (i.e., infected) to this virus, but not in lymphocytes from those not so infected.

The role of cell-mediated immunity in arbovirus infections has been very little studied. It is possible that it may be important in controlling virus persistence and in determining the immunopathological lesions suspected in certain manifestations of arbovirus infection.

8. Patterns of Host Response

8.1. Clinical Features

Inapparent and subclinical human host responses predominate in most arbovirus infections. Clinical illness is frequently the exception rather than the rule. This varies from virus to virus. For example, infection with WEE, SLE, and CE viruses results principally in mild and inapparent infections, whereas in infection with EEE virus, the host response is likely to be clinically apparent and often severe; the reasons for these differences are not known.

The range of host responses to a few of the more frequently encountered arboviruses is seen in Table 7. The responses to individual viruses are shown in Tables 5 and 6 and in Section 10.

8.2. Diagnosis

Cases of arbovirus infections in the United States are not likely to be diagnosed unless there is a high degree of clinical suspicion operating. Outbreaks of encephalitis in horses in summer, caused by EEE, WEE, or VEE viruses, serve to focus attention on febrile illness in humans associated with symptoms or signs indicating involvement of the central nervous system (CNS). Cases with such symptoms and signs occurring in children in the Midwestern states such as Wisconsin, Indiana, Minnesota, and Ohio in late summer should arouse suspicion of CE virus involvement. SLE virus epidemic sweeps have few indicators in the natural scene. Birds, although widely infected, are not clinically ill, and the primary culicine mosquitos involved in transmission are diffusely spread throughout the United States, especially in areas with inadequate disposal of waste

Table 7. Patterns of Host Response to Arbovirus Infections in Man

Response	Examples[a]
Asymptomatic infection	WEE, SLE, CE
Mild febrile illness	WEE, SLE, CE, yellow fever
Influenzalike illness with aching and joint pains	Dengue, chikungunya
Encephalitis, mild	CE, WEE, SLE
Encephalitis, severe	SLE, EEE, WEE, tick-borne encephalitis
Jaundice, proteinuria	Yellow fever
Rash, sometimes with hemorrhagic manifestations	Dengue (chikungunya?)
Shock syndrome	Dengue (following secondary infection with a different dengue serotype)

[a] Certain viruses have been selected for this list particularly to illustrate the range of symptoms that may be seen in populations infected with a single virus. For definitions of abbreviations, see Table 3, footnote a.

water such as slum areas and the outskirts of towns. The risk may thus be generalized and diffuse and the prediction or pinpointing of an actual outbreak impossible.

Recognition of the arbovirus infection acquired by the traveler outside the United States also depends on the alertness of the examining physician. Rapid jet transport now permits exposed overseas travelers to reach home and fall sick even within the short incubation period of such infections. The physician must maintain a high degree of suspicion when seeing CNS infections or influenzalike illnesses occurring in travelers recently returned from areas endemic for arboviruses. Since specific diagnosis depends on the laboratory, if the specific question is not asked, the laboratory is not likely to carry out the tests needed for specific diagnosis.

It should be emphasized that arbovirus infections constitute only a small fraction of the encephalitis cases seen in the United States. For example, of 938 cases of infectious encephalitis reported to the Center for Disease Control (CDC) in 1977, only 10.7% were associated with arboviruses; 3.3% were due to mumps, 5.9% to exanthem viruses, 7.1% to other viruses, and an impressive 72.9% were of indeterminate etiology (Fig. 1).

The laboratory diagnosis depends on the isolation of the virus from the blood and/or a 4-fold rise in titer in a CF, HI, or neutralization of antibody test in sera taken during the acute and during the convalescent phase of illness. Often, the suspicion of an arbovirus infection in individual cases arises too late for virus isolation or for demonstration of a rise in antibody titer. Under these circumstances, the presence of a high antibody titer in a single serum may be significant if the infection is an uncommon one in that region, and particularly if antibody surveys reveal a low antibody prevalence, or if prior surveys have demonstrated the absence of antibody in that community. The appropriate procedure in suspected cases is to (1) notify the health department and seek background epidemiological and clinical data and (2) send acute and convalescent serum samples to the nearest public-health laboratory (usually a state laboratory) with a request for antibody tests for arboviruses and other encephalitis-producing viruses. Some state laboratories may not provide this testing, so a request for transshipment of sera to the CDC might be included. Usually, the specimens should not be shipped directly to the CDC.

9. Control and Prevention

Major control methods include (1) control of the arthropod vector, which may be by elimination of breeding sites or modification of them by application of insecticidal substances, or by direct attack on the adult arthropods through residual insecticide treatment of adult resting places; (2) avoidance of exposure to vector bites by screening of houses, by use of protective clothing, and by application of insect repellent sprays or creams when outside in high-risk areas; (3) immunization, a procedure widely used only for yellow fever and Japanese encephalitis in endemic areas. Specific control measures are discussed in appropriate sections below and

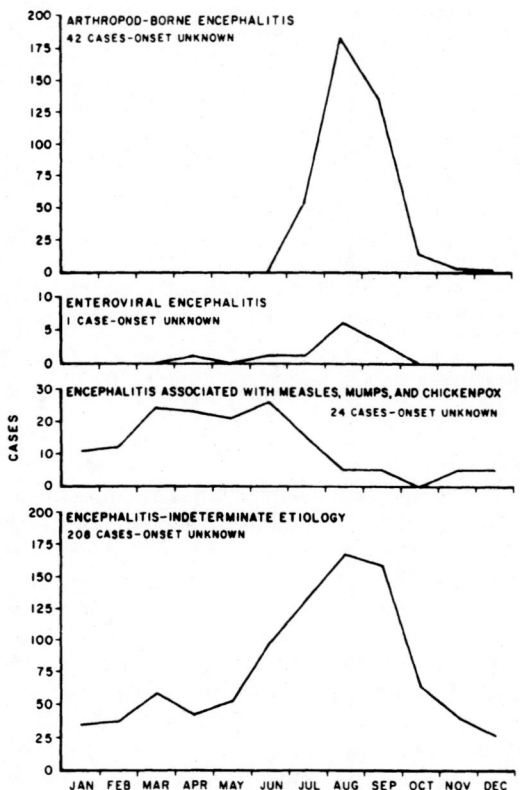

Fig. 1. Reported cases of encephalitis by etiology and month, United States, 1976. Final data not available for 1977.

are listed in Table 5 for arboviruses of importance outside the United States.

Control of vectors through biological approaches ranging from introduction of competing species, of parasites, including protozoa, helminths, bacteria, and viruses, or of genes deleterious to the vector population, or influencing the vector behavior or capacity to be infected with a pathogen is receiving much attention.[84b]

10. Characteristics of Selected Arboviruses

10.1. Arboviruses of Importance in the United States

Five arboviruses are of primary importance in human infections in the United States: eastern equine encephalitis (EEE), western equine encephalitis (WEE), St. Louis encephalitis (SLE), California encephalitis (CE), as subtype LaCrosse (LAC), and Colorado tick fever (CTF) viruses. Brief summaries

of main features for the five viruses are presented in Tables 3, 4, and 6. Powassan (POW), vesicular stomatitis (Indiana) (VSI), and Venezuelan equine encephalitis (VEE) are of minor importance for human disease or of very sporadic occurrence. More detailed presentations for all these viruses can be found in Horsfall and Tamm,[38] but for CE particularly, there is a body of new information in the periodical literature.

10.1.1. Eastern Equine Encephalitis. Involvement of human beings with EEE virus has been sporadic even under epidemic circumstances. Table 2 summarizes available morbidity and mortality data for the United States. Serosurveys of populations, even when focused on population groups estimated to be a greater risk, reveal very low rates of antibody prevalence. However, the high mortality associated with this infection (25–50%) demands continuing epidemiological vigilance. Epidemic outbreaks in equine populations in the Atlantic Seaboard states from Massachusetts to Florida, in the Midwest, and in the Gulf Coast states are kept in check through vaccination using a formalin-inactivated EEE vaccine. Immunization of humans has not been considered as indicated, except for laboratory workers engaged in specific EEE virus manipulation.

Without doubt, the cardinal epidemiological features that serve to protect human populations against outbreaks of EEE relate to the localization and feeding habits of the principal vector, the mosquito *Culiseta melanura*. This mosquito breeds in and remains localized to certain types of deep swamp locations in areas generally remote from human habitation and feeds mainly on small passerine wild birds in such places.[84] Other mosquitos, principally aedines, that feed on wild birds and on larger vertebrates may well be responsible for the occasional and unpredictable movements of virus from wild bird populations to larger vertebrates including equines and man. The movement of EEE virus into penned pheasant flocks is not well understood, but could happen by mosquito bite or by movement of infected wild birds, such as the English sparrow, into inadequately screened pens. Once introduced into penned pheasant populations, the virus can be transmitted from pheasant to pheasant by pecking. Debeaking of penned pheasants to abort such spread is common practice. The peak of occurrence of epidemics and human cases is late summer and early fall. The first heavy frosts signal the termination of transmission. In the southern and midwestern states, *C. melanura* is not found, and the vectors that transmit virus to the wild bird populations include other culicine and aedine species.

The incubation period in human beings is short. The ratio of inapparent or mild infections to severe infections is low (2–4:1). Immunity is probably long-lasting, with no reinfections being described. Fever followed by encephalitis in 1–2 days is the principal clinical feature. The encephalitis is rapidly progressing and often fatal, particularly in small children. Pathological features are those of a diffuse encephalitis with evidence of scattered neuronal destruction. Recovery is usually complete with few or no sequelae.

After initial clinical suspicion, diagnosis is established by virus isolation or more commonly by serological evidence of conversion (CF, HI, or N test) to EEE virus. Evidence of an epidemic involving birds and mosquitos and more particularly equines and human beings in a region should alert clinicians.

10.1.2. Western Equine Encephalitis. Infection of human beings with WEE is much more frequent than with EEE (Table 2), and there is a much higher ratio of inapparent to apparent (diagnosed) infections, estimated in one study as 58:1 in children and 1150:1 in adults.

The major virus activity in the western and southwestern states is closely tied to the presence and behavior of *Culex tarsalis* populations. This mosquito serves to transmit virus among wild birds. Since it also feeds readily on larger vertebrates, it requires no secondary help from other mosquito species to generate an epidemic. Several other mosquito species can also be infected and can transmit infection. The numbers of *C. tarsalis* mosquitos in a region can be augmented greatly by careless irrigation practices, and the major foci of virus activity involving human beings in the West and Southwest relate directly to major areas of crop irrigation. Proper water-management procedures can greatly reduce *C. tarsalis* production, as can the coordinated application of larvicidal measures. Vaccination with an inactivated WEE vaccine is widely used to protect equine populations. An attenuated vaccine strain has been shown to be effective.[9] Immunity conferred by natural infection is long-lasting. Antibody rates in human populations in irrigated regions of the West and Southwest may be high. Although WEE is prevalent on the Eastern Seaboard, infections in human beings are almost unknown. This is probably explainable on the basis of the vector (*Culiseta melanura*), as described for EEE. Reinfection has not been described.

In view of the high ratio of inapparent or mild cases to severe cases, the low figures for human mortality, and the millions of people potentially at risk, vaccination has not been considered necessary in human populations.

After an incubation period of several days, fever is seen, and may be followed by drowsiness and more pronounced signs of encephalitis. A fatal outcome is rare, but sequelae after encephalitis are not uncommon, particularly in small children. Pathological findings are those of a diffuse encephalitis and focal neuronal destruction.

Specific diagnosis is based on virus isolation, and more commonly on serological grounds (CF, HI, or N test), with a fourfold or greater rise in antibodies between early and convalescent specimens considered an adequate criterion. EEE and VEE are the only other antigenically related group A arboviruses in the United States, and the possibilities of confusion resulting from serological cross-reactivity are minimal. The laboratory difficulties are confined to such problems as anticomplementarity of sera (in CF), inadequate extraction of serum inhibitory factors (in HI), or nonreactive antigens (in CF, HI, or N test). Most of these problems can be recognized or resolved by inclusion of adequate controls in the diagnostic tests employed.

The monograph of Reeves and Hammon[56] provides much information on epidemiological studies on WEE in the West.

10.1.3. St. Louis Encephalitis. The first recognized outbreak of SLE in St. Louis in 1932[43] provided epidemiological data that have been added to, but not changed in most essential features, up to the present time.[78,78a]

SLE virus is widely prevalent in wild-bird populations in the southern, southeastern, central, southwestern, and western states in the summer months. There have been outbreaks as far north as New Jersey. The virus is transmitted by a number of culicine mosquitos, including *Culex pipiens, C. quinquefasciatus, C. tarsalis,* and *C. nigripalpus,* and by other mosquitos. In the West and Southwest, it is closely tied in with *C. tarsalis* and irrigation practices, much as is the case with WEE, although SLE may reach peaks of prevalence earlier in the summer season.[56] There is a diffuse endemicity over vast rural areas, with low rates of seropositives in human beings, and only occasional cases of disease recognized. However, there is a more marked concentration of virus activity in irrigated regions, with inapparent infection rates ranging between 10 and 70%.

In the central and southern states, although a diffuse spread of virus undoubtedly occurs, interest focuses on the periodic epidemic flareups on the outskirts of towns and cities. The principal vectors in such outbreaks, *C. pipiens* and *C. quinquefasciatus* (and in Florida *C. nigripalpus*), breed in great numbers under circumstances where there is inadequate disposal of waste water. Conditions are ideal for these vectors in the urban and suburban slum areas on the outskirts of towns and cities. While many communities are at risk annually, and while one or more annual outbreaks can be predicted with near certainty, the site(s) of such outbreak(s) cannot be predicted.

SLE affects all age groups, with a ratio of inapparent to apparent infections reported in one study[11] as 64:1, under circumstances where the attack rate for clinically apparent cases was 280/100,000. In the clinically apparent infections, most cases have a benign course, with fever for a few days, severe headache, and complete recovery. A few cases progress to more pronounced encephalitis, particularly in the older age groups. Remission may be dramatic, and recovery is usually complete. Sequelae, including mental deterioration, personality changes, muscle weakness, and paralysis, are uncommon.

Diagnosis is usually made by serological means. A leukopenia or mild leukocytosis, and slight increase in spinal fluid pressure, cells, and protein, leads to the suspicion of encephalitic involvement, but confirmation must come from virus isolation (very rarely accomplished) or from serological conversion in the CF, HI, or N test to the specific virus antigen. In geographic regions where other group B arboviruses are known to occur or are suspected, the serological conversion demonstrated between the specimen taken early in the course of illness and several weeks later must be evaluated with antigens or immune sera from the other group B viruses of the region included in the test.

There is no vaccine for SLE. Control in the face of an urban epidemic depends on the emergency application of mosquito-control measures. Long-term control for urban and suburban localities depends on good sanitation with respect to drainage and adequate disposal of waste water. In most rural areas, control measures aside from general protection against mosquito bites are not feasible. In more specific rural areas under irrigation, much can be accomplished through water management and directed application of insecticides to keep mosquito populations at a low level.

10.1.4. California Encephalitis. There is a gap of a couple of decades between the first isolation of CE virus from mosquitos in California by Hammon and Reeves[35] and their early recognition of human cases and the finding that the virus is responsible for many cases of "summer encephalitis" in the north central states. Several strains of CE are recognized,[81] but only one of these, the LAC subtype, has been shown to be important in the causation of human disease.[76]

The pattern of disease occurrence, and of human infection in general, is one relating to exposure in sylvan settings. Cases are seen sporadically in inhabitants and workers in forested areas and in picnickers and summer visitors to such areas. This reflects the occurrence of the main vector, *Aedes triseriatus*, a treehole-breeding mosquito of wide distribution, common locally in favorable forest habitats and suburban woodlands. The vector also breeds in water present in old tires in backyards in the LaCrosse area. The virus finds its endemic host in the small-animal populations of such regions. It has been shown in recent studies[80] that the virus can be passed transovarially (vertical transmission) and venereally (horizontal transmission).[77a] in mosquito populations. This may explain virus survival in northern climes, including northwestern Canada and the Yukon, as well as the northeastern states of the United States.

The recognized occurrence of the virus (including subtypes) is wider than the area within which human cases have been reported. The virus has been recovered repeatedly in Connecticut, for example, but no cases in human beings have been identified there despite continuing search.

The clinical features of illness are fever with mild to severe encephalitis.[76] Fatalities are rare; one report of autopsy findings describes diffuse encephalitic changes of neuronal degeneration and patchy inflammatory response in the cortex and in the basal ganglia.[77] Immunity is probably long-lasting. Immunity rates are high only in special population groups with extensive forest exposure.[49] Reinfection probably does not occur. Protective measures are limited to protection of individuals from the bite of mosquitos, through the application of insect repellents. In specific local situations, such as extensively used campgrounds, area disinsectization can be considered. Diagnosis, following initial clinical suspicion, may be by virus isolation, but is much more commonly based on serological procedures (CF or N test) on appropriately spaced serum specimens. There is no difficulty in narrowing diagnosis to the California subset of viruses, but difficulties do remain, only partially resolved as yet, of pinpointing the specific CE subtype unless the virus itself has been isolated, either from the case (the unlikeliest but most desirable situation) or from mosquitoes captured in the vicinity of the infection.

10.1.5. Colorado Tick Fever. CTF, an orbivirus, tick-transmitted and localized to mountainous regions of the western United States, accounts for nearly as much reported morbidity as EEE, WEE, SLE, and CE combined (Table 2), but fortunately it rarely causes serious or fatal illness. Much of the reported morbidity is dependent on the vigilance of individual physicians in the Rocky Mountain area, reporting to and submitting materials for diagnosis to health-department laboratories. There is still undoubtedly much underreporting due to nonrecognition of the disease.

Infection is picked up by hikers, foresters, or vacationers venturing into hilly or mountainous areas populated by various rodents, particularly ground squirrel and chipmunk species, which are in turn infected by immature and adult stages of the wood tick *Dermacentor andersoni*.[13] In diagnosed cases, there is always a history of exposure to ticks, although there is not always a recollection of tick bite.

Overall antibody prevalence is low, as measured by serosurveys of population groups, and despite wide virus distribution in the endemic regions, human infections are usually sporadic and casual. However, one survey of 178 sera from sheepherders revealed 32% seropositives.[29]

Following a tick bite, the incubation period is 3–6 days, with sudden onset of fever, headache, retroorbital pain, and severe muscle pains. A rash is sometimes seen. There may be a brief remission followed by a second bout of fever, and occasionally even three or four exacerbations may be seen. Leukopenia is characteristic, is present by the 3rd day of fever, and becomes pronounced by the 5th or 6th day. Serious complications such as encephalitis or severe bleeding are limited almost exclusively to children. The immunity following recovery is presumably lifelong.

Diagnosis is readily made by isolation of the virus from the blood, the virus being associated with the red blood cells.[39] The resultant viremia is a regular feature throughout the illness. Virus isolation can be made by inoculation of infant mice or of KB or BHK-21 cell cultures. Virus has been isolated from erythrocytes of patients as early as 1 day and as late as 120 days after onset of symptoms.[29] Serological techniques are useful where virus-isolation facilities are lacking. Antibodies appear late, CF antibodies being detectable 4–6 weeks after onset, neutralizing antibodies after 2–4 weeks. An indirect fluorescent-antibody (IFA) test has been shown to be useful,[25] with titers appearing earlier after onset of illness and reaching higher levels than CF titers. An unusual feature of this tick-transmitted orbivirus is that in addition to propagating in various mammalian-cell cultures, the virus also multiplies in a mosquito-cell culture line.[86] This is in decided contrast to most other tick-transmitted arboviruses.

A formalinized vaccine has been described,[75] but has not been licensed. Protection against infection is largely a matter of protection against tick bite (repellents, protective clothing, avoidance of tick-infected regions), and there is no specific therapy.

10.2. Other Arboviruses in the United States That Affect Human Beings

Several other arboviruses capable of causing illness are thus far considered of only minor importance as causative agents of human disease in the United States.

10.2.1. Venezuelan Equine Encephalitis. VEE is an alphavirus (group A arbovirus) responsible for large outbreaks of encephalitis in horses in South and Central America and the West Indies. The first reported horse outbreak in the United States occurred in 1971 in the Southwest, coincident with an extensive outbreak in Mexico. There were 84 laboratory-confirmed human cases. Lord[41] has summarized VEE history in the New World. No epidemic activity has been detected since.

VEE is mosquito-transmitted, with natural reservoirs in small mammals rather than birds.[8] Human cases, diagnosed as encephalitis of mild or moderate severity, are seen in connection with horse outbreaks. Fatal infection of human beings has been described.[24]

A subtype of VEE has been found in southern Florida that is less virulent for horses, and possibly for human beings also. Occasional human infections have been described.[79]

10.2.2. Powassan. POW is the only tick-transmitted virus of the tick-borne encephalitis subgroup of flaviviruses thus far encountered in the New World. It is a relative of tick-borne encephalitis virus, which is an important pathogen in the USSR and northern Europe, and of Kyasanur Forest disease virus, a human pathogen in Mysore State, India. POW virus is widely distributed in Canada and the more northern states of the United States as an infection in various small rodents. It is transmitted by hard ticks (Ixodidae). The original virus isolation was from the brain of a child who died in Ontario in 1959.[48] Since that time, there have been very few human immunes found in extensive antibody surveys, plus a bare smattering of cases in humans, which have been nonfatal.[30]

A factor that limits the invasiveness of the virus for man is undoubtedly the reluctance of the vector ticks, *Ixodes cookei* and *I. marxi*, to attach to and to feed on human beings. Old World counterpart ticks, *I. ricinus* and *I. persulcatus*, do attack human beings readily.

Diagnosis can be accomplished by serological means, taking care to rule out cross-reactions from other flavivirus infections (particularly SLE in the United States). The cardinal step in diagnosis is the initial clinical suspicion, leading to a directed laboratory study.

10.2.3. Vesicular Stomatitis Virus, Indiana Subtype. Epizootics of VSI, a rhabdovirus, have occurred repeatedly in the United States. Mosquitos or *Phlebotomus* flies are suspected as vectors. Recognized infections in human beings are rare. Several infections occurring during an epizootic in Colorado were reported.[27] Widespread immunity to this virus and to VS-New Jersey is reported from Panama,[72] with no evidence of illness in human beings.

Diagnosis would start with suspicion, particularly if an epizootic is in progress, and seroconversion is readily demonstrated by CF.

10.3. Arboviruses Outside the United States That Affect Human Beings

Only a fraction of the over 400 arboviruses now catalogued, possibly only a fifth, are ever involved in causation of recognizable disease in human beings. However, several of the most important and dangerous diseases that afflict mankind are caused by arboviruses. Table 5 gives a very brief summary of the most important exotic (for the United States) arboviruses, plus a selected group of viruses of lesser but still considerable importance. The epidemiologist or physician in the United States will not encounter any of these infections as endemic diseases (with the limited exception of VEE, mentioned earlier). However, with populations as mobile as is the American, there exists the possibility that any of these diseases could enter the country with immigrants or with tourists coming from Africa, Asia, and South America particularly. With the common feature of incubation periods of several days, it not only is possible but also has happened repeatedly that infected individuals, in the incubation period and asymptomatic, can enter the country and proceed to fall ill within the next few days. Also, acutely ill patients may be evacuated from a foreign station for hospitalization in the United States.

The recognition of such illness is complicated by the fact that in the early stages, differential diagnosis is almost impossible. Various causes of febrile illness must be reviewed: malaria, trypanosomiasis, typhoid fever, typhus fever, leptospirosis, hepatitis, gastrointestinal infections with diarrhea and vomiting, and the grab bag of "influenzalike" illnesses. The possibility of arriving at a correct diagnosis is directly dependent on the alertness of the examining physician in uncovering a travel history, guessing at possibilities from such history, and performing or ordering appropriate laboratory examinations (virus isolation attempt, CF, HI, or N test). If the question is not asked, there is small likelihood that appropriate tests will be performed. Not many laboratories, furthermore, are capable of performing the required diagnostic tests.

In general terms, the infections listed in Table 5 are not protracted febrile illnesses, but are acute. Frequently, physicians, baffled by a patient with history of protracted fever, or bouts of fever over a span of weeks, and in hopes of leaving no stone unturned, request examination for possible arbovirus infection. The possibility of an arbovirus causing such an illness is practically nil. However, it can be rewarding to examine serologically a specimen taken several weeks after an acute illness has resolved, even though there may exist no specimen from the acute phase of illness. For example, a positive reaction for chikungunya virus in an American tourist back from a trip to the Far East would be certain evidence of an infection acquired overseas and possibly could be related to an exposure or illness specifically narrowed to the Far East trip.

Several of the arboviruses earlier discussed as occurring in the United States also occur in Central and South America and some of the West Indian islands (EEE, WEE, SLE, and VEE, for example).

10.3.1. Eastern Equine Encephalitis. EEE virus has been recovered from various mosquitos and birds from Canada to the Argentine. Equine outbreaks of large size occasionally occur. Cases in human beings have been seen in Jamaica and the Dominican Republic, associated with EEE strains very closely related to the continental United States strains of virus. Farther to the south, cases have rarely been recognized, yet a serosurvey in one part of the Amazon Delta revealed a high rate of immunity in human beings with no history of encephalitis.[21] It has been noted[18] that Panamanian, Trinidadian, and South American strains of EEE can be distinguished serologically from North American strains. No studies on the comparative pathogenicity of such strains have been made.

10.3.2. Western Equine Encephalitis and St. Louis Encephalitis. WEE and SLE viruses are also widely distributed south of the United States. A very few cases of human disease have been reported in these countries.

10.3.3. Venezuelan Equine Encephalitis. VEE did indeed stage a successful invasion of the United States, even though it was a short-lived one, in 1971. Through the decade of the 1960s and to date, this virus has been responsible for many outbreaks of disease in equines in Latin America. In some of these outbreaks, there have been numerous cases of encephalitis in human beings, with some fatal cases reported. Several substrains of VEE have been described.[85] The relationship of these various substrains to the epidemiological pattern of epidemic and endemic VEE in Latin America is not fully understood as yet.

10.3.4. Yellow Fever. Yellow fever (YF) in urban or jungle form is a continuing threat. The two forms are nonetheless the same virus and the same disease, distinguished on epidemiological grounds. The urban form is transmitted by *Aedes aegypti*, a house-frequenting mosquito of the Old and New World tropics and subtropics. The disease is a threat in mosquito-infested urban and suburban population centers. Urban outbreaks are secondary to the disease cycle in the jungle, where virus transmission occurs in monkey populations, the vectors being *Haemagogus* or aedine mosquitoes. Human beings are involved in the jungle cycle only as they are exposed through working in or entering into the jungles. This is a very real threat highlighted by the reported outbreaks in 1978 of jungle YF in Colombia, South America, and Trinidad, West Indies.

Many cases of YF are so mild as to escape detection. Diagnosis may be suggested by clinical signs in a severe case and confirmed by virus isolation and serological changes.

Control of the disease can be achieved (for the urban cycle) by control of the vector mosquito (*Aedes aegypti*). Human beings can be protected by immunization with YF-17D vaccine (not advised for infants under 1 year of age). A list of the centers in the United States authorized to give the vaccination can be obtained from the Public Health Service.

10.3.5. Dengue and Dengue Hemorrhagic Fever. Dengue viruses are of four recognizable subtypes (DEN types 1, 2, 3, 4) and occur in the Old World and New World tropics and subtropics. One or more of the subtypes may be present wherever the mosquito *Aedes aegypti* abounds and in the Orient may be associated also with *A. albopictus*. The illness is of acute onset, with fever, rash, aching pains of the extremities, and general grippelike features. The fever curve may be of saddleback type. The endemic may be rarely recognized in indigenous populations. The epidemics in due course may become of such size that medical personnel become aware of the situation, although it is certain that large epidemics may go unrecognized, or if recognized go unreported. Fatalities from the basic infection are very rare. However, in recent years, an illness has been described in children in the Orient that begins as a dengue infection by any of the subtypes, progresses through stages with hemorrhagic phenomena (DHF) to a shock syndrome (DSS) and often terminates fatally.[36] Older children and adults are rarely afflicted. Various explanations for this deviant syndrome have been advanced, which are summarized by Halstead.[33] He favors a hypothesis that the serious complications occur in children who have had an earlier dengue infection and who react to a subsequent infection with a different dengue subtype by an exaggerated production of antibodies. A resultant antigen–antibody complexing may then underlie what is essentially a response in the child to the immune complex. This hypothesis has been challenged.[7]

Within the past decade, there have been many outbreaks of dengue in the Caribbean and circum-Caribbean area, including a larger outbreak in Puerto Rico in 1977–1978 that spread to other islands. Dengue types 1, 2, and 3 have been incriminated in these outbreaks. Hemorrhagic manifestations have been rare. A dengue type 1 outbreak occurred in southwestern Texas in 1980.[78b]

Diagnosis of dengue and dengue hemorrhagic fever may be on clinical grounds reinforced by virus isolation or by serological findings in the CF, HI, or N test. Diagnosis of specific dengue type can be done only in a few specialized laboratories.

Treatment of uncomplicated dengue is symptomatic. Treatment of the disease with hemorrhagic manifestations and shock is directed toward immediate and vigorous combating of the shock syndrome. Prompt attention can result in a marked lowering of mortality figures.

Control of dengue is basically control of the vector mosquito, *A. aegypti*, and avoidance of being bitten by mosquitos. Rudnick,[59] working in Malaya, has evidence that forest monkeys may be involved in a "jungle dengue" cycle, with *A. albopictus* serving as a vector. Such a possibility postpones hopes of eventual eradication of the disease. Vaccines for prevention of infection and illness are being investigated.

10.3.6. Chikungunya and O'Nyong Nyong. Chikungunya (CHIK), an alphavirus (group A arbovirus), has been responsible for large outbreaks of denguelike illness in Africa and Asia. It is spread by *Aedes aegypti*. It occurs in the same regions of Asia as does dengue and is possibly responsible for a small proportion of the cases of hemorrhagic fever–shock syndrome. A closely related virus, O'nyong nyong (ONN), associated with epidemics of disease in human beings in East Africa, is spread by anopheline mosquitoes. Wild primates are suspected of being reservoirs for both viruses. Diagnosis may be on clinical grounds, buttressed by the laboratory, including virus isolation and specific serological changes (CF, HI, or N test). Clinically, CHIK infections can be differentiated from dengue, as Carey[14] points out, in that with CHIK, the pains are restricted more to the joints, the febrile period is shorter and not diphasic, and many patients experience persistent residual joint pains following the acute episode.

Such analyses may help in identifying the disease pattern in an epidemic, but it remains of prime importance—with yellow fever, the dengues, chikungunya, and other nonarbovirus infections such as influenza, early smallpox (before the eruption appears), malaria, typhoid fever, rickettsioses and relapsing fever, leptospirosis, Lassa fever, and numerous other endemic and exotic infections—for the diagnostician to remember that the first few days of illness of an individual patient may be accompanied by a disease pattern of quite unspecific character.

No specific treatment exists for CHIK and ONN infections, and control is limited to vector control plus avoidance of being mosquito-bitten.

10.3.7. Japanese Encephalitis. Japanese encephalitis (JE), a mosquito-transmitted flavivirus (group B arbovirus), is closely related to SLE in the New World, to West Nile virus in Africa and the Middle East, and to Murray Valley encephalitis (MVE) virus in Australia–New Guinea. Not only are the viruses close serological relatives, but also the ecological pattern of disease is similar, with mosquito vectors (*Culex* species usually), wild-bird vertebrate reservoirs, and patterns of involvement of human beings with large numbers of inapparent or mild infections for each severe case seen. Nonetheless, JE, affecting huge populations in rice-growing, suburban, and rural regions of the Orient, has been responsible for large outbreaks of encephalitis in Korea, Japan, China, Taiwan, and India, and a more diffuse scattering of cases in Malaysia, Southeast Asia, and Indonesia. The outbreaks occur in the summer months and affect all age groups, but with peak mortality in the younger age groups, pre-teenagers, and the elderly.

Diagnosis is on clinical grounds, reinforced by laboratory findings in serology (CF, HI, or N test).

There is no specific treatment. Control may be through mosquito control. This can be very difficult in extensive rice-growing regions. In recent years, extensive vaccination campaigns have been initiated, in Japan in particular, using an inactivated vaccine prepared from infected infant mouse brains. The vaccination program, concentrating on children, has been accompanied by a marked reduction in the incidence of serious disease.

10.3.8. Murray Valley Encephalitis. MVE is a close serological relative of SLE, JE, and West Nile viruses, with a similar epidemiological pattern. It is localized to the Australian continent and islands to the north. There is a zone of overlap presumably at some latitudinal level in the East Indies (Wallace's line?) with JE from the north and MVE from the south interdigitating. However, the two viruses are so closely related serologically that the precise localization of this level, if there is a precise localization, remains undefined. The first human epidemic of MVE was described by French[28] in 1952, and since that time case reports have been very sporadic. However, in 1974, there was widespread occurrence of cases in humans again in Australia.[54]

10.3.9. Tick-Borne Encephalitis. Tick-borne encephalitis (TBE) is a flavivirus responsible for a tick-transmitted disease of the more northerly Eurasian regions. The disease has been known under several names, including Russian spring–summer encephalitis and Far Eastern encephalitis. The acute illness is often followed by encephalitis with high mortality rates and has been seen in most of the northern European countries, Russia, and Siberia. The endemic virus cycle involves small mammals (and to a lesser extent birds) in forested regions and the vector ticks, *Ixodes ricinus* and *I. persulcatus*. These ticks will feed readily on human beings, if human beings invade the tick ecosystem in forested lands of moderate elevation in the palearctic regions. Most cases are reported in forest and construction workers in newly opened regions, woodsmen, trappers, and farmers. At the western end of distribution of this virus, human disease is not seen, and the tick-transmitted, closely related virus of louping ill has effects only on sheep, with a virus reservoir in the small-mammal population. As mentioned in Section 10.2.2, the closely related virus in the nearctic region, POW, is transmitted by *I. marxi* and *I. cookei*. Fortunately, these two ticks rarely attack man, so the disease in the New World remains essentially a curiosity. Antibodies to TBE have been found in human populations in hilly or mountainous regions of Italy, Greece, and Turkey. The closely related virus that causes Kyasanur Forest disease (KFD) in Mysore State, India, is also tick-transmitted and has a vertebrate host cycle in two monkey species of the region, as well as in small mammals. None of the TBE subset of viruses has been found in countries south of the equator. It is well known that ticks can be transported on birds. With millions of birds flying south each season, in both the Old World and the New World, it is not at all comprehended why foci of infection with TBE have not been established south of the equator. There are recent unpublished data establishing a TBE relative in Australia.

Transovarial transmission of TBE and KFD viruses has been demonstrated in vector ticks.

No specific therapy exists for TBE or KFD infections. Prevention is through control of tick populations, protection against tick bite (repellents, protective clothing), and avoidance of tick habitats. An inactivated vaccine is widely used in the USSR to protect special groups of workers, and inhabitants in known TBE foci. Diagnosis is made on clinical grounds, reinforced by laboratory procedures of virus isolation and serological tests (CF, HI, or N test).

10.3.10. Crimean Hemorrhagic Fever and Congo. Crimean hemorrhagic fever (CHF) was first recognized in the southern USSR as a clinical entity in 1944. The causative virus was not finally isolated until the mid-1960s. In the meantime, workers in the Congo and Uganda had isolated several virus strains from febrile human beings, to which the name "Congo virus" (CON) was applied. Casals[19] showed in 1969 that the two viruses were indistinguishable.

In the southern USSR and Bulgaria, several hundred cases of CHF are seen annually, with a mortality rate as high as 15–20%. The cases present as febrile illness, with pronounced hemorrhagic manifestations in severe cases. Virus isolation and seroconversions (CF particularly) establish the diagnosis, and it has been noted that the seroreactions are more pronounced and elevated titers persist longer in patients with severe illness than in those with mild disease. Cases are seen in rural regions and are almost invariably associated with bite of certain ixodid ticks of the region, which infest small mammals, particularly rabbits. Tick-control measures have been proposed. An immune γ-globulin preparation has been made and is under trial for treatment of cases.

The situation in Africa is still a challenging unknown. After the initial finding of several human cases in the 1950s (one possible fatality), no additional cases have been found. Yet the known range of the virus has been expanded enormously, with numerous isolations from ticks, cattle, goats, and a hedgehog, and from *Culicoides* (biting gnats) in Nigeria and from ticks in Senegal. The disease in man remains to be described in West Africa.

Diagnosis is by clinical criteria (in USSR) buttressed by virus isolation and by serological tests (CF and immunoprecipitin tests). Nosocomial infections have been reported from the USSR in hospital staff and laboratory workers.

10.3.11. Rift Valley Fever Virus. This virus, a phlebovirus transmitted by mosquitoes, has long been recognized as causing serious illness in sheep, and also in man, in countries south of the Sahara. In 1977, it was responsible for a major outbreak of disease in animals and man in Egypt.[84a]

11. Unresolved Problems

Unresolved problems are discussed from several points of view, relating to the viruses, the vectors, the vertebrate hosts, and transmission cycles involving virus, vector, and host. The disease in the vertebrate host, which includes the host response to the pathogen, merits independent consideration. Problems relating to the epidemiology of each specific disease require a synthesis of many specific items, and, finally, effective control exercised at the level of the virus, the vector, or the vertebrate requires thorough understanding of the epidemiological background. Specific examples will help to illustrate problems.

11.1. The Viruses

Much progress has been made in recent years in categorizing the several hundred described arboviruses and determining the biochemical, growth, and morphological characteristics in intact vertebrates, in invertebrates, and in cell-culture systems of vertebrate and invertebrate cells. Yet it is obvious that the surface has barely been scratched. This includes all the arboviruses, even such much-studied models as Sindbis, Semliki Forest, and the vesicular stomatitis viruses. An area still quite unresolved concerns the extent of RNA homology that may exist among the numerous members of a given arbovirus grouping, such as the alphaviruses (group A arboviruses), the flaviviruses (group B arboviruses), the bunyaviruses (Bunyamwera supergroup arboviruses), the rhabdoviruses (of the arbovirus subset), and the orbiviruses.

11.2. The Vectors

The factors that determine specific virus–vector associations are still unknown. A mosquito-transmitted flavivirus (such as YF) will not multiply in ticks, and a tick-transmitted flavivirus (such as TBE) will not multiply in mosquitoes.

There is a continuing need for taxonomic refinements with respect to arthropods, such as the need for more information on both Old World and New World mosquitoes of the genera *Culex* and *Aedes*, and *Phlebotomus* and *Culicoides* sandflies. This need is generated by the increasing realization of their involvement with a large number of arboviruses. The same remarks are pertinent for the tick vectors. The need is equally great for more information on the biology, feeding preferences, longevity, flight range, and distribution of each arthropod species involved. The genetic constitution of each vector species is basic to an understanding of what constitutes a vector, both physiologically and behaviorally, and will become increasingly important as control of vectors through genetic manipulation is considered.

11.3. The Vertebrate Hosts

For most of the arboviruses, the primary vertebrate host, i.e., the host that serves as the basic unit for propagation of the virus, is some creature other than man. For many of the arboviruses, the vertebrate hosts are not yet determined or are recognized on the most tenuous of evidence. Identification of the host(s) is a prime need, and following this a biological profile of the host, involving (as is the case for arthropods also) the full range of biological and ecological considerations, as well as the degree of host susceptibility to the virus.

11.4. Transmission Cycles Involving Virus, Vector, and Vertebrate

Full cycles are known for very few of the arboviruses. A skeptic may ask whether the complete cycle is known with certainty for any arbovirus, even for such extensively studied ones as EEE, WEE, SLE, and YF. The problem of virus persistence in nature is a particularly baffling one. For example, there are many theories and few facts to explain how a given virus manages to overwinter or survive past a long dry season, when vectors may practically disappear, and vertebrate populations decline (or go into hibernation). Such problems have been explored from the angle of vector populations over-

wintering, with some members harboring virus, or vertebrate populations overwintering with some members infected and the infection in a latent phase, awaiting a vernal reactivation stimulus. Transovarial transmission, permitting passage of virus to generation after generation of vector without the need for an intercalated vertebrate host, has received recent stimulation from demonstrations of the phenomenon with LaCrosse,[80a] dengue,[58a] Japanese encephalitis,[58a] and yellow fever[1a] viruses; venereal transmission in mosquitoes has also been demonstrated.[77a]

Reeves[55] discusses the epidemiological problems of overwintering of arboviruses in northern countries, and possible transport via infected vectors on migrating birds, his discussion extending to Old World as well as New World viruses. Lord and Calisher[42] discuss the transport of arboviruses in infected migrating birds along the Atlantic Coast flyway of the United States.

Certain of the tick-transmitted viruses, such as CTF and TBE, utilizing mechanisms of long persistence in ticks plus transovarial transmission of virus, exist in endemic form in defined geographic areas. For mosquito-transmitted viruses such as EEE, WEE, SLE, VEE, and many others, it has been difficult to establish whether a virus is permanently endemic in a region or is periodically reintroduced via vectors or migrant vertebrates.

Studies of transmission cycles are tied in closely with simulation of cycles by models, with carefully defined parameters. Such models may permit computer manipulation and simulation of field conditions by varying the values applied to defined parameters, following which epidemic curves can be generated. Macdonald[45] has provided a model for malaria. A model for an arbovirus with a vertebrate host in addition to man is of necessity much more complex than one for a simple host–parasite relationship. Much further work on models is needed, with hope of eventual prediction of outbreaks.

Specific cycles and the limits of knowledge concerning them are discussed under the various specific viruses in preceding pages.

11.5. Disease in the Vertebrate Host

Infection in the vertebrate host (including man) has in the past received more attention in the fields of pathology and response of the host immune system than in the fields of pathophysiology and host response to immunological states. The dengue hemorrhagic fever–shock phenomena have awakened an interest in the host response to the presence of an immune complex as a contributing factor to illness in the host. Treatment of disease is much more likely to have success in the area of treatment of syndromes that arise from host responses to virus proliferation and antibody production, including the formation of antigen–antibody complexes, than in the area of specific antiviral substances. Studies of the human response to arboviral infections are made difficult since the epidemics that provide numbers of cases for study usually occur unpredictably in time and often far from modern facilities required for detailed clinical investigation.

Recognition of disease in the vertebrate host calls for further development of simple diagnostic techniques, including techniques for virus isolation, detection of immune response, and monitoring of impaired physiological states.

11.6. Control

Virus vaccines are an obvious means of control, yet for man and the arboviruses, there exists only an attenuated yellow fever (17D) vaccine in use on an international scale. Attenuated dengue virus vaccines, TBE vaccines, and vaccines for VEE, WEE, and JE have been developed and tried on a limited scale. Killed vaccines for TBE, EEE, WEE, and JE have been used, in some cases extensively. Hammon[34] provides a detailed discussion of problems.

Development of methodology for fractionation of viruses into component antigens provides hopes for better vaccines. In the arbovirus area, there has been only limited exploration of this potential.

Control at the vector level involves continuing work on methodology for control of arthropods. Development of resistance to various of the chlorinated hydrocarbons used as insecticides has impaired many control programs, and recent action banning the use of residual insecticides has further intensified the need for exploration of alternative methods for vector control. Work in progress at the University of California[6] and elsewhere leads to the hope that isolation of clones of the mosquito *Culex tarsalis* in nature, or the induction of genetic variants in the laboratory, may lead to effective con-

trol strategies. One approach that merits consideration is the introduction into a mosquito population of genes relating to (1) increased insecticide susceptibility, (2) reduced capacity to support virus multiplication and/or to transmit virus, (3) alternatives in host feeding preferences, (4) reduction in numbers through mutations leading to reduction in reproductive success (sterile males, conditional lethal mutants), and (5) subversions of host feeding habits. The possibility of loading mosquito populations with an insect virus innocuous to human beings, with intent to block reproduction of viruses pathogenic for human beings, is also being studied.[58]

Control procedures at the level of the vertebrate reservoir have not received serious consideration in the arbovirus field. Certainly, rodent control has long been successfully applied for plague control, and more recently for control of Bolivian hemorrhagic fever, caused by the arenavirus Machupo. Monkey extermination for yellow fever control and extermination of wild-bird populations for control of EEE, WEE, SLE, or JE are not acceptable procedures within today's society.

12. References

1. ADLDINGER, H. K., STONE, S. S., HESS, W. R., AND BACHRACH, H. L., Extraction of infectious deoxynucleic acid from African swine fever virus, *Virology* **30:**750–752 (1966).

1a. AITKEN, T. H. G., TESH, R. B., BEATY, B., AND ROSEN, L., Transovarial transmission of yellow fever virus by mosquitoes (*Aedes aegypti*), *Am. J. Trop. Med. Hyg.* **28:**119–121 (1979).

2. AMERICAN COMMITTEE ON ARTHROPOD-BORNE VIRUSES, *Catalogue of Arthropod-Borne Viruses of the World*, U.S. Public Health Service Publication No. 1760, Washington, D.C., 1967; 2 ed.: *International Catalogue of Arboviruses Including Certain Other Viruses of Vertebrates*, 1975.

3. AMERICAN COMMITTEE ON ARTHROPOD-BORNE VIRUSES, Catalogue of Arthropod-Borne Viruses of the World, *Am. J. Trop. Med. Hyg. Suppl.* **19:**1082–1160 (1970).

4. AMERICAN COMMITTEE ON ARTHROPOD-BORNE VIRUSES, Catalogue of Arthropod-Borne and Selected Vertebrate Viruses of the World, *Am. J. Trop. Med. Hyg. Suppl.* **20:**1018–1050 (1971).

4a. AMERICAN COMMITTEE ON ARTHROPOD-BORNE VIRUSES, Catalogue of Arthropod-Borne and Selected Vertebrate Viruses of the World, *Am. J. Trop. Med. Hyg. Suppl.* **27:**372–440 (1978).

5. ARDOIN, P., CLARKE, D. H., AND HANNOUN, C., The

preparation of arbovirus hemagglutinins by sonication and trypsin treatment, *Am. J. Trop. Med. Hyg.* **18**:592–598 (1969).

6. ASMAN, S. M., Cytogenetic observations in *Culex tarsalis*: Mitosis and meiosis, *J. Med. Entomol.* **11**:375–382 (1974).

7. BARNES, W. J. S., AND ROSEN, L., Fatal hemorrhagic disease and shock associated with primary dengue infection on a Pacific island, *Am. J. Trop. Med. Hyg.* **23**:495–506 (1974).

7a. BEATY, B. J., SHOPE, R. E., AND CLARKE, D. H. Salt-dependent hemagglutination with Bunyaviridae antigens, *J. Clin. Microbiol.* **5**:548–550 (1977).

8. BIGLER, W. J., VENTURA, A. K., LEWIS, A. L., WELLINGS, F. M., AND EHRENKRANZ, N. J., Venezuelan equine encephalomyelitis in Florida: Endemic virus circulation in native rodent populations of Everglades hammocks, *Am. J. Trop. Med. Hyg.* **23**:513–521 (1974).

9. BINN, L. N., SPONSELLER, M. L., WOODING, W. L., MCCONNELL, S. J., SPERTZEL, R. O., AND YAGER, R. H., Efficacy of an attenuated western encephalitis vaccine in equine animals, *Am. J. Vet. Res.* **27**:1599–1604 (1966).

10. BORDEN, E. C., SHOPE, R. E., AND MURPHY, F. A., Physicochemical and morphological relationships of some arthropod-borne viruses to bluetongue virus—a new taxonomic group: Physicochemical and serological studies, *J. Gen. Virol.* **13**:261–271 (1971).

11. BRODY, J. A., BURNS, K. F., BROWNING, G., AND SCHATTNER, J. D., Apparent and inapparent attack rates for St. Louis encephalitis in a selected population, *N. Engl. J. Med.* **261**:644–646 (1959).

12. BUCKLEY, S. M., Susceptibility of the *Aedes albopictus* and *Aedes aegypti* cell lines to infection with arboviruses, *Proc. Soc. Exp. Biol. Med.* **131**:625–630 (1969).

13. BURGDORFER, W., AND EKLUND, C. M., Studies on the ecology of Colorado tick fever virus in western Montana, *Am. J. Hyg.* **69**:127–137 (1959).

14. CAREY, D. E., Chikungunya and dengue: A case of mistaken identity? *J. Hist. Med. Allied Sci.* **26**:243–262 (1971).

15. CASALS, J., Immunological relationship among central nervous system viruses, *J. Exp. Med.* **79**:341–359 (1944).

16. CASALS, J., The arthropod-borne group of animal viruses, *Trans. N. Y. Acad. Sci.* **19**:219–235 (1957).

17. CASALS, J., Viral encephalitis, in: *Viral Encephalitis: A Symposium* (WILLIAM S. FIELDS AND RUSSELL J. BLATTNER, eds.), pp. 5–21, Charles C. Thomas, Springfield, Illinois, 1958.

18. CASALS, J., Antigenic variants of eastern equine encephalitis virus, *J. Exp. Med.* **119**:547–565 (1964).

19. CASALS, J., Antigenic similarity between the virus causing Crimean hemorrhagic fever and Congo virus, *Proc. Soc. Exp. Biol. Med.* **131**:233–236 (1969).

20. CASALS, J., AND BROWN, E. V., Hemagglutination with arthropod-borne viruses, *J. Exp. Med.* **99**:429–449 (1954).

21. CAUSEY, O. R., AND THEILER, M., Virus antibody survey of sera of residents of the Amazon valley in Brazil, *Am. J. Trop. Med. Hyg.* **7**:36–41 (1958).

22. CLARKE, D. H., AND CASALS, J., Techniques for hemagglutination and hemagglutination-inhibition with arthropod-borne viruses, *Am. J. Trop. Med. Hyg.* **7**:561–573 (1958).

23. DOWNS, W. G., AITKEN, T. H. G., AND ANDERSON, C. R., Activities of the Trinidad Regional Virus Laboratory in 1953 and 1954 with special reference to the yellow fever outbreak in Trinidad, B.W.I., *Am. J. Trop. Med. Hyg.* **4**:837–843 (1955).

24. EHRENKRANZ, N. J., AND VENTURA, A. K., Venezuelan equine encephalitis virus infection in man. *Annu. Rev. Med.* **25**:9–14 (1974).

25. EMMONS, R. W., DONDERO, D. V., DEVLIN, V., AND LENNETTE, E. H., Serologic diagnosis of Colorado tick fever: A comparison of complement-fixation, immuno-fluorescence, and plaque reduction methods, *Am. J. Trop. Med. Hyg.* **18**:796–802 (1969).

26. EVANS, A. S., COX, F., NANKERVIS, G., OPTON, E., SHOPE, R., WELLS, A. V., AND WEST, B., A health and seroepidemiological survey of a community in Barbados, *Int. J. Epidemiol.* **3**:167–175 (1974).

26a. EVANS, A. S., CASALS, J., OPTON, E. M., BORMAN, E. K., LEVINE, L., AND CUADRADO, R. R., A nationwide serum survey of Colombian military recruits, 1966: Description of sample and antibody patterns with arboviruses, polioviruses, respiratory viruses, tetanus, and treponematosis, *Am. J. Epidemiol.* **90**:292–303 (1969).

26b. EVANS, A. S., CASALS, J., OPTON, E. M., BORMAN, E. K., AND CUADRADO, R. R., A nationwide serum survey of Argentinan military recruits, 1965–1966. 1. Description of samples and antibody patterns with arboviruses, polioviruses, respiratory viruses, tetanus and treponematosis, *Am. J. Epidemiol.* **93**:111–121 (1971).

26c. EVANS, A. S., COOK, J. A., KAPIKIAN, A. Z., NANKERVIS, G., SMITH, A. L., AND WEST, B., A serological survey of St. Lucia, *Int. J. Epidemiol.* **8**:327–332, 1979.

27. FIELDS, B. N., AND HAWKINS, K., Human infection with the virus of vesicular stomatitis during an epizootic, *N. Engl. J. Med.* **277**:989–994 (1967).

28. FRENCH, E. L., Murray valley encephalitis, *Med. J. Aust.* **39**:100–103 (1952).

29. GERLOFF, R. K., AND EKLUND, C. M., A tissue culture neutralization test for Colorado tick fever antibody and use of the test for serologic surveys, *J. Infect. Dis.* **104**:174–183 (1959).

30. GOLDFIELD, M., AUSTIN, S. M., BLACK, H. C., TAYLOR, B. F., AND ALTMAN, R., A nonfatal human case of

Powassan virus encephalitis, *Am J. Trop. Med. Hyg.* **22**:78–81 (1973).

31. GRACE, T. D. C., Establishment of a line of mosquito (*Aedes aegypti* L.) cells grown *in vitro*, *Nature (London)* **211**:366–367 (1966).

32. HALLAUER, C., Über den Virusnachweis mit dem Hirst-Test, *Z. Pathol. Bakteriol.* **9**:553–554 (1946).

33. HALSTEAD, S. B., Observations relating to pathogenesis of dengue hemorrhagic fever. VI. Hypotheses and discussion, *Yale J. Biol. Med.* **42**:350–362 (1970).

34. HAMMON, W. M., Present and future of killed and live arbovirus vaccines, in: *First International Conference on Vaccines Against Viral and Rickettsial Infections of Man*, Pan American Health Organization, Washington, D.C., pp. 252–259, 1967.

35. HAMMON, W. M., AND REEVES, W. C., California encephalitis virus, a newly described agent, *Calif. Med.* **77**:303–309 (1952).

36. HAMMON, W. M., RUDNICK, A., AND SATHER, G. E., Viruses associated with epidemic hemorrhagic fever of the Philippines and Thailand, *Science* **131**:1102–1103 (1960).

37. HAMMON, W. M., AND SATHER, G. E., Arboviruses, in: *Diagnostic Procedures for Viral and Rickettsial Infections*, 4th ed. (E. H. LENNETTE AND N. J. SCHMIDT, eds.), American Public Health Association, New York, 1969.

38. HORSFALL, F. L., JR., AND TAMM, I. (eds.), *Viral and Rickettsial Infections of Man*, 4th ed., Lippincott, Philadelphia, 1965.

39. HUGHES, L. E., CASPER, E. A., AND CLIFFORD, C. M., Persistence of Colorado tick fever virus in red blood cells, *Am. J. Trop. Med. Hyg.* **23**:530–532 (1974).

40. LIBÍKOVÁ, H., AND BUCKLEY, S. M., Studies with Kemerovo virus in Singh's *Aedes* cell lines, *Acta Virol.* **15**:393–403 (1971).

41. LORD, R. D., History and geographic distribution of Venezuelan equine encephalitis, *Bull. Pan Am. Health Org.* **8**:100–110 (1974).

42. LORD, R., AND CALISHER, C. H., Further evidence of southward transport of arboviruses by migratory birds, *Am. J. Epidemiol.* **92**:73–78 (1970).

43. LUMSDEN, L. L., St. Louis encephalitis in 1933: Observations on epidemiological features, *Public Health Rep.* **73**:340–353 (1958).

44. L'VOV, D. K., TIMOPHEEVA, A. A., CHERVONSKI, V. I., GROMASHEVSKI, V. L., KLISENKO, G. A., GOSTINSCHIKOVA, G. V., AND KOSTYRKO, I. N., Tyuleniy virus: A new group B arbovirus isolated from *Ixodes* (*Ceratixodes*) *putus* Pick.-Camb. 1878 collected on Tyuleniy Island, Sea of Okhotsk, *Am. J. Trop. Med. Hyg.* **20**:456–460 (1971).

45. MACDONALD, GEORGE, *The Epidemiology and Control of Malaria*, Oxford University Press, Oxford, 1957.

46. MARCHETTE, N. J., HALSTEAD, S. B., AND CHOW, J. S., Replication of dengue viruses in cultures of peripheral

blood leucocyte from dengue-immune rhesus monkeys, *J. Infect. Dis.* **133**:274–282 (1976).

47. MATTINGLY, P. F., Ecological aspects of the evolution of mosquito-borne virus diseases, *Trans. R. Soc. Trop. Med. Hyg.* **54**:97–112 (1960).

48. MCLEAN, D. M., AND DONOHUE, W. L., Powassan virus: Isolation of virus from a fatal case of encephalitis, *Can. Med. Assoc. J.* **80**:708–711 (1959).

49. MONATH, T. P. C., NUCKOLLS, J. G., BERALL, J., BAUER, H., CHAPPELL, W. A., AND COLEMAN, P. H., Studies on California encephalitis in Minnesota, *Am. J. Epidemiol.* **92**:40–50 (1970).

50. MURPHY, F. A., BORDEN, E. C., SHOPE, R. E., AND HARRISON, A., Physicochemical and morphological relationships of some arthropod-borne viruses to bluetongue virus—a new taxonomic group: Electron microscopic studies, *J. Gen. Virol.* **13**:273–288 (1971).

50a. NIEDERMAN, J. C., HENDERSON, J. R., OPTON, E. M., BLACK, F. L., AND SKURNOVA, K. A., A nationwide serum survey of Brazilian military recruits, 1964. II. Antibody patterns with arboviruses, polioviruses, measles, and mumps, *Am. J. Epidemiol.* **86**:319–329 (1967).

51. PLOWRIGHT, W., BROWN, F., AND PARKER, J., Evidence for the type of nucleic acid in African swine fever virus, *Arch. Gesamte Virusforsch.* **29**:289–304 (1966).

52. PLOWRIGHT, W., PERRY, C. T., PIERCE, M. A., AND PARKER, J., Experimental infection of the argasid tick, *Ornithodoros moubata porcinus*, with African swine fever virus, *Arch. Gesamte Virusforsch.* **31**:33–50 (1970).

53. PRINCE, A. M., METSELAAR, D., KAFUKO, G. W., MUKWAYA, L. G., LING, C. M., AND OVERBY, L. R., Hepatitis B antigen in wild-caught mosquitoes in Africa, *Lancet* **2**:247 (1972).

54. QUEENSLAND INSTITUTE OF MEDICAL RESEARCH, 29th Annual Report, p. 3, Brisbane, Australia, 1974.

55. REEVES, W. C., Overwintering of arboviruses, *Prog. Med. Virol.* **17**:193–220 (1974).

56. REEVES, W. C., AND HAMMON, W. M., Epidemiology of the arthropod-borne viral encephalitides in Kern County, California, 1943–1952, *Univ. Calif. Publ. Public Health* **4**:1–257 (1962).

57. RĚHÁČEK, J., AND PESEK, J., Propagation of eastern equine encephalomyelitis virus in surviving tick tissues, *Acta Virol.* **4**:241–254 (1960).

58. RICHARDSON, J., SYLVESTER, E. S., REEVES, W. C., AND HARDY, J. L., Evidence of two inapparent nonoccluded viral infections of *Culex tarsalis*, *J. Invertebr. Pathol.* **23**:213–224 (1974).

58a. ROSEN, L., TESH, R. B., LIEN, J. C., AND CROSS, J. H., Transovarial transmission of Japanese encephalitis virus by mosquitoes, *Science* **199**:909–911 (1978).

59. RUDNICK, A., Studies of the ecology of dengue in Malaysia: A preliminary report, *J. Med. Entomol.* **2**:203–208 (1965).

60. SABIN, A., Antigenic relationship of dengue and yellow fever viruses with those of West Nile and Japanese B encephalitis, *Fed. Proc. Fed. Am. Soc. Exp. Biol.* **8**:410 (1949).

61. SABIN, A. B., AND BUESCHER, E. L., Unique physicochemical properties of Japanese B virus hemagglutinin, *Proc. Soc. Exp. Biol. Med.* **74**:222–230 (1950).

62. SASLOW, A., A survey of encephalitis of unknown etiology in Connecticut June–September, 1967, Thesis for M.P.H., Department of Epidemiology and Public Health, Yale School of Medicine, 1968.

63. SAWYER, W. A., BAUER, J. H., AND WHITMAN, L., Distribution of yellow fever immunity in North America, Central America, West Indies, Europe, Asia and Australia, with special reference to specificity of the protection test, *Am. J. Trop. Med.* **17**:137–161 (1937).

64. SHOPE, R. E., Arboviruses, in: *Manual of Clinical Microbiology*, 2nd ed. (E. H. LENNETTE, E. H. SPAULDING, AND J. P. TRUANT, eds.), pp. 740–745, American Society for Microbiology, Washington, D.C., 1974.

64a. SHOPE, R. E., AND SATHER, G. E., Arboviruses, in: *Diagnostic Procedures for Viral and Rickettsial Infections*, 5th ed. (E. H. LENNETTE AND N. J. SCHMIDT, eds.), pp. 767–814, American Public Health Association, New York, 1979.

65. SINGH, K. R. P., Cell cultures derived from larvae of *Aedes albopictus* (Skuse) and *Aedes aegypti* (L.), *Curr. Sci.* **36**:506–508 (1967).

66. SINGH, K. R. P., AND PAUL, S. D., Multiplication of arboviruses in cell lines from *Aedes albopictus* and *Aedes aegypti*, *Curr. Sci.* **37**:65–67 (1968).

67. SMITH, H. H., Controlling yellow fever, in: *Yellow Fever* (G. K. STRODE, ed.), pp. 539–628, McGraw-Hill, New York, 1951.

68. SMITHBURN, K. C., Differentiation of the West Nile virus from the viruses of St. Louis and Japanese B encephalitis, *J. Immunol.* **44**:25–31 (1942).

69. SMITHBURN, K. C., Antigenic relationships among certain arthropod-borne viruses as revealed by neutralization tests, *J. Immunol.* **72**:376–388 (1954).

70. STOKES, A., BAUER, J. H., AND HUDSON, N. B., Transmission of yellow fever to *Macacus rhesus*: A preliminary note, *J. Am. Med. Assoc.* **90**:253–254 (1928).

71. SURTEES, G., SIMPSON, D. I. H., BOWEN, E. T. W., AND GRANINGER, W. E., Ricefield development and arbovirus epidemiology, Kano Plain, Kenya, *Trans. R. Soc. Trop. Med. Hyg.* **64**:511–518 (1970).

72. TESH, R. B., PERALTA, P. H., AND JOHNSON, K. M., Ecologic studies of vesicular stomatitis virus. I. Prevalence of infection among animals and humans living in an area of endemic VSV activity, *Am. J. Epidemiol.* **90**:255–261 (1969).

72a. TESH, R. B., ROSEN, L., BEATY, B., AND AITKEN, T. H. G., Studies of transovarial transmission of yellow fever and Japanese encephalitis viruses in *Aedes* mos-

quitoes and their implications for the epidemiology of dengue, *Pan. Am. Health Org. Sci. Publ.* **375**:179–182, 1979.

73. THEILER, M., Action of sodium deoxycholate on arthropod-borne viruses, *Proc. Soc. Exp. Biol. Med.* **96**:380–382 (1957).

74. THEILER, M., AND DOWNS, W. G., *The Arthropod-Borne Viruses of Vertebrates*, Yale University Press, New Haven, 1973.

75. THOMAS, L. A., PHILIP, R. N., PATZER, E., AND CASPER, E., Long duration of neutralizing antibody response after immunization of man with a formalinized Colorado tick fever vaccine, *Am. J. Trop. Med. Hyg.* **16**:60–62 (1967).

76. THOMPSON, W. H., AND EVANS, A. S., California encephalitis studies in Wisconsin, *Am. J. Epidemiol.* **81**:230–244 (1965).

77. THOMPSON, W. H., KALFAYAN, B., AND ANSLOW, R. O., Isolation of California encephalitis group virus from a fatal human illness, *Am. J. Epidemiol.* **81**:245–253 (1965).

77a. THOMPSON, W. H., AND BEATY, B. J., Venereal transmission of LaCrosse (California encephalitis) arbovirus in *Aedes triseriatus* mosquitoes, *Science* **196**(4289):530–531 (1977).

78. U.S. DEPARTMENT OF HEALTH, EDUCATION AND WELFARE, Epidemiologic notes and reports: St. Louis encephalitis—Tennessee, *Morbidity Mortality Weekly Rep.* **23**:294, 299 (1974).

78a. U.S. DEPARTMENT OF HEALTH, EDUCATION AND WELFARE, Epidemiologic notes and reports: St. Louis encephalitis—Texas, Louisiana, *Morbidity Mortality Weekly Rep.* **29**:415–416 (1980).

78b. U.S. DEPARTMENT OF HEALTH, EDUCATION AND WELFARE, Epidemiologic notes and reports: Dengue–Texas, *Morbidity Mortality Weekly Rep.* **29**:451,531–532 (1980).

79. VENTURA, A. K., BUFF, E. E., AND EHRENKRANZ, N. J., Human Venezuelan equine encephalitis virus infection in Florida, *Am. J. Trop. Med. Hyg.* **23**:507–512 (1974).

80. WATTS, D. M., THOMPSON, W. H., YUILL, T. M., DEFOLIART, G. R., AND HANSON, R. P., Overwintering of LaCrosse virus in *Aedes triseriatus*, *Am. J. Trop. Med. Hyg.* **23**:694–700 (1974).

80a. WATTS, D. M., PANTUWATANA, S., DEFOLIART, G. R., YUILL, T. M., AND THOMPSON, W. H., Transovarial transmission of LaCrosse virus (California encephalitis group) in the mosquito *Aedes triseriatus*, *Science* **182**:1140–1141 (1973).

81. WELLINGS, F. M., SATHER, G. E., AND HAMMON, W. M., Immunoelectrophoretic studies of the California encephalitis virus group, *J. Immunol.* **107**:252–259 (1971).

82. WHITMAN, L., Arthropod vectors of yellow fever, in:

Yellow Fever (G. K. STRODE, ed.), pp. 229–298, Mc-Graw-Hill, New York, 1951.

83. WHITMAN, L., AND AITKEN, T. H. G., Potentiality of *Ornithodoros moubata* (Murray) (Acarina, Argasidae) as a reservoir-vector of West Nile virus, *Ann. Trop. Med. Parasitol.* **54:**192–204 (1960).

84. WILLIAMS, J. E., YOUNG, O. P., AND WATTS, D. M., Relationship of density of *Culiseta melanura* mosquitoes to infection of wild birds with eastern and western equine encephalitis viruses, *J. Med. Entomol.* **11:**352–354 (1974).

84a. *WHO Weekly Epidemiological Record* **50:**401 (1977); **51:**7–8 (1978).

84b. WRIGHT, J. W., AND PAL, R., *Genetics of Insect Vectors of Disease*, Elsevier, Amsterdam 1967, 794 pp.

85. YOUNG, N. A., AND JOHNSON, K. M., Antigenic variants of Venezuelan equine encephalitis virus: Their geographic distribution and epidemiologic significance, *Am. J. Epidemiol.* **89:**286–307 (1969).

86. YUNKER, C. E., AND CORY, J., Colorado tick fever virus: Growth in a mosquito cell line, *J. Virol.* **3:**631–632 (1969).

13. Suggested Reading

Catalogue of Arthropod-Borne Viruses of the World, U.S. Public Health Service Publication No. 1760 (1967); Supplement No. 1, *Am. J. Trop. Med. Hyg.* **19:**1082–1160 (1970); Supplement No. 2, *Am. J. Trop. Med. Hyg.* **20:**1018–1050 (1971), and 2nd ed., 1975; Supplement, *Am. J. Trop. Med. Hyg.* **27:**372–440 (1978).

HORSFALL, F. L., JR., AND TAMM, I. (eds.), *Viral and Rickettsial Diseases of Man*, 4th ed., Lippincott, Philadelphia, 1965.

SHOPE, R. E., Arboviruses, in: *Manual of Clinical Microbiology*, 2nd ed. (E. H. LENNETTE, E. H. SPAULDING, AND J. P. TRUANT, eds.), pp. 740–745, American Society for Microbiology, Washington, D.C., 1974.

SHOPE, R. E., AND SATHER, G., Arboviruses, in: *Diagnostic Procedures for Viral and Rickettsial Infections*, 5th ed. (E. H. LENNETTE AND N. J. SCHMIDT, eds.), pp. 767–814, American Public Health Association, New York, 1979.

THEILER, M., AND DOWNS, W. G., *The Arthropod-Borne Viruses of Vertebrates*, Yale University Press, New Haven, 1973.

CHAPTER 6

Arenaviruses

Jordi Casals

1. Introduction

Arenavirus is the proposed designation for a set of viruses that have a unique morphology.[76] The virions are round, oval, or pleomorphic, with diameters between 60 and 350 nm, an electron-dense membrane with spikes or projections, and a number of inclusionlike, dense particles that give the virion an aspect of having been sand-sprinkled (*arenosus*). Arenaviruses have an RNA genome, are inactivated by lipid solvents, and share antigenic components. Since the first-recognized member of this group was lymphocytic choriomeningitis (LCM) virus, it is considered the prototype.

2. Historical Background

LCM virus has been known since 1933, and soon afterward it was associated with a disease syndrome in man, acute benign aseptic meningitis. Tacaribe virus, isolated from bats in Trinidad in 1956 and first described in 1963, has not been associated with human disease in nature[23]; since that time, additional viruses of this group have been reported, some of which cause human illness in nature. Junin virus was isolated and characterized in 1958; the virus was isolated from patients with Argentinian hemorrhagic fever (AHF). Five years later, in 1963, Machupo virus was isolated from a fatal case of an illness, Bolivian hemorrhagic fever (BHF), clinically very similar to AHF. Other viruses antigenically related to Tacaribe virus were discovered soon after: Amapari in Brazil in 1964,[71] Latino in Bolivia,[93] Parana in Paraguay,[92] Pichinde in Colombia,[88] and Tamiami in the United States in 1965[16]; none of these has been associated with human illness. Lassa virus was recovered in 1969 from patients suffering a severe disease, Lassa fever, first seen in Nigeria. Subsequently, two more viruses unrelated to human disease were discovered, Mozambique in southeast Africa[100] and another as yet unnamed in Brazil.[71a]

A serological relationship among members of this set was first observed between Junin and Tacaribe viruses in 1963, resulting in the creation of the Tacaribe antigenic group[57]; the other viruses, except LCM and Lassa, were easily shown to be related to Tacaribe and Junin and placed in the group. The similarity of morphology and morphogenesis between LCM and the Tacaribe group viruses was noted in 1969,[62] and soon afterward it was shown that there was an antigenic connection between them.[77] Finally, it was observed in 1970 that Lassa virus was antigenically related to LCM and to some of the Tacaribe-group agents[15] and that its morphology conformed to that described for LCM.[86]

The International Committee on Taxonomy of Viruses[25a] has recommended that the name Arenaviridae with family status be given to this set of viruses.

Jordi Casals · Department of Epidemiology and Public Health, Yale University School of Medicine, New Haven, Connecticut.

3. Methodology

3.1. Mortality

The case-fatality rate of some members of this group is sufficiently high that deaths from the disease give a good idea of the morbidity rate *provided* an accurate diagnosis can be made. For example, the mortality from hospitalized Lassa fever cases is 20–60%; from AHF, 3–15%; and from BHF, 5–30%. However, deaths from LCM are rare. For the most part, these diseases are rare, limited to localized outbreaks, and confined to a very few geographic areas. For those reasons, the official mortality records would be unlikely to reflect their occurrence in a country.

3.2. Morbidity

Epidemiological studies on arenavirus infections of man are hindered by the fact that disease-reporting is uncertain and incomplete. The diagnosis of sporadic cases of LCM is, most likely, not made or is guesswork in nearly all instances unless laboratory aid is sought. Diagnosis of AHF in the area and seasons where the disease is anticipated is confirmed by laboratory studies in about 70% of clinically diagnosed cases[49,54]; how many clinically undiagnosed infections go undetected is not known. Reporting of cases is encouraged by local health authorities and the World Health Organization. Because of the highly specialized type of diagnostic work required for identification of the viruses and antibodies resulting from infection, and because of the risk associated with certain aspects of the laboratory procedures, knowledge of the prevalence of the infections and illnesses caused by the arenaviruses is limited.

3.3. Serological Surveys

The neutralization (N) test is generally employed in serological surveys because of its high specificity and because neutralizing antibody is of long duration.[14,34,40] However, it is more cumbersome and expensive than other serological tests. It should be noted that except for LCM, serological surveys for arenaviruses have been quite limited. The complement-fixation (CF) and fluorescent-antibody (FA) tests are easier to perform and detect antibodies of shorter duration, thus being indicative of recent infection. They are less type-specific than the N test. The CF test, for example, hardly differentiates between Junin and Machupo viral infections of man,[95] but because of the separate geographic distribution of these viruses, this limitation is of little practical significance.

3.4. Laboratory Diagnosis

While a clinical diagnosis of fully developed, typical cases of AHF and BHF can be made with considerable accuracy in the districts where the diseases are endemic at the time of year when they prevail, particularly if several similar cases appear simultaneously, it is most doubtful that a sporadic case of LCM can be accurately diagnosed. A presumptive diagnosis of Lassa fever can be entertained in known endemic areas by experienced physicians faced with a severe or moderately severe case.[59]

A specific diagnosis of these illnesses requires either that the virus be isolated and identified from the patient's blood, excretions, or secretions, usually early during the disease, or that development of specific antibodies be shown to occur late in the disease or in convalescence.

Attempts to isolate virus have not, in general, been made when AHF or LCM is suspected because serology is considered adequate for diagnostic purposes; they are made with BHF, but are successful in a minority of instances. The diagnosis of these diseases is on the whole based on serological tests. With Lassa fever, on the other hand, diagnosis is based on isolation and identification of the virus.[17a]

Prior to the mid 1970s, the CF test had been most useful as a diagnostic aid in these diseases; however, while it continues to be useful, the FA test has been increasingly employed since that time and to a considerable extent has replaced the CF test.[21a, 32a,69a,98] Neither the FA nor the CF test is an early means of diagnosis, since from 15 to 30 days from onset are required to become positive with most patients, perhaps a shorter time with Lassa fever and LCM. The CF and FA tests are not type-specific tests within the arenaviruses, certainly not between Machupo and Junin viruses,[47,95,99] but since these viruses occur in different areas, a diagnostic error between the two is unlikely to occur. On the other hand, difficulties in the interpretation of CF results have arisen in an area where Junin and LCM viruses have infected man simultaneously or sequentially.[49,50] Whether the wide distribution of LCM virus may give rise to diagnostic problems when applying the CF or FA test to the diagnosis of Machupo or to imported cases of Lassa fever or other exotic arenaviruses in Europe remains to be seen.

The N test has been used less for diagnosis of current illnesses and serological surveys—LCM excepted—than for characterization of the viruses themselves; as will be seen in Section 4.3, it is sharply specific.[93]

4. The Viruses

4.1. Biochemical and Physical Properties

Investigations of the biochemical and physical properties of the arenaviruses, beginning with LCM[69] and Pichinde,[74] have now been extended to include other agents, particularly Tacaribe,[30a] Tamiami,[30a] Junin,[5a,83a] and Machupo.[30b] The picture that emerges from the studies in one of remarkable uniformity.

Arenaviruses contain single-stranded, linear RNA, although circular molecules are occasionally observed; compounds that inhibit DNA synthesis, such as halodeoxyuridines (BUdR, FUdR), have no inhibitory effect on these viruses. Analysis of the RNA from Pichinde, LCM, and Junin viruses by polyacrylamide-gel electrophoresis has repeatedly shown the presence of five species: two with sedimentation constant values of 31–33 and 22–25 S, respectively, which are virus-specific, and three with sedimentation constants of 28, 18, and 4–6 S, respectively, which are of host-cell origin, account for 25–50% of the labeled RNA in the LCM virion, and represent ribosomes from the host cell inside the virion.[5a,69,74] The base composition of the viral RNA differs markedly from that of the host-cell RNA. The RNA responsible for viral coded products would be about 3.2×10^6 daltons with Pichinde virus.[74]

Analysis of the viral proteins by electrophoresis in polyacrylamide gels[30a,74,83a] revealed the presence of one major nonglycosylated polypeptide with a molecular weight between 63,000 and 72,000, closely associated with the RNA and functioning as a nucleoprotein, and two major glycosylated polypeptides, one with a similar molecular weight, the other with a weight between 34,000 and 42,000, both being envelope and spike constituents. Up to three additional minor polypeptides have been reported with the different viruses.

Buoyant density in sucrose gradients has been reported as 1.17 or 1.18 g/ml for LCM, Pinchinde, Machupo, Junin, Tacaribe, and Amapari, and between 1.18 and 1.2 g/ml for Parana virus in cesium chloride. A noninfectious CF antigen produced by these viruses has a buoyant density between 1.09 and 1.11 g/ml in a sucrose gradient.[40]

All arenaviruses are easily inactivated by ethyl ether, chloroform, and sodium deoxycholate. Thermal inactivation of LCM virus is accelerated by the presence of divalent cations in the suspending medium. The effect of β-propiolactone on Lassa virus has been reported; the virus infectivity is completely inactivated with a concentration of the drug between 0.1 and 0.15% with preservation of CF activity.[15]

4.2. Morphology and Morphogenesis

The similarities in morphology and morphogenesis are so marked and distinctive that they were the basis for first associating the viruses in the present taxon.[62,76]

Thin-section electron microscopy of Vero cells infected with all arenaviruses shows them to be indistinguishable from each other. Coinciding with the highest infectious titers of the inoculated cultures is the occurrence of a large number of particles. The particles are round, oval, or pleomorphic, 60–280 nm in diameter, have a membranous envelope with surface projections or spikes approximately 6 nm long, and contain a variable number of from two to ten internal electron-dense granules about 20 nm in diameter, strongly resembling ribosomes. No symmetry has been discerned with any of these viruses.[63,64]

The particles mature by budding from plasma membranes. Vero cells infected with each of the viruses contain distinctive intracytoplasmic inclusion bodies, consisting of a smooth matrix in which are embedded dense granules similar to those seen in the virions and indistinguishable from the host-cell ribosomes. These inclusion bodies seem to match in size and location the cytoplasmic inclusions observed under light microscopy in cells infected with the virus.[63,64]

Negative-contrast electron microscopy of virus particles sedimented from infected cell cultures has been reported with these viruses, except for Junin, Machupo, and Lassa; technical considerations or hazard potential prevented their study. The results with the remaining arenaviruses have, again, shown decided uniformity of the viruses, with pleomorphic particles slightly larger than in thin sections, from 90 to 350 nm, pronounced surface projections, and no resolution of internal structure.[64]

Electron-microscopic studies of whole animals infected with arenaviruses[64] have revealed the presence of particles similar to those described above in a number of tissues of Calomys callosus infected as newborn with Machupo and Latino viruses. No such particles have been seen in hamsters infected with Junin virus and only few in the salivary-gland tissue of mice infected with Tacaribe virus. In general, only occasional virus particles have been observed in the brain tissue of mice infected with LCM, Tacaribe, Lassa, or Tamiami virus, while parallel studies indicate the presence of specific antigen.

The particles associated with arenavirus infection of cells in culture have been shown to contain specific antigen material by labeling procedures, at least with LCM virus; whether all size particles are equally infectious cannot be decided by electron microscopy alone.[53] Estimates of infectious-size particles by centrifugation or filtration have given sizes between 37 and 60 nm for LCM virus[43] and by filtration have given sizes between 70 and 140 nm for Lassa virus.[15]

4.3. Antigenic Properties

Early studies with LCM virus demonstrated the existence of a CF antigen distinct and separable from the infective particle by centrifugation; it was designated *soluble antigen*. The nature and properties of this antigen have been the subject of studies[33] that confirm that virion and CF antigen are distinct entities. The latter on inoculation into experimental animals induces formation of antibodies that react *in vitro* with the CF antigen but will not neutralize the virion; furthermore, repeated inoculations of CF antigen fail to induce any protection against subsequent challenge of guinea pigs. These studies, as well as recently acquired information with other arenaviruses, indicate that there are at least two distinct antigenic molecules in the virion. The ri-

bonucleoprotein core appears to be the main CF determinant and is responsible for the group antigenic relationship; the envelope or surface proteins, including the spikes, are associated with virus neutralization and are highly type-specific. No hemagglutinins have been found for the arenaviruses.

The humoral immune response with arenaviruses has certain characteristics that are observed mainly with LCM virus but that may also appear with other agents: CF and neutralizing antibodies and antibodies detected by the FA technique seem to be independent.[35] CF antibodies against LCM in man appear relatively early in the disease, from 8 days to 2 months; neutralizing antibodies are found later, usually not before 2 months after onset, and FA antibodies may be detected earlier than CF antibodies.[35] It is easy to prepare immune sera in mice with Pichinde or Lassa virus, which react with good titers by CF test; the same sera may have little neutralizing capacity when tested in a mouse N test[88] or in a plaque-reduction test.[15,59]

Antigenic relationships among arenaviruses have been mainly detected by the CF and FA tests. Table 1 is a composite table incorporating results from several sources, and it is an attempt to illustrate the relative positions of the viruses in the taxon. Tacaribe, Junin, Machupo, Amapari, Parana, and Latino viruses are very closely related by CF with mouse hyperimmune sera; the available fragmentary evidence shows that Pichinde and Tamiami viruses are not closely related to the others or to each other. LCM and Lassa viruses are very distantly related to the other agents; only when the highest-titered antisera are used can cross-reactions be observed. Results similar to those of the CF test have been observed by the FA test[99] with which the arenaviruses can be divided into New World and Old World subgroups, the latter comprising LCM, Lassa, and Mozambique viruses.

In contrast to the FA and CF tests, the results of N tests, many of them done with samples of the same sera that showed marked crossing by CF, are very specific. In comprehensive plaque-reduction tests[16,37,93] in which sera had homologous titers in the range from 1:32 to 1:2048, generally 1:128–512, no cross-neutralizations have been noted, even between viruses that are very close by CF, such as Machupo, Tacaribe, and Junin. The same marked specificity has been observed when constant serum was used with varying dilutions of virus. Studies

Table 1. Complement Fixation Test with Arenaviruses[a,b]

Antigen	MAC	JUN Ser. 1	JUN Ser. 2	TCR Ser. 1	TCR Ser. 2	AMA	LAT	PAR	PIC	TAM	LAS	LCM
Machupo	*128*	64		128			64	32		0		
Junin	64	*256*	16	256		64	64	32		0	4	8
Tacaribe	64	64		*512*		32	32	32		0	4	8
Amapari		64		32	64	*128*	32	32		8	4	4
Latino	32	32			8	8	*256*	16	8	0		
Parana	32		16		8	16	16	*512*	16	0		
Pichinde							4	64	*256*	4	0	
Tamiami	32	8		8		32	0	32	64	*128*	0	
Lassa		0		0		0			0		*256*	4
LCM		0		0		4				4	16	*256*

[a] Composite table derived from various authors. Values are the reciprocals of serum titers; 0 = no fixation at dilution 1:4 or 1:8.
[b] Italicized values indicate homologous antigen/serum intersections.

with LCM and Lassa viruses are less extensive, but they also show marked specificity in the N test.

4.4. Biological Properties

The natural hosts and reservoirs of the arenaviruses that cause human disease are discussed in the corresponding sections. The remaining viruses have been isolated in nature from the following animals: Tacaribe from *Artibeus* bats, Amapari from *Oryzomys* and *Neacomys* rats, Pichinde from *Oryzomys* and *Thomasomys*, Parana from *Oryzomys*, Latino from *Calomys*, Mozambique from *Mastomys*, the unnamed Brazil isolate from *Oryzomys*, and Tamiami from *Sigmodon* (cotton rat) and *Oryzomys*.* Attempts to isolate these viruses from other natural hosts, including arthropods, have been reported, largely with negative results: Pichinde virus has been isolated

* The genera *Akodon*, *Calomys*, *Neacomys*, *Oryzomys*, *Sigmodon*, and *Thomasomys* are comprised of mouselike and ratlike rodents, in the tribe Hesperomyinae, subfamily Cricetinae, family Cricetidae, and the entire tribe is New World only. The genera *Mus*, *Rattus*, and *Mastomys* are rats and mice in the family Muridae and are found only in the Old World (except for the established New World immigrants in *Mus* and *Rattus*). To the untrained observer, many of the small mouselike or ratlike rodents of the Old and New World are indistinguishable from one another, but habitats, habits, and life histories may vary greatly.

from ectoparasites taken off viremic hosts, Amapari has been isolated from mites (Gamasidae), Tacaribe was reported to have been isolated from a mixed mosquito pool.

Among experimental hosts, 1- to 4-day-old mice develop fatal illness following intracerebral inoculation of most, but not all, arenaviruses. Latino virus does not infect mice, and Parana inoculation results in illness but no death; LCM virus strains, in general, are lethal when inoculated into young adult mice but not when inoculated into newborn mice. Newborn hamsters are lethally infected by Junin, Latino, Machupo, Parana, and Pichinde viruses; guinea pigs are susceptible to LCM and Junin viruses.

All arenaviruses except LCM replicate with production of plaques under agar overlay in Vero-cell monolayers; some have marked cytopathic effect (CPE) in cells in fluid cultures. Other cells, LLCMK$_2$ and HeLa, are susceptible to some of the viruses with CPE development. LCM virus multiplies, reaching high titers in nearly all cells in culture that have been tried, but CPE, including plaque formation, is not a feature of the multiplication of this virus except in rare circumstances and particular systems.[70]

A special property of arenaviruses that cause disease of man, repeatedly described with LCM and Machupo, is their capacity to induce persistent tolerant infection in their natural hosts with no ill effects to the host and in the absence of an immune response; the epidemiological implications of this fact are evident.

5. Pathogenesis and Immunity

LCM virus infection of the adult mouse is the classic example of virus-induced immunopathological disease. Intracerebral inoculation of the adult mouse results in manifest disease and death, while infection before or soon after birth leads to a nonpathogenic lifelong carrier state. In the neonatal mouse during the period of immunological immaturity, the virus does not stimulate an immune response; since the virus is presumably harmless for the mouse, no ill effects result. In the adult mouse that has reached immunological maturity, the virus incorporated in the cells stimulates an immune response from the host; it is this conflict between the host and the virus that results in disease, a fatal choriomeningitis with no evidence of neuronal destruction. Numerous observations[35,43] by many workers have firmly established the aforedescribed pathogenetic mechanism for the disease; it is, furthermore, observed that immunosuppressants protect adult mice against death due to LCM virus infection. Since, among the immunosuppressing treatments, antilymphocytic serum and neonatal thymectomy are effective, it appears that the immune disease is cell-mediated rather than caused by antibodies.

Studies with Tamiami virus[32] showed that suckling mice after intracerebral inoculation of the virus develop an acute CNS disease with cerebellar ataxia and less frequently paralysis, convulsions, and death. Neonatal thymectomy totally prevented the disease despite the presence of virus in high titer in the brain tissue; it was suggested that the acute disease caused by the virus is immunomediated.

With the present state of knowledge, no definite statement can be made concerning the mechanism through which the arenaviruses cause disease in man. There is nothing to indicate that lesions and disease are immunopathological or allergic phenomena, as is so clearly the case in adult mice infected with LCM virus; clinical and pathological observations rather favor the view that direct damage to cells by the virus best explains the disease.

Little is known about the type and localization of lesions in man following LCM virus infection and about the multiplication and distribution of the virus, duration of viremia, and persistence of antibodies. With other arenaviruses, autopsy of ten patients who died of AHF consistently revealed generalized lymphadenopathy on gross examination; microscopically, endothelial swelling in capillaries and arterioles of all organs examined was seen without exception, and lymphocyte depletion in the spleen was generally observed.[30] In another series,[24] it was stressed that lesions in several organs and tissues were probably caused by direct cytotoxic action of the virus on cells, in the absence of conspicuous cellular infiltration. In connection with the diffuse involvement of the endothelium of capillaries and arterioles,[30] it is of interest to mention that disseminated intravascular coagulation has been described in one case of AHF and suggested as a pathogenetic factor in the disease.[5]

The result of a liver biopsy in a fatal case of Lassa fever is highly pertinent to the pathogenesis of the disease.[96] Diffuse hepatocellular damage was evident, with focal necroses; a clear association between damaged liver cells and virus-particle formation and maturation was observed by electron microscopy, while inflammatory response was minimal. These findings suggested that a direct cytopathic effect was responsible for, at least, the hepatic lesions in Lassa fever and that cell-mediated or humoral immunological damage is not a major factor.

The most constantly reported lesion in AHF, and probably in BHF, is a diffuse swelling of the endothelium of capillaries and arterioles in the absence of inflammatory reaction; clinically, there is in nearly all patients an adenopathy, local or generalized; there are also leukopenia, late appearance of antibodies, and the fact that recovery occurs at the time when antibodies begin to build up; biphasic patterns of clinical disease are all but unknown with AHF and BHF. Finally, cell damage, when it occurs in specific organs, appears to be associated with a direct cytopathic action of the virus on the cell, with no cellular infiltration. On the basis of these observations, the following pathogenesis has been suggested[40] for arenavirus infections of man: the virus gains entry by the upper respiratory or alimentary route and is caught in the local lymphoid tissue of lymph nodes, where it first replicates; it then invades the cells of the reticuloendothelial system including all the cells involved in the immune and cellular immune responses, the functions of which are therefore inhibited at this time. The virus causes, directly or indirectly, extensive capillary damage resulting in capillary fragility, hemorrhagic tendency, and hypovolemic shock; the various organ malfunctions are probably due to capillary damage and edema of the parenchyma rather than actual cell damage. When the disease regresses, no permanent damage ensues, since there has been little cell damage; antibodies develop to a high titer. In progressive cases, a direct cytopathic action of the virus on the cells follows; coagulopathy can occur, but immunopathology is at no time evident.

Following overt infection of man with arenaviruses, antibodies develop that have been detected by CF and N tests and, recently, by the FA technique; no hemagglutination-inhibition test is available for these viruses. With LCM, AHF, and BHF, CF antibodies are generally short-lived, with there titers diminishing rapidly between 6 and 12 months from onset, at the end of which period most sera are negative; on the other hand, neutralizing antibodies remain detectable for years.[40,43] No information is available on persistence of neutralizing antibodies in Lassa fever; by the FA test, they have been positive up to 5 years after onset.[13a,98]

Antibodies have been detected in persons in whom no specific diagnosis had been made, perhaps having had only a subclinical infection, particularly with LCM[1,14]; the current view is that clinically inapparent infection is rare with Junin and Machupo viruses.[40]

6. Lymphocytic Choriomeningitis

LCM virus was first isolated in 1933 in the course of investigations on the etiology of an epidemic of encephalitis in St. Louis, Missouri[8]; the virus may have been present in the CNS tissue of a patient who died of that illness or, more likely, derived from monkeys inoculated during the study. An etiological association between the virus and a disease of man, acute aseptic meningitis, was established[75,83] by isolation of the agent and demonstration of development of antibodies. While at an early period it was assumed that LCM virus was the exclusive etiological agent of acute aseptic meningitis, or Wallgren's disease, it soon became apparent

that the virus caused only a small proportion of the cases. Traub[89] reported that a colony of laboratory albino mice was chronically infected with a virus subsequently identified as LCM; this finding was the beginning of a new concept, persistent tolerant virus infections, that has considerable epidemiological implications with respect to LCM virus and other arenavirus infections of man.

6.1. Descriptive Epidemiology

6.1.1. Incidence and Prevalence. Determination of infection or illness caused by LCM virus requires a laboratory-confirmed specific diagnosis; in general, this is not attempted, since the required laboratories are not always available. Efforts to obtain a specific diagnosis usually require special circumstances, such as a large number of clinically suspect cases appearing simultaneously[7] or the continuing interest of groups of investigators.[4,14,58]

Soon after the discovery of the virus and its association with cases of aseptic meningitis, it became apparent that clinical infection of man due to LCM virus was a rare event; later surveys supported the view.

One of the most extensive surveys to determine the prevalence of clinical LCM virus infection in man was conducted in United States military personnel and dependents over an 18-year period, from 1943 to 1960.[4,58] Examination of nearly 1600 CNS illnesses revealed that only 8% were specifically diagnosed as LCM infections; on the average, seven cases a year occurred during the entire period. No estimate can be made of undiagnosed cases or, if they existed, of subclinical infections; a study in the United States[97] showed that 5% of about 1200 sera from residents of various areas had neutralizing antibodies; it is conceivable that a certain degree of nonspecific neutralization of virus may have occurred in that study,[43] so that the results may not be specific.

Investigations in West Germany since 1960 by Ackerman et al.,[2] Scheidt et al.,[81] and Blumenthal et al.[14] indicate the extent of the distribution of LCM virus in that country and the close association between the incidence of infection of man and the presence of virus in the mouse. Early observations by these investigators had shown the rarity of the disease in a number of large hospitals in the country;

furthermore, antibody surveys with sera from selected individuals revealed only about 1% of positives.[1] In a subsequent survey[14] done after the distribution of the virus in mice had been investigated, sera from about 2000 persons from rural districts were tested for neutralizing antibodies; 68 of these sera, or 3.4%, were positive; on the basis of this survey, Ackerman[1] estimates that as many as 1000 new infections per year may occur in a population of about 6 million persons in rural German areas; since only a minute fraction of this number are clinically recognized, the inference is that most LCM virus infections go undiagnosed or are subclinical.

6.1.2. Geographic Distribution. The virus of LCM may well have worldwide distribution, being present in all parts of the world where the house mouse is found. Well-documented proof of the virus's presence has been given for European countries and North and South America; its presence has also been reported in Asia, less convincingly in Africa, and not in Australia.[43]

6.1.3. Age, Sex, and Occupation. Since LCM is not usually reported, the effect of a number of variables on its spread and prevalence is difficult to appraise. A seroepidemiological report from West Germany[14] indicated that the distribution of antibodies was not influenced by sex or occupation—whether farm work or professional or office work; in that survey, few positives were found among persons under 20 years of age. On the other hand, no influence of age was seen in hamster-related outbreaks.[3,7] It is possible that mouse-associated infections are more common in rural populations or in lower socioeconomic urban groups and that hamster-associated cases are found principally in urban centers. Further, a seasonal fluctuation of cases has been suggested in man, more in winter than in summer. Perhaps this is associated with migratory habits of the house mouse[43] and possibly with closer contact with mice in the cold months in the temperate zone.

Special attention should be given to LCM as an occupational disease in laboratory personnel, either in persons who work with the virus or in those who work with other problems but who use animals—mice, hamsters, possibly monkeys—that may be infected. Reported laboratory accidents may well represent only a fraction of all the occurrences; in the

period between 1952 and 1966, 45 laboratory infections with 5 deaths were documented.[87]

6.2. Mechanism and Route of Transmission

6.2.1. Spread of Virus. The only known lifelong carrier of LCM virus is the mouse from which man becomes infected. The hamster may develop a transient carrier state in the course of which it can also infect man. Man-to-man transmission seems unlikely.

The mechanism of transmission from mouse to man cannot be stated with certainty. It would appear that either the airborne route through household dust contaminated with mouse urine and other excretions and secretions or the contamination of food and drink by mouse excretions is the most likely source of human disease. The portal of entry in these instances would be the upper respiratory tract or, possibly, the upper digestive tract; the possibility of transmission through skin abrasions has also been considered.

While airborne transmission appears the logical mode of human infection, acceptance of this hypothesis runs into problems represented by the known lability of LCM virus under unfavorable conditions; however, no other explanation has been put forward to replace airborne or food contamination. Transmission by an arthropod vector has been investigated, but the evidence is against it; it is worthwhile to mention, however, that *Aedes aegypti* has transmitted the infection by bite to monkeys 15 days after feeding on infected guinea pigs.[20]

6.2.2. Reservoir. In nature, the virus has been isolated from various animal hosts in addition to man, who is most likely a dead-end. Chief among these, for epidemiological implications including maintenance of the virus in nature, is the house mouse (*Mus musculus*).

From the first demonstration of LCM virus in house mice trapped in the homes of two persons suffering from nonbacterial meningitis,[9] the abundance of isolations has left no doubt about the close association in nature between the virus and this rodent. Furthermore, it has been shown that experimental mouse colonies can be chronically infected.[90] Studies on the nature of the infection of laboratory mice by LCM virus extending over a period of 30 years have clearly shown that the mouse infected *in utero* or within a few hours after birth develops a tolerant persistent infection; mice thus infected circulate virus in their blood, develop no antibodies, and maintain an active and relatively normal health condition for a period of time representing a good fraction of a normal mouse's life span. The epidemiologically important feature of the tolerant persistent infection is that wild mice so infected shed virus continuously for the duration of their lives by way of urine, feces, and nasal and oral secretions. The virus thus excreted will contaminate households, including food, drink, dust, and fomites; from these, and by ways as yet undetermined, man becomes infected. In addition, new generations of mice become tolerantly infected at birth or *in utero*, thus maintaining the carrier status of the mouse populations; mice so infected may become the source from which other species—hamsters, guinea pigs, monkeys—are infected, and they, in turn, may infect man.

The studies of Ackerman *et al.*[2] and Blumenthal *et al.*[14] are particularly illustrative of the association between infection of mice and infection of man. Of 1795 mice trapped between 1960 and 1962 in 44 of 376 areas in West Germany, 65 were LCM carriers, as shown by virus isolation; nearly all positive trapping areas were in northern and northwestern Germany, none in southern Germany. Serological surveys done at about the same time in which 1371 persons from rural districts were tested by neutralization test showed that of 511 sera from persons in north and northwestern Germany, in or near the places where LCM virus had been isolated from mice, 9.1% had antibodies. The second set of sera from 811 persons was from south Germany, where no LCM virus had been isolated from mice; only 5, or 0.6%, were positive.

In recent years, the Syrian hamster (*Mesocricetus auratus*) has emerged as an important source of human infection and illness caused by LCM virus, if not as a true reservoir. Small outbreaks had occurred in the past involving persons participating in biomedical research work in which hamsters were used.[10,45] Between 1968 and 1971, 47 LCM infections were described in West Germany. These were specifically diagnosed by antibody detection as caused by LCM virus in persons who shortly before their illness had been in contact with pet hamsters; 45 of these infections were clinical, mainly influ-

enzalike or aseptic meningitis, and 2 had no clinical manifestations.[3] Subsequent investigations in West Germany [26] on commercial breeding colonies showed that of 598 animals examined, representing 11 different breeders, LCM virus was isolated from members of 6 different colonies. According to the authors of that study, it is estimated that close to 1 million hamsters are sold annually as pets in West Germany; it is obvious that the importance of this animal as a source of infection of man cannot be overlooked.

Two outbreaks of LCM in man, associated with hamsters, have been observed in the United States. Early in 1973, an episode occurred in a laboratory where hamsters were used for cancer work.[7] The investigation of the outbreak revealed several interesting points. In all, 21 persons became ill with a severe influenzalike illness, of which 14 cases had occurred before LCM infection was suspected. In addition to the 21 clinical cases, confirmed by FA antibodies, there were 17 persons who had antibodies but no illness; in other words, inapparent infections occurred. The association with hamsters was clearly seen in that 75% of 20 persons admitting to having touched the hamsters were seropositive, while only 17% of 61 persons who had no contact other than entering the premises were positive; the latter may have been instances of airborne infections. LCM virus was isolated from 11 of 24 hamsters tested. The animals appear to have been infected from virus present in the tumor line with which they had been inoculated.

In another extended episode, 93 human cases in seven states were diagnosed and specifically confirmed between December 1973 and April 1974.[25] The association with pet hamsters was established in every instance; in some instances, two or three cases occurred in a family. The diagnoses were established by FA and CF tests in man and hamsters; it appears that of several breeders whose animals were tested, only one had an infected colony.

The episodes in the United States and Germany point to the importance of hamsters as a source of human infection with LCM virus; while this animal is not a true lifelong carrier, it can circulate and excrete virus for periods of 2 or 3 months after its infection.

There are additional animals species from which the virus has reportedly been isolated in nature, such as monkeys, guinea pigs, and dogs. The role that these species play in virus dissemination to man is undetermined, but it appears to be unimportant.

6.3. Patterns of Host Response

6.3.1. Clinical Aspects. Infection of man by LCM virus presents different clinical forms, and there may be inapparent infections. Three major clinical forms seem to prevail: aseptic meningitis, influenzalike or non-nervous-system type, and meningoencephalomyelitic type.[43] The influenzalike and meningeal are the most frequent types. The incubation period is believed to be from 6 to 13 days. In the influenzalike (or grippal) type, there are fever, malaise, muscular pains, coryza, and bronchitis; in the meningeal type, which is the most common, there is a "grippe"-like begginning followed by definite signs and symptoms of meningitis, with stiff neck, headache, and nausea, which may remain mild and of short duration or can be pronounced, last for 2 weeks or longer, and lead to considerable prostration.

The great majority of specifically diagnosed, clinical infections follow a benign course; only a few fatal cases have been reported, either following CNS involvement[4] or after systemic generalized illness with hemorrhagic manifestations.[84] Chronic sequelae, although rare, have been reported, including paralyses, headaches, and personality changes; it appears that the documentation of most such cases is ambiguous.[43] The possibility that prenatal infection with LCM virus may result in hydrocephalus and chorioretinitis has been reported.[83b]

6.3.2. Diagnosis. Clinical and routine laboratory analyses are only indicative of aseptic meningitis: the CSF is under increased pressure, with slightly increased protein, normal or slightly reduced sugar, and moderate number of cells, from 150 to 400/mm^3.

The virus in man can be isolated from blood, CSF, and, in fatal cases, brain tissue. The best sources for isolation are blood during the febrile period and CSF during the period of meningeal manifestations; virus can be isolated from the blood and CSF from experimentally infected man for 20–25 days.[13]

The animal of choice for virus isolation is the laboratory albino mouse, 3–5 weeks old; following intracerebral inoculation, the incubation period and signs of illness are nearly pathognomonic. Care must be taken to use mice from a colony known to

be free from the virus. Inoculation of cells in cultures could be used, since most cells support replication of LCM virus; however, since virus replication in general does not cause CPE or plaques, detection of viral antigen in the cells must be made by CF or FA tests.

The techniques employed for detection of antibody development are the CF and the indirect FA tests; it has been reported that FA antibody appears earlier than CF antibody.[35] In recent investigations of antibody determination in man and hamsters, there has been nearly complete agreement between the results of these two tests.[21a] Neutralizing antibodies appear much later after onset; therefore, the N test is not helpful for an early diagnosis; it is most profitably used in serum surveys.[14]

6.4. Treatment and Prevention

There is no specific treatment advocated; in view of the definite association with mice, it would appear that rodent control may minimize the risk. Pet hamsters may be a source of infection, particularly in children. Monitoring of hamster colonies for presence of virus or antibodies or both would be indicated.

7. Argentinian Hemorrhagic Fever

A disease resembling AHF and with the same geographic location seems to have been first recognized in 1943.[72] Arribalzaga[11] gave the first detailed account of the disease and considered it a new nosological entity; his description included extremely accurate clinical and epidemiological observations. The causal agent, Junin virus, was isolated in 1958.[66,73] Annual outbreaks of the disease have occurred since 1958, and the endemic zone has been progressively increasing in area.

7.1. Descriptive Epidemiology

Collection of data concerning clinically diagnosed cases of the disease and laboratory efforts to confirm the clinical diagnosis appear to be efficiently made through local, provincial, and national public-health centers in Argentina.[21,72]

7.1.1. Prevalence in Man. AHF is predominantly a rural disease that affects adult males with agricultural occupations, particularly harvesting of maize; 80% of nearly 1000 cases analyzed in 1973 were of males, and 63% of the total number were in the age group between 20 and 49 years (Maiztegui[49] and personal communication).

7.1.2. Geographic and Seasonal Distribution. The endemoepidemic zone was first recognized in the northwest of Buenos Aires province; by 1958, its area was estimated at 16,000 km². Since that year, the zone has spread west and north to include additional localities in Buenos Aires as well as sections of two adjacent provinces, Córdoba and Santa Fe; the affected area was estimated in 1970 to be 80,000 km², in which lived a population of 800,000 persons.[79] The total number of cases reported from 1958 to 1972 was about 13,000, with annual fluctuations of between 100 and 3500 cases; the mortality rate for laboratory-confirmed cases studied at Pergamino has been from 10 to 20% (Maiztegui[49] and personal communication).

The disease is sharply seasonal, with the outbreaks beginning late in summer (February), reaching a peak in autumn (May), and ending early in winter. The seasonal distribution coincides with the intensification of agricultural labors, particularly harvest of maize, and with an influx of transient farm workers; at the same time, there is an increase in the population of wild rodents, which are considered the principal reservoir of the virus. While AHF is overwhelmingly a rural disease, cases have been observed in an urban setting in the near absence of the main rodent reservoir (*Calomys*) of the virus[51,79]; however, the simultaneous existence of LCM and Junin virus in an area may create diagnostic problems.[50]

7.2. Mechanism and Route of Transmission

7.2.1. Spread to Man. Chronic infection of rodents with associated viruria is the basic mechanism of transmission of the virus to man; there is no evidence implicating arthropod transmission.[40,79] The mode of transmission from wild-infected rodents to man has not been definitely established. It may be airborne, from dust contaminated by the excretions or secretions from rodents, or by the oral route through ingestion of food and drink equally contaminated. Since the disease has been transmitted to human volunteers by injection,[73] it may be possible that the disease is also acquired through skin abrasions in the course of farm work while materials contaminated with rodent excreta are being handled.

Although the virus has been isolated from throat swabs and urine from patients, contact transmission between individuals is exceptional.[78]

7.2.2. Reservoir. The possible connection between wild rodents and AHF was first stated by Arribalzaga.[11] Accumulated observations beginning in 1958 support the close association between disease and rodents in the endemic areas. The main reservoir is two species of Cricetidae, *Calomys laucha* and *C. musculinus*, which are present in farm fields and along hedgerows, the latter species predominating in Córdoba province[79]; Junin virus has also been isolated from *Akodon, Azarae,* and, rarely, *Mus musculus*.[21] Field and laboratory investigations show that Junin virus causes a chronic tolerant infection in *C. musculinus* with persistent viremia and viruria and no development of antibodies[79]; most likely, the virus is maintained in nature by infection of the rodents at birth. Although the virus has been isolated from mites,[68,73] it has not been established that they play a role in transmission between rodents or to man.

7.3. Patterns of Host Response

7.3.1. Clinical Features. The disease presents a syndrome that includes manifestations of renal, cardiovascular, and hematic involvement; pronounced neurological manifestations are also described, but not frequently. The disease lasts from 7 to 14 days and terminates either with complete recovery with no sequelae or with death. After an incubation period estimated at from 7 to 16 days, there is an insidious and gradual onset with chills, asthenia, malaise, headache, retroocular pain, muscular pains often pronounced in the costovertebral angle, anorexia, nausea, and vomiting. The most prevalent signs at the outset are fever with temperatures up to 102–104°F, conjunctival injection, enanthem, exanthem on face, neck, and upper thorax, a few petechiae particularly in the axilla, polyadenopathy, and muscular tenderness at the thigh. Three to five days after onset, the signs and symptoms become more pronounced in the severe cases, with dry tongue, dehydration, oliguria, hypotension, relative bradycardia, and, in the worst cases, hemorrhages from the gums and nasal cavities, also hematemesis, hematuria, and melena; oliguria may develop into anuria. In the severe cases, there are psychosensorial and motor alterations. Death is caused by uremic coma or hypotension and hypovolemic shock due to plasma leakage, not whole-blood loss. In nonfatal cases, the fever diminishes by lysis, and there is marked diuresis and rapid improvement within days; however, convalescence is prolonged. The case-fatality rate has been as high as 20%; usually, it is between 3 and 15% in different outbreaks. Clinically inapparent infections appear to be very rare. [37,55,79]

7.3.2. Simultaneous Occurrence of AHF and LCM. Investigations in areas of the AHF endemic zone to determine the source of virus in an urban setting[52] led to the finding of antibodies against LCM virus in mice (*M. musculus*); at about the same time, a strain of LCM virus was isolated from that species.[80] A reexamination of antibodies in acute and convalescent sera from nearly 3000 cases of AHF, using LCM and Junin antigens, revealed that in a substantial number of instances, AHF occurred in persons who showed evidence of previous infection with LCM virus.[49] Furthermore, there were a few cases previously diagnosed as AHF in which the serological diagnosis was changed to LCM.[49] Additional evidence of the activity of LCM virus in the endemic AHF area is given by the simultaneous admission to a hospital of two agricultural workers with clinical diagnosis of AHF, but with specific serological conversions to Junin virus in one and to LCM virus in the other.[50]

Since only between 60 and 70% of patients clinically diagnosed as having AHF are generally serologically confirmed, it had previously been suspected that other agents were active in the endemic area in epidemic times; serological evidence of infection with group B arboviruses has been reported[54] in a number of persons diagnosed clinically as AHF cases, and St. Louis encephalitis virus was isolated from one.[56]

7.3.3. Diagnosis. Clinical diagnosis of AHF has been confirmed either serologically or by virus isolation in from 60 to 70% of reported cases.[55] In a thorough study involving 2249 reported cases over the period 1965–1972 in the city of Pergamino, the diagnosis was confirmed in 62% and was doubtful in 11% of cases.[48,49]

During the epidemic season of AHF, there appear to occur in the same areas other diseases of viral etiology that at the early phase present clinical manifestations similar to those of AHF.[54,82] A study of signs and symptoms in a number of patients clinically diagnosed as having AHF, in whom laboratory confirmation was sought, showed that during the first week of illness, a combination of asthenia, dizziness, petechiae in the axillary region or anterior chest wall, and conjunctival congestion was present in 71% of confirmed cases but in only 3.5% of nonconfirmed ones. When leukopenia, thrombocytopenia, and casts in the urine are found in addition, the diagnostic accuracy is further increased.[82]

Specific diagnosis is based on isolation of virus or demonstration of serological conversion. The virus is isolated from the blood during the acute period, probably from the 3rd to the 10th days after onset, and, in fatal cases, from liver, spleen, kidney, and clotted blood. The materials are intracerebrally inoculated into newborn mice 1–3 days old, or into guinea pigs by the peripheral or intracerebral route. While Junin virus replicates with CPE in several cells in culture, little has been reported on the use of tissue cultures for isolation of the virus from nature.[79]

The CF has been the test of choice for demonstration of antibody development; more recently,[32a] the indirect FA test has been increasingly used as a diagnostic aid. AHF shares with other diseases caused by arenaviruses the characteristic that CF antibodies develop relatively late after onset; an early serum sample and a second one taken at least 30 days after onset offer the best possibility for detection of serological conversion. The kinetics of development and the persistence of antibodies detected by the FA test remain to be determined.

Recent investigations[49,65] have shown the simultaneous development of CF antibodies against Junin and LCM virus antigens in patients in the AHF endemic zone, clinically diagnosed as cases of AHF, including some from whose acute-phase blood Junin virus was isolated. This fact creates serious difficulties in reaching a definite diagnosis not heretofore encountered with other arenavirus infections of man; as a result, epidemiological evaluation of data may be faulty.

7.4. Treatment, Control, and Prevention

Beneficial results have been reported after the administration of plasma from recovered individuals to patients.[77a] Vaccination of the exposed population has been advocated; however, there is no available vaccine. Efforts to develop a vaccine employing an attenuated strain of Junin virus have been reported; administration of the preparation to a small number of persons on an experimental basis led to the development of antibodies with only relatively minor febrile reactions.[67]

Ecological control to reduce the number of rodents and exposure of man to them appears difficult to implement. The circumstances under which the bulk of the exposed population live and work at the time of harvest will not be likely to change in the near future; increased mechanization of farm work and improvement of housing conditions would undoubtedly reduce morbidity.[21]

8. Bolivian Hemorrhagic Fever

BHF was first recognized in 1959 in two rural areas in the northeastern part of Bolivia, Department of Beni. In late 1962 or early 1963, cases began to appear in a nearby town, San Joaquin, developing into a large outbreak that continued until the middle of 1964; nearly 700 persons were ill, with a mortality of 18%. The disease has continued to appear in the Department of Beni more or less annually in sharply localized outbreaks.[37,40,46] An outbreak that occurred in 1971 in Cochabamba, Bolivia,[40] differed ecologically from previous ones and represented an extension of the virus to a new area.

8.1. Descriptive Epidemiology

8.1.1. Prevalence in Man. Before 1962, the small outbreaks affected mainly adult males, and most cases occurred from April to September, which is the time of highest agricultural activity. From 1963, when the disease appeared in towns and villages and larger numbers of persons sickened, the pattern changed. Adult males still presented somewhat higher rate of morbidity, but all persons were affected, with little relationship to sex, age, and occupation; it was soon apparent that the disease was "house-associated," with the lower socioeconomic groups experiencing the highest incidence of disease. Although a seasonal pattern is evident, with the highest incidence from February to September, cases occur in each month.[37,46]

8.1.2. Geographic Distribution. The main epidemic centers, San Joaquin and Orobayaya, are located in the Department of Beni, in the northeastern section of Bolivia; these centers are on an immense flat plain east of the Andes. The prevailing vegetation type is that of a grassland broken with "islands" of forest and numerous tree-lined rivers and streams.[42] The human settlements where cases have occurred in the past were on slightly elevated sites that generally escape flooding during the heavy rains; the houses are on the edge of the forest, overlooking the grass-covered marshlands. These villages and settlements are heavily infested with *Calomys callosus*, a mouselike rodent that, although pastoral, readily invades and lives in houses in a manner similar to that of the house mouse, *Mus musculus*.[42]

8.2. Mechanism and Route of Transmission

8.2.1. Spread to Man. Transmission from rodent to man is probably by contamination of food, water, or air with infected rodent urine or by inoculation through skin abrasions.[40] Human-to-human transmission can occur in rare cases of close contact,[22] but it is not considered important in the spread of the natural infection. There may be, however, circumstances that promote such type of transmission, as shown in a small outbreak in Cochabamba, Bolivia, which is outside the habitat of the rodent *Calomys callosus*; from an index case, acquired in the endemic area, five secondary cases developed, including family and medical personnel; all cases were fatal except one.[40]

8.2.2. Reservoir. The distribution of cases in a town in the form of clusters definitely associated with certain houses, the absence of evidence of human-to-human transmission, and the equally negative evidence of an arthropod vector led to the inference that a reservoir species might be involved that lived in or near households; soon, the association of disease with a rodent, *Calomys callosus*, was firmly established. This rodent has been trapped in all households where cases have occurred; houses located in sites that did not favor the presence of this rodent were spared; finally, the dramatic termination of the epidemic in San Joaquin in June 1964, 2 weeks after continuous trapping of *C. callosus* had been implemented, left little doubt about the association.[42,46] Fifty percent of *C. callosus* caught wild at the time of that epidemic were infected with the virus[38]; experimental studies with colonized *Calomys* show that on inoculation of Machupo virus, the rodent develops a tolerant infection with persistent viremia and viruria and no development of antibodies.[41] *Calomys* is easily infected by oral and nasal routes, and also by contact with infected cagemates; about 50% develop viremia and viruria for life.[39]

All efforts to isolate the virus from arthropods caught in the epidemic area at the epidemic time have been negative.[42]

8.3. Patterns of Host Response

8.3.1. Clinical Features. The disease is clinically so similar to AHF that a joint description is often given.[36,37] The incubation period is estimated at from 7 to 14 days. The onset is insidious, and the fever, which has been carefully monitored in numerous etiologically confirmed cases, reaches a temperature between 102 and 105°F, with little diurnal variation, remaining at that level for at least 5 days. About 30% of the patients present hemorrhagic manifestations consisting of petechiae on the upper part of the trunk and oral mucous membranes and, on occasion, bleeding from gums, nose, stomach, intestines, and uterus; blood loss is, however, not a threat to life.[40] Nearly half the patients exhibit a fine intention tremor of tongue and hands beginning 4 or 6 days from onset; about one fourth of these may develop a frank and extensive neurological disorder. Somnolence and coma are hardly ever seen, except in very young children. The acute disease can last for 2–3 weeks; convalescence is long, with complaints of severe generalized weakness and manifestations of autonomic dysfunction. Probably owing to the continuously elevated temperature, loss of hair and transverse grooving of the nails are common. The mortality has varied depending on outbreaks, ranging from 5 to 30%; clinically inapparent infection is very rare.

8.3.2. Diagnosis. The clinical diagnosis by an experienced physician, in the endemic area and in moderately severe or severe cases, is fairly accurate; because of the toxic condition of the patient, BHF may resemble typhus or typhoid fever. Certain clinical laboratory data help the clinician: leukopenia, thrombocytopenia, and increased hematocrit—the last indicates a bad prognosis.[40]

A specific diagnosis is based on virus isolation or development of antibodies. The most successful animal for virus isolation has been the newborn hamster, inoculated by the intracerebral or intraperitoneal route. Recovery of Machupo virus from acutely ill patients is, however, quite difficult; only one in five samples, mostly sera, from serologically confirmed cases yielded virus, most frequently between the 7th and 12th days after onset. Virus is rarely isolated from urine or throat swabs. In fatal cases, on the other hand, virus is easily and generally isolated from spleen and lymph nodes.[37]

The most convenient and efficient means for establishing a specific diagnosis are the FA and CF tests. While these tests are group-specific rather than type-specific, no diagnostic problems have arisen with Machupo virus due to its sharply localized geographic location. As with other diseases in this group of viruses, FA and CF antibodies are relatively late in appearing; although they have been found on the 14th day after onset, it is advisable to test a sample of serum between 40 and 60 days after onset.[46,47]

8.4. Treatment, Prevention, and Control

Administration of convalescent plasma has been advocated and used; despite some impressions of favorable clinical responses, its efficacy has not been established or denied, because of insufficient observation.[36]

Rodent control by continued trapping has been the most effective single means for preventing human infection and for terminating an epidemic; however, this approach seems unlikely to be the long-term solution of the problem. Given the sharply localized geographic distribution of the disease, it would seem that vaccination of exposed populations would be the effective answer, but no vaccine is available. Attenuation of a strain of Machupo virus by serial intracerebral passage in suckling mice has been reported and its possible use as source for a vaccine suggested.[40]

9. Lassa Fever

Lassa fever was first observed in 1969, in a missionary nurse stationed at a locality in northeastern Nigeria; following her admission to a hospital in Jos,

Nigeria, two contact cases developed in nurses at that hospital.[27] Because of the circumstances surrounding this outbreak and the fact that two of the three persons affected died, the disease acquired from the outset a reputation for severity that subsequent events amply justified. In addition to the initial episode, four more outbreaks occurred between 1970 and 1974 in Nigeria, Liberia, and Sierra Leone[17,28,61]; furthermore, laboratory accidents have occurred in the United States.[12,44]

9.1. Descriptive Epidemiology

9.1.1. Geographic Distribution. The disease has been observed in several localities in Nigeria since 1969 (Lassa, Jos, Onitsha, Zaria), in Liberia in 1972, and in Sierra Leone since 1970–1972. The number of cases seen, or retrospectively diagnosed, in the outbreaks has varied from 3 to about 60. Recent investigations indicate that the disease at present occurs in an endemoepidemic form in the eastern section of Sierra Leone and that it may have been seen as far back as 1956.[53a] Serological surveys have demonstrated the probable existence of Lassa virus infection in Guinea,[34] Central African Empire, Mali, Senegal, Cameroon, and Benin.[53a]

9.1.2. Epidemic Types: Season, Age, and Sex Distribution. Two types of outbreaks have been observed. The first type, hospital-associated, develops as a result of exposure and spread from a hospitalized index case to other patients, visitors, and medical staff. The index case is usually acquired in the nearby community; between 10 and 20 days after admission to the hospital, a cluster of secondary cases develops.[17,27,61] This type of outbreak has been the rule, with one exception.

The second type of outbreak, of which there is at present only one example (Sierra Leone, 1970–1972), occurs in the community at large. Patients acquire their infection at home or other community surroundings, rather than by exposure or contact in the hospital with another patient. However, there is also the possibility of nosocomial transmission in this type of outbreak, particularly to the hospital staff.[28]

Tertiary cases have been recorded, but with a few exceptions—notably by transmission to medical staff—they have been milder. No evidence has been reported of further propagation of the disease.[17]

The mortality in hospitalized cases has been between 20 and 66% in different outbreaks, with an average of 36%. The mortality following all types of infection as contrasted with severe illness requiring hospitalization, however, appears to be much lower. In the Sierra Leone focus, many persons with antibodies were found who either had not been ill or possibly remembered a mild disease; the overall mortality from Lassa virus infection in that area may have been only 3–5%.[28]

There is a seasonal distribution of hospital-associated outbreaks, which have occurred from January to April, during the dry season; the Sierra Leone cases occurred through the year, with somewhat higher incidence in the wet season.

With respect to age and sex distribution, the Sierra Leone outbreak with its pattern of transmission in the villages revealed no important predilection in morbidity or in case-fatality rates.[28] In the hospital-associated outbreaks, the distribution by sex and age was determined largely by the characteristics of the exposed population; physicians and nurses have been particularly affected. An antibody survey on more than 800 staff members of Liberian hospitals showed that midwifery students and clinical laboratory workers were the groups at highest risk.[27a]

9.2. Mechanism and Route of Transmission

9.2.1. Spread of Virus. The transmission in a hospital setting is undoubtedly from person to person by either the contact or the airborne route, including direct contact, droplet spread, or sharing of drink, food, clinical instruments, objects, and utensils. The same mode of transmission may be at work in contact infections acquired in the home.

In the community-centered outbreak at Sierra Leone, there was definite clustering of illness and seropositivity without illness in certain households; this could be explained either by multiple instances of human infection from the same natural source or by person-to-person transmission following a house index case acquired from the reservoir.[28]

The mode of transmission to man from the natural source or reservoir—a rodent—is still unknown. It may include direct contact with the rodent, its urine and oral secretions, eating of uncooked rodent flesh, or contact with food and drink contaminated by the rodent; it could also be airborne. The possibility of an arthropod vector appears extremely remote to explain transmission to man. Whether ectoparasites can transmit the infection between rodents is not known. Penetration through a cut while performing an autopsy appears to have been the mode of infection of a physician,[94] and infection through a cut on a finger may have occurred in a nurse.[27] Most medical and nursing personnel probably acquire the disease by droplet infection, since it has been established that the virus is present in the throat washings of patients for several days.[15,44,60]

9.2.2. Reservoir. Certain similarities between Lassa fever and the diseases caused by other arenaviruses, as well as the observation that Lassa virus persists for months in the urine of experimentally infected laboratory mice that appear otherwise healthy,[15] support the view that this virus may have a rodent reservoir in nature.

Among the small wild vertebrates collected in the course of investigating the Sierra Leone outbreak (1970–1972), attention was focused on rodents and bats, since these hosts are implicated in the ecology of other arenaviruses. Pooled tissues of heart, lung, spleen, and kidney from 325 field specimens tested for the presence of virus revealed only one infected species of rat, *Mastomys natalensis.* Ten viral isolations were yielded in 46 specimens tested.[6] This species is common and widely distributed in sub-Saharan Africa. In addition to its wild habitat, it is often peridomestic, entering houses, and other buildings; the potential for human contact is considerable.

Additional information is required to settle the question of the reservoir of Lassa fever virus, particularly whether other vertebrate species are involved in the natural cycle. More study is also needed on the dynamics of *Mastomys natalensis* population and its ecology.

9.3. Patterns of Host Response

9.3.1. Clinical Features. Lassa fever is a disease with generalized organ involvement manifested in severe cases by pharyngitis, pneumonitis, myositis, myocarditis, encephalopathy, nephropathy, and hemorrhagic diathesis. The overall spectrum of infection of man is not yet fully known; therefore, it is not possible to estimate the risk of severe illness following infection with the virus. All earlier reports[17,27,61,94] stressed the severity of the disease; however, there is evidence of milder forms, perhaps even inapparent infections.[28]

The incubation period is ordinarily between 6 and 14 days. The disease has an insidious onset; in variable order appear malaise, asthenia, lassitude, headache, sore throat, muscular aches, abdominal pains, loss of appetite, nausea, vomiting, and diarrhea. Fever appears early with somnolence, indifference, and blurred vision; the temperature is in the range from 101 to 104°F, and may reach 107°F. Petechiae may be seen, although the disease is not severely hemorrhagic. There is marked pharyngitis with firmly adherent, white patches on the soft palate, pharynx, and pillars. In severe progressive forms, signs of increase in capillary fragility appear with a suffusion or flush on the skin of face and upper thorax, puffed face, swollen neck, and markedly blurred vision. There are increased oliguria and dysuria. Additional petechiae appear and sometimes larger subcutaneous hemorrhages on the arms, legs, and abdominal walls. Pleural effusions may also occur. The acute febrile state lasts from 7 to 21 days; in fatal cases, death occurs usually during the course of the second week, its immediate cause being sudden cardiovascular collapse. The death rate in hospitalized cases has been from 30 to 60%, overall about 36%.[17,27,44,61,94]

9.3.2. Diagnosis. Lassa fever, unlike the other arenavirus infections, has a marked tendency to spread by human-to-human contagion. Under these circumstances, prompt diagnosis is essential in order to implement strict isolation measures. In the affected geographic areas, a clinical diagnosis is complicated by the occurrence of other diseases that may resemble Lassa fever. These include malaria, yellow fever, and especially typhoid fever. The lack of local laboratory facilities makes a specific diagnosis unavailable. In endemic areas, an illness characterized by unremitting fever with temperatures of 100°F or higher, persisting for 5–7 days or more, unresponsive to antibiotics and antimalarial drugs, accompanied by pharyngitis, malaise, toxic appearance, leukopenia, and, later, by facial edema, must give rise to a strong suspicion of Lassa fever.[59]

It must be remembered that any laboratory carrying out virological or bacteriological procedures on febrile patients in West Africa is under risk of encountering an unsuspected Lassa fever patient, as is also the case with any medical diagnostician seeing patients in the clinics or the wards.

A specific diagnosis is achieved by isolation of the virus, demonstration of antibody development, or both. Virus is isolated from the blood usually between the 3rd and 14th days of illness,[15,60] less frequently from throat washings, pleural effusions, and urine. Because of the recognized danger inherent in handling the virus, work with it including attempts to isolate it is restricted to laboratories with special high-containment facilities.* Development of antibodies between early and late samples of sera, detected by the FA or CF test, is a useful diagnostic procedure but not helpful for an early diagnosis, since antibodies are not usually detected before the 10th day after onset by FA or before the 18th or 20th by CF.

The frequency with which hospital-centered outbreaks have followed admission of a patient with undiagnosed Lassa fever is a paramount reason for an early diagnosis. Currently, the fastest way of establishing a diagnosis is by inoculation of the clinical specimen, usually acute-phase serum, into several Vero-cell cultures followed by daily examination of a culture by the FA test; under favorable circumstances, a positive diagnosis can be reached in 2 days from the moment when the specimen reaches the laboratory.[98] Examination by the FA test of conjunctival scrapings from patients with marked conjunctivitis in an effort to detect the antigen has been used with promising results[53a]; if generally successful, this would be the most rapid diagnostic procedure.

9.4. Treatment and Disposition of Patients

Plasma from recovered patients has been used, with conflicting reports on its efficacy.[7a,19a,41a,44,60, 94] It appears that additional clinical investigations of the efficacy, antibody contents of the plasma given, and risks of serum therapy in this disease are needed.

In view of the frequency with which the Lassa virus is propagated from person to person in a hospital setting, strict measures must be instituted to isolate patients and those suspected of having the disease. This includes the use of gloves, masks, and

* Laboratories equipped with required containment facilities that will on request undertake to isolate and identify Lassa virus from clinical specimens are: Special Pathogens Branch, Virology Division, CDC, Atlanta, Georgia, U.S.A.; and Centre for Applied Microbiology and Research, Porton Down, Wiltshire, England.

gowns by the staff, individual rooms for suspected cases, thorough decontamination of excretions and secretions, and sterilization of instruments, bedpans, and personal utensils.[59,101]

Transportation of suspected Lassa fever patients should be reduced to a minimum compatible with good medical and nursing care. Evacuation and international transportation of expatriate personnel suspected of having Lassa fever cannot be denied to the individual. However, this presents a serious problem to national and international health authorities whose responsibility is to localize the infection and prevent its spread to other areas. Procedures were developed and guidelines suggested after an imported case, including close surveillance of all contacts during the period prior to strict isolation of the suspected case.[101]

9.5. Prevention and Control

Prevention at the individual level is based on strict sanitary precautions; no vaccine is available. Since *Mastomys natalensis* is, thus far, the only known reservoir, measures that minimize contact of this rodent with man and his habitat will be helpful. However, it is unrealistic at this time to base too much hope on the effectiveness of the control of this rodent in the endemic areas. As mentioned above, special precautions must be taken in hospitals to prevent spread to the medical and nursing staff, especially those on obstetrical services with infected mothers.

10. Hemorrhagic Fever with Renal Syndrome

There is no evidence to indicate that this disease is caused by an arenavirus; the disease is described in this chapter because it has a number of clinical and epidemiological characteristics similar to those seen with arenavirus infections.

Hemorrhagic fever with renal syndrome is known by numerous synonyms, among which are "hemorrhagic nephrosonephritis" and "Korean hemorrhagic fever." It appeared to be caused by a virus, on the basis of investigations carried out with human volunteers by Smorodintsev *et al.*[85] in 1940–1941 in the Soviet Union and by Kitano *et al.*

in Manchuria at about the same time as stated by Gajdusek.[29]

Claims that an etiological agent had been maintained in cell cultures were made in 1971.[31] Recent studies[42a] describe the isolation of an agent from acute-phase serum of patients with the disease, which has been serially maintained by experimental inoculations in a rodent, *Apodemus agrarius*; the agent was identified in the viscera of inoculated animals by the FA test using convalescent sera from recovered patients. It appears (G. R. French, 1979, personal communication) that the agent can be maintained serially in a lung-carcinoma-cell culture, has a diameter between 100 and 220 nm, contains RNA, and has not shown an antigenic relationship with any of the arenaviruses.

The disease is prevalent in several sections of the U.S.S.R., principally in the Far East and in the middle Volga region, Bashkiria; between several hundred and several thousand cases occur annually.[18,19] The disease also occurs in Korea, where in the period between 1951 and 1976 it affected over 8000 persons, including United States and Korean army personnel and Korean civilians; the same or a very similar syndrome occurs in Sweden, Finland, and Hungary.

Clinically, the disease has a prodromal stage, followed by sudden onset with chills, fever, lethargy, frontal or retroorbital headache, myalgia, costovertebral pain, suffusion of face and upper part of thorax, petechiae or larger skin hemorrhages, and pronounced renal involvement with proteinuria, oliguria that may end up in anuria, and low fixed specific gravity of the urine; there are leukopenia and thrombocytopenia. Death is associated with shock and occurs in a variable proportion of cases, from 1–2 to 25–30%; the death rate is higher in the Far East than in the European part of the U.S.S.R.[18,19,29]

Extensive epidemiological investigations in the U.S.S.R. appear to have established a definite link—including season, place, occupation, and exposure—between disease and contact of man with various rodents, chief among them being *Clethrionomys glareolus*, *Apodemus sylvaticus*, *A. agrarius*, and *Microtus fortis*.[18] Soviet investigators consider that the rodents suffer a tolerant, persistent infection, excrete virus in the urine, and thus contaminate the human habitat. Support for the view that rodents are a reservoir of the disease agent is given by outbreaks in laboratory personnel who were in contact with collections of wild-caught rodents.[91]

11. Unresolved Questions

11.1. Vaccines

With the exception of LCM virus, which appears to have worldwide distribution, the other arenavirus diseases of man have been found restricted to definite geographic areas that, although showing a tendency to increase, are still easily identifiable. In the case of Lassa virus, although the areas are multiple and possibly more extensive than now known, they are confined to one continent. These geographic considerations, added to the fact that some of the more exposed groups—maize harvesters for AHF and hospital personnel for Lassa fever—are well defined, make these diseases an excellent target for preventive vaccination; however, no vaccines are currently available for any of the arenavirus diseases of man. Control of the reservoirs would undoubtedly be effective in preventing disease or reducing its incidence. At the moment, however, it does not appear to be a realistic solution.

Investigations to develop a vaccine for AHF have been carried out to the point where a large number of volunteers have been inoculated with an experimental vaccine. Efforts to develop an attenuated strain of Machupo virus have been initiated. No attempts to develop a vaccine against Lassa fever virus have been thus far reported. In view of the severity of these diseases, continued efforts to develop safe and effective vaccines are desirable.

11.2. Serum Therapy

Administration of plasma from persons who have recovered from the respective disease to patients in the acute phase of illness has been advocated as specific therapy. A controlled trial involving close to 450 persons has been reported with AHF[77a] with satisfactory results provided the serum was administered within 5 days from onset. Several reports (see Section 9.4) have discussed the use of immune plasma in Lassa fever; early results were on the whole favorable, but later ones point out failures and even deleterious effects. An argument given against administration of immune plasma in Lassa fever is that viremia, which lasts 2 weeks or longer after onset, coincides in part with circulating antibody, which begins to develop in the course of the 2nd week. The simultaneous presence of virus and antibody in the blood during the 2nd week may explain some of the pathology as due to deposit of complexes; added antibody may aggravate the condition. It is conceivable that with this disease, as with AHF, immune plasma of high antibody titer may be most effective and not harmful when given very soon after onset; additional observations are clearly needed to resolve the question.

11.3. Immunopathology

Although LCM in mice is a definite example of immunopathologically induced disease, there is no direct evidence that this is also the case in man. Disseminated intravascular coagulation has been reported in some fatal cases of AHF; viremia in man occurs, the duration of which is not well established but presumably not long, and antibodies develop late, having been hardly ever reported before the end of the 3rd week; while one may entertain the possibility that antigen–antibody complexes are formed, factual proof is not available.

There is evidence that antigen and antibody coexist in the blood in Lassa fever[98]; formation and deposition of complexes may result in immuno-logically mediated lesions by activation of complement and release of products that increase capillary permeability, which is one of the outstanding characteristics of the disease. In a well-documented autopsy,[96] it was concluded that hepatic lesions appeared to be the result of direct cell damage caused by the virus, with no cellular infiltration or other evidence of immunopathology. Studies on the physiopathology of arenavirus diseases of man are urgently needed in order to improve treatment; these studies, however, are made difficult in great part by the risk involved—particularly with Lassa fever—in handling probably contaminated clinical specimens.

11.4. Geographic Distribution

Knowledge of the distribution of the arenaviruses pathogenic for man is mainly based on recognized and specifically diagnosed disease; this knowledge fails to supply information concerning the total actual prevalence of infections including mild forms of disease and inapparent infections. Furthermore, atypical or mild cases in localities not now considered to be within the endemic areas may go unrecognized, particularly if they appear only sporadically.

Seroepidemiological surveys of LCM have been done in the past in Germany and the United States, but not within the past 10 or 15 years; there is no information available with respect to AHF and BHF, and although there are a few reports concerning Lassa fever, much remains to be done even in this disease. Much of the scarcity of information is to be attributed to the lack of practical, sensitive tests by which to assess the immune status of a population. Determination of neutralizing antibodies by plaque-reduction tests is not of much value with Lassa fever, is not an easy test to perform with LCM, and, while feasible, has not been applied to ASH and BHF to any remarkable extent. Since the CF test gives only limited information owing to the short persistence of antibodies detectable by this test, it would appear that the FA test is at the moment the test of choice; enzyme-linked immunosorbent assays (ELISAs) have not as yet been reported with these agents. It is to be hoped that increased seroepidemiological surveys employing available tests or others as may be developed will supply additional information on the distribution of these viruses.

12. References

1. ACKERMAN, R., Epidemiologic aspects of lymphocytic choriomeningitis in man, in: *Lymphocytic Choriomeningitis Virus and Other Arenaviruses* (F. LEHMANN-GRUBE, ed.), pp. 233–237, Springer-Verlag, New York, 1973.
2. ACKERMAN, R., BLOEDHORN, H., KUPPER, B., WINKENS, I., AND SCHEID, W., Über die Verbreitung des Virus der lymphocitaren Choriomeningitis unter den Mausen in Westdeutschland. I. Untersuchungen überwiegend an Hausmausen (*Mus musculus*), *Zentralbl. Bacteriol. Parasitenkd. Infektionskr. Hyg. Abt. 1* **194**:407–430 (1964).
3. ACKERMAN, R., STILLE, W., BLUMENTHAL, W., HELM, E. B., KELLER, K., AND BALDUS, O., Syrische Gold-

hamster als Übertrager von lymphocytaren Choriomeningitis, *Dtsch. Med. Wochenschr.* **45:**1725–1731 (1972).

4. ADAIR, C. V., GAULD, R. L., AND SMADEL, J. E., Aseptic meningitis, a disease of diverse etiology: Clinical and etiologic studies on 854 cases, *Ann. Intern. Med.* **39:**675–704 (1953).

5. AGREST, A., AVALOS, J. C. S., ARCE, M., AND SLEPOY, A., Fiebre hemorragica Argentina y coagulopatia por consumo, *Medicina* **29:**194–201 (1969).

5a. ANON, M. C., GRAU, O., SEGOVIA, Z. M., AND FRANZE-FERNANDEZ, M. T., RNA composition of Junin virus, *J. Virol.* **18:**833–838 (1976).

6. ANONYMOUS, Follow-up on Lassa fever, *Morbidity Mortality Weekly Rep.* **22:**201–202 (1973).

7. ANONYMOUS, Laboratory epidemic traced to hamsters, *J. Am. Med. Assoc.* **228:**815–816 (1974).

7a. ANONYMOUS, Recommendations for initial management of suspected or confirmed cases of Lassa fever, *Morbidity Mortality Weekly Rep. Supplement* **28:**3S–12S (1980).

8. ARMSTRONG, C., AND LILLIE, R. D., Experimental lymphocytic choriomeningitis of monkeys and mice produced by a virus encountered in studies of the 1933 St. Louis encephalitis epidemic, *Public Health Rep.* **49:**1019–1027 (1934).

9. ARMSTRONG, C., AND SWEET, L. K., Lymphocytic choriomeningitis: Report of two cases, with recovery of the virus from gray mice (*Mus musculus*) trapped in the two infected households, *Public Health Rep.* **54:**673–684 (1939).

10. ARMSTRONG, D., FORTNER, J. G., ROWE, W. P., AND PARKER, J. C., Meningitis due to lymphocytic choriomeningitis virus endemic in a hamster colony, *J. Am. Med. Assoc.* **209:**265–267 (1969).

11. ARRIBALZAGA, R. A., Una nueva enfermedad epidemica a germen desconocido, hipertermica, nefrotoxica, leucopenica y enantematica, *Dia Medico* **27:**1204–1210 (1955).

12. ATKINS, J. L., FREEMAN, S., SCHRACK, D. W., JR., DOWNS, W. G., AND CORONA, R. C., Lassa virus infection, *Morbidity Mortality Weekly Rep.* **19:**123 (1970).

13. BLANC, G., BRUNEAU, J., DELAGE, B., AND POITROT, R., Etude comparative de virus de choriomeningite lymphocytaire d'origine humaine (W. E. Armstrong) et animale (pneumopathie du cobaye), *Bull. Acad. Natl. Med. Paris* **135:**520–528 (1951).

13a. BLOCH, A., A serological survey of Lassa fever in Liberia, *Bull. W.H.O.* **56:**811–813 (1978).

14. BLUMENTHAL, W., KESSLER, R., AND ACKERMAN, R., Über die Durchseuchung der ländlichen Bevölkerung in der Bundesrepublik Deutschland mit dem Virus der Lymphocytären Choriomeningitis, *Zentralbl. Bakteriol. Parasitenkd. Infektionskr. Hyg. Abt. 1 Orig.* **213:**36–48 (1970).

15. BUCKLEY, S. M., AND CASALS, J., Lassa fever, a new

virus disease of man from West Africa. II. Isolation and characterization of the virus. *Am. J. Trop. Med. Hyg.* **19:**680–691 (1970).

16. CALISHER, C. H., TZIANABOS, T., LORD, R. D., AND COLEMAN, P. H., Tamiami virus, a new member of the Tacaribe group, *Am. J. Trop. Med. Hyg.* **19:**520–526 (1970).

17. CAREY, D. E., KEMP, G. E., WHITE, H. A., PINNEO, L., ADDY, R. F., FOM, A. L. M. D., STROH, G., CASALS, J., AND HENDERSON, B. E., Lassa fever: Epidemiological aspects of the 1970 epidemic, Jos, Nigeria, *Trans. R. Soc. Trop. Med. Hyg.* **66:**402–408 (1972).

17a. CASALS, J., Arenavirus, in: *Diagnostic Procedures for Viral, Rickettsial and Chlamydial Infections* (E. H., LENNETTE AND N. J. SCHMIDT, eds.) pp. 815–841, American Public Health Association, New York, 1979.

18. CASALS, J., HENDERSON, B. E., HOOGSTRAAL, H., JOHNSON, K. M., AND SHELOKOV, A., A review of Soviet viral hemorrhagic fevers, 1969, *J. Infect. Dis.* **122:**437–453 (1970).

19. CASALS, J., HOOGSTRAAL, H., JOHNSON, K. M., SHELOKOV, A., WIEBENGA, N. H. AND WORK, T. H., A current appraisal of hemorrhagic fevers in the USSR, *Am. J. Trop. Med. Hyg.* **15:**751–764 (1966).

19a. CLAYTON, A. J., Lassa immune serum, *Bull. W.H.O.* **55:**435–439 (1977).

20. COGGESHALL, L. T., The transmission of lymphocytic choriomeningitis by mosquitoes, *Science* **89:**515–516 (1939).

21. *Comision Nacional Coordinadora para Estudio y Lucha Contra la Fiebre Hemorragica Argentina*, Buenos Aires, pp. 1–117 (1966).

21a. DEIBEL, R., WOODALL, J. P., DECHER, W. J., AND SCHRYVER, G. D., Lymphocytic choriomeningitis in man, *J. Am. Med. Assoc.* **323:**501–504 (1975).

22. DOUGLAS, R. G., WIEBENGA, N. H., AND COUCH, R. B., Bolivian hemorrhagic fever probably transmitted by personal contact, *Am. J. Epidemiol.* **82:**85–91 (1965).

23. DOWNS, W. G., ANDERSON, C. R., SPENCE, L., AITKEN, T. H. G., AND GREENHALL, A. H., Tacaribe virus, a new agent isolated from *Artibeus* bats and mosquitoes in Trinidad, West Indies, *Am. J. Trop. Med. Hyg.* **12:**640–646 (1963).

24. ELSNER, B., SCHWARZ, E., MANDO, O., MAIZTEGUI, J., AND VILCHES, A., Patologia de la fiebre hemorragica Argentina, *Medicina (Suppl. No. 1)* **30:**85–94 (1970).

25. EMMONS, R. W., CHIN, J., NAYFIELD, C. L., WATERMAN, G. E., DIUMARA, N. J., FLEMING, D. S., ZISKIN, R., GOLDFIELD, M., ALTMAN, R., WOODALL, J., DEIBEL, R., AND HINMAN, A. P., Follow-up on hamster-associated LCM infection, *Morbidity Mortality Weekly Rep.* **23:**131–132 (1974).

25a. FENNER, F., Classification and nomenclature of viruses, *Intervirology* **7:**1–115 (1976).

26. FÖRSTER, U., AND WACHENDÖRFER, G., Inapparent in-

fection of Syrian hamster with the virus of lymphocytic choriomeningitis, in: *Lymphocytic Choriomeningitis Virus and Other Arenaviruses* (F. LEHMANN-GRUBE, ed.), pp. 113–120, Springer-Verlag, New York, 1973.

27. FRAME, J. D., BALDWIN, J. M., JR., GOCKE, D. J., AND TROUP, J. M., Lassa fever, a new virus disease of man from West Africa. I. Clinical description and pathological findings. *Am. J. Trop. Med. Hyg.* **23**:1131–1139 (1974).

27a. FRAME, J. D., CASALS, J., AND DENNIS, E. A., Lassa virus antibodies in hospital personnel in western Liberia, *Trans. R. Soc. Trop. Med. Hyg.* **73**:219–224 (1979).

28. FRASER, D. W., CAMPBELL, C. C., MONATH, T. P., GOFF, P. A., AND GREGG, M. B., Lassa fever in the Eastern Province of Sierra Leone, 1970–1972. I. Epidemiologic studies, *Am. J. Trop. Med. Hyg.* **23**: 1131–1139 (1974).

29. GAJDUSEK, D. C., Virus hemorrhagic fevers, *J. Pediatr.* **60**:841–857 (1962).

30. GALLARDO, F., Fiebre hemorragica Argentina: Hallazgos anatomopatologicos en diez necropsias, *Medicina (Suppl. No. 1)* **30**:77–84 (1970).

30a. GARD, G. P., VEZZA, A. C., BISHOP, D. H. L., AND COMPANS, R. W., Structural proteins of Tacaribe and Tamiami virions, *Virology* **83**:84–95 (1977).

30b. GANGEMI, J. D., ROSATO, R. B., CONNELL, E. V., JOHNSON, E. M., AND EDDY, G. A., Structural polypeptides of Machupo virus, *J. Gen. Virol.* **41**:183–188 (1978).

31. GAVRILYUK, B. K., NOSKOV, F. S., AND SMORODINTSEV, A. A., Study of haemorrhagic nephroso-nephritis virus by the fluorescent antibody technique, *Acta Virol.* **15**:485–492 (1971).

32. GILDEN, D. H., FRIEDMAN, H. M., KYJ, C. O., ROOSA, R. A., AND NATHANSON, N., Tamiami virus-induced immunopathological disease of the central nervous system, in: *Lymphocytic Choriomeningitis Virus and Other Arenaviruses* (F. LEHMANN-GRUBE, ed.), pp. 287–297, Springer-Verlag, New York, 1973.

32a. GRELA, M. E., GARCIA, C. A., ZANNOLI, V. H., AND BARRERA ORO, J. G., Serologia de la fiebre hemorragica Argentina. II. Comparación de la prueba indirecta de anticuerpos fluorescentes con la fijación de complemento, *Acta Bio-Clin. Latinoamericana* **9**:141–146 (1975).

33. GSCHWENDER, H. H., AND LEHMANN-GRUBE, F., Antigenic properties of the LCM virus: Virion and complement-fixing antigen, in: *Lymphocytic Choriomeningitis and Other Arenaviruses* (F. LEHMANN-GRUBE, ed.), pp. 26–35, Springer-Verlag, New York, 1973.

34. HENDERSON, B. E., GRAY, G. W., JR., KISSLING, R. E., FRAME, J. D., AND CAREY, D. E., Lassa fever: Virological and serological studies, *Trans. R. Soc. Trop. Med. Hyg.* **66**:409–416 (1972).

35. HOTCHIN, J., *Persistent and Slow Virus Infections*, Vol. 3 of *Monographs in Virology* pp. 1–211, S. Karger, New York, 1971.

36. JOHNSON, K. M., Fiebres hemorragicas de America del Sur, *Medicina (Suppl. No. 1)* **30**:99–110 (1970).

37. JOHNSON, K. M., HALSTEAD, S. B., AND COHEN, S. N., Hemorrhagic fevers of Southeast Asia and South America: A comparative appraisal, *Prog. Med. Virol.* **9**:105–158 (1967).

38. JOHNSON, K. M., KUNS, M. L., MACKENZIE, R. B., WEBB, P. A., AND YUNKER, C. E., Isolation of Machupo virus from wild rodent *Calomys callosus*, *Am. J. Trop. Med. Hyg.* **15**:103–106 (1966).

39. JOHNSON, K. M., AND WEBB, P. A., Rodent transmitted hemorrhagic fevers, in: *Diseases Transmitted from Animals to Man* (W. T. HUBBERT, W. F., McCULLOCH, AND T. R. SCHNURRENBERGER, eds.), 6th ed. pp. 911–918, Charles C. Thomas, Springfield, Illinois, 1975.

40. JOHNSON, K. M., WEBB, P. A., AND JUSTINES, G., Biology of Tacaribe-complex viruses, in: *Lymphocytic Choriomeningitis Virus and Other Arenaviruses* (F. LEHMANN-GRUBE, ed.), pp. 241–258, Springer-Verlag, New York, 1973.

41. JUSTINES, G., AND JOHNSON, K. M., Immune tolerance in *Calomys callosus* infected with Machupo virus, *Nature (London)* **222**:1090–1091 (1969).

41a. KEANE, E., AND GILLES, H. M., Lassa fever in Panguma Hospital, Sierra Leone, 1973–76, *Br. Med. J.* **1**:1399–1402 (1977).

42. KUNS, M. L., Epidemiology of Machupo virus infection. II. Ecological and control studies of hemorrhagic fever, *Am. J. Trop. Med. Hyg.* **14**:813–816 (1965).

42a. LEE, H. W., LEE, P. W., AND JOHNSON, K. M., Isolation of the etiologic agent of Korean hemorrhagic fever, *J. Infect. Dis.* **137**:298–308 (1978).

43. LEHMANN-GRUBE, F., *Lymphocytic Choriomeningitis Virus*, Vol. 10 of *Virology Monographs*, Springer-Verlag, New York, 1971, 173 pp.

44. LEIFER, E., GOCKE, D. J., AND BOURNE, H., Lassa fever, a new virus disease of man from West Africa. II. Report of a laboratory-acquired infection treated with plasma from a person recently recovered from the disease, *Am. J. Trop. Med. Hyg.* **19**:677–679 (1970).

45. LEWIS, A. M., ROWE, W. P., TURNER, H. C., AND HUEBNER, R. J., Lymphocytic-choriomeningitis virus in hamster tumor: Spread to hamsters and humans, *Science* **150**:363–364 (1965).

46. MACKENZIE, R. B., Epidemiology of Machupo virus infection. I. Pattern of human infection, San Joaquin, Bolivia, 1962–64, *Am. J. Trop. Med. Hyg.* **14**:808–813 (1965).

47. MACKENZIE, R. B., WEBB, P. A., AND JOHNSON, K. M., Detection of complement-fixing antibody after Bolivian hemorrhagic fever, employing Machupo, Junin and Tacaribe virus antigens, *Am. J. Trop. Med. Hyg.* **14**:1079–1084 (1965).

48. MAIZTEGUI, J. I., Epidemiologia de la fiebre hemorragica Argentina, in: *Proceedings, Quinto Congresso La-*

tino-Americano de Microbiologia, Punta del Este, Uruguay, pp. 71–76 (1971).

49. MAIZTEGUI, J. I., Argentinian hemorrhagic fever (AHF), in: *Proceedings, Ninth International Congress on Tropical Medicine and Malaria,* Athens, Vol. 1, p. 31 (1973).

50. MAIZTEGUI, J. I., AGUIRRE, G. M., SABATTINI, M. S., AND ORO, J. G. B., Actividad de dos "arenavirus" en seres humanos y roedores en un mismo lugar de la zona endemica de fiebre hemorragica Argentina, *Medicina* **31:**509–510 (1971).

51. MAIZTEGUI, J. I., ESTRIBOU, J. P., SABATTINI, M. S., AND ORO, J. G. B., Estudios tendientes a dilucidar el papel del *Mus musculus* en la epidemiologia de la fiebre hemorragica Argentina (FHA), *Rev. Soc. Argent. Microbiol.* **2:**186–187 (1970).

52. MAIZTEGUI, J. I., SABITTINI, M. S., AND ORO, J. G. B., Actividad del virus de la coriomeningitis linfocitica (LCM) en el area endemica de fiebre hemorragica Argentina (FHA), *Medicina* **32:**131–137 (1971).

53. MANNWEILER, K., AND LEHMANN-GRUBE, F., Electron microscopy of LCM virus-infected L cells, in: *Lymphocytic Choriomeningitis Virus and Other Arenaviruses* (F. LEHMANN-GRUBE, ed.), pp. 37–48, Springer-Verlag, New York, 1973.

53a. MCCORMICK, J. B., AND JOHNSON, K. M., Lassa fever: Historical review and contemporary investigation, in: *Ebola Virus Haemorrhagic Fever* (S. R., PATTYN, ed.), pp. 279–285, Elsevier/North-Holland, Amsterdam, 1978.

54. METTLER, N. E., Estudio realizado con los sueros de la epidemia de fiebre hemorragica Argentina (1963) que no presentaron conversion serologica para virus Junin, *Medicina* **26:**161–169 (1966).

55. METTLER, N. E., *Argentine Hemorrhagic Fever: Current Knowledge,* Pan American Health Organization, Scientific Publications No. 183, pp. 1–55 (1969).

56. METTLER, N. E., AND CASALS, J., Isolation of St. Louis encephalitis virus from man in Argentina, *Acta Virol.* **15:**148–154 (1971).

57. METTLER, N. E., CASALS, J., AND SHOPE, R. E., Study of antigenic relationships between Junin virus, the etiological agent of Argentinian hemorrhagic fever, and other arthropod-borne viruses, *Am. J. Trop. Med. Hyg.* **12:**647–652 (1963).

58. MEYER, H. M., JOHNSON, R. T., CRAWFORD, I. P., DASCOMB, H. E., AND ROGERS, N. G., Central nervous system syndromes of "viral" etiology: A study of 713 cases, *Am. J. Med.* **29:**334–347 (1960).

59. MONATH, T. P., AND CASALS, J., Diagnosis of Lassa fever and the isolation and management of patients, *Bull. W.H.O.* **52:**707–715 (1975).

60. MONATH, T. P., MAHER, M., CASALS, J., KISSLING, R. E., AND CACCIAPUOTI, A., Lassa fever in the Eastern Province of Sierra Leone, 1970–1972. II. Clinical ob-

servations and virological studies on selected hospital cases, *Am. J. Trop. Med. Hyg.* **23:**1140–1149 (1974).

61. MONATH, T. P., MERTENS, P. E., PATTON, R., MOSER, C. R., BAUM, J. J., PINNEO, L., GARY, G. W., AND KISSLING, R. E., A hospital epidemic of Lassa fever in Zorzor, Liberia, March–April 1972, *Am. J. Trop. Med. Hyg.* **22:**773–779 (1973).

62. MURPHY, F. A., WEBB, P. A., JOHNSON, K. M., AND WHITFIELD, S. G., Morphological comparison of Machupo with lymphocytic choriomeningitis virus: Basis for a new taxonomic group, *J. Virol.* **4:**535–541 (1969).

63. MURPHY, F. A., WEBB, P. A., JOHNSON, K. M., WHITFIELD, S. G., AND CHAPPELL, W. A., Arenoviruses in Vero cells: Ultrastructural studies, *J. Virol.* **6:**507–518 (1970).

64. MURPHY, F. A., WHITFIELD, S. G., WEBB, P. A., AND JOHNSON, K. M., Ultrastructural studies of arenaviruses, in: *Lymphocytic Choriomeningitis Virus and Other Arenaviruses* (F. LEHMANN-GRUBE, ed.), pp. 273–285, Springer-Verlag, New York, 1973.

65. ORO, J. G. B., MAIZTEGUI, J. I., AND SABATTINI, M. S., Fiebre hemorragica Argentina en la provincia de Sante Fe, *Rev. Asoc. Argent. Microbiol.* **5:**57–58 (1973).

66. PARODI, A. S., GREENWAY, D. J., RUGIERO, H. R., RIVERO, S., FRIGERIO, M., BARRERA, J. M., METTLER, N., GARZON, F., BOXACA, M., GUERRERO, L., AND NOTA, N., Sobre la etiologia del brote epidemico de Junin, *Dia Med.* **30:**2300–2302 (1958).

67. PARODI, A. S., DE GUERRERO, L. B., ASTARLOA, L., CINTORA, A., CAMBACERES, C. G., MAGLIO, G., MAGNONI, C., MILANI, H., RUGGIERO, H., AND SQUASSI, G., Immunizacion contra la fiebre hemorragica Argentina con una cepa atenuada de virus Junin, *Medicina (Suppl. No. 1)* **30:**3–7 (1970).

68. PARODI, A. S., RUGIERO, H. R., GREENWAY, D. L., METTLER, N. E., MARTINEZ, A., BOXACA, M., AND BARRERA, J. M., Aislamiento del virus Junin (FHE) de los acaros de la zona epidemica (*Echinolaelaps echidninus,* Berlese), *Prensa Med. Argent.* **46:**2242–2244 (1959).

69. PEDERSEN, I. R., LCM virus: Its purification and its chemical and physical properties, in: *Lymphocytic Choriomeningitis Virus and Other Arenaviruses* (F. LEHMANN-GRUBE, ed.), pp. 13–23, Springer-Verlag, New York, 1973.

69a. PETERS, C. B., WEBB, P. A., AND JOHNSON, K. M., Measurement of antibodies to Machupo virus by the indirect fluorescent technique, *Proc. Soc. Exp. Biol. Med.* **142:**526–531 (1973).

70. PFAU, C. J., WELSH, R. W., AND TROWBRIDGE, R. S., Plaque assays and current concepts of regulation in arenavirus infections, in: *Lymphocytic Choriomeningitis Virus and Other Arenaviruses* (F. LEHMANN-GRUBE, ed.), pp. 101–111, Springer-Verlag, New York, 1973.

71. PINHEIRO, F. P., SHOPE, R. E., DE ANDRADE, A. H. P.,

BENSABETH, G., CACIOS, G. V., AND CASALS, J., Amapari, a new virus of the Tacaribe group from rodents and mites of Amapa Territory, Brazil, *Proc. Soc. Exp. Biol. Med.* **122:**531–535 (1966).

71a. PINHEIRO, F. P., WOODALL, J. P., TRAVASSOS DA ROSA, A. P. A., AND TRAVASSOS DA ROSA, J. F., Studies on arenaviruses in Brazil, *Medicina (Buenos Aires) (Suppl. No. 3)* **37:**175–181 (1977).

72. PINTOS, I. M., Epidemiologia del "Mal de los Rastrojos," *Separata An. Com. Invest. Cient. Prov. Buenos Aires* **3:**9–102 (1962).

73. PIROSKY, I., ZUCCARINI, J., MOLINELLI, E. A., DiPIETRO, A., ORO, J. G. B., MARTINI, P., AND COPELLO, A. R., *Virosis Hemorragica del Noroeste Bonaerense: Endemo-epidemica, Febril, Enantematica y Leucopenica*, Comision Nacional ad hoc para Estudiar el Brote de 1958, Tallares Graficos del Ministerio de Asistencia Social y Salud Publica, Buenos Aires, 1959.

74. RAWLS, W. E., RAMOS, B. A., AND CARTER, M. F., Biophysical and biochemical studies of Pichinde virus, in: *Lymphocytic Choriomeningitis Virus and Other Arenaviruses* (F. LEHMANN-GRUBE, ed.), pp. 259–272, Springer-Verlag, New York, 1973.

75. RIVERS, T. M., AND SCOTT, T. F. M., Meningitis in man caused by a filterable virus. II. Identification of the etiological agent, *J. Exp. Med.* **63:**415–432 (1936).

76. ROWE, W. P., MURPHY, F. A., BERGOLD, G. H., CASALS, J., HOTCHIN, J., JOHNSON, K. M., LEHMANN-GRUBE, F., MIMS, C. A., TRAUB, E., AND WEBB, P. A., Arenoviruses: Proposed name for a newly defined virus group, *J. Virol.* **5:**651–652 (1970).

77. ROWE, W. P., PUGH, W. E., WEBB, P. A., AND PETERS, C. J., Serological relationship of the Tacaribe complex of viruses to lymphocytic choriomeningitis virus, *J. Virol.* **5:**289–292 (1970).

77a. RUGIERO, H. A., MAGNONI, C., CINTORA, F. A., MILANI, H. A., AND IZQUIERDO, F. P., Tratamiento de la fiebre hemorragica Argentina con plasma de convaleciente, *Prensa Med. Argent.* **59:**1569–1579 (1972).

78. RUGIERO, H. R., PARODI, A. S., GOTTA, H., BOXACA, M., OLIVARI, A. J., AND GONZALEZ, E., Fiebre hemorragica epidemica: Infeccion de laboratorio y passage interhummano, *Rev. Asoc. Med. Argent.* **76:**413–417 (1962).

79. SABATTINI, M. S., AND MAIZTEGUI, J. I., Fiebre hemorragica Argentina, *Medicina (Suppl. No. 1)* **30:**111–128 (1970).

80. SABATTINI, M. S., ORO, J. G. B., MAIZTEGUI, J. I., FERNANDEZ, D., COSTIGIANI, M. S., AND DIAZ, G. E., Aislamiento de un "arenovirus" relacionado con el de la coriomeningitis linfocitica (LCM) a partir de un *Mus musculus* capturado en zona endemica de fiebre hemorragica Argentina (FHA), *Rev. Asoc. Argent. Microbiol.* **2:**182–184 (1970).

81. SCHEIDT, W., ACKERMAN, R., AND FELGENHAUER, K., Lymphocytäre Choriomeningitis unter dem Bild der Encephalitis lethargica, *Dtsch. Med. Wochenschr.* **93:**940–943 (1968).

82. SCHWARZ, E. R., MANDO, O. G., MAIZTEGUI, J. I., AND VILCHES, A. M., Sintomas y signos iniciales de mayor valor diagnostico en la fiebre hemorragica Argentina, *Medicina (Suppl. No. 1)* **30:**8–14 (1970).

83. SCOTT, T. F. M., AND RIVERS, T. M., Meningitis in man caused by a filterable virus. I. Two cases and the method of obtaining a virus from their spinal fluids, *J. Exp. Med.* **63:**397–414 (1936).

83a. SEGOVIA, Z. M., AND DE MITRI, M. I., Junin virus structural proteins, *J. Virol.* **21:**579–583 (1977).

83b. SHEINBERGAS, M. M., Hydrocephalus due to prenatal infection with the lymphocytic choriomeningitis virus, *Infection* **4:**1–7 (1976).

84. SMADEL, J. E., GREEN, R. H., PALTAUF, R. M., AND GONZALES, T. A., Lymphocytic choriomeningitis: Two human fatalities following an unusual febrile illness, *Proc. Soc. Exp. Biol. Med.* **49:**683–686 (1942).

85. SMORODINTSEV, A. A., KAZBINTSEV, L. I., AND CHUDAKOV, V. G., *Virus Hemorrhagic Fevers*, Israel Program for Scientific Translation, Clearing House, Springfield, Virginia, 1964, 245 pp.

86. SPEIR, R. W., WOOD, O., LIEBHABER, H., AND BUCKLEY, S. M., Lassa fever, a new virus disease of man from West Africa. IV. Electron microscopy of Vero cell cultures infected with Lassa virus, *Am. J. Trop. Med. Hyg.* **19:**692–694 (1970).

87. SULKIN, S. E., AND PIKE, R. M., Prevention of laboratory infections, in: *Diagnostic Procedures for Viral and Rickettsial Diseases* (E. H. LENNETTE AND N. J. SCHMIDT, eds.), pp. 66–78, American Public Health Associations, New York, 1969.

88. TRAPIDO, H., AND SANMARTIN, C., Pichinde virus, a new virus of the Tacaribe group from Colombia, *Am. J. Trop. Med. Hyg.* **20:**631–641 (1971).

89. TRAUB, E., A filterable virus recovered from white mice, *Science* **81:**298–299 (1935).

90. TRAUB, E., Epidemiology of lymphocytic choriomeningitis in a mouse stock observed for four years, *J. Exp. Med.* **69:**801–817 (1939).

91. TRENCSENI, T., AND KELETI, B., *Clinical Aspects and Epidemiology of Hemorrhagic Fever with Renal Syndrome*, Akademiai Kiado, Budapest, 1971, 247 pp.

92. WEBB, P. A., JOHNSON, K. M., HIBBS, J. G., AND KUNS, M. L., Parana, a new Tacaribe complex virus from Paraguay, *Arch. Gesamte Virusforsch.* **32:**379–388 (1970).

93. WEBB, P. A., JOHNSON, K. M., PETERS, C. J., AND HIBBS, J. B., Immunological relationships among Tacaribe complex viruses and description of a new serotype from Boliva, Latino virus (personal communication) (1976).

94. White, H. A., Lassa fever: A Study of 23 hospital cases, *Trans. R. Soc. Trop. Med. Hyg.* **66**:390–398 (1972).

95. Wiebenga, N. H., Shelokov, A., Gibbs, C. J., Jr., and Mackenzie, R. B., Epidemic hemorrhagic fever in Bolivia. II. Demonstration of complement-fixing antibody in patients' sera with Junin virus antigen, *Am. J. Trop. Med. Hyg.* **13**:626–628 (1964).

96. Winn, W. C., Jr., Monath, T. P., Murphy, F. A., and Whitfield, S. G., Lassa virus hepatitis: Observations on a fatal case from the 1972 Sierra Leone epidemic, *Arch. Pathol.* **99**:599–604 (1975).

97. Wooley, J. G., Armstrong, C., and Onstott, R. H., The occurrence in the sera of man and monkeys of protective antibodies against the virus of lymphocytic choriomeningitis as determined by the serum-virus protection test in mice, *Public Health Rep.* **52**:1105–1114 (1937).

98. Wulff, H., and Lange, J. V., Indirect immunofluorescence for the diagnosis of Lassa fever infection, *Bull. W.H.O.* **52**:429–436 (1975).

99. Wulff, H., Lange, J. V., and Webb, P. A., Interrelationships among arenaviruses measured by indirect immunofluorescence, *Intervirology* **9**:344–350 (1978).

100. Wulff, H., McIntosh, B. M., Hamer, D. B., and Johnson, K. M., Isolation of an arenavirus closely related to Lassa virus from *Mastomys natalensis* in south-east Africa, *Bull. W.H.O.* **55**:441–444 (1977).

101. Zweighaft, R. M., Fraser, D. W., Hattwick, M. A. W., Winkler, W. C., Jordon, W. C., Alter, M., Wolfe, M., Wulf, H., and Johnson, K. M., Lassa fever: Response to an imported case, *N. Engl. J. Med.* **297**:803–807 (1977).

13. Suggested Reading

Casals, J., and Buckley, S. M., Lassa fever, *Prog. Med. Virol.* **18**:111–125 (1974).

Coto, C. E., Junin virus, *Prog. Med. Virol.* **18**:127–142 (1974).

International Symposium on Arenaviral Infections of Public Health Importance, *Bull. W.H.O.* **52**:381–766 (1975).

Johnson, K. M., Halstead, S. B., and Cohen, S. N., Hemorrhagic fevers of Southeast Asia and South America: A comparative appraisal, *Prog. Med. Virol.* **9**:105–158 (1967).

Lehmann-Grube, F., *Lymphocytic Choriomeningitis Virus*, Vol. 10 of *Virology Monographs*, Springer-Verlag, New York, 1971, 173 pp.

CHAPTER 7

Coronaviruses

Arnold S. Monto

1. Introduction

The coronaviruses are a group of RNA-containing agents that have been associated with respiratory illnesses in man and with a number of other diseases in laboratory and domestic animals. The name for the group was adopted to describe the characteristic fringe of crownlike projections seen around the viruses by electron microscopy; these projections are rounded, rather than sharp or pointed as is the case with the myxoviruses. Like the myxoviruses, the coronaviruses contain essential lipid and are 80–160 nm in diameter.[18] While the animal strains are readily isolated in several different systems, recovery of the human strains has posed major problems. A number of these strains have been isolated only in organ culture of the human respiratory tract. This factor has made it difficult to determine the relationship among isolates and has complicated efforts to understand the role of these viruses in human respiratory illness. Therefore, much of the information on the epidemiology of the agents has come from serological studies.

2. Historical Background

The first human coronaviruses were isolated by different techniques in the United States and Britain

at approximately the same time. The British Medical Research Council's Common Cold Research Unit had been studying fluids collected from persons with natural respiratory infections and by standard cell-culture isolation methods and by inoculating them into human volunteers. Rhinoviruses or other cytopathogenic agents could be recovered from a portion of the fluids.[36] There was an additional substantial portion from which no agents could be isolated but that could still cause colds in the volunteers. Organ cultures of human embryonic trachea or nasal epithelium were then used in an effort to detect the recalcitrant viruses present in the fluids. A specimen, B814, that had been collected in 1960 from a boy with a common cold had not yielded a virus on inoculation into cell culture. After the specimen had been passaged serially three times in human tracheal organ culture, it could still cause colds on inoculation into volunteers, which indicated that replication had taken place.[58]

In Chicago during the winter of 1962, five agents were isolated in primary human kidney-cell cultures from specimens collected from medical students with common colds. The viruses were ultimately adapted to W138 cultures and exhibited a type of cytopathic effect (CPE) not previously seen. A prototype strain, 229E, was selected for characterization and was found to be RNA-containing, ether-labile, and 89 nm in diameter, but distinct serologically from any known myxo- or paramyxoviruses. Sera collected from the five medical students all exhibited a 4-fold rise in neutralizing antibody titer against 229E.[23]

It became clear that these "novel" viruses were

Arnold S. Monto · Department of Epidemiology, School of Public Health, University of Michigan, Ann Arbor, Michigan.

of more than passing significance when organ-culture methods were added to standard cell-culture techniques in a study of acute respiratory infections of adults conducted at the National Institutes of Health (NIH). Six viruses were found that grew in organ but not cell culture and were ether-labile; on electron microscopy, the agents were shown to resemble avian infectious bronchitis virus (IBV) in structure.[39] The B814 and 229E strains were soon also demonstrated to have a similar structure on electron microscopy and to develop in infected cells by budding into cytoplasmic vesicles.[1,2,22] As a result of the similarity of the human agents to IBV and also to mouse hepatitis virus (MHV), they were collectively considered to represent a group of vertebrate viruses distinct from the myxoviruses antigenically and structurally.[3] The name *coronavirus* was adopted for the group to describe the fringe of projections seen around them on electron microscopy.[18]

Except for 229E, none of the human coronaviruses had been successfully propagated in a system other then organ culture. McIntosh *et al.*[37] reported successful adaptation of two of the NIH isolates, OC (organ culture) 38 and OC43, to the brains of suckling mice. These strains were shown to be essentially identical antigenically but quite distinct from MHV. Only OC38 and OC43 could be so adapted; the other four OC strains resisted such attempts. IBV was known to exhibit hemagglutination under certain conditions, but no such phenomenon had been demonstrated for the human strains until OC38 and OC43 were adapted to mice. Kaye and Dowdle[32] found that the infected brain preparations would directly and specifically agglutinate red cells obtained from chickens, rats, and mice. This technique greatly expanded the ability to do epidemiological studies, since it was simple and reproducible.

Other more recent developments have included adaptation of OC38 and OC43 to growth in cell monolayers; either mouse brain or organ-culture material could be used as source of virus.[11] Not only was CPE available for reading of neutralization tests, but also the OC38 and OC43 virus was found to hemadsorb red cells of rats and mice, making available a more precise means of evaluating end points in tests involving these organ-culture-derived strains.[30] The other OC strains that could not be adapted to mouse brain resisted adaptation to

cell culture. Finally, immune electron microscopy has been added to the methods available for identifying the presence of coronaviruses in organ-culture harvests. This highly sensitive technique should improve the ability to detect virus, but it is obviously unsuitable for use in all but the most specialized studies.[31]

3. Methodology

3.1. Sources of Mortality Data

Coronaviruses that infect domestic and laboratory animals produce illnesses that are sometimes fatal. In contrast, there is no documented report yet on record of human coronaviruses being involved in a lethal infection. This situation may be a reflection of the limited number of investigations carried out as yet. It is known that these agents frequently infect small children and reinfect adults, including persons with chronic respiratory disease.[53] It would be logical to assume that deaths could occasionally occur in these most susceptible segments of the population, but they are probably not very frequent.

3.2. Sources of Morbidity Data

Since coronaviruses usually produce respiratory illnesses indistinguishable from those caused by many other types of viruses, it is not possible to obtain data on morbidity in the absence of laboratory identification of infection. The viruses are difficult to isolate, so most workers have relied on serological techniques to increase the numbers that can be studied. Investigations into coronavirus infection have usually formed part of overall evaluations of the role of viruses in general in respiratory illnesses. As indicated in the partial listing in Table 1, a variety of different open and closed populations have been used for these studies. The 229E strain was originally isolated from medical students in Chicago as part of a long-term study of respiratory illnesses in young adults.[21,23] Employee groups have been the source of specimens in the NIH[29,42] and in the studies at Charlottesville, Virginia.[26] Infection has also been evaluated in children's homes[34] and boarding schools,[36] among military recruits,[60] and among children hospitalized for severe respiratory illnesses in various parts of the world.[29] Serological methods

Table 1. Longitudinal Studies on the Epidemiology of Coronavirus Infection in Humans

Location	Population	Virus studied
Chicago, Ill.[21]	Medical students	229E
Washington, D.C.[29,42]	Hospitalized children	229E, OC43
Bethesda, Md.[29,42]	Adult employees	229E, OC viruses
Atlanta, Ga.[34,35a]	Institutionalized children	229E, OC43
Charlottesville, Va.[26]	Working adults	229E, OC43
Tecumseh, Mich.[16,49]	General community	229E, OC43
Brazil[15]	Nonhospitalized children	229E
Denver, Colo.[40]	Hospitalized asthmatic children	229E, OC43
N. and S. Carolina[60]	Military	229E, OC43

have been used to detect occurrence in persons with acute exacerbations of asthma[40] or chronic obstructive respiratory disease.[53] Patterns of coronavirus infection have been identified among the general population residing in the Tecumseh, Michigan, community as part of a longitudinal study of respiratory illness.[16,49] Volunteers have continued to be employed, especially to determine characteristics of illness not yet well defined in natural infection because of problems associated with isolation of the viruses.[7,8]

3.3. Serological Surveys

Although relatively simple serological techniques are now available for two coronaviruses (22E and OC38 or OC43), extensive surveys of antibody prevalence have not been carried out. When done, the surveys have often formed a part of studies directed mainly toward determination of the incidence of infection. Information on the prevalence of antibody is available for populations in the United States,[16,26,42] Britain,[8] and Brazil.[15] A special situation is the presence in man of antibody against coronaviruses of animals. The finding of mouse hepatitis antibodies in military recruits and in children and adults from the general population was surprising when first described in 1964.[25] It is now recognized that this does not indicate past experience with MHV, but rather with human coronavirus strains that are known to cross-react with it. Similarly, antibodies in human sera against the hemagglutinating encephalomyelitis virus of swine and the coronavirus of calf diarrhea also appear to represent cross-reactions with OC43 or related strains.[35b,c] In contrast, in a survey of antibodies to avian IBV, none could be found in a military population. Low-level antibodies were detected only in a portion of subjects who had close contact with poultry.[45] This virus is not known to cross-react with the human strains.

3.4. Laboratory Methods

3.4.1. Viral Isolation. Only the 229E strain was originally isolated in cell culture. It was eventually adapted to human embryonic lung cells (W138), in which it has been maintained.[23] However, this cell line is not a reliable system for primary isolation of 229E-like agents. To date, human embryonic intestine (MA177) has proven the most suitable cell system, but it is available only in limited quantities.[29] All other known human coronaviruses were originally isolated in organ cultures of human trachea or lung.[24,39,58,59] The presence of virus was usually detected by electron microscopy, or sometimes by fluorescent antibody (FA) staining of impression smears.[57] Two strains that are essentially identical, OC38 and OC43, have been adapted to suckling mouse brain and to primary monkey-kidney and BS-C-1 cell cultures.[11,30,37] Another cell system, L132, a heteroploid human lung line, has been reported to be suitable for primary isolation of 229E, a related virus (LP), and the B814, the first-described organ-culture agent.[6,9] This last finding has not been comfirmed by other workers.[11]

It is conceivable that special conditions of cell culture are required for primary isolation of these agents; this would be similar to the strict requirements for propagation of the rhinoviruses before the availability of W138 cells.[52] The situation is in sharp contrast to that found with the coronaviruses of animals. While they are rather species-specific in their *in vitro* growth characteristics, especially on primary isolation, such isolation is easily accomplished.[44,54–56]

3.4.2. Serological Tests. Neutralization (N) tests of varying degrees of complexity can be performed for all described coronavirus types. The most involved procedure must be used for those viruses that up to now have never been adapted to systems other than organ culture.[39] This technique involves incubating serum with known virus and inoculating the mixture into cultures of human trachea. Evidence of N manifest by a reduction in viral yield is determined by electron microscopy. For those coronaviruses adapted to cell cultures, tube- or plaque-reduction N tests are available. W138 or L132 cells may be used for both methods with 229E virus; a number of cell lines including primary monkey kidney and BS-C-1 have been used for N tests involving the OC38–43 virus.[5,9,11] Hemadsorption rather than CPE can be used for identification of end points with the BS-C-1 cell lines.[12,13]

Most seroepidemiological studies have not used N but rather complement-fixation (CF) or hemagglutination-inhibition (HI) tests as sources of their data. The method of preparing a CF antigen for 229E directly from cell-culture harvests was reported along with the original description of the viruses by Hamre and Procknow.[23] By this method, the CF test detected antibody in low titer and only for a short time after infection. This observation was subsequently confirmed in a large study, and it was suggested that the presence of CF antibody in a population could be interpreted as evidence for recent activity of the virus.[15] However, it was also learned that if the antigen was highly concentrated, antibody could be detected at a higher titer, and this antibody persisted in the population so that the CF method could be employed in surveys of prevalence.[5] An indirect HI test for 229E virus using tanned sheep erythrocytes has also been described. The procedure appears to be highly sensitive, and no cross-reactions with OC43 virus were observed.[35]

It was found that CF tests can be satisfactorily performed with OC43 virus using infected suckling mouse brain as antigen.[42] The same mouse-brain material can also be used in the HI test for OC43 antibody. In this test, the hemagglutination titer was higher for rat than for chicken erythrocytes, but

was sufficient with the chicken cells so that they could generally be employed; this is of particular importance in view of the spontaneous agglutination that often complicates working with rat erythrocytes. Serum to be tested did not require treatment with receptor-destroying enzyme, but rather standard heat inactivation at 56°C. The agglutination took place equally at various temperatures including room temperature.[32] In addition, a single radial hemolysis test has been developed. It can be used not only for OC43 but also for the nonhemagglutinating 229E by using chromic cations to attach virus to glutaraldehyde-treated red cells.[28a]

Other serological tests have been developed that have been used more in antigenic analyses of the different coronaviruses than in epidemiological studies. With the indirect FA technique, characteristic cytoplasmic inclusions were demonstrated with 229E, OC43, and even the other coronaviruses grown in organ culture.[49a] The last were prepared for testing by making smears of fragments of the infected trachea.[41] It has also been possible to demonstrate precipitin lines on gel-diffusion tests with coronavirus antigens concentrated 10- to 50-fold. Two or three precipitin lines were observed by Bradburne[5] in tests with hyperimmune animal or human serum, but others have identified only one such line.[33]

4. Biological Characteristics of the Virus

Very little information is available on the relationship of coronavirus structure to patterns of infectivity and antigenicity. The viruses, although originally thought to be similar to the myxoviruses, are in fact quite different. They contain a single continuous strand of RNA, associated with proteins as a ribonucleoprotein. Biochemical studies on both human and animal strains clearly indicate that they are positive-stranded.[36a,b,43a,56a] The spikes of the virus are distinctive in appearance and are reported to contain glycopolypeptides; both HA and CF antigens have been associated with the surface of the virion and are presumably located in the projections. No neuraminidase has been demonstrated, and therefore it has been concluded that the antigens belong to a single species present on the surface. By analogy, antibodies to these antigens should be associated with protection.[28,33]

The total number of serological types that infect man has not been defined. Here again, the problem revolves around the difficulties encountered in isolating the human coronaviruses. Consequently, there is no way of estimating the proportion of existing types that have already been isolated. It is also difficult to determine the separate antigenic identity of types that grow only in organ culture as compared with those that grow in cell culture. N, CF, HI, gel-diffusion, and immunofluorescent techniques have been used in the antigenic analyses by McIntosh et al.,[41] by Bradburne,[5] and by Bradburne and Somerset.[8] As would be expected, results have differed by each of these procedures, with N tests the most specific. However, cross-reactions were commonly demonstrable even by this method using animal antiserum or immune ascitic fluid, indicating that there must be many shared antigens.

An attempt at placing the human coronaviruses in broad groups is shown in Table 2; MHV is included because of its frequent interrelationships with the human strains, and avian IBV is omitted because it is antigenically distinct. The unadapted organ-culture strains have been listed separately; it has not been possible to prepare animal antisera against them, and they have been tested only against pairs of sera obtained either from individuals naturally infected or from volunteers challenged artificially. Such sera would be expected to be considerably less specific than animals antisera. It has been clearly shown in several laboratories that 229E is quite different from OC38 and OC43 not only in growth characteristics but also antigenically; cross-

reactions can be shown by N tests, but these are demonstrable only using very sensitive procedures. LP virus was originally isolated in organ culture and not in cell culture, but is closely related antigenically to 229E. OC43 virus has a low-level cross-reaction with MHV; in some reports, this has been reciprocal and in some one-way. Although B814 virus is quite different from OC43, they both share some antigens in common; again, cross-reactions with 229E are rare. Among the additional viruses, OC44 is closely related antigenically to OC38 and OC43, but has never been successfully adapted to mouse brain or cell cultures. The four other viruses are listed together by exclusion, i.e., not because of any demonstrated relationship to one another, but rather because they are not closely related to viruses in the first three groups. Some low-level reactions with the agents in these three groups have been shown to be present, with OC16 virus being the most distinctly different strain.

As indicated above, much of the information on the behavior of 229E and OC43 viruses has come from CF and HI tests. In view of the sharing of antigens among many of the viruses listed in Table 2, the specificity of these procedures must be carefully considered. Cross-reactions between 229E and OC43 have been reported only rarely when tested by CF against animal sera. With human serum, heterologous rises in antibody titer have been observed occasionally, but not frequently enough to create problems in studies involving significant numbers of specimens.[10] Of greater practical concern is the occurrence of cross-reactions between OC43 and the other organ-culture viruses. It is possible that rises in titer detected when using OC43 antigen in sero-epidemiological studies may result either from OC43 infection itself or from infection with one of these related viruses. Indirect evidence that the infecting agent may not be OC43 itself is the dissociation seen between the CF and HI tests for OC43 during a particular period of time. Rises in titer by CF should usually be accompanied by rises in titer by HI in the same serum pairs. If this does not ordinarily occur during one time period, but does during a second period, it suggests that a related virus but not OC43 was circulating during the first period.[49]

Data that demonstrate the etiological role of coronaviruses in respiratory infections derive from laboratory and field studies. The viruses do interfere

Table 2. Serological Relationships of the Human Coronaviruses

Group	Strains tested with animal antisera		Strains tested with human antisera
I	229E LP	Closely related but not identical	
II	OC38 OC43 MHV	Nearly identical	OC44
III	B814		
Others			OC16 OC37 OC48 EVS

with the action of cilia in tracheal organ culture, which suggests that they should have the same effect *in vivo*. In addition, volunteers have been inoculated with essentially all available strains with production of illness.[7,8] It has also been possible with 229E to demonstrate that natural infection was statistically related to the production of illness. During the 1967 outbreak of 229E infection in Tecumseh, Michigan, illness was significantly more common among those with infection than among matched subjects without infection.[16] Similarly, 229E infection among Chicago medical students was statistically associated with illness when those with rises in titer were used as their own controls.[21]

5. Descriptive Epidemiology

5.1. Incidence and Prevalence

Evidence is steadily mounting that the coronaviruses are of major importance in common respiratory infections of all age groups. The total impact of coronavirus infections on the general population cannot be calculated at present because not all viral types have been identified. Only 229E and OC43 are amenable to large-scale serological studies; infection rates for other distinct types such as OC16 cannot be determined. The assumption must be made that the former two types are typical of the other viruses. Incidence of infection with these agents exhibits a marked cyclical pattern, so it is to be expected that reported rates will vary based on the number of seasons of high viral activity included

in a particular study. Table 3 presents a summary of results obtained in four such studies.

5.1.1. Incidence and Prevalence of 229E Virus. The activity of 229E was found to be of high prevalence in 3 out of 6 years of a study among Chicago medical students. The mean annual incidence of infection during the total period was 15%, based on person-years of observation. The criterion for identification was a reproducible 2-fold seroconversion determined by CF. There was marked year-to-year variation in infection frequency, ranging from a high of 35% of those tested in 1966–1967 to a low of 1% in 1964–1965. However, nearly 97% of the infections occurred during the months from January to May, often at a time when isolation of rhinoviruses was at a low, and seroconversions for 229E were only rarely accompanied by a rise in titer for another respiratory agent.[21]

The serological study of 229E activity in the community of Tecumseh, Michigan, initially covered 2 years, which included one period of high prevalence. As with the study in Chicago, routine blood specimens were collected so that infection rates could be determined; however, the study group was composed of individuals of all ages living in their homes. Over the 2 years, infections were detected in 7.7% of individuals tested by CF, as shown in the curve in Fig. 1. However, this appeared to be an underestimate of the actual activity of the virus. Serum specimens had been collected on a regular basis, 6 months apart; rises in titer by CF occurred most frequently in those pairs in which the second specimen was collected in April 1967, clearly indicating the peak period of viral dissemination. CF-

Table 3. Reported Frequency of Infection or Illness with 229E and OC43 in Four Locations

Study	Mean incidence of infection with	
	229E	OC43
Chicago medical students[21]	15/100/yr	—
Tecumseh, Mich.[16,49]	7.7/100/yr	17.1/100/yr
	Proportion of colds associated with	
	229E	OC43
Charlottesville, Va., employees[26]	1.7% of illnesses	2.4% of illnesses
Atlanta, Ga., children[34,35a]	4.3% of illnesses	3.3% of illnesses

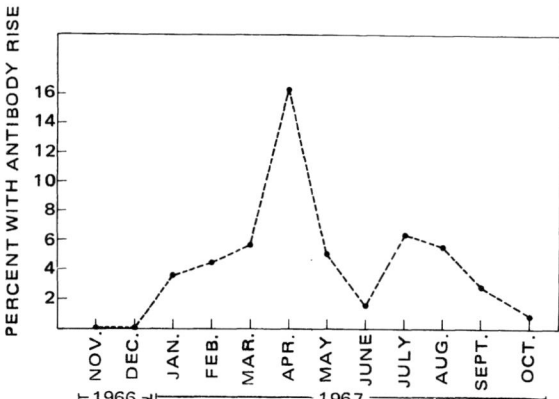

Fig. 1. Serological incidence by CF of infection with 229E virus in Tecumseh, Michigan, 1966–1967.

and the more sensitive N-test results were combined to give an overall infection rate for the population studied; this rate, 34%, was remarkably similar to the 35% observed in Chicago at the same time. Because of the limited period of viral activity, it was possible to compare illness rates of those infected with persons not infected matched by age and sex; it was estimated that 45% of the infections had produced clinical disease. Thus, the rate of 229E-associated illnesses during the outbreak was 15 per 100 persons studied. Activity in all age groups was apparent, including children under 25 years of age.[16]

In other investigations of 229E activity, attention has been directed mainly toward study of associated illnesses; in such studies, sera have been collected before and after the illness, rather than continually on a routine basis as done to determine infection rates. Employees at State Farm Insurance Company in Charlottesville, Virginia, were studied during an 8-year period for rises in titer for both 229E and OC43. By CF, 229E infection could be related to 3% of the colds that occurred in the winter–spring and to 0.4% of colds that occurred in the summer–fall. There was some year-to-year variation in activity, but differences in the number of specimens tested from various years did not permit complete identification of cyclical patterns.[26] Employees of the NIH with respiratory illness were studied by both isolation and serology for 229E infection over a 6-year period. Again, attention was specifically directed toward certain segments of the 6 years, and no specimens were tested during other segments.

Of particular interest once more is the segment from December 1966 to April 1967. Isolation of rhinoviruses and myxoviruses was uncommon at this time, but respiratory illness continued to occur. During this period, 24% of those persons with colds studied had rises in titer for 229E. As part of the same investigation, paired blood specimens collected from infants and children admitted to the hospital with acute lower respiratory disease during the 1967 period of 229E activity were tested for rise in antibody against the virus, but none was found.[29,42] Healthy children institutionalized in Atlanta, Georgia, were studied from 1960 to 1968; antibody response to 229E was determined by the indirect hemagglutination test. The investigation involved collection of serum specimens related to illness and also routine collection of sera from some non-ill individuals. Frequency of infection showed marked variation from year to year. Overall, 4% of colds could be associated with 229E infection, with greatest association in autumn, winter, and spring.[35a]

Surveys of prevalence of 229E antibody have also been carried out to document past history of infection, often as parts of longitudinal studies. A general finding is that antibody is present in a significant portion of adults who, despite possessing this antibody, can go on to have reinfection and illness. Reports of antibody prevalence in adults in the United States have varied from 19 to 41%, depending on the type of test used to determine antibody and the time of collection of serum.[16,26,42] Children under 10 years of age exhibited lower mean antibody titers than older children or adults.[16,42] Individual sera from normal healthy adults collected serially in Britain from 1965 throught 1970 were tested by Bradburne and Somerset.[8] It is of interest that there was a buildup in sera positive by CF from approximately 17% in specimens collected in October–December 1966 to 62% in those collected in July–September 1967. This would suggest that the spring 1967 outbreak that occurred in several parts of the United States may have taken place in Britain as well.

5.1.2. Incidence and Prevalence of OC43 Virus. Populations employed to study infection and illness caused by OC43 virus have generally been the same ones employed to study the occurrence of 229E virus. Kaye et al.[34] used the group of institutionalized children in Atlanta, Georgia, in which to identify infection by means of their HI test. Infections with the agent were detected in all years of the study but with definite cyclical variation. Seasons most involved were the winter and spring. Overall, 3% of the illnesses recorded in the 7-year period could be associated with OC43 infection, with a high of 7% in 1960–1961. Interestingly, testing of the sera collected routinely from non-ill individuals indicated that an additional equal number of OC43 infections were occurring without the production of symptoms.[34] The Charlottesville study of adult employees was of both OC43 and 229E infections. Here, too, the emphasis was on illness, and it was found in all years studied that OC43 was associated with 5% of colds in the winter–spring and with no illnesses in the summer–fall. Again, there was cyclical variation from year to year in the number of rises in titer detected.[26]

The original isolations of OC38 and OC43 were made in December and January 1965–1966 as part of the study carried out among NIH employees with colds. Testing of sera collected from these employees indicated that during this period, up to 29% of the colds studied were accompanied by rise in titer for OC43. In the children hospitalized with lower respiratory disease, up to 10% of illnesses during this period were associated with such a titer rise. However, it was impossible to show that the relationship to disease was truly etiological. This finding was in contrast to that seen with 229E, in which no rises in titer were detected in such cases.[38,42]

In the Tecumseh study, occurrence of OC43 infection was determined in the community population over a 4-year period. CF and HI tests were used on all specimens, and N tests were used as an aid in evaluating these results in selected specimens. During the total period, OC43-related infection was detected in 17.1% of the 910 persons studied for 1 year. Most of the infections took place in the winter–spring months of 1965–1966, 1967–1968, and 1968–1969. The only winter–spring period without such activity was in 1966–1967, when the 229E outbreak had taken place. There was good agreement between the CF and HI tests for the 1965–1966 and the 1968–1969 periods, but not for 1967–1968. The N test was used to clarify the situation. It was found that most rises in titer for the periods in 1965–1966 or 1968–1969, whether they had occurred by CF or HI or both, were also accompanied by rises in N antibody. In 1967–1968, most CF rises in titer were not accompanied by rises in titer in the other test, nor was the reverse true; significant change in N antibody in this period was exceedingly rare. It was concluded that the outbreaks of infection in 1965–1966 and 1968–1969 were probably caused by agents closely related to OC43, while the 1967–1968 activity was due to one of the other OC viruses that share some antigens with OC43 but are more distantly related to it. The 1968–1969 outbreak of OC43 infection was nearly as widespread as the prior 229E outbreak, with 25.6% of the population studied showing evidence of infection. Of special note was the fact that children under 5 years of age had the highest infection rates.[49]

Surveys of antibody prevalence have been conducted in several settings using OC43 antigens. McIntosh et al.[42] found that children began to acquire antibody to this virus in the first year of life. By the third year of life, more than 50% had antibody present. Among adults, 69% could be demonstrated to have antibody; this indicates, in view of the high incidence of infection with the agents in all age groups, the frequency with which such infections must represent reinfection. The high prevalence of antibody has been confirmed in other studies.[26,34] In Britain, Bradburne and Somerset[8] followed prevalence of antibody for OC43 over time, as they also had done with 229E. Each year, the greatest prevalence of antibody was found in the winter–spring period. The single highest point in antibody prevalence was in January–March 1969, at the same time the OC43 outbreak was occurring in some parts of the United States.[8]

5.2. Geographic Distribution

Occurrence of coronavirus infection has been documented, by either isolation or serology, from coast to coast in the United States. In addition to the studies listed in Table 1, a 229E-like virus has been isolated in California, and OC43 and 229E have been demonstrated to be present in Vermont by serological methods.[51,53] Extensive studies have been carried out by the Common Cold Research Unit, which has demonstrated the presence of the agents in Britain. The activity of 229E virus has been documented in Brazil in a study of children and adults with and without respiratory illness. Significant rises in antibody titer accompanied nonhospitalized respiratory infection in the children. Prevalence of antibody was determined by CF, and like the situation in some studies in the North Temperate Zone, children had little antibody, while 26% of adults were antibody-positive.[15] These findings suggest that coronaviruses are worldwide in distribution and cause similar types of illness in different localities; such a situation has been noted with many other repiratory viruses.[47] An attempt was actually made to detect rises in antibody titer for 229E in paired sera collected from small children with lower respiratory infection in many tropical parts of the world. No evidence of infection was found, which is hardly surprising, since no rises in titer were found in similar sera collected as part of the same study in Washington, D.C.[17,29]

5.3. Temporal Distribution

Because most illnesses caused by coronaviruses are similar to those caused by other respiratory viruses, it is impossible to identify epidemic behavior of the viruses. There is, however, great variation in the frequency of infection on both a seasonal and a cyclical basis. Isolation and rises in antibody titer for all types of coronaviruses have been rare events outside the period from December through May. This is the portion of the year in which isolation rates for rhinoviruses and other respiratory viruses often reach their low. In addition, a cyclical pattern may be discerned when individual virus types are considered. In Fig. 2 are summarized data from five longitudinal studies of coronavirus activity carried out in different parts of the United States. In all

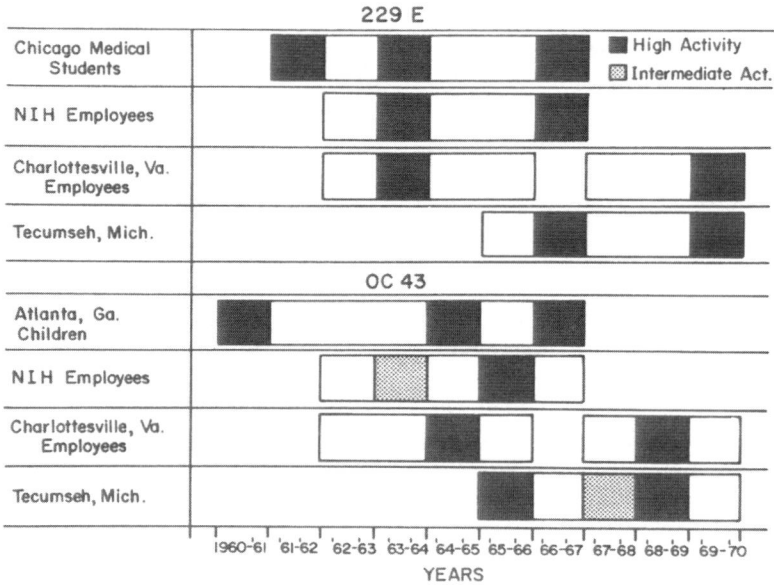

Fig. 2. Cyclic behavior of 229E and OC43 viruses observed in five longitudinal studies.

studies, some sporadic activity did occur in nearly all years studied, but rises in antibody titer were concentrated in certain years that far exceeded the means for the entire studies. Those periods are indicated as solid black boxes in the figure. The times during which specimens were collected in each investigation are indicated in the figure by the white boxes. Activity of 229E was detected in all four studies at the same time, even though two were in the Midwest and two in the eastern United States. It seems possible, on the basis of these data, to postulate a 2- to 3-year cycle for this agent. The greatest number of infections in Chicago was seen in 1967, after absence of the agent for 3 years, which would suggest a role of herd immunity in determining the time of reappearance of the agent.

With OC43, the situation is quite different. As with 229E, in no investigation did two years with high rates of infection or illness follow one another. A possible exception was in the Tecumseh study. However, the agent that caused the rises in titer in 1967–1968 did not appear as closely related serologically to OC43 as the agent involved in the other two outbreaks. This observation indicates a problem in identifying cycling of OC43. The virus undoubtedly shares more antigens with other identified or perhaps unidentified coronaviruses than does 229E (see Table 2), and these other viruses may well have cycles of their own that may confuse the situation. In 1964–1965, high activity occurred in Atlanta and Charlottesville. However, in Bethesda, just a short distance away, high activity was not seen in that year, but in 1965–1966, the same time as high activity occurred in Michigan, many miles away. In 1968–1969, Charlottesville and Tecumseh data did agree with very high activity in both areas. Thus, cycling of the agents was found in all studies, but the cycles did not agree on specific years. This may be a result of actual differences in patterns of occurrence or a result of differences in the serological techniques used to identify infection, which are of greater importance with OC43 because of the problem of cross-reactions. That cycling of coronaviruses does exist and occurs every 2–4 years with production of many infections suggests that the number of truly different coronaviruses may be relatively small. This situation is unlike that seen with the rhinoviruses, in which cycling has been more difficult to demonstrate, in part because of the large number of serotypes.[14]

5.4. Age

All age groups are involved in infection with OC43 virus. High rates have been noted in children and adults during studies separately examining both groups. In the Tecumseh study, a total population group was followed. During the 1968–1969 outbreak, infection rates were relatively uniform for all age groups, varying from a high of 29.2 per 100 person-years in the 0–4 age group to 22.2 in those over 40 years of age.[49] This finding is quite different from the situation that exists with other respiratory agents, such as respiratory syncytial virus, where a more distinct decrease in infection rates can be observed with increase in age.[48] The reversal of the pattern of age-specific infection rates customarily associated with the respiratory viruses becomes complete with 229E. Infection with this virus has been more difficult to demonstrate in small children than in adults. In Tecumseh, during the 1966–1967 outbreak, highest age-specific infection rates by CF were found among those 15–29 years of age, following a steady increase in infection frequency from the 0- to 4-year-olds. However, when neutralization tests were used to detect infection, the 15- to 19-year-olds still had high infection rates, but the serial increase to that point among younger age groups was much less steep.[16] This would suggest that the apparent sparing of small children with 229E may be an artifact resulting from the relative insensitivity of the young to the serological procedures commonly employed. It would be surprising if two different coronavirus serotypes behaved so differently.

5.5. Other Factors

There is little evidence of a sex differential in infections with the coronaviruses simply because the data have rarely been examined in such a manner. In Tecumseh, adult females experienced higher infection rates with OC43 than adult males, which is in conformity with the usual patterns of all respiratory illnesses.[46] In the study by Candeias et al.[15] of antibody prevalence, the results were examined by sex, but no significant differences could be observed. There are no data available data on occupational or racial susceptibility to infection or on the role of socioeconomic status in influencing rates. Occurrence of infection in closed or special populations, such as military recruits or residents of children's institutions, has been reported.[34,36,60] However, it is at present difficult to determine, based on the relative paucity of information on the behavior of the virus in open populations, whether they exhibit any unique features in other settings. There is a suggestion that OC43 virus might cause acute respiratory disease in military recruits.[60] If this finding is confirmed, it would represent a distinct departure from the types of illness customarily associated with that virus in young civilian adults. The role of the school-age child in dissemination of coronavirus has not yet been clearly defined, but it would be surprising if these infections differed in their transmission pattern so markedly from that documented with the other agents. Because of the high frequency of infection in older children and adults, other sites of dissemination may also be of significance. It has been possible to show that the family unit is of importance in transmission, since clustering of 229E and OC43 infections in families was observed in the Tecumseh study.[16]

While nutritional and genetic factors have not been associated with susceptibility to coronavirus infections, there are clear indications that the viruses are associated with exacerbations of chronic obstructive respiratory disease. Such a finding is hardly surprising in view of the high infection rates that have been observed in unselected older adults. It has not yet been demonstrated whether this represents true increased susceptibility to infection or simply a more severe form of expression of the infection when it occurs in an already compromised host. In addition to the situation in older individuals, there is evidence that both OC43 and 229E may trigger acute attacks of wheezing in young asthmatics.[20a,40,53]

6. Mechanisms and Routes of Transmission

The coronaviruses are presumably transmitted by the respiratory route. It has been possible to induce infection experimentally in volunteers by inoculating virus into the nose.[7,59] No other route of transmission for coronaviruses seems involved in man, although animal coronaviruses are infectious by the fecal–oral route.[56] There is currently no direct evidence to aid in identifying the main mechanisms of transmission. However, it is possible to compare the epidemiological behavior of the coronaviruses with that of other respiratory agents the transmission mechanisms of which have been more directly studied. Large-scale outbreaks of coronavirus infections have taken place, as in Tecumseh in 1967.[16] This is much more analogous to the situation seen with influenza than to that with the rhinoviruses. It is likely that the former agent can be transmitted by aerosol in addition to large droplet, which would explain its ability to spread quickly.[19] Rhinoviruses, on the other hand, are thought to be transmitted by large droplet and may at times spread via fomites.[27] It is therefore probable that human coronaviruses can be spread by aerosol as well as by large droplet. Aerosol transmission of avian IBV has actually been documented in poultry.[20]

There is no evidence that any animal reservoir or vector is involved in the maintenance of infection or transmission of the human coronaviruses. Each animal coronavirus appears to be restricted to its own species. The only known exception is the finding of antibody of avian IBV in sera of poultry workers but not of controls.[45]

7. Pathogenesis and Immunity

The incubation period of coronavirus colds is relatively short. In studies involving volunteers, the mean period from inoculation of virus to development of symptoms was from 3.2 to 3.5 days depending on the strain, with a range of 2–4 days.[7,59] Following exposure, the virus apparently multiplies superficially in the respiratory tract in a manner similar to that in which multiplication occurs in vitro. Virus excretion usually reaches a detectable level at the time symptoms begin and lasts for 1–4 days. The duration of the illness is from 6 to 7 days on the average, but with some lasting up to 18 days. Serological response either to induced or to naturally acquired infection has been quite variable depending on the infecting strain and the serological test employed. For example, among those experimentally infected with OC38 or OC43 virus who had a cold produced, only 46% had rises in titer by HI and 23% by CF. Less than half those infected with 229E showed a CF rise. It is not clear how the existence of titer or preinfection antibody affects the magnitude of the response detected by these tests.

Rises in N antibody titer are easier to detect and have been found with sensitive techniques in all volunteers experimentally infected.[5,8]

An important characteristic of the coronaviruses is their apparent high rate of reinfection. In the Tecumseh study, 81.5% of those infected with OC43 actually possessed prior N antibody.[49] Possession of circulating OC43 HI antibody among the Atlanta children did not appear to play a role in modifying severity of a subsequent illness.[34] With 229E virus, Hamre and Beem[21] demonstrated that frequency of rises in titers detected by N was inversely proportional to preinfection levels of N antibody, which would indicate that this antibody exerted some protective effect. However, the importance of this N antibody could not be confirmed when infection was detected by CF. Thus, circulating N antibody as measured at present may bear a relationship to modification of infection, but this association is not a very strong one. Since coronavirus infections involve mainly the surface of the respiratory tract, it is likely that secretory IgA antibody plays a more direct role in protection; this has in fact been demonstrated with a swine coronavirus.[4]

8. Pattern of Host Response

The coronaviruses generally produce a coldlike illness that on an individual basis is difficult to distinguish from illness caused by other respiratory viruses. In both induced and natural infections, the most prominent findings have been coryza and nasal discharge, with the discharge being more profuse than that customarily seen with rhinovirus colds.[7] Sore throat has been somewhat less common and in children has been associated with pharyngeal injection.[34] Experimental colds caused by B814 virus were about as severe as those caused by 229E; however, natural OC43 infections caused illnesses with considerably more cough and sore throat than did 229E infections.[26] The mean duration of coronavirus colds, at 6.5 days, is shorter than that seen in rhinovirus colds, at 9.5 days.[7]

There is no clear evidence yet available that coronaviruses cause severe lower respiratory illness in infants and young children. In fact, such infections were more common in one study among the control group than among the diseased.[42] Mufson

et al.[50] have associated coronavirus 229E and OC43 infection with acute lower respiratory infections in children at Cook County Hospital. The lack of a comparable control group makes assignment of an etiological role to these viruses hazardous at present, but the relationship should be sought in the future. The association of OC43 with the acute respiratory disease (ARD) syndrome in military recruits should also be viewed as tentative.

Clinical disease occurred in no more than 45% of those infected with 229E in Tecumseh during the 1967 outbreak.[16] In Atlanta children, OC43 virus produced illness in about 50% of those infected.[34] It is likely that with increase in age and concomitant experience with these agents, the ratio of clinically apparent to inapparent infection will decrease. As with other respiratory agents, a continuum of severity of symptoms exists among those in whom infection results in disease, and this may also be related to past experience with the viruses.

Coronaviruslike particles have been identified in stools of persons with diarrhea, and therefore a role in etiology of acute enteric disease has been suggested. This would not be surprising in view of the clear involvement of certain strains in severe diarrheal disease of domestic animals.[15a] However, the association with human disease has not been observed in a number of other studies. Coronaviruslike particles have also been observed in renal biopsies from cases of endemic (Balkan) nephropathy. A slow coronavirus infection acquired from pigs has been suggested as being involved.[1a]

9. Control and Prevention

It is premature at present to think in terms of control of coronavirus infection. Not all viral types have been identified, and some known agents cannot be easily propagated in the laboratory. Thus, preparation of vaccines of the conventional types is impossible. The frequency of reinfection observed with these agents is so high that control by vaccination may not be practical, but it is possible that further studies may allow identification of truly protective antibodies. There remains environmental control of infection; such efforts have been useful only rarely for other respiratory agents and they are not likely to be more efficacious for the coronaviruses.[43]

10. Unresolved Problems

The major immediate need in coronavirus research lies in the laboratory. If a practical system can be found for isolation and propagation of the viruses, the gaps in understanding the behavior of these agents would quickly be filled. Only serological tools are available now for most epidemiological studies, and even these can be applied to only two different coronavirus types. Therefore, many of the data that have been so laboriously gained give only partial evidence on the total dimensions of the problem—and the problem is almost certainly a very large one. Coronaviruses have been isolated and outbreaks identified in periods of the winter and spring when rhinoviruses and myxoviruses are uncommon. It appears that during these times, the coronaviruses cause a significant portion of respiratory illnesses. Even discounting suggestions of production of severe disease in young children and those with chronic respiratory disease, the viruses are important pathogens simply in terms of numbers of illnesses produced. Only through further understanding of the behavior of these agents will it be possible to determine the means by which control can be attempted.

11. References

1. ALMEIDA, J. D., AND TYRRELL, D. A. J., The morphology of three previously uncharacterized human respiratory viruses that grow in organ culture, *J. Gen. Virol.* **1**:175–178 (1967).
1a. APOSTOLOV, K., AND SPASIC, P., Evidence of a viral aetiology in endemic (Balkan) nephropathy, *Lancet* **2**:1271–1273 (1975).
2. BECKER, W. B., MCINTOSH, K., DEES, J. H., AND CHANOCK, R. M., Morphogenesis of avian infectious bronchitis virus and a related human virus (strain 229E), *J. Virol.* **1**:1019–1027 (1967).
3. BERRY, D. M., CRUICKSHANK, J. G., CHU, H. P., AND WELLS, R. J. H., The structure of infectious bronchitis virus, *Virology* **23**:403–407 (1964).
4. BOHL, E. H., GUPTA, R. K. P., OLQUIN, M. V. F., AND SAIF, L. J., Antibody responses in serum, colostrum, and milk of swine after infection or vaccination with transmissible gastroenteritis virus, *Infect. Immun.* **6**:289–301 (1972).
5. BRADBURNE, A. F., Antigenic relationships amongst coronaviruses, *Arch. Gesamte Virusforsch.* **31**:352–364 (1970).

6. BRADBURNE, A. F., An investigation of the replication of coronaviruses in suspension cultures of L132 cells, *Arch. Gesamte Virusforsch.* **37**:297–307 (1972).
7. BRADBURNE, A. F., BYNOE, M. L., AND TYRRELL, D. A. J., Effects of a "new" human respiratory virus in volunteers, *Br. Med. J.* **3**:767–769 (1967).
8. BRADBURNE, A. F., AND SOMERSET, B. A., Coronavirus antibody titres in sera of healthy adults and experimentally infected volunteers, *J. Hyg.* **70**:235–244 (1972).
9. BRADBURNE, A. F., AND TYRRELL, D. A. J., The propagation of "coronaviruses" in tissue culture, *Arch. Gesamte Virusforsch.* **28**:133–150 (1969).
10. BRADBURNE, A. F., AND TYRRELL, D. A. J., Coronaviruses of man, *Prog. Med. Virol.* **13**:373–403 (1971).
11. BRUCKOVA, M., MCINTOSH, K., KAPIKIAN, A. Z., AND CHANOCK, R. M., The adaptation of two coronavirus strains (OC38 and OC43) to growth in cell monolayers, *Proc. Soc. Exp. Biol. Med.* **135**:431–435 (1970).
12. BUCKNALL, R. A., KALICA, A. R., AND CHANOCK, R. M., Intracellular development and mechanism of hemadsorption of a human coronavirus, OC43, *Proc. Soc. Exp. Biol. Med.* **139**:811–817 (1972).
13. BUCKNALL, R. A., KING, L. M., KAPIKIAN, A. Z., AND CHANCOK, R. M., Studies with human coronaviruses. II. Some properties of strains 229E and OC43, *Proc. Soc. Exp. Biol. Med.* **139**:722–727 (1972).
14. CALHOUN, A. M., JORDAN, W. S., JR., AND GWALTNEY, J. M., JR., Rhinovirus infections in an industrial population. V. Change in distribution of serotypes, *Am. J. Epidemiol.* **99**:58–64 (1974).
15. CANDEIAS, J. A. N., CARVALHO, R. P. DE S., AND ANTONACIO, F., Seroepidemiologic study of coronavirus infection in Brazilian children and civilian adults, *Rev. Inst. Med. Trop.* **14**:121–125 (1972).
15a. CAUL, E. O., PAVEL, W. K., AND CLARKE, S. K. R., Coronavirus particles in faece from patients with gastroenteritis, *Lancet* **1**:1192 (1975).
16. CAVALLARO, J. J., AND MONTO, A. S., Community-wide outbreak of infection with a 229E-like coronavirus in Tecumseh, Michigan, *J. Infect. Dis.* **122**:272–279 (1970).
17. CHANOCK, R., CHAMBON, L., CHANG, W., GONCALVES FERREIRA, F., GHARPURE, P., GRANT, L., HATEM, J., IMAM, I., KALRA, S., LIM, K., MADALENGOITIA, J., SPENCE, L., TENG, P., AND FERREIRA, W., WHO respiratory disease survey in children: A serological study, *Bull. WHO* **37**:363–369 (1967).
18. Coronaviruses, *Nature (London)* **220**:650 (1968).
19. COUCH, R. B., DOUGLAS, R. G., JR., LINDGREN, K. M., GERONE, P. J., AND KNIGHT, V., Airborne tranmission of respiratory infection with Coxsackievirus A type 21, *Am. J. Epidemiol.* **91**:78–86 (1970).
20. GEILHAUSEN, H. E., LIGON, F. B., AND LUKERT, P. D., The pathogenesis of virulent and avirulent avian in-

fectious bronchitis virus, *Arch. Gesamte Virusforsch.* **40:**285–290 (1973).

20a. GUMP, D. W., PHILLIPS, C. A., FORSYTH, B. R., MCINTOSH, K., LAMBORN, K. R., AND STOUCH, W. H., Role of infection in chronic bronchitis, *Am. Rev. Respir. Dis.* **113:**465–474 (1976).

21. HAMRE, D., AND BEEM, M., Virologic studies of acute respiratory disease in young adults. V. Coronavirus 229E infections during six years of surveillance, *Am. J. Epidemiol.* **96:**94–106 (1972).

22. HAMRE, D., KINDIG, D. A., AND MANN, J., Growth and intracellular development of a new respiratory virus, *J. Virol.* **1:**810–816 (1967).

23. HAMRE, D., AND PROCKNOW, J. J., A new virus isolated from the human respiratory tract, *Proc. Soc. Exp. Biol. Med.* **121:**190–193 (1966).

24. HARNETT, G. B., AND HOOPER, W. L., Test-tube organ cultures of ciliated epithelium for the isolation of respiratory viruses, *Lancet* **1:**339–340 (1968).

25. HARTLEY, J. W., ROWE, W. P., BLOOM, H. H., AND TURNER, H. C., Antibodies to mouse hepatitis viruses in human sera, *Proc. Soc. Exp. Biol. Med.* **115:**414–418 (1964).

26. HENDLEY, J. O., FISHBURNE, H. B., AND GWALTNEY, J. M., JR., Coronavirus infections in working adults, *Am. Rev. Respir. Dis.* **105:**805–811 (1972).

27. HENDLEY, J. O., WENZEL, R. P., AND GWALTNEY, J. M., JR., Transmission of rhinovirus colds by self-inoculation, *N. Eng. J. Med.* **288:**1361–1364 (1973).

28. HIERHOLZER, J. C., PALMER, E. L., WHITFIELD, S. G., KAYE, H. S., AND DOWDLE, W. R., Protein composition of coronavirus OC43, *Virology* **48:**516–527 (1972).

28a. HIERHOLZER, J. C., AND TANNOCK, G. A., Quantitation of antibody to non-hemagglutinating viruses by single radial hemolysis: Serological test for human coronaviruses, *J. Clin. Microbiol.* **5:**613–620 (1977).

29. KAPIKIAN, A. Z., JAMES, H. D., JR., KELLY, S. J., DEES, J. H., TURNER, H. C., MCINTOSH, K., KIM, H. W., PARROTT, R. H., VINCENT, M. M., AND CHANOCK, R. M., Isolation from man of "avian infectious bronchitis virus-like" viruses (coronaviruses) similar to 229E virus, with some epidemiological observations, *J. Infect. Dis.* **119:**282–290 (1969).

30. KAPIKIAN, A. Z., JAMES, H. D., JR., KELLY, S. J., KING, L. M., VAUGHN, A. L., AND CHANOCK, R. M., Hemadsorption by coronavirus strain OC43, *Proc. Soc. Exp. Biol. Med.* **139:**179–186 (1972).

31. KAPIKIAN, A. Z., JAMES, H. D., JR., KELLY, S. J., AND VAUGHN, A. L., Detection of coronavirus strain 692 by immune electron microscopy, *Infect. Immun.* **7:**111–116 (1973).

32. KAYE, H. S., AND DOWDLE, W. R., Some characteristics of hemagglutination of certain strains of "IBV-like" viruses, *J. Infect. Dis.* **120:**576–581 (1969).

33. KAYE, H. S., HIERHOLZER, J. C., AND DOWDLE, W. R.,

Purification and further characterization of an "IBV-like" virus (coronavirus), *Proc. Soc. Exp. Biol. Med.* **135:**457–463 (1970).

34. KAYE, H. S., MARSH, H. B., AND DOWDLE, W. R., Seroepidemiologic survey of coronavirus (strain OC43) related infections in a children's population, *Am. J. Epidemiol.* **94:**43–49 (1971).

35. KAYE, H. S., ONG, S. B., AND DOWDLE, W. R., Detection of coronavirus 229E antibody by indirect hemagglutination, *Appl. Microbiol.* **24:**703–707 (1972).

35a. KAYE, H. S., AND DOWDLE, W. R., Seroepidemiologic survey of coronavirus (strain 229E) infections in a population of children, *Am. J. Epidemiol.* **101:**238–244 (1975).

35b. KAYE, H. S., YARBROUGH, W. B., AND REED, C. J., Calf diarrhoea coronavirus, *Lancet* **2:**509 (1975).

35c. KAYE, H. S., YARBROUGH, W. B., REED, C. J., AND HARRISON, A. K., Antigenic relationship between human coronavirus strain OC43 and hemagglutinating encephalomyelitis virus strain 67N of swine: Antibody responses in human and animal sera, *J. Infect. Dis.* **135:**201–209 (1977).

36. KENDALL, E. J., BYNOE, M. L., AND TYRRELL, D. A. J., Virus isolation from common colds occurring in a residential school, *Br. Med. J.* **2:**82–86 (1962).

36a. KENNEDY, D. A., AND JOHNSON-LUSSENBURG, C. M., Isolation and morphology of the internal component of human coronavirus, strain 229E, *Intervirology* **6:**197–206 (1975/1976).

36b. LOMNICZI, B., AND KENNEDY, I., Genome of infectious bronchitis virus, *J. Virol.* **24:**99–107 (1977).

37. MCINTOSH, K., BECKER, W. B., AND CHANOCK, R. M., Growth in suckling-mouse brain of "IBV-like" viruses from patients with upper respiratory tract disease, *Proc. Natl. Acad. Sci. U.S.A.* **58:**2268–2273 (1967).

38. MCINTOSH, K., BRUCKOVA, M., KAPIKIAN, A. Z., CHANOCK, R. M., AND TURNER, H., Studies of new virus isolates recovered in tracheal organ culture, *Ann. N.Y. Acad. Sci.* **174:**983–989 (1970).

39. MCINTOSH, K., DEES, J. H., BECKER, W. B., KAPIKIAN, A. Z., AND CHANOCK, R. M., Recovery in tracheal organ cultures of novel viruses from patients with respiratory disease, *Proc. Natl. Acad. Sci. U.S.A.* **57:**933–940 (1967).

40. MCINTOSH, K., ELLIS, E. F., HOFFMAN, L. S., LYBASS, T. G., ELLER, J. J., AND FULGINITI, V. A., The association of viral and bacterial respiratory infections with exacerbations of wheezing in young asthmatic children, *J. Pediatr.* **82:**578–590 (1973).

41. MCINTOSH, K., KAPIKIAN, A. Z., HARDISON, K. A., HARTLEY, J. W., AND CHANOCK, R. M., Antigenic relationships among the coronaviruses of man and between human and animal coronaviruses, *J. Immunol.* **102:**1109–1118 (1969).

42. MCINTOSH, K., KAPIKIAN, A. Z., TURNER, H. C., HAR-

TLEY, J. W., PARROTT, R. H., AND CHANOCK, R. M., Seroepidemiologic studies of coronavirus infection in adults and children, *Am. J. Epidemiol.* **91**:585–592 (1970).

43. MCLEAN, R. L., General discussion, International Conference on Asian Influenza, *Am. Rev. Respir. Dis.* **83**(Part 2):36–38 (1961).

43a. MCNAUGHTON, M. R., AND MADGE, M. H., The genome of human coronavirus strain 229E, *J. Gen. Virol.* **39**:497–504 (1978).

44. MEBUS, C. A., STAIR, E. L., RHODES, M. B., AND TWIEHAUS, M. J., Pathology of neonatal calf diarrhea induced by coronavirus-like agent, *Vet. Pathol.* **10**:45–64 (1973).

45. MILLER, L. T., AND YATES, V. J., Neutralization of infectious bronchitis virus by human sera, *Am. J. Epidemiol.* **88**:406–409 (1968).

46. MONTO, A. S., HIGGINS, M. W., AND ROSS, H. W., The Tecumseh study of respiratory illness. VIII. Acute infection in chronic respiratory disease and comparison groups, *Am. Rev. Respir. Dis.* **111**:27–36 (1975).

47. MONTO, A. S., AND JOHNSON, K. M., Respiratory infections in the American tropics, *Am. J. Trop. Med. Hyg.* **17**:867–874 (1968).

48. MONTO, A. S., AND LIM, S. K., The Tecumseh study of respiratory illness. III. Incidence and periodicity of respiratory syncytial and *Mycoplasma pneumoniae* infections, *Am. J. Epidemiol.* **94**:290–301 (1971).

49. MONTO, A. S., AND LIM, S. K., The Tecumseh study of respiratory illness. VI. Frequency of and relationship between outbreaks of coronavirus infection, *J. Infect. Dis.* **129**:271–276 (1974).

49a. MONTO, A. S., AND RHODES, L. M., Detection of coronavirus infection of man by immunofluorescence, *Proc. Soc. Exp. Biol. Med.* **155**:143–148 (1977).

50. MUFSON, M. A., MCINTOSH, K., CHAO, R. K., KRAUSE, H. E., WASIL, R., AND MOCEGA, H. E., Epidemiology of coronavirus infections in infants with acute lower respiratory disease, *Clin. Res.* **20**:534 (1972).

51. OSHIRO, L. S., SCHIEBLE, J. H., AND LENNETTE, E. H., Electron microscopic studies of coronavirus, *J. Gen. Virol.* **12**:161–168 (1971).

52. PELON, W., Classification of the "2060" viruses ECHO28 and further study of its properties, *Am. J. Hyg.* **73**:36–54 (1961).

53. PHILLIPS, C. A., MCINTOSH, K., FORSYTH, B. R., GUMP, D. W., AND STOUCH, W. H., Coronavirus infections in exacerbations of chronic bronchitis, in: *Twelfth Interscience Conference on Antimicrobial Agents and Chemotherapy,* Atlantic City, New Jersey, Abstr. No. 6 (1972).

54. PURCELL, D. A., AND CLARKE, J. K., The replication of infectious bronchitis virus in fowl trachea, *Arch. Gesamte Virusforsch.* **39**:248–256 (1972).

55. SAIF, L. J., BOHL, E. H., AND GUPTA, R. K. P., Isolation of porcine immunoglobulins and determination of the immunoglobulin classes of transmissible gastroenteritis viral antibodies, *Infect. Immun.* **6**:600–609 (1972).

56. STAIR, E. L., RHODES, M. B., WHITE, R. G., AND MEBUS, C. A., Neonatal calf diarrhea: Purification and electron microscopy of a coronavirus-like agent, *Am. J. Vet. Res.* **33**:1147–1156 (1972).

56a. TANNOCK, G. A., AND HIERHOLZER, J. C., Presence of genomic polyadenylate and absence of detectable virion transcriptase in human coronavirus OC-43, *J. Gen. Virol.* **39**:29–39 (1978).

57. TYRRELL, D. A. J., AND ALMEIDA, J. D., Direct electron microscopy of organ cultures for the detection and characterization of viruses, *Arch. Gesamte Virusforsch.* **22**:417–421 (1967).

58. TYRRELL, D. A. J., AND BYNOE, M. L., Cultivation of a novel type of common-cold virus in organ cultures, *Br. Med. J.* **1**:1467–1470 (1965).

59. TYRRELL, D. A. J., BYNOE, M. L., AND HOORN, B., Cultivation of "difficult" viruses from patients with common colds, *Br. Med. J.* **1**:606–610 (1968).

60. WENZEL, R. P., HENDLEY, J. O., DAVIES, J. A., AND GWALTNEY, J. M., JR., Coronavirus infections in military recruits: Three-year study with coronavirus strains OC43 and 229E, *Am. Rev. Respir. Dis.* **109**:621–624 (1974).

12. Suggested Reading

BRADBURNE, A. F., AND TYRRELL, D. A. J., Coronaviruses of man, *Prog. Med. Virol.* **13**:373–403 (1971).

HAMRE, D., AND BEEM, M., Virologic studies of acute respiratory disease in young adults. V. Coronavirus 229E infections during six years of surveillance, *Am. J. Epidemiol.* **96**:94–106 (1972).

KAYE, H. S., MARSH, H. B., AND DOWDLE, W. R., Seroepidemiologic survey of coronavirus (strain OC43) related infections in a children's population, *Am. J. Epidemiol.* **94**:43–49 (1971).

MCINTOSH, K., KAPIKIAN, A. Z., TURNER, H. C., HARTLEY, J. W., PARROTT, R. H., AND CHANOCK, R. M., Seroepidemiologic studies of coronavirus infection in adults and children, *Am. J. Epidemiol.* **91**:585–592 (1970).

MONTO, A. S., AND LIM, S. K., The Tecumseh study of respiratory illness. VI. Frequency of and relationship between outbreaks of coronavirus infection, *J. Infect. Dis.* **129**:271–276 (1974).

Cytomegalovirus

Eli Gold and George A. Nankervis

1. Introduction

Only a small proportion of people throughout the world escape infection with cytomegalovirus (CMV). The age at acquisition, the presence and type of clinical manifestations, and the sites and extent of virus excretion vary, but serological surveys conducted on all continents confirm the ubiquitous distribution of human CMV.

The impression that CMV infection was uniformly associated with severe illness of the newborn and carried a high probability of death or marked damage to the central nervous system has been modified since the availability of laboratory procedures and the performance of prospective studies. It is true that CMV can produce a devastating disease in the newborn, but it has been shown that congenital infection with CMV, although relatively common, is usually clinically inapparent, generally has a benign course, and may be recognized only if laboratory studies are performed.

Most people develop antibody to CMV following unrecognized infection acquired during childhood or the young adult years. A small proportion of normal persons may have a form of infectious mononucleosis or possibly symptoms of a respiratory illness with CMV infection, but clinical disease is much more likely to be evident in those who are immunologically deficient because of neoplastic disease or treatment with immunosuppressants.

Infection with CMV is commonly followed by prolonged, often intermittent periods of virus excretion in the face of high levels of circulating antibody. Dissemination of the agent probably occurs by close contact with an excretor, although spread through the placenta or via blood transfusions accounts for a significant proportion of clinically important infections. The pathogenesis of CMV infection can be deduced only from clinical observations and epidemiological studies, but there is reason to believe that primary infection with CMV carries a greater probability of illness with significant residual effect than does recurrent infection. The factors that determine which infected persons are affected and which have no apparent illness remain unclear.

2. Historical Background

Large inclusion-bearing cells originally found in kidney, lung, or liver of infants who died from various causes were considered to be the result of some strange parasite, possibly a protozoan.[11,26,48] Goodpasture and Talbot[33] noted a similarity between the appearance of these strange cells, which they referred to as "cytomegalia," and the intranuclear inclusions seen in the skin lesions of herpesviruses. Shortly thereafter,[116] the viral etiology of these unusual cells was first postulated. Several years later, Cole and Kuttner[15] were able to transmit the guinea pig form of cytomegalia using filtered

Eli Gold · Department of Pediatrics, University of California, Davis, California. George A. Nankervis · Department of Pediatrics, Medical College of Ohio, Toledo, Ohio.

salivary-gland material, indicating a probable viral etiology. There continued to be many descriptions of typical cells in various tissues of infants, especially those who died in the newborn period of a hemorrhagic disease resembling erythroblastosis and referred to as "inclusion body disease," "cytomegalic inclusion disease" (CID), or "generalized salivary gland virus infection." The reports by Wyatt et al.,[123] Fetterman,[28] Mercer et al.,[78] and Margileth[74] describing typical inclusion-bearing cells in the urine of infants with CID provided a method of diagnosing this disease in nonfatal cases. Finally, in 1956, three laboratories almost simultaneously reported the isolation of the etiological agent employing tissue-culture techniques: Smith[101] from salivary gland, Rowe et al.[95] from cultures of adenoid tissue (thus AD 169), and Weller et al.[120] from a liver biopsy.

3. Methodology

3.1. Mortality

Death from CMV infections is rare, and the cause can usually be recognized only as a result of special virological, serological, or histological examination. Death rates therefore give no indication of the frequency of this disease.

3.2. Morbidity

Since the clinical syndromes associated with CMV infection are not usually clinically distinctive and are usually diagnosed only through laboratory procedures, no estimate can be made of their importance through official health records. Furthermore, most CMV infections are asymptomatic. Such incidence data as are available have come from studies, serological or virological or both, of groups of special risk—pregnant women, neonates, patients undergoing transfusions or organ-transplant surgery, and heterophil-negative patients with a mononucleosislike syndrome.

3.3. Serological Surveys

The complement-fixation (CF) test has been widely used in prevalence studies to determine the experience of different populations with CMV infections[12,23,25,34,46,56,95,99,105] and as an indication of infection in special groups studied prospectively to determine seroconversion (negative to positive) and reinfection rates (4-fold or greater rise in titer) in persons with preexisting antibody.[41,81,83,91,108,113,121] The CF test has been most commonly used for serological surveys or clinical studies because of the relative ease of preparing the reagents and performing the test and because CF antibody is of long duration. The AD 169 strain of CMV has usually been employed as the antigen because of its wide range of reactivity.[77,105] The sensitivity of the test varies depending on the antigen preparation, and antibody levels measured in different laboratories may differ. There are data suggesting the existence of antigenic variants of CMV with which AD 169 does not cross-react, introducing problems with serological surveys based on AD 169 alone.[4,117]

3.4. Laboratory Diagnosis

3.4.1. Virus Isolation. For virus isolation, specimens from the pharynx, buffy coat of peripheral blood, breast milk, urine, stool, tears, cervix, and semen are inoculated onto human fibroblast cultures and observed for 6–8 weeks for the appearance of foci or swollen cells with intranuclear inclusions. Continuous strains of human tonsil, skin–muscle, or fetal lung fibroblasts have been suitable for isolation.

3.4.2. Serological Tests. As mentioned above, the CF test using a single strain of CMV as antigen is widely used to detect antibody to CMV. It is still not possible with existing laboratory methods to determine whether infection with one strain of virus precludes infection with another. In the immunosuppressed patient, it cannot be stated with certainty, for example, whether CMV infection represents reactivation of a latent agent or introduction of a new strain via blood or other route. It is also possible, whether or not cross-immunity develops, that a difference in ability to produce disease exists among the strains of CMV and that virulence of the organism determines the clinical course. Indirect evidence would suggest that such is not the case. In three situations where consecutive pregnancies resulted in congenitally infected infants, only the first in each set showed clinical manifestations.[24,57,102] In addition, one of premature male twins born with congenital CMV infection had generalized CID and died; the other, who shed CMV in saliva and urine-survived and was doing reasonably well on follow-up at 5 months of age.[75]

The neutralization test and platelet-aggregation techniques have also been used but are laborious and often variable in their results.[86,89,118] Several investigators have evaluated the indirect hemagglutination (IHA) method for serological diagnosis of CMV infection.[7,32] There is rather close agreement between the IHA and the carefully performed CF test, but the former appears to be slightly more sensitive and antibody acquisition may be detected earlier in some cases than by the CF method. In addition, it reflects antibody of both the immunoglobulin G (IgG) and IgM types, whereas the CF test reflects principally IgG.

Indirect fluorescent-antibody (FA)[14] and anticomplementary immunofluorescent (ACIF)[91b,102a] tests are useful, being somewhat more sensitive than the CF test and often becoming positive in primary infections before the CF test. The immunoperoxidase (IPA)[32b] test is also convenient once the technique is established and is comparable in sensitivity and specificity to the FA test. Identification of CMV-specific IgM antibody is important in identifying recent infection. It has been measured in an indirect FA test as described by Hanshaw et al.[37] and the more elaborate "sandwich-type" indirect FA test of Schmitz and Haas.[97] The sera from most infants with CID is positive using this test, and it is particularly useful when IgG antibody passively transferred from the mother is present. However, the CMV-specific IgM test has a sensitivity of only 76% for detecting congenital infections based on viruria, and false-positive tests occur in 21% due mostly to the presence of rheumatoid factor[102a]; indeed, tests for rheumatoid factor alone detected 35–45% of CMV congenital infections alone with no false positives.

Another laboratory method employed for diagnosis of CMV infection is the relatively insensitive cytological method of examining tissue, urinary sediment, or smears of respiratory secretion for cytomegalic cells with intranuclear inclusions.

4. Biological Characteristics of the Virus

Individual particles of CMV are morphologically indistinguishable from varicella-zoster, herpes simplex, and other members of the herpesvirus family, but preparations of CMV grown in tissue culture may contain a large proportion of forms incompletely endowed with nucleic acid. These empty or partially empty forms are noninfectious and indicate defective virus synthesis in the in vitro systems. Human strains of CMV appear to replicate in vitro to complete virus only in human tissue, in contrast to the other members of the herpesvirus family. As with the varicella-zoster virus, attempts to infect cultures of human fibroblasts are accompanied by the development of a very characteristic sequence of changes that begins with contraction and rounding of cells, followed by the development of intranuclear and intracytoplasmic inclusions, the enlargement of individual cells, and the eventual formation of large foci of such altered cells, some of which fuse into giant forms.

Virus remains cell-associated, although serial propagation in tissue culture may result in preparations with relatively large amounts of infectious virus in the culture supernate. The agent is labile to low pH, fat solvents, and temperature. Preservation is best achieved by rapid freezing and storage at $-60°$ to $-80°C$, preferably in 30–50% sorbitol. Inactivation at $-20°C$ is more rapid than at $4°C$, making ordinary refrigerator temperature acceptable for short-term storage of specimens.

Virus isolation is best achieved by direct inoculation of fresh materials into cultures of human fibroblasts. Storage even by rapid freezing of suspensions prepared in sorbitol may result in sufficient loss of infectious virus to preclude isolation from samples containing small amounts of virus. Infectivity of specimens is rapidly lost on drying or hard surfaces or in cloth materials such as diapers.

As indicated previously, some evidence for different strains of CMV exists, but the importance of these differences, if any, in the type of clinical syndrome produced, in cross-immunity, and in long-term viral persistence is currently unknown.

As with other herpesviruses, the capacity of CMV to produce latent infections that reactivate under various host settings is an important biological property. The demonstration that CMV can transform hamster cells[1] and produce early antigens[111] suggest potentially oncogenic properties that deserve further study in relation to cancer, especially cervical cancer.[98]

5. Descriptive Epidemiology

The earliest information concerning the occurrence of CMV in man came from pathologists in Holland, the United States, France, Germany, Brazil, Hungary, and elsewhere who reported the finding of typical inclusions either in the salivary gland or generalized in many organs. The proportion of infants in whom such changes were observed varied, but it became apparent that "cytomegalic inclusion disease" could be found throughout the world. More complete data became available with the development of serological methods.

5.1. Prevalence and Incidence

The use of the terms "prevalence" and "incidence" in CMV infections presents difficulties because the presence of virus in the pharynx or urine or of antibody in the blood might represent (1) a primary infection (i.e., incidence), (2) persistence from an earlier infection (prevalence), or (3) reactivation of a latent infection (prevalence plus incidence). The absence of demonstrable antibody from serum does not necessarily mean that prior infection has not occurred, because antibody titers may have dropped to levels not detected by the test used or there may be antigenic differences between the test virus and the infecting virus. The low frequency of clinical response and the lack of a characteristic syndrome associated with primary infection also contribute to the difficulties of interpreting incidence, reinfection, and prevalence data. In infections occurring *in utero*, in newborns, or in infants, the incidence rate of primary infection can be more reliably calculated.

5.1.1. Prevalence. The prevalence of CF antibody to CMV in various population groups has indicated that CMV infection is ubiquitous (Table 1). The differences observed have been related to the speed of acquisition of infection in different geographic and socioeconomic settings. In St. Lucia, a survey of all four herpesviruses revealed by age 5 that 83.8% had CMV antibody but only 7.1% varicella-zoster antibody.[25b] The presence of CMV in the urine, cervix, or breast milk has also been used to reflect infection prevalence in special groups. About 1% of newborns in the United States have CMV in the urine.[8,35,68,103,104] Thirteen percent of women undergoing examination because of sus-

pected venereal disease[49] and 4–28% of pregnant women have CMV in cervical secretions.[79,84,92] Three to six percent of the latter have viruria at the time of delivery,[44,83] and a 27% prevalence of CMV in the breast milk of recently delivered CMV-seropositive Australian mothers has been reported.[40]

5.1.2. Incidence. The incidence of CMV infection and of clinical disease has been determined in prospective studies of special groups as measured by serological or virological tests or both. Table 2 summarizes several of these reports of CMV infection, and the results are discussed below.

a. Pregnant Women. Serological studies have shown that about 60% of women entering the childbearing years have antibody to CMV.[59,83,108] The frequency with which CMV can be isolated from the pregnant woman appears to vary with age, parity, socioeconomic status, site cultured, and time during gestation when she is studied, but in general, viruria has been found in 3–12% of a large number of pregnant women.[27,44,59,79,83,92] In a prospective study of 1089 young pregnant women attending the prenatal clinic of a large general hospital,[83] 65% were found to have CF antibody and 124 (11.4%) excreted CMV in their urine on one or more occasions during their pregnancies. There were 119 living children born to these women; 12, or 10%, were congenitally infected with CMV. Only one of each ten women who excreted virus during pregnancy had an infant with CMV infection.

Further studies attempting to define the factors associated with delivering an infected infant suggest that primary CMV infection during pregnancy may carry a significant risk. A total of 8 pregnant women among over 3000 have had primary CMV infections defined as seroconversion from negative to positive as well as the onset of cytomegaloviruria during the period of the study[82]: 1 in the first trimester, 4 in the second, and 3 in the third. None had accompanying symptoms. The woman with primary CMV in the first trimester had CMV-positive buffy coat cultures during the first and second trimesters and positive urine, throat, and cervical cultures throughout pregnancy, but delivered a normal uninfected infant. The 3 infants born to mothers who acquired infection during the third trimester and 1 of the 4 born to second-trimester converters had congenital CMV infection, but all infants were clinically normal. The infection risk of an infant born to a mother who had primary CMV infection during pregnancy

Table 1. Cytomegalovirus Prevalence by Serological Survey: General Populations

Author	Date	Place	Population	CMV seropositive (%)
Hanshaw[34]	1966	Rochester	0–5 mo	35
			5–24 mo	3
			2–6 yr	6
			6–10 yr	9
			10–17 yr	22
			27–40 yr	38
Rowe et al.[95]	1956	Washington	6–24 mo	14
			5–9 yr	33
			>35 yr	81
Stern and Elek[105]	1965	London	6–60 mo	4
			5–10 yr	15
			>35 yr	54
Carlstrom[12]	1965	Stockholm	6–24 mo	36
			5–10 yr	24
			>50 yr	63
Jack and McAuliffe[46]	1968	Melbourne	6–36 mo	22
			10–15 yr	40
			>35 yr	60
Evans et al.[25]	1974	Barbados	1–5 yr	62
			15–25 yr	77
Embil et al.[23]	1969	Nova Scotia	6–12 mo	12
			10–14 yr	14
			>40 yr	52
Krech and Jung[56]	1970	Tanzania	6–18 mo	80
			5–14 yr	100
			>20 yr	99
Shavrina et al.[99]	1973	Leningrad	7–12 mo	67
			11–15 yr	63
			51–60 yr	80
Evans et al.[25b]	1979	St. Lucia	0–5 yr	83.5
			6–10 yr	94.9
			11–20 yr	92.5
			21–30 yr	96.2
			31–40	100
			>40 yr	96.9

was 4:8 in this series, with the further suggestion that infection late in pregnancy was more likely to be associated with a congenitally infected infant (3 of 3 in the third trimester).

In a prospective study of 1040 pregnant women in London, Stern and Tucker[108] reported that 11 showed antibody evidence of primary infection: 5 in the third trimester, 4 in the second, and 2 in either the late first or early second trimester. The delivery of an infected baby was associated with primary infection early in pregnancy in this study (only 1 of 5 infected infants was born to a mother who had her primary infection in the third trimester.)

In both studies, however, regardless of when during gestation maternal infection was acquired, women excreting virus at the time of delivery were most likely to have infected infants; all 9 mothers of infected infants had positive virus cultures at delivery. The infected babies in both studies were normal except for one infant[108] who showed generalized hypotonia and mental retardation at the age of 6 months.

Table 2. Incidence of Cytomegalovirus Infection in Prospective Studies

Group	Setting	Time period	Number studied	CMV-aby-negative (%)	Initial aby[a] status		Infected	Rate/100/ period of observation	Reference
					Number	Aby[a]			
Pregnant women 1.	All ages in London	6–9 mo	1040	33.4	270	Neg.	11[b]	4.1	Stern and Tucker[108]
2.	Teenagers, Cleveland	Up to 9 mo	1089	35	379	Neg.	5[b]	1.3	Nankervis et al.[83]
Young adults 1.	English colleges	9 mo	1457	70	713	Neg.	10[b]	1.4	UHP[113]
2.	Marine recruits	14 wk	588	69.7	431	Mixed	4[b]	0.9	Wenzel et al.[121]
Surgical patients 1.	Cardiopulmonary bypass	3 mo	212	38.7	82	Neg.	50[b]	61.0	Purcell et al.[91]
					130	Pos.	32[b]	24.6	Henle et al.[41]
2.	Renal transplant	3 mo	44	40.9	18	Neg.	12[c]	66.7	Nankervis et al.[81]
					26	Pos.	18[c]	69.2	

[a] Antibody.
[b] 4× ↑ Aby.
[c] 4× ↑ Aby or CMV culture +.

In Barbados[25] and Tanzania[56] or similar parts of the world where CMV infection is acquired early in life and nearly 100% have antibody by the end of childhood, one would not expect infants to be born with congenital infection, assuming that primary infection during pregnancy is a prerequisite for that event. However, in populations in which the opportunity of exposure is high, the small proportion of women without CMV antibody entering childbearing age appear to have a high risk of contracting primary CMV infection during pregnancy[108] and of delivering an infected infant.

Rates of recovery of CMV from cervix cultures of pregnant women vary from 14% among the Navajo,[79] 18% in Taiwan,[2] 15% in Japan,[84] 12% in Birmingham,[92] 2% in Seattle,[31] to 5% in Pittsburgh.[79] Factors responsible may be racial, seasonal, or more likely socioeconomic. Recovery from the cervix is more frequent than recovery from urine by a factor of 2 or more, and the simultaneous isolation from both sites is uncommon, although this has not been the experience of all investigators.[83] The frequency of positive cultures of the cervix increases as gestation progresses[79,84,92] and appears to be higher[79] in younger mothers with fewer than four pregnancies. Interestingly, infants born to mothers with proved cervical CMV infections are unlikely to have congenital CMV infection, although such infants have a high risk of acquiring CMV infection during the first few months of life. Reynolds et al.[92] offer the hypothesis that the increasing rate of cervical and urinary excretion as gestation proceeds and the high rate of virus excretion in breast milk are the result of reactivation of latent CMV infection perhaps provoked by hormonal influences.

b. Young Adults. Prospective studies of young adults have indicated a very low rate of CMV infection that is usually asymptomatic (Table 2). Among 1457 entering freshman college students in five English colleges and universities, 70% lacked CMV antibody; 713 of the 1026 lacking antibody were retested 7 months later and only 10 were found to have acquired antibody, an infection rate of 1.4% in the susceptible group.[113] Only 1 of these 10 developed a mononucleosislike syndrome. A similar study was made of 588 marine recruits undergoing "boot-camp" training over 14 weeks at Parris Island.[121] On entry, 69.7% lacked CMV antibody. When a group of primarily seronegatives was re-

bled 14 weeks later, 4 had developed CMV antibody, an infection rate of 0.9%. In contrast to CMV, similar surveys for Epstein–Barr virus (EBV) infection in college and military groups have shown seroconversion rates of 12–13% in those lacking EBV antibody, and 25–75% of these infections have been associated with clinical infectious mononucleosis.[66,96,113] It should be noted, however, that CMV mononucleosis occurs more commonly in the 25–35 age group, so that the group at highest risk has not been included in the prospective studies of CMV infections thus far.

c. Transfusion and Postsurgical Groups. The CMV infection rate depends on the initial antibody status of the recipient,[41,91] the evidence of CMV infection in the donor,[81] the number of units transfused,[90] and the immunological status of the recipient. This last is of special significance because a host compromised by natural or drug-induced immunosuppression appears to be at high risk of CMV reactivation. Table 2 presents some representative data. A primary infection rate of 66.7% has been recorded following open-heart surgery in those initially lacking CMV antibody and an antibody rise of 24.6% is now being observed in renal-transplant patients, some of which appears to be temporally associated with kidney rejection, interstitial pneumonia, or hepatitis,[16,17,70,71,81] The amount of actual disease produced by CMV infection in this group is still controversial.

5.2. Geographic Distribution

Antibody to CMV is prevalent in adults throughout the world, ranging from 37% in Rochester, New York,[34] to 50–60% in Nova Scotia,[23] Berlin,[42] London,[105] and Debrecen, Hungary,[114] and rising to greater than 80% in Barbados[25] and Tanzania.[56] The major differences are related to the speed of acquisition of infection in various geographic and socioeconomic settings. Antibody has been detected in all populations thus far tested, including the remote Tiriyo Indians of Brazil, who essentially lack measles and influenza antibody.[9]

5.3. Age and Sex

Plots of antibody prevalence by age and sex show a similar contour for most populations. There is a loss of transplacentally acquired antibody in the first year of life, a gradual acquisition of antibody throughout childhood, a more rapid increase in proportion with antibody during the young adult years, and then a leveling off in the rate of seroconversion. As shown in Table 1, the most striking difference in data from a range of socioeconomic and racial groups is the age at which most persons have their primary CMV infection (i.e., first develop antibody to CMV). Fewer than half the subjects 15 years of age in most of the studies conducted in both the Eastern and the Western hemispheres had CMV antibody, but in Barbados, the figure was approximately 80%, and even 100% in Tanzania.

The age at infection may influence the nature of the clinical syndrome produced. Infection during gestation may result in a congenital CMV syndrome, while infection delayed to age 20 or over may result in cytomegalic mononucleosis syndrome; this latter also occurs after blood transfusion in adults. Regardless of age or sex, the majority of infections with CMV are clinically asymptomatic.

5.4. Temporal Distribution

Seasonal or yearly patterns of CMV infection have not been clearly delineated.

5.5. Occupation

No relationship to occupation *per se* has been shown.

5.6. Race and Socioeconomic Setting

Many variables influence the time at which CMV infections are acquired and the outcome of those infections. People in lower socioeconomic groups, especially if they live in tropical settings, acquire CMV infections earlier in life. In this group, cervical excretion of virus during pregnancy is common, and viruria has a high frequency among neonates.

6. Mechanism of Transmission

Close or prolonged contact with playmates who are excreting virus is probably the most important method of spread of CMV among children. Studies contrasting antibody prevalence among children living together in large groups and those living at home support this view. Children in English boarding schools had antibody prevalence rates 4 times those of children attending day school,[105] and a similar magnitude of difference was demonstrable when Swiss nursery school students were compared with a suitable control group.[56] The high frequency of antibody among children in underdeveloped countries or in lower socioeconomic groups is probably also the result of crowding and poor sanitation. Interestingly, children of migrant farm workers in upper New York State[69] and 1- to 5-year-olds in Egyptian villages[94] had antibody rates similar to those reported for Barbados[25] and Tanzania.[56]

Prolonged excretion of virus in urine, saliva, stool, tears, breast milk, and semen is characteristic following CMV infection whether or not the patient is symptomatic and despite the presence of high levels of circulating antibody. The mechanism responsible for eventually turning off viral synthesis—or, more accurately, turning it off and on, as is frequently observed—is postulated to be related to cell-mediated immune mechanisms, but precise data are not available. Droplet or possibly fecal–oral spread is probably the route by which most postnatal primary CMV infections are acquired, although infection with CMV may occur via blood in the congenital or posttransfusion forms, via transplanted organs such as kidneys, by sexual contact (infected cervix or semen), or by ingestion of breast milk. The presence of CMV in cervix as well as its presence and persistence in semen[62,63] raises the possibility of venereal transmission, and one epidemiological analysis is consistent with this possibility.[49] Virus in the cervix and urine at the time of delivery in many mothers provides a "sea of cytomegalovirus" through which the newborn infant must pass and be placed at high risk of infection.

7. Pathogenesis and Immunity

There appear to be rather marked differences in the consequences of the various forms of CMV infection. Congenital infection carries a significant risk of residual damage, especially to the nervous system, whereas acquired infection, although occasionally associated with illness, is apparently not followed by any disability even when it occurs in the newborn. Although primary infection during pregnancy is associated with a high probability of infection in the newborn, the time during gestation when primary maternal CMV is most likely to involve the fetus has not been defined. Recurrent CMV infection during pregnancy is unlikely to result in the delivery of an infected baby, and probably recurrent infection at any time is unlikely to be of clinical importance except possibly in the immunodeficient patient. The differences in pathogenesis among various types of CMV infections are discussed below.

7.1. Pathogenesis

7.1.1. Neonatal Infection: Congenital.
Early in the course of primary infection, virus is disseminated widely in various organs of the host, as indicated by virus isolation from multiple sites. If the host undergoing primary infection is pregnant, virus may infect the placenta and in some cases penetrate the placenta to infect the fetus. Early studies of infants with CID showed the association between specific clinical manifestations and evidence of infection with CMV.[119] As laboratory methods for demonstrating infection were more widely utilized, the spectrum of changes occurring in congenital CMV broadened and the "expanded syndrome" was described. Later, as information from the prospective study of groups of unselected newborns accumulated, it became apparent that congenital CMV infection is not invariably associated with severe mental or neurological deficit.[6,93,103]

On the basis of the available data, one can make a number of speculations. Maternal viremia is more likely to occur with primary than with recurrent infections, and if it occurs in the latter, the virus titer may be low. Under certain conditions (e.g., trimester of pregnancy, state of placenta), virus in small quantities may cross the placenta and initiate foci of replication in various fetal tissues. Maternal IgG antibody crosses the placenta as it is formed and interacts with the CMV recently synthesized in the fetus. Whether the fetal infection proceeds and whether clinical manifestations of CMV develop may depend on the relative amounts of virus and immune globulin that interact. Much of the time, even with primary maternal infection, virus replication and dissemination may be inadequate to result in fetal infection, but occasionally, even with

recurrent infection, dissemination and fetal infection result, although classic disease is unlikely.

7.1.2. Posttransfusion and Organ Transplant.
The pathogenesis of CMV infection following transfusion or organ transplantation is not clear. The major questions are whether this represents a primary or a reactivated infection, and if the latter, whether the source of virus is the recipient, the blood of blood donors, or the transplanted organs of the donor. In transfusion receipients lacking demonstrable CMV antibody and transfused with blood from antibody-positive donors, some of whom have been shown to harbor CMV in their buffy coats,[19] a primary infection seems most likely. The reservation here is how sensitive the CF test is to identify low-level antibody and whether IgM responses accompany this infection. In the presence of CMV antibody in the recipient, a "mixed-lymphocyte" response between donor and recipient lymphocytes might activate CMV in either. At present, it has not been demonstrated that CMV resides within lymphocytes, although cultured buffy coats reveal CMV after culture on a fibroblast layer[47,64,109]; further, in vitro replication of complete CMV in lymphocytes has not been shown even when stimulated by bromodeoxyuridine, phytohemagglutinin, other lymphocytes, or EBV-infected lymphocytes. In renal-transplant patients, both reactivation and reinfection are probably important. Clear-cut implication of the immunosuppressed recipient or the blood donor as the source of virus has been very difficult. However, at least two studies have indicated that the donor kidney may be the source of virus in many posttransplant patients. Ho et al.[44a] and Nankervis[80a] observed that recipients of kidneys from CMV-seropositive donors had a significantly higher risk of CMV infection than did recipients of kidneys from CMV-negative donors. This was particularly true if the recipients themselves were seronegative.[83a] The presence of immunosuppression in these patients probably contributes to the high risk of CMV infection.

7.1.3. CMV Mononucleosis.
The epidemiology and pathogenesis of CMV mononucleosis pose questions very similar to those about EBV mononucleosis. In both diseases, the host response appears to be associated with primary infection first acquired in young adult life, most likely through intimate exposure to a pharyngeal carrier or acute case. Recent studies indicate that clinical infectious mono-

nucleosis is an immunological response to EBV infection involving T- and B-cell interactions.[100,115] The atypical lymphocyte may represent in part virus-transformed B-type lymphocytes and in part T cells reacting to neoantigens induced by EBV on the B-cell membrane. The similarities of the clinical and hematological picture of CMV mononucleosis to that caused by EBV suggest that a similar immune mechanism may be at play.[91d] The major difference is that CMV infection does not produce heterophil antibody.

7.2. Immunity

Antibody to CMV appears regularly following infection and, although levels may fluctuate, appears to persist for life, with the exception of some congenitally infected children who gradually lose their antibody. The primary immune response to CMV is specific, and infection with another member of the herpesvirus family does not cause the appearance of antibody detectable by the CMV CF test in a previously CMV-antibody-negative subject. Lymphocytes from normal antibody-positive subjects but not from antibody-negative subjects undergo CMV-specific lymphocyte blastogenesis.[89a,95a,110a,116a,125] However, several reports indicate that a specific impairment in cell-mediated immunity to CMV occurs in mothers of infants with CID as well as in the infants themselves.[91c,93a,103b] Thus, a specific defect in cell-mediated immunity may play an important role in the pathogenesis of congenital CMV infection. Further studies are needed to elucidate the role of humoral vs. cell-mediated immunity in protection against primary infection as well as in the prevention of endogenous reactivation.

8. Patterns of Host Response

Most CMV infections are inapparent and asymptomatic and can be detected only by laboratory study. The frequency and nature of the clinical response appear to depend on the age at which infection is acquired, on the route of infection, and on the immune status of the host. The most common forms of associated clinical syndromes are listed in Table 3.

Table 3. Host Responses to Cytomegalovirus Infections

A. Neonatal infections
  1. Congenital
  2. Acquired
B. Infection of children and adults
  1. Hepatitis
  2. Mononucleosis
  3. Posttransfusion CMV infection
  4. Posttransplant syndrome
  5. CMV and malignant disease
  6. Other possible syndromes
    Encephalitis
    (Guillain–Barré syndrome)
    Ulcerative colitis

8.1. Neonatal Infections

8.1.1. Congenital. The risk of infection and the pathogenesis of infection have already been discussed. The association between significant nervous system damage and congenital CMV infection remains unquestioned; what is not known is the frequency with which CMV infection acquired *in utero* leads to immediate or late clinical residua, as well as the factors related to such an outcome. In a follow-up of 20 children with severe CID, most of whom had overt clinical evidence of disease at the time of birth, 4 of 15 who survived were considered to have developed normally, and 2 others showed only equivocal evidence of retardation.[76] Another group of 12 children with clinical and laboratory evidence of congenital CMV infection were evaluated at the age of 3–12 years. Of the 12, 3 were considered of average intelligence, 1 was mildly retarded, 3 were moderately retarded, and 5 were severely retarded.[6]

Several studies indicate that infants with no apparent evidence of CID in the newborn period may develop neurological sequelae. Hanshaw,[34] struck by the association between CID and failure of brain growth observed in early studies, tested sera from physically handicapped children who had no history of CID and found a significantly larger proportion with CMV antibody among the group with microcephaly. Baron *et al.*[4] and Nakao and Chiba[80] were unable to confirm these findings. In further studies,[106] neurological patients with symptoms compatible with possible congenital infection were found to have CMV antibody significantly more frequently than a selected control group. The longitudinal observations of Reynolds *et al.*[93] eliminate many of the hazards of these retrospective studies. Among 267 neonates with elevated umbilical-cord IgM levels, 18 clinically well were found to have laboratory evidence of congenital CMV infection. Of 16 who were followed, 9 developed sensorineural hearing loss. Hanshaw *et al.*[36a] followed 44 children originally identified by elevated specific CMV IgM levels in cord blood. Of the 44 children, 16, or 36.6%, had developmental abnormalities precluding adquate performance in regular school. In addition, 5 of 40 infected children (12.5%) has sensorineural hearing losses as opposed to only 1 of 44 (2.5%) matched controls. Kumar *et al.*[59a] followed 15 children identified at birth by screening newborn urine samples. The mean IQ of 85 at age 4 years was not significantly different from the mean IQ of 86 in a matched control group. Mild high-frequency hearing loss occurred in only 2 of 13 infected children at age 6 years. Other studies indicate that among infants with congenital CMV infection who appear clinically normal in the neonatal period, the presence of elevated IgM levels (not proved to be specific CMV antibody) may predict an increased incidence of late residual effects. In a sample of nearly 2000 unselected newborn infants, 5 with both CMV-specific macroglobulin and elevated total IgM were observed for a period of over 2 years.[35] Of these 5, 2 were microcephalic and severely retarded, 1 showed slow psychomotor development, and 2 were normal. In a similar survey,[8] three infants found to be excreting CMV in their urine within the first 24 hr of life had elevated IgM levels during the first months of life. None of the three had the classic signs of CID, but one developed a mild spasticity in the second year of life and the other two remained normal. In the most unusual situation, where two consecutive pregnancies resulted in the birth of CMV-infected infants, one had elevated cord IgM and became markedly retarded, while the other with normal levels of IgM at birth developed normally.[102] Nankervis *et al.*[83] reported that 4 of 16 infants with clinically inapparent congenital CMV infection had elevated cord IgM levels, but all were apparently normal after a follow-up period averaging 18 months.

The classic syndrome of CID is uncommon, occurring once in 3000–5000 births. However, congenital CMV infection has a frequency of about 1 per 100 live births, and although estimates of the proportion of such infants who eventually develop serious sequelae are based on preliminary data, this figure is about 10%.[35,108] One of every 1000 newborns, at least in England and the United States, will have hearing loss, psychomotor retardation, or neurological defect secondary to congenital CMV infections.

8.1.2. Acquired. It has been observed during the follow-up of infants born to mothers excreting CMV during pregnancy that a significant proportion who were culture-negative at birth became infected with CMV during the first few months of life. In a Cleveland study,[83] 21 infants of over 100 excreting mothers developed viruria, 16 before the age of 14 weeks; others[68,92] have reported similar findings. In one study,[92] infection of the infant during the first few months of life could be correlated with late gestational cervical excretion by the mother, and the conclusion was drawn that the transmission of CMV from the infected cervix during birth is an important route of infection in early life, analogous to that of herpes simplex virus. Transmission of CMV via infected breast milk or from household contacts does not appear to be an important source of infection for the young infants.[84]

Acquired CMV infection in the young infant is, like the congenital form, chronic, and virus excretion in urine or saliva continues for months. Although the patients usually show no symptoms related to their infection, Nankervis *et al.*[83] found that 7 of the 21 infants in the Cleveland study had symptoms that coincided temporally with the first positive urine culture. Three had interstitial pneumonia, two cases being severe enough to require hospitalization. One patient had cervical and inguinal lymphadenopathy associated with a diffuse maculopapular rash, one had mild hepatosplenomegaly with elevated SGOT and SGPT and 17% atypical lymphocytes, one had mild hepatosplenomegaly with a diffuse maculopapular rash, and one had only mild hepatosplenomegaly.

Long-term follow-up with psychometric, neurological, and audiometric testing on infants with acquired disease has not been reported, but preliminary data indicate that they develop normally.[83,92]

8.2. Infection of Children and Adults

Most of the large number of children and adults who have antibody to CMV remain well or have a mild, nonspecific illness when they experience their CMV infection. A small proportion, and this figure is probably considerably less than 1%, may have one of a variety of clinical syndromes that have been shown to occur concurrently with CMV infection. These include hepatitis, an infectious-mononucleosis-like syndrome, various respiratory- or gastrointestinal-tract symptoms, and occasional signs of central nervous system disease. The probability of illness accompanying CMV infection appears greater in the immunodeficient person or in those receiving blood transfusions, but has also been observed in previously well subjects. The syndromes described often overlap, especially in the transplant recipient or patient with malignant disease. The source of infection in patients with the several clinical forms of CMV appears to be exogenous, but in several instances, a number of well-studied cases could have been "reactivated" infections.

8.2.1. Hepatitis. CMV has been associated with liver disease since the original isolation[120] from a biopsy specimen obtained from a child with chorioretinitis, hepatosplenomegaly, and cerebral calcification. Hanshaw et al.[36] evaluated 20 asymptomatic CMV-positive children as well as appropriate controls. Abnormal liver-function tests were 6 times more frequent in virus-positive than in control children. Among a group of 22 children and 1 young adult with enlarged liver or spleen or both for which an explanation was being sought, 9 (39%) had viruria. CMV was also isolated from the liver of 1 child who died. Further studies[104,107] have indicated that liver involvement, which is part of the congenital CMV syndrome, is not uncommon in patients with acquired CMV, although in the latter group, clinical manifestations may vary from mild transient abnormalities in liver function to severe icteric disease difficult to distinguish from other forms of hepatitis. In general, the prognosis of hepatitis associated with CMV is good; a chronic course appears unlikely, and the few deaths recorded have been in patients with abnormal immune systems. Many patients, especially adults, with CMV-related hepatitis have mononuclear cells in their peripheral blood.[112]

8.2.2. Mononucleosis. Klemola and Kaariainen[53] reported a series of patients, all but one of whom were adults, who developed an infectious-mononucleosis-like illness characterized by fever and liver involvement but no pharyngitis or significant cervical adenopathy. Laboratory studies revealed a high percentage of atypical lymphocytes in the smears of peripheral blood, a negative Paul–Bunnell test, an increase in cryoimmunoglobulins, and serological evidence of recent CMV infection. This syndrome has been observed in previously healthy individuals, but occurs more frequently in subjects who have received large volumes of transfused blood, as discussed below. Patients generally improve within 3–6 weeks with a return of normal liver-function tests and the disappearance of atypical lymphocytes from the peripheral blood.

Klemola et al.[54] have provided rather compelling data to relate heterophil-negative mononucleosis to CMV infection. In a series of studies, they found that among 350 patients with infectious diseases of miscellaneous etiology, only 1 showed a rise in antibody to CMV (and that patient had Guillain–Barré syndrome); of 90 patients with Paul-Bunnell-positive infectious mononucleosis, none demonstrated a significant titer elevation, but 13 of 18 individuals with febrile, Paul–Bunnell-negative mononucleosis had a 4-fold or greater rise in level of CMV CF antibody. Overall, CMV mononucleosis was diagnosed in 9% of the patients referred because of "possible mononucleosis." Spontaneous CMV mononucleosis has subsequently been reported from many laboratories[18,50,55,60,73]; overall, it accounts for 5–7% of the infectious-mononucleosis-type syndrome and shows clinical, hematological, and epidemiological features with that due to EBV except that heterophil antibody does not appear.[25a]

8.2.3. Posttransfusion. The syndrome of fever with atypical lymphocytes was initially observed in patients who had undergone cardiac surgery using pump oxygenators,[58,122] and the fresh blood used was suspected as the source of virus. Subsequently, CMV has been recovered from the blood of patients with hepatitis,[109] leukemia,[39,47] and mononucleosis,[50,61,65] and from immunologically depressed transplant recipients,[3,16,29] but only Diosi et al.[19] have been able to isolate CMV from the blood of healthy blood donors (2 of 35 tested). A number of laboratories have been unable to repeat the last results, possibly because of the methods of collecting, storing, or testing of the blood samples.[30,51,87]

In one series of 53 patients who underwent open-heart surgery with an extracorporeal pump,[13] 21 had a rise in CMV antibody, but only 4 developed the typical mononucleosislike syndrome. Other studies[85] have indicated that about a third of such patients show boosts in CMV antibody, with only the occasional patient having an accompanying illness. The volume of blood transfused, the age of the blood, the antibody status of the patient, and the mechanical damage to cells by the pump may all contribute to the possibility of the patient's showing a CMV antibody response, but the relative importance of each factor is difficult to define. Prince et al.[90] reported a rather direct association between the number of units of blood transfused and CMV antibody conversion; 7% of those who received 1 unit of blood but 21% of those given multiple transfusions had significant elevations in CMV antibody titer. The rate was over twice as high in immunosuppressed transplant recipients. Preexisting antibody status or use of fresh blood was of little importance. A boost in CMV antibody followed large-volume transfusions of fresh blood in subjects with no or low titers of preexisting CF antibody but in none who had CF titers of 128 or greater. However, among patients who received stored citrated blood, none had antibody rises regardless of the preoperative level.[85] The lack of preoperative antibody and the rather slow rise in antibody titer suggest that the postperfusion syndrome is associated with a primary infection by CMV derived from donor blood, but in some patients, the antibody status and rapid rise make it difficult to rule out the possibility of reactivation of an old infection with antibody boost. An increased incidence of CMV infection in neonates who have undergone single transfusion[124] or exchange transfusion[72] has also been reported.

8.2.4. Posttransplant. CMV infection following renal transplantation is very common[80a] and may be associated with a variety of clinical manifestations or be completely asymptomatic. The source of the virus is unclear; the virus may be endogenous in origin, introduced with blood, or present in the donor kidney as indicated above.

Autopsy studies of patients who died following renal transplantation during the early days of this procedure were found in many cases to give evidence of pulmonary CMV infection. Kanich and Craighead[52] showed a good correlation between the histological changes diagnosed as CMV and the ability to isolate virus from lung tissue and evidence of generalized CMV infection. They also found that CMV infection was much more likely to occur in the patient given immunosuppressive therapy, that the duration of such therapy affected such probability,

and the immunosuppressive therapy did not prevent a specific antibody response to CMV. Later prospective studies indicated that asymptomatic CMV infection was common in the renal-transplant patient receiving immunosuppressive therapy and that only an occasional patient developed mononucleosis,[3] hepatitis,[71] or pulmonary disease.[16]

There is some suggestion that the patient who acquires primary CMV infection following allograft reception and immunosuppressive therapy has viremia and signs of illness. Armstrong et al.,[3] for example, reported that of four renal transplant recipients with laboratory evidence of primary CMV infection, three had viremia and two became ill, one with mononucleosis and the other with hepatitis. Similarly, Nankervis[80a] reported that 5 of 53 study patients developed fever and chills, leukopenia, and lymphocytosis usually accompanied by an increase in serum creatinine 6 weeks or longer after transplantation. None of the 5 patients had demonstrable CMV CF antibody before transplantation, and 4 of the 5 had virus-positive buffy-coat cultures. However, in the presence of immunosuppressive therapy, it is very likely that reactivation of latent virus and the development of illness can occur and possibly that infection with a second antigenically different strain of CMV may cause illness in the previously infected subject. Studies differentiating primary and recurrent infections and antigenic variants of CMV are required before these points can be clarified.

8.2.5. CMV and Malignant Disease. The patient with malignant disease may have a severe or protracted illness with CMV infection,[10] but may not have an increased risk of acquiring such an infection. Benyesh-Melnick et al.[5] and Dyment et al.,[21] in separate studies, found low rates of CMV in children with leukemia (2%), and Hanshaw and Weller[38] isolated CMV from the urine of 3 patients among 50 with leukemia, lymphoma, or Hodgkin's disease (rate of 6%). Sullivan et al.[110] reported that when seroconversion was used as an indicator of CMV infection, 9 of 16 children had 4-fold antibody rises during the course of leukemia. Henson et al.[43] made the observation, which is difficult to interpret, that among children with leukemia, those excreting CMV had more episodes of pneumonitis or fever with rash but not more episodes of hepatitis, fever without rash, or respiratory-tract infections than those not shedding virus in the urine.

8.2.6. Other Possible Syndromes. There are several case reports in the literature relating specific illnesses such as encephalitis[20] or ulcerative colitis[67] with CMV infection. In most of these studies, a change in antibody status or the excretion of virus is shown to exist concurrently with a particular disease syndrome; in a few, the evidence for the diagnosis of CMV infection consists of the demonstration of typical intranuclear inclusions in various tissues. The variability in antibody titer and the frequency with which virus can be detected in urine or saliva of chronically infected patients make it very hazardous to interpret two concurrent events as being cause and effect. This is emphasized by the authors of many of the articles cited, but it is only by continuing to collect such data that the final question of etiology can be resolved.

9. Immunization

If convincing evidence can be obtained supporting the current impression that primary rather than recurrent CMV infection during pregnancy may result in fetal infection and clinical illness with residual damage, then there is a reasonable basis for considering the use of a vaccine. However, there are two major areas of concern associated with the use of a CMV vaccine. First, there are three reports in the literature documenting congenital CMV infection in consecutive pregnancies.[24,57,102] Although the second infants have been considered to be normal over short periods of evaluation, it is clearly possible for a woman to have two congenitally infected infants in separate pregnancies. Additional data are sorely needed to support or disprove the consistency of normality of the second-born infants in this situation.

The second major area of concern is the malignant potential of the herpesviruses. Members of this group have been clearly implicated as the etiological agents of malignancy in lower animals, and the association between herpes simplex type II and cervical carcinoma in the human is well accepted. In addition, Albrecht and Rapp[1] have shown that irradiated CMV is capable of causing transformation in hamster cells *in vitro*. The transformed cells are oncogenic when inoculated into hamsters. The same group of investigators has recently described *in vitro* growth of human prostate tissue infected *in vivo*

with CMV to passage levels higher than those routinely attained by normal cells.[91a] They have also demonstrated malignant transformation in one cell line derived from a human prostatic adenocarcinoma that possessed CMV antigenic markers.[32a] Nondifferentiated tumors were induced when transformed cells were inoculated subcutaneously into athymic nude mice.

Despite the relatively high titers of CMV that can be obtained in supernatant fluid from roller bottles,[45] this virus probably does not multiply to a high enough titer to make a killed vaccine practical or economically feasible. Thus, an effective live vaccine seems the most reasonable at present, and it may be necessary to use a mixture of several antigenic types or a particular strain that cross-reacts with the overwhelming majority of the common variants.

Elek and Stern[22] have reported results obtained with a live vaccine prepared from AD 169, a standard laboratory strain. The subcutaneous inoculation of this material into 26 seronegative volunteers was followed by the development of antibody in 25. Mild local signs developed at the injection site in half the subjects, and 2 developed tender adenopathy, 1 with reactive lymphocytes. None of the subjects demonstrated any disturbance of liver function tests, and none excreted virus in throat secretions or urine.

Plotkin *et al.*[88a] have developed a live vaccine (Towne strain) by passing an isolate from a congenitally infected infant 125 times in tissue culture. Clinical trials[50b,88,103a] have indicated that vaccinees develop antibodies and manifest a specific cellular immune response not only to the Towne strain, but also to AD 169 and Davis strains of CMV. Local erythema and induration at the site of injection have occurred, but there have been no alterations in blood counts or liver-function tests. Attempts to isolate virus postvaccination from throat, urine, buffy coat, semen, or vaginal tampons have been uniformly negative. Antibody has been demonstrated to persist for at least 4 years postvaccination, although the titers have dropped considerably over that time.[50a] Glazer *et al.*[33a] studied ten vaccinees who underwent renal transplantation subsequent to vaccination. CMV was isolated from six patients after transplantation, but the restriction endonuclease patterns of the viral DNA of the four isolates tested differed significantly from those of the vaccine strain. These data from a very small number of patients suggest that the vaccine strain did not become latent in the host in a form that could be reactivated readily.

Whether antibody stimulated by a live vaccine will persist for many years or is related to subsequent prevention of damaged congenitally infected infants is at present unknown. Clearly, continued studies of the malignant potential of CMV as well as the complex interaction of mother, fetus, and virus must form a crucial background for involvement in the development of a vaccine to protect against such an effective and efficient parasite as the CMV.

10. Unresolved Problems

Unresolved problems include whether there are important biological differences among CMV strains, what the relative importance of various routes of transmission is, whether primary or reactivated CMV is more important clinically, and what the role of humoral and cell-mediated immunity is in both. In addition, the long-term effect of congenital CMV infection needs further study, as does the potential oncogenicity of CMV. Finally, the development of usefulness of a CMV vaccine require further investigation.

11. References

1. ALBRECHT, T., AND RAPP, F., Malignant transformation of hamster embryo fibroblasts following exposure to ultraviolet-irradiated human cytomegalovirus, *Viology* 55:53–61 (1973).
2. ALEXANDER, E. R., Maternal and neonatal infection with cytomegalovirus in Taiwan (abstract), *Pediatr. Res.* 1:210 (1967).
3. ARMSTRONG, D., BALAKRISHNAN, S., STEGIR, L., YU, B., AND STENZEL, K. H., Cytomegalovirus infections with viremia following renal transplantation, *Arch. Intern. Med.* 127:111–115 (1971).
4. BARON, J., YOUNGBLOOD, L., SIEWERS, C. M. F., AND MEDEARIS, D. N., JR., The incidence of cytomegalovirus, herpes simplex, rubella, and toxoplasma antibodies in microcephalic, mentally retarded, and normocephalic children, *Pediatrics* 44:932–939 (1969).
5. BENYESH-MELNICK, M., DESSY, S. I., AND FERNBACH, D. J., Cytomegaloviruria in children with acute leukemia and in other children, *Proc. Soc. Exp. Biol. Med.* 117:624–630 (1964).
6. BERENBERG, W., AND NANKERVIS, G. A., Long-term follow-up of cytomegalic inclusion disease of infancy, *Pediatrics* 46:403–409 (1970).
7. BERNSTEIN, M. T., AND STEWART, J. A., Indirect hemagglutination test for detection of antibodies to cytomegalovirus, *Appl. Microbiol.* 21:84–89 (1971).
8. FIRNBAUM, G., LYNCH, J. I., MARGILETH, A. M., LONERGAN, W. M., AND SEVER, J. L., Cytomegalovirus infections in newborn infants, *J. Pediatr.* 75:789–795 (1969).
9. BLACK, F. L., WOODALL, J. P., EVANS, A. S., LIEBHABER, H., AND HENLE, G., Prevalence of antibody against viruses in the Tiriyo, an isolated Amazon tribe, *Am. J. Epidemiol.* 91:430–438 (1970).
10. CANGIR, A., AND SULLIVAN, M., The occurrence of cytomegalovirus infections in childhood leukemia, *J. Am. Med. Assoc.* 195:616–622 (1966).
11. CAPPELL, D. F., AND MCFARLANE, M. N., Inclusion bodies (protozoan-like cells) in the organs of infants, *J. Pathol. Bacteriol.* 59:385–398 (1947).
12. CARLSTROM, G., Virologic studies on cytomegalic inclusion disease, *Acta Paediatr. Scand.* 54:17–23 (1965).
13. CAUL, E. O., CLARKE, S. K. R., MOTT, M. G., PERHAM, T. G. M., AND WILSON, R. S. E., Cytomegalovirus infections after open heart surgery: A prospective study, *Lancet* 1:777–781 (1971).
14. CHIANG, W., WENTWORTH, B. B., AND ALEXANDER, E. R., The use of an immunofluorescence technique for the determination of antibodies to cytomegalovirus strains in human serum, *J. Immunol.* 104:992–999 (1970).
15. COLE, R., AND KUTTNER, A. G., A filterable virus present in the submaxillary glands of guinea pigs, *J. Exp. Med.* 44:855–873 (1926).
16. COULSON, A. S., LUCAS, Z. J., CONDY, M., AND COHN, R., An epidemic of cytomegalovirus disease in a renal transplant population, *West. J. Med.* 120:1–7 (1974).
17. CRAIGHEAD, J. E., HANSHAW, J. B., AND CARPENTER, C. B., Cytomegalovirus infection after renal allotransplantation, *J. Am. Med. Assoc.* 201:99–102 (1967).
18. DAVIS, L. E., TWEED, G. V., STEWART, J. A., BERNSTEIN, M. T., MILLER, G. L., GRAVELLE, C. R., AND CHIN, D. Y., Cytomegalovirus mononucleosis in a first trimester pregnant female with transmission to the fetus, *Pediatrics* 48:200–206 (1971).
19. DIOSI, P., MOLDOVAN, E., AND TOMESCU, N., Latent cytomegalovirus infection in blood donors, *Br. Med. J.* 4:660–662 (1969).
20. DORFMAN, L. J., Cytomegalovirus encephalitis in adults, *Neurology* 23:136–144 (1973).
21. DYMENT, P. G., ORLANDO, S. J., ISAACS, H., JR., AND WRIGHT, H. T., JR., The incidence of cytomegalovi-

ruria and postmortem cytomegalic inclusions in children with acute leukemia, *J. Pediatr.* **72**:533–536 (1968).

22. Elek, S. D., and Stern, H., Development of a vaccine against mental retardation caused by cytomegalovirus infection *in utero*, *Lancet* **1**:1–5 (1974).

23. Embil, J. A., Haldane, E. V., Mackenzie, R. A. E., and van Rooyen, C. E., Prevalence of cytomegalovirus infection in a normal urban population in Nova Scotia, *Can. Med. Assoc. J.* **101**:730–733 (1969).

24. Embil, J. A., Ozere, R. L., and Haldane, E. V., Congenital cytomegalovirus infection in two siblings from consecutive pregnancies, *J. Pediatr.* **77**:417–421 (1970).

25. Evans, A., Cox, F., Nankervis, G., Opton, E., Shope, R., Wells, A. V., and West, B., A health and seroepidemiological survey of a community in Barbados, *Int. J. Epidemiol.* **3**:167–175 (1974).

25a. Evans, A. S., Infectious mononucleosis and related syndromes, *Am. J. Med. Sci.* **276**:325–339 (1978).

25b. Evans, A. S., Cook, J., Kapikian, A. Z., Nankervis, G., Smith, A., and West, B., A serological survey of St. Lucia, *Int. J. Epidemiol.* **8**:327–332 (1979).

26. Farber, S., and Wolback, S. B., Intranuclear and cytoplastic inclusions ("protozoan-like bodies") in salivary glands and other organs of infants, *Am. J. Pathol.* **8**:123–126 (1932).

27. Feldman, R. A., Cytomegalovirus infection during pregnancy, *Am. J. Dis. Child.* **117**:517–521 (1969).

28. Fetterman, G. H., A new laboratory aid in the clinical diagnosis of inclusion disease of infancy, *Am. J. Clin. Pathol.* **22**:424–425 (1952).

29. Fine, R. N., Grushkin, C. M., Anand, S., Lieberman, E., and Wright, H. T., Cytomegalovirus in children, *Am. J. Dis. Child.* **120**:197–202 (1970).

30. Foster, K. M., and Jack, I., A prospective study of the role of cytomegalovirus in post-transplant mononucleosis, *N. Engl. J. Med.* **280**:1311–1354 (1969).

31. Foy, H. M., Kenny, G. E., Wentworth, B. B., Johnson, W. L., and Grayston, J. T., Isolation of mycoplasma hominis, T-strains, and cytomegalovirus from the cervix of pregnant women, *Am. J. Obstet. Gynecol.* **106**:635–643 (1970).

32. Fuccillo, D. A., Moder, F. A., Traub, R. G., Hensen, S., and Sever, J. L., Micro indirect hemagglutination test for cytomegalovirus, *Appl. Microbiol.* **21**:104–107 (1971).

32a. Geder, L., Sanford, E. J., Rohner, T. J., and Rapp, F., Cytomegalovirus and cancer of the prostate: *In vitro* transformation of human cells, *Cancer Treatment Rep.* **61**:139–146 (1977).

32b. Gerna, G., McCloud, C. J., and Chambers, R. W., Immunoperoxidase technique for detection of antibodies to human cytomegalovirus, *J. Clin. Microbiol.* **3**:364–372 (1976).

33. Goodpasture, E. W., and Talbot, F. B., Concerning the nature of "protozoan-like" cells in certain lesions of infancy, *Am. J. Dis. Child.* **21**:415–421 (1921).

33a. Glazer, J. P., Friedman, H. M., Grossman, R. A., Starr, S. E., Barker, C. F., Perloff, J. L., Huang, E. S., and Plotkin, S. A., Live cytomegalovirus vaccination of renal transplant candidates, *Ann. Intern. Med.* **91**:676–683 (1979).

34. Hanshaw, J. B., Cytomegalovirus complement-fixing antibody in microcephaly, *N. Engl. J. Med.* **275**:476–479 (1966).

35. Hanshaw, J. B., Congenital cytomegalovirus infection: A fifteen year perspective, *J. Infect. Dis.* **123**:555–561 (1971).

36. Hanshaw, J. B., Betts, R. F., Simon, G., and Boynton, R. C., Acquired cytomegalovirus infection association with hepatomegaly and abnormal liver-function tests, *N. Engl. J. Med.* **272**:602–609 (1965).

36a. Hanshaw, J. B., Scheiner, A. P., and Moxley, A. W., School failure and deafness after "silent" congenital cytomegalovirus infection, *N. Engl. J. Med.* **295**:468–470 (1976).

37. Hanshaw, J. B., Steinfeld, H. J., and White, C. J., Fluorescent-antibody test for cytomegalovirus macroglobulin, *N. Engl. J. Med.* **279**:566–570 (1968).

38. Hanshaw, J. B., and Weller, T. H., Urinary excretion of cytomegaloviruses by children with generalized neoplastic disease: Correlation with clinical and histopathologic observations, *J. Pediatr.* **58**:305–311 (1961).

39. Harden, D. G., Elsdale, T. R., Young, D. E., and Ross, A., The isolation of cytomegalovirus from peripheral blood, *Blood* **30**:120–125 (1967).

40. Hayes, K., Danks, D. M., and Gibas, H., Cytomegalovirus in human milk, *N. Engl. J. Med.* **287**:177–178 (1972).

41. Henle, W., Henle, G., Scriba, M., Joyner, C., Harrison, F., von Essen, R., Paloheimo, J., and Klemola, E., Antibody responses to the Epstein–Barr virus and cytomegalovirus after open-heart and other surgery, *N. Engl. J. Med.* **282**:1068–1074 (1970).

42. Henneberg, G., and Antoniadis, G., Serological investigations into the epidemiology of cytomegalovirus infection, International Conference of Cytomegalovirus Infection, St. Gall, April 1–3, 1970.

43. Henson, D., Siegel, S., Fucillo, D. A., Matthew, E., and Levine, S., Cytomegalovirus infections during acute childhood leukemia, *J. Infect. Dis.* **126**:469–481 (1972).

44. Hildebrandt, R. J., Sever, J. L., Margileth, A. M., and Callagan, D. A., Cytomegalovirus in the normal pregnant woman, *Am. J. Obstet. Gynecol.* **98**:1125–1128 (1967).

44a. Ho, M., Suwansirkul, S., Dowling, J. N., Youngblood, L. A., and Armstrong, J. A., The transplanted kidney as a source of cytomegalovirus infection, *N. Engl. J. Med.* **293**:1109–1112 (1975).

45. Huang, E. S., Chen, S. T., and Pagano, J. S., Human cytomegalovirus. I. Purification and characterization of viral DNA, *J. Virol.* **12:**1473–1481 (1973).

46. Jack, I., and McAuliffe, K. C., Sero-epidemiological study of cytomegalovirus infections in Melbourne children and some adults, *Med. J. Aust.* **1:**206–209 (1968).

47. Jack, I., Todd, H., and Turner, E. K., Isolation of human cytomegalovirus from the circulating leukocytes of a leukaemic patient, *Med. J. Aust.* **1:**210–213 (1968).

48. Jesionek, A., and Kiolemenoglou, B., Über einen Befund von protozoenartigen Gebilden in den Organen eines Feten, *Muench. Med. Wochenschr.* **51:**1905–1907 (1904).

49. Jordon, M. C., Rousseau, W. E., Noble, G. R., Stewart, J. A., and Chin, T. D. Y., Association of cervical cytomegalovirus with venereal disease, *N. Engl. J. Med.* **288:**923–934 (1973).

50. Jordon, M. C., Rousseau, W. E., Stewart, J. A., Noble, G. R., and Chin, T. D. Y., Spontaneous cytomegalovirus mononucleosis, *Ann. Intern. Med.* **79:**153–160 (1973).

50a. Just, M., Cytomegalovirus vaccine—Towne strain, Presented at the Experimental Herpesvirus Vaccine Workship, National Institutes of Health, February 8, 1979.

50b. Just, M., Duergin-Wolff, A., Emoedi, G., and Hernandez, F., Immunization trials with live attenuated cytomegalovirus Towne 125, *Infection* **3:**111–114 (1975).

51. Kane, R. C., Rousseau, W. E., Noble, G. R., Tegtmeier, G. E., Wulff, H., Herndon, H. B., Chin, T. D. Y., and Bayer, W. L., A prospective study of cytomegalovirus infection in a volunteer blood donor population, *Infect. Immun.* **11:**719–723 (1975).

52. Kanich, R. E., and Craighead, J. E., Cytomegalovirus infection and cytomegalic inclusion disease in renal homotransplant recipients, *Am. J. Med.* **40:**874–882 (1966).

53. Klemola, E., and Kaariainen, L., Cytomegalovirus as a possible cause of a disease resembling infectious mononucleosis, *Br. Med. J.* **2:**1099–1102 (1965).

54. Klemola, E., Kaariainen, R., von Essen, R., Haltia, K., Koivuniemi, A., and von Bonsdorff, C.-H., Further studies on cytomegalovirus mononucleosis in previously healthy individuals, *Acta Med. Scand.* **182:**311–322 (1967).

55. Krech, U., Jung, M., Jung, F., and Singeisen, C., Virologische und klinische Untersuchungen bei konnatalen und postnatalen Cytomegalien, *Schweiz. Med. Wochenschr.* **98:**1459–1469 (1968).

56. Krech, U. H., and Jung, M., Age distribution of complement-fixing antibodies in Tanzania, 1970, in: *Cytomegalovirus Infections of Man.* pp. 27–28, S. Karger, Basel, 1971.

57. Krech, U., Konjajev, Z., and Jung, M., Congenital cytomegalovirus infection in siblings from consecutive pregnancies, *Helv. Paediatr. Acta* **26:**355–362 (1971).

58. Kreel, I., Zaroff, L. I., Canter, J. W., Krasna, I., and Baronofsky, I. D., Syndrome following total body perfusion, *Surg. Gynecol. Obstet.* **111:**317–321 (1960).

59. Kriel, R. L., Gates, G. A., Wulff, H., Powell, N., Poland, J. D., and Chin, T. D. Y., Cytomegalovirus isolations associated with pregnancy wastage, *Am. J. Obstet. Gynecol.* **106:**885–892 (1970).

59a. Kumar, M. L., Nankervis, G. A., and Gold, E., Inapparent congenital cytomegalovirus infection: A follow-up study, *N. Engl. J. Med.* **288:**1370–1372 (1973).

60. Lamb, S. G., and Stern, H., Cytomegalovirus mononucleosis with jaundice as presenting sign, *Lancet* **2:**1003–1006 (1966).

61. Lang, D. J., and Hanshaw, J. B., Cytomegalovirus infection and the postperfusion syndrome: Recognition of primary infections in four patients, *N. Engl. J. Med.* **280:**1145–1149 (1969).

62. Lang, D. J., and Kummer, J. F., Demonstration of cytomegalovirus in semen, *N. Engl. J. Med.* **287:**756–758 (1972).

63. Lang, D. J., Kummer, J. F., and Hartley, D. P., Cytomegalovirus in semen: Persistence and demonstration in extracellular fluids, *N. Engl. J. Med.* **291:**121–123 (1974).

64. Lang, D. J., and Noren, B., Cytomegaloviremia following congenital infection, *J. Pediatr.* **73:**812–819 (1968).

65. Lang, D. J., Scolnick, E. M., and Willerson, J. T., Association of cytomegalovirus infection with the postperfusion syndrome, *N. Engl. J. Med.* **278:**1147–1149 (1968).

66. Lehane, D. E., A seroepidemiologic study of infectious mononucleosis: The development of EB virus antibody in a military population, *J. Am. Med. Assoc.* **212:**2240–2242 (1970).

67. Levine, R. S., Warner, N. E., and Johnson, C. F., Cytomegalic inclusion disease in the gastrointestinal tract of adults, *Ann. Surg.* **159:**37–48 (1964).

68. Levinsohn, E. M., Foy, H. M., Kenny, G. E., Wentworth, B. B., and Grayston, J. T., Isolation of cytomegalovirus from a cohort of 100 infants throughout the first year of life, *Proc. Soc. Exp. Biol. Med.* **132:**957–962 (1969).

69. Li, F., and Hanshaw, J. B., Cytomegalovirus infection among migrant children, *Am. J. Epidemiol.* **86:**137–141 (1967).

70. Lopez, C., Simmons, R. L., Mauer, S. M., Najarian, J. S., and Good, R. A., Association of renal allograft rejection with viral infections, *Am. J. Med.* **56:**280–289 (1974).

71. LUBY, J. P., BURNETT, W., HULL, A. R., WARE, A. J., SHOREY, J. W., AND PETERS, P. C., Relationship between cytomegalovirus and hepatic function abnormalities in the period after renal transplant, *J. Infect. Dis.* **129**:511–518 (1974).

72. LUTHARDT, T., SIEBERT, H., LOSEL, I., QUEVEDO, M., AND TODT, R., Cytomegalievirus-infektionen bei Kindern mit Blutaustauschtransfusion im Neugeborenenalter, *Klin. Wochenschr.* **49**:81–86 (1971).

73. MANDELL, G. L., Cytomegalovirus mononucleosis, *Del. Med. J.* **43**:155–156 (1971).

74. MARGILETH, A. M., The diagnosis and treatment of generalized cytomegalic inclusion disease of the newborn, *Pediatrics* **15**:270–283 (1955).

75. MCALLISTER, R. M., WRIGHT, H. T., JR., AND TASEM, W. M., Cytomegalic inclusion disease in newborn twins, *J. Pediatr.* **64**:278–281 (1964).

76. MCCRACKEN, G. H., JR., SHINEFIELD, H. R., COBB, K., RAUSEN, A. R., DISCHE, M. R., AND EICHENWALD, H. F., Congenital cytomegalic inclusion disease: A longitudinal study of 20 patients, *Am. J. Dis. Child.* **117**:522–539 (1969).

77. MEDEARIS, D. N., JR., Observations concerning human cytomegalovirus infection and disease, *Bull. Johns Hopkins Hosp.* **114**:181–211 (1964).

78. MERCER, R. D., LUSE, S., AND GUYTON, D. H., Clinical diagnosis of generalized cytomegalic inclusion disease, *Pediatrics* **11**:502–514 (1953).

79. MONTGOMERY, R., YOUNGBLOOD, L., AND MEDEARIS, D. N., JR., Recovery of cytomegalovirus from the cervix in pregnancy, *Pediatrics* **49**:524–531 (1972).

80. NAKAO, T., AND CHIBA, S., Cytomegalovirus and microcephaly, *Pediatrics* **46**:483–484 (1970).

80a. NANKERVIS, G. A., Comments on CMV infections in renal transplant patients, *Yale J. Biol. Med.* **49**:27–28 (1976).

81. NANKERVIS, G. A., BRAUN, W. E., COOPER, A. R., KUMAR, A., AND GOLD, E., A prospective study of cytomegalovirus infection in renal transplant recipients (in prep.) (1981).

82. NANKERVIS, G. A., KUMAR, M. L., AND GOLD, E., Primary infection with cytomegalovirus during pregnancy (abstract), *Pediatr. Res.* **8**:427 (1974).

83. NANKERVIS, G. A., KUMAR, M. L., COX, F. E., AND GOLD, E., A prospective study of maternal cytomegalovirus infection and its effect on the fetus (in prep.) (1981).

83a. NARAQI, S., JACKSON, G. G., JONASSON, O., AND RUBENIS, M., Search for latent cytomegalovirus in renal allografts, *Infect. Immun.* **19**:699–703 (1978).

84. NUMAZAKI, Y., YANO, N., MORIZUKA, T., TAKAI, S., AND ISHIDA, N., Primary infection with human cytomegalovirus: Virus isolation from healthy infants and pregnant women, *Am. J. Epidemiol.* **91**:410–417 (1970).

85. PALOHEIMO, J. A., VON ESSEN, R., KLEMOLA, E., KAARIAINEN, L., AND SILTANEN, P., Subclinical cytomegalovirus infections and cytomegalovirus mononucleosis after open heart surgery, *Am. J. Cardiol.* **22**:624–630 (1968).

86. PENTTINEN, K., KAARIAINEN, L., AND MYLLYLA, G., Cytomegalovirus antibody assay by platelet aggregation, *Arch. Gesamte Virusforsch.* **29**:189–194 (1970).

87. PERHAM, T. G. M., CAUL, E. O., CONWAY, P. J., AND MOTT, M. G., Cytomegalovirus infection in blood donors—A prospective study, *Br. J. Haemotol.* **20**:307–320 (1971).

88. PLOTKIN, S. A., FARQUHAR, J., AND HORNBERGER, E., Clinical trials of immunization with the Towne 125 strain of human cytomegalovirus, *J. Infect. Dis.* **134**:470–475 (1976).

88a. PLOTKIN, S. A., FURUKAWA, T., ZYGRAICH, N., AND HUYGELEN, C., Candidate cytomegalovirus strain for human vaccination, *Infect. Immun.* **12**:521–527 (1975).

89. PLUMMER, G., AND BENYESH-MELNICK, M., A plaque reduction neutralization test for human cytomegalovirus, *Proc. Soc. Exp. Biol. Med.* **117**:145–150 (1964).

89a. POLLARD, R. B., RAND, K. H., ARVIN, A. M., AND MERIGAN, T. C., Cell-mediated immunity to cytomegalovirus infection in normal subjects and cardiac transplant patients, *J. Infect. Dis.* **137**:541–549 (1978).

90. PRINCE, A. M., SZMUNESS, W., MILLIAN, S. J., AND DAVID, D. S., A serologic study of cytomegalovirus infections associated with blood transfusions, *N. Engl. J. Med.* **284**:1125–1131 (1971).

91. PURCELL, R. H., WALSH, J. H., HOLLAND, P. V., MORROW, A. G., WOOD, S., AND CHANOCK, R. M., Seroepidemiological studies of transfusion-associated hepatitis, *J. Infect. Dis.* **123**:406–413 (1971).

91a. RAPP, F., GEDER, L., MURASKO, D., LAUSCH, R., LADDA, R., HUANG, E., AND WEBBER, M. M., Long term persistence of cytomegalovirus genome in cultured cells of prostatic origin, *J. Virol.* **16**:982–990 (1975).

91b. REYNOLDS, D. W., Development of early nuclear antigen in cytomegalovirus infected cells in the presence of RNA and protein synthesis inhibitors, *J. Gen. Virol.* **40**:475–480 (1978).

91c. REYNOLDS, D. W., DEAN, P. H., PASS, R. F., AND ALFORD, C. A., Specific cell-mediated immunity in children with congenital and neonatal cytomegalovirus infection and their mothers, *J. Infect. Dis.* **140**:493–499 (1979).

91d. RINALDO, C. R., JR., CARNEY, W. P., RICHTER, B. S., BLACK, P. H., AND HIRSCH, J. S., Mechanism of immunosuppression in cytomegaloviral mononucleosis, *J. Infect. Dis.* **141**:488–495 (1980).

92. REYNOLDS, D. W., STAGNO, S., HOSTY, T. S., TILLER, M., AND ALFORD, C. A., JR., Maternal cytomegalo-

virus excretion and perinatal infection, *N. Engl. J. Med.* **289**:1–5 (1973).

93. REYNOLDS, D. W., STAGNO, S., STUBBS, K. G., DAHLE, A. J., LIVINGSTON, M. M., SAXON, S. S., AND ALFORD, C. A., Inapparent congenital cytomegalovirus infection with elevated cord IgM levels, *N. Engl. J. Med.* **290**:291–296 (1974).

93a. ROLA-PLESZCZYNSKI, M., FRENKEL, L. D., FUCILLO, D. A., HENSEN, S. A., VINCENT, M. M., REYNOLDS, D. W., AND BELLANTI, J. A., Specific impairment of cell-mediated immunity in mothers of infants with congenital infection due to cytomegalovirus, *J. Infect. Dis.* **135**:386–391 (1977).

94. ROWE, W. A., Adenovirus and salivary gland virus infections in children, in: *Viral Infections of Infancy and Childhood* (H. M. ROSE, ed.), pp. 205–214, Hoeber, New York, 1960.

95. ROWE, W. P., HARTLEY, J. W., WATERMAN, S., TURNER, H. C., AND HUEBNER, R. J., Cytopathogenic agent resembling human salivary gland virus recovered from tissue cultures of human adenoids, *Proc. Soc. Exp. Biol. Med.* **92**:418–424 (1956).

95a. RYTEL, M. W., AGUILAR-TORRES, F. G., BALAZ, J., AND HEIM, L. R., Assessment of the status of cell-mediated immunity in cytomegalovirus-infected renal allograft recipients, *Cell. Immunol.* **37**:31–40 (1978).

96. SAWYER, R. N., EVANS, A. S., NIEDERMAN, J. C., AND MCCOLLUM, R. W., Prospective studies of a group of Yale University freshmen. I. Occurrence of infectious mononucleosis, *J. Infect. Dis.* **123**:263–270 (1971).

97. SCHMITZ, H., AND HAAS, R., Determination of different cytomegalovirus immunoglobulins (IgG, IgA, IgM) by immunofluorescence, *Arch. Gesamte Virusforsch.* **37**:131–140 (1972).

98. SCHWARTZ, R. S., Immunoregulation, oncogenic viruses, and malignant lymphomas, *Lancet* **1**:1266–1269 (1972).

99. SHAVRINA, L. V., ASHER, D. M., ILYENKO, V. I., AND SMORODINTSEV, A. A., Antibodies of cytomegalovirus in the population of Leningrad, *Vopr. Virusol.* **2**:156–159 (1973).

100. SHELDON, P. J., PAPAMICHAIL, M., HEMSTED, E. H., AND HOLBOROW, E. J., Thymic origin of atypical lymphoid cells in infectious mononucleosis, *Lancet* **1**:1153–1155 (1973).

101. SMITH, M. G., Propagation in tissue cultures of a cytopathogenic virus from human salivary gland virus (SGV) disease, *Proc. Soc. Exp. Biol. Med.* **92**:424–430 (1956).

102. STAGNO, S., REYNOLDS, D. W., LAKEMAN, A., CHARAMELLA, L. J., AND ALFORD, C. A., Congenital cytomegalovirus infection: Consecutive occurrence due to viruses with similar antigenic compositions, *Pediatrics* **52**:788–794 (1973).

102a. STAGNO, S., PASS, R. F., REYNOLDS, D. W., MOORE, M. A., NAHMIAS, A. J., AND ALFRED, C. A., Comparative study of diagnostic procedures for congenital cytomegalovirus infection, *Pediatrics* **65**:251–257 (1980).

102b. STAGNO, S., VOLANAKIS, J. E., REYNOLDS, D. W., STROUD, R., AND ALFORD, C. A., Immune complexes in congenital and natal cytomegalovirus infections of man, *J. Clin. Invest.* **60**:838–845 (1977).

103. STARR, J. G., BART, R. D., JR., AND GOLD, E., Inapparent congenital cytomegalovirus infection: Clinical and epidemiologic characteristics in early infancy, *N. Engl. J. Med.* **282**:1075–1077 (1970).

103a. STARR, S. E., FRIEDMAN, H. M., GLAZER, J. P., GARRABRANT, T., AND PLOTKIN, S. A., Immune responses to live cytomegalovirus vaccine (Towne strain) in normal and immunosuppressed volunteers (Abstract No. 805), Interscience Conference on Antimicrobial Agents and Chemotherapy (1979).

103b. STARR, S. E., TOLPIN, M. D., FRIEDMAN, H. M., PAUCKER, K., AND PLOTKIN, S. A., Impaired cellular immunity to cytomegalovirus in congenitally infected children and their mothers, *J. Infect. Dis.* **140**:500–505 (1979).

104. STERN, H., Isolation of cytomegalovirus and clinical manifestations of infection at different ages, *Br. Med. J.* **1**:665–669 (1968).

105. STERN, H., AND ELEK, S. D., The incidence of infection with cytomegalovirus in a normal population: A serologic study in greater London, *J. Hyg.* **63**:79–87 (1965).

106. STERN, H., ELEK, S. D., BOOTH, J. C., AND FLECK, D. G., Microbial causes of mental retardation: The role of prenatal infections with cytomegalovirus, rubella virus, and toxoplasma, *Lancet* **2**:443–448 (1969).

107. STERN, H., AND TUCKER, S. M., Cytomegalovirus infection in the newborn and in early childhood: Three atypical cases, *Lancet* **2**:443–448 (1969).

108. STERN, H., AND TUCKER, S. M., Prospective study of cytomegalovirus infection in pregnancy, *Br. Med. J.* **2**:268–270 (1973).

109. STULBERG, C. S., ZUELZER, W. W., PAGE, R. H., TAYLOR, T. E., AND BROUGH, Cytomegalovirus infections from lymph node and blood, *Proc. Soc. Exp. Biol. Med.* **123**:976–982 (1966).

110. SULLIVAN, M. P., HANSHAW, J. B., CANGIR, A., AND BUTLER, J. J., Cytomegalovirus complement-fixation antibody levels of leukemic children, *J. Am. Med. Assoc.* **206**:569–574 (1968).

110a. TENNAPEL, C. H. H., THE, T. H., BIJKER, J., DEGAST, G. C., AND LANGENHUYSEN, M. M. A. C., Cytomegalovirus directed lymphocyte reactivity in healthy adults tested by a CMV-induced lymphocyte transformation test, *Clin. Exp. Immunol.* **29**:52–60 (1977).

111. THE, T. H., KLEIN, G., AND LANGENHUYSEN, M. M.

A. C., Antibody reactions to virus-specific early antigens (EA) in patients with cytomegalovirus (CMV) infections, *Clin. Exp. Immunol.* **16**:1–12 (1974).

112. TOGHILL, P. J., BAILEY, M. E., WILLIAMS, R., ZEEGEN, R., AND BOWN, R., Cytomegalovirus hepatitis in the adult, *Lancet* **1**:1351–1354 (1967).

113. UNIVERSITY HEALTH PHYSICIANS AND P. H. L. S. LABORATORIES, Infectious mononucleosis and its relationship to EB virus antibody, *Br. Med. J.* **4**:643–646 (1971).

114. VACZI, L., GONCZOLL, E., LEHEL, F., AND GEDER, L., Isolation of cytomegalovirus and incidence of complement-fixing antibodies against cytomegalovirus in different age-groups, *Acta Microbiol. Acad. Sci. Hung.* **12**:115–121 (1965).

115. VERLAINEN, M., ANDERSSON, L. C., LALLA, M., AND VON ESSEN, R., T-lymphocyte proliferation in mononucleosis, *Clin. Immunol. Immunopathol.* **2**:114–120 (1973).

116. VON GLAHN, W. C., AND PAPPENHEIMER, A. M., Intranuclear inclusions in visceral disease, *Am. J. Pathol.* **1**:445–465 (1925).

116a. WANER, J. L., AND BUCNICK, J. E., Blastogenic response of human lymphocytes to human cytomegalovirus, *Clin. Exp. Immunol.* **30**:44–49 (1977).

117. WANER, J. L., WELLER, T. H., AND KEVY, S. V., Patterns of cytomegaloviral complement-fixing antibody activity: A longitudinal study of blood donors, *J. Infect. Dis.* **127**:538–543 (1973).

118. WELLER, T. H., HANSHAW, J. B., AND SCOTT, D. E., Serologic differentiation of viruses responsible for cytomegalic inclusion disease, *Virology* **12**:130–132 (1960).

119. WELLER, T. H., AND HANSHAW, J. B., Virologic and clinical observations on cytomegalic inclusion disease, *N. Engl. J. Med.* **266**:1233–1244 (1962).

120. WELLER, T. H., MACAULEY, J. C., CRAIG, J. M., AND WIRTH, P., Isolation of intranuclear inclusion producing agents from infants with illnesses resembling cytomegalic inclusion disease, *Proc. Soc. Exp. Biol. Med.* **94**:4–12 (1957).

121. WENZEL, R. P., McCORMICK, D. P., DAVIES, J. A., BERLING, C., AND BEAM, W. E., JR., Cytomegalovirus infection: A seroepidemiologic study of a recruit population, *Am. J. Epidemiol.* **97**:410–414 (1973).

122. WHEELER, E. O., TURNER, J. D., AND SCANNELL, J., G., Fever, splenomegaly and atypical lymphocytes: Syndrome observed after cardiac surgery utilizing pump oxygenator, *N. Engl. J. Med.* **266**:454–456 (1962).

123. WYATT, J. P., SAXTON, J., LEE, R. S., AND PINKERTON, H., Generalized cytomegalic inclusion disease, *J. Pediatr.* **36**:271–294 (1950).

124. YEAGER, A. S., Transfusion-acquired cytomegalovirus infection in newborn infants, *Am. J. Dis. Child.* **128**:478–483 (1974).

125. ZAIA, J. A., LEARY, P. L., AND LEVIN, M. J., Specificity of the blastogenic response of human mononuclear cells to herpes virus antigens, *Infect. Immun.* **20**:646–651 (1978).

12. Suggested Reading

HANSHAW, J. B., Congenital cytomegalovirus infection: A fifteen year perspective, *J. Infect. Dis.* **123**:555–561 (1971).

HO, M., Cytomegalovirus infections and diseases, *Dis.-Mon.* **24**(12):1–61 (1978).

KRECH, U., JUNG, M., AND JUNG, F., *Cytomegalovirus Infections of Man*, S. Karger, Basel, 1971.

KUMAR, M. L., AND NANKERVIS, G. A., Cytomegalovirus infections, *South. Med. J.* **72**:854–861 (1979).

WELLER, T. H., Cytomegaloviruses: The difficult years, *J. Infect. Dis.* **122**:532–539 (1970).

WELLER, T. H., The cytomegaloviruses: Ubiquitous agents with protean clinical manifestations, *N. Engl. J. Med.* **285**:203–214, 267–274 (1971).

WRIGHT, H. T., JR., Cytomegaloviruses, in: *The Herpesviruses* (ALBERT S. KAPLAN, ed.), Academic Press, New York, 1973.

CHAPTER 9

Enteroviruses

Joseph L. Melnick

1. Introduction

The enterovirus group, named in 1957,[31] brought together polioviruses, coxsackieviruses, and echoviruses, all of which inhabit the human alimentary tract. These viruses share a number of clinical, epidemiological, and ecological characteristics as well as physical and biochemical properties.

Enteroviruses of human origin include the following:

1. Polioviruses: types 1–3.
2. Coxsackieviruses A: 23 types and several variants [coxsackieviruses Al–A24 (coxsackievirus type A23 is the same virus as echovirus9)].
3. Coxsackieviruses B: types B1–B6.
4. Echoviruses: 31 types [types 1–33 (echovirus 10 has been reclassified as reovirus type 1 and echovirus 28 as rhinovirus type 1A)].
5. Enterovirus types 68–71: These viruses would formerly have been classed as either coxsackievirus or echovirus types (see Section 2).

In 1963, the name *picornavirus* (*pico* = small; *rna* = ribonucleic acid genome) was introduced as a larger grouping[131] to which not only the enteroviruses but also the rhinoviruses would belong by reason of fundamental similarities in many of their properties. With the advancement of viral classification on the basis of further knowledge of biophysical and biochemical characteristics, the Inter-

national Committee on Nomenclature of Viruses has officially assigned family status (Picornaviridae) to this larger taxon, with *Enterovirus* as one genus, *Rhinovirus* as another, and two other genera chiefly infecting lower animals—*Aphthovirus* and *Cardiovirus*, including, respectively, the agents of foot-and-mouth disease of cattle and encephalomyocarditis virus of rodents.[35,147]

Another important virus, hepatitis A virus (HAV), is considered an enterovirus, and is expected to be formally classed with this genus. In Table 1, the properties that have been recently determined for HAV are listed alongside the properties of the first known enterovirus, poliovirus type 1. Now that HAV is considered as an enterovirus, we can make certain predictions about its other properties, the most significant of which are the following: (1) One would not expect there to be chronic carriers of HAV, since carriage of an enterovirus is usually limited to a few weeks. (2) One would not expect HAV to cause posttransfusion hepatitis, since enterovirus viremia is rarely detected and never lasts longer than 1 or 2 days.

New enteroviruses continue to be recognized. In 1978, an enterovirus unrelated to any presently established serotype was isolated in South Africa. About 25 isolations were made, mainly from patients with the clinical diagnosis of poliomyelitis but from whom poliovirus could not be recovered. The new virus failed to grow in cell cultures and had to be isolated and passaged in suckling mice.

In addition, certain plant and insect viruses (e.g., tomato bushy stunt, turnip yellow mosaic, acute bee paralysis viruses) have properties similar to those

Joseph L. Melnick · Department of Virology and Epidemiology, Baylor College of Medicine, Houston, Texas.

18

Table 1. Comparative Biophysical Properties of Hepatitis Type A Virus and Poliovirus Type 1

Physicochemical characteristics of major virus-particle population	Hepatitis type A virus	Poliovirus type 1
Morphology		
Diameter	28 nm	28 nm
Envelope	None	None
Sedimentation rate	160 S	160 S
Density (CsCl)	1.34 g/ml	1.34 g/ml
Nucleic acid		
Type	Single-stranded RNA	Single-stranded RNA
Length[a]	1.7 μm	2.3 μm
Molecular weight	1.9×10^6	2.6×10^6
Polypeptides (major)—	22,000[b]	24,000
molecular weights	24,000	25,000
	29,000	34,000

[a] As measured by electron microscopy.
[b] Values of 23,000, 25,500, and 34,000 have also been reported.

of the picornaviruses—as do some of the RNA-containing bacteriophages.

Many enteroviruses cause diseases in man ranging from severe and permanent paralysis to minor undifferentiated febrile illnesses. For all members of the group, however, subclinical infection is far more common than clinically manifest disease. Although certain enteroviruses have been more frequently responsible for epidemics involving a specific syndrome, the same serotypes may at other times and in other places be associated with sporadic infections having different clinical manifestations or producing no symptoms. On the other hand, different viruses may produce the same syndrome. For these reasons, clinical disease is not a satisfactory basis for classification or—as a rule—for diagnosis.

Poliomyelitis is an acute infectious disease that in its serious form affects the CNS. The destruction of motor neurons in the spinal cord results in flaccid paralysis.

The coxsackieviruses produce a variety of illnesses, including aseptic meningitis, herpangina, epidemic myalgia (pleurodynia, Bornholm disease), hand, foot, and mouth disease, myocarditis, pericarditis, pneumonia, rashes, and common colds. They may also have a role in some congenital malformations and perhaps in some forms of diabetes.

Aseptic meningitis, febrile illnesses with or without rash, and common colds are among the diseases caused by echoviruses.

Among the newer enterovirus types, enterovirus 68 has caused lower respiratory illnesses, enterovirus 70 is the agent of widespread epidemics of acute hemorrhagic conjunctivitis, and enterovirus 71 has caused aseptic meningitis and encephalitis and hand, foot, and mouth disease in a number of countries. (Further details of clinical manifestations of enterovirus infections are given in Section 8.1).

Because polioviruses can cause the most severe disease of any for which enteroviruses are responsible, these agents have received the most comprehensive study and have served as models in studies of other enteroviruses. In this chapter, therefore, poliovirus studies are used frequently as illustrative of phenomena that also hold true for other enteroviruses.

2. Historical Background

A wealth of detailed information on the development of knowledge about the enteroviruses is available in earlier reviews and textbooks.[9, 42,80,121–123,176] Consequently, only a few of the historic advances in knowledge of the enteroviruses will be mentioned here; for more information, see Paul.[169]

Although crippling disease retrospectively recognizable as paralytic poliomyelitis appears in records of early antiquity, it began to be described as a clinical entity only in the late 18th and early 19th centuries and became the subject of intensified study after increasingly severe epidemics began to appear in Europe and North America. Experimental work became possible with the successful transmission of the disease to monkeys in 1908 by Landsteiner and Popper.[100] During the next 40 years, it was shown that the virus was regularly present in stools of patients, that subhuman primates could be infected by the alimentary route, and that strains could be adapted to growth in laboratory rodents, permitting an expansion of laboratory studies. Significant antigenic differences among poliovirus strains were documented, resulting in their separation into three serological types, and it was discovered that polioviruses can be isolated and cultivated *in vitro*, in cell cultures derived from primate nonneural tissue.

The first strains of what are now known as coxsackievirus subgroup A were isolated by inoculation of infant mice with fecal material from two children suffering from paralysis during an epidemic of poliomyelitis in 1948 in Coxsackie, New York.[43] Additional types, including the first of the coxsackieviruses of subgroup B,[142] were discovered shortly thereafter. Coxsackievirus B agents were associated with a syndrome like nonparalytic poliomyelitis (aseptic meningitis) and also with epidemic myalgia and pleurodynia.[39] Group A and B coxsackieviruses were distinguished by their differing pathological effects in baby mice (see Section 4).

As soon as cultures of human and monkey cells began to be used to search for polioviruses in stool specimens of patients,[47] still more unknown viruses were found that, unlike polioviruses and the newly recognized coxsackieviruses, were not pathofor laboratory animals but produced cytopathic effects in cultured cells.[128,177]

It soon became apparent that these agents could be isolated from healthy children[70,75,128,173] as well as from patients with aseptic meningitis[119,177] and that multiple types existed.[119,173] Because the relationship of these newly recognized agents to human disease was unknown, and because they failed to produce illness in laboratory animals, they were called "orphan" viruses or human enteric viruses; later they became known as ECHO (enteric cytopathogenic human orphan) viruses,[30] a name subsequently simplified to "echoviruses."

In addition to their characteristic mouse pathogenicity, certain of the coxsackieviruses were found to grow readily in tissue cultures; other strains, serologically identical with the mouse-pathogenic prototype, failed to produce paralysis in baby mice. Conversely, certain strains of echoviruses were found to be pathogenic for mice. As instances of such overlapping properties accumulated, blurring the initial distinction made between coxsackieviruses and echoviruses, it was recommended[179] that subsequently, as new enterovirus types were discovered, they would simply be assigned sequential numbers, as enterovirus 68, enterovirus 69, etc. The currently accepted serotypes thus assigned are listed in Table 8 (Section 8).

3. Methodology Involved in Epidemiological Analysis

3.1. Sources of Mortality Data

In the United States, paralytic poliomyelitis, aseptic meningitis, encephalitis, and any poliovirus that is isolated are "notifiable," i.e., regularly required to be reported to local, state, and national health officers. But among fatalities due to enteroviruses, only poliomyelitis is generally confirmed by virus isolation. Thus, in deaths due to infections by other enteroviruses (such as encephalomyocarditis in infants), the virus responsible may not be recognized unless testing facilities are available. Information reported to the U.S. Center for Disease Control (CDC) is regularly and promptly circulated in the CDC publication *Morbidity and Mortality Weekly Report* and in special annual CDC surveillance summaries on poliomyelitis, on aseptic meningitis and encephalitis, and on the viruses being isolated and identified.

In worldwide surveillance and reporting programs of the World Health Organization (WHO), also, the most consistently investigated enterovirus-associated fatalities are those involving poliomyelitis. However, increasingly broad and useful information is becoming available on other enterovirus diseases (see Sections 3.2 and 5).

The case-fatality rate for poliovirus infection is not easily determined because of the difficulties in diagnosing nonparalytic infections. In years of high prevalence, the case-fatality rate may appear lower than in years of low prevalence because of the likelihood that nonparalytic poliomyelitis is diagnosed more readily at times of epidemic prevalence. The usual rate varies between 5 and 10% and is highest in the older age groups. In recent epidemics, in which a third of the cases occurred in patients over 15 years old, two thirds of the deaths were in this age group.

3.2. Sources of Morbidity Data

The sources of morbidity data for enteroviruses are generally far from ideal in that most studies, necessarily conducted in localized or special groups, can only suggest what may occur in the population generally. Results depend on the industriousness of the individual investigator, the specific type of situation (e.g., military or institutional), the means of data collection, and the investigator's knowledge of prior reports in the literature and his ability to relate his findings to them.

Many fruitful enterovirus studies have centered around patients as they came to medical attention or have been occasioned by outbreaks of illness; others have entailed observations of special populations or have consisted of challenge experiments with volunteers. Such investigations can yield valuable knowledge of routes of transmission, types and severity of clinical illness that can be associated with infection, sites and duration of virus excretion, and antibody responses.

But with a group of agents such as the enteroviruses, these studies have certain limitations; large proportions of enterovirus infections are subclinical and do not reach the attention of a physician; a single enterovirus serotype may produce a variety of syndromes, and a similar syndrome may be produced by a number of different enteroviruses as well as by members of other virus groups. In special environments, especially in closed populations— e.g., children's homes or military training centers where close contact, age homogeneity, and unusual stresses are often involved—the patterns of spread of infection may be atypical.

Of considerable significance in filling this gap in the knowledge of viral ecology are studies typified by the Virus Watch Programs,[51,52,90] under which families living in normal circumstances have been observed longitudinally over a period of years, with regular sampling, surveillance, and testing procedures. In an open population, enlisted families with children (or, in later periods of the programs, those with a newborn infant) are maintained under continuing virological surveillance. The principal objectives are to describe the occurrence of enteric and respiratory viral infections and/or possibly related illnesses and, by analysis of such descriptive information, to determine for specific viruses or virus groups the mode and pattern of intrafamilial spread, the relationship of age and immune status to both infection and disease, the nature of associated disease, and the frequency with which it follows infection.

Virus Watch Programs serve as an important guide for experimental design in which the family is taken as the basic epidemiological unit and in which infection, rather than solely overt illness, is the focus of study. Some of the findings are included in Section 5.

Another important source of information concerning virus infections on a global scale was initiated in 1963, in the WHO system for collecting and distributing laboratory and epidemiological information. Virus infections diagnosed by isolation or serology are reported by WHO Reference Centers and national virus laboratories around the world; the data have been consolidated and analyzed by the WHO Virus Unit, Geneva, and distributed in *WHO Weekly Epidemiological Records, WHO Quarterly* and *Annual Reports on Virus Isolations*, and in other special reports. By the end of 1975, 119 laboratories in 47 countries were participating in this scheme. From 1967 through 1975, more than 280,000 reports on viral infections were collected in the WHO virus data file. The volume of data increased from about 20,500 reports received in 1967 to more than 55,000 in 1975. Despite the limitations imposed by a wide diversity of laboratory methods, selective interests and responsibilities of various laboratories (e.g., a necessary sampling bias toward persons with overt illness), and other problems inherent in a program of this scope, these data yield indications of temporal trends in viral infections, marked linkages of certain serotypes to specific clinical syndromes, trends in age incidence, and other new knowledge about enteroviral infections. A report by Assaad and Cockburn[1] on the nonpolio enteroviruses reported during the 4-yr period 1967–1970 illustrates the very useful analyses which can be developed on the basis of these WHO records (see Section 5). An up-dating of these analyses, extending the covered period to 8 years (1967–1974), appears in a review by Grist, Bell and Assaad.[65]

Clinical surveys also have a place in providing information about the occurrence of at least one enteroviral illness: paralytic poliomyelitis. Surveys of residual paralysis in young children have provided useful data on the recent history of poliomyelitis in a community, as suggested by Payne.[171] Since the sequelae of paralytic poliomyelitis seem to be distinctive, they have been used as a measure of prior prevalence of the disease. A survey of lameness among children of school age in Ghana in 1974 yielded information on the disease in both rural and urban communities.[156,161] The results of a survey of this type for lameness in Ghana are given in Section 5.2.

3.3. Serological and Clinical Surveys

The science of serological epidemiology has reached a high degree of sophistication in a relatively short time, thanks to the pioneers who developed this field under exceedingly difficult conditions and with only crude tests available.

Even before the three serotypes of poliovirus were completely delineated, and when tests for antibodies could be conducted only in monkeys, literature reports and serological surveys of a variety of populations around the globe were compared with respect to antibody patterns. Throughout the early studies of poliomyelitis, serological surveys continued to add essential pieces to the puzzle of poliovirus transmission, susceptibility, widely varying geographic and socioeconomc patterns of infection, duration of type-specific immunity, and the shift of populations from endemic to epidemic experience with the polioviruses.[167,168] It was found that the highest percentages of persons possessing poliovirus antibodies were recorded among normal adolescents and adults in tropical areas where some contemporary "authorities" of the period believed that poliomyelitis did not exist.

Today, serological surveys continue to have an important role in maintaining protection against resurgence of epidemic poliomyelitis, by making possible the surveillance of immunity levels. Continuing serological surveillance is needed to answer such questions as the following: Are significant proportions of the susceptible age group being reached and protected by vaccination? Do the results of serosurveys parallel the estimates from surveys of immunization history? How well are antibodies induced by vaccination persisting over the years in comparison with their duration after natural infection? Since the answers to these questions may vary from one locality to another[76] and even within different population sectors of the same community,[124] local immunity patterns must be monitored to locate the specific age groups and sectors of the community in which declining antibody levels or failure to

obtain vaccination (particularly among disadvantaged inner-city children) is resulting in "protection gaps" (see Sections 5 and 9).

Furthermore, despite the increasing availability of effective poliomyelitis vaccines, there remain a number of developing countries in which vaccination is not yet widely used. Serological surveys can determine whether patterns of naturally acquired immunity are changing and thus can alert the national-health authorities to the growing need for vaccination before this need is made disastrously clear by the occurrence of large epidemics.

Serological surveys of varying scope have contributed data from which the history of local exposure to enteroviruses can be read. For example, the tests with serum collected from Eskimos in northern Alaska[2] revealed a population heavily exposed to coxsackieviruses A4 and A10, less experienced with A1, and having no detectable previous experience with coxsackieviruses B1 and B2. In the early years of investigation of the nonpolio enteroviruses, when only a few serotypes were known, the proportion of seroconversions occurring in various age groups during a single year could be obtained by serological surveys conducted in a community before and after the summer–fall season. The serological data, analyzed in conjunction with virus isolations and monitoring of concurrent illness patterns, yielded much of the information now available concerning the age patterns, the ease and routes of dissemination, and the ratio of inapparent infections to clinical illness.[137]

At present, however, general serological screening to detect seroconversions or rises in antibody titer against all possible enteroviruses is a virtual impossibility, for such a general screening would require tests against more than 70 enterovirus antigens, in combined tissue-culture and mouse systems (see Section 3.5). Epidemiological studies to learn the current pattern of infection with enteroviruses in a community can be conducted much more easily by means of virus isolation and typing, since the availability of reference antiserum pools has vastly reduced the number of tests required to identify an isolate.

In instances where an epidemic due to a single serotype is in progress, serological surveys can be usefully incorporated into well-planned and specifically targeted prospective or retrospective epidemiological studies and can provide timely guidance for physicians in making presumptive diagnoses of current illnesses.

3.4. Virus Isolation from Surface Waters as an Indicator of Community Infections

The enteroviruses are excreted so regularly and abundantly in feces that their presence in sewage can provide a great deal of information about the circulation of these viruses in a community. As early as 1940–1945,[117] consecutive tests of sewage samples reflected the seasonal prevalence of polioviruses, showed that these viruses remain infective in flowing sewage for many hours, and demonstrated that the viruses may be continually present in sewage over a period of several months. Taken together with the incidence of clinical polio in the community, the findings also provided a basis for estimating the ratio of inapparent poliovirus infections to clinical poliomyelitis. From the data obtained in New York City, this ratio turned out to be well over 100:1.[117]

Numerous studies[4,8,25,64,87,99,112,133] in developed countries have readily demonstrated the presence of enteroviruses of all subgroups in contaminated streams, in sewage, and in effluents from sewage-treatment plants. In some localities, wild polioviruses have continued to be present long after the introduction of oral poliovirus vaccine. In one metropolitan area, at the same time as virulent polioviruses were revealed in the city streams, there was a small outbreak of paralytic poliomyelitis among unimmunized infants in the area.[87] Of special note is the fact that although methods currently used for sewage treatment may slightly reduce the amount of viruses present, they do not eliminate them from the effluent. In some cases, the concentration of virus in the effluent equals that in the influent sewage or even exceeds it because of disaggregation of virus particles from clumps.

Sampling of sewage reflects not only the presence of enteroviruses but also the changes in predominant serotypes from one period to another[87,133] and has been used recently to assess the impact of oral poliovirus vaccine on the circulation of nonpolio enteroviruses.[77] Isolation of virus from an open lake swimming area served as confirmation of a coxsackievirus B5 epidemic at a summer camp[73] and provided an indication of the extent of the infections.

Portable apparatus and methods amenable to use in the field have been developed for concentrating virus from sewage and from surface water.[134,213] These methods have as their ultimate purpose the monitoring of the viral content of sewage and of water sources, so as to protect communities from viral disease that might be transmitted through drinking and recreational waters. This may become more crucial as water recycling becomes increasingly necessary.[5,224] An important by-product of this work is providing a more accurate index of the kinds and amounts of enteroviruses present within the community.

3.5. Laboratory Methods

Detailed descriptions of standard laboratory principles and procedures for investigation of enterovirus infections are available in reference books and texts.[103,104,146,192,195] Background information and details on development of procedures utilizing monkeys as well as tissue cultures may be found in earlier editions of the American Public Health Association textbook (1956 and 1964).[103]

Epidemiological knowledge of the enterovirus group—with its numerous members, frequency of silent infection, and variability of clinical manifestations when these do occur—must depend in large part on investigators' ability to identify the viruses isolated and to communicate accurately with others studying the same or similar enteroviruses. This in turn rests on the establishment of a common nomenclature for the viruses and on the development of standard reagents, both reference virus strains and type-specific antisera. Early in studies of enteroviruses, it was recognized that cooperative development of standard reagents was requisite to progress in understanding of enteroviral disease.[30] During the past 25 years, there has followed a steadily broadening series of collaborative studies among working virologists around the world to develop such reagents. These developments have been reviewed recently.[125] At present, two sets of lyophilized pools of collaboratively evaluated and standardized equine antisera are available (see Section 3.5.1). These are eight pools (A–H) of antisera against 42 enteroviruses that grow readily in cell cultures and seven pools (J–P) of antisera against 19 coxsackie virus A serotypes, including those that do not grow in cell culture and can be cultivated only in newborn mice. Use of these pools greatly facilitates the identification of enterovirus isolates.

3.5.1. Virus Isolation and Identification. The usual specimens are stools, rectal swabs, throat swabs, or throat washings. In addition, cerebrospinal fluid (CSF) yields virus frequently in cases of aseptic meningitis due to coxsackieviruses or echoviruses, but seldom if this syndrome is due to a poliovirus (nonparalytic poliomyelitis). Polioviruses, and some coxsackieviruses and echoviruses, have been detected in blood specimens taken very early in infection. Virus may also be isolated from vesicle fluids, urine, conjunctival swabs (enterovirus 70), and nasal secretions (which yield coxsackievirus A21 isolates more readily than specimens from the throat). Virus may be recovered from throat swabs taken during the first few days of illness (or of silent infection) and from rectal swabs or stools for several weeks. Most echoviruses are excreted for shorter periods than the other enteroviruses.

In fatal cases of suspected enteroviral etiology, virus should be sought in the organ system affected (e.g., in spinal cord and medulla in polio; in myocardium, endocardium, and pericardial fluid in cardiac illnesses), as well as in colon contents.

Not all agents recovered from feces or oropharynx are enteroviruses. Others that might be recovered are reoviruses, adenoviruses, rhinoviruses, and measles, mumps, rubella, and herpes simplex viruses. Many of these agents produce peculiar cytopathic effect (CPE), which at once differentiates them from enteroviruses. Several evoke fatal encephalitis in newborn mice.

If the virus laboratory has experienced personnel, a presumptive diagnosis of enteroviral infection can often be made on the basis of the nature of the associated illness (if any), the time of year when the specimen was obtained, the tissue-culture (or mouse) system in which the virus isolate grew, and the characteristic CPE observed in the cultures or the characteristic pathology induced in the mice. There is often value in reporting a presumptive identification without waiting for specific typing of the isolate. Even though specific antiviral therapy is lacking at present, early recognition of probable enteroviral infection can provide information for the management of a patient or of a community outbreak of similar illnesses and may serve to contraindicate administration of unnecessary or undesirable antibiotic therapy and to assist in narrowing the scope of diagnostic tests undertaken during an outbreak of compatible illnesses.

Most of the common enterovirus serotypes that are cytopathogenic can be recovered by inoculation of specimens into primary and passage cultures of monkey-kidney cells, but at least one human tissue-culture system must also be included if recovery of all possible types is being attempted. In addition, inoculation of newborn mice must be used if one is to detect those coxsackieviruses of group A that cannot be cultivated in cell cultures. Among the human-cell cultures that have been reported as most sensitive for a broad range of enteroviruses are WI-38 (a cell line from human embryonic lung), HEK (primary human embryonic kidney), and various local cell strains. For example, WI-38 cultures more readily support growth of echovirus 30 isolates, as well as a number of other echovirus serotypes[32,46,69,85]; however, in initial isolation of polioviruses and coxsackievirus B types, HEK cultures far surpassed either WI-38 or combined HeLa cell and monkey-kidney-cell culture systems.[32] The RD cell line, derived from a human rhabdomyosarcoma,[115] has been shown to support replication of a number of the coxsackievirus group A strains, including types A5 and A6, which previously had been grown only in newborn mice, and several other types that would grow only to low titers in other cell cultures.[38,193] Fortunately, several types that do not grow in RD cells are cultivable in HeLa or other human cell cultures.[193] It should be noted that with RD cells, most strains tested required a second passage to obtain clear-cut CPE. With utilization of RD cell cultures, only coxsackieviruses A1, A19, and A22 remain as types that require newborn mice for their cultivation. The BGM line of African green monkey kidney cells has been reported[40] as offering greater sensitivity than primary rhesus or green monkey kidney cells for titration of certain enterovirus types and also for recovery of plaque-forming enteric viruses from sewage and water. Comparative tests with clinical specimens in another laboratory indicated that the line may have limitations in sensitivity for routine isolation of a variety of echovirus types, as compared to primary rhesus monkey kidney and human fetal diploid kidney cells.[194] One potential variable is that the BGM cells obtained commercially and used in testing the clinical specimens may have been less sensitive to virus because of mycoplasma contamination.

It may not be in the best interest of the community or of an individual patient to attempt to identify the specific serotype for every enterovirus isolate. The decision to proceed with type identification should be made after weighing the specific need that would be served. At present, it is probably sufficient in many instances for the physician or health officer to know simply that an enterovirus has been isolated.

For most enteroviruses, specific identification of the serotype rests with serum neutralization testing, although hemagglutination-inhibition (HI), complement-fixation (CF), immunofluorescence, precipitin, and other antigen–antibody reactions may be used in some instances. While the isolation of an enterovirus is simple and relatively rapid, its specific identification may be slow and expensive, if only monospecific hyperimmune sera are used. However, identification of isolates has been considerably simplified by the development of internationally standardized hyperimmune equine antisera[135] that are now incorporated into combination antiserum pools constituted in a pattern proposed by Lim and Benyesh-Melnick[109] (LBM) in such a way that a given antiserum appears either in one pool, in two pools, or in three pools. An unknown enterovirus may be identified by its pattern of neutralization by the pool or pools containing its homotypic antiserum. Pools A–H were the first sets of these LBM pools to become available. They can be obtained in lyophilized form from the Research Resources Branch (RRB), National Institute of Allergy and Infectious Diseases, Bethesda, Maryland, or from WHO Virus Reference Centers. By use of the pools in accordance with standardized directions, together with five monovalent antisera, 42 enteroviruses that grow readily in cell cultures can be correctly identified.[141] Standardized equine monovalent antisera against the mouse-grown types of coxsackievirus group A are also available through the RRB. These have also been combined into additional sets of pools (J–P), incorporating 19 coxsackievirus A antisera in a scheme parallel to that described above, and are available in lyophilized form.[143] Although these pools are available in substantial amounts, it is prudent to conserve them; therefore, if an epidemic due to a single serotype is in progress, use of the single

monovalent hyperimmune serum to identify most isolates is indicated.

In use of the LBM pools to identify field isolates, some strains require special attention. For example, echovirus type 9 antiserum—particularly that prepared against the prototype strain—may not give solid neutralization of all field strains of this serotype. In such instances, it is important to make early readings to get a clue as to the probable identity of the virus. Neutralization of the virus at this early stage may be followed by later breakthrough with some strains. It may be desirable to confirm the identity of the isolate with monovalent echovirus type 9 antiserum.

With certain strains, efforts at identification by neutralization have been complicated by aggregation of viral particles or other factors, which reduce the accessibility of the virus to specific antibody. For example, as recognized soon after the discovery of the enteroviruses, the prototype echovirus 4 strain (Pesascek) is poorly neutralized by homologous antisera. The Du Toit strain is much more sensitive and is preferred for neutralization tests. The poor neutralization of the Pesascek strain was shown to be due to aggregation of viral particles; virus in nonneutralizable aggregates was found to constitute up to 30% of untreated Pesascek stock preparations, but only 0.1% of Du Toit. With monodispersed virus obtained by filtration through Millipore membranes of appropriate porosity, efficient neutralization of Pesascek strain can be obtained.[212]

This phenomenon is still encountered with enteroviruses, as illustrated by the fact that better neutralization of coxsackievirus A isolates has been obtained by treatment with sodium deoxycholate, to increase the accessibility of the virus to antibody, most likely by disaggregation of the virus particles. Isolates of enterovirus 71, also, are often difficult to neutralize, and this has produced problems in recognition of this important pathogen. Successful neutralization of the Swedish strains of enterovirus 71 depended on the use of monodispersed virus,[7] and the etiological agents of the serious epidemics in Bulgaria and Hungary were identified as strains of this serotype only in special testing of the isolates through cooperative endeavors of WHO Centres for Virus Reference and Research in Moscow, Sofia, Budapest, Berkeley, and Houston.[144] Problems with neutralization of enterovirus 71 strains and also other enterovirus isolates have been met not only by filtration but also by treatment with sodium deoxycholate, ethyl ether, and chloroform. Kapsenberg *et al.*[85a] have found chloroform treatment to be the treatment of choice for routine typing of enterovirus 71 and coxsackievirus types A7 and A16, since much virus is lost by filtration, sodium deoxycholate is cytotoxic and can be used only with virus suspensions of high titer, and removal of the imflammable ethyl ether can be difficult and hazardous. Chloroform treatment was found to be effective with virus suspensions of low titer; chloroform is nonflammable and heavier than water, and it can be removed by simple centrifugation.

A possible mechanism for the development and the elimination of a "nonneutralizable fraction" can be postulated on the basis of certain recent investigations with poliovirus. In the course of studies dealing with synthetic lipid vesicles as vehicles for introduction of foreign materials into eukaryotic cells, it has been shown that poliovirus particles can be experimentally encapsulated within synthetic large phospholipid vesicles and that such encapsulated particles are then resistant to type-specific antiserum and are infectious for cells that normally resist infection because of a membrane restriction.[219a] In light of these findings, it is a speculative possibility that the occurrence of such encapsulation during viral replication in nature may be the underlying mechanism causing virus aggregation and the observation of a "nonneutralizable fraction" of picornaviruses. Virus particles entirely or partly covered with cell-membrane materials would have an increased tendency to aggregate and would have decreased accessibility to neutralization by antibody. Such a situation would be compatible with the effects mentioned above in disaggregation of enteroviruses.

In other instances of neutralization problems, neutralization tests based on plaque reduction can be used to detect antibodies even in the presence of nonneutralizable fractions of virus.

HI and CF tests have also been used to identify enterovirus serotypes. Only about one third of enteroviruses agglutinate erythrocytes, and this limits the usefulness of this test for routine use. Likewise, all enteroviruses cannot be identified by the CF test.

A brighter hope for rapid identification of enterovirus isolates may rest with immunofluorescent staining of viral antigens.[200] A new technique utilizes combination antiserum pools in conjunction with indirect immunofluorescence to detect type-specific enteroviral antigens in CSF leukocytes of patients with aseptic meningitis.[202] The results could be available within hours after procurement of the CSF. In addition to speed, this method has the advantage of associating the enteroviral isolate more closely with the illness than would isolation from stool or throat. The fluorescent-antibody assay method for polioviruses has been made more rapid (18-hour total) and quantitative by use of tragacanth gum.[86]

If a virus isolate cannot be identified, it may represent a new enterovirus or a mixture of viruses. Therefore, plaque-purification or purification by terminal dilution passages should be carried out.

3.5.2. Tests for Antibody. Testing for presence of type-specific antibody against enteroviruses is feasible only when (1) a known enterovirus isolate from the patient is available and confirmation of the infecting serotype is necessary; (2) a clinical picture such as pleurodynia clearly implicates a small number of antigens (in this case, usually group B coxsackieviruses) against which serum should be tested; (3) an epidemic due to a single serotype is in progress; or (4) a seroepidemiological survey is being conducted to determine the community or study-group history of experience with a particular serotype or group (e.g., polioviruses). Otherwise, for initial determination of a current infection in a patient or a locality, virus isolation is far simpler and is recommended.

For any purpose except a serological survey, paired serum specimens are required; the first sample must be taken as early as possible in the course of the illness or infection, the second 3–4 weeks later.

The neutralization test is accurate and type-specific and is at present the test commonly used for most enteroviruses [for polioviruses, the CF test has some advantages (see below)]. Acute and convalescent sera are usually tested simultaneously, using various dilutions of serum against a constant amount of the specific virus. Serum titers are calculated on the basis of the dilution of serum that neutralizes a given amount of virus, and a 4-fold or greater rise in antibody titer is considered significant—indicative of an infection during the period covered. However, it should be noted that neutralizing antibody titers may already be high at the time of onset of clinical symptoms, making interpretation difficult; if neutralizing antibody titers are found to be equally high in both acute and convalescent specimens, the infection might have taken place either recently or many years before, since neutralizing antibody to any of the enteroviruses persists for years if not for life. In addition to the homologous antibody, antibodies against other enterovirus types may appear transiently and at low levels. In poliovirus infections, neutralizing antibody also may be found in the urine.

Other serological tests that may be used include CF, HI, immunofluorescence, and passive hemagglutination.

CF antibodies appear during the course of an infection, but may disappear or drop to a low level within a few months. For most enteroviruses, the CF test has little value because of major heterotypic cross-reactions among the enterovirus antigens and because many persons fail to develop homotypic CF antibody. The test has, however, been used successfully in the diagnosis of poliovirus infections.

N (native) and H (heated) CF antigens of poliovirus are described in Section 4.3. In the course of poliomyelitis infection, H antibodies form before N antibodies, and subsequently the level of H antibodies declines first. Early acute-stage sera thus contain H antibodies only; 1–2 weeks later, both N and H antibodies are present; in late convalescent sera, only N antibodies are present. Only first infection with poliovirus produces strictly type-specific CF responses. Subsequent infections with heterotypic polioviruses recall or induce antibodies, mostly against the heat-stable antigenic components shared by all three types of poliovirus, i.e., against the poliovirus group antigen. Very high CF antibody levels against a poliovirus are strongly suggestive of a recent infection.

After a coxsackievirus infection, patients may develop CF antibodies to a number of both group A and group B agents, and heterotypic echovirus CF antibody responses also are common.

The HI test is relatively easy to perform, and patients who become infected with an enterovirus that hemagglutinates do develop homotypic antibody, which may persist for years. They also may develop heterotypic antibody, making the test somewhat nonspecific. The major drawback to the HI test,

however, is that only about one third of the known enteroviruses agglutinate erythrocytes; even within a single serotype, some strains may hemagglutinate while others do not.

It is possible to detect and titrate serum antibody against enteroviruses by use of an immunofluorescence technique. Infected coverslip cultures for use as a source of antigen may be prepared and kept frozen at −20°C for at least 1 year, making this test readily available for rapid diagnosis.[13,195]

Another test, originally developed to screen for rises in antibody to rhinoviruses,[49] has been found to be effective for detecting rises in antibody titer to enteroviruses. This test, a passive hemagglutination test, relies on the use of a coupling reagent, chromic chloride, to attach proteins to indicator erythrocytes. It has made possible the hemagglutination of red blood cells by antigens that otherwise do not demonstrate this property. Although enteroviruses cross-react in this test and thus specific enterovirus serotypes cannot be distinguished, it can serve for rapid, simple, and useful screening to detect rises in antibody to an enterovirus—i.e., to indicate that an enterovirus infection is present even though the serotype is not known. Such information can be useful, for example, in a community outbreak of illness caused by a single enterovirus serotype that has already been identified. The technique has been utilized as a screening test using paired sera collected during an epidemic of coxsackievirus B5 infections.

4. Biological Characteristics of the Virus That Affect the Epidemiological Pattern

4.1. General Properties

Enteroviruses share the basic properties of Picornaviridae including a genome of single-stranded RNA, small size (diameter 22–30 nm), lack of an envelope (i.e., a "naked" nucleocapsid), and insensitivity to ether and other lipid solvents, indicating lack of essential lipids. The molecular weight of the nucleic acid is 2.3–2.8 million, constituting about 30% of the particle mass. It has been estimated that picornaviruses have 12 genes, in contrast to 400 estimated for the large poxviruses. The virus matures in the cytoplasm. Infective nucleic acid has been extracted from several enteroviruses and rhinoviruses. Because it is freed of the surface protein antigen, such RNA cannot be neutralized by antiserum against the intact virus.

Although cardioviruses can infect humans, the picornaviruses that infect man are almost always enteroviruses or rhinoviruses. These genera differ in a number of properties, but the most useful and reliable feature in distinguishing them is sensitivity to acid: enteroviruses are stable at acid pH (3–5) for 1–3 hr, whereas rhinoviruses are acid-labile. Rhinoviruses multiply chiefly in the nose and throat and can be recovered from these sites, but only rarely from fecal specimens, while enteroviruses, inhabitants of the alimentary tract, may be isolated from the lower intestine or the throat. Enteroviruses grow readily in stationary cultures at 36–37°C, but initial growth of rhinoviruses in primary fetal-cell cultures is favored when cultures are incubated on roller drums at 33°C. Among the enteroviruses that are cytopathogenic [polioviruses, echoviruses, some coxsackieviruses, and the new enterovirus types (68–71)], growth can usually be obtained readily in primary cultures of human and monkey-kidney cells and in certain cell lines (such as HeLa or, for some serotypes, WI-38); in contrast, most rhinoviruses of man can be recovered initially only in cells of human origin (embryonic human kidney, human diploid-cell strains). In cesium chloride, enteroviruses have a density of 1.34 g/ml, whereas rhinoviruses have a density of 1.4 g/ml. Enteroviruses and some rhinoviruses can be stabilized by magnesium chloride against thermal inactivation.

4.2. Reactions to Chemical and Physical Agents

Enteroviruses are resistant to all known antibiotics and chemotherapeutic agents. Laboratory disinfectants, such as 70% alcohol, 5% Lysol, or 1% quaternary ammonium compounds (Roccal), are ineffective. The viruses are insensitive to ether, deoxycholate, and various detergents, which destroy other viruses (e.g., arboviruses, myxoviruses). Treatment with 0.3% formaldehyde, 0.1 N HCl, or free residual chlorine at a level of 0.3–0.5 ppm causes rapid inactivation, but the presence of extraneous organic matter protects the virus from inactivation.[207] Thus, caution must be exercised before carrying over laboratory findings on the chlorination of enteroviruses, often in purified form, to chlorination under natural conditions. Another caution-

ary note has been raised by a recent study[234] showing that after treatment of a dispersed suspension of echovirus type 1 with chlorine, a significant part of the lost infectivity titer (as measured by the plaque method) was regained if the pH of the medium was adjusted to 4.5, inducing aggregation of the virus. Apparently, individual virions were not repaired, but rather there was a multiplicity-related increase in the plaquing efficiency when several damaged virions in a clump were received by the host cell.

Enteroviruses are inhibited from propagating in cell cultures by 2-(α-hydroxybenzyl) benzimidazole (HBB), with the exception of group A coxsackieviruses 7, 11, 13, 16, and 18 and echoviruses 22 and 23.[205] Guanidine is also a potent inhibitor of polioviral (and other enteroviral) synthesis in cell cultures. However, viral progeny grown in the presence of guanidine become resistant to the drug[132] and further passage results in selection of strains that are drug-dependent.[199]

Exposure of these viruses to a temperature of 50°C destroys them rapidly. However, in the presence of molar magnesium chloride, virtually no detectable inactivation occurs in 1 hr at 50°C.[210] Enteroviruses are stable at freezing temperatures for many years and remain viable for weeks at icebox temperatures (4°C) and for days at room temperature. Their inactivation at all temperatures is inhibited by magnesium chloride; this property has led to the widespread use of $MgCl_2$ as a stabilizer of oral poliovirus vaccine.

Enteroviruses are rapidly inactivated by ultraviolet light and usually by drying, unless special conditions are observed. Vital dyes (neutral red, acridine orange, proflavine), when incorporated into the structure of these viruses, render them readily susceptible to visible light.[190,211]

4.3. Antigenic Characteristics

Poliovirus types 1 and 2 share common antigens. Intratypic strain differences are known for all three poliovirus serotypes, and pronounced intratypic variation has been encountered among both coxsackie- and echoviruses. The considerable differences in antigenic structure among strains within each poliovirus serotype have been further emphasized in a study in which intratypic serodifferentiation of polioviruses was performed by neutralization or immunodiffusion tests utilizing strain-specific antisera prepared by cross-adsorption with the heterologous strain.[208] The technique is very useful in distinguishing vaccine and nonvaccine poliovirus strains. Since marked differences could also be demonstrated among wild strains, the technique should also be helpful in epidemiological studies. By the application of this method, the type 1 poliovirus strains isolated from patients and carriers in the 1978 Netherlands poliomyelitis outbreak were compared with various type 1 strains and were found to be similar antigenically to the virulent Mahoney strain and also to wild strains recently isolated in Kuwait and in France. The type 1 strains from an epidemiologically associated outbreak in Canada also resembled the Netherlands isolates.[55]

With some enteroviruses, antigenic variation resulting in the appearance of prime strains is encountered.[120] The prime strain is poorly neutralized by antiserum to the originally characterized (prototype) strain, but it induces the production of antibody that neutralizes the prime strain and the prototype strain equally well. The prime strains, however, share complement-fixing (CF) antigens with their prototypes.

Another problem has been the difficulty of demonstrating neutralization of certain strains arising not from antigenic differences but from aggregation of virus particles, as discussed in Section 3.5.1.

A number of cross-relationships exist between several enteroviruses, for example, coxsackieviruses A3 and A8, A11 and A15, A13 and A18; echoviruses 1 and 8, 12 and 29, 6 and 30; and polioviruses 1 and 2 to a minor degree. The cross-reactions that have been previously observed between echovirus types 1 and 8, chiefly in the serum neutralization test, have been documented in detail recently, along with antigenic diversity of strains within each of these serotypes. Investigation of a number of strains of each type by means of double-diffusion gel precipitation tests now indicates that strains of both types share a common antigen and that, in addition, some strains possess a second antigen relating them more closely to one or the other of the prototype strains.[72] The reaction is not like that of the classic prime relationship, but is similar to antigenic variations described for echoviruses 4 and 9. As indicated in Section 3.5.1, these variations have to be taken into account in identifying field strains through the use of the LBM combination antiserum pools.

For enteroviruses, there has been little documentation of any long-term trends in antigenic alterations of serotypes like those seen with influenza viruses. Such a trend may be suggested, however, by observations that strains of coxsackievirus B5 isolated in 1973 from patients in the United Kingdom are very different antigenically from the prototype B5 virus (Faulkner strain) isolated in 1952. Not only were wide differences observed in immunodiffusion and neutralization tests, but also RNA hybridization procedures showed current human strains to have 100% homology with each other, but only 50% homology with the prototype Faulkner strain,[11] a difference of the same order as that found between different serotypes of poliovirus. In addition, an enterovirus that causes swine vesicular disease has been shown to be closely related antigenically to human coxsackievirus B5.[10,11,62] In RNA hybridization tests, the porcine virus showed about 50% homology with human strains. The serological relationship, together with evidence indicating that the virus has only recently infected swine, has led to the suggestion that the swine virus may have originated rather recently, by transmission of a human B5 strain to the porcine species.[62]

Associated with the RNA genomic changes described above are changes in the polypeptide composition of newer coxsackievirus B5 isolates compared to the 1952 prototype virus. Similarly, such differences exist in the swine viruses of 1966–1971 and those of 1972–1973. In the same year, however, a swine virus from France and a human isolate of coxsackievirus B5 have shown virtually identical patterns.[71] Further work is necessary to establish the pathological and epidemiological significance of these variations.

CF antigens are known for each of the three poliovirus serotypes. They may be prepared from tissue culture or infected CNS. Inactivation of the virus by formalin, heat, or ultraviolet light liberates a soluble CF antigen. This antigen is cross-reactive and fixes complement with heterotypic poliomyelitis antibodies. A type-specific precipitin reaction occurs when virus in sufficient concentration is used with immune animal or convalescent human sera. Two type-specific antigens are contained in poliovirus preparations and can be detected by precipitin and CF tests. They are called D (or N) and C (or H). The D antigen occurs as a band in the more dense regions of a sucrose density gradient and comprises most of the virus infectivity. The upper band containing the C antigen has little infectivity. The virus in the D zone appears intact in electron micrographs and contains 20–25% RNA, whereas that in the C zone is damaged and contains little or no RNA. There is a direct relationship between the amount of D antigen, measured by CF, and the number of intact physical particles of poliovirus as counted by electron microscopy. The two antigens are also known as N (native) and H (heated). Heat changes N (or D) preparations from complete virus particles to empty particles when viewed in the electron microscope.

Several coxsackieviruses and echoviruses agglutinate human type O erythrocytes. The hemagglutinins are associated with the infectious viral particles: both are sedimented together by ultracentrifugation and are also adsorbed together by red cells during hemagglutination. About one third of the known enteroviruses have this property, and antibodies against the virus can be measured by hemagglutination inhibition.[61,178]

4.4. Host Range *in Vivo* and *in Vitro*

The host range of the enteroviruses varies greatly from one type to the next and even among strains of the same type. They may be readily induced, by laboratory manipulation, to yield variants that have host ranges and tissue tropisms different from those of certain wild strains; this has led to the development of attenuated polio vaccine strains.

Polioviruses have a very restricted host range among laboratory animals. Most strains will infect only monkeys and chimpanzees. Infection is initiated most readily by direct inoculation into the brain or spinal cord. Chimpanzees and cynomolgus monkeys can also be infected by the oral route; in chimpanzees, the infection thus produced is usually asymptomatic. The animals become intestinal carriers of the virus; they also develop a viremia that is quenched by the appearance of antibodies in the circulating blood. Unusual strains have been transmitted to mice or chick embryos.

Most strains can be grown in primary or continuous cell-line cultures derived from a variety of human tissues or from monkey kidney, testis, or muscle.

Coxsackieviruses are highly infective for newborn mice. Certain strains (B1–B6, A7, A9, A16) also grow in monkey-kidney-cell culture. Some group A strains grow in human amnion cells, HeLa cells, or the RD cell line.[115,193] Coxsackieviruses A1, A19, and A22 have not yet been grown successfully in any cultures and must be cultivated in newborn mice. Chimpanzees and cynomolgus monkeys can be infected subclinically; virus appears in the blood and throat for short periods and is excreted in the feces for 2–5 weeks. Type A14 produces poliomyelitis-like lesions in adult mice and in monkeys, but in suckling mice, this type produces only myositis. Type A7 strains produce paralysis and severe CNS lesions in monkeys.[41,209]

Group A viruses produce widespread myositis in the skeletal muscles of newborn mice, resulting in flaccid paralysis without other observable lesions. Group B viruses can produce a myositis that is more focal in distribution than that produced by viruses of group A, but they also give rise to a necrotizing steatitis involving principally the maturing fetal fat lobules (e.g., interscapular pads, cervical and cephalic pads). Encephalitis is found at times; the animals die with paralysis of the spastic type. Some B strains also produce pancreatitis, myocarditis, endocarditis, and hepatitis in both suckling and adult mice. The corticosteroids may enhance the susceptibility of older mice to infection of the pancreas. Normal adult mice tolerate infections with group B coxsackieviruses, but in mice subjected to sustained postweaning undernutrition (marasmus), B3 virus produces severe disease, including persistence of infective virus in the heart, spleen, liver, and pancreas. Lymphoid tissues are markedly atrophic in marasmic animals. Transfer of lymphoid cells from normal mice immunized against the virus provides virus-infected marasmic mice with significant protection against the severe sequelae. These observations support the hypothesis that lymphocyte-mediated defense mechanisms may play an important role in normal recovery from primary viral infections.

To be included in the echovirus group, prototype strains must fail to produce disease in suckling mice, in rabbits, or in monkeys. However, different strains can produce variants that exhibit animal pathogenicity. A number of the echoviruses have produced inapparent infections in monkeys, with mild lesions in the CNS.[215] In the chimpanzee, no apparent illness is produced, but infection can be demonstrated by the presence and persistence of virus in the throat and in the feces and by type-specific antibody responses.[81]

Most of the common echoviruses can be isolated in primary monkey-kidney-cell cultures, but strains of a number of the echovirus serotypes grow more readily in human cell cultures (see Section 3.5).

Initially, echoviruses were distinguished from coxsackieviruses by their failure to produce pathological changes in newborn mice, but echovirus 9 can produce paralysis in newborn mice. Conversely, strains of some coxsackievirus types (especially A9) lack mouse pathogenicity and thus resemble echoviruses. This variability in biological properties is the chief reason that new enteroviruses are no longer being subclassified as echo- or coxsackieviruses.

There are four new enteroviruses, types 68–71, all of which grow in monkey-kidney-cell cultures. Three of these are known to cause human disease (types 68, 70, and 71). Enteroviruses 70 and 71 were isolated in human cell cultures and subsequently adapted to monkey-kidney cultures (see Table 8 and Section 8.1 for details). Some strains of enterovirus 70 are adaptable to cultivation in the L strain of murine cells.[201] Some strains of enterovirus 71 grow better in suckling mice than in cultured primate cells.

The growth of enteroviruses in monolayers of cultured cells is generally associated with a characteristic cytopathic effect.[175] Infected cells round up, show shrinkage and marked nuclear pyknosis, become refractile, and eventually degenerate and fall off the glass surface. In cell cultures covered by fluid nutrient medium, virus may spread via the fluid bathing the cells. Under agar overlay, which confines the spread of virus to a cell-to-adjoining-cell route, plaques of degenerating cells are formed by various members of the enterovirus group in cultures of susceptible cells. Methods that utilize plaque formation have provided very precise quantification of infective virus, required for many laboratory research studies of enteroviruses.[78]

The factors underlying cell susceptibility to enteroviruses are basic to understanding host susceptibility to infection. Human cells possess a receptor for poliovirus and can therefore be infected and killed by the virus. Rodent cells do not possess the receptor and cannot be infected by polioviruses unless the viruses have been altered by laboratory cultivation. But in human–rodent hybrid cells, possession of a human gene for the poliovirus receptor was found to be sufficient to enable the virus nucleic acid to enter the cell, and once this first step had been taken, the virus then multiplied without the mediation of any further human gene products, the rodent genetic apparatus being sufficient for its needs. The human chromosome carrying the gene concerned with poliovirus reception was identified by making use of human–rodent hybrid cells that differ in their complement of human chromosomes. In these studies, it was found that some of the human chromosomes were shed after hybridization. Only when chromosome 19 was lost did the cells lose their susceptibility to poliovirus.[148] This implies that chromosome 19 carries all the information necessary for acceptance of poliovirus by a human cell and suggests that only a single gene codes for the receptor protein.

4.5. Replication of Enteroviruses

The replication of poliovirus provides useful insights into its transmission, its *in vivo* and *in vitro* host range, and its relatedness to other enteroviruses. The essential theme of viral replication is that specific messenger RNA (mRNA) must be transcribed from the viral nucleic acid for successful expression and duplication of genetic information. Once this is accomplished, viruses use cell components to translate the mRNA. In the replication of poliovirus, all steps are independent of host DNA and occur in the cell cytoplasm.

Polioviruses adsorb to cells at specific cell receptor sites. This is evidenced by the fact that intact poliovirus infects only primate cells in culture, whereas the isolated RNA will also infect nonprimate cells (rabbit, guinea pig, chick) and complete one cycle of multiplication. Multiple cycles of infection are not observed in nonprimate cells because the resulting progeny possess protein coats and will again infect only primate cells. After attachment, the virus particles are taken into the cell, and the viral RNA is uncoated. The single-stranded genomic RNA can then serve as its own messenger RNA (mRNA). This mRNA is translated, resulting in the formation of an enzyme, RNA polymerase, that is necessary for the formation of a replicative intermediate and then a replicative form—which is a double-stranded molecule consisting of the positive parental RNA strand and a complementary negative strand—and also for the formation of inhibitors that turn off the synthesis of cellular RNA and protein. The number and nature of these inhibitors are not known. Single-stranded viral RNA molecules, positive strands, are then synthesized from the replicative form. The newly synthesized positive-strand RNA molecules perform any of the three following functions: (1) serve as mRNA for synthesis of structural proteins; (2) serve as template for continued RNA replication; or (3) become encapsidated, resulting in mature progeny virions. The synthesis of viral capsid proteins is initiated at about the same time as RNA synthesis.

The entire poliovirus genome acts as its own mRNA and is translated to form a single large polypeptide that is subsequently cleaved to produce the various viral capsid polypeptides. Thus, the poliovirus genome serves as a polycistronic messenger molecule. Completion of encapsidation produces mature virus particles that are then released when the cell undergoes lysis.

Despite the relatively limited information on which the establishment of the enterovirus group was originally based and its subgroups were defined, the validity of these groupings has been borne out by recent studies utilizing sophisticated techniques of modern molecular virology. Comparison of the genomes of representative polioviruses, coxsackieviruses of subgroups A and B, and echoviruses by RNA hybridization has shown at least 5% of the genome to be shared by all enteroviruses tested.[233] In these recent studies, the polynucleotide sequence relationships were consistent with the biological classification of enteroviruses into subgroups (polioviruses, coxsackieviruses A and B, and echoviruses). In general, 30–50% of the nucleotide sequences were shared by different serotypes tested within each subgroup, whereas among the different groups, there was less than 20% homology. However, the coxsackievirus B studied (B4) appeared to be more closely related to echoviruses than to group A coxsackieviruses, while polioviruses were related only distantly to any of the other enteroviruses tested.

Other investigations into the mechanisms and the intermediate products of replication of enteroviruses and of other picornaviruses have been conducted. On the basis of some of these data, the picornavirus family has been divided into four major subgroups: (1) the enteroviruses, (2) the rhinoviruses, (3) the cardioviruses [encephalomyocarditis

(EMC)], and (4) foot-and-mouth disease viruses (now named aphthoviruses) of cattle. Several laboratories have been involved in identifying the virus-specific polypeptides of poliovirus and other picornaviruses and the posttranslational mechanisms by which they are produced. Several lines of evidence suggest that the picornaviral RNA possesses a single initiation site and that, once initiated, each ribosome completes translation of the entire viral RNA. This property has facilitated the genetic mapping of these viruses.[16,89a]

The genetic map has been determined wholly or in part for EMC virus, rhinovirus, and poliovirus, and recently a comparative study was conducted with these three viruses in terms of the genetic map of each, the molecular weights of the different viral polypeptides, and the rates of cleavage of several analogous polypeptides.[16,33] Previous work has shown that there are three main families of EMC-virus-specific polypeptides. Translation of the EMC viral ribonucleic acid generates at least three primary products, termed polypeptides A, F, and C. Polypeptide A undergoes successive cleavages to produce the four major capsid polypeptides. Polypeptide F is stable, and polypeptide C cleaves to form polypeptide D, which in turn cleaves to form polypeptide E. Comparison of EMC virus with rhinovirus and poliovirus indicates that evolutionary pressures on these different members of the picornavirus family have resulted in extensive differences in antigenicity of the virions; furthermore, each profile had polypeptides that were unique to that particular virus, and analogous cleavages proceeded at considerably different rates for the different viruses studied. But as judged by the results of this study, many common features have been retained in the evolution of these viruses, including the general mechanism of synthesis and the size and genetic order of the three principal families of polypeptides.

Double neutralization of virus particles obtained from mixed infections has been observed. Usually—and particularly for antigenically distinct virus types such as influenza viruses A and B or polioviruses types 1 and 2—the doubly antigenic virus proved to be unstable on passage, suggesting that the phenomenon could be explained by phenotypic mixing. Phenotypic mixing has also been found to occur between an echovirus and a coxsackievirus.[82] Virus particles containing antigens of both viruses were obtained that on passage segregated into parental types. The phenotypically mixed particles may be regarded as having an additional surface antigen heterologous to the genetic core or mosaic surface antigens composed of the two parental types. A single particle with two distinct genetic cores (one of each virus) and mixed antigenic coats would also be expected to behave like a phenotypic mixture, i.e., to be doubly neutralizable but on passage breed the pure parental types. Recently, the protein of a plant virus (cowpea chlorotic mottle virus) has been shown to be able to encapsidate *in vitro* the genome of poliovirus, to form a particle known as a pseudovirion. When assayed in the presence of DEAE–dextran to facilitate entrance into susceptible human cells in cultures, the polio pseudovirions were about 50 times more infectious than poliovirus RNA itself. This suggests that the encapsidation of the polio genome in a foreign coat protected the RNA from destruction by cellular nucleases.

In the course of work that led to the control of poliomyelitis through vaccination, a great deal was learned about the molecular biology of the virus. Although this knowledge did not contribute directly to the vaccine's success, it turned poliovirus into a useful model for studies in molecular biology. Even if wild polioviruses were completely eradicated, and polio vaccines were 100% effective, polioviruses would continue to be agents of great interest and usefulness to virologists. Because they have been so fully studied and because they are small and relatively simple viruses, they have served and will continue to serve as models for understanding the nature of viruses and their structure, function, replication, and genetics.[33,34] Translation of virus-specific mRNA has been reported under conditions where host-cell translation is stopped. Cell-free protein-synthesizing systems that initiate on endogenous mRNA have been developed from uninfected and poliovirus-infected human cells. Poliovirus double-stranded (replicative) RNA was found to be an inhibitor of protein synthesis in these extracts, both of cell-directed and of virus-specific protein synthesis.[19]

Polioviruses are included among the agents that during their replication produce deletion mutants called "defective interfering" particles that interfere with the growth of the normal virus from which they are derived. Defective interfering particles have potential clinical significance, since they may play a role in limiting acute viral infections; furthermore,

they are present in high concentrations in oral polio vaccines, suggesting the possibility that their presence may be a factor in attenuation.[28]

5. Descriptive Epidemiology

5.1. General Epidemiology of Enteroviruses

5.1.1. Incidence and Prevalence. The epidemiological markers of the *diseases* associated with the enteroviruses are based on the occurrence of a clinical syndrome sufficiently characteristic to be recognized, such as paralysis of poliomyelitis or the lesions of the hand, foot, and mouth syndrome of echovirus 16, or on the occurrence of an outbreak of aseptic meningitis or of an exanthem in which the causative enterovirus has been isolated. The epidemiological markers of the presence in the community of *infection* due to enteroviruses include the prevalence of the virus in the stools of healthy persons or in the sewage from the area and the prevalence of antibody as determined by serological surveys.

In considering enterovirus epidemiology, it is important to reemphasize that by far the most common form of infection with any of these viruses is a mild or silent episode and that severe manifestations are rare. Paralytic poliomyelitis remained an epidemiological enigma until this concept was developed.[18,217] It must also be kept in mind that clinical features presented by infections with the different serotypes may be similar and that manifestations of infections with the same serotype may vary widely.

The pattern of incidence and prevalence, the age at the time of infection, and the nature of the host response are the consequences of a number of interdependent variables the common denominator of which is probably the opportunity for exposure, along with the hygienic level under which such exposure occurs. These interdependent variables include geographic area, climate, and socioeconomic setting.

5.1.2. Epidemic and Endemic Behavior. In the prevaccine era, epidemics of poliomyelitis occurred with great frequency in the economically advanced countries of the world. In the United States, the first sizable outbreak was recognized in Vermont in 1894 and involved 132 cases; it was by far the largest number of cases ever reported in any one year anywhere in the world up to that time. In the first half of the 20th century, recurrent outbreaks involved the "developed countries" of the world, such as the United States, Canada, Australia, and European and Scandinavian countries.

Great reductions in epidemic incidence occurred after the introduction of poliovaccine in 1955. In the period 1951–1955, an average of almost 38,000 cases of poliomyelitis (approximately 21,000 paralytic) were reported annually in the United States; from 1961 to 1965, the annual average was 570 cases (460 paralytic). After live attenuated vaccines were widely administered in the United States during 1962–1963, even further reductions took place (see Section 5.2.3). Similar reductions from 1951–1955 to 1961–1965 followed vaccination in other countries: in the United Kingdom, from 4381 to 322; in Australia, from 2187 to 154; in Denmark, from 1614 to 77; in Sweden, from 1526 to 28; and in Czechoslovakia, from 1081 to 0. In these areas, the numbers of cases have continued to fall. During 1971–1975, only 15 cases occurred in the United States, 8 cases in the United Kingdom, 2 in Australia, and none in Denmark or Czechoslovakia.[63,223,225]

Outbreaks of infection with coxsackieviruses and echoviruses have occurred frequently in a wide variety of places and years and continue to do so. Among the enterovirus isolations reported through the WHO virus reporting system during the 8-year period 1967–1974,[65] the most frequently reported types were, for coxsackieviruses of group A, types 9 and 16; for members of group B, types 3 and 5; and for echoviruses, types 6, 9, 11, and 30. A large number of strains of both coxsackieviruses and echoviruses have been involved in epidemics; enteroviruses 70 and 71 have also been responsible for epidemics in various parts of the world. These outbreaks have been mostly localized to one area, although one epidemic of echovirus 9 infections in the late 1950s had almost worldwide distribution, and enterovirus 70 spread explosively in Asia and Africa during 1969–1973. In 1981, epidemics reappeared in Asia and Africa, and also spread to the Western Hemisphere.

In the United Kingdom, during the first 34 weeks of 1978, 449 echovirus type 11 infections were diagnosed—more than the annual totals reported in any of the previous 8 years. Most infections were reported in infants and children and slightly more cases in males than females. In 51% of the cases,

the nervous system was affected (mainly aseptic meningitis), 33% of the patients had fever or respiratory symptoms, and 10% had gastrointestinal disorders. There were 13 patients with Bornholm disease (epidemic pleurodynia). Ten fatal cases were reported, all in children under 5 years of age, including five neonates.

During 1969–1971, a pandemic of acute hemorrhagic conjunctivitis (AHC) occurred in Africa, Southeast Asia (including Singapore), Japan, and India, involving tens of millions of people. The cause of this widespread disease was recognized as a new enterovirus[94,229] and was designated enterovirus type 70.[145,149] The disease, generally localized to the eye, is characterized by subconjunctival hemorrhage. The eye disease has a short incubation period and sudden onset, and recovery is generally complete within 10 days. Rarely, neurological complications, in the form of a poliolike motor paralysis, may develop some time after the episode of eye disease—up to several weeks later[92,93] (see Section 8.1.7). Enterovirus 70 is highly contagious, spreading rapidly under crowded and unhygienic conditions; warm, humid coastal climates seem particularly favorable to its transmission. Intrafamilial spread is common. Some localized outbreaks, especially in developed countries, have centered around eye clinics. AHC seems to have appeared in man first during 1969, in Ghana,[24] and soon thereafter in other African countries. An Asian focus in Java was observed as early as mid-1970. Large epidemics occurred during 1971 in Japan,[94] Singapore,[229] and Morocco.[155] Small outbreaks were seen in Europe beginning in 1971, and later reported European outbreaks were in 1973 in Yugoslavia and in France.[91] Serological surveys in Japan, Ghana, and Indonesia confirmed that the virus was not prevalent before the pandemic and that after the outbreaks antibodies appeared in the populations involved.[95] Multiple epidemics have occurred within a 5-year period in the same regions, particularly in Southeast Asia, suggesting that immunity may be short-lived. Until 1981, Australia and the Americas had been free of the disease. In more than 1000 sera collected in 1971–1974 from residents of the United States, only 3 had antibodies to the virus.[74]

A new enterovirus was recovered from the stool of a patient with CNS disease in a 1969–1970 outbreak in California during which an identical strain was recovered from the brain of a patient with fatal encephalitis.[196] The new agent was designated as enterovirus 71.[145] In the years following 1970, this newly recognized virus has moved about the world and has been associated with different clinical manifestations in different regions: a 1972 outbreak in Australia in which aseptic meningitis predominated[88] and 1973 outbreaks in Japan (hand, foot, and mouth disease with some aseptic meningitis cases, and some patients with both syndromes)[68,150a] and in Sweden (aseptic meningitis with some hand, foot, and mouth disease cases also).[7] A very severe epidemic occurred in Bulgaria in 1975, with 700 cases including numerous polioencephalitis cases as well as meningitis[144]; about 21% of the 700 patients developed paralysis, and there were 44 fatalities. In the summer of 1978, a large outbreak with some 1000 cases occurred in Hungary; clinical manifestations were predominantly aseptic meningitis, but there were some cases of encephalitis and some fatalities (see Section 8.1). In 65 cases from the Bulgarian outbreak, 92 virus strains of the same serological type were isolated from CNS, from mesenteric lymph nodes and tonsils, and from feces.[144]

With most nonpolio enteroviruses, the pattern of infection for a specific serotype in a particular locality resembles that of poliomyelitis: (1) There may be local serotypes that are endemic, constantly circulating among the few nonimmunes; these are mostly very young children, since virtually all the older children and adults already have protective antibody from previous infections. (2) Or specific serotypes may be completely absent from a particular locality or very limited in dissemination for a number of years (see examples below); a population of susceptibles then builds up, and a wave of wide and rapid spread of the virus may occur, reaching a large proportion of all age groups. Dissemination of different serotypes may thus occur in waves, with one predominant type in an area succeeding another from one year to the next or even within the same summer–fall season.

An example of waves of infection with different enterovirus serotypes can be seen in data from the United Kingdom and the Republic of Ireland during 1960–1969. A number of echovirus types were isolated sporadically and in relatively small numbers.[225] In 1968, continuing into 1969, there was an epidemic of type 6 infections, and type 6 was by far the one most frequently recovered during 1968 (about 40%

of all echovirus isolates reported); in 1969, echovirus type 9 also became epidemic, accounting for about 40% of the echovirus isolates in that year. In the latter epidemic, one fourth to one third of all the cases occurred in Scotland. In 1971, however, about 60% of the echovirus isolates in the United Kingdom were echovirus type 4, which in previous years had been responsible for only about 5% of the echovirus reports. These infections were confined mainly to northern and northwestern regions of England and to Scotland and Ireland. Significantly, in view of the limited previous circulation of echovirus 4, a large share of the isolations were from older children and young adults. It should be noted that the infections selected for laboratory investigation may be biased toward significant illnesses; it seems probable that the younger children were also experiencing widespread infection but that overt illness more frequently brought the older groups to clinical attention. In 1971, echovirus 6 accounted for only 3% of all United Kingdom isolates; echovirus 9 accounted for 2%.

During this period, coxsackievirus A9 was almost always the serotype most frequently reported in the United Kingdom, constituting 35–55% of the group A isolates. Coxsackievirus A16 was frequently reported in most years, but tended toward epidemic prevalence every 3 years: peaks of dissemination were recorded in 1964, 1967, 1970, and again in 1973. In 1970, about 57% of the coxsackie A isolates were of the A16 type. Coxsackieviruses B2, B3, B4, and B5 also appeared to be somewhat cyclical in the United Kingdom, in periods of 3–6 years; B1 did not share this periodicity and usually was isolated in lower numbers, although an epidemic due to this virus occurred in 1970; type B6 was rarely reported. Periodicity in enterovirus infections in a particular region can be clearly seen in the data on virus isolations at the Regional Virus Laboratory, Ruchill Hospital, Glasgow, covering a 20-year period, 1957–1976 (Table 2).[65] Although the Glasgow laboratory may isolate 25 or more different enterovirus serotypes in any one year, certain types clearly tend to recur at quite regular intervals. For example, echovirus 9 tended to recur at 4-year intervals, whereas echoviruses 4 and 30 were absent for 7–9 years between outbreaks. As indicated above, the serotypes (echoviruses 4 and 30, in this case) recurring at the longer time intervals and in large epidemics are those for which higher proportions of

Table 2. Infections by Selected Enteroviruses in the Glasgow Area during 20 Years[a,b]

Virus	Year																			
	1957	1958	1959	1960	1961	1962	1963	1964	1965	1966	1967	1968	1969	1970	1971	1972	1973	1974	1975	1976
Coxsackie A7	0	0	0	0	0	0	15	0	0	0	9	1	6	0	0	0	1	0	0	0
Coxsackie B5	2	1	8	5	10	0	0	4	37	0	0	0	2	0	10	2	0	2	1	8
Echo 4	0	0	0	0	0	0	42	12	0	0	0	0	0	0	73	37	0	0	0	0
Echo 6	1	0	3	1	2	22	1	2	9	1	16	34	14	0	1	0	1	8	6	0
Echo 9	3	0	0	119	2	0	0	44	2	0	0	9	38	1	5	0	49	4	0	1
Echo 17	0	0	0	0	0	0	0	0	0	0	1	0	2	23	0	0	0	0	0	0
Echo 19	0	0	0	0	5	0	0	0	0	3	15	20	0	0	4	1	0	9	10	10
Echo 30	0	0	74	6	0	0	0	1	2	92	0	0	0	1	0	1	0	0	19	9

[a] From Grist et al.[(65)] Used with permission.
[b] Figures represent infections detected by virus isolation at the Regional Virus Laboratory, Ruchill Hospital, Glasgow.

infections have been reported in older children and in adults. That is, in the absence of early childhood exposure, many persons remained susceptible into these older age groups during the longer interval. These parallel age–incidence data can be seen in world-wide virus-isolation data for 1967–1974, collected and collated by the WHO (Table 3).[65]

An example of very rapid succession of different enterovirus serotypes in a small community has been well documented.[157,230] In the course of 1968–1971, six outbreaks of febrile viral disease with respiratory and gastrointestinal symptoms occurred in an Israeli kibbutz of about 450 members and were differentiated by correlated clinical, epidemiological, and laboratory study. In a single summer, there was an extensive outbreak of febrile illnessess, characterized by respiratory and abdominal symptoms, which began in May 1970 and continued without interruption until the beginning of August. During this period, 21 children were ill on two occasions and 6 were sick three times, with some of the episodes giving the clinical impression of relapses in a disease caused by a single agent. However, these illnesses were found to be due to successive and overlapping large outbreaks of coxsackievirus B4 and echovirus 9 infections, in which 43 persons were shown to have been infected by both viruses in sequence, at intervals of 3–4 weeks. Echovirus 16 was also found to be involved in a small number of the early illnesses.

5.1.3. Geographic Distribution and Climate. Enteroviruses are found in all parts of the world. In tropical and semitropical regions, they are widely distributed throughout the year. In temperate climates, they are present at low levels in winter and spring, but are encountered far more commonly during summer and fall. Some outbreaks of enteroviral infection have continued from fall into winter months; winter outbreaks have been recorded, but they are rare.

Climate appears to be an important factor in the circulation and prevalence of enteroviruses. Even within the climate range represented in the continental United States, healthy children in southern cities harbor a greater abundance of enteroviruses and a wider variety of antigenic types than do those of comparable age in northern cities. Repeated tests on the stools of 136 healthy preschool children in Charleston, West Virginia, over a period of 29 months indicated that 90% of the cytopathogenic

enteroviruses were recovered during the summer and the autumn months and that the incidence was 3–6 times higher in the lower socioeconomic than in the middle to upper middle class districts; 52% of the viruses recovered belonged to the echovirus group[120] (see Table 6). In areas farther south, such as Phoenix, Arizona,[120] and Louisiana,[58] the prevalence of enteroviruses among healthy children was more evenly distributed throughout the year but still markedly higher during the months of May to October. Subsequent studies on enterovirus excretion rates in young children in Seattle, San Francisco, Minneapolis, Buffalo, Atlanta, and Miami[54,59] have confirmed and extended the earlier results: higher levels of endemicity and longer periods of prevalence were found in the southern cities.

Among the Atlanta and Miami children studied in 1960–1963 and in the earlier investigations in Charleston and Phoenix,[120] average annual virus excretion rates were 7–14%, and far larger numbers of enterovirus serotypes were commonly prevalent than in northern cities. In the normal population under study in the New York Virus Watch Program,[90] only four to six serotypes of cytopathogenic enteroviruses were prevalent at any given period, and the enterovirus isolation rate in fecal specimens from young children (0–5 years of age) was only 2.4%.

Among children living in warm climates and poor hygienic conditions, the incidence of infection with one or more enterovirus serotypes may exceed 50%, and mixed infections are common. In a study of infants in Karachi, Pakistan–almost all of whom were less than 2 years of age–approximately 80% of those tested yielded at least one enterovirus.[166] Additional virus serotypes were recovered by mixing a portion of the original swab specimen with type-specific antiserum to block the virus type or types previously isolated from the swab and then inoculating the mixture into tissue cultures. If an isolate was obtained, it was first confirmed as a new type by retesting against antiserum to the previously recovered type or types; if confirmed as new, the serotype was then identified. Of 116 rectal-swab specimens restudied for multiple virus isolation, approximately 45% were positive for at least two different viruses, 14% for three viruses, and each of two infants had four different viruses in a single swab specimen.[166] Mixed infections may also occur in children living under good socioeconomic circum-

Table 3. Number of Reports of Echovirus Infections by Age (WHO Data 1967–1974)[a]

Age (yr)	Echovirus type																				Total	
	1	3	4	5	6	7	9	11	12	13	14	16	17	18	19	20	21	22	25	30	n	%
<1	132	148	156	66	390	300	505	648	112	68	304	58	63	147	169	46	50	353	72	119	3906	16.9
1–4	132	290	182	87	978	671	1146	937	96	124	348	74	124	193	204	130	89	186	163	391	6545	28.4
5–14	65	208	660	84	1451	326	1804	727	57	43	203	46	146	251	311	57	78	27	99	1170	7813	33.9
All children	329	646	998	237	2819	1297	3455	2312	265	235	855	178	333	591	684	233	217	566	334	1680	18264	79.3
15–24	23	33	277	20	415	68	472	185	12	11	46	11	35	105	110	18	25	3	27	345	2241	9.7
25–59	30	49	235	28	367	90	580	247	16	22	42	24	30	111	158	16	20	10	28	295	2398	10.4
≥60	2	3	7	1	30	7	24	21	4	0	3	0	2	3	3	3	1	2	3	6	125	0.5
All adults	55	85	519	49	812	165	1076	453	32	33	91	35	67	219	271	37	46	15	58	646	4764	20.7
TOTALS:	384	731	1517	286	3631	1462	4531	2765	297	268	946	213	400	810	955	270	263	581	392	2326	23028	100.0

[a] From Grist et al.[65] Used with permission.

stances in temperate areas,[32] but they are less frequent.

In some isolated groups, such as certain Eskimo communities,[2] the whole population may lack antibodies to some serotypes (see Fig. 1). In the survey depicted, not even the oldest persons, up to 72 years of age, had any serological evidence of past infection with either coxsackievirus B1 or coxsackievirus B2; coxsackievirus A1 apparently had been present some years previously, and coxsackieviruses A4 and A10 were currently present or had been in the very recent past.

On the other hand, a study conducted in the Accra area of Ghana, at a time before polio vaccination was introduced in that country to any significant extent, indicated that infants and young children were experiencing widespread infections with all three types of polioviruses,[164] a pattern typical for a dense population living under poor hygienic conditions. Even among children less than

3 years old, 77% had antibody to poliovirus type 1 and only slightly lower proportions to type 2 and to type 3; 80% were immune to all three types by the age of 6 years. In the same children, coxsackievirus A9 antibody developed at almost the same rate as poliovirus, antibodies, and 79% infected by 3 years of age, and 94% by the age of 6. Coxsackievirus B3, however, was less widespread, infecting only 52% of the children by 4–6 years of age.

The beginnings of a global picture of nonpolio enterovirus prevalence were drawn by Assaad and Cockburn,[1] who analyzed the reports received by WHO for the 4-year period 1967–1970 from laboratories around the world that participate in the WHO reporting system. This analysis was extended to cover 8 years, 1967–1974, by Grist et al.[65] Because few tropical countries had yet joined the reporting scheme, chiefly temperate regions were represented in these reports. The reports used for the 8-year analysis included about 5200 coxsackievirus A iso-

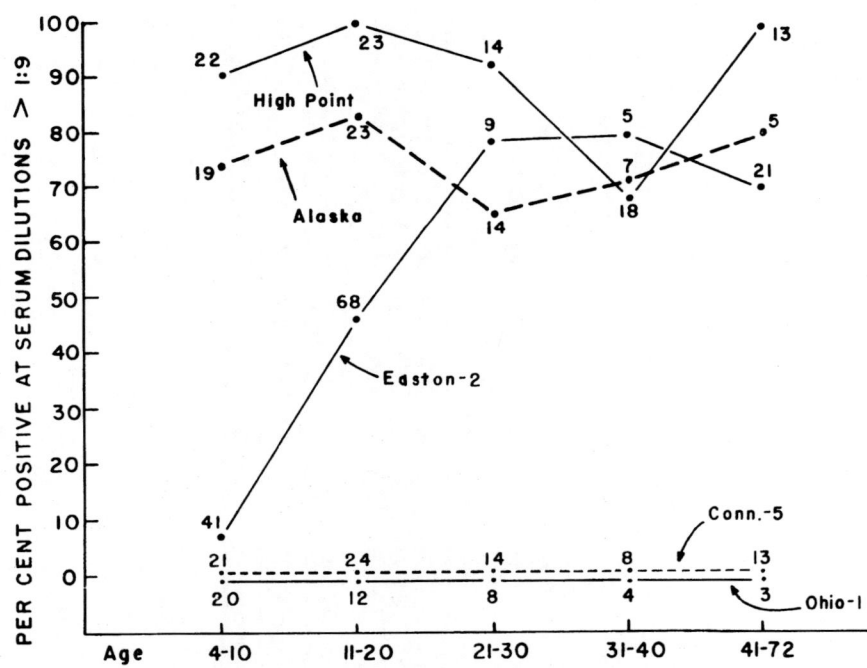

Fig. 1. Results of neutralization tests with local Eskimo sera and coxsackieviruses expressed in terms of percentages of sera positive against five coxsackievirus strains. The serotypes represented are High Point (coxsackievirus A4), Alaska (coxsackievirus A10), Easton-2 (coxsackievirus A1), Conn.-5 (coxsackievirus B1), and Ohio-1 (coxsackievirus B2). The numerals at each point show the number of sera tested in the indicated age group. From Banker and Melnick.[2]

lates, more than 13,000 coxsackievirus B, and more than 23,000 echoviruses.

These investigators were able to draw comparisons concerning infections by these agents despite the limitations implicit in the nature of the reports—particularly the underrepresentation of coxsackievirus A isolates, since relatively few laboratories now include mice in their isolation systems.

Most of the infections reported to WHO in 1967–1974[65] were in children under 15 years of age: 85% of the coxsackievirus A isolates came from this age group, 79% of the coxsackieviruses B, and 79% of the echoviruses. These overall percentages were virtually identical in both the 4-year periods, the total 8-year data changing by only 1 or 2 percentage points from those reported for 1967–1970.

With all the coxsackieviruses (both A and B groups) that were isolated in sufficient numbers for inclusion in the 8-year tabulation, and with most of the echovirus serotypes also, the number of isolates from younger children (0–4 years) was greater than that for the 5- to 14-yr-old group and constituted 62% of all the coxsackievirus A isolations reported, 54% of the coxsackievirus B, and 45% of the echovirus isolations. However, with echovirus types 4, 6, 9, and 30, the younger children accounted for a smaller share of the infections, while the 5- to 14-year-old group had 44, 40, 40, and 50%, respectively, of the isolations of these types, and the adults, 34, 22, 24, and 28% (see Table 3). Adults and older children also had a significant share of the coxsackievirus B infections reported (types 1–5).

Among the five group B coxsackieviruses under study, B3 and B5 were the most frequently isolated.

No regular yearly pattern, worldwide, was observed in the recurrence of specific types. With each serotype analyzed, the number of reported isolations fluctuated greatly from year to year, and even larger fluctuations were observed for individual countries, e.g., of 154 coxsackievirus A9 infections reported by Japan during the period 1967–1970, all but 8 were concentrated in 1967.

In this worldwide survey, which tended to focus on virus isolations from sick persons, the clinical manifestations usually included aseptic meningitis, respiratory disease, skin eruptions, undifferentiated febrile illnesses, or gastroenteritis. In the combined reports for the 8-year period 1967–1974, disease of the CNS—commonly aseptic meningitis—was associated with 28% of the coxsackievirus A infections (and with nearly 50% of those identified as A9 infections), with 34% of the coxsackievirus B infections (42% of those identified as infections with B5), and with 56% of the echovirus infections (with much higher percentages of the infections with types 4, 6, 9, and 30: 81, 63, 68, and 83%, respectively). The previously recognized associations of specific syndromes to specific serotypes were also observed, e.g., Bornholm disease (pleurodynia) and myocarditis associated with coxsackieviruses B—particularly in persons over 15 years of age. Although cardiac involvement was more frequently associated with coxsackieviruses B as a group, representing 3.2% of the coxsackievirus B isolations reported, a few cases of cardiac illness were reported with all the coxsackievirus A types tabulated by Grist et al.[65] and with most echovirus types, including 3% of the isolates of echovirus 22. Skin eruptions were the most frequent disease associations of coxsackievirus A isolates (especially hand, foot, and mouth disease, seen mainly in children under 5 years of age); 33% of the coxsackievirus A group infections generally, but 82% of A16 infections, 44% of A5, and 41% of A10 infections were associated with disease of the skin or mucosa or both. Respiratory illnesses accounted for about 20% of the coxsackievirus B isolations, but only about 12% of the coxsackievirus A and the echovirus infections; however, with echoviruses 1, 11, 13, and 22, about 25% of the isolations were associated with respiratory disease. There were also small numbers of cases of paralytic CNS disease reported in association with many of the types of each group.

Irrespective of virus type, the largest number of cases of CNS disease was in children under 15 years of age, although substantial numbers of adults also had neurological involvement. The largest number of cases of respiratory illness was in children under 5 years of age.

5.1.4. Age and Sex. Children are the prime targets of these viruses and thus serve as the chief vehicle for their spread. In warmer lands and in families living under unsanitary and poor socioeconomic conditions in temperate zones, children are infected very early in life, and more than 90% may have already experienced infections with a number of the locally prevalent enteroviruses before the age of 5 years. In such settings, paralytic poliomyelitis is rarely recognized and epidemics generally do not occur. When infection is delayed to older childhood and young adult life, the incidence of paralytic poliomyelitis rises, as does the frequency of the more severe manifestations of the other enterovirus infections.

The pattern of age distribution of the nonpolio enteroviruses can be defined by serological studies. For example, an examination of antibodies to coxsackievirus A9 and coxsackieviruses B1–B5 was made in sera obtained from New York Virus Watch families[90] on entry into the program. The results are shown in Table 4. Although comparison by age among virus types can only be suggested on the basis of the relatively small sample, it is clear that coxsackievirus B2, B4, and B5 antibodies were infrequent in the youngest children at the beginning of the Virus Watch observation period. This relative vacuum in immunity was partially filled by subsequent outbreaks of infection with these viruses.

For those enteroviruses on which data have been obtained, the patterns of exposure and spread and of increasing development of antibodies along with increasing age are generally similar. Sex appears to play no important role in infection with most enteroviruses, although childhood paralytic poliomyelitis is twice as common in boys as in girls.

5.1.5. Occurrence in Families and Closed Ecological Units. Enterovirus infections are highly communicable. Within a community, the viruses generally spread horizontally via preschool children and are found more frequently in families of large size and lower socioeconomic level. However, once an agent has invaded a family, regardless of family size or circumstances, nonimmune family members readily become infected. In the New York Virus Watch Program, spread of coxsackieviruses to susceptible members of the household was high (76%), while that of echoviruses was considerably lower (43% of the susceptibles) (Table 5). In addition to infecting those without prior type-specific antibody, coxsackieviruses also spread to and reinfected one half the siblings under the age of 10 years who already had specific antibody. Only one echovirus reinfection was observed. The frequency of intrafamilial infection may be related in part to the duration of virus excretion by the young index child; in the New York Virus Watch, with a 2-week interval between routine collections, only 16% of those infected with echoviruses yielded virus on more than one occasion, while coxsackievirus excretion for more than 1 day was found in 44% of the infections, and excretion for more than a month was not uncommon.

Rapid and extensive spread also occurs in familylike close associations such as those in children's institutions, in cabin groups in summer camps,[73] and in the environment of a small kibbutz.[157,230]

Wide dissemination, in which overt illnesses represent only a "very small tip of a very large iceberg"

Table 4. New York Virus Watch: Prevalence of Neutralizing Antibodies to Coxsackieviruses on Entrance to Observation, in Subsequently Invaded and Control Households,[a] by Age and Virus Type[b]

| | Serum neutralizing antibodies by age (yr) | | | | | | | |
| | 0–4 | | 5–19 | | 20+ | | All ages | |
Coxsackievirus type	Number of persons	Percent positive	Number of persons	Percent positive	Number of persons	Percent positive	Number of persons	Percent positive
A9	56	23	57	35	69	59	182	40
B1	10	(20)[c]	2	(0)[c]	14	14	26	15
B2	36	3	37	16	37	30	110	16
B3	14	14	14	36	20	40	48	40
B4	22	5	27	33	24	58	73	33
B5	33	3	53	11	62	24	148	15
All	171	14	190	24	226	41	587	27

[a] Control households were selected because no member had yielded the virus in question and because they were being observed during the period of maximum incidence of infection with the specified virus. The members examined were selected for age (preference given to children) and availability of paired or serial sera bracketing the desired period.
[b] From Kogen et al.[90] Used with permission.
[c] Parentheses are used for percentages based on ten or fewer observations.

Table 5. New York Virus Watch: Age Distribution of Infections[a]

Virus group	Percentage infected (number observed) by age in years						
	0–1	2–5	6–9	10–19	Mothers	Fathers	All ages
Coxsackie[b]	74 (39)	85 (54)	88 (40)	67 (18)	78 (37)	47 (30)	76 (218)
Echo	43 (7)	68 (25)	58 (24)	22 (18)	24 (17)	24 (17)	43 (108)

[a] From Kogen et al.[90] Used with permission.
[b] The coxsackieviruses sought included only those that could be grown in cell cultures at the time of the studies.

first described for poliovirus infections, has been repeatedly documented for a number of enteroviruses. During an epidemic in which 149 inhabitants of a city of 740,000 were hospitalized with echovirus 9 disease, approximately 6%, or 44,000 persons, had an illness compatible with infection due to this agent.[186] Among families that had been invaded by the virus, the rate of inapparent or unrecognized infection (based on recovery of the virus) was 18%; however, among 107 persons in families where no illness was observed, only one person yielded the virus from a stool specimen.

When outbreaks of aseptic meningitis and related illnesses due to echovirus type 30 began to spread along the Pacific Coast in 1968, the arrival of the virus in the Washington area coincided with the initiation of the Seattle Virus Watch Program, and extraordinary opportunities were available to observe infection and illness among the regularly studied Virus Watch families as related to the community pattern of illness.[69] Sixty-four such families containing 291 members underwent continuing virological surveillance in this period. By virus isolation or serology or both, infection was documented in 70 (79%) of 88 members of 18 families; in the total observed Virus Watch population, the rate was 24%. The invaded families were of slightly larger size, included more children 5–9 years of age, and included only three persons (two adults and one young child) who had antibody prior to the epidemic. (The families escaping infection were by no means totally immune, but prior antibody was present in 13, 14, and 17% of the children in the age groups 2–4, 5–9, and 10–19, respectively.) Of the persons observed to shed virus, 47% reported possibly related mild febrile illnesses, few of which were serious enough to require medical attention; one father in an invaded family did develop aseptic meningitis, almost certainly due to echovirus 30,

although virus could not be isolated from his specimens. Thus, on the basis of the Virus Watch family experiences, there must have been many thousands of echovirus 30 infections in the Seattle area, more than half of which were completely without symptoms, during the period when 44 virologically confirmed cases of echovirus 30 aseptic meningitis occurred in Seattle.[206]

In the normal middle-class families of the New York Virus Watch Program,[90] all the coxsackievirus- and echovirus-associated illnesses observed throughout the study period were mild, and the largest number consisted of upper respiratory disease with or without accompanying enteric illness, rash, or other signs and symptoms. CNS involvement, pleurodynia, pericarditis, and herpangina were not observed. To arrive at an estimate of the number of illnesses attributable to the infection with which they were temporally associated, allowance was made for illnesses "expected" had the observed concurrent infection not been present. For this correction, two types of controls were used: the illness records of matched but virus-free controls and the subject's own illness record before and after the episode of viral infection. For the coxsackievirus infections, these corrected rates of attributable illnesses were 24 or 19% (depending on which type of control is used), and for the echoviruses, 9 or 18%. The observation of respiratory illness in association with coxsackievirus infections has numerous parallels in other studies, particularly in relation to coxsackieviruses of group B. A number of echovirus serotypes have also been incriminated in respiratory or respiratory–enteric diseases.

The mildness of the illnesses associated with infection in the Virus Watch families is noteworthy. Many of the reports on which the more severe disease associations were based have been derived from patient-centered or epidemic-centered investigations. As the authors indicate, the absence of more serious enteroviral disease in this study suggests either that the more severe syndromes are rare—as with poliovirus infections—or that strains infecting the Virus Watch families were of unusually low virulence.

5.1.6. Socioeconomic Setting. The close correlation between low socioeconomic settings and the early acquisition of infection with the enteroviruses has been repeatedly emphasized in both tropical and temperate environments and reflects the general level of hygiene of the group. Fox[50] has predicted that in parallel with the transition of poliomyelitis from endemic to epidemic, the frequency of severe disease associated with coxsackievirus and echovirus infections may increase as levels of hygiene and sanitation improve. More individuals may escape infection as young children, only to experience more serious clinical manifestations if they become infected in later childhood or adulthood. That this may in fact be occurring is suggested by the increase in reports of epidemics of enterovirus-caused aseptic meningitis, which does not seem to be merely due to the increase in reporting because of the growing numbers and improved capabilities of virus-diagnostic laboratories around the world.[65]

5.2. Epidemiological Patterns of Poliomyelitis

Poliomyelitis can be viewed as having three major epidemiological phases: endemic, epidemic, and postvaccination. All these coexist at the present time, in different regions of the world. In some crowded, developing areas, chiefly in the tropics, paralytic poliomyelitis continues to be a disease of infancy (truly "infantile paralysis") that is seen only sporadically. In these populations, virtually all children over 4 years of age are already immune. With the almost universal presence of antibody to all three poliovirus types in women of childbearing age, passive immunity is transferred from mother to offspring, and many infants subsequently experience their first poliovirus infections while maternal antibodies still provide some protection. In addition, the ratio of inapparent to apparent infections is highest in infants and young children, and paralytic disease is thus relatively rare despite the abundance of circulating virus. In the past, the rarity of clinical poliomyelitis in the tropics had led many to believe that no poliovirus infections were present

in such areas, when in fact the reverse was true: polioviruses were highly endemic, but the infections were largely asymptomatic. Despite the rarity of reports of poliomyelitis in such areas, some paralytic cases do occur and may indeed be increasing more rapidly than had been believed. Recent studies have utilized surveys of residual paralysis in school-age children (see Section 3.3). By gathering information on the prevalence among these children of types of lameness compatible with a history of paralytic poliomyelitis, investigators have estimated the annual incidence of paralytic poliomyelitis during the years just prior to the survey.

In 1974, although there was no record of poliomyelitis epidemics occurring in the previous few years, the observed prevalence of lameness in Ghana among school-age children was 7 per 1000; the annual incidence of paralytic polio was estimated to be at least 28 per 100,000 population.[161] These figures are comparable to those in the United States and Europe before the introduction of polio vaccines. Somewhat similar surveys conducted in Burma, Egypt, and the Philippines indicated that the recent prevalence of paralytic poliomyelitis in children had been much higher than was believed from case reports. In each survey, it was concluded that a vigorous and extensive vaccination campaign should be initiated.

5.2.1. Behavior in Temperate Zones and Developed Countries. In many areas of the temperate zones with better standards of community and household hygiene, poliomyelitis during the first half of the 20th century underwent a transition from the endemic phase to one in which increasingly larger and more severe epidemics of the paralytic disease occurred. The generally accepted explanation, borne out by numerous studies, is that improved sanitation and hygiene reduced the opportunities for infection among the very young. Therefore, increasing numbers of persons encountered poliovirus for the first time in later childhood or in adult life, at ages when poliovirus infections are more likely to take the paralytic form. The delay in infection also resulted in a buildup of susceptibles in the population to a point at which there was a "critical mass" sufficient to support wide and rapid circulation of the viruses. Thus, epidemics began to occur, sometimes in an abrupt shift, sometimes after gradual increases in the annual case rates of "sporadic" poliomyelitis. For example, in the United

States, just before inactivated polio vaccine became generally available, the average annual number of cases of paralytic poliomyelitis was approximately 21,000. In epidemics, the peak age incidence was in the 5- to 9-year-olds, and about one third of the cases and two thirds of the deaths occurred in persons over 15 years of age. This was a marked change from the pattern in the great 1916 epidemic, in which approximately 80% of cases were in children under 5 years of age.[102]

In the first half of the 20th century, not only was it the "advantaged" nations that experienced epidemic polio, but it was also the socioeconomically advantaged sectors of the population within these nations that were most at risk. Even within the same city, wider circulation of the wild polioviruses in lower socioeconomic areas with poorer sanitation and hygiene provided more children with immunizing infections at an earlier age and reduced their chances of eventually developing paralytic disease.[136,139] The last outbreaks in the United States before polio vaccine became available included families living in good socioeconomic conditions; the spread of the virus through the community could be traced through young children who might or might not manifest illness; however, a high incidence of paralytic cases occurred among susceptible parents exposed to their virus-carrying children.[116,138,158]

5.2.2. Behavior in Tropical Areas and Developing Countries. This changing pattern of occurrence of paralytic poliomyelitis is now being seen in developing countries with rising levels of sanitation, particularly in tropical and semitropical areas. Of 71 tropical and semitropical countries, 45 reported an overall incidence of poliomyelitis in 1966 that was 3 times greater than the average annual incidence for the period 1951–1955. In such areas, if comprehensive and regular vaccination programs are not yet being carried out, outbreaks of paralytic poliomyelitis continue to occur. For example, in Ghana, the average annual number of reported cases was only 9 during 1951–1955, but increased to 36 in 1961–1965 and to 53 in 1966–1970; this increase accelerated during 1971–1975 to an annual average of 162, and 313 cases were reported in 1976.[223] (On the basis of lameness surveys, it has been estimated that this may represent no more than 10% of the actual cases that occurred.[156,161]) Oral poliovaccine had been administered to only a small proportion

of urban Ghanian children since about 1966 (estimated at about 20% of the children in Accra). In Upper Volta, a similar increase occurred over the same period: from 15 cases in 1951–1955 to 129 in 1971–1975, and 113 in 1976, followed by 388 cases in 1977. In some Central and South American countries where, with or without some vaccination program, the disease has not yet been controlled, a similar trend has been seen. In Honduras, for example, in the years from 1969 to 1973, the endemic level of poliomyelitis was reported as being 20 to 66 cases each year. Then, in late 1976, after more than a year without a single case being reported, there were 29 cases in 3 months, and during the first 3 months of 1977 there were 109 paralytic cases with 5 deaths. Most of the patients were young children, 73% of them less than 3 years old, 32% less than 1 year old. Only 2 patients were older than 7 years. Although some vaccine had been used in Honduras, 72% of the patients had never received any vaccine, and only 9% had received more than a single dose. Until vaccination programs are implemented on a regular basis, these countries should anticipate—and indeed may already be experiencing—rates of incidence of paralytic poliomyelitis such as those that occurred in the temperate countries before the introduction of the vaccine.

Payne[170] and others have shown that there tends to be an inverse relationship between infant mortality rates and the incidence of clinical poliomyelitis. Paul[167] pointed out that when the infant mortality rate in a country drops below 75 per 1000 live births, the incidence of reported polio can be expected to increase. Thus, epidemic polio was a disease of affluent societies in the first half of the 20th century and is now an unwelcome concomitant of improved living standards in developing nations, unless it is controlled by vaccination.

5.2.3. Behavior in the Postvaccine Era. The postvaccine era for most countries in Europe, North America, and Oceania, and some countries in other regions of the world, began after 1955 when inactivated polio virus vaccine was introduced and particularly after 1959 when live attenuated vaccines became available on a large scale. These areas experienced a marked reduction in the incidence of poliomyelitis; rarely was a serious disease controlled so quickly and dramatically.

In 1955, 17,364 cases of poliomyelitis were reported in the U.S.S.R., 27,343 in 23 other European countries, and 31,582 in the United States, Canada, Australia, and New Zealand—a total of over 76,000. In these same countries in 1967, only 1013 cases were recorded—a reduction of 99% in 12 years.

Even further reductions have followed. In 22 industrialized European countries, the total average annual number of poliomyelitis cases in 1966–1970 was 751, and in 1971–1975, this figure was 357; in 1976, there were 151 cases, and in 1977, 145. Adding to these, for the same periods, the data from Australia, Canada, Japan, New Zealand, and the United States, the total annual case rate—in these 27 industrialized countries around the world (containing a total of approximately 680 million persons)—was 807 cases for 1966–1970, 377 in 1971–1975, 165 in 1976, and 169 in 1977.[223]

In the United States following the introduction of live poliovirus vaccine during 1961–1965, the annual number of paralytic cases decreased to 465. In subsequent years, the rates averaged 40 to 50 cases annually, decreasing to 18 cases in 1969. In 1970, however, 31 cases were reported, including 22 from an epidemic in Texas among unimmunized persons. During 1971–1975, the average annual number of cases was 15; in 1976, there were 14 cases, and in 1977, 18 cases were reported, with 2 deaths. Among the 1977 patients, 2 had contracted the illness outside the country. Three of the cases were in recent vaccine recipients, and 10 were in close contacts of recently vaccinated persons. The remaining 3 patients were persons "without known vaccine association." In 1977, none of the cases in the United States was in individuals with cellular and/or humoral deficiency states. In 1978, only 3 cases of paralytic poliomyelitis were reported in the United States. (The data in this paragraph were derived chiefly from CDC reports[20,21] and Gregg.[63])

Now, in the well-vaccinated areas of the world, "postvaccine" epidemiological patterns of poliomyelitis are emerging. These patterns differ from one country to another and to some extent even within the same country.

a. Virus Isolation. In a few areas, where repeated mass vaccination campaigns are conducted regularly and are implemented so as to reach virtually all young children, wild polioviruses are rarely identified; almost all isolates now closely resemble the vaccine strains and are generally presumed to be vaccine progeny. Vaccine viruses are abundantly excreted by the vaccinee and infect unvaccinated

contacts.[77] The rare cases of poliomyelitis that do appear may be due to imported wild viruses or may in some instances be vaccine-associated (see Section 9). Results of recent studies, for example, suggest that wild polioviruses have been almost completely eradicated from Japan. Since 1964, infants in Japan between the ages of 3 months and 18 months have been vaccinated with two doses of trivalent live virus vaccine, in routine administration at local health centers over short periods in spring or autumn. Since 1962, a collaborative study, conducted under sponsorship of the Ministry of Health and Welfare, has included serological surveys for levels of antibody against polioviruses and virological studies for isolation and identification of polioviruses from the feces of healthy children in periods when vaccine campaigns were not under way. Since no comparable study is being carried out in the United States, isolation from fecal specimens obtained in 1962–1968 from healthy children in Japan 2 months or more after routine vaccination periods[204] are here compared to American findings of more than a decade earlier (in 1951–1953)[120] made in surveys of healthy preschool children in Charleston, West Virginia, and Phoenix, Arizona, during the period prior to the development of polio vaccines. The results are shown in Tables 6 and 7. The rates of occurrence for nonpolio enteric viruses in Japan were of the same order of magnitude as those found earlier in the United States cities, but the effect of systematic widespread vaccination is clearly reflected in greatly reduced prevalence of polioviruses. Most of the poliovirus isolates studied in Japan were vaccine-like in their properties and were considered to be vaccine virus progeny.[203]

b. Is Poliomyelitis Being Eradicated? In a number of well-vaccinated countries, there have been almost no poliomyelitis cases reported for several years, and (as indicated above) studies of virus isolates indicate that most of the poliovirus strains extant in these countries may be vaccine progeny. Virtual eradication of wild polioviruses has been reported in some European countries. In the United States, if we subtract imported cases and vaccine-associated cases, then only 7 endemic cases occurred during the 5-year period 1973–1977. Yorke *et al.*[232] have postulated that the pool of susceptible individuals in the United States has already dropped below the level required for perpetuation of wild polioviruses and that a break in the historic chain of infection

Table 6. Distribution of Enteroviruses Isolated from Healthy Children in Populations of Contrasting Socioeconomic Levels during a Nonepidemic Period (1951–1953)[a]

Population group	Number of specimens tested	Percentage yielding viruses			
		Polioviruses	Coxsackieviruses	Echoviruses	All enteroviruses
Charleston, W.Va.					
Lower	597	2.3	2.3	3.7	8.4
Upper	1028	0.5	1.5	0.8	2.7
Phoenix, Ariz.					
Lower	943	3.0	2.0	8.3	13.3
Upper	399	1.0	1.0	0.3	2.3
Total					
Lower	1540	2.8	2.1	6.6	11.4
Upper	1427	0.6	1.3	0.6	2.6

[a] From Melnick.[120] Used with permission.

has been achieved. However, wild poliovirus, if reintroduced into a well-vaccinated population, may still seek out susceptibles in a narrow stream of transmission, as illustrated in the Netherlands and Canada in 1978[55,222] and in the United States in 1979.[22] Considerations of whether, how, and where eradication can be accomplished will be a focal point of international discussions in the next few years. As of this writing, there are at least 40 developing countries in the world in which—with or without some use of vaccination—poliomyelitis has not yet been brought under control; the total population in these countries is almost 400 million. Tens of thousands of cases of polio are still reported each year, and doubtless many more go unreported. As long as wild polioviruses continue to circulate widely in a large part of the world, efforts at immunization must be maintained and strengthened before eradication can become a practical international goal. The WHO Expanded Programme for Immunization (EPI) was initiated recently with the objective of reducing morbidity and mortality from six target diseases, including polio, by providing immunization against them for every child in the world by 1990. The programme activities depend heavily on technical cooperation with and among developing countries. As of May 1978, 42 countries had been identified as actively participating in the EPI.[223] The program is as yet too new for the results to be measurable, or distinguishable from natural year-to-year fluctuations in polio incidence, but the next 5 years should bring significant progress.

c. *Breadth of Immunity.* In some field studies, children immunized previously with one strain of type 3 vaccine virus were more susceptible to another vaccine strain of the same serotype (heterologous, but homotypic) than they were to the homologous strain.[84] The neutralizing antibody response was higher after administration of the heterologous vaccine virus than after administration of a second dose of the homologous strain.

The success of live poliovirus vaccination programs in many countries of the world has reduced substantially the wild poliovirus circulation in these areas, so that there are now increasing numbers of people whose immunological experience is limited to a single vaccine strain of each type. This change in immunity status of populations has brought a new question into focus.

It is conceivable that the changed ecological situation could act on wild poliovirus populations as a selective mutational pressure toward wide antigenic divergence from the attenuated vaccine strains, bringing about significant antigenic shifts—although there is no evidence as yet that such a selection is actually taking place. If such shifts occur, and if they permit silent circulation of heterologous wild strains to increase, individuals who for some reason lack sufficient vaccine-induced immunity *might* be at risk to paralytic poliomyelitis. In anticipation of such problems, an appropriate subject for further investigation is whether successive infections with two different attenuated polioviruses of the same type could provide a broadening of ali-

Table 7. Poliovirus Isolation from Fecal Specimens from Healthy Children Collected Not Less than 2 Months after the Routine Vaccination[a]

Year	Time of specimen collection	Number of specimens examined	Number of cytopathogenic agents isolated[b]	Poliovirus isolated Number[b]	Type 1	Type 2	Type 3	Other cytopathogenic agents[b]
1962	Late summer–early autumn	974	31 (3.2)	1 (0.1)	0	1	0	30 (3.1)
1963	Late summer–early autumn	4954	127 (2.6)	5 (0.1)	0	4	1	122 (2.5)
1964	Late summer–early autumn	2299	81 (3.5)	10 (0.4)	1	2	7	71 (3.1)
	Late autumn–early winter	1803	18 (1.0)	17 (0.9)	4	11	2	1 (0.1)
1965	Late summer–early autumn	2069	174 (5.7)	1 (0.05)	0	1	0	173 (5.6)
	Late autumn–early winter	1770	41 (2.3)	1 (0.06)	0	1	0	40 (2.3)
1966	Late summer–early autumn	3048	107 (5.2)	5 (0.2)	1	1	3	102 (5.0)
	Late autumn–early winter	1831	19 (1.4)	6 (0.3)	1	1	4	13 (0.7)
1967	Late summer–early autumn	1962	131 (6.7)	0	0	0	0	131 (6.7)
	Late autumn–early winter	1833	20 (1.1)	2 (0.1)	2	0	0	18 (1.0)
1968	Late summer–early autumn	1504	114 (7.6)	2 (0.1)	2	0	0	112 (7.4)
	Late autumn–early winter	1583	32 (2.0)	3 (0.2)	0	1	2	29 (1.8)

[a] From Takatsu et al.[204] Used with permission.
[b] The figures in parenthesis indicate the percentage of the total number of specimens examined.

mentary-tract resistance to wild homotypic viruses. Other aspects of vaccination including social failure are discussed in Section 9.

6. Mechanisms and Route of Transmission

Man is the only known reservoir for members of the human enterovirus group, and close human contact appears to be the primary avenue of spread. For almost all these agents, virus can be recovered from the oropharynx and intestine of individuals infected either clinically or subclinically and is generally shed for longer periods (up to a month or more) in stools than in secretions of the upper alimentary tract. Thus, fecal contamination (fingers, table utensils, foodstuffs, milk) is the usual source of infections. However, droplets or aerosols from coughing or sneezing can also be a source of direct or indirect contamination. Coxsackievirus A21 has been shown to be more abundant in nasal secretions than in those from the throat and has been experimentally transmitted from infected volunteers by airborne aerosols produced by natural coughing.[36] Enterovirus 70, the newly recognized agent of acute hemorrhagic conjunctivitis,[149] has thus far been found almost exclusively in conjunctival and throat specimens, but fecal isolations have been reported.

Warm weather favors the spread of virus by increasing human contacts, the susceptibility of the host, or the dissemination of the virus by extrahuman sources. The viruses are most readily spread within the family, and the extent of intrafamilial infection appears to be closely related to duration of virus shedding, particularly by young children.

During periods of epidemic prevalence, in both rural and urban areas, houseflies (*Musca domestica*) and filth flies (*Phormia regina, Phaenicia sericata, Sarcophaga* species) may be found contaminated with enteroviruses and may act as mechanical carriers. The importance of flies in transmission is not easily evaluated, although it is important to note that poliovirus has been found in food naturally contaminated by flies. As described in Section 3.4, enteroviruses are also present in urban sewage during periods when subclinical or clinical disease is prevalent. Sewage may serve as a source of contamination of flies or of water supplies used for drinking or bathing, or through its use as fertilizer. Enteroviruses have been isolated frequently from sewage. Until recently, they had never been recovered from open recreational water not obviously contaminated by sewage. During an epidemic of coxsackievirus B5 infections in a boys' summer camp on Lake Champlain, the virus was isolated from water from the lake swimming area.[73] Although in this outbreak the clustering of infection in cabins suggests the principal mode of spread to be person to person, an oral–water–oral route is possible, as well as a rectal–water–oral route.

A strain of coxsackievirus A6, originally obtained from mosquitos in Fiji, has been found to survive in mosquitos experimentally infected by injection or by feeding on viremic mice, and a small number of transmissions to baby mice by bite were obtained. The function of the mosquito as a true vector was not demonstrated, however, for virus did not multiply within the insect; in both fed and injected mosquitos, virus titers never exceeded the original level.[114]

7. Pathogenesis and Immunity

7.1. Pathogenesis

The portal of entry of enteroviruses is believed to be the alimentary tract via the mouth. The incubation period (defined as the time from exposure to onset of disease) is usually between 7 and 14 days, but may be 2–35 days. After initial and continuing multiplication, probably in lymphoid tissue of the pharynx and gut, viremia may occur and in turn lead to further virus proliferation in the cells of the reticuloendothelial system and finally to involvement of the target organs (spinal cord and brain, meninges, myocardium, skin). Usually, the virus is excreted in the stools for several weeks and is present in the pharynx 1–2 weeks postinfection in individuals having either clinical or subclinical infection. Enteroviruses have been isolated from feces, pharyngeal washings, cerebrospinal fluid (CSF), heart, blood, the CNS, urine, conjunctivae, and lesions of skin or mucous membrane.

Two or more enteroviruses may propagate simultaneously in the alimentary tract,[166] but under many circumstances, multiplication of one virus may interfere with growth of the heterologous type. Interference with the growth ("take") of live polio vaccine by other concurrent enterovirus infections is now well established.

Pathogenesis has been studied more thoroughly for poliomyelitis, the most serious disease caused by any of the enteroviruses.[9,176] The status may be summarized as follows:

Poliovirus may be found in the blood of patients with the abortive form ("minor illness") and can be detected several days before onset of clinical signs of CNS involvement in patients who develop nonparalytic or paralytic poliomyelitis. In orally infected monkeys and chimpanzees, viremia is also regularly present in the preparalytic phase of the disease. Antibodies to the virus appear early in the natural infection and also early in orally infected experimental animals. They are usually present by the time paralysis appears. In man, viremia has been demonstrated regularly following ingestion of type 2 oral poliovaccine. Free virus is present in the serum between days 2 and 5 after vaccination, and virus bound to antibody can be detected for an additional few days.[140] Bound virus is detected by acid treatment, which inactivates the antibody and liberates active virus.

These findings led to the view that the virus first multiplies in the tonsils, the lymph nodes of the neck, Peyer's patches, and the small intestine. The CNS may then be invaded by way of the circulating blood. In monkeys infected by the oral route, small amounts of antibody prevent the paralytic disease, whereas large amounts are necessary to prevent passage of the virus along nerve fibers. In man also, antibody in low titer in the form of γ-globulin may prevent paralysis if given before exposure to the virus.

In the experimental infection in monkeys, poliovirus can spread along axons of peripheral nerves to the CNS, and there it continues to progress along the fibers of the lower motor neurons to increasingly involve the spinal cord or the brain. Neural spread may also occur in children who have inapparent infections at the time of tonsillectomy. In this situation, poliovirus present in the oropharynx may enter nerve fibers exposed during surgery and spread to the brain, resulting in bulbar paralysis. A similar mechanism of virus spread along neural pathways may be responsible for the rare instances of paralysis in a limb recently injected with an irritating material during a period of high poliovirus prevalence. An alternative mechanism for the adverse effects of tonsillectomy has been suggested (see Section 7.2).

Poliovirus invades certain types of nerve cells, and in the process of its intracellular multiplication, it may damage or completely destroy these cells. The anterior horn cells of the spinal cord are most prominently involved, but in severe cases, the intermediate gray ganglia and even the posterior horn and dorsal root ganglia are often affected. Lesions are found as far forward as the hypothalamus and thalamus. In the brain, the reticular formation, the vestibular nuclei, the cerebellar vermis, and the deep cerebellar nuclei are most often affected. The cortex is virtually spared, with the exception of the motor cortex along the precentral gyrus.

Poliovirus does not multiply in muscle *in vivo*. Its chief site of action is in the neuron, and the changes that occur in peripheral nerves and voluntary muscles are secondary to destruction of the nerve cell. Changes occur rapidly in nerve cells, from mild chromatolysis to neuronophagia and complete destruction. Cells that are not killed, but that lose their function temporarily as a result of edema, may recover completely. Inflammation occurs secondary to the attack on the nerve cells; the focal and perivascular infiltrations are chiefly lymphocytes, with some polymorphonuclear cells, plasma cells, and microglia. In addition to pathological changes in the nervous system, hyperplasia and inflammatory lesions of lymph nodes and of Peyer's patches and other lymph follicles in the intestinal tract are frequently observed; interstitial infiltration of the myocardium with leukocytes is common, but necrotizing myocarditis is rare.

7.2. Immunity

Immunity to the poliovirus type causing the infection is permanent. There may be a low degree of heterotypic resistance induced by infection, especially between type 1 and type 2 polioviruses. This may account for the observation that second attacks of polio have most often involved types 1 and 3.

Passive immunity is transferred from mother to offspring. The maternal antibodies gradually disappear during the first 6 months of life. Passively administered antibody lasts only 3–5 weeks.

Virus-neutralizing antibody forms within a few days after exposure to the virus, often before the onset of illness, and persists, apparently, for life. Its formation early in the infection is a result of viral multiplication in the intestinal tract and deep lymphatic structures before invasion of the nervous system. Since antibodies must be present in the blood to prevent the dissemination of virus to the brain and are not effective after this has already occurred, immunization is of value only if it precedes the onset of symptoms referable to the nervous system.

A decrease in resistance to poliovirus accompanies removal of tonsils and adenoids. Preexisting secretory antibody levels in the nasopharynx decrease sharply following operation (particularly in young male children) without any change in antibody levels in serum. Local antibody levels remain low or absent for as long as 7 months. In seronegative children, nasopharyngeal antibody response to polio vaccine develops significantly later and to lower titers in children previously tonsillectomized than in those with intact tonsils. Thus, surgery of this type may eliminate a valuable source of immunocompetent tissue of importance in resistance to poliovirus.

Strains of coxsackievirus studied by cross-protection tests in infant mice born of immunized mothers show the same type-specificity as that observed in neutralization and complement-fixation (CF) tests. The immunity conferred by mother's milk is also type-specific. In humans, a passive transfer of neutralizing and CF antibodies from the mother to the offspring also occurs.

Circulating serum antibody against enteroviruses is not the only source of protection against infection. The nature of the so-called local or cellular immunity, which is manifested by protection against intestinal reinfection after recovery from a natural infection or after immunization with the live polio vaccine, has not been satisfactorily elucidated. Locally produced antibodies, or perhaps interferon, are more likely to be responsible than are nonhumoral factors. Local or secretory antibody is increasingly recognized as having an important role in defense against enteroviral infections.[162,163,182]

It had been thought that individuals with defects of the humoral immune system who retained cell-mediated immunity, e.g., individuals with a defect in immunoglobulin synthesis, would not be unduly susceptible to most viral infections or experience unusual complications. In administration of live poliovirus vaccines, therefore, inclusion of such persons had not been emphatically warned against (in contrast to the strong cautions concerning vaccination of persons with combined immunodeficiency disease). However, it is being recognized increasingly that viral infections (including infections with live attenuated poliovirus vaccine) do carry a considerably increased risk for persons with various immunodeficiencies in either humoral or cell-mediated immunity. In such persons, poliovirus infection—either by wild virus or by vaccine strains—may develop in an atypical manner, with an incubation period longer than 28 days, a high mortality rate after a long chronic illness, and unusual lesions in the CNS. A few such persons are included among the vaccine-associated paralytic poliomyelitis cases that have been reported in the United States (see Section 9.2.2). In addition to the devastating consequences to some of these individuals after infection by polioviruses, recent studies have documented a number of persistent or fatal infections of immunodeficient persons by echoviruses of several types (echovirus types 30, 19, 9, 33, and 11).[218,235] In most of the patients in these studies, the chief deficit was in the B-cell functions associated with humoral immunity, and the T-cell function was normal (or only secondarily defective). The patients had been regularly treated with reasonable success—some of them from birth into the mid-teens—by administration of human immune serum globulin. A prominent feature of the echovirus infections was the patients' inability to eradicate the virus from the CSF; some continued to yield virus from CSF for up to 3 years.

8. Patterns of Host Response and Diagnosis

8.1. Clinical Syndromes

In Tables 8–12 are listed the prototype strains of the known enteroviruses, together with the illness (if any) in the person yielding the prototype virus. In Sections 8.1.1 through 8.1.12 are described the various host responses to enteroviruses, including the major clinical manifestations associated with enteroviruses and the serotypes most frequently associated with them. It should be noted that Section 8.1.1—Asymptomatic Infections—is purposely included below to emphasize the frequency with which no apparent illness is manifested by the individual infected with an enterovirus. The listing of clinical syndromes in the subsequent sections is not exhaustive, since additional serotypes have been sporadically associated with other syndromes. Further details concerning enteroviral diseases may be found in several reviews on the role of nonpolio enteroviruses in human disease,[65,89,146] viral myocardiopathies,[101,107,108] coxsackievirus infections of newborns,[57] virus diseases associated with cutaneous eruptions,[216] respiratory disease viruses,[83] congenital malformations associated with maternal viral infection,[6] and the possible role of viruses in diabetes mellitus.[37,159]

8.1.1. Asymptomatic Infections. By far the most common form of infection by any enteroviruses is asymptomatic, or is manifest by no more than minor malaise. This is true not only for poliovirus infection, but also for infections by coxsackieviruses, echoviruses, and the newly recognized enterovirus serotypes. Nonetheless, serious clinical syndromes can be associated with many of these agents. The more common of these are discussed in the paragraphs which follow.

Table 8. New Enterovirus Types

Type	Prototype strain	Geographic origin	Illness in person yielding prototype virus	Investigator(s)
68	Fermon	California	Lower respiratory illness (pneumonia and bronchiolitis)[a]	Schieble et al.[191]
69	Toluca-1	Mexico	None[b]	Rosen et al.[180]
70	J670/71	Japan and Singapore	Acute hemorrhagic conjunctivitis (AHC)[c]	Kono et al.,[94] Yin-Murphy and Lim,[229] Mirkovic et al.[149]
71	BrCr	California	Meningitis[d]	Schmidt et al.[196]

[a] Prototype isolated from throat swabs.
[b] Prototype isolated from rectal swabs.
[c] Prototype isolated from conjunctival swabs.
[d] Prototype virus recovered from stool; an identical strain was isolated from the brain of a fatal encephalitis case in the same local outbreak of CNS disease, which occurred in California in 1970. Strains of the same serotype have since been isolated from patients during epidemics of polioencephalitis, meningitis, and hand, foot, and mouth disease.[7,68,88,144,150a]

8.1.2. Poliomyelitis. When an individual susceptible to infection is exposed to poliovirus, one of the following responses may occur: (1) inapparent infection without symptoms, (2) mild (minor) illness, (3) aseptic meningitis, (4) paralytic poliomyelitis. As the disease progresses, one response may merge with a more severe form, often resulting in a biphasic course: a minor illness, followed first by a few days free of symptoms and then by the major, severe illness. Only about 1% of infections result in recognized clinical illness.

a. Abortive Poliomyelitis. Abortive poliomyelitis is the most common form of the disease. The patient has only the minor illness, characterized by fever, malaise, drowsiness, headache, nausea, vomiting, constipation, or sore throat in various combinations. The patient recovers in a few days. The diagnosis of abortive poliomyelitis cannot be made with assurance, even during an epidemic, except when the virus is isolated or antibody development is measured.

b. Nonparalytic Poliomyelitis (Aseptic Meningitis). In addition to the aforementioned symptoms and signs, the patient with the nonparalytic form presents stiffness and pain in the back and neck. The disease lasts 2–10 days, and recovery is rapid and complete. In a small percentage of cases, the disease advances to paralysis. Poliovirus is only one of many viruses that produce aseptic meningitis.

c. Paralytic Poliomyelitis. In the absence of virological diagnosis, poliovirus must be suspected if disease occurs in persons associated with paralytic patients, since paralysis is rare in other enterovirus infections. In poliomyelitis, the major illness, when it occurs, may follow the minor illness described above, particularly in young children, but it usually occurs without the antecedent first phase. The predominating sign is flaccid paralysis resulting from lower motor neuron damage. However, incoordination secondary to brainstem invasion and painful spasms of nonparalyzed muscles may also occur. The amount of damage and destruction varies from

Table 9. Polioviruses[a]

Type	Prototype strain	Geographic origin	Illness in person yielding prototype virus	Investigator(s)
1	Brunhilde	Maryland	Paralytic polio[b]	Howe and Bodian
2	Lansing	Michigan	Fatal paralytic polio[c]	Armstrong
3	Leon	California	Fatal paralytic polio[c]	Kessel

[a] From Melnick et al.[146] Used with permission.
[b] Virus recovered from feces.
[c] Virus recovered from spinal cord.

Table 10. Group A Coxsackieviruses[a,b]

Type	Prototype strain	Geographic origin	Illness in person yielding prototype virus[c]	Investigator
1	Tompkins	Coxsackie, N.Y.	Poliomyelitis[d]	Dalldorf
2	Fleetwood	Delaware	Poliomyelitis[d]	Dalldorf
3	Olson	New York	Meningitis	Dalldorf
4	High Point	North Carolina	(Sewage of polio community)	Melnick
5	Swartz	New York	Poliomyelitis	Dalldorf
6	Gdula	New York	Meningitis	Dalldorf
7	Parker	New York	Meningitis	Dalldorf
8	Donovan	New York	Poliomyelitis	Dalldorf
9	Bozek	New York	Meningitis	Dalldorf
10	Kowalik	New York	Meningitis	Dalldorf
11	Belgium-1	Belgium	Epidemic myalgia	Curnen
12	Texas-12	Texas	(Flies in polio community)	Melnick
13	Flores	Mexico	None	Sickles
14	G-14	South Africa	None	Gear
15	G-9	South Africa	None	Gear
16	G-10	South Africa	None	Gear
17	G-12	South Africa	None	Gear
18	G-13	South Africa	None	Gear
19	NIH-8663	Japan	Guillain–Barré syndrome	Huebner
20	IH-35	New York	Infectious hepatitis	Sickles
21	Kuykendall; Coe	California	Poliomyelitis[d]; mild respiratory disease[e]	Lennette
22	Chulman	New York	Vomiting and diarrhea	Sickles
24	Joseph	South Africa	None	Gear

[a] From Melnick et al.[146] Used with permission.
[b] Cross-reactivity has been observed between A3 and A8, A11 and A15, and A13 and A18.
[c] All isolates were from stools, except for prototypes of A4 and A12 which were isolated from sewage and flies, as indicated. Numerous strains of each of these types were isolated from stools also.
[d] When coxsackieviruses have been isolated from patients with paralytic poliomyelitis, the patient has often been found to have a dual infection, the polioviruses presumably being responsible for the paralytic illness.
[e] The Coe virus was isolated from throat washings.

case to case. Muscle involvement is usually maximal within a few days after the paralytic phase begins. The maximal recovery usually occurs within 6 months, but it may take longer.

8.1.3. Meningitis and Mild Paresis. Fever, malaise, headache, nausea, and abdominal pain are common early symptoms. One to two days later there may be signs of meningeal irritation with stiffness of the neck or back; vomiting may also appear. The disease sometimes progresses to mild muscle weakness that is often confused clinically with paralytic poliomyelitis. Patients almost always recover

Table 11. Group B Coxsackieviruses[a]

Type	Prototype strain	Geographic origin	Illness in person yielding prototype virus[b]	Investigator
1	Conn-5	Connecticut	Meningitis	Melnick
2	Ohio-1	Ohio	Summer grippe	Melnick
3	Nancy	Connecticut	Minor febrile illness	Melnick
4	JVB	New York	Chest and abdominal pain	Sickles
5	Faulkner	Kentucky	Mild paralytic disease with residual atrophy	Steigman
6	Schmidt	Philippine Islands	None	Hammon

[a] From Melnick et al.[146] Used with permission.
[b] All isolates were from stools.

Table 12. Echoviruses[a,b]

Type	Prototype strain	Geographic origin	Illness in person yielding prototype virus[c]	Investigator(s)
1	Farouk	Egypt	None	Melnick
2	Cornelis	Connecticut	Meningitis	Melnick
3	Morrisey	Connecticut	Meningitis	Melnick
4	Pesascek	Connecticut	Meningitis	Melnick
5	Noyce	Maine	Meningitis	Melnick
6	D'Amori	Rhode Island	Meningitis	Melnick
6'	Cox	Ohio	None	Ramos-Alvarez, Sabin
6"	Burgess	Connecticut	Meningitis	Melnick
7	Wallace	Ohio	None	Ramos-Alvarez, Sabin
8	Bryson	Ohio	None	Ramos-Alvarez, Sabin
9	Hill	Ohio	None	Ramos-Alvarez, Sabin
11	Gregory	Ohio	None	Ramos-Alvarez, Sabin
12	Travis	Philippine Islands	None	Hammon, Ludwig
13	Del Carmen	Philippine Islands	None	Hammon, Ludwig
14	Tow	Rhode Island	Meningitis	Melnick
15	CH 96-51	West Virginia	None	Ormsbee, Melnick
16	Harrington	Massachusetts	Meningitis	Kibrick, Enders
17	CHHE-29	Mexico City	None	Ramos-Alvarez, Sabin
18	Metcalf	Ohio	Diarrhea	Ramos-Alvarez, Sabin
19	Burke	Ohio	Diarrhea	Ramos-Alvarez, Sabin
20	JV-1	Washington, D.C.	Fever	Rosen
21	Farina	Massachusetts	Meningitis	Enders, Kibrick
22	Harris	Ohio	Diarrhea	Sabin
23	Williamson	Ohio	Diarrhea	Sabin
24	DeCamp	Ohio	Diarrhea	Sabin
25	JV-4	Washington, D.C.	Diarrhea	Rosen
26	Coronel	Philippine Islands	None	Hammon
27	Bacon	Philippine Islands	None	Hammon
29	JV-10	Washington, D.C.	None	Rosen
30	Bastianni	New York	Meningitis	Plager, Duncan, Lennette
31	Caldwell	Kansas	Meningitis	Wenner, Lennette, von Magnus
32	PR-10	Puerto Rico	Meningitis	Branche
33	Toluca-3	Mexico	None	Rosen, Kern
34	DN-19[d]	Texas	Infantile diarrhea	Melnick

[a] From Melnick et al.[(146)] Used with permission.
[b] Types 1 and 8 share antigens, type 1 having the broader spectrum.
[c] All isolates were from stools.
[d] DN-19 antiserum partially neutralizes coxsackievirus A24, but A24 antiserum does not neutralize DN-19 virus, although it reacts with the virus in CF and gel diffusion tests. Thus, DN-19 should be considered a prime strain of coxsackievirus A24, rather than as a distinct echovirus.

completely from nonpoliovirus paresis. However, with a number of enteroviruses, there is a small risk of serious neurological sequelae among infants infected during their first year of life.[(198)]

As indicated in the preceding section, poliovirus infection frequently is manifested as meningitis or as transient mild paresis.

Almost all coxsackieviruses of both A and B groups, as well as most echoviruses, have been associated to some degree with meningitis and (in very rare instances) with paralytic CNS disease. However, the chief types associated with CNS disease among coxsackieviruses are B1–B6, A7, and A9.

Echoviruses 4, 6, 9, 11, 14, 16, and 30 have been the ones repeatedly associated with meningitis;

types 3, 18, and 19 have also been responsible for some outbreaks of this syndrome. Other types (including 2 and 5) have been associated with meningitis only in sporadic cases. With echoviruses 6 and 9, muscle weakness and mild transient paralysis have been observed; echovirus 9 has been recovered in high titer from the medulla of a fatal case.

Among the newer enteroviruses, type 70, the agent of acute hemorrhagic conjunctivitis (AHC), in rare instances has been involved in neurological complications inducing poliomyelitis-like illnesses.[92,93] An important feature of infections with enterovirus 71 has also been meningitis. Enterovirus 71 has exhibited a variety of clinical manifestations in different regions of the world and at different times. In the California outbreak from which the prototype strain was reported, meningitis predominated, but there were other CNS manifestations including a fatal encephalitis case.[196] Meningitis also predominated in a 1972 outbreak in Australia[88] and a 1973 outbreak in Sweden[7]; however, there were some cases of hand, foot, and mouth disease in the Swedish outbreak, and this latter syndrome predominated in a Japanese outbreak that

occurred in the same year.[68] In some areas of Japan in 1973, a number of the patients had concomitant hand, foot, and mouth symptoms and meningitis symptoms.[150a] The most severe epidemic to date was the one in 1975 in Bulgaria,[144] in which, among 700 patients, about 21% developed poliomyelitis-like paralysis and 44 died. The 1978 Hungarian outbreak included chiefly meningitis cases, but some encephalitis, with some fatalities, occurred among the 1000 patients.

The associations of nonpolio enteroviruses with neurological disease have been tabulated by Grist et al.[65] and are shown in Table 13.

8.1.4. Pleurodynia (Epidemic Myalgia, Bornholm Disease). Pleurodynia is generally caused by group B coxsackieviruses, rarely by echoviruses (notably types 6 and 9). Fever and chest pain are almost invariably present together; they are usually abrupt in onset, but are sometimes preceded by malaise, headache, and anorexia. The chest pain may be located on either side or substernally, is intensified by movement, and may last from 2 days to 2 weeks. Abdominal pain resulting from involvement of the diaphragm occurs in approximately half

Table 13. Neurological Disease Associations of Coxsackieviruses, Echoviruses, and "New" Enteroviruses[a]

Syndrome or clinical feature	Virus types[b]
Meningitis	Coxsackieviruses A1, **2**, 3, **4**, **5**, **6**, 7*, 8, 9*, **10**, 11, **14**, **16**, 17, 18, **22**, 24
	Coxsackieviruses B1*, **2***, **3***, **4***, **5***, 6
	Echoviruses 1, **2***, **3***, **4***, **5**, 6, **7***, **9***, **11***, 12, 13, **14***, **15**, **16***, **17***, **18***, **19***, 20, 21, 22, 23, **25***, 27, **30***, **31**, **33***
	Enterovirus 71*
Paralytic disease	Coxsackieviruses A4, 6, 7, 9, 11, 14, 21
	Coxsackieviruses B1, **2**, 3, 4, 5, 6
	Echoviruses 1, **2**, 3, **4**, 6, 7, **9**, **11**, 14, **16**, 18, **19**, **30**
	Enterovirus 70, **71**
Encephalitis	Coxsackieviruses A2, 5, 6, 7, **9**
	Coxsackieviruses B1, 2, 3, **5**, **6**
	Echoviruses 2, 3, 4, **6**, 7, **9**, 11, 14, **17**, 18, **19**, 25
	Enterovirus **71**
Ataxia	Coxsackieviruses A4, 7, 9
	Echovirus 9

[a] From Grist et al.[65] Used with permission.
[b] Boldfaced figures indicate virus isolation from cerebrospinal fluid or other parenteral source.
[c] Asterisk indicates outbreaks reported with this type.

the cases; in children, this often takes the place of chest pain and may be the chief complaint. The illness is self-limited and recovery is complete, although relapses are common.

Coxsackieviruses A have been associated with Bornholm disease less often; the serotypes involved have been A4, A6, and A10. A9 has been associated with this syndrome and also with chronic diseases of muscles and joints.[65] Several reports of pseudocrystalline arrays of picornavirus-like particles in the myocytes of patients with chronic muscle dis-

eases suggest that enteroviruses might have a role in these diseases.[67] (see Figure 2).

8.1.5. Herpangina. Herpangina is caused chiefly by coxsackievirus group A types 1, 2, 3, 4, 5, 6, 8, 10, and 22.[65] The illness is characterized by an abrupt onset of fever and sore throat. There may be anorexia, dysphagia, vomiting, and abdominal pain. The pharynx is usually hyperemic, and a few (not more than 10–12) characteristic tiny discrete vesicles with a red areola occur on the anterior pillars of the fauces, the posterior pharynx, the palate, uvula,

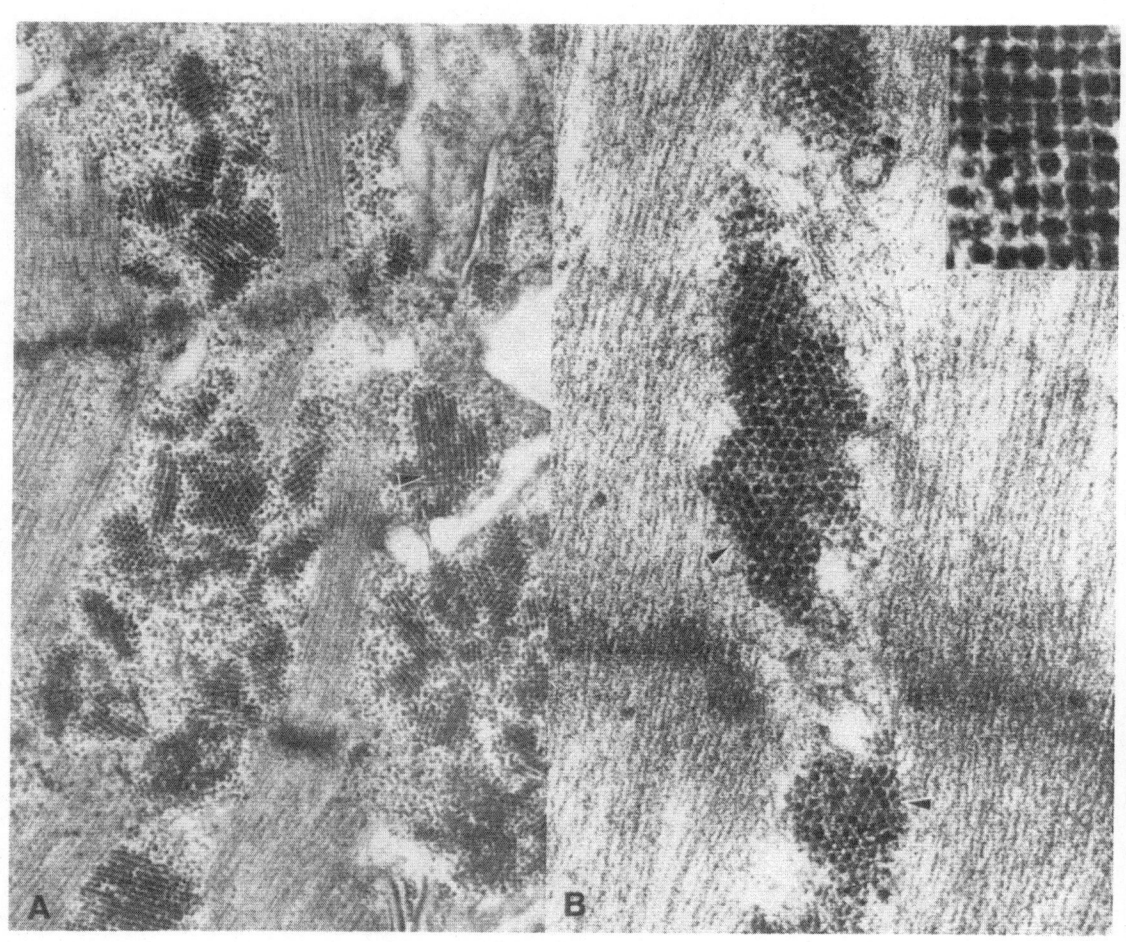

Fig. 2. High-magnification electron micrographs of muscle biopsy from a patient with a disease resembling Parkinsonism. Particles vary from round to hexagonal and are localized within muscle cells (see arrowheads). (A) × 43,000; (B) × 78,000. *Inset:* The individual particles within an array have a center-to-center distance of approximately 23 nm. × 190,000. Reproduced with permission from *Intervirology* (Gyorkey *et al.*[67]).

tonsils, or tongue. The illness is self-limited and occurs most frequently in small children.

8.1.6. Hand, Foot, and Mouth Disease. Hand, foot, and mouth disease has been associated particularly with coxsackievirus A16—which continues to predominate as the cause of numerous outbreaks—but A4, A5, A9, and A10 have also been implicated, as well as coxsackieviruses B2 and B5. Enterovirus 71 has caused a number of outbreaks of this syndrome since this virus made its appearance in the 1970s. Virus may be recovered not only from the stool and pharyngeal secretions but also from vesicular fluid. A combined syndrome has also been reported, in which vesicular lesions and pneumonia are both present.

8.1.7. Respiratory Illnesses. A number of enteroviruses have been associated with mild upper respiratory illness; among these are coxsackieviruses A2, A10, A21, A24, and B2–B5. Coxsackieviruses have also been implicated in mild lower respiratory infections, particularly in young children. There have been reports—although rare—of fatal pneumonia caused by coxsackievirus A7, in which the virus has been isolated from the lung postmortem.

Echoviruses have also been isolated in association with respiratory illnesses; these include types 1, 11, 19, 20, and 22. Except in epidemic conditions, a clear-cut causative association of the virus with the illness often cannot be established. The most certain association is with outbreaks in very young children, in whom serious or even fatal lower respiratory tract disease may be involved.

Enterovirus 68 has been associated with pneumonia and bronchiolitis in children.[191]

8.1.8. Eye Disease. Infections with some coxsackieviruses and echoviruses have been accompanied by conjunctivitis. During an epidemic in Sweden, Sandelin *et al.*[188a] recovered seven isolates of echovirus type 7 from conjunctivae; in sporadic cases, other enteroviruses (coxsackievirus B2, echovirus 11) have been recovered from eye specimens. In 1970, however, a large epidemic of acute conjunctivitis occurred in Singapore, with 60,000 cases reported; the agent was identified as a variant of coxsackievirus A24.[110,150] A similar coxsackievirus A24 outbreak was later reported to have taken place in Hong Kong in 1971.[228] This coxsackievirus A24 variant characteristically induces mild to severe conjunctivitis, but only in a minority of cases does subconjunctival hemorrhage occur; recovery is usually complete after 1–2 weeks. This virus was isolated

from conjunctival swabs or scrapings and also from throat swabs. Again in 1975, outbreaks of coxsackievirus A24 conjunctivitis were observed in Singapore[111] and in Hong Kong.[23]

In the same period as the first outbreaks of coxsackievirus A24 conjunctivitis were taking place, during 1969–1971, a pandemic of a different form of conjunctivitis was occurring in Africa, Southeast Asia (including Singapore), Japan, and India, involving tens of millions of people. The cause of this widespread disease, termed acute hemorrhagic conjunctivitis (AHC), was recognized as a new enterovirus[94,229] and was designated enterovirus type 70.[145,149] The disease is generally localized to the eye and is characterized by subconjunctival hemorrhage ranging from discrete petechiae to large blotches of frank hemorrhage covering the bulbar conjunctiva. Corneal involvement, in the form of epithelial keratitis, may occur, but is transient. The incubation period is about 24 hr, onset is sudden, and recovery is usually complete within less than 10 days. Rarely, neurological complications (acute lumbar radiculomyelopathy, cranial nerve involvement) have been observed. Motor paralysis resembling poliomyelitis is the most striking feature, and in some patients there is residual paralysis and muscle atrophy. The neurological symptoms develop up to several weeks after the onset of AHC.[92,93] In connection with this complication, it is important to note that enterovirus 70 has been shown to be neurovirulent for laboratory primates.[96] This neurological aspect occurs chiefly in adults, in contrast to the age pattern of poliomyelitis in most of the populations affected, where poliomyelitis remains a disease of early childhood. Worldwide, about 100 cases have been reported—a small number among the tens of millions of AHC cases. However, cases doubtless have gone unreported because they were unrecognized as being related to the AHC episode some weeks earlier. In any case, the potential for neurovirulence calls for careful attention to any outbreak of enterovirus 70 infection.

8.1.9. Cardiac Diseases. The etiological role of the enteroviruses in acute myocarditis and pericarditis is well established, and there are new leads that some chronic cardiovascular diseases may result from coxsackievirus B infections (see also Section 8.1.10).

a. Acute Myocardiopathy and Pericardiopathy. Coxsackievirus B infections are increasingly recognized as a cause of primary myocardial disease in adults as well as in children.[101,107] In some series, up to 39% of persons infected with coxsackievirus B5 developed cardiac abnormalities. Coxsackieviruses of group A and echoviruses have also been implicated, but to a lesser degree. In one series of patients with a clinical diagnosis of pericarditis (148 patients), myocarditis (92 patients), or pleurodynia (19 patients), 27% had IgM antibody to one of the group B coxsackieviruses—indicative of current or recent infection—as compared with 8% of the control group.[197]

Evidence for a high degree of association of virus with disease has been obtained, usually at autopsy, by demonstration of virus localized in the myocardium, endocardium, and pericardial fluid; the presence of virus at the sites of pathological change has been demonstrated by immunofluorescence, peroxidase-labeled antibody, or ferritin-labeled antibody. It has been estimated that about 5% of all symptomatic coxsackievirus infections induce heart disease. The virus may affect the endocardium, pericardium, myocardium, or all three. Acute myocardiopathies have been shown to be caused by coxsackieviruses A4, A14, A16, B1–B5, and others, and also by echovirus types 9 and 22 and others.

Monkeys infected with coxsackievirus B4 develop pancarditis, with a pathological picture strikingly similar to that of rheumatic heart disease. In experimental animals, the severity of acute viral myocardiopathy is greatly increased by vigorous exercise, hydrocortisone, alcohol consumption, pregnancy, and undernutrition and is greater in males than in females. In human illnesses, these factors may similarly increase the severity of the disease.

b. Chronic Cardiovascular Disease. After acute coxsackievirus carditis, lasting heart damage has been reported with the persistence, in diseased tissue, of viral antigen detectable by immunofluorescence. These antigens have been reported in diseased heart tissues[15] and other tissues,[14] suggesting viral persistence in the cardiovascular system. Animal studies have been more revealing. Findings in weanling mice experimentally infected with coxsackievirus B3 suggest that continuing inflammation observed following infection with this virus is an immunopathological process,[219] resulting from the cytotoxicity of immune spleen cells (T lymphocytes) against virus-infected target cardiac cells.[220] A continuing cardiac myonecrosis results from sensitized lymphocytes. (B lymphocytes and macrophages do not appear to have an important role in this process.)[106,220]

8.1.10. Neonatal Disease. Several reviews have dealt with neonatal infections by enteroviruses and also with fetal developmental defects in association with maternal enterovirus infections.[6,57,89] Neonatal infection with group B coxsackieviruses may be acquired transplacentally or—more commonly—in the birth canal or as a contact infection in the newborn nursery. The range of response is from inapparent infection to severe and even fatal disease. In the symptomatic infant, onset may be marked by lethargy, feeding difficulty, and vomiting with or without fever. In severe cases, myocarditis or pericarditis or both may develop within the first 8 days of life. Cardiac and respiratory embarrassment are indicated by tachycardia, dyspnea, cyanosis, and changes in the electrocardiogram. The clinical course may be rapidly fatal, or the patient may progress to complete recovery. Myocarditis has also been caused by some group A coxsackieviruses and echoviruses.

Studies in Colorado[98] and in Italy[154] have reemphasized coxsackievirus B infection of the neonate as having potential for severe, generalized, and fatal disease. Hemorrhagic manifestations in many organs were prominent features of necropsy findings in these studies. Myocarditis, a major feature of many early reports of neonatal coxsackievirus B infection, has been less constantly seen in recent studies, and some outbreaks have had meningitis or other disturbances as the predominant feature.

Coxsackievirus A serotypes have rarely been associated with neonatal illnesses, but echoviruses have been reported frequently in both nursery outbreaks and sporadic infections. Among the echovirus types incriminated are echoviruses 4, 9, 11, 17, 18, 19, 20, 22, and 31. Fatalities have been associated with types 9, 11, 17, 19, and 31. In 1977–1978, fatal infections with echovirus 11—several of them having an unusual pathological picture not previously reported with this virus—occurred in outbreaks in two different special-care baby units in the United Kingdom.[44,151] In several of the fatal echovirus 11 infections, necropsy showed severe hemorrhagic features.

As concerns a possible role of enteroviruses in developmental defects of the fetus, a large prospective study[12] examined enteroviral seroconversions of women during their pregnancy in relation to anomalies in their infants. In comparison to matched controls, a higher rate of infection (largely inapparent) was found in women whose offspring were abnormal; there was suggested evidence of an association between maternal infections with coxsackieviruses B2 and B4 and urogenital abnormalities and between coxsackievirus A9 infection and defects of the digestive system. Cardiovascular anomalies were associated with maternal infections by coxsackieviruses B3 and B4, and multiple infections with coxsackieviruses during pregnancy increased the likelihood of congenital heart disease in the infant. However, others found no significant associations of coxsackievirus group B infections with developmental anomalies.[181]

8.1.11. Gastrointestinal Diseases. *a. Diarrhea.* Gastrointestinal upset is commonly reported among associated symptoms in infections by a number of enteroviruses in which other clinical features predominate. In many outbreaks, the enterovirus reported may be merely a passenger virus unrelated to the illness itself. Some enteroviruses (notably echoviruses 4, 11, 14, 18, and 19) have been documented[89] in relation to outbreaks to diarrhea, but diarrhea was not invariably present in those infected. Echovirus type 20 has been associated with a febrile disease involving both the respiratory and enteric tracts. Rotaviruses are more significant in causing diarrheal disease.

b. Hepatitis. Hepatitis is known to be a part of many severe generalized infections of neonates by coxsackieviruses or other enteroviruses. Hepatitis A virus, now considered a probable member of the enterovirus group (see Table 1), is of course an important cause of this disease. It is discussed in detail in Chapter 12.

c. Pancreatitis. Pancreatitis may be a part of generalized infections of infants with coxsackievirus B agents. In one study, pancreatic damage was suggested by raised amylase levels in 31% of coxsackievirus B5 infections and 25% of coxsackievirus A9 infections, but not in infections with echovirus type 4 or 6.[153] In experimental infections of mice with coxsackieviruses of the B group, pancreatitis is a long-recognized effect.

d. Diabetes. Attention is periodically directed to the possible role of enteroviruses (particularly group B coxsackieviruses) in insulin-dependent diabetes mellitus, on the basis of reports concerning diabetic children and also of studies in experimentally infected animals.[28a,37,56,159] Although the evidence in

man is not altogether convincing as yet, coxsackie B4 has been isolated from a fatal case of diabetes in a 10-year-old boy, and the disease has been experimentally reproduced in mice with the virus isolated.[159a]

8.1.12. Summer Minor Illnesses with or without Exanthems. Enteroviruses are often isolated from patients with acute febrile illnesses of short duration and without distinctive features, occurring during the summer or fall. With some coxsackievirus serotypes, the illness in young children may be accompanied by a rubelliform rash on the face, neck, and chest; it is maculopapular, is not pruritic, and does not desquamate.

Rash is also a common manifestation of infection with echovirus type 9 (less frequently with type 4 and others); the incidence is high in young children and decreases with age. Conjunctivitis may also be present. Echovirus type 16 has been responsible for outbreaks of the maculopapular rash that characterizes "Boston exanthem disease."

8.2. Diagnosis

In view of the wide range of host response to any single enterovirus serotype, from the most common form—silent infection—to the severe diseases that may occur, diagnosis must rest on virus isolation and identification and on type-specific antibody response, as described in Section 3.5. The significance of enterovirus isolations in association with illness must be critically evaluated, for enteroviruses circulate abundantly, particularly among young children, and coincidental associations are inevitable in some instances. For example, in a series of surveys conducted in Glasgow, enteroviruses were isolated from feces of one fifth to one half of well day-nursery children less than 5 years of age, even though most specimens were obtained in nonepidemic periods.[66]

Differential diagnosis can present even greater difficulties when a community is invaded simultaneously by several enteroviruses and by other viruses with similar symptomatology, especially when some individuals are infected by both viruses, e.g., St. Louis encephalitis (SLE) virus and an enterovirus. For example, the distinction between an aseptic meningitis or encephalitis due to SLE virus and that due to an enterovirus often cannot be made on clinical grounds; firm diagnosis of singly infected patients, as well as of those with dual enterovirus–SLE infections, can be made only by utilizing the virus laboratory.[172]

To establish etiological association of an enterovirus with disease, the following criteria can be used: (1) There is a much higher rate of recovery of virus from patients with the disease than from healthy individuals of the same age and socioeconomic level living in the same area at the same time. (2) Antibodies against the virus develop during the course of the disease. If the clinical syndrome can be caused by other known agents, then virological or serological evidence must be negative for concurrent infection with such agents. (3) The virus is isolated in significant concentrations from body fluids or tissues manifesting lesions, e.g., from the cerebrospinal fluid in cases of aseptic meningitis.

9. Control and Prevention of Poliomyelitis

Both live and killed poliovirus vaccines have been used widely in the past 25 years. Formalin-killed vaccine (Salk),[187] prepared from virus grown in monkey-kidney cultures, is now little used in the United States and is extensively used only in a few European countries (Finland, Sweden, Holland) and in some parts of Canada. The inactivated polio vaccine (IPV) continues to be available in the United States in small amounts, for use under special circumstances (see Sections 9.1.1 and 9.2.2). With vaccines of the potency of those prepared in the 1950s when intensive studies were made, four inoculations were required for primary immunization, the first three at 4- to 6-week intervals and the fourth 6–12 months later. A booster dose was necessary every 2–3 years subsequently to maintain immunity. IPV induces circulating (humoral) antibodies and thus protects the CNS against subsequent invasion by wild virus. Local secretory IgA antibody or cell-mediated immunity is not induced by the killed-virus vaccine; hence, wild poliovirus can still multiply in the gut and be a source of infection to others.

After the widespread administration of killed vaccine from 1956 to 1961, paralytic poliomyelitis was greatly reduced, and many thousands of cases of paralytic disease were prevented by its use in various parts of the world. The incidence dropped dramatically in the United States, from 21,000 cases

annually seen in prevaccine years (until 1956). However, a few localized epidemics continued to occur, the cases being concentrated in slum areas among unvaccinated preschool children. Some cases continued to occur even in the vaccinated; in a study of several thousand paralytic cases, 17% were in triply vaccinated children. In 1960, despite extensive use of the killed vaccine for almost 5 years, there were still 2545 paralytic cases reported in the United States.

During 1952–1954, some of the first papers were published on attenuation of wild poliovirus for vaccine purposes,[48,118,185] and live virus vaccine candidates were then developed by a number of workers. These efforts came to fruition in 1955–1959, and large-scale field trials were held in many countries under a variety of conditions.[165] Routine use of live oral poliomyelitis vaccines was begun in many countries during the spring of 1960, and vaccines made from the Sabin strains[184] were licensed in the United States in 1961–1962. In the early years of live vaccine immunization, monovalent vaccines incorporating each serotype separately were the most commonly used, but trivalent vaccine is now used widely. Following extensive administration of live polio vaccine, cases in the United States were dramatically reduced, to an average annual total of 15 in1971–1975, and even further since that period, to 8 cases in 1976, 18 in 1977, and only 9 in 1978.

In the United States, the current recommendations for immunization against poliomyelitis are as follows: Primary immunization with trivalent oral poliovaccine (TOPV) for infants should begin at 2 months of age simultaneously with the first diphtheria–pertussis–tetanus (DPT) inoculation. The second and third doses should be given at 2-month intervals thereafter and a fourth dose at 1½ years of age. A trivalent booster is recommended for all children entering elementary school. No further boosters are recommended at present. The primary immunization schedule for children and adolescents consists of two doses of trivalent vaccine at 8-week intervals followed by a third dose 6 months to a year later.

Routine immunization for adults residing in the continental United States is not felt to be necessary because of the small risk of exposure. However, adults who are at increased risk because of contact with a patient or who are planning travel to an epidemic or endemic area should be immunized. Pregnancy is neither an indication for nor a contraindication to required immunization.

Special precautions (see below and Section 9.2.2) should be noted in considering vaccination of any person known or suspected to have a defective immune system or of the household contacts of such a person.

Both live and killed poliomyelitis virus vaccines have been used extensively over many years and have been both safe and effective. Nevertheless, a healthy respect should be maintained for the poliovirus strains used as vaccine sources, and great care must be exercised by those undertaking the manufacture or the administration of either vaccine.

No medical intervention is absolutely risk-free. Even the most common drugs carry some degree of risk. A public-health or medical judgment must be made on the basis of balancing the values and the problems of one procedure against those of another procedure and against the risks of doing nothing at all. There are advantages and disadvantages, risks and benefits, with either the killed or the live polio vaccine.

9.1. Killed Polio Vaccine (see Table 14)

9.1.1. Advantages. Properly prepared and administered, killed vaccine induces good levels of humoral antibodies in a satisfactory proportion of those receiving sufficient dosage and thus protects the vaccinee against paralytic poliomyelitis. It can also provide protection to whole populations and is believed to have limited the circulation of polioviruses in several nations that use it. However, the countries that have used it exclusively with a considerable degree of success are small nations with excellent public-health systems, where coverage by

Table 14. Killed Poliovaccine: Advantages and Problems[a]

Advantages	Problems
Confers humoral immunity in satisfactory proportion of vaccinees, if sufficient numbers of doses are given.	Several studies have indicated a disappointing record in percentage of vaccinees developing antibody after three doses.[b]
Can be incorporated into regular pediatric immunization, with other vaccinees (DPT).	Generally, repeated boosters have been required to maintain detectable antibody levels.[b]
Abscence of living virus excludes potential for mutation and reversion to virulence.	Does not induce local (intestinal) immunity in the vaccinee; hence, vaccinees do not serve as a block to infection with wild polioviruses.
Absence of living virus permits its use in immunodeficient or immunosuppressed individuals and their households.	More costly than live vaccine, in single-dose cost, administration expense, and total amount required, including boosters.
Appears to have greatly reduced the spread of polioviruses in small countries where it has been properly used (wide and frequent coverage).	Subject to problems from present and growing scarcity of monkeys (but could be resolved if high-titer virus could be grown in human diploid cells and shown in field tests with adequate numbers of persons to be free of any problems resulting from *injection* of virus grown in human cells.
May prove especially useful in certain tropical areas where live vaccine has failed to "take" in young infants.	Use of virulent polioviruses as vaccine seed creates potential for tragedy if a single failure in virus inactivation were to occur in a lot of released vaccine.

[a] From Melnick.[127] Used with permission.
[b] Some of the disappointing results in the decade after killed vaccine was introduced may have been due in part to problems that may now have been corrected.

the killed vaccine has been wide and frequent, reaching 90% or more of the target population.

Killed vaccine, since it contains no living virus, cannot mutate toward increasing virulence. Because living virus is absent, it is safe to administer killed vaccine to persons with immune deficiency diseases and to their families and to persons undergoing immunosuppressive therapy. Killed vaccine might be combined with DPT vaccines and incorporated into an immunization schedule for infants and young children. Such a combination program of "quadruple" vaccine administration can be especially helpful in certain tropical areas where there have been failures of live poliomyelitis vaccine to "take" in infants.[126] Although the killed-virus vaccine may not confer intestinal resistance to carriage and spread of virulent live virus in the community, the neutralizing antibody it elicits would provide protection against paralysis even if vaccinated children were to become infected with a wild virulent virus. On a philosophical level, it has the advantage of not introducing into the community any living virus that can spread in an uncontrolled fashion to persons other than those who have sought or agreed to receive the live vaccine.

9.1.2. Disadvantages. The licensing of killed vaccine was preceded by an immense nationwide trial in the United States, in which vaccine was administered to several hundred thousand children. Yet immediately after the success of the trial had been reported and the vaccine licensed, 61 cases of paralytic poliomyelitis appeared in vaccine recipients and 80 cases in their family contacts. These cases were epidemiologically linked to certain lots of vaccine subsequently found to contain small amounts of live, virulent poliovirus that had been undetected by the manufacturer. The breakdown in safety procedures that allowed the live virus to remain in the final vaccine was due to problems of transferring laboratory procedures to manufacturing production processes, particularly of extrapolating inactivation data. These problems were resolved, and there have been no further reports of any residual live-virus problems with any inactivated poliomyelitis vaccines manufactured according to well-standardized procedures.

In some studies, disappointingly low proportions of vaccinees developed antibodies after three inoculations of the killed vaccine. Some of these problems with immunogenicity may have been due primarily to difficulties that have now been corrected in the areas still using inactivated vaccines. For example, after the early manufacturing defect that sometimes allowed residual live virus to be present, an extra filtration step was included in the processing. This reduced the concentration of viral antigen in the vaccines, and consequently diminished their potency, during the 1950s.

Killed vaccines have usually required continued administration of booster doses at various intervals. This situation is conducive to a decline of immunity levels in the population over a period of time because the required booster schedule may be neglected or overlooked by families, and by physicians also, particularly in relatively mobile populations like that of the United States. Booster doses also add to the cost of the vaccine and its administration.

In Sweden, Finland, The Netherlands, and two provinces of Canada (Ontario and Nova Scotia), the current poliomyelitis immunization programs rely on killed vaccine alone. A survey in 1969 and 1970 in Ontario indicated serious gaps in the antibody protection of children who had received only IPV, while almost all those who had received both killed and live vaccines had antibodies to all three poliovirus types.[113] The investigators predicted that immunity in the school-age population would decline to a dangerous level unless live vaccine were used after immunization with killed vaccine.

One argument often given for the use of killed-virus vaccine is that although serum antibody may be at very low or even undetectable levels, there is an enduring "immunological memory." This state, not measured by antibody tests, is said to enable the vaccinee to make a very quick and high-titer antibody response on further exposure to the virus.[188] Lack of serum antibody indeed may not indicate complete lack of protection against clinical illness. However, serum antibodies do contribute to the prevention of viremia and therefore minimize the possibility that the nervous system will be invaded. It is therefore risky to assume that protection exists when serum antibody cannot be demonstrated.

Another problem associated with immunity following the administration of killed poliomyelitis vaccine is that although humoral antibodies are induced, local (intestinal) immunity is not. Hence, wild polioviruses can still multiply in the intestinal tract of the vaccinees and be a source of infection to others.

There had been several reports that killed vaccine alone could provide complete protection to whole national populations. However—as mentioned above—these reports were based on the experience of small countries with excellent national-health programs covering the entire population and ensuring administration of full primary vaccination and frequent booster dosage. In Finland and Sweden up to 1977, no paralytic poliomyelitis had been reported for more than a decade, and in the Netherlands, for a number of years only rare sporadic cases had been seen—in unvaccinated persons, chiefly within religious communities having low vaccine acceptance rates because of their religious beliefs. It has been suggested that the reason so little poliovirus has been found in these nations is that they are adjacent to countries where live vaccine continues to be widely distributed and that opportunities for the importation of wild polioviruses are thus reduced.

However, early in 1977, two cases occurred in Sweden, and a number of poliovirus carriers were detected in the area. The patients had no history of vaccination; this was also true of most of the carriers. And in 1978, the Netherlands experienced an epidemic of type 1 poliomyelitis, in which a total of 110 cases were reported[222]; 80 patients had paralysis; of these 67 had spinal paralysis, 7 had bulbar paralysis, and 6 had both bulbar and spinal involvement. All patients were members of a religious group that had refused vaccination. This outbreak occurred in a country with a very high polio vaccine acceptance rate; of persons under 27 years of age, 93% had received between three and six doses of killed-poliovirus vaccine. No cases were reported among vaccinated persons. Until 1978, cases in the Netherlands had occurred only in municipalities with overall vaccination acceptance rates lower than 50–60%. However, some of the municipalities involved in the 1978 outbreak had high vaccine acceptance rates, that is, some of the cases occurred in areas where a high degree of herd immunity in the general population might have been thought to protect unvaccinated individuals. However, the 70,000 persons in the religious group that refused vaccine perhaps should be viewed as a single co-herent population, because of their frequent in-group contacts. It should be noted that all the cases in 1978 occurred among this particular group of unvaccinated persons and that no polio cases were reported in the far larger number of 350,000 unvaccinated persons scattered throughout the country who are not members of these religious groups. It is also noteworthy that in nursery and primary schools in the affected communities, about 24% of the vaccinated and 71% of the nonvaccinated children tested were excreting the wild poliovirus.

Clearly, a great deal of population protection has been conferred in the Netherlands by their immunization program. But despite the high vaccination rate in the general population, virulent wild type 1 poliovirus was able to enter the country and travel in a narrow stream among susceptibles within these close-knit subpopulations. In unvaccinated members of this same religious group in Canada, there were also several paralytic type 1 cases in 1978, and a number of persons investigated in the patients' households and communities were also infected with this virus—one found to belong antigenically to the same subtype as the Dutch strains.[55,208] Two of the Canadian patients were known to have been in close contact with visitors from the affected communities in The Netherlands.

9.2. Live Attenuated Polio Vaccine (see Table 15)

9.2.1. Advantages. This vaccine is given by the oral route. It infects, multiplies, and thus immunizes. In simulating the natural poliovirus infection, it confers long-lasting (possibly even lifelong) immunity. Like the natural infection, it quickly stimulates the development of circulating antibody.

In addition to inducing humoral immunity, live poliovaccine also induces a state of resistance of the intestinal tract, which subsequently tends to block the spread of circulating poliovirus in the community. Indeed, it is postulated[232] that because of this intestinal resistance, the administration of live polio vaccine has already brought about a break in the chain of transmission of polioviruses within the United States, halting the perpetuation of wild polioviruses in this country. Intestinal resistance after administration of live virus vaccine seems to be dependent on the extent of initial vaccine virus

Table 15. Live Poliovaccine: Advantages and Problems[a]

Advantages	Problems
Confers both humoral and intestinal immunity, like natural infection.	Being living viruses, the vaccine viruses do mutate, and in rare instances have reverted toward neurovirulence sufficiently to cause paralytic polio in recipients or their contacts.
Immunity induced may be lifelong.	
Induces antibody very quickly in a large proportion of vaccinees.	
Oral administration is more acceptable to vaccinees than injection and easier to accomplish.	Vaccine progeny virus spreads to household contacts.[b]
Administration does not require use of highly trained personnel.	Vaccine progeny virus also spreads to persons in the community who have not agreed to be vaccinated.[b]
When stabilized, can retain potency under difficult field conditions with little refrigeration and no freezers.	In certain warm-climate countries, induction of antibodies in a satisfactorily high proportion of vaccinees has been difficult to accomplish unless repeated doses are administered. In some areas, even repeated administration has not been effective.
Under epidemic conditions, not only induces antibody quickly but also rapidly infects the alimentary tract, blocking spread of the epidemic virus.	
Is relatively inexpensive, both to produce the vaccine itself and to administer it, and does not require continued booster doses.	Contraindicated in those with immunodeficiency diseases, and in their household associates, as well as in persons undergoing immunosuppressive therapy.
Can be prepared in human cells, thus is not dependent on continuing large supplies of scarce monkeys. This also eliminates theoretical risk of including monkey virus contaminants in the vaccine.	

[a] From Melnick.[127] Used with permission.
[b] Some people consider this spread into the community to be an advantage, but the progeny virus excreted and spread by vaccinees is often a mutated virus. Obviously, it cannot be a safety-tested vaccine, licensed for use in the general population.

multiplication in the alimentary tract, rather than on serum antibody level.

Under epidemic conditions, live vaccine has the advantage of inducing immunity rapidly.[231] Furthermore, by quickly infecting the enteric tract, the vaccine strains tend to preempt this site in many persons in the population, interfering with and halting further spread of the epidemic virus—often within a matter of days, even before the vaccine-induced immunity becomes fully effective.

In a well-vaccinated country, repeated booster doses of live vaccine after the initial childhood series are seldom considered necessary. Since the live vaccine is given orally, it is easy and inexpensive to administer and is more acceptable in many populations. It is also more practical for mass administration and can be readily taken to remote areas and given rapidly without requiring the services of large numbers of skilled personnel. Furthermore, it is much less expensive than the inactivated vaccine, both in terms of single-dose costs and administration and in terms of the total amount needed to establish and maintain adequate immunity.

For use in warm countries under conditions of mass administration and in remote field clinics where refrigeration is limited or nonexistent, stabilizers are available to protect the potency of live poliovirus vaccines against thermal inactivation.[129]

Another advantage of live vaccine is that it does not depend on a supply of scarce monkeys, except for neurovirulence testing. Initially, oral poliomyelitis vaccine was prepared in monkey-kidney cultures, but more recently human diploid-cell cultures have been used, and human diploid-cell lines are now licensed for vaccine production. This is desirable because of the possibility that the supply of suitable monkeys from the wild may be greatly curtailed. Also, the use of monkey tissues carries possible hazards (e.g., unknown viral contaminants such as the dangerous Marburg virus) that would not exist with human cells. The most thoroughly studied human diploid-cell lines are WI-38 and MRC-5; these cells have been found free of microbial contamination and can be held frozen until needed for vaccine production. Safety testing of such a cell stock can be far more complete than the testing that is possible within the relatively brief life-span of primary cultures such as those from monkey kidney. However, current studies with monkeys bred in captivity, in which the kidneys of newborn animals are used for vaccine production, indicate another economically feasible option.

9.2.2. Disadvantages. While the spread of live vaccine virus from the vaccinee to household and community contacts is considered by some to be an advantage, in that it may provide "free immunization" to larger numbers of persons, the fact remains that the virus that spreads to the contacts is not a licensed vaccine. Vaccine virus progeny excreted by the vaccinees is known to mutate, and it is theoretically possible that it could revert sufficiently toward neurovirulence to cause paralytic poliomyelitis in the contacts of the vaccinee. All strains of poliovirus, regardless of how highly attenuated, retain the property of multiplying in and destroying cells in the monkey spinal cord—the crucial test used to determine whether a strain is sufficiently attenuated and safe for vaccine use. The degree to which monkey neurotropism is retained, however, varies over an enormous (millionfold) range from the virulent strains to the highly attenuated ones suitable for vaccine seed. The techniques used in recognizing and certifying vaccine strains for safety are such that different degrees of neurotropism, even among attenuated strains, can be detected. For example, it has been found that vaccine progeny virus after multiplication in the vaccinees, although still attenuated, would no longer pass the safety tests required of the vaccine itself. The viruses, particularly type 3, do mutate in the course of their multiplication in vaccinated children, and rare cases of paralytic poliomyelitis have occurred in recipients or in their household contacts. It is for this reason that when a developed nation or region begins administration of oral poliomyelitis vaccines, the initial program should be conducted in intensive campaigns designed for mass immunization of the entire population of an area at the same time; thus, the polioviruses that would infect virtually the entire population of all ages would be the certified and tested vaccine viruses themselves, rather than untested progeny viruses excreted by vaccinees. At the minimum, all susceptible members of a family, including the parents, should be vaccinated simultaneously. Once the bulk of the population in an area has been immunized, subsequent routine immunizations can be limited to babies and young children. This procedure should be sufficient, so long as a large proportion of the children (80–90%) do indeed receive the complete course.

When a developing country begins administration of oral poliomyelitis vaccine, the initial program should be conducted in intensive campaigns designed to immunize the entire child population of 3–24 months of age at the same time. If serological surveys or clinical disease indicate risk to younger or older children, the age limits of the populations to be vaccinated may be altered accordingly, from 1 to 36 months of age.

Epidemiological data indicate that the instances in which the live vaccine virus has reverted to neurovirulence and attacked vaccinees or their close contacts are exceedingly rare. Recently, in the United States, new discussions and arguments have arisen from proposals that killed vaccines be reestablished for general use in this country. The argument for killed vaccines has included reference to the "dangers" of the live vaccine. It is important to reemphasize what has repeatedly been stated by many different national and international groups of experts: a vaccine that in the United States produces, at most, 1 case per 11.5 million vaccinees (and 1 case per 3.9 million contacts) is far from "dangerous," but rather is outstandingly safe, as well as effective. Corresponding figures calculated for the United Kingdom since 1967 are similar—about 1 case in a recipient and 2 cases in contacts per 10 million doses distributed.[29] Indeed, the actual number of vaccine-induced cases is probably even smaller than these figures indicate, for the assignment of "vaccine-associated" status to a paralytic case means only that on the basis of the temporal relationship of vaccination and onset of the illness, the vaccine *cannot be ruled out* as a possible cause.

Because of the need to monitor the characteristics

of polioviruses isolated from persons who have received live vaccine—and particularly from those few who develop paralytic poliomyelitis or whose contacts develop poliomyelitis—there have been many efforts to design laboratory tests capable of indicating whether a poliovirus isolate is vaccine-derived or is a wild virus. A number of such "marker" tests have been used, but their results cannot give absolute answers and some investigators consider them of little help, at least in deciding whether a particular case of poliomyelitis is vaccine-derived. They can contribute toward designating a particular virus excreted by a vaccinee or a contact as "vaccine-like" or "non-vaccine-like," but the former does not necessarily mean that the virus was derived from the vaccine virus, for there are wild polioviruses with similar "marker" properties. Results of the currently available marker tests cannot, by themselves, indicate whether vaccine virus progeny caused the illness. At best, such markers can be used only by highly experienced investigators, together with other information about the history of a particular poliomyelitis case, to make an informed judgment as to whether the case was "probably vaccine-caused" or "probably caused by a wild virus." [152] Among the methods for intratypic differentiation of poliovirus strains that have been collaboratively evaluated in WHO laboratories, antigenic characterization with cross-adsorbed immune sera was the most dependable. [208] As regards determining the degree of virulence of a poliovirus strain (whether vaccine-derived or wild), the monkey neurovirulence test, conducted by inoculating monkeys and evaluating the results according to precise and standardized procedures, is the only test that can truly distinguish virulent and attenuated strains.

A detailed study has been under way since 1969, conducted by a WHO Committee specifically charged "to investigate the possible relationship between acute persisting spinal paralysis and the use of poliomyelitis vaccine (oral)." In reporting on the first 5 years of their studies, the group states: "The findings of this report confirm . . . that poliomyelitis vaccines (oral) made from the Sabin attenuated strains are among the safest vaccines in use today. . . ." [221]

The classification of cases, in general closely following the pattern used in the Neurotropic Viral Diseases Surveillance program of the U.S. Center for Disease Control, includes "recipient" vaccine-associated case (one in which illness begins 7–30 days after receiving the vaccine), "contact" vaccine-associated case (one in which the patient is known to have been in contact with a vaccinee and becomes ill 7–60 days after the vaccinee received the vaccine), "possible contact" case (no known contact with a vaccinee but occurring in an area and time of mass vaccination), and "no known contact" case (paralysis occurring with no known contact in an area where intensive vaccination is not in progress or where routine vaccination can be given any time during the year).

In an evaluation of the study, a coherent picture has begun to emerge, despite different methods of investigation and reporting among the participating countries. During the first 5 years of the study, 360 cases of paralytic poliomyelitis were assessed; 155 were classed as "no known contact" and appeared to have been due to wild viruses still circulating in these communities. In the participating countries (in which more than 191 million doses of vaccine were given during the period under review), there remained 205 cases that had at least a possible association with live poliomyelitis vaccines. The rates in recipients and contacts were usually less than 1 per million doses distributed. Most of the cases in the recipient groups occurred in children under 5 years of age, but in the contact groups, there was a difference in the age grouping of the cases between short-campaign countries and countries conducting vaccination throughout the year: in the countries such as the United States that vaccinate throughout the year, many of the contact cases occurred in the nonimmune parents of recently vaccinated infants, whereas in the short-campaign countries, most contact cases occurred in children under 5 years of age. However, the pattern of parents as contact cases may be changing, since in 1977 none of 50 reported vaccine-associated cases was in an adult. The shift in age distribution was striking in that more than half the reported cases were in infants less than 1 year old, and all but two of the others were 1–4 years of age.

In warm-climate countries, there is some evidence that live poliomyelitis vaccines do not induce antibody production in as high a proportion of vaccinees as in areas with more temperate climates. This lower rate of vaccine "take" has been ascribed to various possible factors, including interference from other enteric viruses already present in the intestinal tract.

Interference can be an important problem in warm-climate regions where enteroviruses are abundant.[166] Other factors that have been suggested as possibly responsible for this problem are: the presence of antibody in breast milk, the presence of cellular resistance in the intestinal tract owing to previous exposure to naturally circulating polioviruses (or perhaps related viruses), or the presence of an inhibitor (saliva) in the alimentary tract of infants in these areas that acts against multiplication of the vaccine virus.[26,45]

For the present, practical experience has shown that a high level of population immunity can be achieved in some warm-climate countries by use of repeated doses of standard live vaccine alone, if given on a regular basis to infants and young children. Furthermore, live vaccine has been shown to be as effective a means of cutting short an epidemic in a warm-climate country as it is in a temperate-climate country when given, preferably in repeated doses, to a high proportion of the presumed susceptible population in an epidemic area.[26,231] However, in certain areas where multiple doses of live vaccine have not succeeded in adequately immunizing infants, a program for inoculating killed vaccine, or for administering killed vaccine together with scheduled feedings of live vaccine, should be considered for use until this special problem can be overcome.[60,126] Early indications suggest that the combination of vaccines can be successful in controlling poliomyelitis in such areas.

In making recommendations for vaccination, and also in evaluating vaccine-associated cases, it is important to emphasize the hazards of administering live vaccines to persons with immune-system problems. These include not only patients with immunodeficiency disease but also persons with altered immune states resulting from other diseases or from immunosuppressive therapeutic procedures. In the United States during 1961–1971, there were 73 poliomyelitis cases among vaccine recipients and 37 cases among contacts. Nearly 10% of these cases were in persons with immune-system disorders, an incidence almost 10,000 times greater than in normal persons.[227] Cases associated with vaccination in persons with immune-system problems have continued to be reported, with 10 additional patients identified in the nation through 1976.[21,226]

Without discounting the tragedy involved for the individual child and family who suffer in the ex-ceedingly rare instance when an immunodeficient individual encounters and succumbs to infection by vaccine or vaccine progeny virus, it must be recognized that some of these children are notoriously subject to infection—which is frequently fatal—by a wide variety of normally benign or avirulent agents.[218,235] Clearly, if compromised immune-system function is known or even suspected in potential vaccinees or their siblings, live poliomyelitis vaccine should not be given. However, unless other circumstances have brought the condition to light, such an immune-system problem is usually not known by the time the first routine vaccine doses are given at about 2 months of age.

9.3. Conclusions on Polio Vaccines and Their Future Use

The advantages and disadvantages of killed and live polio vaccines need to be weighed with respect to the particular setting in which a vaccine is used. Since killed vaccine has proved to be effective in preventing poliomyelitis outbreaks in small countries with very competent and thorough vaccination programs, there seems to be no reason for them to change. But by the same token, since live virus vaccines have been working superbly for 20 years in the United States, the U.S.S.R., most other European countries, the United Kingdom, Australia, and Japan, as well as in many other countries around the world, it would be unwise to interfere with these programs, which involve hundreds of millions of persons.

If a national-health service elected to recommend a change from live to killed vaccine, then a new and untried situation would exist in that country's defenses against poliomyelitis. Urgent new questions would have to be raised that have never been fully answered in the particular national settings concerned, especially in large countries with voluntary health systems: Would individuals maintain their immunity adequately by returning for repeated booster injections? Would immunity induced by killed vaccine, even if sufficient to protect the individual from paralytic poliomyelitis, be able to block the circulation of wild viruses in large and mobile populations as effectively as the live vaccine? Would the extra costs for vaccine, for its administration, and for repeated booster inoculations be justified? In nations where live vaccine has already proved to be effective and safe, are there not other health programs far more urgently in need of the extra funds that would be required for implementation of a killed polio vaccine program?

There is a considerable question whether the United States could ever achieve the high levels of over 90% polio vaccine acceptance that have been characteristic of those countries that depend on killed virus vaccine. In the United States, immunization ultimately depends on the initiative of the family in seeking care either from a private physician or from a public-health clinic. Furthermore, it is difficult to hope that so large a proportion of families would maintain the needed schedule for repeated killed vaccine doses and boosters in a mobile population where a young family is quite likely to move several times during a child's preschool years, changing physicians at each move.

In some tropical areas where it is known that repeated administration of live virus vaccines has not provided full protection, killed vaccine should be incorporated into the initial phases of the poliovirus vaccination programs.

Some new techniques are being explored toward improving killed-virus vaccines. One approach has been to obtain a very high concentration of virus, purify it, and then prepare a subunit vaccine that contains no viral nucleic acid but only selected polypeptides that are antigenically active. This would not really be a killed-virus vaccine but an alternative to either killed-virus or live-virus vaccine. It would be a vaccine made up of a purified antigenic component, containing virtually no extraneous material except the precise components needed to stimulate good immunity. Just such a polypeptide preparation is being studied in one of the promising approaches to a vaccine against hepatitis B.

Recombinant DNA techniques have recently opened the way to prepare, in *Escherichia coli*, polypeptide vaccines containing only the essential immunogenic components. For a DNA virus like hepatitis B, the essential portion of the viral genetic material can be inserted into an *E. coli* plasmid or phage.[53] For an RNA virus like poliovirus, the *complementary* DNA (cDNA) of the virus is first prepared from viral RNA by use of the reverse transcriptase enzyme. The entire cDNA of poliovirus—or a part of it—is then inserted into the phage for replication in *E. coli*. Subsequent transcription and translation of the viral genetic material under controlled conditions will yield the desired polypeptide vaccine free of any potentially infectious poliovirus nucleic acid.

9.4. Current Status of Immunity against Poliomyelitis in the United States

Following the introduction of live poliovirus vaccine, during 1961–1965, the annual number of paralytic cases in the United States decreased to 465, and in subsequent years, the rates have ranged from 50 to as low as 9 in 1978.

The general trends established with the introduction of polio vaccines are overwhelmingly favorable, and eradication of poliomyelitis has been discussed as a conceivable future goal. But serological surveys as well as surveys of vaccination status in the United States have revealed a downward trend since 1964 in the percentage of young children (1–4 years of age) who have antibody to all three poliovirus types and in the percentage who have been fully vaccinated. Whereas 87% of this age group had received a full course of vaccine in 1964, this declined to only 67% in 1971. The problem of susceptibility is even more pronounced among preschool children who live in the inner-city and other areas where the environment is characterized by poverty and associated deficiencies of health care. Surveys in 1971 showed that only 40% of this population had been fully vaccinated; in nonpoverty areas, only 68% had received adequate immunization. Again in 1976, a national survey by interview revealed that 38% of children of ages 1–4 years in the United States had no history of primary vaccination against poliomyelitis; the vaccination rates among infants and young children in disadvantaged urban and rural areas were even lower.[21]

The risks that are implied by these vaccination deficits apparently have been somewhat alleviated by the fact that—like it or not—live-virus polio vaccine does spread to unvaccinated contacts. A higher degree of population protection against wild polioviruses has been observed than would be expected on the basis of vaccination histories. The decline in poliovirus vaccination rates in the United States has been roughly paralleled by a decrease in rates of vaccination against measles. Following this decline in vaccination delivery, the incidence of measles has greatly increased, but no such increased incidence has occurred with poliomyelitis, and the numbers of poliomyelitis cases continue to be exceedingly low—averaging less than 10 per year since 1973. The circulation of wild polioviruses, known to be imported regularly—chiefly from Mexico—seems to have been effectively blocked, an effect consonant with greater population immunity than could be expected from the numbers of vaccinees alone. However, with the likelihood of virulent poliovirus importations continuing to exist, vigilance cannot be relaxed, and high levels of vaccination remain a necessity to ensure that paralytic poliomyelitis does not reemerge.

The prevalence and levels of poliovirus antibody in the population are not reassuring. The magnitude of danger that can exist is indicated in Figure 3, in which the percentages of children *lacking* antibody in various age groups are shown both for 1963, shortly after a large community-wide vaccination program had been conducted, and for 1968, after 5 years in which there had been no widely publicized mass campaign. The children studied were from low-income families to whom polio vaccine is freely available provided that they attend public health clinics and ask for it and were from the same population sector in both years. Immunization histories obtained in 1968 showed that the sole polio vaccination experience of many children, even those of school age, consisted of the single series of monovalent vaccines they had received during the 1962 mass campaign. Three paralytic poliomyelitis cases occurred in the Houston area in late 1968 and early 1969, all in nonvaccinated infants less than 1 year of age, from the low-income group.

Marked decline of antibody titers to low levels has been documented in some follow-up studies of individual vaccinees,[3,17,105] but studies in other areas and groups have shown high antibody prevalence among young children in some localities[76] and persistence of antibodies, although at low titers, 8–10 years after vaccination.[183,189] Where antibodies persist, there may well have been reinforcement of immunity by exposure to circulating virus, either wild or vaccine strains, within the community.

Most evaluations of current immune status have focused on children or on those previously vaccinated in their early childhood. There is now some reason for concern that the immune status of the general population could be tending toward hazard in the postvaccine era, contrary to the hopes that older persons would be protected by the barrier of herd immunity and by indirect immunization through spread of attenuated virus from vaccinees. Some of the reports of vaccine-associated cases of poliomyelitis have been in adult contacts, particularly the parents, of young vaccinees. Poliovirus antibody prevalence and levels found in sera from persons of all age groups in Tecumseh, Michigan, indicate several problems in this regard.[160] Disturbing proportions of children were susceptible to at least one poliovirus type, and significantly more 5- to 9-year-olds were susceptible in 1971 (40%) than in 1966 (25%). Fewer susceptibles were found in those between 10 and 29 years of age, but in those 30 years of age and older, there was seen a progressive increase in susceptibles with age, up to 60%, and in those who did possess antibody, titers were very low. The greater protection among those 10–29 years old may reflect sources of immunization that are not necessarily continuing with the same intensity at the present time: immunization by broadly circulating wild poliovirus in their prevaccine childhood, special attention as priority vaccinees during the periods of enhanced emphasis immediately after the inactivated and then the live vaccine became available, and indirect immunization or boostering by spread of vaccine virus from their own young children. The decreased antibody among the older groups in the Michigan study probably reflects not only smaller numbers who have ever received vaccine but also longer periods of time since either naturally acquired or vaccine-induced immunity has been reinforced by reexposure to circulating virus.

Decline of antibody levels after 5 or 6 years has also been reported among 175 children who were studied in 1974 at the time of receiving a booster dose of TOPV at various intervals (less than 6 months up to more than 9 years) after their primary series. Prior to the booster, antibody was at undetectable levels (less than 1:2) in a number of the children, and postbooster antibody responses of those with low prior titers indicated that intestinal infection by the booster vaccine virus had taken place.[3] The antibody in the postbooster sera was IgG in those tested, precluding initial vaccine failure as the cause of the low titers. Because the vaccine virus was able to multiply in the intestinal tracts of a number of these vaccinees, the authors speculate that wild polioviruses might also be able to multiply in vaccinees whose antibody levels had greatly declined with time. Whether the virus could also pro-

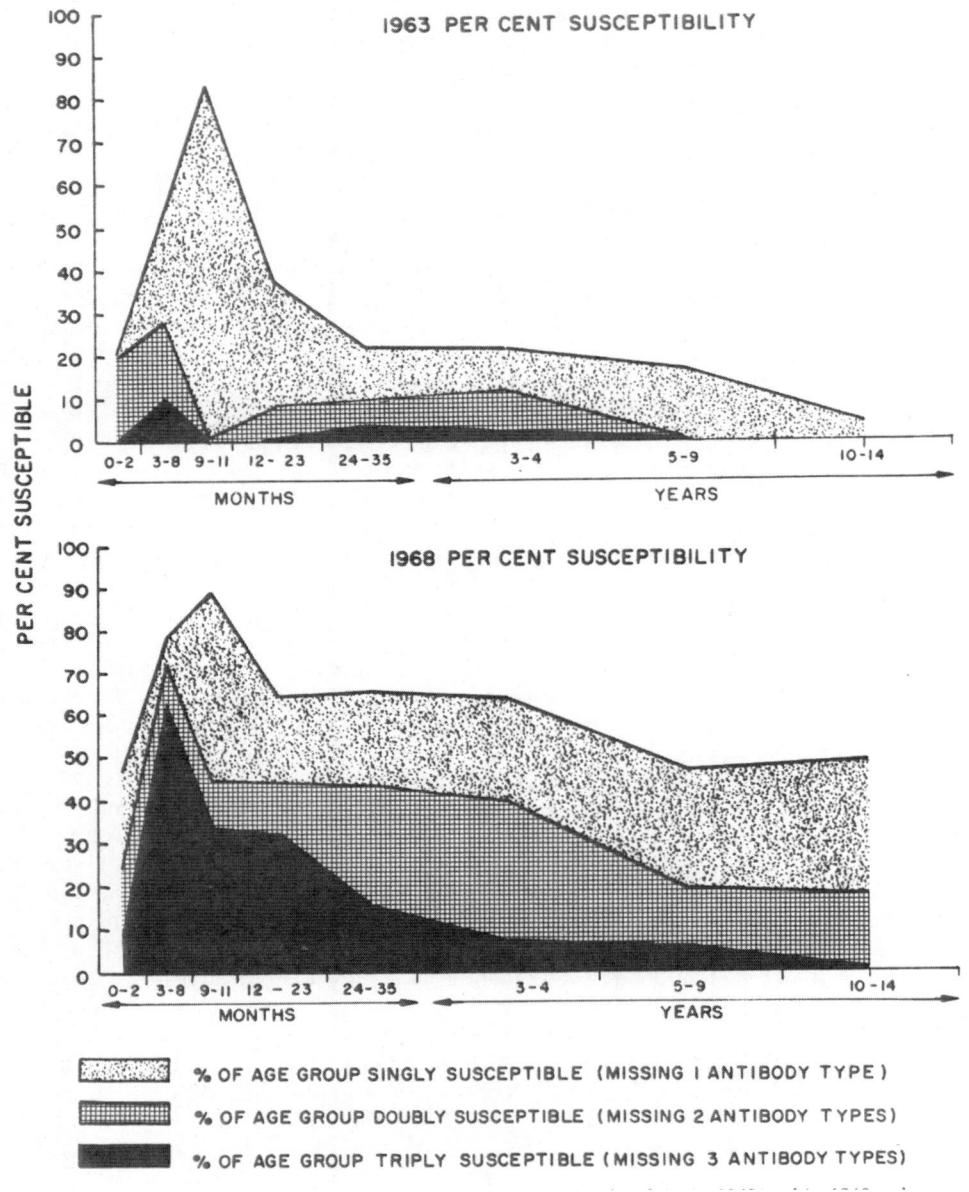

Fig. 3. Percentage of each age group in low-income Houston families, in 1963 and in 1968, who were susceptible to one or more types of poliovirus, as measured by lack of type-specific antibody. From Melnick et al.[130]

duce viremia and even invade the CNS of the vaccinee is not known, but in any case, the frequency of intestinal susceptibility serves as a warning: those vaccinated in the past with live poliovaccine do not necessarily maintain antibody sufficient to constitute an impermeable barrier to the spread of wild virus that might be introduced into the community. On the basis of these findings, consideration should be given to administering a booster vaccination of TOPV 5–6 years after the last dose received.

A survey of 268 U.S. Army recruits in 1976 indicated that 8.2, 8.6, and 11.6% lacked serum neutralizing antibodies to poliovirus types 1, 2, and 3, respectively; 20.9% of those studied lacked antibody to at least one type.[15a] It is not clear from these data whether the lack of antibody resulted entirely from lack of adequate immunization or was due in part to waning of antibody levels with time since vaccination. In view of the susceptibility of about 20% of the new recruits to at least one type of poliovirus and the recognized laxity of vaccination practices among the civilian population of the United States, it has been recommended that the current practice be continued for administering a primary immunization sequence of oral poliovaccine to all new armed forces recruits and that surveillance of immunity to polioviruses be maintained.

Passive immunization by administration of γ-globulin can provide protection for a few weeks against the paralytic disease, but does not prevent subclinical infection. The dose is about 0.14 ml per lb, intramuscularly. γ-Globulin is effective only if given shortly before infection; it is of no value after clinical symptoms of the disease are apparent.

9.5. "Social Failures" of Polio Vaccine Administration

most countries in which polio vaccine is widely used, circulation of wild polioviruses has been suppressed, but these viruses have not been eliminated from the world. In the United States within the past decade, virulent wild polioviruses have been detected in sewage[64] and also, unfortunately, in paralyzed children.[130] The presence in the world of virulent wild polioviruses that can be imported all too easily into even the most fully vaccinated countries was also demonstrated once again in the 1978 outbreak in the Netherlands, which spread to Canada,[55,227] and the early 1979 infections in the United

States[22]—all in populations unvaccinated or inadequately vaccinated because of religious beliefs. Even if the future may hold hope for worldwide eradication of poliomyelitis, virulent polioviruses, still endemic in many parts of the world and producing many tens of thousands of cases each year, remain a very real and present threat.

In the United States, in contrast to the prevaccine epidemic phase of poliomyelitis (in which older groups were chiefly affected), the postvaccine era is marked by the young age of the polio victims, who mostly are unimmunized infants and preschool children, often those in "inner-city" or other poverty areas. Thus, in some parts of this country, vaccination has not established sufficient "herd immunity" of the general population to constitute a solid barrier that would fully block circulation of wild viruses and thereby indirectly protect even unvaccinated susceptibles. Instead, it has reduced wild-virus circulation sufficiently to minimize the early natural infections that might otherwise have immunized these same disadvantaged children. Children of higher socioeconomic groups are no longer unprotected because almost all are fully vaccinated in infancy: these advantaged children now become victims of polio only in extraordinary circumstances, such as refusal of vaccination because of religious beliefs.[97,214] But in the absence of more effective efforts to provide early and complete vaccination for infants and young children of lower socioeconomic groups, large numbers of such children are not now receiving adequate vaccination. These children are growing up susceptible and are at risk to paralytic poliomyelitis should they encounter virulent polioviruses—even if these viruses may now be entirely imported, or mutated vaccine virus progeny, as has been speculated.[232]

As indicated above, serious deficits have been documented in regard both to immunization histories and to antibody levels in the United States. A similar picture is seen in some of the other "well-vaccinated" countries. For example, in the early 1970s in the United Kingdom, only 49% of 75 nursery-school children surveyed in one district of Glasgow had antibody to all three types of poliovirus; 54% of the children with a history of immunization lacked triple immunity.[174] Immunization acceptance rates have continued to be low in some sectors of the United Kingdom population, and antibody protection is also low. Among the 26 victims of paralytic poliomyelitis reported in the United Kingdom for the two years 1976 and 1977, most (19) had never received any vaccine or were incompletely vaccinated.[29] In one study of polio immunity, tests were made of more than 1000 sera collected during a 10-month period in 1976–1977 from persons of all age groups in England and Wales.[27] Among children 1–5 years of age, only 43% had antibody to all three poliovirus types, and 25% lacked antibody to any poliovirus type. Among those 5–19 years of age, 40% were triply immune, and 17% were completely lacking in poliovirus antibody. In all adult age groups except those 30–39 years of age, at least 15% entirely lacked polio antibodies, and the proportion of triply immune persons ranged from just under to just over 50% of each group.

Lack of serum antibody may not indicate complete lack of protection against clinical illness. Antibody may be present but at low levels undetectable by commonly used testing methods, or local secretory antibodies may afford protection in the absence of detectable circulating antibody.[162] However, serum antibodies do contribute to the prevention of viremia and therefore minimize the possibility of invasion of the CNS (see Section 7). It is thus misleading to assume that adequate protection is present when serum antibody cannot be demonstrated.

Thus, at least two factors contribute to the development of deficiencies in the immune status of populations: (1) failure to obtain proper vaccination, which can lead to the development of pockets of susceptibles even within a "well-vaccinated" community; and (2) decline of antibody levels in individuals with passage of time after vaccination. Declining antibody titers may become even more common if virus circulation is indeed greatly reduced. If the trend continues or increases for less solid immunity among children, the way could become open for introduction and wide circulation of wild polioviruses in the general population, with outbreaks in which paralytic poliomyelitis could once again become prevalent among nonimmune adolescents and adults.

Immunity levels in all age groups can and should be monitored by periodic serological surveys to detect conditions of risk before poliomyelitis epidemics reappear. Because a large proportion of poliovirus infections are silent and subclinical, imported viruses could become widely disseminated before the first sign of their presence appeared in the form of paralyzed children and adults. Such epidemics would be even more tragic than those of the 1940–1950 era, for now—with the means of prevention readily at hand—a resurgence of paralytic poliomyelitis would reflect not "vaccine failures" but social failures. The central-city poverty areas depend chiefly on the public sector for health-care delivery. More effective efforts of both public and private-practice health professionals are needed to contribute toward community awareness of what care is available, when and how it can be obtained, and why it is needed. Cross-cultural failures of communication contribute significantly to these serious deficits. Some successes in overcoming these problems seem to be coming through community-based, decentralized immunization and surveillance programs with substantial support and assistance from the larger community.[79]

In a number of developing nations with populations that are entering the epidemic phase of poliomyelitis, determined efforts in immunization programs are yielding good results in reducing the incidence of paralytic poliomyelitis. In nations that are not yet conducting effective programs of vaccination, wild virulent polioviruses will continue to be actual or potential threats to health.

9.6. Nonspecific Control Measures for Poliomyelitis

It is not possible to list rules for the prevention of poliomyelitis other than vaccination. Quarantine either of patients or of exposed family or intimate contacts is ineffective in controlling the spread of the disease. This is understandable in view of the large number of inapparent and therefore unrecognized infections that occur during an epidemic.

During epidemic periods, children with fever should be given bed rest. Undue exercise or fatigue should be avoided, especially if there is any suspicion of involvement of the nervous system. Elective nose and throat operations and dental extractions should be avoided. Children should not travel unnecessarily to or from epidemic areas. Food and human excrement should be protected from flies. Once the poliovirus type responsible for the epidemic is determined, type-specific monovalent oral polio vaccine should be administered to susceptible persons in the population.

Patients with poliomyelitis can be admitted to

general hospitals provided that the hospital regulations are followed. All pharyngeal and bowel discharges are considered infectious.

10. Control of Other Enterovirus Infections

For the nonpolio enteroviruses, no specific control measures are known. Avoidance of contact with patients exhibiting acute febrile illness, especially those with a rash, is advisable for very young children. Members of institutional staffs responsible for caring for infants should be tested to determine whether they are carriers of enteroviruses. This is particularly important during outbreaks of diarrheal disease among infants.

There have been several reports of severe and even fatal echovirus 11 infections of newborns in special-care baby units.[44,151] Hospital personnel need to be particularly alert to even "minor illnesses" compatible with enterovirus infections in mothers delivering babies who enter newborn nurseries or special units, and the staff members of these units also need to be constantly aware of the possible significance of their own "minor illnesses."

11. Control of Enteroviruses in Water

The presence of human enteric viruses in water has been recognized for several decades, but the full health significance of this pollution has yet to be determined. Studies have shown that enteric viruses can easily survive present sewage treatment procedures and that many can persist for several months in natural waters. Viruses have been found at times in the drinking water supplies of some large cities of the world, even though these water supplies have been treated by conventional methods considered sufficient for protection against pathogenic bacterial contaminants. The bacterial agents that traditionally had been considered adequate indicators of pollution (and are still used in evaluating the safety of most potable water supplies) now are recognized to be inadequate markers of the possible presence of viruses in these waters. The procedures that had been believed to eliminate pollutants (e.g., percolation through soil, treatment processes used for water and for wastewater) remove the traditional

indicator bacteria much more readily than they do viruses. Caution is also indicated by recent findings that chlorine-inactivated echovirus could regain infectivity if the pH was adjusted to induce aggregation of the virus particles.[234]

In relatively few instances has it been possible to obtain adequate evidence for or against water-borne transmission of enteric viruses as the source of massive outbreaks of illness. However, continual exposure of large groups of people to even relatively small amounts of enteric virus contaminants in water may initiate human-to-human transmission in the community. Standards of water safety should include sufficiently sensitive monitoring and effective treatment methods to assure that drinking water and recreational water are essentially free of viral pathogens.[5,224] A related problem is the entry of viral contaminants into the food chain because of the concentration of viruses from streams, lakes, and seawater by food animals, notably shellfish.[134]

These problems are not merely speculative ones that might present hazards some years in the future. In view of the increasing demand for water, some countries are already seriously considering the intentional recycling of wastewater that originally contains a heavy load of viruses, often reaching 10^4–10^5 infectious units per liter. This intentional recycling obviously carries with it inherent dangers. However, indirect reuse, in which the treated sewage effluent is supplied to lakes, rivers, or groundwater, is often considered safe because the water undergoes some natural purification and subsequent plant processing at the point of reuse. But such indirect reuse, particularly in the case of heavily polluted rivers carrying 50% or more of virus-polluted sewage effluent, may present essentially the same degree of health risk as that associated with direct reuse. As we move toward ever greater amounts of deliberate recycling of water to conserve this finite resource, control of viral contamination becomes increasingly important.[5,224]

12. Unresolved Problems

Although many of the unresolved problems concerning the enteroviruses are described or implied in the foregoing presentation, this section is included to emphasize their importance to persons concerned with public health and epidemiology, who may be ideally situated to contribute uniquely toward solutions for the numerous problems that still remain.

Answers are needed to the "social failures" of vaccine delivery; to the epidemiological consequences of a highly successful polio vaccine program for one segment of the population while another segment is placed at higher risk by reduction of natural infection at an early age; to the present and potential problems of viruses in drinking and recreational water and the need for public awareness and support of new water-treatment methods that would permit safe recycling of this limited and dwindling resource; and to the possible association of enteroviruses with diseases of unknown etiology, such as diabetes. We must be alert to the possibility that infections with nonpolio enteroviruses might undergo a shift in age incidence, involving a consequent increase in severity of the illnesses that they cause, in parallel with that which took place with the polioviruses in the late 19th and early 20th centuries. For example, enteroviruses that appear to be increasingly involved with CNS disease, such as enterovirus 71 and certain echoviruses, will need to be studied more fully and watched epidemiologically.

The freedom that the Western Hemisphere had thus far enjoyed from acute hemorrhagic conjunctivites (an enterovirus-70 disease) cannot be taken for granted—as was demonstrated in 1981 (see Section 5.1.2). Health care personnel—most particularly those dealing with eye examinations—must be alert for the onset of any outbreak. In any large pandemic of this infection, besides the temporarily incapacitating eye disease, the likelihood of a certain small proportion of more serious CNS complications must also be recognized.

Despite the availability of effective vaccines, poliomyelitis can be expected to be an increasing problem in developing countries in tropical areas as well as in low socioeconomic groups of developed countries. Even in countries where vaccine is being widely introduced, there remains the question of how successful "takes" of the vaccine can be achieved in the face of interference by other enteroviruses or by inhibitors or other unknown factors that limit vaccine effectiveness. The epidemiologist must recognize that the major determinants of poliomyelitis infection and disease are now not the result of natural infection but depend on the public-health immunization practices of the country and the degree to which effective and long-lasting immunity has been induced in all segments of the population. Eradication of poliomyelitis is beginning to be viewed as a possible future goal, but this should not lead to slackening of immunization efforts. At present, wild virulent polioviruses can all too easily be imported into a supposedly polio-free country, and vigilant maintenance and expansion of vaccination programs will be required for a long time yet. Monitoring to ensure that levels of immunity remain sufficient should not consist merely of being alert for the occurrence of "sentinel" clinical cases, but instead should be determined by periodic serum surveys to determine the distribution and level of antibody in the population.

Development of vaccines for selected nonpolio enteroviruses is technically possible. It may be wise to look toward having such vaccines available for certain of these agents, particularly coxsackieviruses of the B group, that have a recognized role in myo-carditis of infants and that may well prove, if the proper studies are conducted, to be responsible for a significant share of adult cardiovascular disorders—perhaps including chronic as well as acute cardiac disease. Such vaccines may not appear to be required for widespread use in any entire population, but could be important for specifically targeted groups at high risk.

ACKNOWLEDGMENT

The able assistance of Miss Verle Rennick in the preparation of this chapter is gratefully acknowledged.

13. References

1. ASSAAD, F., AND COCKBURN, W. S., Four-year study of WHO virus reports on enteroviruses other than poliovirus, *Bull. WHO* **46:**329–336 (1972).
2. BANKER, D. D., AND MELNICK, J. L., Isolation of Coxsackie virus (C virus) from North Alaskan Eskimos, *Am. J. Hyg.* **54:**383–390 (1951).
3. BASS, J. W., HALSTEAD, S. B., FISCHER, G. W., PODGORE, J. K., AND WIEBE, R. A., Oral polio vaccine: Effect of booster vaccination one to 14 years after primary series, *J. Am. Med. Assoc.* **239:**2252–2255 (1978).

4. BERG, G. (ed.), *Transmission of Viruses by the Water Route*, Wiley, New York, 1967.

5. BERG, G., BODILY, H., LENNETTE, E. H., MELNICK, J. L., AND METCALF, T. G. (eds.), *Viruses in Water*, American Public Health Association, Washington, D.C., 1976.

6. BLATTNER, R. J., WILLIAMSON, A. P., and HEYS, F. M., Role of viruses in the etiology of congenital malformations, *Prog. Med. Virol.* **15**:1–41 (1973).

7. BLOMBERG, J., LYCKE, E., AHLFORS, K., JOHNSSON, T., WOLONTIS, S., AND VON ZEIPEL, G., New enterovirus type associated with epidemic of aseptic meningitis and/or hand, foot, and mouth disease, *Lancet* **2**:112 (1974).

8. BLOOM, H. H., MACK, W. N., KRUEGER, B. J., AND MALLMANN, W. L., Identification of enteroviruses in sewage, *J. Infect. Dis.* **105**:61–68 (1959).

9. BODIAN, D., AND HORSTMANN, D. M., Polioviruses, in: *Viral and Rickettsial Infections of Man*, 4th ed. (F. L. HORSFALL, JR., AND I. TAMM, eds.), pp. 430–473, Lippincott, Philadelphia, 1965.

10. BROWN, F., TALBOT, P., AND BURROWS, R., Antigenic differences between isolates of swine vesicular disease virus and their relationship to Coxsackie B5 virus, *Nature (London)* **245**:315–316 (1973).

11. BROWN, F., AND WILD, F., Variation in the coxsackievirus type B5 and its possible role in the etiology of swine vesicular disease, *Intervirology* **3**:125–128 (1974).

12. BROWN, G. C., AND KARUNAS, R. S., Relationship of congenital anomalies and maternal infection with selected enteroviruses, *Am. J. Epidemiol.* **95**:207–217 (1972).

13. BROWN, G. C., AND O'LEARY, T. P., Fluorescent antibody responses of cases and contacts of hand, foot, and mouth disease, *Infect. Immunol.* **9**:1098–1101 (1974).

14. BURCH, G. E., SHEWEY, L. L., AND HARB, J. M., Coxsackie B4 viruses and atrial myxoma, *Am. Heart J.* **88**:634–639 (1974).

15. BURCH, G. E., SUN, S. C., CHU, K. C., SOHAL, R. S., AND COLCOLOUGH, H. L., Interstitial and coxsackievirus B myocarditis in infants and children: A comparative histologic and immunofluorescent study of 50 autopsied hearts, *J. Am. Med. Assoc.* **203**:1–8 (1968).

15a. BURKE, D. S., GAYDOS, J. C., HODDER, R. A., AND BANCROFT, W. H., Seroimmunity to polioviruses in U.S. Army recruits, *J. Infect. Dis.* **139**:225–227 (1979).

16. BUTTERWORTH, B. E., A comparison of the virus-specific polypeptides of encephalomyocarditis virus, human rhinovirus-1A, and poliovirus, *Virology* **56**:439–453 (1973).

17. CABASSO, V. J., NOZELL, H., RUEGSEGGER, J. M., AND COX, H. R., Poliovirus antibody three years after oral trivalent vaccine (Sabin strain), *J. Pediatr.* **68**:199–203 (1966).

18. CAVERLY, C. S., Notes of an epidemic of acute anterior poliomyelitis, *J. Am. Med. Assoc.* **26**:1–5 (1896).

19. CELMA, M. L., AND EHRENFELD, E., Effect of poliovirus double-stranded RNA on viral and host-cell protein synthesis, *Proc. Natl. Acad. Sci. U.S.A.* **71**:2440–2444 (1974).

20. CENTER FOR DISEASE CONTROL, Reported morbidity and mortality in the United States, 1973, in: *Morbidity and Mortality Weekly Report*, Annual Supplement, 1973, Vol. 22, No. 53 (July 15, 1974).

21. CENTER FOR DISEASE CONTROL, Poliomyelitis surveillance summary 1974–76, October 1977.

22. CENTER FOR DISEASE CONTROL, Poliomyelitis—Pennsylvania, Maryland, *Morbid. Mortal. Weekly Rep.* **28**:49–50 (1979).

23. CHANG, W. K., LIU, K. C., FOO, T. C., LAM, M. W., AND CHAN, C. F., Acute haemorrhagic conjunctivitis in Hong Kong 1971–1975, *Southeast Asian J. Trop. Med. Public Health* **8**:1–6 (1977).

24. CHATTERJEE, S., QUARCOOPOME, C. O., AND APENTENG, A., Unusual type of epidemic of conjunctivitis in Ghana, *Br. J. Ophthalmol.* **54**:628–630 (1970).

25. CLARKE, N. A., AND KABLER, P. W., Human enteric viruses in sewage, *Health Lab. Sci.* **1**:44–49 (1964).

26. COCKBURN, W. C., AND DROZDOV, S. G., Poliomyelitis in the world, *Bull. WHO* **42**:405–417 (1970).

27. CODD, A. A., AND WHITE, E., Protection against poliomyelitis, *Lancet* **2**:1078 (1977).

28. COLE, C. N., Defective interfering (DI) particles of poliovirus, *Prog. Med. Virol.* **20**:180–207 (1975).

28a. COLEMAN, T. J., GAMBLE, D. R., AND TAYLOR, K. W., Diabetes in mice after Coxsackie B4 virus infection, *Br. Med. J.* **3**:25–27 (1973).

29. COLLINGHAM, K. E., POLLOCK, T. M., AND ROEBUCK, M. O., Paralytic poliomyelitis in England and Wales, 1976–77, *Lancet* **1**:976–977 (1978).

30. COMMITTEE ON THE ECHO VIRUSES, Enteric cytopathogenic human orphan (ECHO) viruses, *Science* **122**:1187–1188 (1955).

31. COMMITTEE ON THE ENTEROVIRUSES, National Foundation for Infantile Paralysis, The enteroviruses, *Am. J. Public Health* **47**:1556–1566 (1957).

32. COONEY, M. K., HALL, C. E., AND FOX, J. P., The Seattle Virus Watch. III. Evaluation of isolation methods and summary of infections detected by virus isolations, *Am. J. Epidemiol.* **96**:286–305 (1972).

33. COOPER, P. D., Genetics of picornaviruses, in: *Comprehensive Virology*, Vol. 9 (H. FRAENKEL-CONRAT AND R. WAGNER, eds.), pp. 130–207, Plenum Press, New York, 1977.

34. COOPER, P. D., STEINER-PRYOR, A., AND WRIGHT, P. J., A proposed regulator for poliovirus: The equestron, *Intervirology* **1**:1–10 (1973).

35. COOPER, P. D., *et al.* (Study Group on Picornaviridae, Vertebrate Virus Subcommittee, International Committee on Taxonomy of Viruses), Picornaviridae: Second Report, *Intervirology* **10**:165–180 (1978).

36. COUCH, R. B., DOUGLAS, R. G., JR., LINDGREN, K. M., GERONE, P. J., AND KNIGHT, V., Airborne transmission of respiratory infection with coxsackievirus A type 21, *Am. J. Epidemiol.* **91**:78–86 (1970).

37. CRAIGHEAD, J. E., The role of viruses in the pathogenesis of pancreatic disease and diabetes mellitus, *Prog. Med. Virol.* **19**:161–214 (1975).

38. CROWELL, R. L., AND GOLDBERG, B., Propagation and assay of group A coxsackieviruses in RD cells, *Abstr. Annu. Meet. Am. Soc. Microbiol.* **44**:208 (1974).

39. CURNEN, E. C., SHAW, E. W., AND MELNICK, J. L., Disease resembling nonparalytic poliomyelitis associated with a virus pathogenic for infant mice, *J. Am. Med. Assoc.* **141**:894–901 (1949).

40. DAHLING, D. R., BERG, G., AND BERMAN, D., BGM, a continuous cell line more sensitive than primary rhesus and African green monkey kidney cells for the recovery of viruses from water, *Health Lab. Sci.* **11**:275–282 (1974).

41. DALLDORF, G., Neuropathogenicity of group A Coxsackie viruses, *J. Exp. Med.* **106**:69–76 (1957).

42. DALLDORF, G., AND MELNICK, J. L., Coxsackieviruses, in: *Viral and Rickettsial Infections of Man*, 4th ed. (F. L. HORSFALL, JR., AND I. TAMM, eds.), pp. 474–512, Lippincott, Philadelphia, 1965.

43. DALLDORF, G., SICKLES, G. M., PLAGER, H., AND GIFFORD, R., A virus recovered from the feces of "poliomyelitis" patients pathogenic for suckling mice, *J. Exp. Med.* **89**:567–582 (1949).

44. DAVIES, D. P., HUGHES, C. A., MACVICAR, J., HAWKES, P., AND MAIR, H. J., Echovirus-11 infection in a special-care baby unit, *Lancet* **1**:96 (1979).

45. DÖMÖK, I., BALAYAN, M. S., FAYINKA, O. A., ŠKRTIĆ, N., SONEJI, A. D., AND HARLAND, P. S. E. G., Factors affecting the efficacy of live poliovirus vaccine in warm climates, *Bull. WHO* **51**:333–347 (1974).

46. DUNCAN, I. B. R., A comparative study of 63 strains of echovirus type 30, *Arch. Virusforsch.* **25**:93–104 (1968).

47. ENDERS, J. F., WELLER, T. H., AND ROBBINS, F. C., Cultivation of the Lansing strain of poliomyelitis virus in cultures of various human embryonic tissues, *Science* **109**:85–87 (1949).

48. ENDERS, J. F., WELLER, T. H., AND ROBBINS, F. C., Alteration in pathogenicity for monkeys of Brunhilde strain of poliomyelitis virus following cultivation in human tissues, *Fed. Proc. Fed. Am. Soc. Exp. Biol.* **11**:467 (1952).

49. FAULK, W. P., VYAS, G. N., PHILLIPS, C. A., FUDENBERG, H. H., AND CHISM, K., Passive hemagglutination test for anti-rhinovirus antibodies, *Nature (London) New Biol.* **231**:101–104 (1971).

50. FOX, J. P., Epidemiological aspects of coxsackie and echo virus infections in tropical areas, in: *Proceedings of the 7th International Congresses on Tropical Medicine and Malaria*, Vol. 3, pp. 212–213, 1964.

51. FOX, J. P., Family-based epidemiologic studies: The Second Wade Hampton Frost Lecture, *Am. J. Epidemiol.* **99**:165–179 (1974).

52. FOX, J. P., HALL, C. E., COONEY, M. K., LUCE, R. E., AND KRONMAL, R. A., The Seattle Virus Watch. II. Objectives, study population and its observation, data processing and summary of illnesses, *Am. J. Epidemiol.* **96**:270–285 (1972).

53. FRITSCH, A., POURCEL, C., CHARNAY, P., AND TIOLLAIS, P., Clonage du génome du virus de l'hépatite B dans *Escherichia coli*, *C. R. Acad. Sci. Paris* **287**:1453–1456 (1978).

54. FROESCHLE, J. E., FEORINO, P. M., AND GELFAND, H. M., A continuing surveillance of enterovirus infection in healthy children in six United States cities. II. Surveillance enterovirus isolates 1960–1963 and comparison with enterovirus isolates from cases of acute central nervous system disease, *Am. J. Epidemiol.* **83**:455–469 (1966).

55. FURESZ, J., ARMSTRONG, R. E., AND CONTRERAS, G., Viral and epidemiological links between poliomyelitis outbreaks in unprotected communities in Canada and the Netherlands, *Lancet* **2**:1248 (1978).

56. GAMBLE, D. R., TAYLOR, K. W., AND CUMMING, H., Coxsackie viruses and diabetes mellitus, *Br. Med. J.* **4**:260–262 (1973).

57. GEAR, J. H. S., AND MEASROCH, V., Coxsackievirus infections of the newborn, *Prog. Med. Virol.* **15**:42–62 (1973).

58. GELFAND, H. M., FOX, J. P., AND LEBLANC, D. R., The enteric viral flora of a population of normal children in southern Louisiana, *Am. J. Trop. Med.* **6**:521–531 (1957).

59. GELFAND, H. M., HOLGUIN, A. H., MARCHETTI, G. E., AND FEORINO, P. M., A continuing surveillance of enterovirus infections in healthy children in six United States cities. I. Viruses isolated during 1960 and 1961, *Am. J. Hyg.* **78**:358–375 (1963).

60. GERICHTER, C. B., LASCH, E. E., SEVER, I., EL-MASSRI, M., AND SKALSKA, P., Paralytic poliomyelitis in the Gaza Strip and West Bank during recent years, International Symposium on Standardization and Use of *Vaccines in the Developing Countries: Developments in Biological Standardization*, Vol. 41, (R. H. REGAMEY, ed.), pp. 173–177, S. Karger, Basel, 1978.

61. GOLDFIELD, M. S., SRIHONGSE, S., AND FOX, J. P., Hemagglutinins associated with certain human enteric viruses, *Proc. Soc. Exp. Biol. Med.* **96**:788–791 (1957).

62. GRAVES, J. H., Serological relationship of swine vesicular disease virus and coxsackie B5 virus, *Nature (London)* **245**:314–315 (1973).

63. GREGG, M. B., Poliomyelitis in the United States since 1955, Presented at the American Academy of Pediatrics, Evanston, Illinois, August 11–12, 1975.

64. GRINSTEIN, S., MELNICK, J. L., AND WALLIS, C., Virus isolations from sewage and from a stream receiving effluents of sewage treatment plants, *Bull. WHO* **42**:291–296 (1970).

65. GRIST, N. R., BELL, E. J., AND ASSAAD, F., Enteroviruses in human disease, *Prog. Med. Virol.* **24**:114–157 (1978).

66. GRIST, N. R., BELL, E. J., AND REID, E., The epidemiology of enteroviruses, *Scot. Med. J.* **20**:27–31 (1975).

67. GYORKEY, F., CABRAL, G. A., GYORKEY, P. K., URIBE-BOTERO, G., DREESMAN, G. R., AND MELNICK, J. L., Coxsackievirus aggregates in muscle cells of a polymyositis patient, *Intervirology* **10**:69–77 (1978).

68. HAGIWARA, A., TAGAYA, I., AND YONEYAMA, T., Epidemic of hand, foot and mouth disease associated with enterovirus 71 infection, *Intervirology* **9**:60–63 (1978).

69. HALL, C. E., COONEY, M. K., AND FOX, J. P., The Seattle Virus Watch Program. I. Infection and illness experience of Virus Watch families during a community-wide epidemic of echovirus type 30 aseptic meningitis, *Am. J. Public Health* **60**:1456–1465 (1970).

70. HAMMON, W. McD., LUDWIG, E. H., SATHER, G., AND YOHN, D. S., Comparative studies on patterns of family infections with polioviruses and ECHO virus type 1 on an American military base in the Philippines, *Am. J. Public Health* **47**:802–811 (1957).

71. HARRIS, T. J. R., AND BROWN, F., Correlation of polypeptide composition with antigenic variation in the swine vesicular disease and coxsackie B₅ viruses, *Nature (London)* **258**:758–760 (1975).

72. HARRIS, L. F., HAYNES, R. E., CRAMBLETT, H. G., CONANT, R. M., AND JENKINS, G. R., Antigenic analysis of echoviruses 1 and 8, *J. Infect. Dis.* **127**:63–68 (1973).

73. HAWLEY, H. B., MORIN, D. P., GERAGHTY, M. E., TOMKOW, J., AND PHILLIPS, C. A., Coxsackievirus B epidemic at a boys' summer camp: Isolation of virus from swimming water, *J. Am. Med. Assoc.* **226**:33–36 (1973).

74. HIERHOLZER, J. C., HILLIARD, K. A., AND ESPOSITO, J. J., Serosurvey for "acute hemorrhagic conjunctivitis" virus (enterovirus 70) antibodies in the southeastern United States, with review of the literature and some epidemiologic implications, *Am. J. Epidemiol.* **102**:533–544 (1975).

75. HONIG, E. I., MELNICK, J. L., ISACSON, P., PARR, R., MYERS, I. L., AND WALTON, M., An epidemiological study of enteric virus infections: Poliomyelitis, Coxsackie, and orphan (ECHO) viruses isolated from normal children in two socio-economic groups, *J. Exp. Med.* **103**:247–262 (1956).

76. HORSTMANN, D. M. Need for monitoring vaccinated populations for immunity levels, *Prog. Med. Virol.* **16**:215–240 (1973).

77. HORSTMANN, D. M., EMMONS, J., GIMPEL, L., SUBRAHMANYAN, T., AND RIORDAN, J. T., Enterovirus surveillance following a community-wide oral poliovirus vaccination program: A seven-year study, *Am. J. Epidemiol.* **97**:173–186 (1973).

78. HSIUNG, G. D., *Diagnostic Virology: An Illustrated Handbook*, 2nd ed., Yale University Press, New Haven, 1973.

79. IMPERATO, P. J., PINCUS, L., HWA, C. L., AND CHAVES, A. D., The control of measles in New York City, *Bull. N. Y. Acad. Med. 2nd Ser.* **50**:602–619 (1974).

80. INTERNATIONAL POLIOMYELITIS CONFERENCES: Poliomyelitis: Papers and discussions presented at the First through Fifth International Poliomyelitis Conferences (M. FISHBEIN, ed.), Lippincott, Philadelphia, 1949, 1952, 1955, 1958, 1961.

81. ITOH, H., AND MELNICK, J. L., The infection of chimpanzees with ECHO viruses, *J. Exp. Med.* **106**:677–688 (1957).

82. ITOH, H., AND MELNICK, J. L., Double infections of single cells with ECHO 7 and Coxsackie A9 viruses, *J. Exp. Med.* **109**:393–406 (1959).

83. JACKSON, G. G., AND MULDOON, R. L., Viruses causing common respiratory infections in man, *J. Infect. Dis.* **127**:328–408 (1973).

84. JANDA, Z., ADAM, E., AND VONKA, V., Properties of a new type 3 attenuated poliovirus. VI. Alimentary tract resistance in children fed previously with type 3 Sabin vaccine to reinfection with homologous and heterologous type 3 attenuated poliovirus, *Arch. Virusforsch.* **20**:87–98 (1967).

85. KAPLAN, G. J., CLARK, P. S., BENDER, T. R., FELTZ, E. T., LIST-YOUNG, B., NEVIUS, S. E., AND CHIN, T. D. Y., Echovirus type 30 meningitis and related febrile illness: Epidemiologic study of an outbreak in an Eskimo community, *Am. J. Epidemiol.* **92**:257–265 (1970).

85a. KAPSENBERG, J. G., RAS, A., AND KORTE, J., Improvement of enterovirus neutralization by treatment with sodium deoxycholate or chloroform, *Intervirology* **12**:329–334 (1979).

86. KEDMI, S., AND KATZENELSON, E., A rapid quantitative fluorescent antibody assay of polioviruses using tragacanth gum, *Arch. Virol.* **56**:337–340 (1978).

87. KELLY, S., WINSSER, J., AND WINKELSTEIN, W., JR., Poliomyelitis and other enteric viruses in sewage, *Am. J. Public Health* **47**:72–77 (1957).

88. KENNETT, M. L., BIRCH, C. J., LEWIS, F. A., YUNG, A.

P., LOCARNINI, S. A., AND GUST, I. D., Enterovirus type 71 infection in Melbourne, *Bull. WHO* **51**:609–615 (1974).

89. KIBRICK, S., Current status of Coxsackie and ECHO viruses in human disease, *Prog. Med. Virol.* **6**:27–70 (1964).

89a. KITAMURA, N., SEMLER, B. L., ROTHBERG, P. G., LARSEN, G. R., ADLER, C. J., DORNER, A. J., EMINI, E. A., HANECAK, R., LEE, J. J., VAN DER WERF, S., ANDERSON, C. W., AND WIMMER, E. Primary structure, gene organization and polypeptide expression of poliovirus RNA, *Nature* **291**:547–553 (1981).

90. KOGON, A., SPIGLAND, I., FROTHINGHAM, T. E., ELVEBACK, L., WILLIAMS, C., HALL, C. E., AND FOX, J. P., The Virus Watch Program: A continuing surveillance of viral infections in metropolitan New York families. VII. Observations on viral excretion, seroimmunity, intrafamilial spread and illness association in coxsackievirus and echovirus infections, *Am. J. Epidemiol.* **89**:51–61 (1969).

91. KONO, R., Apollo 11 disease or acute hemorrhagic conjunctivitis: A pandemic of a new enterovirus infection of the eyes, *Am. J. Epidemiol.* **101**:383–390 (1975).

92. KONO, R., MIYAMURA, K., TAJIRI, E., SASAGAWA, A., PHUAPRADIT, P., ROONGWITHU, N., VEJJAJIVA, A., JAYAVASU, C., THONGCHAROEN, P., WASI, C., AND RODPRASSERT, P., Virological and serological studies of neurological complications of acute hemorrhagic conjunctivitis in Thailand, *J. Infect. Dis.* **135**:706–713 (1977).

93. KONO, R., MIYAMURA, K., TAJIRI, E., SHIGA, S., SASAGAWA, A., IRANI, P. F., KATRAK, S. M., AND WADIA, N. H., Neurologic complications associated with acute hemorrhagic conjunctivitis virus infection and its serologic confirmation, *J. Infect. Dis.* **129**:590–593 (1974).

94. KONO, R., SASAGAWA, A., ISHII, K., SUGIURA, S., OCHI, M., MATSUMIYA, H., UCHIDA, Y., KAMEYAMA, K., KANEKO, M., AND SAKURAI, N., Pandemic of new type of conjunctivitis, *Lancet* **1**:1191–1194 (1972).

95. KONO, R., SASAGAWA, A., MIYAMURA, K., AND TAJIRI, E., Serologic characterization and sero-epidemiologic studies on acute hemorrhagic conjunctivitis (AHC) virus, *Am. J. Epidemiol.* **101**:444–457 (1975).

96. KONO, R., UCHIDA, N., SASAGAWA, A., AKAO, Y., KODAMA, H., MUKOYAMA, J., AND FUJIWARA, T., Neurovirulence of acute-haemorrhagic-conjunctivitis virus in monkeys, *Lancet* **2**:1191–1194 (1972).

97. KRAUS, G., Details of poliomyelitis outbreak, *N. Engl. J. Med.* **288**:1357–1358 (1973).

98. LAKE, A. M., LAUER, B. A., CLARK, J. C., WESENBERG, R. L., AND McINTOSH, K., Enterovirus infections in neonates, *J. Pediatr.* **89**:787–791 (1976).

99. LAMB, G. A., CHIN, T. D. Y., AND SCARCE, L. E., Isolations of enteric viruses from sewage and river water in a metropolitan area, *Am. J. Hyg.* **80**:320–327 (1964).

100. LANDSTEINER, K., AND POPPER, E., Übertragung der Poliomyelitis acuta auf Affen, *Z. Immunitaetsforsch. Orig.* **2**:377–390 (1909).

101. LANSDOWN, A. B. G., Viral infections and diseases of the heart, *Prog. Med. Virol.* **24**:70–113 (1978).

102. LAVINDER, C. H., FREEMAN, A. W., AND FROST, W. H., Epidemiologic studies of poliomyelitis in New York City and northeastern United States during the year 1916, *Public Health Bull.* No. 91, July, 309 pp. (1918).

103. LENNETTE, E. H., General principles underlying laboratory diagnosis of viral and rickettsial infections, in: *Diagnostic Procedures for Viral and Rickettsial Infections*, 4th ed. (E. H. LENNETTE AND N. J. SCHMIDT, eds.), pp. 1–65, American Public Health Association, New York, 1969.

104. LENNETTE, E. H., MELNICK, J. L., AND MAGOFFIN, R. L., Clinical virology: Introduction to methods in: *Manual of Clinical Microbiology*, 2nd ed. (E. H. LENNETTE, E. H. SPAULDING, AND J. P. TRUANT, eds.), pp. 667–677, American Society for Microbiology, Washington, D.C., 1974.

105. LEPOW, M. L., NANKERVIS, G. A., AND ROBBINS, F. C., Immunity of school children two years after oral poliomyelitis vaccination, *J. Am. Med. Assoc.* **202**:121–125 (1967).

106. LERNER, A. M., Coxsackievirus myocardiopathy, *J. Infect. Dis.* **120**:496–499 (1969).

107. LERNER, A. M., Myocarditis and pericarditis, in: *International Textbook of Medicine* (A. I. BRAUDE, ed.), pp. 1520–1530, W. B. Saunders, Philadelphia, 1981.

108. LERNER, A. M., AND WILSON, F. M., Virus myocardiopathy, *Prog. Med. Virol.* **15**:63–91 (1973).

109. LIM, K. A., AND BENYESH-MELNICK, M., Typing of viruses by combinations of antiserum pools: Application to typing of enteroviruses (Coxsackie and echo), *J. Immunol.* **84**:309–317 (1960).

110. LIM, K. H., AND YIN-MURPHY, M., An epidemic of conjunctivitis in Singapore in 1970, *Singapore Med. J.* **12**:247–249 (1971).

111. LIM, K. H., AND YIN-MURPHY, M., The aetiologic agents of epidemic conjunctivitis, *Singapore Med. J.* **18**:41–43 (1977).

112. LUND, E., HEDSTRÖM, C.-E., AND STRANNEGÅRD, O., A comparison between virus isolations from sewage and from fecal specimens from patients, *Am. J. Epidemiol.* **84**:282–286 (1966).

113. MACLEOD, D. R. E., ING, W. K., BELCOURT, R. J.-P., PEARSON, E. W., AND BELL, J. S., Antibody status to poliomyelitis, measles, rubella, diphtheria and tet-

anus, Ontario, 1969–70: Deficiencies discovered and remedies required, *Can. Med. Assoc. J.* **113**:619–623 (1975).

114. MAGUIRE, T., The laboratory transmission of Coxsackie A6 virus by mosquitoes, *J. Hyg.* **68**:625–630 (1970).

115. MCALLISTER, R. M., MELNYK, J., FINKELSTEIN, J. Z., ADAMS, E. C., JR., AND GARDNER, M. B., Cultivation *in vitro* of cells derived from a human rhabdomyosarcoma, *Cancer* **24**:520–526 (1969).

116. MCCARROLL, J. R., MELNICK, J. L., AND HORSTMANN, D. M., Spread of poliomyelitis infection in nursery schools, *Am. J. Public Health* **45**:1541–1550 (1955).

117. MELNICK, J. L., Poliomyelitis virus in urban sewage in epidemic and in non-epidemic times, *Am. J. Hyg.* **45**:240–253 (1947).

118. MELNICK, J. L., Variation in poliomyelitis virus on serial passage through tissue culture, *Cold Spring Harbor Symp. Quant. Biol.* **18**:278–279 (1953).

119. MELNICK, J. L., Application of tissue culture methods to epidemiological studies of poliomyelitis, *Am. J. Public Health* **44**:571–580 (1954).

120. MELNICK, J. L., Echo viruses, in: *Cellular Biology, Nucleic Acids and Viruses*, Special Publication of the New York Academy of Sciences, Vol. 5, pp. 365–381 (1957).

121. MELNICK, J. L., Advances in the study of the enteroviruses, *Prog. Med. Virol.* **1**:59–105 (1958).

122. MELNICK, J. L., Echoviruses, in: *Viral and Rickettsial Infections of Man*, 4th ed. (F. L. HORSFALL, JR., AND I. TAMM, eds.), pp. 513–545, Lippincott, Philadelphia, 1965.

123. MELNICK, J. L., Enteroviruses: Vaccines, epidemiology, diagnosis, and classification, *CRC Crit. Rev. Clin. Lab. Sci.* **1**:87–118 (1970).

124. MELNICK, J. L., Periodic serological surveillance, in: *Serological Epidemiology* (J. R. PAUL AND C. WHITE, eds.), pp. 143–154, Academic Press, New York, 1973.

125. MELNICK, J. L., Reference materials in virology: The enterovirus example, in: *Proceedings of the International Conference on Standardization of Diagnostic Materials*, pp. 213–235, CDC Monograph, Center for Disease Control, Atlanta, Georgia, 1974.

126. MELNICK, J. L., Report to the World Health Organization: Recommendations for the control of poliomyelitis in Israel, West Bank and Gaza Strip. Report No. EM/VIR/7, EPID/54. World Health Organization, Geneva, 1977.

127. MELNICK, J. L., Advantages and disadvantages of killed and live poliomyelitis vaccines, *Bull. WHO* **56**:21–38 (1978).

128. MELNICK, J. L., AND ÅGREN, K., Poliomyelitis and Coxsackie viruses isolated from normal infants in Egypt, *Proc. Soc. Exp. Biol. Med.* **81**:621–624 (1952).

129. MELNICK, J. L., ASHKENAZI, A., MIDULLA, V. C., WALLIS, C., AND BERNSTEIN, A., Immunogenic potency of MgCl$_2$-stabilized oral poliovaccine, *J. Am. Med. Assoc.* **185**:406–418 (1963).

130. MELNICK, J. L., BURKHARDT, M., TABER, L. H., AND ERCKMAN, P. N., Developing gap in immunity to poliomyelitis in an urban area, *J. Am. Med. Assoc.* **209**:1181–1185 (1969).

131. MELNICK, J. L., COCKBURN, W. C., DALLDORF, G., GARD, S., GEAR, J. H. S., HAMMON, W. McD., KAPLAN, M. M., NAGLER, F. P., OKER-BLOM, N., RHODES, A. J., SABIN, A. B., VERLINDE, J. D., AND VON MAGNUS, H., Picornavirus group, *Virology* **19**:114–116 (1963).

132. MELNICK, J. L., CROWTHER, D., AND BARRERA-ORO, J., Rapid development of drug-resistant mutants of poliovirus, *Science* **134**:557 (1961).

133. MELNICK, J. L., EMMONS, J., COFFEY, J. H., AND SCHOOF, H., Seasonal distribution of Coxsackie viruses in urban sewage and flies, *Am. J. Hyg.* **59**:164–184 (1954).

134. MELNICK, J. L., GERBA, C. P., AND WALLIS, C., Viruses in water, *Bull. WHO* **56**:499–508 (1978).

135. MELNICK, J. L., AND HAMPIL, B., WHO collaborative studies on enterovirus reference antisera: Fourth report, *Bull. WHO* **48**:381–396 (1973).

136. MELNICK, J. L., AND LEDINKO, N., Social serology: Antibody levels in a normal young population during an epidemic of poliomyelitis, *Am. J. Hyg.* **54**:354–382 (1951).

137. MELNICK, J. L., AND LEDINKO, N., Development of neutralizing antibodies against the three types of poliomyelitis virus during an epidemic period: The ratio of inapparent infection to clinical poliomyelitis, *Am. J. Hyg.* **58**:207–222 (1953).

138. MELNICK, J. L., MCCARROLL, J. R., AND HORSTMANN, D. M. A winter outbreak of poliomyelitis in New York City: The complement-fixation test as an aid in rapid diagnosis, *Am. J. Hyg.* **63**:95–114 (1956).

139. MELNICK, J. L., PAUL, J. R., AND WALTON, M., Serologic epidemiology of poliomyelitis, *Am. J. Public Health* **45**:429–437 (1955).

140. MELNICK, J. L., PROCTOR, R. O., OCAMPO, A. R., DIWAN, A. R., AND BEN-PORATH, E., Free and bound virus in serum after administration of oral poliovirus vaccine, *Am. J. Epidemiol.* **84**:329–342 (1966).

141. MELNICK, J. L., RENNICK, V., HAMPIL, B., SCHMIDT, N. J., AND HO, H. H., Lyophilized combination pools of enterovirus equine antisera: Preparation and test procedures for the identification of field strains of 42 enteroviruses, *Bull. WHO* **48**:263–268 (1973).

142. MELNICK, J. L., SHAW, E. W., AND CURNEN, E. C., A virus from patients diagnosed as non-paralytic poliomyelitis or aseptic meningitis, *Proc. Soc. Exp. Biol. Med.* **71**:344–349 (1949).

143. MELNICK, J. L., SCHMIDT, N. J., HAMPIL, B., AND HO,

H. H., Lyophilized combination pools of enterovirus equine antisera: Preparation and test procedures for the identification of field strains of 19 group A coxsackievirus serotypes, *Intervirology* 8:172–181 (1977).

144. MELNICK, J. L., SCHMIDT, N. J., MIRKOVIC, R. R., CHUMAKOV, M. P., LAVROVA, I. K., AND VOROSHILOVA, M. K. Identification of Bulgarian strain 258 of enterovirus 71, *Intervirology* 12:297–302 (1979).

145. MELNICK, J. L., TAGAYA, I., AND VON MAGNUS, H., Enteroviruses 69, 70, and 71, *Intervirology* 4:369–370 (1974).

146. MELNICK, J. L., WENNER, H. A., AND PHILLIPS, C. A., Enteroviruses, in: *Diagnostic Procedures for Viral, Rickettsial, and Chlamydial Infections*, 5th ed. (E. H. LENNETTE AND N. J. SCHMIDT, eds.) pp. 471–534, American Public Health Association, Washington, 1979.

147. MELNICK, J. L. *et al.* (Study Group on Picornaviridae, Vertebrate Virus Subcommittee, International Committee on Taxonomy of Viruses), Picornaviridae, *Intervirology* 4:303–316 (1974).

148. MILLER, D. A., MILLER, O. J., VAITHILINGAM, G. D., HASHMI, S., TANTRAVAHI, R., MEDRANO, L., AND GREEN, H., Human chromosome 19 carries a poliovirus receptor gene, *Cell* 1:167–173 (1974).

149. MIRKOVIC, R. R., KONO, R., YIN-MURPHY, M., SOHIER, R., SCHMIDT, N. J., AND MELNICK, J. L., Enterovirus type 70: The etiologic agent of pandemic acute haemorrhagic conjunctivitis, *Bull. WHO* 49:341–346 (1973).

150. MIRKOVIC, R. R., SCHMIDT, N. J., YIN-MURPHY, M., AND MELNICK, J. L., Enterovirus etiology of the 1970 Singapore epidemic of acute conjunctivitis, *Intervirology* 4:119–127 (1974).

150a. MIWA, C., YAMADA, F., MATSUURA, A., AND YOSHIZAWA, K., Epidemic of hand, foot and mouth disease in Gifu prefecture in 1973, *Virus* 28:78–86 (1978).

151. NAGINGTON, J., WREGHITT, T. G., GANDY, G., ROBERTON, N. R. C., AND BERRY, P. J., Fatal echovirus 11 infections in outbreak in special-care baby unit, *Lancet* 2:725 (1978).

152. NAKANO, J. H., HATCH, M. H., THIEME, M. L., AND NOTTAY, B., Parameters for differentiating vaccine-derived and wild poliovirus strains, *Prog. Med. Virol.* 24:178–206 (1978).

153. NAKAO, T., Coxsackie viruses and diabetes, *Lancet* 2:1423 (1971).

154. NARDI, G., BARONI, M., TANZI, M. L., GRANDI, D., BEVILACQUA, G., AND TEDESCHI, F., Epidemic due to group B Coxsackie viruses in a newborn infants' department, *Ann. Sclavo* 18:793–808 (1976).

155. NEJMI, S., GAUDIN, O. G., CHOMEL, J. J., BAAJ, A., SOHIER, R., AND BOSSHARD, S., Isolation of a virus responsible for an outbreak of acute haemorrhagic conjunctivitis in Morocco, *J. Hyg.* 72:181–183 (1974).

156. NICHOLAS, D. D., KRATZER, J. H., OFOSU-AMAAH, S., AND BELCHER, D. W., Is poliomyelitis a serious problem in developing countries?—the Danfa experience, *Br. Med. J.* 1:1009–1012 (1977).

157. NISHMI, M., AND YODFAT, Y., Successive overlapping outbreaks of a febrile illness associated with coxsackie virus type B4 and echo virus type 9 in a kibbutz, *Isr. J. Med. Sci.* 9:895–899 (1973).

158. NOLAN, J. P., WILMER, B. J., AND MELNICK, J. L., Poliomyelitis: Its highly invasive nature and narrow stream of infection in a community of high socioeconomic level, *N. Engl. J. Med.* 253:945–954 (1955).

159. NOTKINS, A. L., Virus-induced diabetes mellitus, *Arch. Virol.* 54:1–17 (1977).

159a. YOON, JI-WON, AUSTIN, M., ONODERA, T., AND NOTKINS, A. L., Virus-induced diabetes mellitus. Isolation of a virus from the pancreas of a child with diabetic ketoacidosis, *New Engl. J. Med.* 300:1173–1179 (1979).

160. OBERHOFER, T. R., BROWN, G. C., AND MONTO, A. S., Seroimmunity to poliomyelitis in an American community, *Am. J. Epidemiol.*, 101:333–339 (1975).

161. OFOSU-AMAAH, S., KRATZER, J. H., AND NICHOLAS, D. D., Is poliomyelitis a serious problem in developing countries?—Lameness in Ghanaian schools, *Br. Med. J.* 1:1012–1014 (1977).

162. OGRA, P. L., AND KARZON, D. T., Formation and function of poliovirus antibody in different tissues, *Prog. Med. Virol.* 13:156–193 (1971).

163. OGRA, P. L., OGRA, S. S., AL-NAKEEB, S., AND COPPOLA, P. R., Local antibody response to experimental poliovirus infection in the central nervous system of rhesus monkeys, *Infect. Immun.* 8:931–937 (1973).

164. PACSA, S., AND WERBLINSKA, J., Natural immunity of Ghanaian children to polio and coxsackieviruses: Brief report, *Arch. Gesamte Virusforsch.* 33:192–193 (1971).

165. PAN AMERICAN HEALTH ORGANIZATION, *Live Poliovirus Vaccines*, Special Publications of the Pan American Health Organization, Nos. 44 (1959) and 50 (1960).

166. PARKS, W. P., QUEIROGA, L. T., AND MELNICK, J. L., Studies of infantile diarrhea in Karachi, Pakistan. II. Multiple virus isolations from rectal swabs, *Am. J. Epidemiol.* 85:469–478 (1967).

167. PAUL, J. R., Endemic and epidemic trends of poliomyelitis in Central and South America, *Bull WHO* 19:747–758 (1958).

168. PAUL, J. R., Development and use of serum surveys in epidemiology, in: *Serological Epidemiology* (J. R. PAUL AND C. WHITE, eds.), pp. 1–13, Academic Press, New York, 1973.

169. PAUL, J. R., *A History of Poliomyelitis*, Yale University Press, New Haven, 1971.

170. PAYNE, A. M.-M., Poliomyelitis as a world problem, Papers and discussions presented at the Third In-

ternational Poliomyelitis Conference, pp. 393–400, Lippincott, Philadelphia, 1955.

171. PAYNE, A. M.-M., Immunization against poliomyelitis in the light of existing immunity of populations, Papers and discussions presented at the Fourth International Poliomyelitis Conference, pp. 157–164, Lippincott, Philadelphia, 1958.

172. PHILLIPS, C. A., MELNICK, J. L., BARRETT, F. F., BEHBEHANI, A. M., AND RIGGS, S., Dual virus infections: Simultaneous enteroviral disease and St. Louis encephalitis, J. Am. Med. Assoc. 197:169–172 (1966).

173. RAMOS-ALVAREZ, M., AND SABIN, A. B., Characteristics of poliomyelitis and other enteric viruses recovered in tissue culture from healthy American children, Proc. Soc. Exp. Biol. Med. 87:655–661 (1954).

174. REID, D., BELL, E. J., AND GRIST, N. R., Poliomyelitis: A gap in immunity?, Lancet 2:899–900 (1973).

175. REISSIG, M., HOWES, D. W., AND MELNICK, J. L., Sequence of morphological changes in epithelial cell cultures infected with poliovirus, J. Exp. Med. 104:289–304 (1956).

176. RIVERS, T. M., AND HORSFALL, F. L., JR. (eds.), Viral and Rickettsial Infections of Man, 3rd ed., Lippincott, Philadelphia, 1959.

177. ROBBINS, F. C., ENDERS, J. F., WELLER, T. H., AND FLORENTINO, G. L., Studies on the cultivation of poliomyelitis viruses in tissue culture. V. The direct isolation and serologic identification of virus strains in tissue culture from patients with nonparalytic and paralytic poliomyelitis, Am. J. Hyg. 54:286–293 (1951).

178. ROSEN, L., AND KERN, J. K., Hemagglutination and hemagglutination-inhibition with coxsackie B viruses, Proc. Soc. Exp. Biol. Med. 107:626–628 (1961).

179. ROSEN, L., MELNICK, J. L., SCHMIDT, N. J., AND WENNER, H. A., Subclassification of enteroviruses and echovirus type 34, Arch. Gesamte Virusforsch. 30:89–92 (1970).

180. ROSEN, L., SCHMIDT, N. J., AND KERN, J., Toluca-1, a newly recognized enterovirus, Arch. Gesamte Virusforsch. 40:132–136 (1973).

181. ROSS, C. A. C., BELL, E. J., KERR, M. M., AND WILLIAMS, K. A. B., Infective agents and embryopathy in the West of Scotland 1966–70, Scott. Med. J. 17:252–258 (1972).

182. ROSSEN, R. D., KASEL, J. A., AND COUCH, R. B., The secretory immune system: Its relation to respiratory viral infection, Prog. Med. Virol. 13:194–238 (1971).

183. ROUSSEAU, W. E., NOBLE, G. R., TEGTMEIER, G. E., JORDAN, M. C., AND CHIN, T. D. Y., Persistence of poliovirus neutralizing antibodies eight years after immunization with live, attenuated-virus vaccine, N. Engl. J. Med. 289:1357–1359 (1973).

184. SABIN, A. B., Oral poliovirus vaccine, J. Am. Med. Assoc. 194:872–876 (1965).

185. SABIN, A. B., HENNESSEN, W. A., AND WINSSER, J.,

Studies on variants of poliomyelitis virus. I. Experimental segregation and properties of avirulent variants of three immunologic types, J. Exp. Med. 99:551–576 (1954).

186. SABIN, A. B., KRUMBIEGEL, E. R., AND WIGAND, R., ECHO type 9 virus disease: Virologically controlled clinical and epidemiologic observations during 1957 epidemic in Milwaukee with notes on concurrent similar diseases associated with Coxsackie and other ECHO viruses, Am. J. Dis. Child. 96:197–219 (1958).

187. SALK, J. E., Poliomyelitis: Control, in: Viral and Rickettsial Infections of Man, 3rd ed. (T. M. RIVERS AND F. L. HORSFALL, JR., eds.), pp. 499–518, Lippincott, Philadelphia, 1959.

188. SALK, J., AND SALK, D., Control of influenza and poliomyelitis with killed virus vaccines, Science 195:834–847 (1977).

188a. SANDELIN, K., TUOMIOJA, M., AND ERKKILÄ, H., Echovirus type 7 isolated from conjunctival scrapings, Scand. J. Infect. Dis. 9:71–73 (1977).

189. SANDERS, D. Y., AND CRAMBLETT, H. G., Antibody titers to polioviruses in patients ten years after immunization with Sabin vaccine, J. Pediatr. 84:406–408 (1974).

190. SCHAFFER, F. L., Binding of proflavine by and photoinactivation of poliovirus propagated in the presence of the dye, Virology 18:412–425 (1962).

191. SCHIEBLE, J. H., FOX, V. L., AND LENNETTE, E. H., A probable new human picornavirus associated with respiratory disease, Am. J. Epidemiol. 85:297–310 (1967).

192. SCHMIDT, N. J., Tissue culture technics for diagnostic virology, in: Diagnostic Procedures for Viral and Rickettsial Infections, 4th ed. (E. H. LENNETTE AND N. J. SCHMIDT, eds.), pp. 79–178, American Public Health Association, New York, 1969.

193. SCHMIDT, N. J., HO, H. H., AND LENNETTE, E. H., Propagation and isolation of group A coxsackieviruses in RD cells, J. Clin. Microbiol. 2:183–185 (1975).

194. SCHMIDT, N. J., HO, H. H., AND LENNETTE, E. H., Comparative sensitivity of the BGM cell line for isolation of enteric viruses, Health Lab. Sci. 13:115–117 (1976).

195. SCHMIDT, N. J., AND LENNETTE, E. H., Advances in the serodiagnosis of viral infections, Prog. Med. Virol. 15:244–308 (1973).

196. Schmidt, N. J., LENNETTE, E. H., AND HO, H. H., An apparently new enterovirus isolated from patients with disease of the central nervous system, J. Infect. Dis. 129:304–309 (1974).

197. SCHMIDT, N. J., MAGOFFIN, R. L., AND LENNETTE, E. H., Association of group B coxsackieviruses with cases of pericarditis, myocarditis, or pleurodynia by demonstration of immunoglobulin M antibody, Infect. Immun. 8:341–348 (1973).

198. SELLS, C. J., CARPENTER, R. L., AND RAY, C. G., Sequelae of central-nervous-system enterovirus infections, *N. Engl. J. Med.* **293**:1–4 (1975).

199. SERGIESCU, D., HORODNICEANU, F., AND AUBERT-COMBIESCU, A., The use of inhibitors in the study of picornavirus genetics, *Prog. Med. Virol.* **14**:123–199 (1972).

200. SOMMERVILLE, R. G., Rapid diagnosis of viral infections by immunofluorescent staining of viral antigens in leukocytes and macrophages, *Prog. Med. Virol.* **10**:398–414 (1968).

201. STANTON, G. J., LANGFORD, M. P., AND BARON, S., Effect of interferon, elevated temperature, and cell type on replication of acute hemorrhagic conjunctivitis viruses, *Infect. Immun.* **18**:370–376 (1977).

202. TABER, L. H., MIRKOVIC, R. R., ADAM, V., ELLIS, S. S., YOW, M. D., AND MELNICK, J. L., Rapid diagnosis of enterovirus meningitis by immunofluorescent staining of CSF leukocytes, *Intervirology* **1**:127–134 (1973).

203. TAGAYA, I., NAKAO, C., HARA, M., AND YAMADERA, S., Characterization of poliovirus isolates in Japan after the mass vaccination with live oral poliomyelitis vaccine (Sabin), *Bull. WHO* **48**:547–554 (1973).

204. TAKATSU, T., TAGAYA, I., AND HIRAYAMA, M., Poliomyelitis in Japan during the period 1962–68 after the introduction of mass vaccination with Sabin vaccine, *Bull. WHO* **49**:129–137 (1973).

205. TAMM, I., AND EGGERS, H. J., Differences in the selective virus-inhibitory action of 2-(α-hydroxybenzyl)-benzimidazole and guanidine·HCl, *Virology* **18**:439–447 (1962).

206. TORPHY, D. E., RAY, C. G., THOMPSON, R. S., AND FOX, J. P., An epidemic of aseptic meningitis due to echovirus type 30: Epidemiological features and clinical laboratory findings, *Am. J. Public Health* **60**:1447–1455 (1970).

207. TRASK, J. D., MELNICK, J. L., AND WENNER, H. A., Chlorination of human, monkey-adapted and mouse strains of poliomyelitis virus, *Am. J. Hyg.* **41**:30–40 (1945).

208. VAN WEZEL, A. L., AND HAZENDONK, A. G., Intratypic serodifferentiation of poliomyelitis virus strains by strain-specific antisera, *Intervirology* **11**:2–8 (1979).

209. VOROSHILOVA, M. K., AND CHUMAKOV, M. P., Poliomyelitis-like properties of AB-IV-Coxsackie A7 group of viruses, *Prog. Med. Virol.* **2**:106–170 (1959).

210. WALLIS, C., AND MELNICK, J. L., Cationic stabilization—A new property of enteroviruses, *Virology* **16**:683–700 (1961).

211. WALLIS, C., AND MELNICK, J. L., Photodynamic inactivation of enteroviruses, *J. Bacteriol.* **89**:41–46 (1965).

212. WALLIS, C., AND MELNICK, J. L., Virus aggregation as the cause of the non-neutralizable persistent fraction, *J. Virol.* **1**:478–488 (1967).

213. WALLIS, C., HOMMA, A., AND MELNICK, J. L., A portable virus concentrator for testing water in the field, *Water Res.* **6**:1249–1256 (1972).

214. WEINSTEIN, L., Poliomyelitis—A persistent problem, *N. Engl. J. Med.* **288**:370–372 (1973).

215. WENNER, H. A., The ECHO viruses, *Ann. N. Y. Acad. Sci.* **101**:398–412 (1962).

216. WENNER, H. A., Virus diseases associated with cutaneous eruptions, *Prog. Med. Virol.* **16**:269–336 (1973).

217. WICKMAN, I., Studien über Poliomyelitis acuta; zugleich ein Beitrag zur Kenntnis der Myelitis acuta, 1905 (English translation, Nervous and Mental Disease Monograph Series, No. 16, Karger, Berlin, 1913).

218. WILFERT, C. M., BUCKLEY, R. H., MOHANAKUMAR, T., GRIFFITH, J. F., KATZ, S. L., WHISNANT J. K., EGGLESTON, P. A., MOORE, M., TREADWELL, E., OXMAN, M. N., AND ROSEN F. S., Persistent and fatal central-nervous-system echovirus infections in patients with agammaglobulinemia, *N. Engl. J. Med.* **296**:1485–1489 (1977).

219. WILSON, F. M., MIRANDA, Q. R., CHASON, J. L., AND LERNER, A. M., Residual pathologic changes following murine coxsackie A and B myocarditis, *Am. J. Pathol.* **55**:253–265 (1969).

219a. WILSON, T., PAPAHADJOPOULOS, D., AND TABER, R., Biological properties of poliovirus encapsulated in lipid vesicles: Antibody resistance and infectivity in virus-resistant cells, *Proc. Natl. Acad. Sci. U.S.A.* **74**:3471–3475 (1977).

220. WONG, C. Y., WOODRUFF, J. J., AND WOODRUFF, J. F., Generation of cytotoxic T lymphocytes during coxsackievirus B-3 infection. II. Characterization of effector cells and demonstration of cytotoxicity against viral-infected myofibers, *J. Immunol.* **118**:1165–1169 (1977).

221. WORLD HEALTH ORGANIZATION COMMITTEE ON POLIOMYELITIS, The relation between acute persisting spinal paralysis and poliomyelitis vaccine (oral): Results of a WHO enquiry, *Bull. WHO* **53**:319–331 (1976).

222. WORLD HEALTH ORGANIZATCON, Poliomyelitis Surveillance, *Weekly Epidemiol. Rec.*, No. 42, p. 304 (20 October 1978).

223. WORLD HEALTH ORGANIZATION, Poliomyelitis in 1977, *Weekly Epidemiol. Rec.*, No. 45, pp. 321–327 (10 November 1978).

224. WORLD HEALTH ORGANIZATION SCIENTIFIC GROUP, Human viruses in water, wastewater, and soil, *WHO Tech. Rep. Ser.*, No. 639 (1979).

225. WORLD HEALTH ORGANIZATION, WHO Weekly Epidemiological Records, during the 1960s and 1970s.

226. WRIGHT, P. F., HATCH, M. H., KASSELBERG, A. G., LOWRY, S. P., WADLINGTON, W. B., AND KARZON, D. T., Vaccine-associated poliomyelitis in a child with

sex-linked agammaglobulinemia, *J. Pediatr.* **91:**408–412 (1977).

227. WYATT, H. V., Hypothesis: Poliomyelitis in hypogammaglobulinemics, *J. Infect. Dis.* **128:**802–806 (1973).

228. YIN-MURPHY, M., Viruses of acute haemorrhagic conjunctivitis, *Lancet* **1:**545–546 (1973).

229. YIN-MURPHY, M., AND LIM, K. H., Picornavirus epidemic conjunctivitis in Singapore, *Lancet* **2:**857–858 (1972).

230. YODFAT, Y., AND NISHMI, M., Epidemiologic and clinical observations in six outbreaks of viral disease in a kibbutz, 1968–1971, *Am. J. Epidemiol.* **97:**415–423 (1973).

231. YOFE, J., GOLDBLUM, N., EYLAN, E., AND MELNICK, J. L., An outbreak of poliomyelitis in Israel in 1961 and the use of attenuated type 1 vaccine in its control, *Am. J. Hyg.* **76:**225–238 (1962).

232. YORKE, J. A., NATHANSON, N., PIANIGIANI, G., AND MARTIN, J., Seasonality and the requirements for perpetuation and eradication of viruses in populations, *Am. J. Epidemiol.* **109:**103–123 (1979).

233. YOUNG, N. A., Polioviruses, coxsackieviruses, and echoviruses: Comparison of the genomes by RNA hybridization, *J. Virol.* **11:**832–839 (1973).

234. YOUNG, D. C., AND SHARP, D. G., Partial reactivation of chlorine-treated echovirus, *Appl. Environ. Microbiol.* **37:**766–773 (1979).

235. ZIEGLER, J. B., AND PENNY, R., Fatal echo 30 virus infection and amyloidosis in X-linked hypogammaglobulinemia, *Clin. Immunol. Immunopathol.* **3:**347–352 (1975).

14. Suggested Reading

GEAR, J. H. S., AND MEASROCH, V., Coxsackievirus infections of the newborn, *Prog. Med. Virol.* **15:**42–62 (1973).

GRIST, N. R., BELL, E. J., AND ASSAAD, F., Enteroviruses in human disease, *Prog. Med. Virol.* **24:**114–157 (1978).

LANSDOWN, A. B. G., Viral infections and diseases of the heart, *Prog. Med. Virol.* **24:**70–113 (1978).

MELNICK, J. L., Advantages and disadvantages of killed and live poliomyelitis vaccines, *Bull. WHO* **56:**21–38 (1978).

MELNICK, J. L., Combined use of live and killed vaccines to control poliomyelitis in tropical areas. *Dev. Biol. Standard.* **47:**265–273 (1981).

MELNICK, J. L., GERBA, C. P., AND WALLIS, C., Viruses in water, *Bull. WHO* **56:**499–508 (1978).

MELNICK, J. L., WENNER, H. A., AND PHILLIPS, C. A., Enteroviruses, in: *Diagnostic Procedures for Viral, Rickettsial, and Chlamydial Infections*, 5th ed. (E. H. LENNETTE AND N. J. SCHMIDT, eds.), pp. 471–534, American Public Health Association, Washington, 1979.

PAUL, J. R., *A History of Poliomyelitis*, Yale University Press, New Haven, 1971.

CHAPTER 10

Epstein–Barr Virus

Alfred S. Evans and James C. Niederman

1. Introduction

Epstein–Barr virus (EBV), a member of the herpes group of viruses, is the cause of heterophile-positive infectious mononucleosis, of most heterophile-negative cases, and of occasional cases of tonsillitis and pharyngitis in childhood. Rarely, it may involve the liver or central nervous system as primary manifestations. This virus is strongly implicated as having a causal relationship to African Burkitt lymphoma and to nasopharyngeal cancer. High antibody titers are also present in 30–40% of cases of Hodgkin's disease, in some patients with sarcoidosis, and in systemic lupus erythematosus.

This chapter will deal with the epidemiology of EBV infections and the epidemiology of infectious mononucleosis. Infectious mononucleosis can be defined as an acute febrile illness involving children and young adults characterized clinically by sore throat and lymphadenopathy, hematologically by lymphocytosis of 50% or more, of which 10% or more are atypical, and serologically by an elevated absorbed heterophile-antibody titer and the development of EBV immunoglobulin M (IgM) and other EBV antibodies. This chapter also mentions the relationship of high antibody titers to certain chronic and malignant diseases, but the major discussion of Burkitt lymphoma and of nasopharyngeal cancer will be found in later chapters of this book.

Alfred S. Evans · WHO Serum Reference Bank, Section of International Epidemiology, Department of Epidemiology and Public Health, Yale University School of Medicine, New Haven, Connecticut. **James C. Niederman** · Department of Epidemiology and Public Health, Yale University School of Medicine, New Haven, Connecticut.

2. Historical Background

In 1889, Emil Pfeiffer of Wiesbaden, Germany, described a condition called *Drüsenfieber* (glandular fever), characterized by fever, adenopathy, mild sore throat, and in severe cases enlargement of the liver and spleen.[63,126] Since Pfeiffer's original description, as well as Filatov's,[53,54] a Russian, in 1892, antedated by some 30–50 years recognition of the hematological changes and the heterophile antibody, it is uncertain whether these were true infectious mononucleosis. However, his description of this febrile syndrome in older children and young adults seems best to fit this diagnosis. There is little doubt about the classic description of the disease made by Sprunt and Evans,[139] from Johns Hopkins, in 1920. They described the disorder in young adults as we now know it, named the disease "infectious mononucleosis," and reported in detail the hematological changes. This description was followed rapidly by similar reports from other workers.[12,14,22,96,108] A definitive presentation of hematological changes was made by Downey and McKinlay[28] in 1923. The next major development was the discovery in 1932 of the heterophile antibody by John R. Paul and William W. Bunnell[121] of Yale University. Their report was based on an accidental observation while studying the occurrence of heterophile antibodies in rheumatic fever. This search had been initiated because of the clinical similarity of rheumatic fever and serum sickness and because of the work of Davidsohn[24] describing the presence of heterophile antibodies in serum sickness. Among the control subjects for rheumatic fever patients was one who had infectious mononucleosis and was found to have a much higher heterophile antibody titer than present in any other condition. Paul and Bunnell then continued these observations in 3 additional cases of infectious mononucleosis and utilized 275 controls for comparison. Their paper also describes what they believed to be a false-positive heterophile antibody occurring in a patient with aplastic leukemia. A review of the details of this case[43] reveals that the heterophile antibody occurred about 20 days after the administration of several units of blood, and therefore this patient may represent the first case of transfusion infectious mononucleosis. Soon after the discovery of the presence of heterophile antibodies, Davidsohn and Walker[23] reported on the use of guinea pig kidney and of beef cells to absorb serum prior to heterophile testing in order to increase the specificity of the test. Both these procedures have withstood the test of time well and still constitute one of the major criteria of diagnosis. Regular alterations in various liver-function tests during acute infectious mononucleosis were recognized in several laboratories in the late 1940s and 1950s,[13,35,86] even though only 5% of patients had clinical jaundice. This was followed by the discovery of alterations in serum glutamic oxalacetic transaminase (SGOT) and other hepatic enzymes during the course of disease.[6,131,158]

Search for the etiological agent of infectious mononucleosis began in the 1920s, but met with little success until 1942, when Wising[156] reported the successful transmission of classic infectious mononucleosis to a female medical student volunteer who received 250 ml of blood from a patient ill with the acute disease. This successful experiment was not reproducible by Wising in several other attempts, nor by Bang,[4] who carried out a similar set of volunteer experiments. In 1947 and again in 1950, additional efforts of this sort were carried out at Yale University using whole blood, serum, or throat washings. The results provided suggestive but inconclusive evidence of transmission.[34,36] A third effort without success was reported from Yale University in 1965.[112] Subsequent EBV antibody tests on the sera from these last experiments in 1968 revealed that all volunteers had actually been immune to infection prior to the experiment as indicated by the presence of antibody.[111]

Repeated attempts in the 1950s to isolate an infectious agent from the throat or blood of patients with infectious mononucleosis using several tissue-culture systems, long-term cultures of lymphocytes on a feeder layer, and fluorescent antibody techniques to identify an agent were unsuccessful.[37] Epidemiologically, the key events during this time were the observations of Hoagland, who suggested that the disease might be transmitted by kissing[79] and that the incubation period was of the order of 30–49 days.[81]

Early in 1968, evidence first appeared that EBV was the cause of infectious mononucleosis.[72,114] This virus, isolated by Epstein et al.[33] from a culture of African Burkitt tumor tissue,[128] was found to be a new member of the herpes group of viruses. While working with this agent, a technician in the Henles' laboratory in Philadelphia developed infectious mononucleosis. Her serum, which lacked antibody several months prior to disease, developed EBV antibody during illness, and her lymphocytes, which had previously failed to be cultivated successfully, now grew well in tissue culture and were shown to contain EBV antigen.[72] This serendipitous observation was rapidly confirmed and extended at that time by the Henles in conjunction with Niederman and McCollum[114] of Yale and later in several other prospective studies carried out by the Yale team[50,113,132] and in one English study.[148] Subsequent investigations established the presence and persistence of EBV in the throat during and after acute infectious mononucleosis,[19,59,103] the occurrence of EBV-specific IgM,[3,66,114b,133] and the reproduction of some features of mononucleosis by inoculation of EBV into monkeys.[135,154] Fuller details of the history of infectious mononucleosis have been published elsewhere.[16,43]

3. Methodology

3.1. Mortality Data

Infectious mononucleosis is rarely a fatal disease; only about 50 fatalities have been reported.[39] Examination of autopsy records or of international indexes of causes of death would therefore give little indication of the occurrence of the disease even though its pathological features are quite characteristic.

3.2. Morbidity Data

Infectious mononucleosis is not a reportable disease in most states and in most countries. Exceptions are the state of Connecticut, where it has been reportable since 1948,[21] and the United States armed forces, which collect hospitalization data on all diseases.[41] Unless strong emphasis is placed on the need for fulfilling clinical, hematological, and serological criteria for diagnosis before reporting, the reliability of morbidity data from these sources must be seriously questioned. This requirement is emphasized by the fact that even for the 15–25 age group—in which the disease has its highest incidence, its most characteristic clinical features, and the highest frequency of elevated heterophile antibody tests—only one-third of the serum samples sent to a state laboratory for diagnosis of suspected cases were heterophile antibody positive.[38]

To collect morbidity data, special surveys of selected populations for infectious mononucleosis have been carried out in college infirmaries,[50,83a,113,132] community medical care groups,[69] and general practitioners' offices,[83] and by physicians and laboratories serving defined communities.[29a,36,68,131a] The Center for Disease Control (CDC) also periodically publishes a Surveillance Report on infectious mononucleosis based on data derived from 19 colleges.[18]

The problems of data derived from such surveys are related to the extent to which the numerator or case report reflects the proper diagnosis and whether adequate surveillance has been carried out with respect to the denominator—the population at risk.

3.3. Serological Surveys

Up to 1968, when the causal association of EBV with infectious mononucleosis was discovered, the heterophile antibody constituted the only serological approach to diagnosis and survey work. Because this is an IgM-type antibody and is transient in nature, it can be used as a serological tool only for incidence data—i.e., during the acute illness—and as an essential diagnostic feature.[114] The specificity of a properly performed quantitative heterophile-antibody test is high provided that the serum has been preabsorbed with guinea pig kidney in the sheep and horse red cell tests or that the beef hemolysin test has been used. In a test performed in this way, an elevated titer quite accurately reflects the occurrence of infectious mononucleosis even in the absence of clinical and hematological data and has been utilized as an indicator of infectious mononucleosis in sera sent to hospitals and state laboratories.[38] The major limitation of this approach is the extent to which physicians have sent sera from suspected cases to the diagnostic laboratory for analysis. The increasing use of simple laboratory kits for identifying heterophile-antibody elevations in the physician's office probably results in much less utilization of state and hospital laboratories, so that morbidity data from these sources may greatly underestimate the occurrence of the disease. Thus, utilization of the heterophile antibody as an epidemiological tool to identify the acute illness has high reliability and specificity but low sensitivity. Heterophile-positive cases diagnosed in the Connecticut State Public Health Laboratory alone represented 74.5% of all the reported cases in the state in 1972.

Since the discovery of EBV as the cause of infectious mononucleosis in 1968, many serological surveys in different countries have been made for the presence of antibody to this virus in sera collected from healthy persons, usually employing the indirect immunofluorescence test[70] for viral capsid antigen (VCA). This IgG antibody persists for many years, perhaps for life.[113,114] These studies yield prevalence data on prior EBV *infection*, but give no direct indication of the occurrence of clinical infectious mononucleosis. More recently, the EBV-specific IgM antibody has been included in surveys to identify recent infection.[144a]

The most accurate information on the *incidence* of both EBV infections and clinical infectious mononucleosis has come from prospective seroepidemiological studies of defined populations with close clinical surveillance for the occurrence of suspected cases of infectious mononucleosis and other illnesses. Sera taken at the start of the observation period are tested to define the number of susceptibles, i.e., those lacking EBV antibody; samples showing seroconversion at the end of the observation period will identify the total EBV infection rate; those collected during interim illnesses and tested for EBV and heterophile antibodies will delineate the number and spectrum of clinical illnesses, such as infectious mononucleosis, associated with EBV infection.

3.4. Laboratory Methods

3.4.1. EBV Isolation. The virus cannot be grown in the usual tissue cultures employed for other herpesviruses. The currently available isolation technique is tedious, difficult, and usually confined to research laboratories. It is based on the ability of EBV to transform uninfected human leukocytes into continuous cell lines and the identification of this effect as due to EBV.[19,103] Leukocytes derived from the cords of newborn infants or from persons lacking EBV antibody are employed to ensure absence of EBV antigen in the lymphocytes. Throat washings or other materials to be tested are usually filtered to remove debris and bacteria, then added to the leukocytes, and placed on a placental fibroblast feeder layer. If EBV is present, evidence of transformation is indicated by an abrupt increase in the total number of cells, the production of acid, growth of cells in clumps, and the development of the capacity to be subcultured indefinitely. Usually, transformation occurs 30–90 days after addition of the throat washing.

The presence of EBV-associated nuclear antigen (EBNA) can be demonstrated in acetone-fixed smears of transformed cord cells using an indirect complement-fixation (CF) fluorescence technique,[129] but VCA cannot be demonstrated by ordinary immunofluorescence methods, presumably because the virus does not mature sufficiently in such cells. EBV-transformed leukocytes may also be grown further in culture to prepare a CF antigen as a means of identification; however, this is a laborious method. More sensitive methods of antigen detection, chemical means of enhancing the rapidity of viral multiplication to shorten the long observation time, or discovery of a more sensitive cell line will be needed before viral isolation will be practical in the diagnostic laboratory. Robinson and Miller[129a] have demonstrated that DNA stimulation occurs early in EBV-infected cord cells and can be detected by increased uptake of radio-labeled thymidine.

3.4.2. EBV Antibody. A wide variety of techniques to measure EBV antibody have been developed. Five antibody methods based on immunofluorescence have been used.[73a] First, for epidemiological purposes, the indirect immunofluorescence test of the Henles[70] for VCA has been widely employed in serological surveys as a reliable indicator of susceptibility and immunity to infectious

mononucleosis. However, it has not proved very useful as a diagnostic test for infectious mononucleosis because antibody is usually present by the time the patient seeks medical care and rises in titer are detectable in only 15–20% of cases. Second, antibody to "early antigen" is also identified by immunofluorescence techniques,[74,76] and its presence is indicative of recent or active infection. Unfortunately, from a diagnostic standpoint, it is demonstrable only in about 75% of patients with infectious mononucleosis[77]; it also occurs in the sera from patients with Burkitt lymphoma and nasopharyngeal cancer. Third, antibodies to EBNA are detectable by an immunofluorescence technique based on CF; these usually arise only 1 month or more after onset of infectious mononucleosis and after primary infections and probably persist for life.[73] Their late appearance impairs their usefulness in routine diagnosis. Fourth, there is an indirect immunofluorescence test for EBV-specific IgM antibody, and this is the most useful procedure for the diagnosis of heterophile-negative infectious mononucleosis[29,114b,133]; however, in its present form, this test is technically difficult to perform, and it is not currently available in most diagnostic laboratories. Finally, a membrane fluorescence test has been developed by Klein et al.[88–90] Other antibody tests include CF using either the virus[1] or soluble antigens,[56,57] neutralization tests based on contact inhibition,[78,105] and immunodiffusion tests.[116]

3.4.3. Heterophile Antibody Tests. Three general methods are employed: (1) the classic Paul–Bunnell test[121] using sheep or horse red cells after absorption of the serum with guinea pig kidney as developed by Davidsohn and Walker[23]; (2) the beef-cell hemolysin test of Bailey and Raffel[2] adopted for diagnostic use by Mason,[98] which does not require absorption of sera with guinea pig kidney because beef-cell hemolysins are absent or at very low titers in normal sera; and (3) the enzyme test of Wöllner,[157] in which red-cell receptors for heterophile antibody are specifically removed by treatment with papain or a similar enzyme. Recent evidence suggests that heterophile-antibody titers may reach diagnostic levels even after mild or asymptomatic EBV infections provided serial specimens are tested over a month or so by the horse-cell differential test.[52] The test is also useful in childhood EBV infections, which are often mild. Most state and large diagnostic laboratories employ either the Davidsohn differential absorption test or the beef-cell hemolysin test; the former, using horse cells, is more sensitive, and heterophile antibody to this antigen often persists at diagnostic levels for as long as a year or so.[52,93] The beef hemolysin test is more specific but less sensitive, and disappears in 3 months or less; it is perhaps the most reliable test to diagnose infectious mononucleosis during the acute illness. A new immunoadherence test of high sensitivity is also promising.[94c]

A number of commercial testing kits for the diagnosis of infectious mononucleosis in the physician's office are now available. Most are slide agglutination tests, usually performed at a single dilution and commonly based on the agglutination of formalinized horse cells. Some of these employ guinea pig kidney to remove nonspecific agglutinins from the serum prior to testing. Other tests employ papain-treated red cells in the agglutination test. A spot test using horse red cells and absorption procedures is recommended. Such tests are useful if carried out by trained personnel.

4. Biological Characteristics of the Agent

4.1. The Virus

EBV is a distinctive member of the herpes group of viruses. On electron microscopy, EBV appears similar to other herpes-group viruses.[33] Currently, two laboratory strains of EBV have been identified,[106] but the sophisticated techniques needed to differentiate strain differences as small as exist between herpes types I and II are not yet available. Definitive evidence of differences in EBV isolates from nature have not yet been found, although minor variations exist.[59a] The virus has been cultivated only in suspension cultures of primate lymphocytes, and most cultures yield only small amounts of extracellular virus. These limitations have made characterization of the physical and chemical properties of EBV very difficult. EBV is a lymphotropic virus and infects B lymphocytes, which have EBV receptors on their surface[85a] near to or identical with the C3 receptors[154a]; new membrane antigens are induced to which T cells respond. All lymphocytes in continuous cultures established from infectious mononucleosis blood or Burkitt lymphoma biopsies contain the EBV genome as demonstrated

by DNA hybridization or EBNA tests, but only 1–3% have demonstrable VCA[115,117,129,160]; cell clones grown from such cultures show a similar low percentage of complete virus.[99,159] One line of cells from Burkitt lymphoma, the P3J line of Pulvertaft,[128] and its cloned derivative, the HR1K, produce more extracellular virus than other lines but fail to induce transformation.[106] Another line, B95-8, derived from EBV-infected marmoset cells by Miller and Lipman,[102] releases about 1000 times more transforming virus but about the same number of viral particles as HR1K. It has been useful in viral characterization.[68c,d]

Some of the biological properties of EBV are important epidemiologically. The capacity for persistence of a lytic infection in the throat provides a source of potential transmission; the low yield of extracellular virus may bear on the need for intimate, oral contact for transmission in young adults.[114b] The reasons for the higher efficiency of transmission of EBV infection in young children than in adults are unknown, but might include the production of more infectious virus in the pharynx of children, more intense exposure, or indirect spread by saliva in settings with poor hygiene.

The capacity for persistence and latency of EBV in a *nonproductive* form sets the stage for later reactivation under conditions of immunosuppression (e.g., malaria, therapeutic immunosuppression in renal transplants). African Burkitt lymphoma and nasopharyngeal cancer may be expressions of this reactivation. The long-term persistence of EBV in lymphocytes is of importance epidemiologically in the transmission of infection during blood transfusions to susceptible recipients. Of great importance is the capacity of EBV to transform uninfected primate lymphocytes, inducing in them the potential for unlimited proliferation; this property was termed "immortalization" by Miller,[100] and the lymphocytes that result are termed "I lymphocytes." The EBV-transformed and -infected cells are B-type lymphocytes.[118,119] Viral induction of new antigens (or unmasking of preexisting ones) such as the membrane antigen of Klein et al.[88] may have immunological consequences in the development of new antibodies, in a graft-vs.-host response, and in the induction of cytotoxic T lymphocytes.[83b,131c]

A better understanding of the dynamics and effects of EBV activity at molecular and cellular levels ("molecular epidemiology") and of the responses of the host of them under varied conditions of age, concomitant infection, immune status, and genetic constitution will be needed before the full spectrum of clinical response is known.

4.2. Proof of Causation of Infectious Mononucleosis

The causation of heterophile-positive infectious mononucleosis by EBV has been established beyond any reasonable doubt. The proof is based on seroepidemiological and virological evidence and also on partial success in the experimental transmission of infection to monkeys and man.

Seroepidemiological investigations have repeatedly shown that *antibody* to EBV of the IgG type has been consistently absent in sera taken prior to the onset of infectious mononucleosis, regularly appears during illness, and persists for years thereafter.[50,65,114,132,148] The presence of this antibody indicates immunity to clinical infectious mononucleosis, and its absence indicates susceptibility to the disease. Table 1 summarizes 11 prospective studies involving over 5000 children and young adults in support of this relationship. No other virus has been found that induces a similar antibody, and no other viral antibody has been demonstrated during heterophile-positive infectious mononucleosis. The occurrence of some heterophile-negative cases of infectious mononucleosis due to EBV has also been noted in prospective studies.[50,65] Other mono-like syndromes are due to cytomegalovirus and other agents.[44a,92]

EBV-specific antibody of the IgM class has been demonstrated during acute infectious mononucleosis and found to disappear during convalescence, thus indicating that this is a primary response to EBV infection.[4,29,66,133] Both the IgG and IgM EBV-specific antibodies of infectious mononucleosis are distinct from the heterophile antibody.

The virological evidence consists of the appearance of EBV in the oropharynx and in the circulating lymphocytes of patients with acute infectious mononucleosis. The agent has been regularly demonstrated in the pharynx of over 80% of patients during the acute illness[19,59,103,125] and may be multiplying in epithelial cells.[94a] In addition, EBV antigens have been found in tonsillar lymphocytes.[149a,b] They persist for many months and in several cases have persisted for as long as a year or so. A chronic carrier state may exist, as suggested by the presence of virus in the oropharynx of 15–20% of healthy adults.[20,59,143]

EBV has been regularly demonstrated in lymphocyte cultures from patients with acute infectious mononucleosis, where it may remain in a latent form for years and may be a source of transfusion mononucleosis.[26,58,75] EBV has now been demonstrated in *fresh* B lymphocytes from patients with acute infectious mononucleosis[90a,130a]: up to 0.5% of circulating mononuclear leukocytes are EBV-infected during the acute illness.[130a] The appearance and persistence of EBV in the oropharynx following mild or asymptomatic infections provides a large pool of healthy carriers capable of transmitting infection through appropriate exposure.

Efforts to transmit infectious mononucleosis to volunteers using blood, throat washings, or stools from acutely ill patients were made prior to the discovery of EBV in 1968; the results were largely inconclusive or unsuccessful, probably because of the presence of prior immunity in those inoculated.

Table 1. Summary of 11 Prospective Studies of Epstein–Barr Virus Infection in Children and Young Adults[a]

EBV antibody status at start	Number	Percentage	Subsequent rate/100 per year	
			EBV infection	Clinical infectious mononucleosis[b]
With antibody	3733	70.7	0	0
Without antibody	1547	29.3	16.4	7.1
TOTALS:	5280	100	4.6	2.0

[a] From ten studies carried out by Yale investigators[50,132,148] and one by an English team.[148]
[b] Clinical infectious mononucleosis was recognized in 47% of those infected with EBV.

However, there are a few exceptions. Wising[156] successfully transmitted the full-blown disease to a female volunteer by transfusion. Evans[37] and Taylor[145] reported suggestive evidence of successful transmission by inoculation of pooled sera from patients with acute infectious mononucleosis into patients with acute leukemia as a therapeutic effort to induce a remission; the young age of this group probably meant that some were susceptible because they had not been previously exposed. About 50 other experiments in humans were equivocal or unsuccessful.[3,34,36,112] Similarly, earlier efforts to induce infectious mononucleosis in monkeys were not rewarding.[49,137]

Recent studies with this virus in humans have been very limited because of concern for the oncogenicity of EBV. Grace *et al.*[61] repeatedly inoculated partially purified EBV into a terminal cancer patient who lacked prior antibody; both EBV and heterophile antibodies developed. Inoculation of EBV-infected lymphocytes into gibbons has resulted in an exudative tonsillitis and the appearance of EBV antibody.[154] Shope and Miller[135] have induced transient EBV and heterophile antibody in squirrel monkeys inoculated with virus-transformed leukocytes. The current evidence of successful transmission of infectious mononucleosis to monkeys must be regarded as incomplete at this time.

In summary, the results of seroepidemiological, virological, and transmission studies in man and monkeys indicate that EBV is the cause of all cases of heterophile-positive mononucleosis and most heterophile-negative cases.[40,42,44a]

5. Descriptive Epidemiology

5.1. Prevalence and Incidence

The *prevalence of antibody* to the VCA of EBV has been determined in many countries and in many age groups.[42] Figure 1 indicates the percentage of children in several areas of the world with EBV antibody. In developing and tropical areas, most children have been infected by age 6 years. Because infections with EBV are often mild and asymptomatic in young children, infectious mononucleosis may not be commonly recognized as a clinical entity in such countries. However, more intensive clinical and serological studies, especially employing newer diagnostic techniques, have permitted identification of both heterophile-positive and heterophile-negative cases of infectious mononucleosis in children in such settings as Singapore[12a] and Brazil.[117a] The prevalence of EBV antibody in young adults living in different parts of the world is depicted in Fig. 2. A similar socioeconomic pattern exists. It is only when a significant percentage of the population reaches ages 15–25 before exposure to and infection with EBV that infectious mononucleosis emerges as an important clinical entity. This delay in exposure is largely limited to nations with high economic and hygienic levels and to middle and upper socioeconomic classes in any country. The most susceptible college group tested thus far were entering freshman students at Yale University in the period 1958–1963, when nearly 75% were at risk to infectious mononucleosis because they lacked antibody;

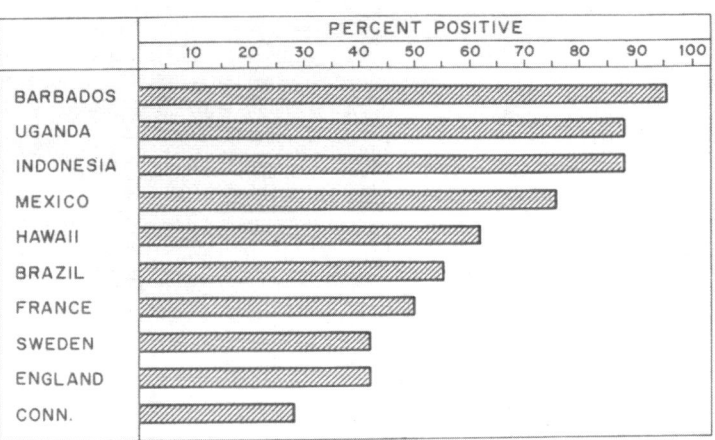

Fig. 1. EBV antibody prevalence at age 4–6 years in different populations. Adapted from Evans.[42]

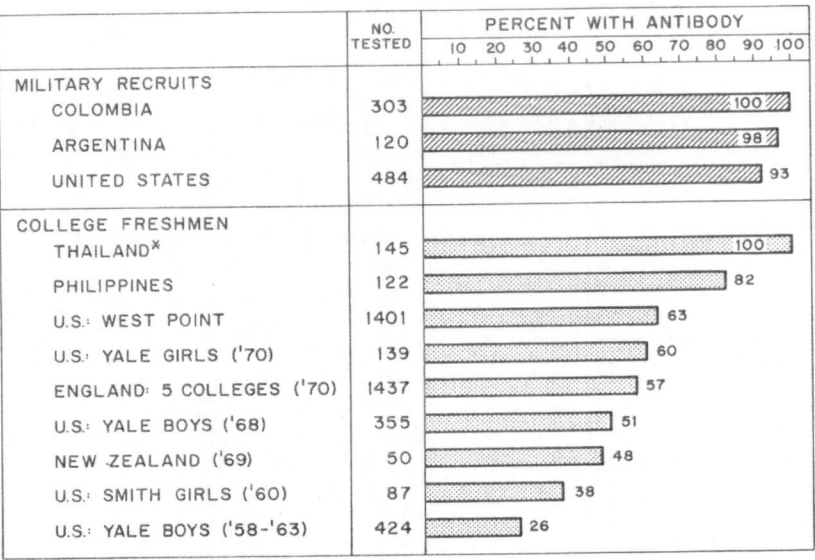

Fig. 2. EBV antibody prevalence in young adults in different populations. (×) Student nurses. Adapted from Evans.[42]

coincident with programs that broadened admission to include students with widely differing socioeconomic backgrounds, among them many minority groups, the susceptibles decreased to 40–50%. In contrast, under 20% of undergraduate students at the University of Philippines lacked EBV antibody, and all of 145 freshman student nurses in Thailand had antibody.

Hospitalization rates for infectious mononucleosis in the armed forces range from 148 to 250 per 100,000.[41] In the Navy and Marine Corps, for which comparative data are available, it ranks as the fifth most common infectious disease and the fourth most common cause of days lost.

The incidence of clinical infectious mononucleosis is not well documented, since reporting is not obligatory in most states in the United States, and the available data have usually been derived from special surveys such as the community survey in Atlanta, Georgia, where a rate of 45 per 100,000 of heterophile-positive cases was found, and in Olmstead County, which includes the Mayo Clinic, where resident rates were 200 per 100,000. In Denmark, the rate of notified cases is 60 per 100,000.[131a] The state of Connecticut requires reporting of infectious mononucleosis, and rates of 48 per 100,000

were recorded in 1972.[21] In 1979, a simplified report form and an aggressive surveillance system were initiated for all reportable diseases, resulting in a rate for infectious mononucleosis of 137.7 per 100,000.[21a] This rate of infectious mononucleosis is surpassed only by chicken pox and gonorrhea among reportable diseases in Connecticut for 1979 and greatly exceeds mumps, rubella, measles, and hepatitis (Table 2). As comparison, the United States rates for these communicable diseases per 100,000 in 1978 were as follows: gonorrhea, 464.7; chicken pox, 80.4; hepatitis A, 13.5; measles, 12.3; primary and secondary syphilis, 10.0; and rubella, 8.4. Among college students, the rates of infectious mononucleosis are very high, averaging 840 per 100,000 students in 19 colleges in 1971–1972.[18]

The most accurate measure of EBV infection and of disease has been obtained in prospective serological and clinical studies, where the number of susceptibles, the infection (seroconversion) rate, and the clinical attack rate can be critically defined. Comparative data are available from three prospective investigations of freshman students: at Yale University,[132] at five English colleges and universities,[148] and at the U.S. Military Academy at West Point, New York.[65] As depicted in Table 3, the

Table 2. Reported Cases and Cases per 100,000 Population for Infectious Mononucleosis and Other Reportable Diseases in Connecticut for 1979[a]

Disease	Reported cases	Cases/100,000[b]
Chicken pox	11,525	363.0
Gonorrhea	9,627	303.2
Infectious mononucleosis	4,371	137.7
Rubella	258	8.1
Mumps	231	7.3
Hepatitis B	213	6.7
Hepatitis A	185	5.8
Measles	4	0.1

[a] Derived from data provided by the Connecticut State Department of Health.
[b] Based on a population of 3,174,784.

incidence rate of EBV *infection* was strikingly similar in all three settings: 12–13% of *susceptible* students were infected with EBV during the freshman year, and of those with known EBV infection, 27.7–74.0% developed clinical infectious mononucleosis. At the U.S. Military Academy, where a prospective investigation was carried on in a single cohort of freshmen over 4 years, the EBV infection rate in susceptible cadets was 12.4% in the first year, 24.4% in the second year, 15.1% in the third year, and 30.8% in the fourth college year.[65] Over the 4-year period, 45.9% of susceptible cadets were infected with EBV, and 26.4% of these were known to have clinical infectious mononucleosis; others may have been ill but not have reported to the clinic for treatment. The reasons for the varying rates of clinical expression among EBV-infected young adults in similar settings are not known. The variation may be related to the intensity of clinical surveillance, the students' attitude toward the health service, the average time of hospitalization, or various host factors. Some ev-

idence on the influence of psychological factors is emerging[88a] (see Section 5.11).

5.2. Epidemic Behavior

True epidemics of infectious mononucleosis that fulfill appropriate diagnostic criteria have not occurred in modern times.[38,82] Earlier, many purported epidemics were described, of which the most impressive are those described by West[155] in the United States in 1896, by Moir[107] in the Falkland Islands in 1930, and by Carlson *et al.*[15] in Wisconsin in 1926. More recent and suggestive outbreaks have been described from an Emergency Medical Hospital[64] and from Oxford, England, reported by Hobson *et al.*[83] A small outbreak involving 9 of 29 staff members in an outpatient clinic was recently reported by Ginsburg *et al.*[59c]; however, the source of the outbreak and means of spread were not identified.

The high incidence in military camps during World War II probably reflects the rapid turnover of large numbers of men.[46,149,153] Some reported hospital "outbreaks" are suggestive of a true outbreak,[64,83] but in general do not fully meet diagnostic criteria. On a hypothetical basis, the early acquisition of immunity to infectious mononucleosis by mild and inapparent infections with EBV in childhood and the probable route of transmission via intimate oral contact in young adults weigh heavily against the occurrence of "epidemic infectious mononucleosis."

The high prevalence rates of EBV antibody in children in developing countries,[42,48] in nurseries,[124] and in orphanages[147] suggest that EBV spreads effectively in young children under circumstances of crowding and poor hygiene to reach almost all susceptibles. However, the contagiousness of infectious mononucleosis has been notoriously low in young adult populations; secondary cases have

Table 3. Epstein–Barr Virus Infection Rates during Freshman Year and Percentage Clinically Expressed in Different Colleges

Place	Number in study	Susceptible (%)	Infection rate in susceptibles (%)	Clinical infectious mononucleosis (%)
U.S. Military Academy[65]	1401	36	12.3	27.7
Five English schools[148]	1487	43	12.0	59.1
Yale University[132]	355	49	13.1	74.0

been rare in roommates of index cases,[37,65,79] in college dormitories,[37,45,132] aboard ship,[122] and on Polaris submarines.[142] The low contagiousness in college populations has been confirmed in recent studies employing the status of EBV antibody as a marker of susceptibility and of infection. Among susceptible and exposed roommates of Yale freshmen with infectious mononucleosis, no evidence of increased risk was found over the susceptible population as a whole[132]; however, there tended to be some aggregation of cases in social clusters in dormitories. In a more critical analysis of this issue at the U.S. Military Academy over a period of 4 years, no evidence of increased spread of EBV infection to susceptible roommates exposed to an index case was detected as compared with susceptible roommates not so exposed.[65] In a family setting, about 10% of exposed and susceptible members will develop EBV infection.[71,85,151]

This low level of contagiousness of EBV infection in older children and in young adults of the same sex may be related to a high level of existing immunity and to the need for intimate oral contact. The rate of infection among susceptible persons who are known to have had intimate oral contact with patients who have infectious mononucleosis or with established pharyngeal carriers of EBV has not yet been defined; it may well be high.

5.3. Geographic Distribution

Infection with EBV is worldwide. Antibody to EBV has been demonstrated in every population thus far tested, including very isolated tribes in Brazil,[11] Alaska,[147] and other remote areas[57] where measles and influenza antibody are often lacking. Infection occurs earlier in life in developing countries.

Clinical infectious mononucleosis occurs most commonly in those hygienic and socioeconomic areas where exposure to and infection with EBV are delayed until older childhood and young adult life. This includes Australia, Canada, England, many European countries, New Zealand, Scandinavian countries, and the United States.[42] In contrast, at the University of the Philippines, not a single case was recorded among 5000 admissions to the college infirmary, where laboratory facilities existed[47]; EBV antibody determinations in this college population

revealed a very high level of prior immunity. The disease is now being recognized with more careful clinical and diagnostic scrutiny in developing countries.[12a,117a] The prevalence of EBV antibody had been found to vary in young adults entering the U.S. Military Academy from different areas of the United States.[65] The highest rate of 81.5% was found in cadets resident for 6 years or more in the East South Central States and the lowest prevalence rate of 51.9% in the West North Central States. Since admission to the academy is based on competitive academic, athletic, and achievement values rather than on any social or economic considerations, a broad range of backgrounds would be expected.

5.4. Temporal Distribution

There is no clear-cut evidence of yearly fluctuations in the incidence of infectious mononucleosis, although appropriate morbidity data are not available to determine this accurately. Since 1948 in Connecticut, a yearly increase in incidence has been noted from 3.9 cases per 100,000 initially to 46.7 in 1967[21]; this probably reflects increased reporting rather than actual changes in incidence. In one Swedish hospital where the same population was served and the same diagnostic criteria were presumably applied over a period from 1940 to 1957, the hospitalization rate increased from 12 cases per year in 1940–1942 to 110 per year in 1955–1957.[144] Caution must be observed in interpreting hospital data in which there is no defined denominator. No changes in the incidence rates of infectious mononucleosis were noted at Yale University over a 5-year period[50] or in a careful study with a defined population base in Rochester, Minnesota, over the period 1950–1969.[69]

Earlier studies of college students at the U.S. Military Academy[82] and at the University of Wisconsin[37] showed a peak in February, some 4–6 weeks after Christmas vacation, presumably due to increased exposure at these times. However, no clear-cut seasonal pattern has been seen in the CDC Surveillance Reports from 19 colleges and universities.[18] In a recent community study in Atlanta, Georgia,[68] two peaks were found, one in early fall and a larger one in later winter and early spring, but in Rochester, Minnesota,[69] no seasonal peak was observed.

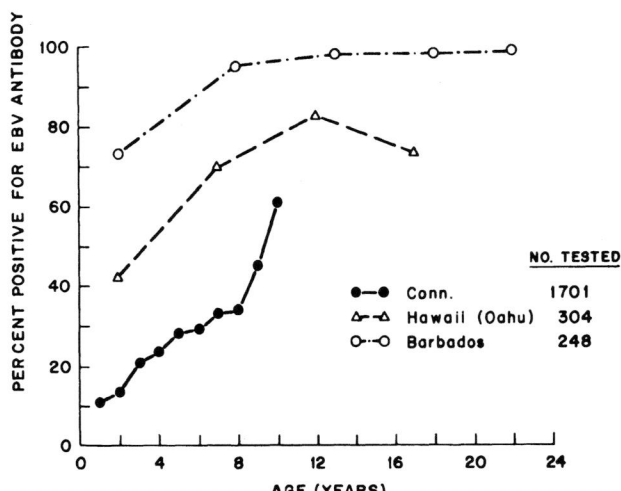

Fig. 3. Acquisition of EBV antibody by age in three different areas. Data derived in part from Evans[42] and Jennings.[84]

5.5. Age

The acquisition of EBV antibody by age is shown in Fig. 3 for three different geographic areas. Antibody occurs early in life in economically underdeveloped countries, often reaching close to 100% immunity by age 10. In a prospective study of EBV infections in newborns living in Accra, Ghana, 81% had acquired antibody by age 21 months,[10a] but none showed evidence of clinical infectious mononucleosis.[10b] In contrast, clinical infectious mononucleosis is clearly a disease of older children and young adults in economically developed countries, with its highest incidence in the 15- to 25-year-old age group. This has been true of data based on hospitalized cases in the United States,[55,68,69,95,110]

France,[138] and Denmark,[146] on heterophile-positive cases identified in state public-health laboratories,[25,38,108a,109,131a] and on recent community surveys in which the population at risk can be defined.[68,69] In results from the Atlanta community survey based on 575 heterophile-positive cases, the highest rate, 345.2 per 100,000, occurred in the 15–19 age group and the next highest, 122.8, in the 20–24 age group; 27 heterophile-positive cases occurred in the 5–9 age group, and 4 in the 0–4 age group. Figure 4 shows the distribution of cases in this study. A similar age distribution was observed in the Wisconsin State laboratory data based on elevated antibody titers in sera from suspected cases sent in for heterophile testing.[38] The peak frequency was in the 20–24 age group, in which 29.6%

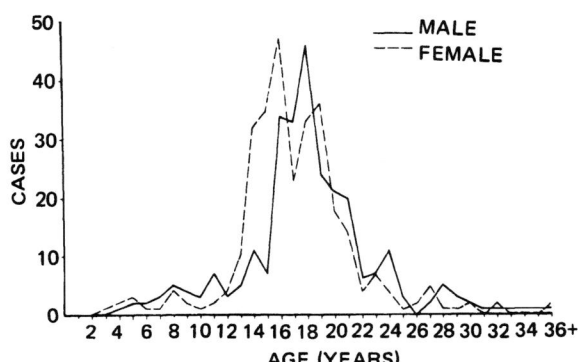

Fig. 4. Cases of infectious mononucleosis, by age and sex, metropolitan Atlanta, Georgia, 1968.

of the sera were positive. Some cases occurred at the extremes of age: 11.9% of the sera from suspected cases were positive in the 5–9 age group and 5.8% in the 65–69 age group. Use of more sensitive heterophile tests and of the EBV IgM tests now permits an increasing number of cases to be identified in childhood.[54a,59b,117a] The mean age of mononucleosis cases was 18.4 years in Wisconsin[38] and 19.3 years in Norway.[108a]

The age pattern described is that of developed countries. In developing countries, the age distribution will be shifted downward because of the small number of children who escape infection until an age when the host response is that of recognizable infectious mononucleosis. In a recent study in São Paulo, Brazil, the average age of 15 heterophile-negative patients was 4.7 years and that of 31 heterophile-positive cases was 13.2 years.[117a] The oldest case was age 15; 5 cases occurred in the 0–2 age group. In this setting, over 90% of the population has EBV antibody by age 10.[17]

5.6. Sex

No difference in EBV-antibody prevalence rates by sex have been noted in population surveys.

Infectious mononucleosis occurs equally in both sexes, although girls appear to develop the disease earlier than boys,[68,69] with a peak occurring in girls at age 16 and boys at age 18 (see Fig. 4).

5.7. Race

EBV *infection* occurs in all ethnic groups; no evidence of differential susceptibility has been found.

Infectious mononucleosis in developed countries has been rare in blacks, but this probably reflects socioeconomic levels and earlier acquisition of infection rather than any difference in susceptibility. The incidence of the disease in whites in Atlanta, Georgia, was 30 times higher than in blacks.[68] Antibody prevalence to EBV among entering black cadets at the U.S. Military Academy was 85% as compared with 65% among whites.[65] In an analysis of prevalence rates among different ethnic groups in Hawaii,[84] higher rates were observed in Hawaiians and Filipinos than in Caucasians of the same age. However, socioeconomic levels, hygienic habits, and varying cultural practices in the home cannot be separated from the ethnic backgrounds.

5.8. Occupation

Infectious mononucleosis is most often a disease of the college student and of the white-collar worker.[55,110] It is these persons who are likely to escape infection until young adult life because of higher socioeconomic level or hygienic standards or both. It is also common in the military.[30,41]

5.9. Occurrence in Different Settings

The original cases of Pfeiffer[126] suggested that the disease had a familial pattern, and this has been partially borne out by subsequent studies. Analyses of sera from the Cleveland family study[27,71] produced evidence of several cases in three of seven families. There appeared to be a paucity of EBV infections in the 6–12 year age group in this setting, with higher rates observed in children under 6 and over 12. Among 75 Canadian families, Joncas and Mitnyan[85] identified 67 persons lacking EBV antibody; in follow-up over approximately 2 years, only 10.5% of these susceptible persons developed EBV antibody. In Sweden, Wahren et al.[151] found EBV antibody increases in 7 of 21 members exposed to an index case; 6 of the 21 contacts lacked EBV antibody initially, and 3 of these seroconverted.

The high rates of infectious mononucleosis in college and military settings have already been noted. However, during the early recruit-training period in the armed forces, infectious mononucleosis is not a common disease, unlike adenovirus, *Mycoplasma pneumoniae*, and other respiratory infections. This is probably due both to a high level of preexisting immunity among recruits and to the long incubation period of about 4–7 weeks, so that cases usually develop after the end of the usual training period and after dispersal of recruits to other military assignments. The former point is supported by the finding of an antibody prevalence rate of 85% in entering Marine recruits at Parris Island[94] and of 93% in Army recruits at Fort Jackson, South Carolina.[51] Among the Marine recruits at Parris Island whose sera lacked antibody, the infection rate was 18.5 per 1000 over the 16-week training period; in those returning from a 13-month overseas assignment, the EBV infection rate was estimated at 23.8 per 1000. Among the 34 Fort Jackson recruits who lacked EBV antibody, 3 recruits developed EBV antibody during the 16 weeks of basic and advanced training,[51] a rate of 88 per 1000 recruits.

5.10. Socioeconomic Factors

Socioeconomic settings influence the incidence of both EBV infection and infectious mononucleosis, but in opposite directions. Low socioeconomic groups have high rates of EBV infection early in life, but little clinical infectious mononucleosis; high socioeconomic groups have low levels of EBV infection early in life, but a high rate of clinical disease that occurs in the 15- to 25-year-old group. Two examples illustrate this effect on infection rates. At the U.S. Military Academy at West Point, the EBV-antibody prevalence rate was 77.1% in cadets coming from families earning under $6000 and only 58.6% among those from families with incomes of over $30,000.[65] In New Haven, the antibody prevalence among first-graders in three schools serving a low socioeconomic group was 84.8%, and in three schools serving a high socioeconomic group, it was 37.8%.[136] A second serum sample collected from these same children 4–5 years later revealed an EBV seroconversion rate of 50% among susceptible children from lower socioeconomic areas and only 2.4% in susceptible children in the higher socioeconomic group.

5.11. Other Factors

Little is known of the role of nutritional and genetic factors in relation either to EBV infections or to infectious mononucleosis. However, it is recognized that ABO blood groups are not correlated with susceptibility to infection or to clinical disease.[65,132] The relationship to HLA antigens has not been clearly established.[132b] It seems likely that genetic control of the immune response plays a role in the severity of clinical illness, in the persistence of virus, and in possible oncogenic sequelae as suggested in recent studies of EBV infections in the X-linked lymphoproliferative syndrome.[128a,b]

Psychological and behavioral factors may influence the frequency with which clinical infectious mononucleosis develops after EBV infection. By correlation of psychological scores taken on entry into the school and subsequent academic achievement with the prospective serological and clinical data collected in cadets at the United States Military Academy at West Point,[65] the following factors were found to be significantly associated with an increased risk of development of *clinical* infectious

mononucleosis in cadets infected with EBV[88a]: (1) having fathers who were "overachievers"; (2) having a strong commitment to a military career; (3) ascribing strong values to various aspects of the training and military career; (4) scoring poorly on indices of relative academic performance; and (5) having strong motivation and doing relatively poorly academically. The same factors seemed to influence development of heterophile antibody during mild or inapparent EBV infections, a result free of bias toward seeking medical care.

6. Mechanism and Route of Transmission

The major route of transmission of infectious mononucleosis in young adults is probably through intimate oral contact in kissing with the exchange of saliva, as first suggested by Hoagland[79] in 1955. This concept is supported by three types of circumstantial evidence: First, close personal contact without kissing, as in roommates of infected patients[132] or in such confining environments as a destroyer[122] or a Polaris submarine, rarely leads to secondary cases[142]; this has been true even when the exposed roommate is known to lack EBV antibody and is followed closely over 2 months for the appearance of antibody or of clinical symptoms.[65] Second, a history of intimate oral contact within the appropriate incubation period is common in young adults who develop infectious mononucleosis[79] and occurs statistically more frequently than in healthy controls or patients with acute respiratory infections.[37] Third, the presence of EBV has been demonstrated in the pharynx during acute illness and during convalescence for periods of many months (Table 4).[19,59,103,114a] In addition, cross-sectional studies of presumably healthy adults have also shown EBV pharyngeal excretion in 15–20% of young adults.[59,143] One investigation found a leukocyte-transforming factor, presumably EBV, in the throats of 18% of 368 patients attending an outpatient clinic.[20] Transmission of EBV infection may also occur via blood transfusions, usually without illness.[58,75,150]

This prolonged carrier state after clinical infectious mononucleosis and following inapparent EBV infection may serve as the principal source of exposure in young adults. The long duration of virus excretion may explain the difficulties in tracing

Table 4. Recovery of Epstein–Barr Virus from Oropharyngeal Excretions of 32 Patients with Infectious Mononucleosis

| | Throat washings | | |
| | | Positive | |
Days after onset	Number tested	Number	%
0–6	5	1	20.0
7–14	20	15	75.0
15–21	8	5	62.5
22–28	10	6	60.0
29–60	13	8	61.5
61–150	12	11	91.7
>150	19	6	31.6
TOTALS:	87	52	59.7

transmission of disease from case to case. Virus excretion occurs in the presence of circulating antibody, which suggests that humoral antibody does not have a major role in the regulation of oropharyngeal shedding. Clearly, identification of the specific oropharyngeal cells that produce infectious virus remains an important area for further investigation. EBV was not found in the urine of 10 acute cases or in the cervix of 175 pregnant or postpartum women.[149c]

The mechanism of transmission accounting for the rapid and high rate of acquisition of EBV antibody in nurseries and in young children in low socioeconomic circumstances[59a,124,147] is not definitely known. Presumably, transfer of infected saliva on fingers, toys, and other inanimate objects in settings of poor hygiene can account for much of the spread of infection. Perhaps more cell-free virus is released in childhood infections. A recent report of hepatitis due to EBV in a hemodialysis unit raises the possibility of airborne spread.[21b]

From a practical standpoint, the low contagiousness of the disease in young adults eliminates the need for strict isolation procedures.

7. Pathogenesis and Immunity

The incubation period of infectious mononucleosis is 4–7 weeks[37,81] in college students. This esti-

mate is based on well-defined, often single contacts between an index case and a member of the opposite sex involving intimate oral contact.

Studies of the recovery of EBV from oropharyngeal secretions of patients with infectious mononucleosis have revealed that virus shedding occurs during acute illness and from several weeks to months after onset, but the type of cells involved in viral maturation and release is unknown. Transformation of umbilical-cord leukocytes into continuous cell lines has been the assay system used for demonstration of the virus, and this transformation has been neutralized by sera containing EBV antibody, but not affected by sera lacking this antibody.[103] In addition, transformed leukocytes acquire EBV genome, demonstrated by nucleic acid hybridization, and express EBV-associated antigens. The virus has been detected in throat washings for prolonged periods and as indicated in Table 4 is regularly recovered several months after clinical illness. In 6 of 19 patients, the agent was still present over 5 months after disease had occurred and in 1 case was detected 24 months after onset. No special clinical characteristics have as yet been identified in those cases associated with prolonged oropharyngeal virus shedding.

Prior to the onset of definite symptoms in young adults, there is frequently a history of ill-defined complaints, such as malaise and easy fatigue. It has been suggested that an early, abortive infection of this type may occur in children without subsequent development of classic infectious mononucleosis.[37] In an analysis of 100 presumed heterophile-negative cases of infectious mononucleosis involving the 0–9 year age group studied in England,[83] the incubation period was shorter than for adults and estimated at 4–10 days.

The pathogenesis of infectious mononucleosis is intriguing not only because the self-limited clinical disease is manifested primarily in young adults but also because of the suspected oncogenicity of the virus and its relationship to African Burkitt lymphoma and to nasopharyngeal carcinoma.[32a] An understanding of what immunological mechanisms turn infectious mononucleosis on and what mechanisms turn it off is important in this context.

Transient depression of delayed hypersensitivity has been described during acute infectious mononucleosis,[10,62] and depressed T-cell stimulation[134] by phytohemagglutinin has been recorded. Recently, profound alterations in cell-mediated immunity were demonstrated by intradermal skin tests, *in vitro* lymphocyte stimulation, and enumeration of absolute numbers of peripheral-blood T and B cells.[97] Lymphocyte responsiveness to a variety of mitogens and antigens was found to be depressed during the first weeks of illness. Serial studies of the interaction of T- and B-cell populations during acute disease indicated that peripheral-blood B cells increase during the first week of illness and return to normal levels several weeks later. In contrast, T cells reach peak values during the second week of disease and remain elevated for approximately 5 weeks.[97]

Recent investigations indicate that both T and B cells may be transformed into atypical lymphocytes characteristic of this disease.[31,60,97,120] These observations suggest that B cells may be transformed by infection with EBV and T cells transformed as an immunological response to the viral antigen itself or to altered antigens on the surface of the B cells.

A schematic diagram of the possible pathogenesis of infectious mononucleosis (Fig. 5) summarizes a hypothetical concept. EBV enters the oropharynx through salivary transfer, probably by kissing in young adults or saliva-contaminated objects in young children. It multiplies locally, presumably in epithelial cells,[94a] possibly cells of the salivary gland.[94a,107b] A sore throat accompanies this, often with exudative pharyngotonsillitis. A persistent, intermittent oropharyngeal excretion over many years occurs in 15–20% following either apparent or inapparent EBV infection,[20,114b] which may be greatly increased during immunosuppression.[143] The local lymphatics are probably invaded, resulting in cervical lymphadenopathy. The virus enters the bloodstream from one of these sources, involves B lymphocytes, and spreads hematologically to the liver, producing hepatitis, and to the spleen, causing splenomegaly; involvement of the brain, lung, or other organs occurs rarely.

EBV has at least three functional effects on B lymphocytes, although it is not known whether sepa-

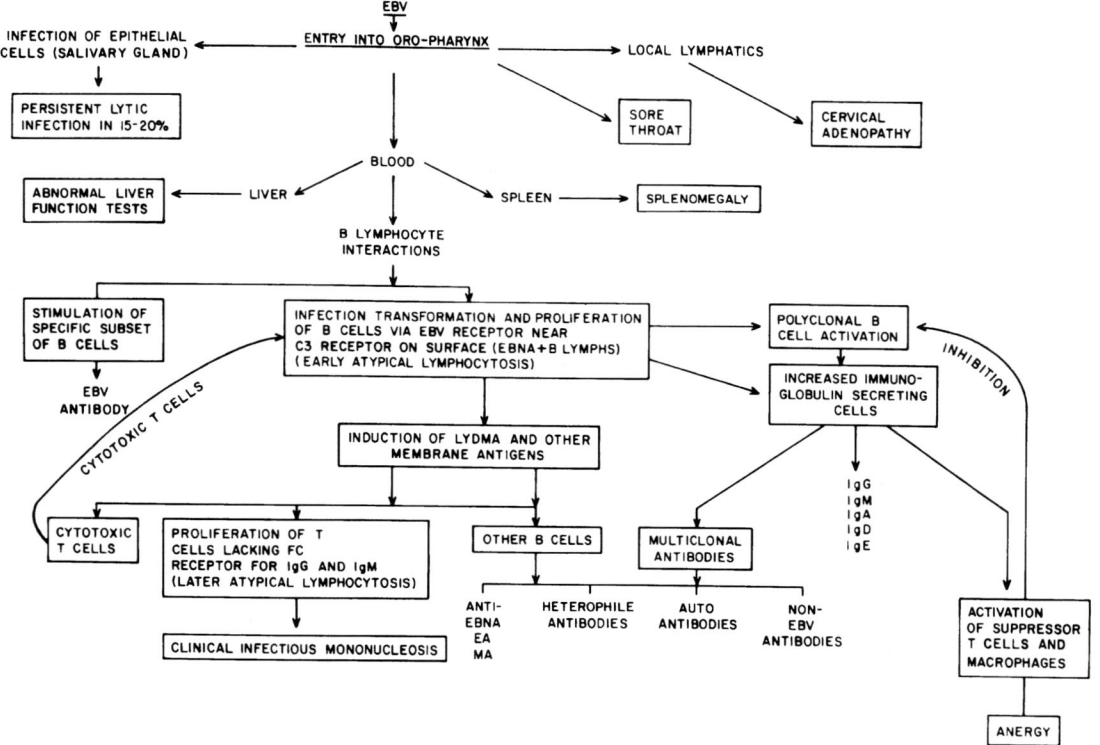

Fig. 5. Hypothetical pathogenesis of EBV infection.

rate B-cell populations are involved. One is due to the action of virus on a subset of specific antibody-producing cells, the second results from infection and transformation, and the third is a consequence of polyclonal B-cell activation. The first leads to the production of EBV antibody. The second is a complex event related to the existence of EBV receptors on the surface of B cells near receptors for C_3[85b]; the virus enters and multiplies in the B cell, producing EBNA-positive cells and a variety of antigens such as early antigen, VCA, and EBNA, against which specific antibodies are produced via other B cells. The EBNA-positive B cell transforms and proliferates, and this constitutes most of the early atypical lymphocytosis of infectious mononucleosis.[97] *In vitro*, the transformed B cell is "immortalized"— i.e., made capable of continual multiplication.[100a] EBV induces neoantigens on the surface of some infected B cells, more from adults than children and not in cord cells.[100a] These antigens include lymphocyte-determined membrane antigen (LDMA) and possibly heterophile antigen of the Paul–Bunnell type, antibodies to which are formed by other B cells. The neoantigens stimulate a B–T cell interaction similar to a graft-vs.-host response, which may account for some of the clinical symptoms of the disease. The mechanism of production of the clinical features of infectious mononucleosis is not well understood, but might result from these B–T cell interactions, from immune complex deposition or other immunopathological events, from direct effects of EBV on cells, or from some combination of these mechanisms. The rarity of classic infectious mononucleosis in early childhood might be related to the failure of EBV to evoke some of these immunological responses, such as induction of neoantigens on the B-cell surface. The T cells that respond to such neoantigens in older children and young adults represent the atypical lymphocytosis that characterizes the later stages of the acute clinical disease and are composed largely of proliferating T cells that lack the Fc receptor for IgG and IgM.[68b] As in other viral infections, some T cells are cytotoxic and lyse infected cells,[7,67,83b,87,140] limiting their proliferation and accounting for the low percentage of EBNA-positive B cells demonstrable in the peripheral blood during the acute disease.[90a,130a] Very early, there may be 15–20% EBNA-positive B cells, which are reduced early by cytotoxic cells and later by suppressor T cells to 1–2% or less. A sufficient

number survive, however, to initiate long-term *in vitro* cultures years later.[32] The third functional effect of EBV on B cells is similar to that of pokeweed mitogen, but is probably due to infection of B cells, rather than a surface effect, and results in a polyclonal B-cell proliferation; an increase in immunoglobulin-secreting cells then occurs, synthesizing IgA early, with IgD, then later IgM and IgG. Multiclonal antibodies are stimulated via other B cells such as sheep-cell antibodies of the Forssman, and possibly of the Paul–Bunnell, type, plus other antibodies unrelated to EBV.[87a,147a] These antibodies are probably not produced directly by EBNA-positive B cells. In the wake of these B–T cell interactions, there appear suppressor T cells, and perhaps macrophages, which inhibit the proliferation of B cells[68a,147a] and probably underlie the severe anergy that occurs in infectious mononucleosis. To date, EBV-specific suppressor T cells have not been demonstrated, but they may exist.

While the appearance of transformed and proliferating B cells and of cytotoxic and suppressor T cells has been documented, their origin, specificity, interrelationship, and relationship to EBV await clarification. The proliferation of B cells, and the acute disease itself, are limited by cytotoxic T cells, suppressor cells, and humoral antibody. The development of specific cell-mediated immunity to EBV during infectious mononucleosis has been demonstrated.[114b] A failure of these immune mechanisms, either on a genetic basis, as in the X-linked lymphoproliferative syndrome of males,[128a,b] or due to acquired immunodeficiencies, as possible in a fatal case in a 4-year-old girl,[129b] can permit uncontrolled B-cell proliferation, leading to an immunoblastic B-cell sarcoma or to other lymphoproliferative responses (Burkitt lymphoma, ?Hodgkins disease). Such severe, often fatal, oncogenic and sometimes lytic consequences of EBV infection are of great importance in terms of both human life and an understanding of their pathogenesis. A registry has been set up in Massachusetts to record and study them.[65a]

The mechanism of heterophile-antibody production is still unexplained, as is the source of the antigen that produces it, but knowledge that its appearance is most common in EBV infections of young adults[42] and that the degree of expression and release of EBV *in vitro* varies in lymphocytes from donors of different ages suggests avenues of investigation. For example, EBV-infected fetal lymphocytes do not have demonstrable VCA, but do contain EBNA by the EBNA test[101,129] and CF antigen.[101,104] In lymphocytes from adults and from marmosets, EBV may mature more fully, resulting in release of EBV antigens to other lymphocytes. Heterophile antibody may occur in response to membrane-induced antigens of EBV expressing themselves more fully in lymphocytes of young adults than in those of younger children or in fetal lymphocytes. There is preliminary evidence of heterophile-antibody production by lymphocytes cultured from acute cases of infectious mononucleosis,[107a] and the various possible mechanisms of its appearance have been reviewed by Kano and Milgrom.[87a]

While the presence of antibody to the VCA of EBV has been shown to indicate protection against infectious mononucleosis and its absence indicates susceptibility,[44,50,65,113,132] the actual antibody that provides immunity is probably the neutralizing antibody for which tests have recently been developed.[78,105] One attack of infectious mononucleosis confers a high degree of durable immunity to subsequent attacks of clinical infectious mononucleosis.[16,50,105] Presumably, subclinical or inapparent EBV infections also confer lasting immunity. One fairly well-documented case of clinical recurrence has been reported,[9] and a resurgent anamnestic heterophile response after infectious mononucleosis has also been noted in patients who subsequently develop a respiratory infection.[8,80] Reinfection with or without clinical illness has not yet been fully documented by appropriate heterophile and EBV antibody tests, but asymptomatic endogenous reactivation was found in 32% of renal-transplant recipients.[1a]

8. Patterns of Host Response

8.1. Clinical Features

When infection with EBV occurs in childhood, a mild, nonspecific illness or an inapparent infection may develop, both of which are associated with the appearance and persistence of antibody to EBV. If exposure and primary infection are delayed until adolescence or young adulthood, the characteristic clinical picture usually occurs. This consists of fever,

pharyngitis, and cervical lymphadenopathy, accompanied by splenomegaly in 50% and hepatomegaly in 10%. The pharyngitis is often associated with a whitish or a gray-green exudate having an offensive odor. The eyelids may be swollen, and petechiae occur on the hard palate in 25% of cases.

Abnormalities of liver-function tests are a regular feature of infectious mononucleosis, and clinically recognizable jaundice occurs in 5% of cases. Rare manifestations include a variety of central nervous system syndromes (encephalitis, meningoencephalitis, Guillain–Barré syndrome), pneumonitis and pneumonia, thrombocytopenic purpura, myocarditis, and nephritis.[39,82] Hepatitis and central nervous system involvement may occur in the absence of other features of infectious mononucleosis.[29a,61a] The major complications include splenic rupture and airway obstruction from exudative pharyngotonsillitis. About 50 deaths have been reported due mostly to central respiratory failure; recently, cell-associated EBV was detected in the cerebrospinal fluid of a case with complicating meningoencephalitis.[132a] An immunological deficit, especially in cell-mediated immunity, may influence the severity of the clinical response, as suggested by the report of two deaths in a family[5] and a recent severe illness in a women with a T-cell defect.[136a] An X-linked recessive lymphoproliferative syndrome in which EBV has been implicated has also been described by Purtilo et al.[128a,b] Both lytic and proliferative manifestations have appeared in one kindred. These include fatal infectious mononucleosis, malignant lymphoma, and agammaglobulinemia.

The frequency with which EBV infections are expressed as clinical illness in young adults has varied in different populations. In a study of a cohort of U.S. Military Academy cadets over a 4-year period, only 26.4% of 201 infected with this agent developed heterophile-positive clinical infectious mononucleosis.[65] The apparent : inapparent EBV infection ratio in different years ranged from 1:1 to 1:2.6 in this population. Comparison of the frequency of clinically expressed infectious mononucleosis in freshman students in three different settings is presented in Table 3 (Section 5.1). As mentioned, the reasons for the differences are not known, by may relate to the motivation to seek medical care, physical fitness, psychological factors, or concern about the effect of hospitalization on academic and school activities.

The relationships between clinical features and antibody levels in a typical heterophile-positive case in an 18-year-old student are shown in Fig. 6. Following a prodromal period associated with fatigue, fever, and headache over several days, the onset of sore throat, cervical adenopathy, and recurrent fever developed during the second week. Characteristic blood changes were present on the 3rd day after onset, and on culture the patient's lymphocytes contained EBNA CF antigens in a nuclear location. The heterophile-antibody titer was negative on the first day of symptoms, rose to 1:14 after guinea pig absorption 2 days later, and then increased to 1:896 on the 15th day. In contrast, Epstein–Barr VCA antibodies of IgG type, undetectable on the 3rd day of illness, were present on the 8th day and rose to a level of 1:320 by the 2nd week. EBV-specific IgM antibodies were demonstrable on the 8th day at a titer of 1:2.5, which then increased to 1:10 by the 15th day.

No direct correlation has been found between the levels of Epstein–Barr VCA and heterophile antibodies or between VCA, early antigen, and EBNA antibody levels and the severity of clinical symptoms and hematological changes.[73,77,114] Neither does their persistence correlate with the duration of clinical illness.

8.2. Diagnosis

The diagnosis of infectious mononucleosis is based on a typical clinical picture with the triad of fever, sore throat, and cervical lymphadenopathy, the occurrence of at least 50% lymphocytosis with at least 10% atypical lymphocytes, and the appearance of heterophil antibodies. The presence of IgM or early antigen antibodies to EBV, or both, is an absolute requirement in doubtful or heterophile-negative cases. Antibody to VCA is usually present at the time the physician first sees the patient, and only 15–20% of patients will show a subsequent rise in titer; antibodies to early antigen appear later, but are present in only 75% of typical cases.[77] Antibodies to EBNA usually arise 1 month or more after illness and probably persist for life.[73] EBV-specific IgM antibodies are demonstrable in 85% of cases during acute illness. Figure 7 depicts the course of EBV-specific IgG and IgM antibodies during the course of illness. IgG antibodies persist for years, perhaps for life; IgM antibodies usually disappear in 3–6 months. At present, the EBV-VCA-IgM is the best antibody test for diagnosis in cases that are heterophile-antibody negative[29,52,59b,114c]; the presence of false positives due to rheumatoid factor must be excluded.

The main reliance in diagnosis must be placed on the heterophile antibodies, which are of the IgM type. Methods in most common use are the sheep- and horse-cell agglutination tests after absorption of the serum with guinea pig kidney to remove Forssman antibody, and the beef-cell hemolysin test, which does not require absorption. The appearance and persistence of these tests during acute

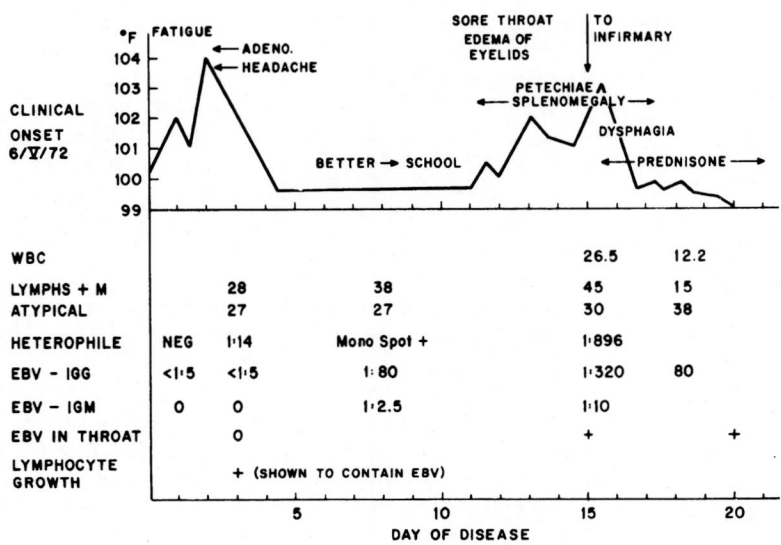

Fig. 6. Relationship between clinical and laboratory features of infectious mononucleosis in an 18-year-old male.

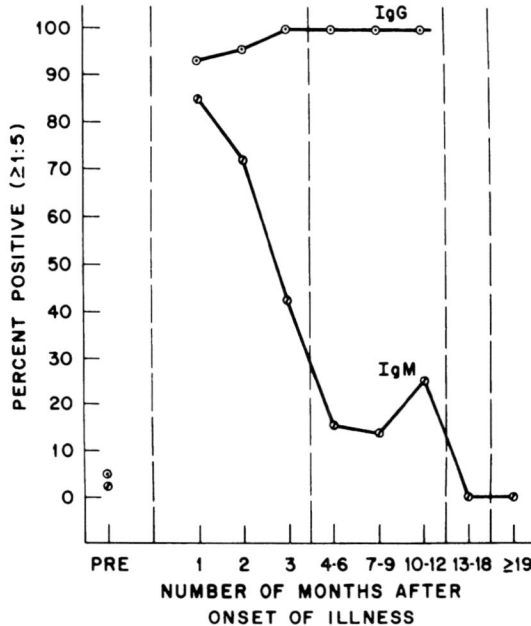

Fig. 7. Appearance and duration of IgG and IgM antibodies specific for EBV during infectious mononucleosis. From Evans *et al.*[52]

and convalescent infectious mononucleosis are shown in Fig. 8. The beef hemolysin test is the most specific but has a short duration; the horse-cell test is the most sensitive and most persistent, with positive tests present for a year or more in 75%.[52] The appearance and persistence of antibody to horse cells have been found to follow mild and subclinical episodes of infectious mononucleosis provided that sera are collected over a long enough time. This test is useful in childhood infections with EBV, which

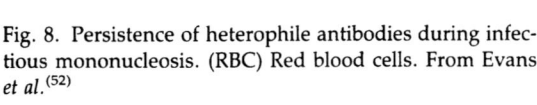

Fig. 8. Persistence of heterophile antibodies during infectious mononucleosis. (RBC) Red blood cells. From Evans *et al.*[52]

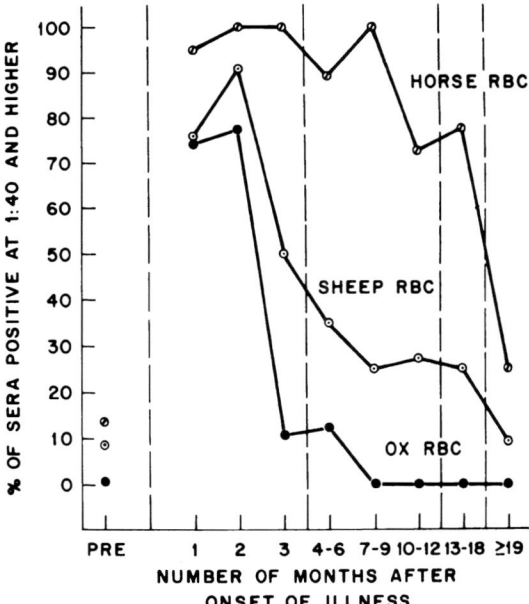

are often heterophile-negative by other tests or when inadequately followed. A new immune adherance heterophile test may also be very useful in childhood infections.[54a,94c]

Development of EBV antibody has also been shown in cases where the clinical and hematological characteristics are those of infectious mononucleosis but the heterophile antibody remains persistently negative.[50,114b] These heterophile-negative, EBV-antibody-positive cases appear to be common in infants and children, but are rare in adults.[10a,b,59a] Infection with cytomegalovirus (CMV) may produce a clinical picture of heterophile-negative mononucleosis that is hard to distinguish from classic infectious mononucleosis; however, it usually occurs at a later age, and adenopathy and exudative pharyngitis are rare.[91] EBV may possibly be reactivated during the course of other herpesvirus infections, especially CMV.[94b] Infection with EBV can result in development of a false-positive CMV-IgM-antibody response; however, the reverse does not occur. *Toxoplasma gondii*, adenovirus, rubella, and hepatitis A infections may also resemble heterophile-negative infectious mononucleosis, but the lymphocytosis is relative and not absolute. The infectious-mononucleosis-like syndromes have recently been reviewed.[44a]

9. Control and Prevention

Attempts to control infectious mononucleosis and EBV infections by interrupting the presumed chain of transmission in young adults seem neither realistic nor perhaps desirable in light of our current knowledge. If salivary exchange represents the major route of spread, there seems little likelihood of interdicting this practice. If poor hygienic conditions promote the spread of EBV infections in young children, then improvement in hygienic and socioeconomic circumstances might reduce their incidence. Unfortunately, control of spread at this time when infection is largely mild and asymptomatic might simply delay exposure to later childhood and young adult life when the majority of EBV infections are expressed as clinical infectious mononucleosis.

The high degree of protection against infectious mononucleosis provided by natural infection with EBV suggests that a vaccine capable of evoking similar humoral, cell-mediated, and local immunity might be highly effective. An attenuated live vaccine administered orally would be the most desirable. However, the apparent limitation of viral multiplication *in vitro* to primate lymphocyte suspension cultures and the low yield of infectious virus released are formidable technical obstacles at present. Work on EBV-membrane antigens is under way to circumvent some of these problems.[123,128c]

If an effective vaccine were available, it might best be given on entrance to high school to permit natural infection with little clinical illness to occur before that and then to prevent clinical illness in the young adult. It would be useful only in developed countries with a high incidence of infectious mononucleosis.

The oncogenic and transforming potential of EBV poses a serious question of risk for use of a vaccine. The numerous problems associated with long-term surveillance for possible complications would be considerable, but these risks in developed countries may not be great. The association between EBV and cancer is evident primarily in Burkitt lymphoma in Africa and in nasopharyngeal carcinoma (NPC) patients of Chinese descent in the Far East. In these settings, clinical infectious mononucleosis is too rare a disease to merit vaccination. Furthermore, tumor development is associated with malaria in African Burkitt lymphoma and immunogenetic susceptibility to NPC in Chinese. In the absence of malaria and genetic susceptibility, as in the United States, both these tumors are very rare. Such considerations suggest that if the technical problems of viral attenuation and vaccine production can be overcome, oncogenicity would be a hazard of negligible magnitude in the United States and other countries where clinical infectious mononucleosis is a common and disabling disease.

10. Unsolved Problems

The problems that remained to be solved concerning the nature of EBV infections are summarized in Table 5. While EBV is well established as the cause of heterophile-positive infectious mononucleosis and "turns on" the immunological events that are involved in the pathogenesis of the clinical disease, we need more information as to what

Table 5. Unsolved Questions Concerning Epstein–Barr Virus

1. What turns infectious mononucleosis off and makes it a self-limited disease?
2. What cell supports pharyngeal multiplication of EBV?
3. What is the route of transmission in young children?
4. Where does heterophile antibody originate?
5. Can the EBV-IgM-antibody test be simplified for routine diagnostic use?
6. What causes different responses to EBV at different ages?
7. Is an infectious mononucleosis vaccine possible?
8. Does EBV cause cancer?
9. Why are EBV antibody titers high in some chronic diseases?
10. What accounts for the geographic distribution of Burkitt lymphoma and nasopharyngeal cancer?

"turns off" the lymphoproliferative cycle and makes the disease a benign, self-limited one.

The persistence of EBV in circulating lymphocytes following infection and the presence of a small number of "atypical lymphocytes" in healthy persons suggest that the proliferative process is not fully "turned off" but held under careful control and immunological surveillance; the continued presence of anti-VCA, anti-EBNA, CF, and other viral antibodies supports the concept of continued antigenic stimulation. Viral excretion in the pharynx certainly continues long after infection, perhaps intermittently for life, but the cells supporting this multiplication are at present unknown. The source of heterophile antibody and of the variety of other nonviral antibodies that appear during the course of infectious mononucleosis remains a mystery; whether these antibodies appear in milder EBV infections in smaller amounts and at a later time is not known, but recent evidence suggests this may be so. A simple EBV-IgM antibody test is needed in the diagnostic laboratory to confirm presumably heterophile-negative cases. An explanation is lacking for the observation that a more severe clinical response to EBV infection occurs when exposure is delayed until later childhood and young adult life, similar to the more frequent occurrence of jaundice in hepatitis and paralysis in poliomyelitis infections in adults. If the clinical syndrome of infectious mononucleosis is primarily an immunological response of T cells to EBV-induced neoantigens on the B-cell membrane, then one can speculate that induction of membrane antigens occurs more commonly in lymphocytes from mature persons in whom more complete virus is formed than in lymphocytes from young children; this idea is supported by the failure of EBV-infected cord cells to produce VCA or membrane antigens. The possibility of a vaccine has already been discussed, and the relationship of EBV to cancer is explored in other chapters of this book. Infectious mononucleosis continues to be an important model for studying the immunological and virological events involved in a persistent and possibly neoplastic infection.

11. References

1. ARMSTRONG, D., HENLE, G., AND HENLE, W., Complement-fixation tests with cell lines derived from Burkitt's lymphoma and acute leukemias, *J. Bacteriol.* 91:1257–1262 (1966).
1a. ARMSTRONG, J. A., EVANS, A. S., RAO, N., AND HO, M., Viral infections in renal transplant recipients, *Infect. Immun.* 14:970–975 (1976).
2. BAILEY, G. H., AND RAFFEL, S., Hemolytic antibodies for sheep and ox erythrocytes in infectious mononucleosis, *J. Clin. Invest.* 14:228–244 (1935).
3. BANATVALA, J. E., BEST, J. M., AND WALLER, D. K., Epstein–Barr virus-specific IgM in infectious mononucleosis, Burkitt lymphoma, and nasopharyngeal carcinoma, *Lancet* 1:1205–1208 (1972).
4. BANG, J., Forsoeg paa at overfoere mononucleosis infectiosa til mennesket, *Ugeshkr. Laeg.* 105:499–504 (1943).
5. BAR, R. S., DELOR, J., CLAUSEN, K. P., HURTUBISE, P., HENLE, W., AND HEWETSON, J. F., Fatal infectious mononucleosis in a family, *N. Engl. J. Med.* 290:363–367 (1974).
6. BARONDESS, J. A., AND ERLE, H., Serum alkaline phosphatase activity in hepatitis of infectious mononucleosis, *Am. J. Med.* 29:43–54 (1960).
7. BAUSCHER, J. C., AND SMITH, R. T., Studies of Epstein–Barr virus–host-relationship: Autochthonous and allogeneic lymphocyte stimulation by lymphoblast cell lines in mixed cell culture, *Clin. Immunol. Immunopathol.* 1:270–281 (1973).

8. BENDER, C. E., Interpretation of hematologic and serologic findings in the diagnosis of infectious mononucleosis, *Ann. Intern. Med.* **49**:852–865 (1958).

9. BENDER, E. C., Recurrent mononucleosis, *J. Am. Med. Assoc.* **182**:954–956 (1962).

10. BENTZON, J. W., The effect of certain infectious diseases on tuberculin allergy, *Tubercle* **34**:34–41 (1953).

10a. BIGGAR, R. J., HENLE, W., FLEISCHER, G., BÖCKER, J., LENNETTE, E. T., AND HENLE, G., Primary Epstein–Barr virus infections in African infants. I. Decline of maternal antibodies and time of infection, *Int. J. Cancer* **22**:239–243 (1978).

10b. BIGGAR, R. J., HENLE, G., BÖCKER, J., LENNETTE, E. T., FLEISCHER, G., AND HENLE, W., Primary Epstein–Barr virus infections in African infants. II. Clinical and serological observations during seroconversion, *Int. J. Cancer* **22**:244–250 (1978).

11. BLACK, F. L., HIERHOLZER, W. J., PINHEIRO, DeP., EVANS, A. S., WOODALL, J. P., OPTON, E. M., EMMONS, J. E., WEST, B. S., EDSALL, G., DOWNS, W. G., AND WALLACE, G. D., Evidence for persistence of infectious agents in isolated human populations, *Am. J. Epidemiol.* **100**:230–250 (1974).

12. BLOEDORN, W. A., AND HOUGHTON, J. E., The occurrence of abnormal leucocytes in the blood in acute infections, *Arch. Intern. Med.* **27**:315–325 (1921).

12a. BOON, W. H., MUI, C. L. Y., AND TOO, M., Infectious mononucleosis in Singapore, *J. Singapore Pediatr. Soc.* **19**:153–161 (1977).

13. BROWN, J. W., CLIFFORD, J. E., SIMS, J. L., AND WHITE, E., Liver function during infectious mononucleosis, *Am. J. Med.* **6**:321–328 (1949).

14. CABOT, R. C., The lymphocytosis of infection, *Am. J. Med. Sci.* **145**:335–339 (1913).

15. CARLSON, G. W., BROOKS, E. H., AND MARSHALL, V. F., Acute glandular fever: Recent epidemic, report of cases, *Wis. Med. J.* **25**:176–178 (1926).

16. CARTER, R. L., AND PENMAN, H. G., The early history of infectious mononucleosis and its relation to "glandular fever," in: *Infectious Mononucleosis* (R. L. CARTER AND H. G. PENMAN, eds.), Blackwell, Oxford, 1969.

17. CARVALHO, R. P. S., EVANS, A. S., FROST, P., DALLDORF, G., CAMARGO, M. E., AND JARMA, M., EBV infection in Brazil. I. Occurrence in normal persons, in lymphomas and in leukemias, *Int. J. Cancer* **11**:191–201 (1973).

18. CENTER FOR DISEASE CONTROL, Infectious Mononucleosis Surveillance, November 1972.

19. CHANG, R. S., AND GOLDEN, H. D., Transformation of human leucocytes by throat washings from infectious mononucleosis patients, *Nature (London)* **234**:359–360 (1971).

20. CHANG, R. S., LEWIS, J. P., AND ABILDGAARD, C. F., Excretors of leucocyte-transforming agents among a human population, *N. Engl. J. Med.* **289**:1328–1329 (1973).

21. CHRISTINE, B. W., Infectious mononucleosis, *Conn. Health Bull.* **82**:115–119 (1968).

21a. CONNECTICUT STATE HEALTH DEPARTMENT, Personal communication.

21b. COREY, L., STAMM, W. E., FEORINO, P. M., BRYAN, J. A., WESELEY, S., GREGG, M. B., AND SOLANGI, K., HB$_s$ AG-negative hepatitis in a hemodialysis unit: Relation to Epstein–Barr virus, *N. Engl. J. Med.* **293**:1273–1278 (1975).

22. CROSS, J. G., Conditions simulating an acute leukemia (acute benign leukemia), *Minn. Med.* **5**:579–581 (1922).

23. DAVIDSOHN, I., AND WALKER, P. H., The nature of the heterophilic antibodies in infectious mononucleosis, *Am. J. Clin. Pathol.* **5**:455–465 (1935).

24. DAVIDSOHN, I., Heterophile antibodies in serum sickness, *J. Immunol.* **16**:259–273 (1929).

25. DAVIDSOHN, R. J. L., A survey of infectious mononucleosis in the North-East Regional Hospital Board area of Scotland, 1960–9, *J. Hyg.* **68**:393–400 (1970).

26. DIEHL, V., HENLE, G., HENLE, W., AND KOHN, G., Demonstration of a herpes group virus in cultures of peripheral leukocytes from patients with infectious mononucleosis, *J. Virol.* **2**:663–669 (1968).

27. DINGLE, J. H., BADGER, G. F., AND JORDAN, W. S., JR., *Illness in the Home: A Study of 25,000 Illnesses in a Group of Cleveland Families*, The Press of Western Reserve, Cleveland, 1964.

28. DOWNEY, H., AND MCKINLAY, C. A., Acute lymphadenosis compared with acute lymphatic leukemia, *Arch. Intern. Med.* **32**:82–112 (1923).

29. EDWARDS, J. M. B., AND McSWIGGAN, D. A., Studies on the diagnostic value of an immunofluorescence test for EB virus specific IgM, *Clin. Pathol.* **27**:647–651 (1974).

29a. EDWARDS, J. M. B., VANDERVELDE, E. M., COHEN, B. J., AND McSWIGGAN, D. A., Laboratory diagnosis of EB virus infection in some cases presenting as hepatitis, *J. Clin. Pathol.* **31**:179–182 (1978).

30. ELLENBOGEN, C., AND REINARZ, J. A., The Epstein–Barr virus and its relationship to infectious mononucleosis in air force recruits, *Mil. Med.* **140**:371–373 (1974).

31. ENBERG, R. N., EBERLE, B. J., AND WILLIAMS, R. C., Peripheral blood T and B cells in infectious mononucleosis, *J. Infect. Dis.* **130**:104–111 (1974).

32. EPSTEIN, M. A., AND ACHONG, B. G., Various forms of Epstein–Barr virus infection in man: Established facts and a general concept, *Lancet* **2**:836–839 (1973).

32a. EPSTEIN, M. A., AND ACHONG, B. G., Pathogenesis of infectious mononucleosis, *Lancet* **2**:1270–1278 (1977).

33. EPSTEIN, M. A., ACHONG, B. G., AND BARR, Y. M.,

Virus particles in cultured lymphoblasts from Burkitt's lymphoma, *Lancet* **1**:702–703 (1964).

34. EVANS, A. S., Experimental attempts to transmit infectious mononucleosis to man, *Yale J. Biol. Med.* **20**:19–26 (1947).

35. EVANS, A. S., Liver function tests in infectious mononucleosis, *J. Clin. Invest.* **27**:106–110 (1948).

36. EVANS, A. S., Further experimental attempts to transmit infectious mononucleosis to man, *J. Clin. Invest.* **29**:508–512 (1950).

37. EVANS, A. S., Infectious mononucleosis in University of Wisconsin students: Report of a five-year investigation, *Am. J. Hyg.* **71**:342–362 (1960).

38. EVANS, A. S., Infectious mononucleosis: Observations from a public health laboratory, *Yale J. Biol. Med.* **34**:261–276 (1961/1962).

39. EVANS, A. S., Complications of infectious mononucleosis: Recognition and management, *Hosp. Med.* **3**:24–25, 28–33 (1967).

40. EVANS, A. S., Infectious mononucleosis: Recent developments, *Gen. Pract.* **60**:127–134 (1969).

41. EVANS, A. S. Infectious mononucleosis in the armed forces, *Mil. Med.* **135**:300–304 (1970).

42. EVANS, A. S., New discoveries in infectious mononucleosis, *Mod. Med.* **1**:18–24 (1974).

43. EVANS, A. S., The history of infectious mononucleosis, *Am. J. Med. Sci.* **267**:189–195 (1974).

44. EVANS, A. S., Commentary—EB virus, infectious mononucleosis and cancer: The closing of the web, *Yale J. Biol. Med.* **47**:113–122 (1974).

44a. EVANS, A. S., Infectious mononucleosis and related syndromes, *Am. J. Med. Sci.* **276**:325–339 (1978).

45. EVANS, A. S., AND ROBINTON, E. D., An epidemiologic study of infectious mononucleosis in a New England college, *N. Engl. J. Med.* **242**:492–496 (1950).

46. EVANS, A. S., AND PAUL, J. R., Infectious mononucleosis, in: *Preventive Medicine in World War II*, Vol. V: *Communicable Diseases* (J. B. COATES, JR., ed.), Office of the Surgeon General, Department of the Army, Washington, D.C., 1960.

47. EVANS, A. S., AND CAMPOS, L. E., Acute respiratory diseases in students at the University of the Philippines, *Bull. WHO* **45**:103–112 (1971).

48. EVANS, A. S., CARVALHO, R. P. S., AND GROSSMAN, L., EBV infections in Brazil. III. Infectious mononucleosis, Unpublished (1974).

49. EVANS, A. S., EVANS, B. K., AND STURTZ, V., Standards for hepatic and hematologic tests in monkeys: Observations during experiments with hepatitis and mononucleosis, *Proc. Soc. Exp. Biol. Med.* **82**:437–440 (1953).

50. EVANS, A. S., NIEDERMAN, J. C., AND McCOLLUM, R. W., Seroepidemiological studies of infectious mononucleosis with EB virus, *N. Engl. J. Med.* **279**:1121–1127 (1968).

51. EVANS, A. S., JENSEN, R., NIEDERMAN, J. C., AND WALLACE, D. K., Studies of EBV antibody in Fort Jackson military recruits, Unpublished data (1974).

52. EVANS, A. S., NIEDERMAN, J. C., CENABRE, L. C., WEST, B., AND RICHARDS, V. A., A prospective evaluation of heterophile and Epstein–Barr virus-specific IgM antibody tests in clinical and subclinical infectious mononucleosis: Specificity and sensitivity of the tests and persistence of antibody, *J. Infect. Dis.* **132**:546–554 (1975).

53. FILATOV, N. F., *Semiotik and Diagnotik de Kinderkrankheiten*, Verlag von Ferdinand Enke, Stuttgart, 1892.

54. FILATOV, N. F., Lektuse ob ostrikh infektsion nikh lolieznyak (Lectures on acute infectious diseases of children), Moscow, U Deitel, 1885; cited by Wising, P. J., *Acta Med. Scand. Suppl.* **133**:1–102 (1942).

54a. FLEISCHER, G., LENNETTE, E. T., HENLE, G., AND HENLE, W., Incidence of heterophile antibody responses in children with infectious mononucleosis, *J. Pediatr.* **94**:723–728 (1979).

55. GARDNER, H. T., AND PAUL, J. R., Infectious mononucleosis at the New Haven Hospital, 1921–46, *Yale J. Biol. Med.* **19**:839–853 (1947).

56. GERBER, P., AND DEAL, D. R., Epstein–Barr virus-induced viral and soluble complement-fixing antigens in Burkitt lymphoma cell cultures, *Proc. Soc. Exp. Biol. Med.* **134**:748–751 (1970).

57. GERBER, P., AND ROSENBLUM, E. N., The incidence of complement-fixing antibodies to herpes simplex and herpes-like viruses in man and rhesus monkeys, *Proc. Soc. Exp. Biol. Med.* **128**:541–546 (1968).

58. GERBER, P., PURCELL, R. H., ROSENBLUM, E. N., AND WALSH, J. H., Association of EB-virus infection with the post-perfusion syndrome, *Lancet* **1**:593–596 (1969).

59. GERBER, R., GOLDSTEIN, L. I., LUCAS, S., NONOYAMA, M., AND PERLIN, E., Oral excretion of Epstein–Barr viruses by healthy subjects and patients with infectious mononucleosis, *Lancet* **2**:988–989 (1972).

59a. GERBER, P., NKRUMAH, F. K., PRITCHETT, R., AND KIEFF, E., Comparative studies of Epstein–Barr virus strains from Ghana and the United States, *Int. J. Cancer* **17**:71–81 (1976).

59b. GINSBURG, C. M., HENLE, W., HENLE, G., AND HORWITZ, C. A., Infectious mononucleosis in children: Evaluation of Epstein–Barr virus specific serological data, *J. Am. Med. Assoc.* **237**:781–785 (1977).

59c. GINSBURG, C. M., HENLE, G., AND HENLE, W., An outbreak of infectious mononucleosis among the personnel of an outpatient clinic, *Am. J. Epidemiol.* **104**:571–575 (1976).

60. GIULANO, V. J., JASIN, H. E., AND ZIFF, M., The nature

of the atypical lymphocyte in infectious mononucleosis, *Clin. Immunol. Immunopathol.* **3**:90–98 (1974).

61. GRACE, J. T., BLAKESLEE, J., AND JONES, R., Induction of infectious mononucleosis in man by the herpestype virus (HTV) in Burkitt lymphoma cells in tissue culture, *Proc. Am. Assoc. Cancer Res.* **10**:31 (1969).

61a. GROSE, C., HENLE, W., HENLE, G., AND FEORINO, P. M., Primary Epstein–Barr infections in acute neurologic disease, *N. Engl. J. Med.* **292**:392–393 (1975).

62. HAIDER, S., COUTINHO, M. D., AND EMOND, R. T. D., Tuberculin anergy and infectious mononucleosis, *Lancet* **2**:74 (1973).

63. HAINEBACH, J., II. Beitrag zur Aetiologie des Pfeiffer'schen Drüsenfiebers, *Dtsch. Med. Wochenschr.* **26**:419–420 (1899).

64. HALCROW, J. P. A., OWEN, L. M., AND ROGER, N. O., Infectious mononucleosis with an account of an epidemic in E.M.S. hospital, *Br. Med. J.* **2**:443–447 (1943).

65. HALLEE, T. J., EVANS, A. S., NIEDERMAN, J. C., BROOKS, C. M., AND VOEGTLY, J. H. Infectious mononucleosis at the U.S. Military Academy: A prospective study of a single class over four years, *Yale J. Biol. Med.* **47**:182–195 (1974).

65a. HAMILTON, J. K., SULLIVAN, J. L., MAURER, H. S., CRUZI, F. G., PROIRSON, A. J., STENKE, K., FINKELSTEIN, G. Z., LANDING, B., GRUNNET, M., AND PURTILO, D. T., X-linked lymphoproliferative syndrome registry report, *J. Pediatr.* **4**:669–673 (1980).

66. HAMPAR, B., HSU, K. C., MARTOS, L. M., AND WALKER, J. L., Serologic evidence that a herpes-type virus is the etiologic agent of heterophile-positive infectious mononucleosis, *Proc. Natl. Acad. Sci. U.S.A.* **68**:1407–1411 (1971).

67. HARDY, D. A., AND STEEL, C. M., Cytotoxic potential of lymphocytes stimulated with autochthonous lymphoid cell lines, *Experientia* **27**:1336–1338 (1971).

68. HEATH, C. W., BRODSKY, A. L., AND POTOLSKY, A. I., Infectious mononucleosis in a general population, *Am. J. Epidemiol.* **95**:46–52 (1972).

68a. HAYNES, B. F., SCHOOLEY, R. T., PLAYING-WRIGHT, C. R., GROUSE, J. E., DOLIN, R., AND FAUCI, A. S. Emergence of suppressor cells of immunoglobulin synthesis during acute Epstein–Barr-virus-induced infectious mononucleosis, *J. Immunol.* **123**:2095–2101 (1979).

68b. HAYNES, B. F., SCHOOLEY, R. T., GROUSE, J. E., PLAYING-WRIGHT, C. R., DOLIN, R., AND FAUCI, A. S., Characterization of thymus-derived lymphocyte subsets in acute Epstein–Barr virus induced infectious mononucleosis, *J. Immunol.* **122**:699–702 (1979).

68c. HENDERSON, E., MILLER, G., ROBINSON, J., AND HESTON, L., Efficiency of transformation of lymphocytes by Epstein–Barr virus, *Virology* **76**:152–163 (1977).

68d. HENDERSON, E., HESTON, L., GROGAN, E., AND MILLER, G., Radiobiological inactivation of Epstein–Barr virus, *J. Virol.* **25**:51–59 (1978).

69. HENKE, C. E., KURLAND, L. T., AND ELVEBACK, L. R., Infectious mononucleosis in Rochester, Minn., 1950 through 1969, *Am. J. Epidemiol.* **98**:483–490 (1973).

70. HENLE, G., AND HENLE, W., Immunofluorescence in cells derived from Burkitt's lymphoma, *J. Bacteriol.* **91**:1248–1256 (1966).

71. HENLE, G., AND HENLE, W., Observations on childhood infections with Epstein–Barr virus, *J. Infect. Dis.* **121**:303–310 (1970).

72. HENLE, G., HENLE, W., AND DIEHL, V., Relation of Burkitt's tumor-associated herpes-type virus to infectious mononucleosis, *Proc. Natl. Acad. Sci. U.S.A.* **59**:94–101 (1968).

73. HENLE, G., HENLE, W., AND HORWITZ, C. A., Antibodies to Epstein–Barr virus-associated nuclear antigen in infectious mononucleosis, *J. Infect. Dis.* **130**:231–239 (1974).

73a. HENLE, W., HENLE, G., AND HORWITZ, C. A., Epstein–Barr virus specific diagnostic tests in infectious mononucleosis, *Hum. Pathol.* **5**:551–565 (1974).

74. HENLE, G., HENLE, W., AND KLEIN, G., Demonstration of two distinct components in the early antigen complex of Epstein–Barr virus-infected cells, *Int. J. Cancer* **8**:272–282 (1971).

75. HENLE, W., HENLE, G., HARRISON, F. S., JOYNER, C. R., KLEMOLA, E., PALOHEIMO, J., SCRIBA, M., AND VON ESSEN, F., Antibody responses to the Epstein–Barr virus and cytomegaloviruses after open-heart and other surgery, *N. Engl. J. Med.* **282**:1068–1074 (1968).

76. HENLE, W., HENLE, G., PEARSON, G., SCRIBA, M., WAUBKE, R., AND ZAJAC, B. A., Differential reactivity of human serums with early antigens induced by Epstein–Barr virus, *Science* **169**:188–190 (1970).

77. HENLE, W., HENLE, G., NIEDERMAN, J. C., HALTIA, K., AND KLEMOLA, E., Antibodies to early antigens induced by Epstein–Barr virus in infectious mononucleosis, *J. Infect. Dis.* **124**:58–67 (1971).

78. HEWETSON, J. F., ROCHI, G., HENLE, W., AND HENLE, G., Neutralizing antibodies to Epstein–Barr virus in healthy populations and patients with infectious mononucleosis, *J. Infect. Dis.* **128**:283–389 (1973).

79. HOAGLAND, R. J., The transmission of infectious mononucleosis, *Am. J. Med. Sci.* **229**:262–272 (1955).

80. HOAGLAND, R. J., Resurgent heterophil-antibody reaction after infectious mononucleosis, *N. Engl. J. Med.* **269**:1307–1308 (1963).

81. HOAGLAND, R. J., The incubation period of infectious mononucleosis, *Am. J. Public Health* **54**:1699–1705 (1964).

82. HOAGLAND, R., *Infectious Mononucleosis,* Grune and Stratton, New York, 1967.

83. HOBSON, F. G., LAWSON, B., AND WIGFIELD, M., Glandular fever, a field study, *Br. Med. J.* **1**:845–852 (1958).

83a. HOSKINS, T. W., FLETCHER, W. B., BLAKE, J. M., PEREIRA, M. S., AND EDWARDS, J. M. B., EB virus antibody and infectious mononucleosis in a boarding school for boys, *J. Clin. Pathol.* **29**:42–45 (1976).

83b. HUTT, L. M., HUANG, Y. T., DASCOMB, H. E., AND PAGANO, J. S., Enhanced destruction of lymphoid cell lines by peripheral blood leucocytes taken from patients with acute infectious mononucleosis, *J. Immunol.* **115**:243–248 (1975).

84. JENNINGS, E., Prevalence of EB virus antibody in Hawaii, M.D. thesis, Yale University School of Medicine, 1973.

85. JONCAS, J., AND MITNYAN, C., Serological response of the EBV antibodies in pediatric cases of infectious mononucleosis and in their contacts, *Can. Med. Assoc. J.* **102**:1260–1263 (1970).

85a. JONDAL, M., AND KLEIN, G., Surface markers on human B and T lymphocytes. II. Presence of Epstein–Barr virus receptors on B lymphocytes, *J. Exp. Med.* **138**:1365–1378 (1973).

85b. JONDAL, M., KLEIN, G., OLDSTONE, M. B. S., BOKISH, V., AND YEFENOF, E., Surface markers on human B and T lymphocytes. VII. Association between complement and Epstein–Barr virus receptors on human lymphoid lines, *Scand. J. Immunol.* **5**:401–410 (1976).

86. JORDAN, W. S., AND ALBRIGHT, R. W., Liver function tests in infectious mononucleosis, *J. Lab. Clin. Med.* **35**:688–698 (1950).

87. JUNGE, U., DEINHARDT, F., AND HOEKSTRA, J., Stimulation of peripheral lymphocytes by allogeneic and autochthonous mononucleosis lymphocyte cell lines, *J. Immunol.* **106**:1306–1315 (1971).

87a. KANO, K., AND MILGROM, F., Heterophile antigens and antibodies in medicine, *Current Top. Microbiol. Immunol.* **77**:43–69 (1977).

88. KLEIN, G., KLEIN, E., CLIFFORD, P., AND STERNSWARD, G., Search for tumor specific immune reactors in Burkitt lymphoma patients by the membrane immunofluorescence reaction, *Proc. Natl. Acad. Sci. U.S.A.* **55**:1628–1635 (1966).

88a. KASSL, S. V., EVANS, A. S., AND NIEDERMAN, J. C. Psychosocial risk factors in the development of infectious mononucleosis, *Psychosom. Med.* **41**:445–466, 1979.

89. KLEIN, G., LINDAHL, T., JONDAL, M., LEIBOLB, W., MENÉZES, J., NILSSON, K., AND SUNDSTRÖM, C., Continuous lymphoid cell lines with characteristics of B cells (bone-marrow-derived) lacking the Epstein–Barr virus genome, and derived from three human lymphomas, *Proc. Natl. Acad. Sci. U.S.A.* **71**:3283–3286, (1974).

90. KLEIN, G., DIEHL, V., HENLE, G., HENLE, W., PEARSON, G., AND NEIDERMAN, J. C., Relations between Epstein–Barr viral and cell membrane immunofluorescence in Burkitt tumor cells. II. Comparison of cells and sera from patients with Burkitt's lymphoma and infectious mononucleosis, *J. Exp. Med.* **128**:1021–1030 (1968).

90a. KLEIN, G., SVEDMVY, E., JONDAL, M., AND PERSSON, P. O., EBV-determined nuclear antigen (EBNA)-positive cells in the peripheral blood of infectious mononucleosis patients, *Int. J. Cancer* **17**:21–26 (1976).

91. KLEMOLA, E., HENLE, G., HENLE, W., AND VON ESSEN, R., Infectious mononucleosis-like disease with negative heterophile agglutination test: Clinical features in relation to Epstein–Barr virus and cytomegalovirus antibodies, *J. Infect. Dis.* **121**:608–614 (1970).

92. LANG, D. J., AND HANSHAW, J. B., Cytomegalovirus infection and the postperfusion syndrome: Recognition of primary infection in four patients, *N. Engl. J. Med.* **280**:1145–1149 (1969).

93. LEE, C. L., DAVIDSOHN, I., AND SLABY, R., Horse agglutinins in infectious mononucleosis. *Am. J. Clin. Pathol.* **49**:3–11 (1968).

94. LEHANE, D. E., A seroepidemiologic study of infectious mononucleosis: The development of EB virus antibody in a military population, *J. Am. Med. Assoc.* **212**:2240–2242 (1970).

94a. LEMON, S. M., HUTT, L. M., SHAW, J. C., LI, J. H., AND PAGANO, J. H., Replication of EBV in epithelial cells during infectious mononucleosis, *Nature (London)* **268**:268–270 (1977).

94b. LEMON, S. M., HUTT, L. M., HUANG, Y., BLUM, J., AND PAGANO, J. H., Simultaneous infection with multiple herpesviruses, *Am. J. Med.* **66**:270–276 (1979).

94c. LENNETTE, E. T., HENLE, G., HENLE, W., AND HOROWITZ, C. A., Heterophil antigen in bovine sera detectable by immune adherence hemagglutination with infectious mononucleosis sera, *Infect. Immun.* **19**:923–927 (1978).

95. LIEBOWITZ, S., *Infectious Mononucleosis*, Grune and Stratton, New York, 1953.

96. LONGCOPE, W. T., Infectious mononucleosis (glandular fever), with a report of ten cases, *Am. J. Med. Sci.* **164**:781–807 (1922).

97. MANGI, R., NIEDERMAN, J. C., KELLEHER, J. E., DWYER, J. M., EVANS, A. S., AND KANTOR, F. S., Depression of cell-mediated immunity during acute infectious mononucleosis, *N. Engl. J. Med.* **291**:1149–1153 (1974).

98. MASON, K. L., An ox cell hemolysin test for the diagnosis of infectious mononucleosis, *J. Hyg.* **49**:471–481 (1951).

99. MAURER, B. A., IMAMURA, T., AND WILBERT, S. M., Incidence of EB virus containing cells in primary and

secondary clones of several Burkitt lymphoma cell lines, *Cancer Res.* **30**:2870–2875 (1970).

100. MILLER, G., The oncogenicity of Epstein–Barr virus, *J. Infect. Dis.* **130**:187–205 (1974).

100a. MILLER, G., Biology of Epstein–Barr virus, in: *Viral Oncology* (G. KLEIN, ed.), pp. 713–738, Raven Press, New York, 1980.

101. MILLER, G., AND HESTON, L., Expression of Epstein–Barr viral capsid, complement fixing and nuclear antigens in stationary and exponential phase cultures, *Yale J. Biol. Med.* **47**:123–135 (1974).

102. MILLER, G., AND LIPMAN, M., Release of infectious Epstein–Barr virus by transformed marmoset leucocytes, *Proc. Natl. Acad. Sci. U.S.A.* **70**:190–194 (1973).

103. MILLER, G., NIEDERMAN, J. C., AND ANDREWS, L. L., Prolonged oropharyngeal excretion of Epstein–Barr virus after infectious mononucleosis, *N. Engl. J. Med.* **288**:229–232 (1973).

104. MILLER, G., MILLER, M. H., AND STITT, D., Epstein–Barr viral antigen in single cell clones of two human leucocytic lines, *J. Virol.* **6**:699–701 (1970).

105. MILLER, G., NIEDERMAN, J. C., AND STITT, D. A., Infectious mononucleosis: Appearance of neutralizing antibody to Epstein–Barr virus measured by inhibition of formation of lymphoblastoid cell lines, *J. Infect. Dis.* **125**:403–406 (1972).

106. MILLER, G., ROBINSON, J., HESTON, L., AND LIPMAN, M., Differences between laboratory strains of Epstein–Barr virus based on immortalization, abortive infection and interference, *Proc. Natl. Acad. Sci. U.S.A.* **71**:4006–4010 (1974).

107. MOIR, J. I., Glandular fever in the Falkland Islands, *Br. Med. J.* **2**:822–823 (1930).

107a. MORI, T., KANO, K., AND MILGROM, F., Formation of Paul Bunnell antibodies by cultures of lymphocytes from infectious mononucleosis, *Cell. Immunol.* **34**:289–298 (1977).

107b. MORGAN, D. G., NIEDERMAN, J. C., MILLER, G., SMITH, H. W., AND DOWALIBY, J. M., Site of Epstein–Barr virus replication in the oropharynx, *Lancet* **2**:1154–1157 (1979).

108. MORSE, P. F., Glandular fever, *J. Am. Med. Assoc.* **77**:1403–1404 (1921).

108a. MUÑOZ, N., DAVIDSON, R. J. K., WITTHOFF, B., ERICSSON, J. E., AND DE THE, G., Infectious mononucleosis and Hodgkin's disease, *Int. J. Cancer* **22**:10–13 (1978).

109. NEWALL, K. W., The reported incidence of glandular fever, and analysis of a report of the Public Health Laboratory Service, *J. Clin. Pathol.* **10**:20–22 (1957).

110. NIEDERMAN, J. C., Infectious mononucleosis at the Yale-New Haven Medical Center, 1946–1955, *Yale J. Biol. Med.* **28**:629–643 (1956).

111. NIEDERMAN, J. C., The presence of EBV antibody in

sera from volunteers in infectious mononucleosis transmission attempts prior to inoculation, Unpublished work (1969).

112. NIEDERMAN, J. C., AND SCOTT, R. B., Studies on infectious mononucleosis: Attempts to transmit the disease to human volunteers, *Yale J. Biol. Med.* **38**:1–10 (1965).

113. NIEDERMAN, J. C., EVANS, A. S., MCCOLLUM, R. W., AND SUBRAHMANYAN, L., Prevalence, incidence and persistence of EB virus antibody in young adults, *N. Engl. J. Med.* **282**:361–365 (1970).

114. NIEDERMAN, J. C., MCCOLLUM, R. W., HENLE, G., AND HENLE, W., Infectious mononucleosis: Clinical manifestations in relation to EB virus antibodies, *J. Am. Med. Assoc.* **203**:205–209 (1968).

114a. NIEDERMAN, J. C., MILLER, G., PEARSON, H. A., PAGANO, J. S., AND DOWALIBY, J. M., Infectious mononucleosis: Epstein–Barr shedding in saliva and the oropharynx, *N. Engl. J. Med.* **294**:1355–1359 (1976).

114b. NIKOSKELAINEN, J., LEIKOLA, J., AND KLEMOLA, E., IgM antibodies specific for Epstein–Barr virus in infectious mononucleosis without heterophile antibodies, *Br. Med. J.* **4**:72–75 (1974).

114c. NIKOSKELAINEN, J. J., ABLASHI, D. V., ISENBERG, R. A., NEEL, E. U., MILLER, R. G., AND STEVENS, D. A., Cellular immunity in infectious mononucleosis. II. Specific reactivity to Epstein–Barr virus antigens and correlation with clinical and hematologic parameter, *J. Immunol.* **121**:1239–1244 (1978).

115. NONOYAMA, M., AND PAGANO, J. S., Homology between Epstein–Barr virus DNA and viral DNA from Burkitt's lymphoma and nasopharyngeal carcinoma determined by DNA-DNA reassociation kinetics, *Nature (London)* **242**:44–47 (1973).

116. OLD, L. J., CLIFFORD, P., BOYSE, E. A., DEHARVEN, E., GEERING, G., OETTGEN, H. F., AND WILLIAMSON, B., Precipitating antibody in human serum to an antigen present in cultured Burkitt lymphoma cells, *Proc. Natl. Acad. Sci. U.S.A.* **56**:1699–1704 (1966).

117. PAGANO, J. S., The Epstein–Barr viral genome and its interactions with human lymphoblastoid cells and chromosomes, in: *Viruses, Evolution and Cancer* (K. MARAMOROSCH AND E. KURSTAK, eds.), 79–116, Academic Press, New York, 1974.

117a. PANNUTI, C. S., CARVALHO, R. P. S., EVANS, A. S., CENABRE, L. C., NETO, A., CAMARGO, M., ANGELO, M. J. P., AND TAKIMOTO, S., A prospective clinical study of the mononucleosis syndrome in a developing country, *Int. J. Epidemiol.* **9**:349–353 (1980).

118. PATTENGALE, P. K., GERBER, P., AND SMITH, R. W., Selective transformation of B lymphocytes by EB virus, *Lancet* **2**:1153–1155 (1973).

119. PATTENGALE, P. K., GERBER, P., AND SMITH, R. W., B-cell characteristics of human peripheral and cord

blood lymphocytes transformed by Epstein–Barr virus, *J. Natl. Cancer Inst.* **52**:1081–1086 (1974).

120. PATTENGALE, P. K., SMITH, R. W., AND PERLIN, E., Atypical lymphocytes in acute infectious mononucleosis, *N. Engl. J. Med.* **291**:1145–1148 (1974).

121. PAUL, J. R., AND BUNNELL, W. W., The presence of heterophile antibodies in infectious mononucleosis, *Am. J. Med. Sci.* **183**:91–104 (1932).

122. PAUL, O., Mononucleosis on board a destroyer, *U.S. Naval Med. Bull.* **44**:614–617 (1945).

123. PEARSON, G., DEWEY, F., KLEIN, G., HENLE, G., AND HENLE, W., Relation between neutralization of Epstein–Barr virus and antibodies to cell membrane antigens induced by the virus, *J. Natl. Cancer Inst.* **45**:989–995 (1970).

124. PEREIRA, M. S., BLAKE, J. M., AND MACRAE, A. D., EB virus antibody at different ages, *Br. Med. J.* **4**:526–527 (1969).

125. PEREIRA, M. S., FIELD, A. M., BLAKE, J. M., RODGERS, F. G., BAILEY, L. A., AND DAVIES, J. R., Evidence for oral excretion of E.B. virus in infectious mononucleosis, *Lancet* **1**:710–711 (1972).

126. PFEIFFER, E., DRÜSENFIEBER, *Jahrb. Kinderheilkd.* **29**:257–264 (1889).

127. POPE, J. H., HORNE, M. K., AND WETTERS, E. J., Significance of a complement-fixing antigen associated with herpes-like virus and detected in the Raji cell line, *Nature (London)* **228**:186–187 (1969).

128. PULVERTAFT, R. J. X., Cytology of Burkitt's tumor (African lymphoma), *Lancet* **1**:238–240 (1964).

128a. PURTILO, D. T., BHAWAN, J., HUTT, L. M., DE NICOLA, L., SZYMANSKI, I., YANG, J. P. S., BOTO, W., MAIER, R., AND THORLEY-LAWSON, D., Epstein–Barr virus infections in the X-linked recessive lymphoproliferative syndrome, *Lancet* **1**:798–801 (1978).

128b. PURTILO, D. T., HUTT, L., BHAWAN, J., YANG, J. P. S., CASSEL, C., ALLEGRO, S., AND ROSEN, F. S., Immunodeficiency to the Epstein–Barr virus in the X-linked recessive lymphoproliferative syndrome, *Clin. Immunol. Immunopathol.* **9**:147–156 (1978).

128c. QUALTIERE, L. F., AND PEARSON, G. R., Solubilization of Epstein–Barr virus induced membrane antigen by limited papain digestion, *Fed. Proc. Fed. Am. Soc. Exp. Biol.* **37**:1817 (1978).

129. REEDMAN, B. M., AND KLEIN, G., Cellular localization of an Epstein–Barr virus (EBV) associated complement-fixing antigen in producer and non-producer lymphoblastoid cell lines, *Int. J. Cancer* **11**:499–520 (1973).

129a. ROBINSON, J., AND MILLER, G., Assay for Epstein–Barr virus based on stimulation of DNA synthesis in mixed leukocytes from human umbilical cord blood, *J. Virol.* **15**:1065–1072 (1975).

129b. ROBINSON, J. E., BROWN, N., ANDIMAN, W., HALLIDAY, K., FRANCKE, U., ROBERT, M. F., ANDERSSON-

ANVRET, M., HORSTMANN, D., AND MILLER, G., Diffuse polyclonal B-cell lymphoma during primary infection with Epstein–Barr virus, *New Engl. J. Med.* **320**:1293–1296 (1980).

130. ROCCHI, G., HEWETSON, J., AND HENLE, W., Specific neutralizing antibodies in Epstein–Barr virus associated diseases, *Int. J. Cancer* **11**:637–647 (1973).

130a. ROCCHI, G., DE FELICI, A., RAGONA, G., AND HEINZ, A., Quantitative evaluation of Epstein–Barr-virus-infected mononuclear peripheral blood leukocytes in infectious mononucleosis, *N. Engl. J. Med.* **296**:132–134 (1977).

131. ROSALKI, S. B., LWYNN, J. T., AND VERNEY, P. T., Transaminase and liver function studies in infectious mononucleosis, *Br. Med. J.* **1**:929–932 (1960).

131a. ROSDAHL, N., LARSEN, S. O., AND THAMDRUP, B., Infectious mononucleosis in Denmark: Epidemiological observations based on positive Paul–Bunnell reactions 1940–1969, *Scand. J. Infect. Dis.* **5**:163–170 (1973).

131b. ROSEN, A., GERGELY, P., JONDAL, M., AND KLEIN, G., Polyclonal Ig production after Epstein Barr virus infection of human lymphocytes *in vitro*, *Nature (London)* **267**:52 (1977).

131c. ROYSTON, I., SULLIVAN, J. L., PERIMAN, P. O., AND PERLIN, E., Cell-mediated immunity to Epstein–Barr virus-transformed lymphoblastoid cells in acute infectious mononucleosis, *N. Engl. J. Med.* **293**:1159–1163 (1975).

132. SAWYER, R. N., EVANS, A. S., NIEDERMAN, J. C., AND McCOLLUM, R. W., Prospective studies of a group of Yale University freshmen. I. Occurrence of infectious mononucleosis, *J. Infect. Dis.* **123**:263–269 (1971).

132a. SCHIFF, J., SCHAEFFER, J., AND ROBINSON, J., Cell-associated Epstein–Barr virus in the cerebrospinal fluid of a patient with meningoencephalitis complicating infectious mononucleosis, Personal communication (1978).

132b. SCHILLER, J., AND DAVEY, F. R., Human leukocyte locus A (HL-A antigens and infectious mononucleosis, *Am. J. Clin. Pathol.* **62**:325–328 (1974).

133. SCHMITZ, H., AND SCHERER, M., IgM antibodies to Epstein–Barr virus in infectious mononucleosis, *Arch. Gesamte Virusforsch.* **37**:332–339 (1972).

134. SHELDON, P. J., HEMSTED, E. H., HOLBOROW, E. J., AND PAPAMICHAEL, M., Thymic origin of atypical lymphocytes in infectious mononucleosis, *Lancet* **2**:1153–1155 (1973).

135. SHOPE, T., AND MILLER, G., Epstein–Barr virus, heterophile responses in squirrel monkeys inoculated with virus-transformed autologous leucocytes, *J. Exp. Med.* **137**:140–147 (1973).

136. SHOPE, T., EVANS, A. S., AND HORSTMANN, D. M., Seroconversion rates of EBV antibody in New Haven

school children by socio-economic level, Unpublished studies (1973).

136a. SMITH, H., AND DENMAN, A. M., A new manifestation of infection with Epstein–Barr virus, *Br. Med. J.* **2**:248–249 (1978).

137. SOHIER, R., LEPINE, P., AND SAUTTER, V., Recherches sur la transmission experimentale de la mononucleose au singe et a l'homme, *Ann. Inst. Pasteur* **65**:50–62 (1940).

138. SOHIER, R., *La Mononucleose Infectieuse*, Masson et Cie, Paris, 1943.

139. SPRUNT, T. P., AND EVANS, F. A., Mononuclear leukocytosis in reaction to acute infections (in infectious mononucleosis), *Bull. Johns Hopkins Hosp.* **31**:410–417 (1920).

140. STEEL, C. M., AND LING, N. R., Immunopathology of infectious mononucleosis, *Lancet* **2**:861–862 (1973).

141. STEVENSON, E. M. K., AND BROWN, T. G., Infectious mononucleosis: Preliminary investigation of a series of cases, *Glasgow Med. J.* **140**:139–150 (1943).

142. STORRIE, M. D., SAWYER, R. N., SPHAR, R. L., AND EVANS, A. S., Seroepidemiological studies of Polaris submarine crews. II. Infectious mononucleosis, *Mil. Med.* **141**:30–33 (1976).

143. STRAUCH, B., ANDREWS, L., MILLER, G., AND SIEGEL, N., Oropharyngeal excretion of Epstein–Barr virus by renal transplant recipients and other patients treated with immunosuppressant drugs, *Lancet* **1**:234–237 (1974).

144. STRÖM, J., Infectious mononucleosis—Is the incidence increasing?, *Acta Med. Scand.* **168**:35–39 (1960).

144a. SUMAYA, C. V., Primary Epstein–Barr virus infections in children, *Pediatrics* **59**:16–21 (1977).

145. TAYLOR, A. W., Effects of glandular fever in acute leukemia, *Br. Med. J.* **1**:589–593 (1953).

146. THOMSEN, S., *Studier over Mononucleosis Infectiosa*, Munksgaard, Copenhagen, 1942.

146a. THORLEY-LAWSON, D. A., CHESS, L., AND STROMINGER, J. L., Suppression of *in vitro* Epstein–Barr virus infection: A new role for adult human T lymphocytes, *J. Exp. Med.* **146**:495–507 (1977).

147. TISCHENDORF, P., BALAGTAS, R. C., DEINHARDT, F., KNOSPE, W. H., MAYNARD, J. E., NOBLE, G. R., AND SHRAMEK, G. J., Development and persistence of immunity to Epstein–Barr virus in man, *J. Infect. Dis.* **122**:401–409 (1970).

147a. TOSATO, G., MAGRATH, I., KOSKI, I., DOOLEY, N., AND BLAESE, M., Activation of suppressor T cells during Epstein–Barr-virus induced infectious mononucleosis, *N. Engl. J. Med.* **301**:1133–1137 (1979).

148. UNIVERSITY HEALTH PHYSICIANS AND P.H.L.S. LABORATORIES, A joint investigation: Infectious mononucleosis and its relationship to EB virus antibody, *Br. Med. J.* **4**:643–646 (1971).

149. VANDERMEER, R., LUTTERLOH, C. H., AND PILOT, J., Infectious mononucleosis: An analysis of 26 clinical and 340 subclinical cases, *Am. J. Med. Sci.* **210**:765–774 (1945).

149a. VELTRI, R. W., McCLUNG, J. E., AND SPRINKLE, P. M., EBV antigens in lymphocytes of patients with exudative tonsillitis, infectious mononucleosis and Hodgkin's disease, *Int. J. Cancer* **21**:683–687 (1978).

149b. VELTRI, R. W., McCLUNG, J. E., AND SPRINKLE, P. M., Epstein–Barr nuclear antigen (EBNA) carrying lymphocytes in human palatine tonsils, *J. Gen. Virol.* **32**:455–460 (1976).

149c. VISINTINE, A. M., GERBER, P., AND NAHMIAS, A. J., Leucocyte transforming agent (Epstein–Barr virus) in newborn infants and older individuals, *J. Pediatr.* **89**:571–575 (1976).

150. VIROLAINEN, M., ANDERSON, L. C., LALLA, M., AND VON ESSEN, R., T-lymphocyte proliferation in mononucleosis, *Clin. Immunol. Immunopathol.* **2**:114–120 (1973).

151. WAHREN, B., ESPMARK, A., LANTORP, K., AND STERNER, G., EBV antibodies in family contacts of patients with infectious mononucleosis, *Proc. Soc. Exp. Biol. Med.* **133**:934–939 (1970).

152. WALTERS, M. K., AND POPE, J. H., Studies of the EB virus-related antigens of human leucocyte cell lines, *Int. J. Cancer* **8**:32–40 (1971).

153. WECHSLER, H. F., ROSENBLUM, A. H., AND SILLS, C. T., Infectious mononucleosis: Report of an epidemic in an army post, *Ann. Intern. Med.* **25**:113–133, 236–265 (1946).

154. WERNER, J., HAFF, R. F., HENLE, G., HENLE, W., AND PINTO, C. A., Responses of gibbons to inoculation of Epstein–Barr virus, *J. Infect. Dis.* **126**:678–681 (1972).

154a. YEFENOF, E., BAKACS, T., EINHORN, L., ERNBERG, I., AND KELIN, G., Epstein–Barr virus (EBV) receptors, complement receptors and EBV infectibility of different lymphocyte fractions of human peripheral blood, *Cell. Immunol.* **35**:34–42 (1978).

155. WEST, J. P., An epidemic of glandular fever, *Arch. Pediatr.* **13**:889–900 (1896).

156. WISING, P. J., A study of infectious mononucleosis (Pfeiffer's disease) from the etiological point of view, *Acta Med. Scand. Suppl.* **133**:1–102 (1942).

157. WÖLLNER, D., Ueber die serologische Diagnose der infektiosen Mononukleose nach Paul–Bunnell mit nativen und fermentierten Hammel Erythrocyten. 2, *Immunitaets Forsch.* **112**:290–308 (1955).

158. WROBLEWSKI, F., Increasing clinical significance of alterations in enzymes in body fluids, *Ann. Intern. Med.* **50**:62–93 (1959).

159. ZAJAC, B. A., AND KOHN, G., Epstein–Barr virus antigens, marker chromosomes, and interferon production in clones derived from cultured Burkitt tumor cells, *J. Natl. Cancer Inst.* **45**:399–406 (1970).

160. ZUR HAUSEN, H. H., CLIFFORD, P., HENLE, G., HENLE, W., KLEIN, G., SANTESSON, L., AND SCHULTE-HOL-

THAUSEN, H., EB-virus DNA in biopsies of Burkitt tumors and anaplastic carcinomas of the nasopharynx, *Nature (London)* **228**:1056–1057 (1970).

161. ZUR HAUSEN, H., DORRIER, K., EGGER, H., SCHULTE-HOLTHAUSEN, H., AND WOLF, H., Attempts to detect virus-specific DNA in human tumors. II. Nucleic acid hybridizations with complementary RNA of human herpes group viruses, *Int. J. Cancer* **13**:657–664 (1974).

12. Suggested Reading

CARTER, R. L., AND PENMAN, H. G. (eds.), *Infectious Mononucleosis*, Blackwell, Oxford, 1969.

CHERVENICK, P. A., Infectious mononucleosis, *Dis.-Mon.* 1–56 (December 1974).

EVANS, A. S., Infectious mononucleosis and related syndromes, *Am. J. Med. Sci.* **276**:325–339 (1978).

GLADE, P. R. (ed.), *Infectious Mononucleosis*, Lippincott, Philadelphia, 1973.

HENLE, W., AND HENLE, G., Epstein–Barr virus, *Sci. Am.* **241**:48–59 (1979).

HOAGLAND, R., *Infectious Mononucleosis*, Grune and Stratton, New York, 1967.

KLEIN, G., *The Epstein–Barr Virus in Herpesviruses* (A. S. KAPLAN, ed.), Academic Press, New York, 1973.

MILLER, G., Epstein–Barr virus and infectious mononucleosis, *Prog. Med. Virol.* **20**:84–112 (1975).

CHAPTER 11

Viral Gastroenteritis

Albert Z. Kapikian, Harry B. Greenberg,
Richard G. Wyatt, Anthony R. Kalica, Hyun Wha Kim,
Carl D. Brandt, William J. Rodriguez, Robert H. Parrott,
and Robert M. Chanock

1. Introduction

Nonbacterial gastroenteritis is a syndrome that affects a broad segment of the population throughout the world. In the developed countries, it is a major cause of morbidity in infants and young children, whereas in the developing countries, it is a major cause of both morbidity and mortality in this same age group. In the Cleveland Family Study, which included some 25,000 illnesses over an approximate 10-year period, infectious gastroenteritis was the second most common disease experience and accounted for 16% of all illnesses.[58] In addition, a

Albert Z. Kapikian, Harry B. Greenberg, Richard G. Wyatt, Anthony R. Kalica, Hyun Wha Kim, Carl D. Brandt, William J. Rodriguez, Robert H. Parrott, and Robert M. Chanock · Laboratory of Infectious Diseases, National Institute of Allergy and Infectious Diseases, National Institutes of Health, Bethesda, Maryland; Children's Hospital National Medical Center of Washington, D.C.; and George Washington University School of Medicine and Health Sciences, Department of Child Health and Development, Washington, D.C.

winter survey of a sample of United States physicians engaged in pediatric practice revealed that "GI disturbance" was the second most common disease for which children were brought to the physicians' offices, accounting for 9.5% of all visits.[3] On the global scale, the impact of diarrheal diseases is staggering; World Health Organization (WHO) statistics have revealed that diarrheal diseases account for a large proportion of the total reported deaths in many countries.[280] An estimate of the total number of diarrheal episodes in 1975 in children less than 5 years of age in Asia, Africa, and Latin America revealed that over 450 million episodes of diarrhea would occur, and of these 1–4% would be fatal, resulting in the deaths of 5–18 million infants and young children in this 1-year period.[217] In a recent report on a strategy for disease control in developing countries, it was estimated that in Africa, Asia, and Latin America in a 1-year period (1977–1978), there would be 3–5 billion cases of diarrhea and 5–10 million deaths; diarrheas were ranked number one in frequency in the categories of disease and mortality.[271]

Despite the great importance of this problem,

studies failed to reveal an etiological agent for the majority of diarrheal illnesses.[51] However, discoveries made since 1972 of two new groups of viruses—the "parvoviruslike" group, of which the 27-nm Norwalk particle is the prototype, and the 70-nm rotavirus group—have brought forth an abundance of new information about viral gastroenteritis.[21,135,136] The Norwalk group has been associated with gastroenteritis outbreaks occurring in school, community, and family settings affecting school-aged children, adults, family contacts, and some young children as well.[102,136] The 70-nm rotaviruses have been associated with 39–63% of the acute diarrheal diseases of infants and young children requiring hospitalization in several developed countries in different parts of the world and appear to be important ethiological agents of severe acute infantile gastroenteritis in developing countries also. This chapter will deal primarily with these two new groups of viruses; in addition, other viral agents that do play a role or may also play a role in this syndrome will be discussed at the end of the chapter.

2. Historical Background

Diarrhea in humans has been documented since pre-Hippocratic times. Discoveries made in the past century in the fields of bacteriology and parasitology resulted in the elucidation of the etiology of a portion of the diarrheal syndromes. However, it soon became apparent that despite the bacteriological and parasitic discoveries, a significant proportion of epidemic and infantile gastroenteritis could not be ascribed to any etiological agent. By exclusion, it was assumed that many of these infectious gastroenteritides were due to viruses. In 1945, Reimann, Price and Hodges[206] described the transmission of gastroenteric illness to volunteers following administration by the respiratory route of nebulized bacteria-free filtrates of throat washings or fecal suspensions from gastroenteritis patients. Gordon et al.,[96] in 1947, induced an afebrile diarrheal illness in volunteers by the oral administration of bacteria-free fecal filtrates and throat washings from gastroenteritis patients; this infectious inoculum was designated the Marcy strain, since it was derived from pooled diarrheal stools obtained from two patients in a gastroenteritis outbreak at Marcy State Hospital near Utica, New York.

In 1948, Kojima et al.[140] induced gastroenteric illness in volunteers following oral administration of bacteria-free fecal filtrates derived from diarrhea cases in the Niigata Prefecture and other districts; serial passage was achieved, and short-term immunity was demonstrated on challenge with a single strain. Yamamoto et al.,[292] in 1948, also induced diarrheal illness in volunteers (and cats as well) with bacteria-free fecal filtrates derived from an epidemic of gastroenteritis in the Gumma Prefecture. Later, in 1957, Fukumi et al.[92] reported on the relationship between the Niigata Prefecture strain (derived from a pool of stools of several patients with diarrhea as described above and shown to have been infectious in volunteers) and the Marcy strain. In cross-challenge studies Niigata and Marcy strains were found to be related.

In 1953, Jordan, Gordon, and Dorrance reported the induction of a febrile gastroenteric illness in volunteers following the oral administration of a bacteria-free fecal filtrate derived from a patient with gastroenteritis who was enrolled in the Cleveland Family Study (FS) cited in Section 1; the agent, which was designated the FS strain, was serially passaged in volunteers.[117] Cross-challenge studies in volunteers revealed that the Marcy and FS strains were not antigenically related; in addition, the incubation period of and clinical illness induced by the two strains were somewhat different.[117]

Studies on the etiology of severe infantile gastroenteritis also failed to reveal an etiological agent in the majority of instances. However, in 1943, Light and Hodes[151] were able to induce diarrhea in calves with a filterable agent derived from diarrheal stools obtained from infants who developed diarrheal illness during outbreaks of such illness in premature or full-term nurseries. A calf stool that had been lyophilized and stored for over 30 years was recently examined by electron microscopy (EM) and found to contain rotavirus.[112] Whether this represented a true calf rotavirus or the human strain passaged in calves could not be determined conclusively; in recent studies, the agent was not infectious when administered to a gnotobiotic calf.[112,281]

In 1972, application of the technique of immune electron microscopy (IEM) led to the discovery of 27-nm particles in stool material derived from a gastroenteritis outbreak in Norwalk, Ohio[135] (Fig. 1A).

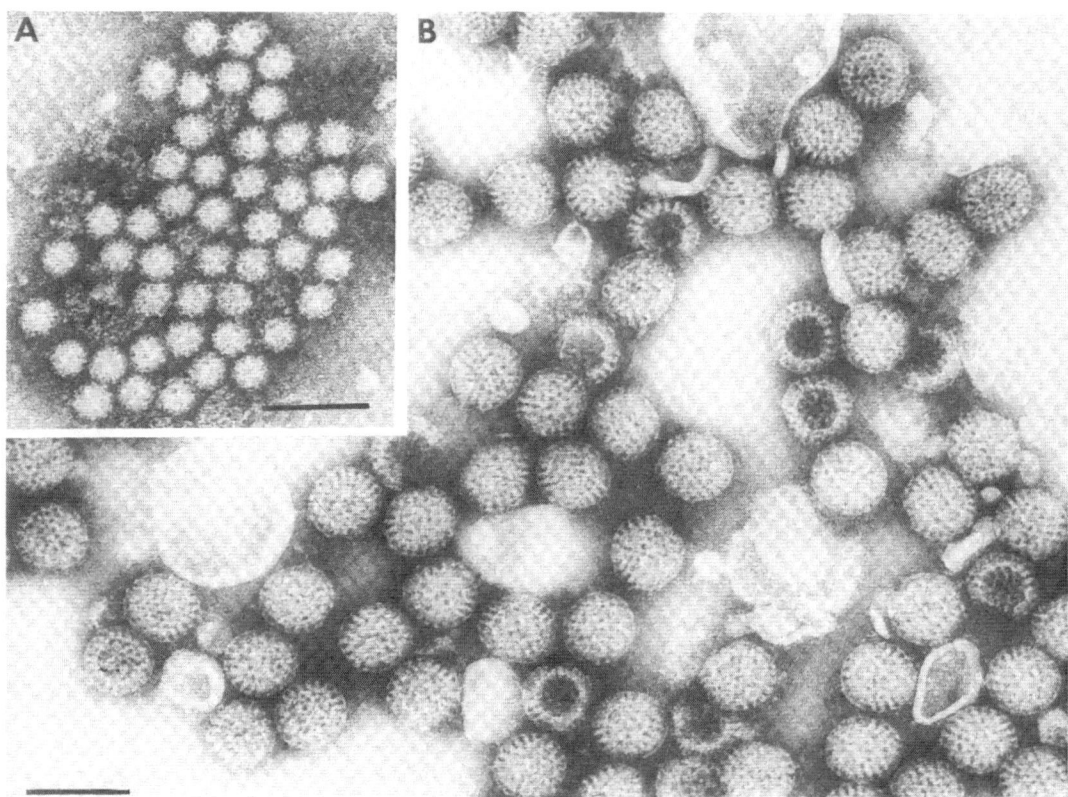

Fig. 1. (A) A group of Norwalk virus particles observed after incubation of 0.8 ml of Norwalk stool filtrate (prepared from a stool of a volunteer administered the Norwalk agent) with 0.2 ml of a 1:5 dilution of a volunteer's prechallenge serum and further preparation for EM. The quantity of antibody on these particles was rated as 1+. Scale bar: 100 nm. From Kapikian *et al.*[135] (bar added). (B) Human rotavirus particles observed in a stool filtrate (prepared from a stool of an infant with gastroenteritis) after incubation with phosphate-buffered saline and further preparation for EM. The particles appear to have a double-shelled capsid. Occasional "empty" particles are seen. Scale bar: 100 nm. From Kapikian *et al.*[134]

This technique, which had actually been described in 1939 but not used to its fullest potential until recently, might be considered as the direct observation of antigen–antibody interaction by EM.[7,8,12,129] The 27-nm particles were visualized in a known infectious stool filtrate derived from a volunteer who had developed illness following administration of the Norwalk agent[135]; the particle-positive specimen had also induced illness in other volunteers on serial passage.[60] The particles were recognized following reaction of the known infectious stool filtrate with a volunteer's convalescent serum prior to preparation for examination by IEM.[135] Serological evidence of infection with this particle was also demonstrated by IEM in certain experimentally and naturally infected individuals and from these and other data it was concluded that the 27-nm particle was the etiological agent of the Norwalk outbreak.[135] Particles morphologically similar to Norwalk virus—such as the Hawaii, Montgomery County, Ditchling, "W," cockle, Parramatta, and Marin County agents—were later detected from patients in outbreaks of gastroenteritis by IEM or conventional EM.[9,11,48,193,256]

It soon became apparent from other studies that a 70-nm particle—formerly known by various names such as orbivirus, orbiviruslike, reoviruslike agent, duovirus, and infantile gastroenteritis virus but now officially designated rotavirus—was indeed the major etiological agent of infantile diarrhea.[21,54,66, 86,104,107a,133,165,201] The human rotavirus was discovered in 1973 by Bishop et al.[20,21] by examination by thin-section EM of duodenal biopsies obtained from infants and young children hospitalized with acute gastroenteritis in Australia. Subsequently, it was found to be readily detectable in stool preparations by EM.[19,83] In a relatively short time, laboratories from all over the world reported in rapid succession the presence of rotavirus in stool specimens from infants and young children with diarrheal illness, and it thus became apparent that this virus was indeed the long-sought major viral etiological agent of diarrhea of infants and young children (Fig. 1B).

Two final notes of historical interest: In 1963, Adams and Kraft,[1] using thin-section EM to study intestinal tissue from mice infected with epizootic diarrhea of infant mice virus, described particles very similar to those first observed in 1973 in infants and young children in Australia. In 1969, Mebus et al.[174] described the presence of reoviruslike particles in stools obtained from calves with a diarrheal illness. Later, both the mouse and calf viruses were found to be antigenically related to human rotavirus.[86,126,127,134] It is of interest that both the Norwalk and rotavirus groups could have been discovered much sooner than they were if the concept of "direct virology" using EM had been applied to appropriate specimens.[136]

3. Methodology Involved in Epidemiological Analysis

3.1. Sources of Mortality Data

Age-specific mortality data are available in the United States in the Vital Statistics Report prepared by the National Center for Health Statistics of the Office of Health Research Statistics and Technology, Public Health Service, Hyattsville, Maryland. One of the causes of death enumerated in this report is "enteritis and other diarrheal diseases." Another is "bacillary dysentery and amebiasis." Since the clin-ical manifestations of viral diarrheas are not distinctive enough to permit differentiation from many other causes of diarrhea, and since the laboratory diagnosis of infection with viral gastroenteritis agents remains essentially a research tool, it is not yet possible to estimate the role of specific viruses in overall mortality from diarrhea. On a worldwide scale, mortality data for diarrheal diseases are available in WHO and Pan American Health Organization publications. Vital statistics from around the world give the overall importance of diarrhea as a cause of death, but, for the same reasons noted above, do not specify the role of the newly discovered viruses. However, with the emergence of rotaviruses as a major cause of infantile diarrhea, it is generally assumed that this group of agents is of importance as a cause of mortality from diarrheal diseases in the developing countries. However, its relative importance in this regard in comparison to bacterial agents has not yet been ascertained.

3.2. Sources of Morbidity Data

Since the clinical manifestations of viral gastroenteritis are indistinguishable in individual cases from many other forms of gastroenteritis, it is not possible to obtain specific morbidity data without the aid of laboratory diagnosis, and as yet such diagnosis remains essentially a research tool. Recently, the National Institute of Allergy and Infectious Diseases initiated an enteric-diseases program that has as one of its aims the collection of gastroenteritis morbidity data from an epidemiological as well as an etiological view point. This program now includes studies in families, day-care centers, health-plan members, and other groups, and already some information has emerged on gastroenteritis morbidity associated with the new agents. With rare exceptions, such as the longitudinal study of infection with gastroenteric viruses in a Guatemalan village,[291] most of the data on morbidity associated with gastroenteritis viruses comes from cross-sectional hospital-based studies of infants and young children admitted for diarrheal illness and from studies of outbreaks of gastroenteritis. Such studies undoubtedly provide only a limited view of the total morbidity associated with these viruses, since they include only patients sick enough to come to the hospital or ill persons in selected outbreaks.

3.3. Serological Surveys

Serological surveys have been carried out with the rotaviruses and the Norwalk agent to elucidate the prevalence of infection, the pattern of antibody acquisition by age, and the geographic distribution of these agents.[100,127,131,286,302] Rotavirus serology has relied heavily on the complement-fixation (CF) and enzyme-linked immunosorbent assay (ELISA) techniques.[126,127,302] Until very recently, large-scale serological surveys could not be carried out with Norwalk virus, since the only assay available was immune electron microscopy (IEM); this technique was not practical for such studies, since it not only was very time-consuming but also required relatively large amounts of antigen, which was in short supply. However, the development of an immune adherence hemagglutination assay (IAHA) and a radioimmunoassay (RIA) has now made it possible to perform serological surveys with Norwalk virus.[104,131] Such surveys have not been carried out with other members of the Norwalk group, since the only available serological assay for them is still IEM.

3.4. Laboratory Methods

3.4.1. Norwalk Group of Viruses

a. *Antigen Detection.* Since this group of viruses has not yet been cultivated in any *in vitro* system, EM remains a mainstay for their recognition from stool specimens. IEM entails the reaction of antibody (such as that present in the patient's convalescent serum or in pooled immune serum globulin) with virus in the patient's stool preparation.[128,136] Following centrifugation, the pellet (which contains the antigen–antibody complex) is prepared for examination by negative-stain EM. Antibodies directed against the particle are seen on the surface of the particle, and under appropriate conditions, antibodies induce aggregation of the particles. However, aggregation *per se* is not indicative of the presence of antibody, since nonspecific aggregating may occur. The presence of antibodies on the particle with or without aggregation enables its differentiation from nonspecific matter. The specificity of the reaction must be determined in additional IEM experiments, since stools contain a large amount of particulate matter that may cause considerable confusion. Thus, a serological test as outlined in Section

3.4.1b below must be carried out with the putative particle as antigen and paired acute (or pre-) and postinfection sera as the source of antibody to determine whether an increase in antibody to the particle occurred. Such paired sera may be from the patient, another subject in the outbreak, or a subject with a response to a known agent. Such a study should routinely be done under code. The direct examination of stool material without addition of serum may also be carried out if sufficient antigen is present; however, identification or determination of the significance of such a particle should be carried out by IEM as outlined above.[128,136]

An RIA for detection of the prototype strain of the Norwalk group of agents has recently been developed[99,104] that is even more efficient than IEM. The test is essentially a research tool, since suitable reagents are not generally available. An IAHA has also been developed for the Norwalk agent,[131] but is not efficient for its detection in clinical specimens. RIA and IAHA techniques are not available for the other members of the Norwalk group; thus, EM and IEM remain the only methods for their detection and IEM the only method for their identification.

The Norwalk group of agents has not been shown to produce illness in any experimental animal.[25,60,61,136,284,287] However, the Norwalk virus has been found to infect chimpanzees by the alimentary route as indicated by shedding of antigen and a serological response.[104,284]

b. *Serological Studies.* As noted above, IEM remains a mainstay for studying this group of agents. In this technique, the stool material that contains the particle is incubated with a standard dilution of an acute, or pre-, and postillness serum specimen, and the amount of antibody coating the particle is scored on a 0–4 + scale.[128,129,135,136] An example of a seroresponse to the Norwalk virus by a volunteer who developed illness following oral administration of Norwalk virus is shown in Fig. 2. The difference in the amount of antibody coating the Norwalk virus following its incubation with the volunteer's prechallenge serum and his postchallenge serum is clearly evident. Since numerous spherical particles are detected in stool by EM, it is essential to establish the significance of these objects by IEM employing appropriate paired sera. After a viruslike particle has been detected, a seroresponse should be demonstrated as an initial step in associating this particle with infection.

The development of an RIA-blocking test for measurement of Norwalk virus antibody has greatly facilitated epidemiological study of this agent.[100,101,102] This assay is as efficient as IEM for detecting a seroresponse but is much more practical, since it is much less time-consuming and also requires much less antigen and antibody. In addition, an IAHA for detection of Norwalk virus antibody has been developed.[131] It is not quite as efficient as either IEM or RIA, but is, of course, more practical than IEM. Both the RIA-blocking and IAHA techniques remain

essentially research tools because of the paucity of appropriate Norwalk antigen. Neither an RIA-blocking nor an IAHA technique is available for other members of the Norwalk group of agents.

3.4.2. Rotavirus

a. Antigen Detection. Since the human rotavirus in clinical specimens does not grow readily in tissue culture or in small laboratory animals, it cannot be detected by conventional cultivation techniques.[286,288] Thus, in the early studies, EM was the

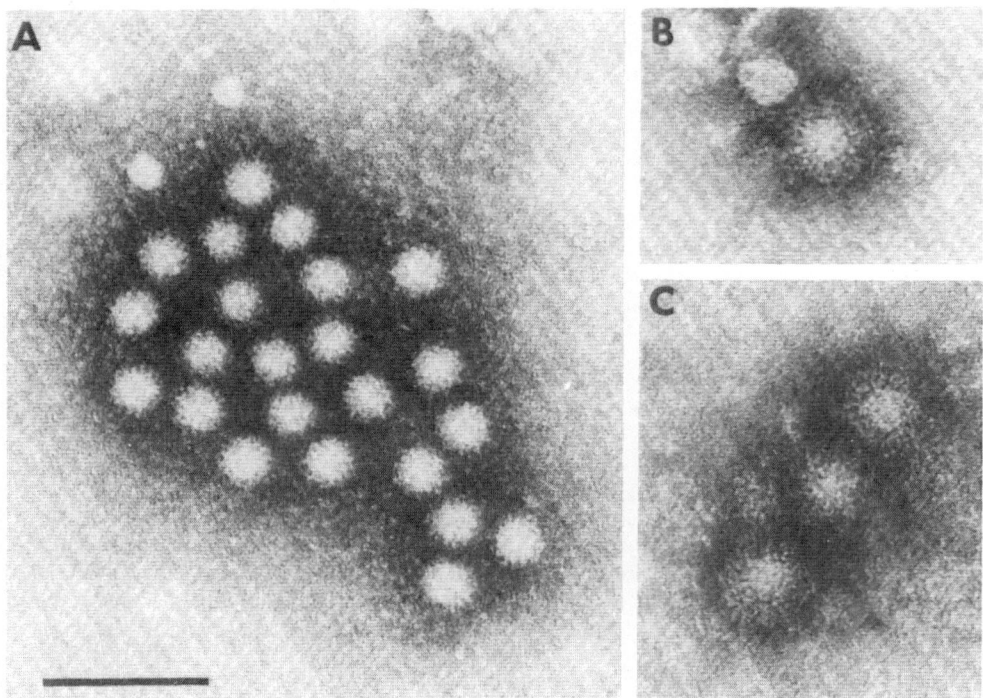

Fig. 2. (A) An aggregate observed after incubation of 0.8 ml of Norwalk (8FIIa) stool filtrate with 0.2 ml of a 1:5 dilution of a volunteer's prechallenge serum and further preparation for electron microscopy. This volunteer developed gastroenteritis following challenge with a second passage Norwalk filtrate which had been heated for 30 minutes at 60°C.[60] The quantity of antibody on the particles in this aggregate was rated 1−2−2+ and this prechallenge serum was given an overall rating of 1−2+. (B) A single particle and (C) three single particles observed after incubating 0.8 ml of the Norwalk (8FIIa) stool filtrate with 0.2 ml of a dilution of the volunteer's postchallenge convalescent serum and further preparation for EM. These particles are very heavily coated with antibody. The quantity of antibody on these particles was rated 4+ and the serum was given an overall rating of 4+ also. The difference in the quantity of antibody coating the particles in the prechallenge and post challenge sera of this volunteer is clearly evident. The bar = 100 nm and applies to A, B, and C. From: Kapikian *et al.*[129]

Table 1. Efficiency and Practicality of Methods Available for Detection of Human Rotaviruses from Stool Specimens[a]

Method	Efficiency[b]	Practicality for large-scale epidemiological studies (assuming 4+ efficiency)
Electron microscopy (EM)[19,83,134,182,202]	4+	1+
Immune electron microscopy (IEM)[133,134]	4+	1+
Complement-fixation (CF) (conventional)[95,141,182,228,240,265]	1+	4+
Human fetal intestinal organ culture [with immunofluorescence (IF)][288]	1+	0
Counterimmunoelectroosmophoresis[10,97,180,240,241,264]	3–4+	4+
Fluorescent virus precipitin test[91,199,299]	4+	1+
Cell culture (cytopathic effect)[186,283]	1+	2–3+
Cell culture (with IF)[6,186,204,283]	1+	1+
Cell culture (with EM)[6,204,283]	1+	1+
Centrifugation onto cell culture (with IF)[15,38,259,263]	3–4+	1+
Gel diffusion[278]	1+	4+
Smears (with IF)[274]	1+	4+
Radioimmunoassay (RIA)[24,53,119,179]	4+	3–4+
Enzyme-linked immunosorbent assay (ELISA)[294,296,300]	4+	4+
Immune adherence hemagglutination assay (IAHA)[164]	3+	2–3+
RNA electrophoresis patterns in gels[78]	3+	1+
Modified CF[304]	3–4+	2–3+
Enzyme-linked fluorescence assay (ELFA)[297]	4+	3+
Ultrasensitive enzymatic radioimmunoassay (USERIA)[110]	4+	3+
Solid-phase aggregation of coupled erythrocytes (SPACE)[31]	3–4+	3–4+

[a] From Kapikian et al.[136] with additions.
[b] On a scale of 1–4+, where 1+ indicates a low degree of efficiency or practicality and 4+ indicates a high degree of efficiency or practicality.

mainstay for detection of rotavirus in stool specimens. Although IEM was also employed, the addition of antibody was not essential, since in contrast to the Norwalk group, rotaviruses have a quite distinct morphological appearance as shown in Fig. 1B.[134] However, various simpler and more readily available methods for rotavirus detection have been developed as practical alternatives to EM for diagnosis and for research epidemiological studies. Table 1 shows numerous methods that have been described for rotavirus detection and presents a rating for each on a 1–4+ scale, with 1+ indicating a low degree of efficiency or practicality and 4+ a high degree. Though EM and IEM are very efficent, they are not practical, but nevertheless remain the "supreme court" of rotavirus detection, since questionable results by any of the assays can usually be resolved by examination of the specimen by EM. In our laboratory, the method of choice at present is the ELISA, since it is practical and efficient and does not require sophisticated equipment. However,

with this assay, all "positive" specimens detected by the conventional ELISA must be confirmed by an appropriate blocking test, or alternatively and more practically appropriate positive and negative sera should be employed in the initial detection system so that a confirmatory test is done at the time of virus detection.[136,296] Recently, a modification of this test called the enzyme-linked fluorescence assay (ELFA) was described as being even more sensitive than the conventional ELISA: a special substrate is employed that is examined for the degree of fluorescence (rather than for the degree of color change as in the conventional ELISA).[297] An even more sensitive assay designated as ultrasensitive enzymatic radioimmunoassay (USERIA) has also been described recently.[110] Another assay that has been described as being efficient for rotavirus detection—solid-phase aggregation of coupled erythrocytes (SPACE)—has recently been introduced.[31] The selection of technique will depend on the investigator's capabilities and experience and

Table 2. Efficiency and Practicality of Methods Available for Detecting Serological Evidence of Human Rotavirus Infection[a]

Method	Efficiency[b]	Practicality for large-scale epidemiological studies (assuming 4+ efficiency)
Immune electron microscopy (IEM)[30,84,133,134,141]	4+	<1+
Complement-fixation (CF)[30,66,74,106,107,126,127,133,134]	3–4+	4+
Immunofluorescence (IF)[56,74,86,127,139,186,194,285,288]	4+	1+
Gel diffusion[278]	Not known	2+
Counterimmunoelectroosmophoresis[52,180]	Variable	2+
Neutralization of calf rotavirus in cell culture[86,108,124,127,262,278]	2+	1+
Radioimmunoassay (RIA)[24]	Not known	3+
Enzyme-linked immunosorbent assay (ELISA)[234,295,298,301,302]	4+	3–4+
Inhibition (neutralization) of fluorescent foci[38,74,257,259,285]	Not known	1+
Immune adherence hemagglutination assay (IAHA)[131,162,164]	3–4+	4+
Hemagglutination-inhibition (HI)[80,233,242]	2–3+	4+

[a] After Kapikian et al.[136] with certain reference changes.
[b] On a scale of 1–4+, where 1+ indicates a low degree of efficiency or practicality and 4+ indicates a high degree of efficiency or practicality.

the availability of appropriate reagents. Regardless of the methods employed, it is striking that almost all the rotavirus-detection methods do not require *in vitro* cultivation, but rather employ "direct virology"—a simple concept that, as so often occurs in medical research, could have been employed years ago but has been applied only recently.[136]

b. *Serological Studies.* Numerous assays have been described for detection of rotavirus antibody. Since the agent could not be grown in cell cultures, initial studies of serological responses relied on IEM, utilizing human rotavirus-positive stools as antigen.[134] However, this time-consuming method was soon superseded by the development of a CF test in which particle-rich human stools were used as antigen.[126,127,134] This method was limited by the paucity of human stools containing sufficient particles for the CF assay. It was soon discovered, however, that animal and human rotaviruses shared a common CF antigen and thus that animal strains could be used as substitute CF antigens for detection of infection with human rotavirus.[126,127] This antigenic relationship was of special importance, since certain animal rotaviruses such as a few calf strains, simian strain SA-11, and the "O" agent (from intestinal washings of sheep and cattle) had been propagated efficiently in cell cultures[158,169]; thus the quantity of CF antigen was virtually unlimited. Moreover, the recent efficient propagation of human rotavirus strain Wa (see Section 4.2) should make

sufficient human rotavirus antigen available for this and other assays.[285] A variety of other serological assays have been developed to detect serological evidence of rotavirus infection, such as immunofluorescence (IF), IAHA, hemagglutination-inhibition (HI), and ELISA. A summary of the relative efficiency and practicality of serological methods for rotavirus is presented in Table 2. The ELISA blocking and binding assays are more efficient than CF for detecting rotavirus infection in infants less than 6 months of age and also in adults.[298,301] The CF and ELISA methods are comparable in efficiency for infants and young children 6–24 months of age. IF is almost as efficient as ELISA for rotavirus antibody detection.[298] Thus, ELISA appears to be the most efficient of the available methods; however, it is not quite as practical as CF in laboratories where the latter is used routinely for other agents. CF may be employed with confidence if its limits of efficiency are recognized and alternate tests are employed when needed. The ELISA has an additional advantage over CF in that the former permits the measurement of immunoglobulin classes.[295,301] It is noteworthy that in most of the serological assays shown in Table 2 in which human rotavirus was used as antigen, the approach of "direct virology," which obviates *in vitro* cultivation of an agent, was quite successful.[136] Of course, a source of antigen such as particle-rich stools was essential for these serological assays.

4. Biological Characteristics

4.1. Norwalk Group of Viruses

This group of agents is comprised of several viruses that (1) were detected in the stool of patients with gastroenteritis, (2) have not been propagated *in vitro*, (3) share a morphological appearance similar to that of picorna- or parvoviruses and in certain preparations to the caliciviruses also, and (4) have a buoyant density in $CsCl_2$ of 1.37–1.41 g/cm³.[9,11,130,135,136,256,287] The Norwalk virus represents the prototype strain of this group of agents.[135]

There are several other members of the group the origins and epidemic features of which are shown in Table 3 and described later in this section. The Norwalk and Hawaii viruses were shown to be distinct by cross-challenge and immune-electron-microscopic (IEM) studies, the Norwalk and Montgomery County to be related, and the relationship of Hawaii and Montgomery County to be inconclusive.[135,282] The Ditchling and W agents appear to be related but distinct from Norwalk and Hawaii by IEM.[9,129] The cockle agent is distinct from Norwalk virus, but its relationship to other agents is inconclusive.[11]

Some of the biochemical or biophysical characteristics of two of these viruses have been elucidated in volunteer studies in which the ability of a treated stool filtrate to induce illness was determined. The Norwalk virus was found to be acid-stable (pH 2.7 for 3 hr at room temperature) and relatively heat-stable, and both the Norwalk and "W" viruses were ether-stable (20% ether at 4°C for 24 hr).[50,60]

This group has not yet been classified into any family of viruses. However, it has been suggested that the Norwalk virus was "parvoviruslike" since it shared certain characteristics with this group such as morphology by negative-stain EM, density in CsCl, and ether, acid, and relative heat stability.[60,135] This suggestion was quite tentative, since the nucleic acid content of the Norwalk virus as well as of the other agents in this group was not known. Recent studies of the polypeptides of Norwalk virus suggest that it may be caliciviruslike because a single primary virion-associated protein with molecular weight of 59,000 was detected; in addition, a single soluble protein with a molecular weight of 30,000 was also found.[102] Caliciviruses also have a single structural protein with a molecular weight of about 65,000[35,223b,224]; in addition, a small virion-associated protein with a molecular weight of about 15,000, as well as a nonstructural virus-associated protein with a molecular weight of 29,000 have been described.[35,223b]

As shown in Table 3, other potential members of this group include the Parramatta,[48] the Colorado (Snow Mountain)[185,193] and Marin County agents.[98,193] The Parramatta and Marin County agents were readily visualized by EM and IEM, respectively; only a few 27-nm particles were visualized in a filtrate of the Colorado agent. The density of each of these particles has not been described.

Evidence for the etiological role of the Norwalk group of agents in gastroenteritis differs for each member. In one study, the Norwalk agent was shown to induce illness in 30 (58%) of 52 volunteers[282]; serological evidence of infection has been demonstrated in most of a sample of volunteers who developed illness as well as in certain subjects in the original outbreak.[104,131,135] Further evidence of an etiological association was the demonstration that volunteers who developed illness after Norwalk challenge had a close temporal relationship between virus shedding and illness, with maximal shedding occurring at the onset of experimental illness.[255] Only short-term immunity characteristically occurs in volunteers who develop illness after initial challenge[60,197,282]; prechallenge serum antibody titers could not be correlated with susceptibility to illness.[197] Volunteers have also developed illness following administration of stool filtrates containing the Hawaii, Montgomery County, "W," and Colorado agents.[50,185,282] IEM seroresponses were observed in volunteers challenged with the Hawaii and Montgomery County agents.[135,256] Homologous seroresponses also occur in most individuals who develop illness associated with the Parramatta or Marin County agents.[48,193]

4.2. Rotaviruses

Human rotavirus has been detected in stools of about 30–60% of infants and young children hospitalized with acute gastroenteritis and much less often in older children and adults with this disease,[33,54,102,133,136,141] as well as in stools of numerous animals. Rotaviruses have been identified with a diarrheal illness in the calf,[169,174,276] infant mouse,[187] piglet,[148,168,210,254,277] foal,[85] lamb,[238] young rabbit,[39,203] monkey,[247] newborn deer,[268] newborn antelope,[205] young chimpanzee,[13] young go-

Table 3. Characteristics of Norwalk, Norwalklike, and Possibly Related Agents Associated with Acute Epidemic Nonbacterial Gastroenteritis in Humans

Agent	Size (nm)	Buoyant density in cesium chloride (g/cm³)	Growth in cell culture	Administration[a] of agent induces illness in: Humans	Administration[a] of agent induces illness in: Animal(s)	Particle detected by	Serological studies by	Antigenic relationships
Norwalk[60,61,104,130,131,135,255,284]	27 × 32[b]	1.38–1.41	No	Yes	No	IEM[c]	IEM; RIA, AHA	Distinct
Hawaii[62,135,256,282]	26 × 29[b]	1.37–1.39	No	Yes	No	IEM	IEM	Distinct
Montgomery County[135,256,282]	27 × 32[b]	1.37–1.41	No	Yes	No	IEM	IEM	Related to Norwalk agent by IEM and cross-challenge studies.
Ditchling[9]	25–26	1.38–1.40	No	N.T.[d]	No	EM	IEM	Ditchling and "W" agents related to each other, but appear to be distinct from Norwalk and Hawaii agents by IEM.
"W"[9,50,129]	25–26	1.38–1.40	No	Yes	N.T.	EM	IEM	
Cockle[11]	25–26	1.40	No	N.T.	N.T.	EM	IEM	Appears to be distinct from Norwalk agent by IEM.
Parramatta[48]	23–26	N.T.	No	N.T.	N.T.	EM	IEM	Distinct from Norwalk agent by IEM.
Colorado (Snow Mountain)[98,185,193]	c	N.T.	No	Yes	N.T.	IEM	IEM	Distinct from Norwalk, Hawaii, and Marin County[f] agents by IEM or RIA or both.
Marin County[99a,193]	27	N.T.	No	Yes	No	IEM	IEM	Distinct from Norwalk, Hawaii, and Colorado[f] agents by IEM or RIA.

[a] By alimentary route. [b] Shortest × longest diameter. [c] Immune electron microscopy. [d] Not tested. [e] IEM and RIA tests with paired sera from a Colorado-agent-infected volunteer. [f] IEM test with paired sera from a Colorado-agent-infected volunteer.

rilla,[13] young turkey,[16,167] chicken,[116] young goat,[231] and young kitten[235]; pneumoenteric illness has been found in the newborn impala,[79] newborn addax,[74] and newborn gazelle.[79] The offal ("O") agent was derived from mixed intestinal washings from abattoir waste,[158] and a rotavirus has been derived from dogs with no known illness.[218] Of all these rotaviruses, human rotavirus Wa (discussed later in this Section), the calf, piglet, and monkey isolates, and the "O" agent from sheep and calf intestines have been successfully carried through two or more passages in cell cultures. Further descriptions of these animal rotaviruses have been recently reviewed.[286] With the exception of the SA-11 strain of simian rotavirus, canine rotavirus, and the "O" agent that was derived from mixed intestinal washings from an abattoir waste, each of the others has been associated with naturally occurring diarrheal (or pneumoenteric, as already noted) illness in newborns of each respective group.

As shown in Fig. 1B, rotaviruses have a distinctive morphological appearance. Complete particles possess a double-shelled capsid and measure about 70 nm in diameter; single-shelled particles measure about 55 nm in diameter, whereas the core has a diameter of about 37 nm.[75,88,114,159,196,200,231] The term rotavirus comes from the Latin word *rota*, meaning wheel, and was suggested because the sharply defined circular outline of the outer capsid gives the appearance of the rim of a wheel placed on short spokes radiating from a wide hub.[82,86] Rotaviruses resemble orbiviruses and reoviruses morphologically, but differ characteristically in their fine structure.[192,286]

The rotavirus genome is comprised of 11 segments of double-stranded RNA,[118,120,121,192,211,225,260] which distinguishes them from reoviruses and orbiviruses, both of which possess only 10 RNA segments.[89,286] The migration patterns of the RNA segments of rotaviruses as determined by polyacrylamide-gel electrophoresis are of importance not only in the biophysical characterization of these agents but also as epidemiological probes; they have served as one of the methods of differentiating human and animal rotaviruses as well as various human rotavirus strains.[118,120] The distinctive RNA migration pattern of rotaviruses has also been used for detection and identification of rotavirus strains from clinical specimens.[78] Rotaviruses contain eight to ten polypeptides, with five or six associated with

the inner shell and three or possibly four with the outer shell of the double-shelled capsid.[191,192,211,212,260] Complete particles have a density of 1.36 g/cm³ in CsCl₂ and a sedimentation coefficient of 520–530 S.[127,132,200,201,211,212,253] Particles that lack the double capsid (core particles) have a density of approximately 1.38 g/cm³, whereas "empty" particles that have been penetrated by negative stain have a density of approximately 1.29–1.30 g/cm³.[75,211,253]

Since rotaviruses share certain properties with the reoviruses and orbiviruses and yet are distinct serologically and in certain biophysical aspects, they have been officially classified as a new genus in the family Reoviridae.[165] This family now contains six genera: reovirus, orbivirus, rotavirus, phytoreovirus, Fijivirus, and an as yet unnamed group comprising the cytoplasmic polyhedrosis viruses.[165] Certain members of the first three infect humans, whereas the phytoreoviruses and Fijiviruses infect plants and the cytoplasmic polyhedrosis viruses infect insects.[165]

Antigenically, rotaviruses are distinct from reoviruses by complement-fixation (CF) and IEM and from those orbiviruses tested by CF.[56,88,119,126,127,134] By neutralization assay, there are at least 3 human rotavirus serotypes.[15a,88a,98,98a,281,285] Rotaviruses can also be separated into at least 2 distinct subgroups by IEM, specific CF, ELISA, and IAHA.[33,70a,90,118a,125a,215,302,303] It has recently been shown that the neutralization and the subgroup specificities are coded for by different genes.[118a] As noted earlier, the various animal and human rotaviruses are morphologically similar and possess common CF and fluorescent-antibody antigens[5,86,126,127,278]; however, by enzyme-linked immunosorbent assay (ELISA) blocking and by neutralization of immunofluorescent (IF) focus formation in cell culture, human rotavirus may be differentiated from various animal rotaviruses, and various animal rotaviruses may be distinguished from one another.[259,278,293]

The human rotaviruses are rather fastidious agents, and until very recently, not a single strain had been propagated efficiently in any cell- or organ-culture system. However, a few strains had been cultivated to a limited extent with only a small percentage of cells exhibiting evidence of infection.[6,79,283,288] Recently, human rotavirus Wa, a subgroup 2 virus was adapted to grow efficiently in primary African green monkey kidney (AGMK) cells following 11 serial passages of a strain in gnotobiotic piglets.[285] Pretreatment of porcine-grown virus with trypsin was required for optimal growth of this strain in AGMK cells; low-speed centrifugation of the virus inoculum onto cell cultures was also employed. The availability of this cell-culture-adapted strain has implications for vaccine development, for the production of specific antigens for use in various immunological assays and for assessment of the relationships among rotaviruses by neutralization in tissue culture. In addition, recently noncultivatable human rotaviruses were successfully rescued following mixed infection of cell cultures with noncultivatable human rotavirus and cultivatable bovine rotavirus, and application of various selective pressures.[98a] The cultivatable reassortants had mixed genotypes, but also had the neutralization specificity of human rotavirus. Also, efficient propagation of human rotaviruses in cell cultures has recently been reported.[65,223a]

Experimentally, human rotavirus induces a diarrheal illness in various newborn animals including gnotobiotic calves, gnotobiotic and conventional piglets, rhesus monkeys, and gnotobiotic lambs.[118,147,148,173,181,184,237,261,262,290]; subclinical infections also occur in newborn puppy dogs.[267] Particle-positive stools from calves have been an important source of human rotavirus for biophysical and serological studies.

Firm evidence exists for the association of rotavirus with gastrointestinal illness. The virus has been detected significantly more often in stools from patients 6–24 months old with gastroenteritis than in those without gastroenteritis[33,54] in both hospitalized patients and outpatients. Serological evidence of rotavirus infection has also been observed significantly more often in hospitalized gastroenteritis patients than in hospitalized "controls."[133] The virus is detectable predominantly during the acute phase of illness.[54] In addition, illness has been induced in volunteers with a stool filtrate containing human rotavirus D strain.[124] Serum antibody appeared to be associated with resistance.

5. Descriptive Epidemiology

5.1. Norwalk Group of Viruses

5.1.1. Incidence and Prevalence Data. Specific incidence data for the Norwalk group in the general population are not available. Estimates of the importance of this group of agents are suggested from various sources. Infectious gastroenteritis was the second most common disease experience in the Cleveland Family Study over an approximate 10-year period.[58] and the Norwalk group was probably associated with at least some of these illnesses, especially in the adults. About one third of all outbreaks of nonbacterial gastroenteritis studied are associated with Norwalk virus infection.[101,102] It is probable that other members of the group are also responsible for a portion of epidemic gastroenteritis, but appropriate tests are not available to confirm this. In children in developed countries, the Norwalk group is probably not an important cause of severe gastroenteritis. Thus, 27-nm virus particles were present in less than 2% of infants and children hospitalized with diarrhea at the Children's Hospital, Washington, D.C., a value not significantly different from that observed in controls,[33] nor was serological evidence of Norwalk virus infection detected in selected diarrhea patients from this study.[131]

Prevalence data are available for the Norwalk virus, since the development of both an immune adherence hemagglutination assay (IAHA) and a radioimmunoassay (RIA) has permitted the study of serum specimens from different age groups and from different locations. By IAHA, the acquisition of antibody to Norwalk virus and rotavirus was compared in infants and young children in the metropolitan Washington, D.C., area, young adults at the University of Maryland, and adults in the metropolitan Washington, D.C., area.[131] As shown in Fig. 3, the pattern of antibody acquisition differed markedly for these two viruses. There was a gradual acquisition of Norwalk antibody beginning slowly in childhood and accelerating in the adult period, so that by the 5th decade of life, 50% of the subjects possessed Norwalk antibody. In contrast, rotavirus antibody was acquired early in life so that by the 36th month of age over 90% had such antibody. The gradual acquisition of Norwalk antibody is similar to that observed with hepatitis A virus and certain rhinovirus serotypes in comparable populations.[107,250,251] This pattern of antibody acquisition in a major metropolitan area of a developed country suggests that Norwalk virus is not an important cause of gastroenteritis in infants and young children, but rather is associated most often with such illness in older persons. A comparison of the prevalence of IAHA Norwalk and rotavirus an-

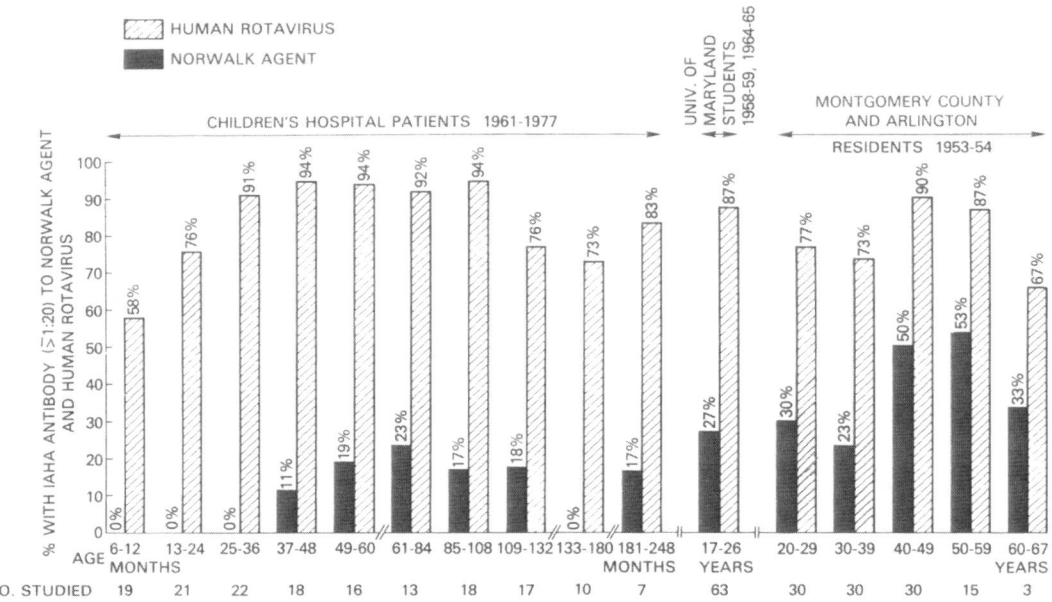

Fig. 3. Prevalence of antibody to Norwalk agent and rotavirus by IAHA in three groups. From Kapikian *et al.*[131]

tibody in a welfare institution for homeless but otherwise normal children yielded a pattern similar to that just described.[131] In a very limited study, IAHA antibody to Norwalk agent was also detected in infants, children, and adults in Bangladesh, but the Norwalk antibody prevalence was markedly less than that of rotavirus.[131]

The prevalence of Norwalk antibody was studied in subjects from various parts of the world with the RIA-blocking assay.[100] As shown in Fig. 4, the prevalence rates in adults in the United States and in certain European and less developed countries were similar, with at least a majority of subjects from each country possessing such antibody. An exception was a highly isolated Ecuadorian Indian tribe in Gabaro in which none of the adults studied had evidence of prior Norwalk infection. This was in marked contrast to three other less isolated Ecuadorian villages, where approximately 90% had Norwalk antibody. The prevalence of Norwalk antibody in adult male and female homosexuals in the United States was approximately equal (57 and 65%, respectively) and not appreciably different from adult blood donors in the United States studied by

RIA or from adults studied by IAHA as described above.[100]

Children from the United States and to a lesser extent Yugoslavia acquired antibody more slowly than did children from less well developed countries such as Ecuador and Bangladesh (Fig. 5).[100] The high antibody prevalence in the pediatric age group in Bangladesh and Ecuador was unexpected and indicates that the Norwalk or an antigenically related virus infects early in life in at least these parts of these less developed countries; its importance as an etiological agent of clinical gastroenteritis in this age group remains to be determined. Prevalence data are not available for the other members of the Norwalk group, since suitable serological assays have yet to be developed.

5.1.2. Epidemic Behavior. The Norwalk group of agents is associated with epidemic viral gastroenteritis that occurs in family, school, group, institutional, or community-wide outbreaks affecting adults, school-aged children, family contacts, and some young children as well. Although the term "winter vomiting disease" has been applied to certain outbreaks of epidemic viral gastroenteritis, a clear-cut

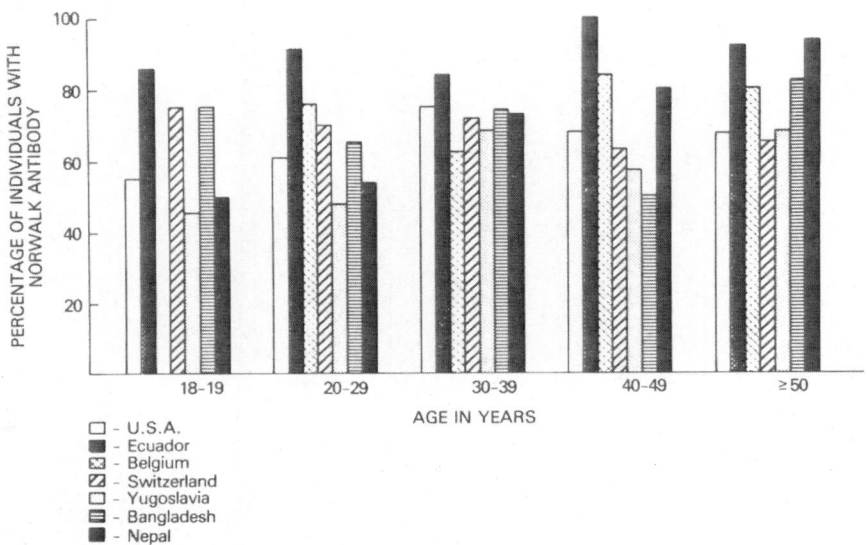

Fig. 4. Prevalence by age of serum antibody to Norwalk virus in healthy adults from various parts of the world..Note that no specimens were tested in the 18- to 19-year age group from Belgium. From Greenberg et al.[100]

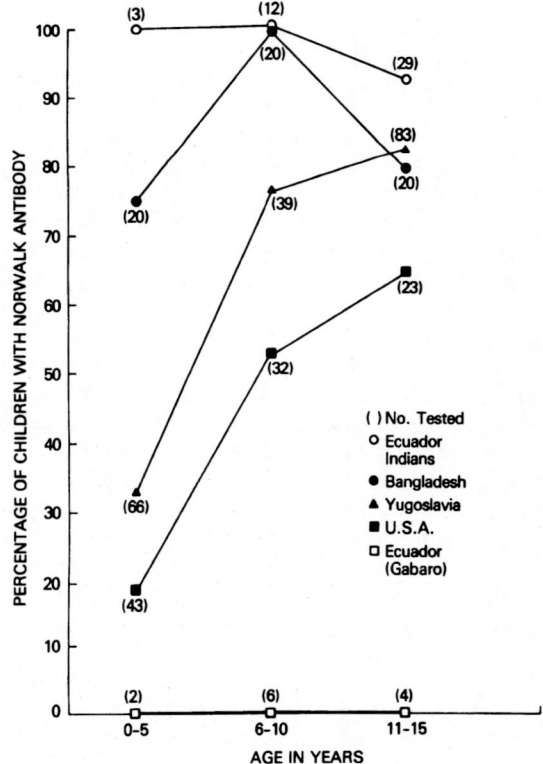

Fig. 5. Age-related prevalence of serum antibody to Norwalk virus in children from various countries. From Greenberg et al.[100]

seasonality does not appear to occur, at least for Norwalk virus-associated outbreaks.[2,101,102,302a]

A summary of several outbreaks of gastroenteritis associated with the Norwalk group of viruses (Table 4) indicates primary attack rates of 24–55% and secondary household attack rates of 11–32%. Some outbreaks have been brief, others extended over several months. The incubation period, where measured, was short, with an average of 48 hr in secondary cases in the Norwalk, Ohio, outbreak. The Hawaii and Montgomery County agents were obtained in family outbreaks.[256,282] A "cockle" agent derives its name from two outbreaks of gastroenteritis in England that occurred 24–30 hr after the ingestion of cockles.[11] In Australia, a large outbreak, in which a portion of the cases was associated with Norwalk agent, occurred in the winter months of June–July 1978 in over 2000 persons after ingestion of oysters.[102,105,189]

In a systematic study of selected paired sera from 23 outbreaks of nonbacterial gastroenteritis over a 12-year period employing the RIA-blocking assay, 6 outbreaks appeared related to Norwalk virus.[102] The outbreaks involved two cruise ships, two groups of college students (one affecting over 1000 students), a family, and a primary school in Japan in which over 100 students were ill with an attack rate of 40%. If the Norwalk, Hawaii, and Montgomery County family outbreaks studied by immune electron microscopy[135,256] are added to the 23 studied by RIA, then 8 of 26, or 31%, were Norwalk-virus-associated. Recent serological studies by RIA, including the 23 cited above, incriminated Norwalk agent in 24 of 70 outbreaks (34%).[102] Of the 24 outbreaks, 4 occurred in each of four settings: recreational camps, cruise ships, contaminated drinking or swimming water, and a community or family; 3 involved elementary or college students; 2, nursing homes; 1, shellfish; and 2 others, adults in other settings. The Norwalk-related outbreaks occurred in both the cooler and the warmer months. The association of such a high percentage of nonbacterial gastroenteritis outbreaks with a single member of this group of viruses was unexpected; however, it is thus possible that a majority might have a recognizable etiology when satisfactory serological as-

Table 4. Summary of Outbreaks of Norwalk Group Gastroenteritis

Agent	Group involved	Number at risk	Attack rate (%)	Dates of outbreak	Other information
Norwalk[2]	Students and teachers in elementary school, Norwalk, Ohio	232	50	Oct. 30–31, 1968	Incubation period 12–24 hr Secondary attack rate in families 32%; with an average incubation period 48 hr
"W"[50]	Students in boys' boarding school, England	830	24	Mar. 14–22, 1963	Only 1 teacher and kitchen staff ill. Attack rate: higher in younger boys than in older boys
Ditchling[9]	Students in primary school, Ditchling, England	138	24	Oct. 3–7, 1975	Related to "W" agent
Parramatta[48]	Students and teachers in primary school in Sydney, Australia	381	54	July 18–Aug. 18, 1977	9 of 18 teachers ill
Marin County[193]	Elderly residents and employees of convalescent home in Marin, California	187	51	Mar.–May, 1978	7% of employees also ill
Colorado (Snow Mountain)[185]	Persons at a resort camp in Colorado	760	55	Dec. 1976	Contaminated water supply suspected; secondary attack rate in households 11%

says are available for the other members or possible members of the Norwalk group of agents.

5.1.3. Geographic Distribution. Norwalk virus appears to have a worldwide distribution because antibody has been detected in populations in the United States, Belgium, Switzerland, Yugoslavia, Bangladesh, Nepal, Japan, Ecuador, Indonesia, and Australia.[100–102, 104,105,131] The only population studied that lacked detectable antibody was the very isolated Gabaro Ecuadorian Indians, who also lacked antibody to hepatis B virus (anti-HBc negative).[100] In contrast, they were found to have serum antibody to rotavirus, respiratory syncytial virus, and hepatitis A virus.[100]

5.1.4. Temporal Distribution. In developed countries, illness with the Norwalk group of agents was believed to occur predominantly in outbreaks during the cooler months of the year, from the fall through the spring seasons; however, recent studies have revealed that 9 of 24 Norwalk outbreaks occurred during the warmer months of the year.[102] The temporal distribution in tropical countries is not known.

5.1.5. Age. In developed countries, the Norwalk agents appear to induce illness in all age groups. During outbreaks, the peak incidence is observed in school-aged children and adults who are in close contact in various group settings.[102] However, close contact is not always essential, since outbreaks have occurred after ingestion of contaminated water or seafood.[11,102,105,185,189] In the United States, antibody-prevalence data indicate that the Norwalk virus is not an important cause of gastroenteritis in infants and young children,[131] nor has it played an important role in diarrheal illness of early life serious enough to require hospitalization.[33,131,133] Its overall importance in the developing countries is not known, but in parts of Bangladesh and Ecuador, Norwalk virus infection is common in infants and young children, suggesting that it may cause gastroenteritis in this age group.[100] Further studies are needed to answer this question.

5.1.6. Sex, Race, and Occupation. There is no evidence of differential susceptibility to this group of agents on the basis of sex, race, or occupation.

5.1.7. Occurrence in Different Settings. Illnesses associated with the Norwalk group of agents tend to occur in sharp outbreaks in families, schools, institutions, or communities and to affect adults, school-aged children, and family contacts, as well as some young children. Overall, this epidemic characteristic is one of the main epidemiological features that differentiates the Norwalk group from the rotaviruses, since the latter are characteristically associated with sporadic gastroenteritis of infants and young children and only infrequently affect older age groups.

5.1.8. Socioeconomic Status. In developed countries, there is no evidence of differential susceptibility to the Norwalk group on the basis of socioeconomic standing. However, the greater prevalence of Norwalk antibody in the pediatric age group in Bangladesh and in certain groups in Ecuador in comparison to that in developed countries may reflect a role of crowding or other socioeconomic factors in facilitating the spread of this agent.[100]

5.1.9. Other Factors. The influence of factors such as malnutrition on susceptibility to infection with the Norwalk group is not known. It has been suggested that genetic factors may play a role in determining susceptibility or resistance to infection with Norwalk virus.[197] These are discussed in greater detail in Section 7.1.3.

5.2. Rotaviruses

5.2.1. Incidence and Prevalence Data. Rotaviruses have emerged as the major etiological agents of serious diarrheal disease in infants and children under 2 years of age in practically all areas of the world where this disease has been studied etiologically. [68–70,73] The illness rate among family contacts of patients with rotavirus gastroenteritis is low, although subclinical infections in contacts occur frequently.[133,139,252,266] In the metropolitan Washington, D.C. area, the pattern of acquisition of rotavirus antibody contrasted sharply to that of the Norwalk agent.[131] By the end of the 3rd year of life, over 90% of infants and young children had acquired rotavirus antibody, a pattern similar to that observed for respiratory syncytial and parainfluenza 3 viruses.[131,138a,198] A high prevalence of antibody was maintained into adulthood, probably as a result of frequent reinfection with these agents. In other studies, the acquisition of rotavirus antibody has followed a similar pattern.[74,106,115,127,302] In the metropolitan Washington, D.C., area study, acquisition of antibody to both rotavirus serotypes followed a similar pattern, so that by the 3rd year of life, over 90% of infants and young children tested had antibody to type 1 and type 2 rotaviruses.[302]

In a cross-sectional study of patients admitted with a diarrheal illness to Children's Hospital National Medical Center in Washington, D.C., from January 1974 to June 1978, 39% of 604 patients shed rotavirus in a stool or rectal swab specimen (Fig. 7).[33] The major role of rotaviruses in diarrheal illnesses requiring hospitalization has also been observed in many other countries of the world, including Australia, Canada, England, and Japan.[37, 54,142,182,183] For example, in an Australian study that embraced a period of 1 year, 52% of 378 patients admitted with gastroenteritis shed rotavirus.[54] In a Japanese study that covered three peaks of rotavirus prevalance, December 1974 through March 1977, rotavirus was detected in stools of 320 (63%) of 506 infants and young children.[142] A characteristic temporal pattern of rotavirus infections has been observed in temperate climates and is discussed in Sections 5.2.2 and 5.2.4. In the Children's Hospital, Washington, D.C., study, each of the 313 rotavirus strains was subgrouped by ELISA: 238 (76%) were subgroup 2, and 75 (24%) were subgroup

1.[33,302] The greater frequency of subgroup 2 infections in hospitalized patients may indicate that serotypes in this subgroup have a greater pathogenic potential than those of subgroup 1. Further evidence to support this view was observed in a longitudinal study of Guatemalan infants and young children studied during the first 3 years of life. Each of 16 infections with a subgroup 2 virus was associated with diarrheal illness, whereas only 6 of 11 subgroup 1 infections were associated with such disease.[291] Sequential infections with human rotavirus have been documented in 9 infants and young children: 8 of the 9 shed a different subgroup virus during each of the sequential infections, and all but 1 of the 8 developed a diarrheal illness during the second infection, suggesting that infection with one subgroup does not protect against illness associated with the other subgroup.[302] Neutralization assays with specific serotypes within each subgroup are needed to clarify the implications of such sequential infections.

The relative role of rotaviruses and bacterial agents in the etiology of gastroenteritis was recently summarized for 6352 patients for a 1-year period, February 1978–January 1979, at the Matlab Treatment Center in Bangladesh.[22,102] This study showed

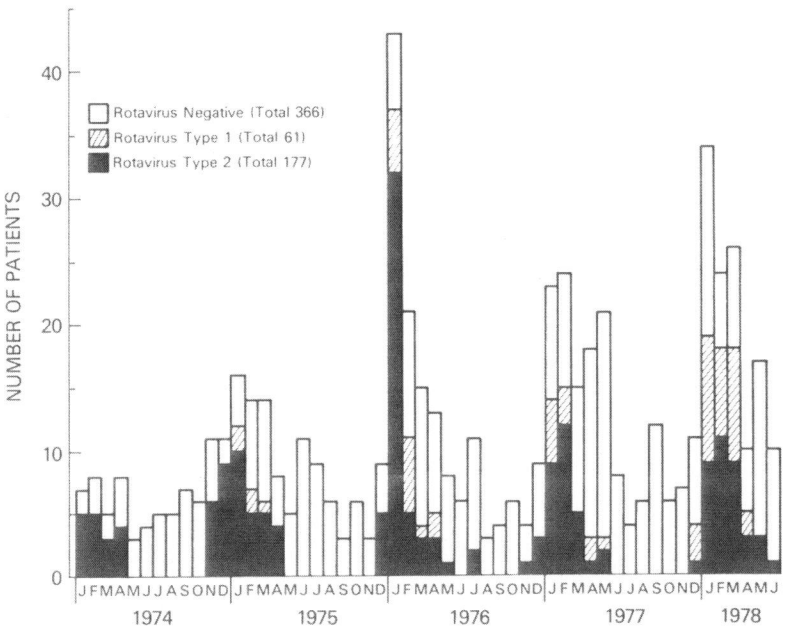

Fig. 6. Temporal distribution of rotavirus subgroup 1 and subgroup 2 infections in 604 infants and young children hospitalized with gastroenteritis at Children's Hospital National Medical Center, Washington, D.C., Jan. 1974(partial)–June 1978. From Brandt et al.[33]

that 46% of the patients under 2 years of age shed rotavirus and that 28% shed toxigenic *Escherichia coli.* In the 2-year-and-over age group, bacterial agents were detected more frequently than rotaviruses.

Although rotaviruses have been implicated during cross-sectional studies as a major cause of gastroenteritis necessitating hospitalization of infants and young children, rates of hospitalization were not available, since it was not possible to define accurately the population base from which the hospitalized patients had come. Recently, however, the incidence of hospitalization was estimated in the Washington, D.C., area.[214] Medical care for the population under study was provided by Group Health Association, Inc., and almost all pediatric hospitalizations of the group occurred at the Children's Hospital National Medical Center, which had an ongoing study of the etiology of gastroenteritis. Between January 1977 and March 1979, which included three periods of rotavirus prevalence, about 29,000 patients less than 15 years of age were under surveillance each year or part of a year. Of the 38 children hospitalized, 31 were under 2 years old. Of 30 studied microbiologically, 19 (63%) shed rotavirus, and 1 who did not, developed serological evidence of infection. From this analysis, it was calculated that 1 in 272 (3.7/1000) subjects less than 1 year of age and 1 in 451 (2.2/1000) 12–24 months of age were hospitalized for rotavirus gastroenteritis; this rate dropped precipitously in the 25- to 60-month age group (1 in 5519), and such illness was not observed after 5 years of age. In total, rotavirus infection was associated with 62% of the pediatric hospitalizations for gastroenteritis in this population over a 2¼-year period. Other agents played a minor role in comparison to the rotaviruses. In the 12- to 24-month age group, 1 of every 3.4 children on the average made an outpatient visit to the clinic for gastroenteritis during each year of the study, and in the less than 12-month age group, 1 of every 7.8 infants. The incidence declined sharply in the 25-month-to-15-year age group.[214] Longitudinal studies that are in progress should provide additional data, including the incidence of subclinical rotavirus infections that do not require a visit to a clinic.

An incidence of about 1.1 rotavirus diarrheal episodes per child during the first 3 years of life was estimated in a group of 24 infants and young children residing in the Guatemalan highland village of Santa Maria Cauque[291] on the basis of selected

ciated with bacterial and parasitic pathogens (about 42%) and those from whom stools were not available for study (about 5%). The true incidence may thus actually be greater than this estimate. It should be noted that specimens were not examined for enterotoxigenic *E. coli.*

5.2.2. Epidemic Behavior. Unlike the situation with the Norwalk group, true outbreaks of rotavirus gastroenteritis are rare. In the temperate climates, rotavirus infections have characteristically demonstrated a consistent temporal pattern similar to that observed in studies at Children's Hospital, Washington, D.C., during 1974–1978 (Fig. 6),[33,37,54,133,142,182] which was characterized by a large number of hospitalizations in infants and young children for gastroenteritis during the cooler months of each year.[33] Rotaviruses were also associated with milder bouts of gastroenteritis not requiring hospitalization. For example, in the Children's Hospital study 22% of 200 outpatients with gastroenteritis studied from November 1975 through June 1978 shed rotavirus. Community outbreaks of rotavirus illness occur rarely if at all, since most adults appear to be immune, most likely by virtue of previous rotavirus infection(s). However, subclinical rotavirus infections occur quite commonly in adults.[133,139,252,266] In one study, 22 (55%) of 40 adult contacts of patients hospitalized with gastroenteritis which was associated with rotavirus infection had serological evidence of rotavirus infection at or about the time of their child's admission, whereas only 4 (17%) of 24 control adults whose children also had gastroenteritis, but were not infected with rotavirus were found to be infected with this agent.[139] Only 3 of the 26 adult contacts with rotavirus infection gave a history of an associated gastrointestinal illness. It appears that older siblings or parents might be a source of rotavirus infection for young persons. The frequency of rotavirus infection in contacts also demonstrates the highly contagious nature of rotavirus infection.[71,139,252,266]

Although community outbreaks of rotavirus gastroenteritis are rare, one unusual outbreak involving not only children and mothers in a playgroup but also fathers and grandparents was recently described[216]: all 9 children 15 months through 5 years of age, 3 of 5 mothers who shared playgroup activities, 4 of 5 fathers, and each of 2 grandparents developed gastroenteritis. The incubation period was

24–48 hr. The index cases were most likely non-playgroup siblings who had been cared for (about 48 hr prior to the playgroup meeting) by the mother at whose home the playgroup met. The suspected index cases had gastroenteritis, the mother who took care of the index cases developed diarrhea 24 hr before the playgroup met, and her daughter had onset of diarrhea just before the playgroup met, and vomited during the playgroup meeting. In all, 18 of 21 persons developed gastroenteritis, and evidence of rotavirus infection was demonstrated in 10 of 11 persons tested for virus in stools or for a serological response, or for both. This unusual outbreak further attests to the contagiousness of rotavirus infection.

5.2.3. Geographic Distribution. Rotavirus infection has been detected in virtually all parts of the world. In developed countries where the etiology of gastroenteritis of infants and young children has been studied, rotaviruses have emerged as the major etiological agents of diarrheal illnesses severe enough to warrant hospitalization. In each locality, the pattern was similar to that described for Washington, D.C.[68–70,73] In less developed countries, such as Bangladesh and Guatemala, rotaviruses have been shown to be important etiological agents of severe diarrheal illness in infants and young children[111,157,220,291]; however, it appears that toxigenic *E. coli* also play an important role in underdeveloped countries such as Bangladesh where intensive etiological studies have been pursued.[22,67,102,149] Further studies must be carried out in the developing countries to determine the relative importance of the rotavirus and toxigenic *E. coli*. In practically every area of the world studied, rotaviruses have exhibited an important role in acute gastrointestinal disease of the young.

5.2.4. Temporal Distribution. In developed countries in the temperate climates, rotavirus infections display a characteristic temporal pattern that peaks in the cooler months of the year. The pattern for Washington, D.C., is shown in Fig. 6[5,33,37,54,133, 141,182]: during five Januarys, from 1974 (partial) through 1978, 87 (71%) of 123 patients admitted for diarrheal illness were found to be shedding rotavirus;[33] similarly, during three Januarys, from 1976 to 1978, 21 (62%) of 34 gastroenteritis outpatients were rotavirus-positive.[33] In Japanese studies, rotavirus was detected in stools of 288 (79%) of 365 hospitalized gastroenteritis patients during the cooler months (December to March) in a 28-month study.[142]

The reason for this striking seasonal pattern of infection is not known.

The pattern of infection with rotavirus strains belonging to subgroups 1 or 2 from 1974 to 1978 in the Children's Hospital, Washington, D.C., study is also shown in Fig. 6.[33] Viruses in subgroup 2 were first observed in January 1974 and during each succeeding yearly winter peak; 75% of the rotavirus strains detected over the 4½-year period belonged to subgroup 2. Strains belonging to subgroup 1 rotavirus were first observed in January 1975 and then detected yearly thereafter in December or January. Although this subgroup represented only about 25% of the 238 strains detected over the 4½-year period, a marked fluctuation in the temporal distribution of rotavirus subgroups was observed. For example, whereas subgroup 1 strains accounted for 14% of the total from October 1974 to September 1976, in the last epidemic year reported, subgroup 1 strains were identified in 31 (46%) of the 68 rotavirus-positive patients studied. Also, clustering of subgroups was observed in shorter periods within some of the seasons. The distribution of subgroups in gastroenteritis outpatients was similar to that observed for inpatients. The overall distribution of subgroups in populations in Guatemala, Costa Rica, Belgium, England, Australia, Asia, and Africa was also similar to that in the Washington, D.C., study in that rotavirus subgroup 2 strains predominated over subgroup 1 strains, ranging from a low of 62% (16 of 26) of the strains in Guatemala to a high of 100% in Costa Rica (10 of 10) and England (25 of 25).[302] It will be important to ascertain the pattern of infection of specific serotypes (as determined by neutralization) within each subgroup. Such studies have not been feasible until very recently because of the fastidious nature of rotaviruses.

The striking seasonal pattern of rotavirus infections described above is not observed in all situations, since a significant number of rotavirus infections has been observed throughout the year in South Africa, during the summer in Taiwan, during the "small rains" in Ethiopia, during most months in the tropical climates but with peak periods during the slightly cooler months, during the summer in a newborn nursery in England, and in all seasons in a newborn nursery in Australia.[14,66,111,157,160,188, 227,228,246,263,270] In both the nursery studies, most rotavirus-positive infants were symptom-free, a finding that has yet to be explained satisfactorily.

Studies of the frequency of rotavirus infections in relation to the amount of rainfall have led to variable results.[111,160,270]

5.2.5. Age. In studies from various parts of the world, infants and young children, characteristically from about 6 months to 2 years of age, experience the highest frequency of rotavirus gastroenteritis that requires hospitalization[33,37,54,142]; infants under 6 months of age have the next highest frequency. An unexplained paradox in the epidemiology of rotavirus infection is the low rate of clinical illness in neonates who shed rotavirus.[14,188,263] In one study, breast-fed infants shed rotavirus significantly less often than those who were not breast fed; however, the effect of breast feeding on illness could not be determined, since most of the rotavirus infections in both the breast-fed and bottle-fed neonates were subclinical.[263]

Rotavirus strains in subgroups 1 and 2 were found in the Children's Hospital (D.C.) study to have quite different patterns of infection in relation to age: the number of subgroup 1 infections declined with increasing age during the first year of life and was quite low thereafter, whereas the number of subgroup 2 infections peaked at 10–12 months and gradually declined thereafter.[33] The percentage of gastroenteritis patients who had infections with subgroup 1 viruses showed relatively little variation with increasing age, whereas the percentage with infections with subgroup 2 viruses increased steadily, with a peak at 13–15 months of age. The largest number of rotavirus infections with either subgroup 1 or subgroup 2 viruses was observed in the 10- to 12-month age group, and the group with the greatest percentage of rotavirus infections was 13–15 months of age. Rotavirus gastroenteritis has been reported in older children and adults, who, as noted earlier, may be important in the transmission of infection to infants and young children.[28–30,108,109,133, 139,176,195,266,305]

5.2.6. Sex. A somewhat larger number of males (335) than females (269) (M/F = 1.2) was hospitalized for gastroenteritis, irrespective of age, in the Children's Hospital of Washington, D.C., study.[33] This was also reflected in the number of males or females positive for each of the rotavirus serotypes, but this difference was not striking.[33] A higher frequency of hospitalization of males for acute gastroenteritis was also observed in a Canadian study.[183]

5.2.7. Race and Socioeconomic Status. In the Children's Hospital study, 1974–1978, the age distribution of patients admitted to the hospital for gastroenteritis of any etiology was quite different among black and nonblack patients: 59% of all black patients admitted for gastroenteritis were less than 6 months of age.[33] This difference was reflected in hospitalizations for gastroenteritis associated with either subgroup 1 or subgroup 2 rotavirus, since black patients were about 6 months younger than nonblacks with respect to each subgroup. The median age of black vs. nonblack patients for rotavirus subgroup 1 was 5 months vs. 11.5 months; for subgroup 2 rotavirus, it was 8 months vs. 14 months. Also, D.C. residents and Medicaid recipients who were hospitalized with rotavirus infection tended to be younger than non-D.C. residents and non-Medicaid recipients. In addition, there was a tendency for rotavirus illness to occur earlier in the course of the outbreak in blacks and in D.C. residents. Transmission of rotavirus might be facilitated by crowding and poor sanitation, and this may explain the earlier appearance of rotavirus infection in D.C. when compared to the suburbs, in blacks as compared to nonblacks, and in Medicaid recipients as compared to non-Medicaid recipients.[33]

Malnutrition is probably an important factor in increasing the susceptibility of an infant or young child to develop severe clinical manifestations following rotavirus infection. In addition, it has been suggested that repeated diarrheal infections may be a prelude to the development of malnutrition by various mechanisms including damage to the intestinal mucosa so that absorptive cells are compromised over an extended period.[161]

5.2.8. Occurrence in Different Settings. Rotavirus gastroenteritis occurs predominantly in infants and young children; rotavirus infection has been observed by the 36th month of age in almost all children studied who were residing in a family setting.[26,74,106,131] Family contacts are also frequently infected with rotavirus, but usually subclinically.[133,139,252,266] Rotavirus infections have also been observed for extended periods in newborn nurseries as described above.[5,14,263] In addition, nosocomial rotavirus infections occur commonly.[183,219] In one study, 10 (17%) of the 60 children admitted to the hospital without diarrhea (but during a period of rotavirus prevalence) developed diarrheal illness associated with rotavirus infection while hospitalized.[219] In another hospital study, over a 1-year period, about 1 of every 5 rotavirus infections appeared to be hospital-acquired.[183] Outbreaks of rotavirus gastroenteritis have been observed in school-aged children, in a home playgroup setting, and in a military group, but characteristically, rotavirus illness occurs sporadically and not in widespread community outbreaks as does the Norwalk group of agents.[29,30,108,109,176,216] Thus, rotavirus illness is not common beyond the first few years of life.

6. Mechanisms and Route of Transmission

6.1. Norwalk Group of Viruses

Infection with the Norwalk group of agents is most likely spread from person to person by the fecal–oral route. Volunteer studies have established that the Norwalk, Hawaii, "W," and Colorado agents can be transmitted via the oral route, i.e., following the ingestion of stool material containing the infectious agent.[60,61,150,185,282] It is unlikely that this group of agents is transmitted by the respiratory route. In one study, nasopharyngeal washings from a volunteer acutely ill with experimentally induced Norwalk illness failed to induce illness in three volunteers.[60] Recently, Norwalk virus has been detected in vomitus from certain infected volunteers.[103]

The explosive nature of some of these outbreaks in which large numbers of people develop illness in a cluster within 24–48 hr has suggested that a common-source exposure should also be considered in certain outbreaks. Indeed, in the Colorado outbreak, 61% of the 418 cases had onset of illness on a single day.[185] Epidemiological analysis revealed that the attack rate increased with consumption of water or ice-containing beverages and that the water supply of the camp was not only inadequately chlorinated but also contaminated by a leaking septic tank; it was thus suggested that a waterborne agent was responsible for the outbreak. In the Norwalk, Ohio, outbreak, 50% of the students and teachers of an elementary school developed gastroenteritis; it was striking that such illnesses occurred during a 2-day period.[2] Although a com-

mon-source exposure was sought, none could be established. However, secondary cases among family contacts were observed, and the Norwalk particle was derived from a rectal swab of one such secondary case. Ingestion of contaminated seafood such as cockles (cockle agent) and oysters (Norwalk agent) has also been described as a mode of transmission of this group of agents.[11,72,105,189] In addition, outbreaks of Norwalk gastroenteritis have now been associated with ingestion of contaminated drinking water and with swimming in a contaminated lake.[43,44,102]

6.2. Rotaviruses

Rotaviruses are also transmitted by the fecal–oral route. Volunteer studies have clearly demonstrated that oral administration of rotavirus-positive stool material can induce a diarrheal illness.[124] The rapid acquisition of rotavirus antibody in the first few years of life in all populations studied has led to the suggestion that rotaviruses might also be transmitted by the respiratory route.[26,74,106,115,127,131] No experimental evidence for this exists. Throat gargles obtained from volunteers with an experimentally induced rotavirus diarrheal illness failed to yield rotavirus.[124] Although the possibility of common-source exposure to rotavirus, such as a contaminated water supply, has been suggested, it is unlikely that such exposure plays an important role in its transmission.

The source of infection for the young infant who is not normally in contact with other infants and young children with gastroenteritis is not known with certainty. However, a substantial proportion of parents of rotavirus-infected infants and young children were infected with rotavirus at or about the time of their child's illness; most of these adult infections were subclinical.[133,139,252,266] Thus, an older sibling or family member who is undergoing subclinical rotavirus infection may be the source of infection for the infant or young child with whom he has contact. The highly contagious nature of rotavirus infection may be due in part to the rotavirus' high degree of stability, as demonstrated by the retention of infectivity of calf rotavirus-positive feces that had been kept at room temperature for 7 months.[84] It is likely that human rotavirus is also quite stable and may remain viable in the environment unless destroyed by careful disinfection. The persistence of rotavirus infections in certain newborn nurseries and the high frequency of nosocomial rotavirus infection in hospitals provide additional evidence for this possibility. Effective disinfection of contaminated material and care in hand-washing may be important measures in containing rotavirus infection, especially in a hospital setting.[139,219]

The role, if any, of animals in transmitting rotaviruses to humans is not known. Although rotaviruses are established causes of diarrhea in newborn animals of many species, there is no evidence of transmission of an animal rotavirus to humans. On the other hand, human rotavirus has been shown to induce a diarrheal illness in various newborn animals under experimental conditions.[118,147,148,173, 181,184,237,261,262,290] It appears unlikely, however, that even if animal-to-human transmission of rotavirus could be documented, such transmission would account for an appreciable number of infections.

7. Pathogenesis and Immunity

7.1. Norwalk Group of Viruses

7.1.1. Incubation Period. From studies of outbreaks associated with this group of agents, the incubation period is estimated to be 24–48 hr.[2,9,11,185] The incubation period in volunteer studies with the Norwalk agent ranged from 10 to 51 hr, and the illness usually lasted less than 48 hr.[25,60,61,282] Norwalk virus shedding as determined by immune electron microscopy coincided with the onset of illness and usually could not be detected after 72 hr following onset.[255]

7.1.2. Pathogenesis. The pathogenesis of Norwalk- and Hawaii-induced illness studied in volunteers by light microscopy of biopsies of the proximal small intestine has characteristically revealed broadening and blunting of villi, with mucosa itself being intact histologically; mononuclear cell infiltration and cytoplasmic vacuolization were also observed.[4,62,229,230] Transmission electron microscopy of the proximal small intestine showed intact epithelial cells with shortening of microvilli.[4,62,229,230] The extent of the small-intestinal involvement is not known, since studies have included only the proximal small intestine. Histological lesions were not observed in the gastric fundus and antrum or the colonic mucosa of normal volunteers challenged with the Norwalk agent.[273] Brush-border small-intestinal enzyme levels (including alkaline phosphatase, sucrase, and trehalase) were decreased during illness; adenylate cyclase activity was not elevated.[4,81,150,222] Recently, it was found that volunteers with Norwalk-induced gastroenteritis or the characteristic small-intestinal pathological changes, or both, experienced marked delays in gastric emptying.[175]

7.1.3. Immunity. Volunteer studies with the Norwalk agent have raised rather perplexing questions about the mechanism of immunity to the Norwalk agent. It appears that two forms of clinical immunity to Norwalk-virus-induced illness exist—one with a short-term and the other with a long-term immunity.[60,197,282] The former seems to be serotype-specific. For example, volunteers who become ill following administration of Norwalk virus are characteristically resistant to challenge with this virus 6–14 weeks later. In contrast, they are not resistant to challenge with the Hawaii virus, nor are Hawaii-virus-infected volunteers later resistant to challenge with Norwalk virus.[60,282]

The situation with regard to long-term immunity is different, as indicated when 12 volunteers were challenged with the Norwalk agent on two separate occasions 27–42 months apart[197] and 4 were rechallenged again 4–8 weeks after the second challenge. Of these 12 volunteers, 6 developed illness following challenge and again after rechallenge 27–42 months later. In contrast, 6 of the other volunteers failed to become ill after initial challenge or after rechallenge 31–34 months later. Of the 6 volunteers who developed illness after each of the two sequential challenges, 4 were inoculated a third time with the same inoculum, but only 1 became ill. Serological studies carried out to clarify this unusual pattern of susceptibility and resistance to Norwalk virus failed to reveal a consistent relationship between the presence or absence of antibody and the subsequent occurrence of illness following challenge. Thus, it seems that serum antibody is not a critical factor in immunity to Norwalk gastroenteritis. It is also difficult to explain these findings on the grounds that local intestinal IgA antibody is of prime importance in long-term resistance, since this supposes the existence of two cohorts of subjects, one able and the other unable to sustain the production of local antibody essential for long-term resistance. It has been suggested that other factors that are genetically determined may influence susceptibility to Norwalk infection. For example, there may be a genetically determined specific receptor essential for entry of the Norwalk virus into epithelial cells of the small intestine.[197]

Further evidence for the possible role of nonimmunological factors in resistance to Norwalk illness was observed when the prechallenge serum and local jejunal antibody levels in 23 volunteers were studied by the radioimmunoassay (RIA)-blocking technique.[102] Neither the geometric mean Norwalk antibody titer in serum nor that in jejunal fluid correlated with resistance to illness after challenge. Paradoxically, the prechallenge geometric mean Norwalk antibody titer of jejunal fluid was significantly greater, and such antibody titer of serum tended to be greater in volunteers who became ill after challenge than in those who did not become ill.[102] A similar paradoxical relationship between prechallenge serum antibody titer and lack of resistance to Norwalk illness in volunteers was reported in another study in which antibody was measured also by RIA.[23]

7.2. Rotaviruses

7.2.1. Incubation Period.
From clinical studies, rotavirus diarrheal illness has been estimated as having an incubation period of less than 48 hr.[54] In volunteer studies in which four adults developed a diarrheal illness after oral administration of an untitered stool filtrate containing rotavirus, the incubation period ranged from 2 to 4 days. Virus shedding began the 2nd, 3rd, or 4th day after inoculation and lasted a total of at least 6 days.[124]

7.2.2. Pathogenesis.
Limited studies of biopsies from the proximal small intestine of a few infants and children hospitalized with rotavirus infections have shown shortening of the villi, mononuclear-cell infiltration in the lamina propria, distended cisternae of the endoplasmic reticulum, mitochondrial swelling, and sparse, irregular microvilli.[114,248] Impaired D-xylose absorption was also observed.[166] In addition, some patients had depressed disaccharidase levels (maltase, sucrase, and lactase).[21]

The pathogenesis of human rotavirus D strain, a subgroup 2 virus, infection was studied experimentally in newborn gnotobiotic colostrum-deprived calves that developed illness following intraduodenal administration of this virus.[172] Morphological changes in the small intestine proceeded in a cephalocaudad direction: within $\frac{1}{2}$ hr of experimentally-induced diarrhea, morphological changes such as denuding of villi and flattening of epithelial cells were observed in the upper small intestine, but rotavirus antigens were not detected by immunofluorescence [fluorescent-antibody (FA) test]; at this time, the lower small intestine was intact, but abundant rotaviral antigens were observed by FA test in swollen epithelial cells. Moreover, 7 hr after onset of diarrhea, the lower small intestine demonstrated morphological changes such as denuded villi that were similar to those observed in the upper small intestine earlier; rotaviral antigens could not be detected by FA test. The intestine appeared relatively normal 48 hr after onset of diarrhea. When diarrhea was induced in piglets by human rotavirus, certain functional alterations were observed in the villous epithelial cells of the small intestine: glucose-coupled Na^+ transport was impaired, sucrase activity diminished, and thymidine kinase activity increased. In contrast, adenylate cyclase and cyclic AMP were not stimulated.[55,93]

7.2.3. Immunity.
Epidemiological observations, as well as experimental studies in animals and humans, have helped in understanding certain mechanisms involved in rotavirus immunity.[34,124,148,171, 237,239,279] The observation was made that newborn calves frequently develop rotavirus diarrhea despite a high level of circulating rotavirus antibody acquired from ingestion of colostrum.[279] This was confirmed experimentally in calves challenged with calf rotavirus, and additionally it was shown that antibody in the lumen of the small intestine was of prime importance in protection.[34,279]

A similar study in gnotobiotic lambs also examined the relative role of local and systemic rotavirus antibody by evaluating the clinical response of two groups of lambs to challenge with lamb rotavirus.[237,238,239] From these and other studies in animals, it appears that antibody in the lumen of the intestine was of prime importance in resistance to rotavirus illness in animals.[148,179]

The mechanism of immunity was also studied in 18 volunteers who were administered a human rotavirus by the oral route.[124] Of these 18, 5 shed rotavirus, and 4 of these 5 developed a diarrheal illness. Examination of the relationship of prechallenge rotavirus antibody measured by immunofluorescence (IF), neutralization (to bovine rotavirus), complement-fixation, and to the development of diarrheal illness revealed that the absence of IF antibody was significantly associated with the development of illness, whereas a similar trend was observed with antibodies measured by other assays. The role of local intestinal rotavirus antibody needs further evaluation. Two volunteers who developed illness following initial challenge were rechallenged with the same inoculum 19 months later; neither developed a diarrheal illness, although one had mild clinical manifestations.

Reinfections with rotavirus occur commonly in adult contacts of patients with rotavirus illness; however, most of these reinfections are subclinical.[133,139,252,266] Whether those that are manifested clinically are the result of a low level or absence of local intestinal rotavirus IgA antibody is not known. Sequential rotavirus illnesses have been observed in infants and young children.[90,215,291,302] However, such sequential illnesses have thus far been associated with strains belonging to different subgroups, suggesting that immunity does develop. The duration of such immunity, however, is not known. However, neutralization assays with specific serotypes within each subgroup are needed to clarify immune mechanisms in rotavirus infections.

One of the perplexing areas in the study of rotavirus epidemiology has been the unexplained relative sparing of neonates from rotavirus illness despite frequent infection in this age group.[5,14,263] In one study of newborn babies, rotavirus infections occurred significantly less often in breast-fed infants than in bottle-fed infants. The effect of breast feeding on illness could not be determined, since most of the infections in the breast-fed and bottle-fed infants were subclinical.[14,263] Whether high levels of circulating rotavirus antibody acquired transplacentally play a role in resistance to disease during early life is not known. However, rotavirus illnesses are observed with moderate frequency in infants less than 6 months of age but beyond the neonatal period, a time when passively acquired circulating antibody is still present but not at as high a level as in neonates.[33,133]

8. Patterns of Host Response

8.1. Norwalk Group of Viruses

8.1.1. Clinical Features. Clinical features observed in the original Norwalk outbreak from which the Norwalk particle was derived are characteristic of those observed with this group of agents. Of the 604 subjects tabulated as primary or secondary cases, 85% had nausea, 84% vomiting, 62% abdominal cramps, 57% lethargy, 44% diarrhea, 32% fever, and 5% chills.[2] The duration of clinical manifestations was 12–24 hr; none of the affected subjects was hospitalized. These clinical findings are similar but not identical to those observed in a report describing 31 of 52 volunteers who developed definite or probable illness following administration of the Norwalk agent.[282] Of the 31 volunteers, 45% had fever (≥ 99.4°F), 81% diarrhea, 65% vomiting, 68% abdominal discomfort, 90% anorexia, 81% headache, and 58% myalgias; clinical manifestations usually lasted 24–48 hr. The diarrheal stools characteristically do not contain gross blood, mucus, or white blood cells.[59] Of 16 volunteers who became ill following Norwalk- or Hawaii-agent challenge, 14 developed a transient lymphopenia.[63] The illness observed in volunteers was generally mild and self-limited, although one volunteer who vomited about 20 times within a 24-hr period required parenteral fluids.[25,60,61,282] A graphic summary of signs and symptoms of illness observed in two volunteers who developed illness following administration of the Norwalk agent is shown in Fig. 7.[61] The difference in clinical manifestations in these two volunteers who received the same inoculum is striking, since one vomited but did not have diarrhea and the other developed diarrhea but not vomiting. Shedding of Norwalk virus by volunteers as determined by immune electron microscopy (IEM) was maximal around the onset of illness and was rarely detected after 3 days following onset.[255] A valid estimate of the ratio of subclinical to clinical Norwalk infections has not been made. However, serologically proven infection without definite gastroenteric illness has been observed.[123,245]

8.1.2. Diagnosis. A specific diagnosis of infection with the Norwalk group is not possible on the basis of a patient's clinical manifestations. Thus, since this group of agents does not grow in cell culture or produce disease in an experimental ani-

Fig. 7. Response of two volunteers to oral administration of stool filtrate derived from a volunteer who received original Norwalk rectal-swab specimen. The height of the curve is directly proportional to the severity of the sign or symptom. Volunteer 1 had severe vomiting without diarrhea, while volunteer 2 had diarrhea without vomiting, although both received the same inoculum. From Dolin et al.[61]

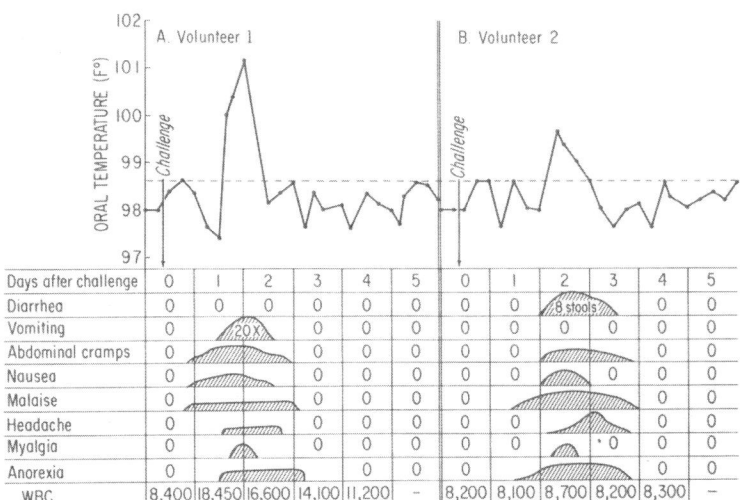

Days after challenge	0	1	2	3	4	5	0	1	2	3	4	5
Diarrhea	0	0	0	0	0	0	0	0	8 stools	0	0	
Vomiting	0	20X	0	0	0	0	0	0	0	0	0	
Abdominal cramps	0			0	0	0	0	0		0	0	
Nausea	0			0	0	0	0	0		0	0	
Malaise	0			0	0	0	0			0	0	
Headache	0			0	0	0	0	0		0	0	
Myalgia	0		0	0	0	0	0	0	• 0	0	0	
Anorexia	0			0	0	0	0			0	0	
WBC	8,400	8,450	16,600	14,100	11,200	–	8,200	8,100	8,700	8,200	8,300	–

mal, diagnosis of infection remains essentially a research procedure. For virus detection and identification, IEM remains the mainstay procedure for the group as a whole[128,129,135,136]; however, for the Norwalk virus, a recently developed radioimmunoassay (RIA) has been shown to be even more sensitive than IEM for detection of Norwalk antigen in clinical specimens.[99,104] Direct EM examination of negatively stained stool material with or without prior concentration may also be attempted.[32] Although EM examination of stools is a simple and relatively rapid procedure, caution must be used in interpreting the significance of "particles" visualized, since stools contain a myriad of small objects that have no relationship to the illness being studied.[128] It is for this reason that carefully controlled IEM studies with appropriate paired sera should be carried out under code to determine the significance of the particles observed. Ideally, a patient's paired sera should show an IEM antibody increase with the particle that has been visualized being used as the antigen (see Fig. 2); in addition, if paired sera are not available, careful IEM studies with γ-globulin, paired sera from other subjects in the same outbreak or from other outbreaks, or antisera to morphologically similar agents should be studied to determine the significance of the particle in question. Simple aggregation of particles by a serum should not be taken as evidence of a specific response, since certain particles, such as Norwalk, demonstrate aggregation without the addition of serum. These nonspecific aggregates may appear to be coated with a small or moderate amount of antibody. Thus, it is essential to determine the amount of antibody coating the particles even if they are aggregated. If there is any question about the significance of aggregation, the concentration of antigen or antibody may be varied. Such maneuvers should affect both the size of the aggregates and the amount of antibody coating the particles as the reaction proceeds from antigen excess to antibody excess.[128,136] Awareness of specificity of aggregation is essential, since certain stools contain groups of 22-nm particles that characteristically appear in "aggregate" form with little or no "antibody" on them and that have had no known relationship to the illness being studied.[128,136] These aggregates generally appear similar with paired acute or convalescent sera. IEM remains the only method for detecting serological evidence of infection for other members of the group not antigenically related to the Norwalk virus. Serological diagnosis of Norwalk infection can of course be made by IEM, but recently a practical RIA-blocking test has been developed for this agent.[23,104] The development of an RIA-blocking test has permitted the study of a large number of serum specimens from outbreaks in different localities and thus paved the way to an understanding of the epidemiology of this virus.[102,104] An immune adherence hemagglutination assay has also proved useful for detecting serological evidence of Norwalk infection, but it is not quite as sensitive as RIA and also uses larger amounts of antigen.[131] Although practical, these assays are limited to use in research laboratories, since reagents are not generally available.

8.2. Rotaviruses

8.2.1. Clinical Features. Clinical characterization of rotavirus illness in infants and young children has been heavily weighted toward disease severe enough to warrant hospitalization. The three major clinical manifestations observed in rotavirus gastroenteritis in such studies are vomiting, diarrhea, and dehydration. A comparison was made of signs and symptoms observed in 72 patients hospitalized with a diarrheal illness associated with rotavirus and 78 patients hospitalized with a diarrheal illness that could not be associated with rotavirus[213] (Table 5). The rotavirus group experienced both vomiting and

dehydration significantly more often then the nonrotavirus group. The dehydration was isotonic in 95% of the patients in the rotavirus group and in 77% of the rotavirus-negative group. As determined from history and hospital records, the mean duration of vomiting was also longer in the rotavirus than in the nonrotavirus group (2.6 vs. 0.9 days). Diarrhea began later but lasted longer than vomiting in the rotavirus group (mean duration 5 days vs. 2.6 days). Once the patient was hospitalized, diarrhea continued for an average of 2.6 days (range 1–9 days) in the rotavirus group and 3.8 days (range 1–16 days) in the nonrotavirus group. The duration of hospitalization ranged from 2 to 14 days (mean 4 days) for the rotavirus group. The greatest frequency of rotavirus diarrhea was in the 6- to 24-month age group.

Notable laboratory findings were related to the degree of dehydration.[213] Elevated BUN (>18 mg/dl) and urine specific gravity (>1.025) were observed in 58 and 71%, respectively, of the rotavirus group, frequencies significantly greater than those observed in the nonrotavirus group.

Table 5. Clinical Characteristics of 150 Children Hospitalized with Acute Gastroenteritis[a]

	Percentage having each clinical finding	
Clinical finding	Rotavirus infection detected (72 patients)	Rotavirus infection not detected (78 patients)
Vomiting	96[b]	58[b]
Fever (°C)		
37.9–39	46	29
>39	31	33
Total	77	61
Dehydration	83[c]	40[c]
Hypertonic	5	16
Isotonic	95	77
Hypotonic	0	6
Irritability	47	40
Lethargy	36	27
Pharyngeal erythema	49	32
Tonsillar exudate	3	3
Rhinitis	26	22
Red tympanic membrane with loss of landmarks	19	9
Rhonchi or wheezing	8	8
Palpable cervical lymph nodes	18	9

[a] From Rodriguez et al.[213] with minor changes.   [b] $p < 0.01$.   [c] $p < 0.01$.

Deaths have been reported in infants and young children with rotavirus infection.[40,54,177,178,182,183] In a Canadian study, 21 deaths were reported in infants and young children with rotavirus infection from May 1972 to March 1977. Of these 21 children, 10 were dead on arrival at the hospital, while 10 were moribund and could not be successfully resuscitated on arrival.[40] One child was already in the hospital when he acquired the disease; this patient had congestive cardiomyopathy that contributed to his death. All except this patient and one other had been healthy previously. The patients with fatal disease ranged in age from 4 to 30 months, with a mean of 11 months. The deaths occured 1–3 days after onset of symptoms. The major factor causing death was believed to be dehydration and electrolyte imbalance in 16 cases, aspiration of vomitus in 3 cases, and in the remaining 2, seizures were a contributing factor. It is striking that the parents of 16 of the 20 children brought to the hospital moribund or already dead had had some contact with a physician during the course of the illness.[40]

Rotavirus infection has also been observed in pediatric patients with intussusception and with self-limited gastrointestinal bleeding.[57,143] One of the patients in the latter group had clinical findings compatible with Henoch–Schoenlein purpura. One patient with rotavirus gastroenteritis was observed to develop a fatal Reye's syndrome with severe CNS manifestations.[223] Another patient with rotavirus gastroenteritis developed encephalitis with severe CNS manifestations and was making a slow recovery.[223] Hemolytic uremic syndrome or disseminated intravascular coagulation have been reported in several children with rotavirus infection[207]; one child with rotavirus gastroenteritis developed severe neurological sequelae after marked dehydration and intravascular coagulation.[183] Elevated serum transaminases have also been reported in patients with rotavirus-associated gastroenteritis.[64,252] The relationship or frequency, or both, of rotavirus infection with these unusual clinical manifestations should be clarified in future studies. Growth of rotavirus has also been described in tissue cultures inoculated with filtrates prepared from intestinal tissue of patients with Crohn's disease, but this observation could not be confirmed.[125,272]

In the volunteer studies in which the D strain, a subgroup 2 human rotavirus was administered orally to volunteers, four developed a diarrheal illness that began 2–4 days after inoculation.[124] Two of the four volunteers with diarrhea also vomited, one the day after inoculation (2 days before the onset of diarrhea) and the other 3 days after inoculation (the day of onset of diarrhea). Average duration of diarrhea was 2.5 days, with a range of 1–4 days. The number of diarrheal stools per illness ranged from 1 to 24 stools, with one volunteer having a maximum of 11 in one day. Thus, under experimental as well as natural conditions, adults can develop a rotaviral diarrheal illness. However, subclinical rotavirus infection in adults appears to be much more common, as demonstrated in one study in which 22 of 50 family contacts of pediatric patients hospitalized with rotavirus gastroenteritis themselves developed serological evidence of rotavirus infection at or about the time of their children's hospitalization[139]; however, only 3 infected parents had a gastroenteric illness at or about the time of their children's illnesses.

8.2.2. Diagnosis. As with the Norwalk group, specific diagnosis of infection with human rotavirus is not possible on the basis of clinical manifestations. Even though rotavirus infection follows a predictable seasonal pattern of recurrent high prevalence during the "winter" or cooler months in temperate climates, a laboratory diagnosis is essential, since other agents may also cause gastroenteritis even during peak rotavirus periods.

The human rotaviruses do not grow readily in tissue culture or in conventional laboratory animal models.[286] However, numerous assays have been developed for the detection of rotaviruses, as outlined previously in Table 1. The most widely applied methods are able to detect rotavirus in stool specimens by direct visualization or by immunological assay ("direct virology").[136] EM has the distinct advantage of being highly specific, since the rotavirus has such a characteristic morphological appearance; it is limited, however, by the requirement for an electron microscope as well as a capable operator. EM is the most rapid method of diagnosis when dealing with only a few specimens. Other efficient but more practical assays for large numbers of specimens include counterimmunoelectroosmophoresis, RIA, and enzyme-linked immunosorbent assay (ELISA). The ELISA is probably the most practical diagnostic method for large-scale studies and is limited only by the availability of suitable reagents. False-positive reactions may occur, and the laboratory should be able to confirm all positive samples by appropriate methods. Thus, there are several efficient and practical methods for detecting rotaviruses; the method of choice will vary according to the resources and experience of individual laboratories.

Serological evidence of rotavirus infection may be detected by a variety of techniques (see Table 2). Complement fixation is efficient and practical when testing sera from pediatric patients about 6–24 months of age.[136,298] However, it is not as efficient as certain other techniques when testing sera from patients less than 6 months of age and from adults.[298] Serological evidence of rotavirus infection may be detected in these age groups by ELISA or immunofluorescence. ELISA has also been employed to measure specific immunoglobulin responses in rotavirus infection.[301] As long as the limitations of the various methods are recognized, the method of choice will vary according to the resources and experience of individual laboratories.

9. Control and Prevention

9.1. Norwalk Group of Viruses

There are no methods available for the prevention or control of infection or illness with the Norwalk group of agents. Since this group of agents is highly contagious and transmitted by the fecal–oral (or vomitus–oral) route, it is possible that in a family or group setting where one member is ill with this form of gastroenteritis, effective hand-washing and disposal or disinfection of contaminated material could decrease the likelihood of transmission. Increased vigilance concerning the purity of drinking water or of water in swimming pools might also limit the number of outbreaks due to these agents.

Treatment of gastroenteritis caused by the Norwalk group characteristically consists of replacement of fluid loss by the administration of liquids orally. Parenteral intravenous fluid therapy is only rarely necessary in this form of generally self-limited gastroenteritis.[59–61] The impact of this group of agents in debilitated hosts has not been evaluated extensively. In addition, it should be noted that recent volunteer studies with the Norwalk agent revealed that oral administration of bismuth subsalicylate after onset of symptoms significantly reduced

the severity and duration of abdominal cramps and the median duration of gastrointestinal symptoms. This treatment did not significantly affect the number, weight, or water content of stools.[245]

Neither the need for the development of a vaccine for this group nor the techniques required for such a vaccine (such as propagation of these agents in cell culture) have been established. For example, the number of serotypes in this group and their overall importance in epidemic gastroenteritis must be understood before immunoprophylaxis can be considered. Furthermore, the unusual aspects of Norwalk virus immunity require more precise definition. This represents a clear priority in view of the apparent nonimmunological basis for long-term immunity. Thus, it is premature to consider immunoprophylaxis for the Norwalk group of agents.

9.2. Rotaviruses

In both the developed and developing countries, rotaviruses represent a major cause of severe diarrhea of infants and young children. Thus, it is clear that a rotavirus vaccine is needed. Although diarrheal illnesses are not a major cause of mortality in the developed countries, such illnesses are the leading cause of death in infants and young children in many developing countries. The role of rotaviruses in the estimated 5–10 million fatal diarrheal illnesses that occur in developing countries each year[271] has not been established, although their major importance in the etiology of severe gastroenteritis in these populations is now well documented. Moreover, rotaviruses are known to cause a severe dehydrating diarrheal illness, and such illness if untreated can be fatal. Indeed, in a Canadian study, 21 deaths associated with rotavirus gastroenteritis were observed.[40] All but one of the fatalities occurred in infants and young children who died on the way to the hospital or in the emergency clinic at the time of hospitalization. Although rotavirus infections can be fatal, it is not known what the impact of an effective rotavirus vaccine would be on the staggering death toll from diarrheal disease in the developing countries. Recently, it has been suggested that enterotoxigenic *E. coli* may be a more important cause of death from diarrhea in developing countries than rotavirus.[67,149] For example, in the United States in New York City in the early 1900s, these authors note that there was a staggering infant mortality rate with a large proportion of deaths attributable to outbreaks of summer diarrhea in slum tenements.[149] The infant death rate declined markedly in the next decades, and it has been suggested that this decline was not because of better medical management of summer diarrhea, but rather was the result of development of improved sanitary conditions such as iceboxes, flush toilets, and water supply, which limited bacterial contamination.[149] Indeed, despite the advanced sanitary conditions and high standards of living in the United States today, almost all persons still undergo rotavirus infection by the end of the 3rd year of life, though mortality from diarrheal illnesses is infrequent in the United States. Decline in mortality from diarrheal diseases in developed countries is due in part to the availability of fluid replacement therapy and possibly better nutrition, but undoubtedly other factors have played a major role, such as the decline of incidence of bacterial diarrheas as sanitation improved.[149] The relative role of bacteria, the rotaviruses, and other agents in infant mortality from diarrheal illness in developing countries needs intensive investigation.

Animal studies cited earlier clearly indicate that antibody in the intestinal lumen plays a major role in resistance to rotavirus disease. In experimentally infected animals, serum rotavirus antibody in the absence of intestinal antibody was not effective in preventing rotavirus illness. Thus, one approach in the control of rotavirus illness may be the encouragement of breast feeding as a means of providing local antibody to the young infant. Colostrum and milk contain IgA rotavirus antibody, and it may be that such antibody would exert some protective role against rotavirus illness in the infant and young child.[295] If a successful rotavirus vaccine were developed, it might be beneficial to immunize the mother to raise the level of antibodies in her breast milk for transfer to the intestine of the infant. One discouraging aspect of this approach is the frequency of diarrheal diseases, including those associated with rotavirus, in countries where infants and young children are breast fed almost exclusively for extended periods. However, the nutritional status of the nursing mother may be a critical factor.

It is likely that a rotavirus vaccine would be most effective if administered orally to stimulate local IgA antibody, since this antibody may be a major determinant of resistance to rotavirus illness.

The aim of a successful vaccine would be to prevent serious illness during the first 2 years of life, when the outcome of such infection may be especially serious or fatal. Thus, the vaccine would be administered within the first 6 months of life with a possible need for boosters at appropriate intervals.[45] With the recent successful cultivation of the Wa strain rotavirus, the development of a vaccine against at least one serotype appears possible.[285] It will be essential to propagate other rotavirus serotypes, since a vaccine should probably contain prevalent serotypes. Approaches to the development of a vaccine center about the development of mutants that have lost their ability to induce illness but are capable of inducing immunity. Such a vaccine would be tested initially in experimental animals for safety, antigenicity, and protective effect. If the vaccine were shown to be safe, immunogenic, and protective, studies would be carried out in adult volunteers initially. If safe, immunogenic, and protective in adult volunteers, the vaccine would be tested for safety and immunogenicity in a stepwise progression in younger age groups with the ultimate aim of a small field trial for efficacy.

Another approach to vaccine development takes advantage of the antigenic relatedness of human and animal rotavirus strains.[126,127,163,278] Thus, if an animal rotavirus, such as a bovine rotavirus, can be shown capable of infecting humans and inducing immunity without causing illness, such a strain might be an ideal vaccine candidate, especially if it protected against prevalent serotypes. The feasibility of this approach has been tested in calves. Calves were inoculated *in utero* with calf rotavirus or with placebo (or nothing).[289] Shortly after birth, the calves were challenged with the strain D of human rotavirus and it was found that *in utero* infection with calf rotavirus induced resistance to disease caused by challenge with this human rotavirus strain; in contrast, animals that had received placebo (or nothing) developed illness on challenge with human rotavirus D strain soon after birth. Thus, cross-protection between the calf and human rotavirus was demonstrated, indicating that the bovine virus was sufficiently related antigenically to human rotavirus D strain, a subgroup 2 virus, to induce protection, a finding that warrants further evaluation. Of course, prior to human studies, extensive safety tests would have to be performed.

Thus, it is hoped that an effective immunogen will be developed for rotavirus. However, it should be stressed that since a human rotavirus vaccine has not yet been developed, effective treatment for rotavirus diarrhea is available in the form of fluid and electrolyte replacement therapy by the oral or parenteral route of administration.[190,221] Thus, one means of controlling the severe morbidity and mortality from rotavirus diarrhea would be to make available fluids and electrolytes necessary for rehydration. In addition, since this agent is transmitted by the fecal–oral route, careful attention to hand-washing, disinfection, and disposal of contaminated material would appear to be one way of limiting the spread of this highly contagious agent, especially in nurseries and hospitals, where nosocomial infections are common.

10. Unresolved Problems

10.1. Norwalk Group and Miscellaneous Enteric Agents

Numerous unresolved problems remain for the Norwalk group. Intensive efforts are needed to determine the number of serotypes of agents responsible for epidemic viral gastroenteritis. Such studies entail careful electron-microscopic (EM) or immune-EM (IEM) studies for detection of viral particles. IEM must then be used to determine the significance of any particles observed and their antigenic relatedness to previously recognized viruses of the group. The development of a radioimmunoassay for Norwalk virus has permitted the study of the epidemiological importance of this agent. Such a practical assay is needed for the other known agents of this syndrome, such as the Hawaii, Ditchling, cockle, Parramatta, Marin County, and Colorado agents. It is conceivable that the etiology of most of epidemic viral gastroenteritis could be accounted for by the known members of the Norwalk group.

Efforts are also needed to find a suitable cell-culture system to propagate these agents. Such a system would facilitate epidemiological studies and assist in further characterization of these agents. For example, it is not yet known whether the Norwalk agent is an RNA or a DNA virus.

Studies of immunity to Norwalk agent have raised rather perplexing questions, since there appears to be one cohort of individuals who demonstrates immunity to Norwalk infection and illness, whereas there is another who characteristically demonstrates short-term but not long-term immunity. One explanation for this phenomenon postulates a genetic factor, such as a receptor for Norwalk virus, that is lacking in one cohort and present in the other.[197] The role of local IgA antibody should also be explored further.

Finally, a major unresolved area in the etiology of epidemic viral gastroenteritis is the role of other agents such as astroviruses, caliciviruses, minireoviruses, and other small, round viruses.[10,36,37,54,66, 77,83,87,144–146,152–156,166,177,184,226,236] Some of these agents, such as the astroviruses, have been studied rather intensively: for example, astroviruses, which are 28 nm in diameter and derive their name from the five- or six-pointed star-shaped configuration observed by negative staining in certain particles,[152] have been administered to volunteers and found to induce a diarrheal illness in 1 of 17 volunteers but to infect a substantial number[145]; studies of the prevalence of astrovirus antibody have demonstrated a rather rapid acquisition of antibody, so that by the 10th year, 75% of persons have antibody.[144] Astroviruses have also been detected in stools of lambs with diarrhea and in calves without diarrhea.[236,275] The lamb astrovirus has been shown to induce illness in lambs under experimental conditions, whereas the calf astrovirus did not induce illness under such conditions. Caliciviruslike particles, which are about 32–40 nm in diameter and have characteristic cuplike configurations on their surface,[152] have also been studied rather intensively. For example, gastroenteritis in infants and young children in Japan, England, and Canada has been associated with such particles.[47,52a,243a,249] As noted earlier, recent evidence suggests that the Norwalk agent may be a calicivirus.[102] Another particle 34–38 nm in diameter with a density of 1.35–1.37 g/cm³ has been associated with an outbreak of gastroenteritis in a work-training facility for mentally deficient persons 15 years of age or older. These particles were believed to be different from caliciviruses and astroviruses morphologically.[269] The classification of all these particles needs further study.

Two other groups that have no morphological similarity to Norwalk agent are the adenoviruses and the coronaviruses. Fastidious adenoviruses that do not grow readily in cell culture have been observed in stools of infants and young children hospitalized with diarrhea.[18,37,54,66,133,265] In the Washington, D.C., Children's Hospital study, adenoviruses were detected by EM significantly more often in stools or rectal-swab specimens of patients hospitalized with gastroenteritis than in those hospitalized for other than diarrheal illness (5.1 vs. 1.9%).[33] A large proportion of these adenoviruses could not be cultivated in cell culture. In addition, gastroenteritis outpatients were also found to shed adenoviruses significantly more often than nongastroenteritis outpatients (2.5 vs. 0.3%).[33] Adenoviruses have also been detected in stools of 15% of patients hospitalized with gastroenteritis in a Canadian study.[208] In addition, adenoviruses were associated with the deaths of two infants who had dehydration from severe gastroenteritis; adenovirus antigen was detected in their jejunal cells by immunofluorescence.[208] Adenoviruses have also been associated with a gastroenteritis outbreak in a long-stay children's ward.[84] Adenoviruses have also been found in small-intestinal fluid of pediatric patients with gastroenteritis[166]; in such patients, D-xylose absorption appears to have been impaired. Overall, the contribution of adenoviruses to etiology of pediatric gastroenteritis appears to be small. Adenovirus infection has also been associated with intussusception.[49,94]

Coronaviruses are established as etiological agents of diarrheal disease in many animals, but they have not yet been implicated conclusively in published reports as etiological agents of infantile gastroenteritis.[17,27,76,122,138,170,209,244] Coronaviruses have been reported to have been detected by EM in stools obtained from three outbreaks of gastroenteritis in adults, and the particles in a stool from one of the outbreaks were propagated in organ and cell cultures.[41,42] In February, 1980, enteric coronaviruses were described as associated with an outbreak of severe hemorrhagic enterocolitis in newborn infants in France, with two deaths.[46] In addition, the occurrence of enteric coronavirus in epidemics of diarrhea in 4- to 30-month-old patients was described.[46] Human serum has been shown to contain neutralizing antibody to calf coronavirus; however, since the human respiratory coronavirus organ culture (OC)43 and the calf coronavirus share some antigenic relationship, it is not certain whether this antibody is related to OC43 or to another human co-

ronavirus.[137,232] Thus, a major area of future research involves delineation of the role of these miscellaneous enteric agents in viral gastroenteritis.

10.2. Rotaviruses

There are numerous unresolved problems relating to the epidemiology of rotaviruses. The impact of rotavirus diarrhea on the staggering mortality rate from diarrheal diseases in the developing countries must be elucidated. Although rotaviruses are an important cause of severe diarrheal illness, the role of rotaviruses in infant mortality needs to be elucidated.

The incidence of rotavirus diarrhea in the general population in the United States and worldwide is not yet known. It is anticipated that in the United States, this information will be gathered from ongoing longitudinal studies, whereas worldwide information will be obtained from a recently launched WHO diarrheal diseases control program.

The paradox of rotavirus infections that are predominantly subclinical in neonates in certain nurseries has not been explained. The mechanism of this overall decreased susceptibility should be elucidated. In addition, the effect of such neonatal infection on future response to rotavirus should be determined.

Another area of interest is an understanding of the possible reservoirs of rotaviruses. Practically every animal studied has been found to have an indigenous rotavirus capable of causing diarrhea. However, there is no documented evidence of natural spread of an animal rotavirus to humans or vice versa. It is known, however, that the human rotavirus can induce diarrhea in piglets, calves, and monkeys under experimental conditions.

The inability to propagate rotavirus efficiently from clinical material remains a hindrance to the study of this agent. However, as described in Section 4.2, recently important advances have been made in this regard. Efficient cultivation of all prevalent serotypes in cell cultures is a major research goal.

The question of the number of rotavirus serotypes must also be resolved. There is agreement on at least two serotypes; however, the existence of up to five serotypes has been reported. The number of serotypes and their importance epidemiologically should be elucidated.

Another area to be resolved concerns the role of rotavirus infection in malnutrition and the effect of malnutrition on rotavirus infection. The possible role of breast milk in prevention of rotavirus diarrhea must also be evaluated. Although there is evidence that breast milk can exert an effect on rotavirus shedding, its role in the prevention of rotavirus diarrhea remains to be established.

The synergism, if any, between rotaviruses and bacteria should be studied. In animals, it is described that the presence of certain bacteria acts synergistically with rotavirus to cause more severe illness than if either were present alone.

Finally, with the worldwide importance of rotaviruses as a cause of diarrhea established, there is an ever-increasing demand for reagents for study of these agents. Suitable reagents for ELISA for detecting human rotavirus are available from various sources. The availability of such reagents should facilitate worldwide study of rotavirus.

11. References

1. ADAMS, W. R., AND KRAFT, L. M., Epizootic diarrhea of infant mice: Identification of the etiologic agent, *Science* **141:**359–360 (1963).
2. ADLER, I., AND ZICKL, R., Winter vomiting disease, *J. Infect. Dis.* **119:**668–673 (1969).
3. ALDRICH, R. A., Introduction to pediatrics: The change from pediatrics to child health and human development, in: *Brennemann's Practice of Pediatrics* (V. C. KELLEY, ed.), pp. 1–28, Harper and Row, Hagerstown, Maryland, 1972.
4. AGUS, S. G., DOLIN, R., WYATT, R. G., TOUSIMIS, A. J., AND NORTHRUP, R. S., Acute infectious nonbacterial gastroenteritis: Intestinal histopathology. Histologic and enzymatic alterations during illness produced by the Norwalk agent in man, *Ann. Intern. Med.* **79:**18–25 (1973).
5. ALBREY, M. B., AND MURPHY, A. M., Rotavirus and acute gastroenteritis of infants and children, *Med. J. Aust.* **1:**82–85 (1976).
6. ALBREY, M. B., AND MURPHY, A. M., Rotavirus growth in bovine monolayers, *Lancet* **1:**753 (1976).
7. ALMEIDA, J. D., AND WATERSON, A. P., The morphology of virus antibody interaction, *Adv. Viral Res.* **15:**307–338 (1969).
8. ANDERSON, T. F., AND STANLEY, W. M., A study by means of the electron microscope of the reaction between tobacco mosaic virus and its antiserum, *J. Biol. Chem.* **139:**339–344 (1941).
9. APPLETON, H., BUCKLEY, M., THOM, B. T., COTTON, J. L., AND HENDERSON, S., Virus-like particles in winter vomiting disease, *Lancet* **1:**409–411 (1977).
10. APPLETON, H., AND HIGGINS, P. G., Viruses and gastroenteritis in infants, *Lancet* **1:**409–411 (1977).
11. APPLETON, H., AND PEREIRA, M. S., A possible virus etiology in outbreaks of food-poisoning from cockles, *Lancet* **1:**780–781 (1977).
12. ARDENNE, M. V., FRIEDRICH-FRESKA, H., AND SCHRAMM, G., Electronenmikrokopischen Untersuchung der Präcipitinreaktion von Tabakmosaik Virus mit Kaninchenanti-serum, *Arch. Gesamte Virusforsch.* **2:**80–86 (1941).
13. ASHLEY, C. R., CARL, E. O., CLARK, S. K. R., CORNER, B. D., AND DUNN, S., Rotavirus infections of apes, *Lancet* **2:**477 (1979).
14. BANATVALA, J. E., CHRYSTIE, I. L., AND TOTTERDELL, B. M., Rotaviral infections in human neonates, *J. Am. Vet. Med. Assoc.* **173:**527–530 (1978).
15. BANATVALA, J. E., TOTTERDELL, B., CHRYSTIE, I. L., AND WOODE, G. N., In vitro detection of human rotaviruses, *Lancet* **2:**821 (1975).
15a. BEARDS, G. M., PILFOLD, J. N., THOULESS, M. E., AND FLEWETT, T. H., Rotavirus serotypes by serum neutralization *J. Med. Virol.* **5:**231–237 (1980).
16. BERGLUND, M. E., MCADARAGH, J. P., AND STOTZ, I., Proceedings of the 26th Western Poultry Disease Conference at University of California, Davis, pp. 129–130, 1966.
17. BINN, L. N., LAZAR, E. C., KEENAN, K. P., HUXSOLL, D. L., MARCHWICKI, R. H., AND SRANO, A. J., Recovery and characterization of a coronavirus from military dogs with diarrhea, Proceedings of the 78th Annual Meeting of the U.S. Animal Health Association, pp. 359–366, 1974.
18. BIRCH, C. J., LEWIS, F. A., KENNETT, M. L., HOMOLA, M., PRITCHARD, H., AND GUST, I. D., A study of prevalence of rotavirus infection in children with gastroenteritis admitted to an infectious diseases hospital, *J. Med. Virol.* **1:**69–77 (1977).
19. BISHOP, R. F., DAVIDSON, G. P., HOLMES, I. H., AND RUCK, B. J., Detection of a new virus by electron microscopy of fecal extracts from children with acute gastroenteritis, *Lancet* **1:**149–151 (1974).
20. BISHOP, R. F., DAVIDSON, G. P., HOLMES, I. H., AND RUCK, B. J., Evidence for viral gastroenteritis, *N. Engl. J. Med.* **289:**1096–1097 (1973).
21. BISHOP, R. F., DAVIDSON, G. P., HOLMES, I. H., AND RUCK, B. J., Virus particles in epithelial cells of duodenal mucosa from children with acute gastroenteritis, *Lancet* **2:**1281–1283 (1973).
22. BLACK, R. E., MERSON, M. H., MIZANUR RAHMAN, A. S. M., YANUS, M. D., ALIM, A. R. M. A., HUQ, I., YOLKEN, R. H., AND CURLIN, G. T., A 2 year study of bacterial, viral, and parasitic agents associated

with diarrhea in rural Bangladesh, *J. Infect. Dis.* **142**:660–664 (1980).

23. BLACKLOW, N. R., CUKOR, G., BEDIGIAN, M. K., ECH-EVERRIA, P., GREENBERG, H. B., SCHREIBER, D. S., AND TRIER, J. S., Immune response and prevalence of antibody to Norwalk enteritis virus as determined by radioimmunoassay, *J. Clin. Microbiol.* **10**:903–909 (1979).

24. BLACKLOW, N. R., CUKOR, G., PANJAVANI, Z., CA-POZZA, F., AND BEDNAREK, F., Simplified radioim-munoassay for detection of rotavirus in pediatric and adult stools, for assessment of duration of antibody to rotavirus in human breast milk (abstract), Fourth International Congress for Virology, The Hague, p. 464, 1978.

25. BLACKLOW, N. R., DOLIN, R., FEDSON, D. S., DUPONT, H., NORTHRUP, R. S. HORNICK, R. B., AND CHANOCK, R. M., Acute infectious nonbacterial gastroenteritis: Etiology and pathogenesis (A combined clinical staff conference at the Clinical Center of the National In-stitutes of Health), *Ann. Intern. Med.* **76**:993–1008 (1972).

26. BLACKLOW, N. R., ECHEVERRIA, P., AND SMITH, D. A., Serological studies with reovirus-like enteritis agent, *Infect. Immun.* **13**:1563–1566 (1976).

27. BOHL, E. H., Transmissible gastroenteritis, in: *Di-seases of Swine*, 3rd ed. (H. W. DUNNE, ed.), pp. 158–176, Iowa State University Press, Ames, 1970.

28. BOLIVAR, R., CONKLIN, R. H., VOLLETT, J. J., PICK-ERING, L. K., DUPONT, H. L., WALTERS, D. L., AND KOHL, S., Rotavirus in travelers' diarrhea: Study of an adult student population in Mexico, *J. Infect. Dis.* **137**:324–327 (1978).

29. BONSDORFF, C. H. VON, HOVI, T., MAKELA, P., HOVI, L., AND TEVALUSTO-AARNIO, M., Rotavirus associated with acute gastroenteritis in adults, *Lancet* **2**:423 (1976).

30. BONSDORFF, C. H. VON, HOVI, T., MAKELA, P., AND MORTTINEN, A., Rotavirus infections in adults in as-sociation with acute gastroenteritis, *J. Med. Virol.* **2**:21–28 (1978).

31. BRADBURNE, A. F., ALMEIDA, J. D., GARDNER, P. S., MOOSAI, R. B., NASH, A. A., AND COOMBS, R. R. A., A solid phase system (SPACE) for the detection and quantification of rotavirus in faeces, *J. Gen. Virol.* **44**:615–623 (1979).

32. BRANDT, C. D., KIM, H. W., RODRIGUEZ, W. J., THOMAS, L., YOLKEN, R. H., ARROBIO, J. O., KAPI-KIAN, A. Z., PARROTT, R. H., AND CHANOCK, R. M., Comparison of direct electron microscopy, immune electron microscopy, and rotavirus enzyme-linked immunosorbent assay for detection of gastroenteritis viruses in children, *J. Clin. Microbiol.* **13**:976–981 (1981).

33. BRANDT, C. D., KIM, H. W., YOLKEN, R. H., KAPIKIAN,

A. Z., ARROBIO, J. O., RODRIGUEZ, W. J., WYATT, R. G., CHANOCK, R. M., AND PARROTT, R. H., Compar-ative epidemiology of two rotavirus serotypes and other viral agents associated with pediatric gastroen-teritis, *Am. J. Epidemiol.* **110**:243–254 (1979).

34. BRIDGER, J. C., AND WOODE, G. N., Neonatal calf diarrhea: Identification of a reovirus-like (rotavirus) agent in feces by immunofluorescence and immune electron microscopy, *Br. Vet. J.* **131**:528–535 (1975).

35. BURROUGHS, J. N., AND BROWN, F., Presence of a con-alently linked protein in calicivirus RNA, *J. Gen. Virol.* **41**:443–446 (1978).

36. BRUCE-WHITE, G. B., ASHTON, C. I., ROBERTS, C., AND PARRY, H. E., "Rotavirus" in gastroenteritis, *Lancet* **2**:726 (1974).

37. BRYDEN, A. S., DAVIES, H. A., HADLEY, R. E., FLEW-ETT, T. H., MORRIS, C. A., AND OLIVER, P., Rotavirus enteritis in the West Midlands during 1974, *Lancet* **2**:241–243 (1974).

38. BRYDEN, A. S., DAVIES, H. A., THOULESS, M. E., AND FLEWETT, T. H., Diagnosis of rotavirus infection by cell culture, *J. Med. Microbiol.* **10**:121–125 (1977).

39. BRYDEN, A. S., THOULESS, M. E., AND FLEWETT, T. H., Rotavirus in rabbits, *Vet. Rec.* **99**:232 (1976).

40. CARLSON, J. A. K., MIDDLETON, P. J., SZYMANSKI, M., HUBER, J., AND PETRIC, M., Fatal rotavirus gastroen-teritis: An analysis of 21 cases, *Am. J. Dis. Child.* 132:477–479 (1978).

41. CAUL, E. O., AND EGGLESTONE, S. I., Further studies on human enteric coronaviruses, *Arch. Virol.* **54**:107–117 (1977).

42. CAUL, E. O., PAVER, W. K., AND CLARKE, S. K. R., Coronavirus particles in faeces from patients with gastroenteritis, *Lancet* **1**:1192 (1975).

43. CENTER FOR DISEASE CONTROL, Viral gastroenteritis—Pennsylvania, *Morbid. Mortal. Weekly Rep.* **27**:403–404 (1978).

44. CENTER FOR DISEASE CONTROL, Gastroenteritis asso-ciated with lake swimming—Michigan, *Morbid. Mor-tal. Weekly Rep.* **28**:413–416 (1979).

45. CHANOCK, R. M., WYATT, R. G., AND KAPIKIAN, A. Z., Immunization of infants and young children against rotavirus gastroenteritis: Prospects and problems, *J. Am. Vet. Med. Assoc.* **173**:570–572 (1978).

46. CHANY, C., Discussion at Perspectives in Virology, XI Meeting, *Perspect. Virol.* **11**:185–187 (1981).

47. CHIBA, S., SAKUMA, Y., KOGASAKA, R., AKIHARA, M., HORINO, K., NAKAO, T., AND FUKUI, S., An outbreak of gastroenteritis associated with caliciviruses in an infant home. *J. Med. Virol.* **4**:249–254 (1979).

48. CHRISTOPHER, P. J., GROHMANN, G. S., MILLSOM, R. H., AND MURPHY, A. M., Parvovirus gastroenteri-tis—a new entity for Australia, *Med. J. Aust.* **1**:121–124 (1978).

49. CLARKE, E. J., JR., PHILLIPS, I. A., AND ALEXANDER,

E. R., Adenovirus infection in intussusception in children in Taiwan, *J. Am. Med. Assoc.* **208:**1671–1674 (1969).

50. CLARKE, S. K. R., COOK, G. T., EGGLESTONE, S. I., HALL, T. S., MILLER, D. L., REED, S. E., RUBENSTEIN, D., SMITH, A. J., AND, TYRRELL, D. A. J., A virus from epidemic vomiting disease, *Br. Med. J.* **3:**86–89 (1972).

51. CONNOR, J. D., AND BARRETT-CONNOR, E., Infectious diarrheas, *Pediatr. Clin. North Am.* **14:**197–221 (1967).

52. COOK, D. A., ZBITNEW, A., DEMPSTER, G., AND GERRARD, J. W., Detection of antibody to rotavirus by counterimmunoelectrophoresis in human serum, colostrum and milk, *J. Pediatr.* **93:**967–970 (1978).

52a. CUBITT, W. D., McSWIGGAN, D. A., AND MOORE, W., Winter vomiting disease caused by calicivirus. *J. Clin. Pathol.* **32:**786–793 (1979).

53. CUKOR, G., BERRY, M. K., AND BLACKLOW, N. R., Simplified radioimmunoassay for detection of human rotavirus in stools, *J. Infect. Dis.* **138:**906–910 (1978).

54. DAVIDSON, G. P., BISHOP, R. F., TOWNLEY, R. R. W., HOLMES, I. H., AND RUCK, B. J., Importance of a new virus in acute sporadic enteritis in children, *Lancet* **1:**242–245 (1975).

55. DAVIDSON, G. P., BUTLER, D. G., GALL, D. G., PETRIC, M., AND HAMILTON, J. R., Ion transport in enteritis caused by human rotavirus, *American Society for Microbiology Annual Meeting*, abstract A-20/1043, May 1977, American Society of Microbiology, Washington, D.C., 1977.

56. DAVIDSON, G. P., GOLLER, I., BISHOP, R. F., TOWNLEY, R. R. W., HOLMES, I. H., AND RUCK, B. J., Immunofluroesecence in duodenal mucosa of children with acute enteritis due to a new virus, *J. Clin. Pathol.* **28:**263–266 (1975).

57. DELAGE, G., McLAUGHLIN, B., AND BETHAUME, L., A clinical study of rotavirus gastroenteritis, *J. Pediatr.* **93:**455–457 (1978).

58. DINGLE, J. H., BADGER, G. F., AND JORDAN, W. S., *Illness in the home: A Study of 25,000 Illnesses in a Group of Cleveland Families*, p. 19, The Press of Western Reserve Univerity, 1964.

59. DOLIN, R., Norwalk-like agents of gastroenteritis, in: *Principles and Practices of Infectious Diseases* (G. L. MANDELL, R. G. DOUGLAS, JR., AND J. E. BENNETT, eds.) pp. 1364–1370, John Wiley, New York, Chichester, Brisbane, Toronto, 1979.

60. DOLIN, R., BLACKLOW, N. R., DuPONT, H., BUSCHO, R. J., WYATT, R. G., KASEL, J. A., HORNICK, R., AND CHANOCK, R. M.: Biological properties of Norwalk agent of acute infectious nonbacterial gastroenteritis, *Proc. Soc. Exp. Biol. Med.* **140:**578–583 (1972).

61. DOLIN, R., BLACKLOW, N. R., DuPONT, H., FORMAL, S., BUSCHO, R. F., KASEL, J. A., CHAMES, R. P., HORNICK, R., AND CHANOCK, R. M., Transmission of acute infectious nonbacterial gastroenteritis to volunteers by oral administration of stool filtrates, *J. Infect. Dis.* **123:**307–312 (1971).

62. DOLIN, R., LEVY, A. G., WYATT, R. G., THORNHILL, T. S., AND GARDNER, J. D., Viral gastroenteritis induced by the Hawaii agent: Jejunal histopathology and seroresponse, *Am. J. Med.* **59:**761–767 (1975).

63. DOLIN, R., REICHMAN, R. C., AND FAUCI, A. S., Lymphocyte populations in acute viral gastroenteritis, *Infect. Immun.* **14:**422–428 (1976).

64. DOMINICK, H. C., AND MAASS, G., Rotavirus Infectionen im Kindersalter, *Klin. Paediatr.* **191:**33–39 (1979).

65. DROZDOV, S. G., SHEKOYAN, L. A., KOROLEV, M. B., AND ANDZHAPARIDZE, A. G., Human rotavirus in cell culture: Isolation and passaging, *Vopr. Virusol.* **4:**389–392 (1979).

66. ECHEVERRIA, P., HO, M. T., BLACKLOW, N. R., QUINNAN, G., PORTNOY, B., OLSON, J. G., CONKLIN, R., DuPONT, H. L., AND CROSS, J. H., Relative importance of viruses and bacteria in the etiology of pediatric diarrhea in Taiwan, *J. Infect. Dis.* **136:**383–390 (1977).

67. EDELMAN, R., AND LEVINE, M. M., Acute diarrheal infections in infants. II. Bacterial and viral causes, *Hosp. Pract.* **15:**96–104 (1980).

68. Editorial, Reovirus-like agent as a cause of human diarrheal disease, *South. Med. J.* **70:**390–392 (1977).

69. Editorial, Rotavirus gastroenteritis, *Br. Med. J.* **2:**784–785 (1977).

70. Editorial, Rotaviruses of man and animals, *Lancet* **1:**257–259 (1975).

70a. Editorial, Towards a rotavirus vaccine, *Lancet* **2:**619–620 (1981).

71. Editorial: Viral cross-infections in wards, *Lancet* **1:**1391–1393 (1976).

72. Editorial, Viruses from shellfish, *Lancet* **2:**1224–1225 (1979).

73. Editorial, Viruses of infantile gastroenteritis, *Br. Med. J.* **3:**555–556 (1975).

74. ELIAS, M. M., Distribution and titers of rotavirus antibodies in different age groups, *J. Hyg. (Cambridge)* **79:**365–372 (1977).

75. ELIAS, M. M., Separation and infectivity of two particle types of human rotavirus, *J. Gen. Virol.* **37:**191–194 (1977).

76. ELLENS, D. J., AND DeLEEUW, P. W., ELISA for detection of bovine coronavirus in faeces, Abstract of the International Congress for Virology, No. 627, The Hague, 1978.

77. ESPARZA, J., VIERA DE TORRES, B., PINERO, A., CARMONA, F. O., AND MAZZALI DE ILIA, R., Rotavirus in Venezuelan children with gastroenteritis, *Am. J. Trop. Med. Hyg.* **26:**148–151 (1977).

78. ESPEJO, R. T., CALDERON, E., AND GONZALEZ, N.,

Distinct reovirus-like agents associated with acute infantile gastroenteritis, *J. Clin. Microbiol.* **6**:502–506 (1977).

79. EUGSTER, A. K., STROTHER, J., AND HARTFIELD, D. A., Rotavirus (reovirus-like) infection of neonatal ruminants in a zoo nursery, *J. Wildl. Dis.* **14**:351–354 (1978).

80. FAUVEL, M., SPENCE, L., BABIUK, L. A., PETRO, R., AND BLOCH, S., Hemagglutination and hemagglutination inhibition studies with a strain of Nebraska calf diarrhea virus (bovine rotavirus), *Intervirology* **9**:95–105 (1978).

81. FIELD, M., Modes of action of enterotoxins from *Vibrio cholerae* and *Escherichia coli*, *Rev. Infect. Dis.* **1**:918–925 (1979).

82. FLEWETT, T. H., Diagnosis of enteritis virus, *Proc. R. Soc. Med.* **69**:693–696 (1976).

83. FLEWETT, T. H., BRYDEN, A. S., AND DAVIES, H., Virus particles in gastroenteritis, *Lancet* **2**:1497 (1973).

84. FLEWETT, T. H., BRYDEN, A. S., AND DAVIES, H., Epidemic viral enteritis in a long-stay children's ward, *Lancet* **1**:4–5 (1975).

85. FLEWETT, T. H., BRYDEN, A. S., AND DAVIES, H., Virus diarrhea in foals and other animals, *Vet. Rec.* **97**:477 (1975).

86. FLEWETT, T. H., BRYDEN, A. S., DAVIES, H., WOODE, G. N., BRIDGER, J. C., AND DERRICK, J. M., Relation between viruses from acute gastroenteritis of children and newborn calves, *Lancet* **2**:61–63 (1974).

87. FLEWETT, T. H., AND DAVIES, H., Caliciviruses in man, *Lancet* **1**:311 (1976).

88. FLEWETT, T. H., DAVIES, H., BRYDEN, A. S., AND ROBERTSON, M. J., Diagnostic electron microscopy of faeces. II. Acute gastroenteritis associated with reovirus-like particles, *J. Clin. Pathol* **27**:608–614 (1974).

88a. FLEWETT, T. H., THOULESS, M. E., POLFOLD, J. N., BRYDEN, A. S., AND CANDEIAS, J.ˈA. N., More serotypes of human rotavirus, *Lancet* **2**:632 (1978).

89. FLEWETT, T. H., AND WOODE, G. N., The rotaviruses (brief review), *Arch. Virol.* **57**:1–23 (1978).

90. FONTEYNE, J., ZISSIS, G., AND LAMBERT, J. P., Recurrent rotavirus gastroenteritis, *Lancet* **1**:983 (1978).

91. FOSTER, L. G., PETERSON, H., AND SPENDLOVE, R. S., Fluorescent virus precipitin test, *Proc. Soc. Exp. Biol. Med.* **150**:155–160 (1975).

92. FUKUMI, H., NAKAYA, R., HATTA, S., NORIKI, H., YUNOKI, H., AKAGI, K., SAITO, T., UCHIYAMA, K., KOBARI, K., AND NAKANISHI, R., An indication as to identity between the infectious diarrhea in Japan and the afebrile infectious non-bacterial gastroenteritis by human volunteer experiments, *Jpn. M. Med. Sci. Biol.* **10**:1–17 (1957).

93. GALL, D. G., Pathophysiology of viral diarrhea, in: Proceedings of the 73rd Ross Conference on Pediatric Research: Etiology, Pathology, and Treatment

of Acute Gastroenteritis, Ponte Vedra Beach, Florida, March 20–22, 1977.

94. GARDNER, P. S., KNOX, E. G., COURT, S. D. M., AND GREEN, C. A., Virus infection and intussusception in childhood, *Br. Med. J.* **2**:697–700 (1962).

95. GOMEZ-BARRETO, J., PALMER, E., NAHMIAS, A. J., HATCH, M. N., Acute enteritis associated with reovirus-like agents, *J. Am. Med. Assoc.* **235**:1857–1860 (1976).

96. GORDON, I., INGRAHAM, H. S., AND KORNS, R. F., Transmission of epidemic gastroenteritis to human volunteers by oral administration of fecal filtrates, *J. Exp. Med.* **86**:409–422 (1947).

97. GRAUBALLE, P. C., GENNER, J., MEYLING, A., AND HORNSLETH, A., Rapid diagnosis of rotavirus infections: Comparison of electron microscopy and immunoelectro-osmophoresis for detection of rotavirus in human infantile gastroenteritis, *J. Gen. Virol.* **35**:203–218 (1977).

98. GREENBERG, H. B., et al., Unpublished studies.

98a. GREENBERG, H. B., KALICA, A. R., WYATT, R. G., JONES, R. W., KAPIKIAN, A. Z., AND CHANOCK, R. M., Rescue of noncultivatable human rotavirus by gene reassortment during mixed infection with ts mutants of a cultivatable bovine rotavirus, *Proc. Nat. Acad. Sci. USA* **78**:420–424 (1981).

99. GREENBERG, H. B., AND KAPIKIAN, A. Z., Detection of Norwalk agent antibody and antigen by solid-phase radioimmunoassay and immune adherence hemagglutination assay, *J. Am. Vet. Med. Assoc.* **173**:620–623 (1978).

99a. GREENBERG, H. B., SINGH, N., OSHIRO, L., LONDON, W. T., SLY, D. L., unpublished studies.

100. GREENBERG, H. B., VALDESUSO, J., KAPIKIAN, A. Z., CHANOCK, R. M., WYATT, R. G., SZMUNESS, W., LARRICK, J., KAPLAN, J., GILMAN, R. H., AND SACK, D. A., Prevalence of antibody to the Norwalk virus in various countries, *Infect. Immun.* **26**:270–272 (1979).

101. GREENBERG, H. B., VALDESUSO, J., YOLKEN, R. H., GANGAROSA, E., GARY, W., WYATT, R. G., KONNO, T., SUZUKI, H., CHANOCK, R. M., AND KAPIKIAN, A. Z., Role of Norwalk virus in outbreaks of nonbacterial gastroenteritis, *J. Infect. Dis.* **139**:564–568 (1979).

102. GREENBERG, H. B., WYATT, R. G., KALICA, A. R., YOLKEN, R. H., BLACK, R., KAPIKIAN, A. Z., AND CHANOCK, R. M., New insights in viral gastroenteritis, *Perspect. Virol.* **11**:163–187 (1981).

103. GREENBERG, H. B., WYATT, R. G., AND KAPIKIAN, A. Z., Norwalk virus in vomitus, *Lancet* **2**:55 (1979).

104. GREENBERG, H. B., WYATT, R. G., VALDESUSO, J., KALICA, A. R., LONDON, W. T., CHANOCK, R. M., AND KAPIKIAN, A. Z., Solid-phase microtiter radioimmunoassay for detection of the Norwalk strain of acute nonbacterial epidemic gastroenteritis virus and its antibodies, *J. Med. Virol.* **2**:97–108 (1978).

105. GROHMANN, G. S., GREENBERG, H. B., WELCH, B. M., AND MURPHY, A. M., Oyster-associated gastroenteritis in Australia: The detection of Norwalk virus and its antibody by immune electron microscopy and radioimmunoassay, *J. Med. Virol.* **6**:11–19 (1980).

106. GUST, I. D., PRINGLE, R. C., BARNES, G. L., DAVIDSON, G. P., AND BISHOP, R. F., Complement-fixing antibody response to rotavirus infection, *J. Clin. Microbiol.* **5**:125–130 (1977).

107. GWALTNEY, J. M., JR., Medical reviews: Rhinoviruses, *Yale J. Biol. Med.* **48**:17–45 (1975).

107a. HAMILTON, J. R., GALL, D. G., KERZNER, B., BUTLER, D. G., AND MIDDLETON, P. J., Recent developments in viral gastroenteritis, *Pediatr. Clin. N. Am.* **22**:747–755 (1975).

108. HARA, M., MUKOYAMA, J., TSURUHARA, T., ASHIWARA, Y., SAITO, Y., AND TAGAYA, I., Acute gastroenteritis among school children associated with reovirus-like agent, *Am. J. Epidemiol.* **107**:161–169 (1978).

109. HARA, M., MUKOYAMA, J., TSURUHARA, T., SAITO, Y. AND TAGAYA, I., Duovirus in school children with gastroenteritis, *Lancet* **1**:311 (1976).

110. HARRIS, C. C., YOLKEN, R. H., KROKAN, H., AND HSU, I. C., Ultrasensitive enzymatic radioimmunoassay: Application to detection of cholera toxin and rotavirus, *Proc. Nat. Acad. Sci. USA* **76**:5335–5339 (1979).

111. HIEBER, J. P., SHELTON, S., NELSON, J. D., LEON, J., AND MOHS, E., Comparison of human rotavirus disease in tropical and temperate settings, *Am. J. Dis. Child.* **132**:853–858 (1978).

112. HODES, H. L., American Pediatric Society Presidential Address, *Pediatr. Res.* **10**:201–204 (1976).

113. HOLMES, I. H., Viral gastroenteritis, *Prog. Med. Virol.* **25**:1–36 (1979).

114. HOLMES, I. H., RUCK, B. J., BISHOP, R. F., AND DAVIDSON, G. P., Infantile enteritis viruses: Morphogenesis and morphology, *J. Virol.* **16**:937–943 (1975).

115. JESUDOSS, E. S., JOHN, T. J., MATHAN, M., AND SPENCE, L., Prevalence of rotavirus antibody in infants and children, *India J. Med. Res.* **68**:383–386 (1978).

116. JONES, R. C., HUGHES, C. S., AND HENRY, R. R., Rotavirus infection in commercial laying hens, *Vet. Rec.* **104**:22 (1979).

117. JORDAN, W. S., GORDON, I., AND DORRANCE, W. R., A study of illness in a group of Cleveland families. VII. Transmission of acute nonbacterial gastroenteritis to volunteers: Evidence for two different etiologic agents, *J. Exp. Med.* **98**:461–475 (1953).

118. KALICA, A. R., GARON, C. F., WYATT, R. G., MEBUS, C. A., VANKIRK, D. H., CHANOCK, R. M., AND KAPIKIAN, A. Z., Differentiation of human and calf reovirus-like agents associated with diarrhea using polyacrylamide gel electrophoresis of RNA, *Virology* **74**:86–92 (1976).

118a. KALICA, A. R., GREENBERG, H. B., WYATT, R. G., FLO-

RES, J., SERENO, M. M., KAPIKIAN, A. Z., AND CHANOCK, R. M., Genes of human (strain Wa) and bovine (strain UK) rotaviruses that code for neutralization and subgroup antigens, *Virology* **112**:385–390 (1981).

119. KALICA. A. R., PURCELL, R. H., SERENO, M. M., WYATT, R. G., KIM, H. W., CHANOCK, R. M., AND, KAPIKIAN, A. Z., A microtiter solid phase radioimmunoassay for detection of the human reovirus-like agent in stools, *J. Immunol.* **118**:1275–1279 (1977).

120. KALICA, A. R., SERENO, M. M., WYATT, R. G., MEBUS, C. A., CHANOCK, R. M., AND KAPIKIAN, A. Z., Comparison of human and animal rotavirus strains by gel electrophoresis of RNA, *Virology* **87**:247–255 (1978).

121. KALICA, A. R., WYATT, R. G., AND KAPIKIAN, A. Z., Detection of differences among human and animal rotaviruses using analysis of viral RNA, *J. Am. Vet. Med. Assoc.* **173**:531–537 (1978).

122. KAPIKIAN, A. Z., The coronaviruses, in: *CRC Chemoprophylaxis and Virus Infections of the Respiratory Tract*, Vol II, 9th ed. (G. S. OXFORD, ed.), pp. 95–117, CRC Press, Cleveland, 1977.

123. KAPIKIAN, A. Z., Unpublished studies.

124. KAPIKIAN, A. Z., WYATT, R. G., LEVINE, M. M., YOLKEN, R. H., VAN KIRK, D. H., DOLIN, R., GREENBERG, H. B., AND CHANOCK, R. M., Oral administration of a human rotavirus to volunteers: Induction of illness and correlates of resistance (manuscript submitted).

125. KAPIKIAN, A. Z., BARILE, M. F., WYATT, R. G., YOLKEN, R. H., TULLY, J. G., GREENBERG, H. B., KALICA, A. R., AND CHANOCK, R. M., Mycoplasma contamination in cell culture of Crohn's disease material, *Lancet* **2**:466–467 (1979).

125a. KAPIKIAN, A. Z., CLINE, W. L., GREENBERG, H. B., WYATT, R. G., KALICA, A. R., BANKS, C. E., JAMES, H. D., JR., FLORES, J., AND CHANOCK, R. M., Antigenic characterization of human and animal rotaviruses by immune adherence hemagglutination assay (IAHA): Evidence for distinctness of IAHA and neutralization antigens, *Infect. Immun.* **33**:415–425 (1981).

126. KAPIKIAN, A. Z., CLINE, W. L., KIM, H. W., KALICA, A. R., WYATT, R. G., VANKIRK, D. H., CHANOCK, R. M., JAMES, H. D., JR., AND VAUGHN, A. L., Antigenic relationships among five reovirus-like (RVL) agents by complement-fixation (CF) and development of a new substitute CF antigen for the human RVL agent of infantile gastroenteritis, *Proc. Soc. Exp. Biol. Med.* **152**:535–539 (1976).

127. KAPIKIAN, A. Z., CLINE, W. L., MEBUS, C. A., WYATT, R. G., KALICA, A. R., JAMES, H. D., JR., VAN KIRK, D., CHANOCK, R. M., AND KIM, H. W., New complement-fixation test for the human reovirus-like agent of infantile gastroenteritis: Nebraska calf diarrhea virus used as antigen, *Lancet* **1**:1056–1069 (1975).

128. KAPIKIAN, A. Z., DIENSTAG, J. L., AND PURCELL, R

H., Immune electron microscopy as a method for the detection, identification, and characterization of agent not cultivable in an *in vitro* system, in: *Manual of Clinical Immunology*, 2nd. ed. (N. R. ROSE AND H. FRIEDMAN, eds.), pp. 70–83, American Society for Microbiology, Washington, D.C., 1980.

129. KAPIKIAN, A. Z., FEINSTONE, S. M., PURCELL, R. H., WYATT, R. G., THORNHILL, T. S., KALICA, A. R., AND CHANOCK, R. M., Detection and identification by immune electron microscopy of fastidious agents associated with respiratory illness, acute nonbacterial gastroenteritis, and hepatitis A, *Perspect. Virol.* **9**:9–47 (1975).

130. KAPIKIAN, A. Z., GERIN, J. L., WYATT, R. G., THORNHILL, T. S., AND CHANOCK, R. M., Density in cesium chloride of the 27-nm "8FIIa" particle associated with acute infectious nonbacterial gastroenteritis: Determination by ultracentrifugation and immune electron microscopy, *Proc. Soc. Exp. Biol. Med.* **142**:874–877 (1974).

131. KAPIKIAN, A. Z., GREENBERG, H. B., CLINE, W. L., KALICA, A. R., WYATT, R. G., JAMES, H. D., JR., LLOYD, N. L., CHANOCK, R. M., RYDER, R. W., AND KIM, H. W., Prevalence of antibody to Norwalk agent by a newly developed immune adherence hemagglutination assay, *J. Med. Virol.* **2**:281–294 (1978).

132. KAPIKIAN, A. Z., KALICA, A. R., SHIH, J. W., CLINE, W. L., THORNHILL, T. S., WYATT, R. G., CHANOCK, R. M., KIM, H. W., AND GERIN, J. L., buoyant density in cesium chloride of the human reovirus-like agent of infantile gastroenteritis by ultracentrifugation, electron microscopy, and complement-fixation, *Virology* **70**:564–569 (1976).

133. KAPIKIAN, A. Z., KIM, H. W., WYATT, R. G., CLINE, W. L., ARROBIO, J. O., BRANDT, C. D., RODRIGUEZ, W. J., SACK, D. A., CHANOCK, R. M., AND PARROTT, R. H., Human reovirus-like agent as the major pathogen associated with "winter" gastroenteritis in hospitalized infants and young children, *N. Engl. J. Med.* **294**:965–972 (1976).

134. KAPIKIAN, A. Z., KIM, H. W., WYATT, R. G., RODRIGUEZ, W. J., ROSS, S., CLINE, W. L., PARROTT, R. H., AND CHANOCK, R. M., Reovirus-like agent in stools: Association with infantile diarrhea and development of serologic tests, *Science* **185**:1049–1053 (1974).

135. KAPIKIAN, A. Z., WYATT, R. G., DOLIN, R., THORNHILL, T. S., KALICA, A. R., AND CHANOCK, R. M., Visualization by immune electron microscopy of a 27 nm particle associated with acute infectious nonbacterial gastroenteritis, *J. Virol.* **10**:1075–1081 (1972).

136. KAPIKIAN, A. Z., YOLKEN, R. H., GREENBERG, H. B., WYATT, R. G., KALICA, A. R., CHANOCK, R. M., AND KIM, H. W., Gastroenteritis viruses, in: *Diagnostic Procedures for Viral, Rickettsial, and Chlamydial Infections*, 5th ed. (E. H. LENNETTE AND N. J. SCHMIDT,

eds.), pp. 927–995, American Public Health Association, Washington, D.C., 1979.

137. KAYE, H. S., YARBROUGH, W. B., AND REED, C. J., Calf diarrhea coronavirus, *Lancet* **2**:509 (1975).

138. KEENAN, K. P., JERVIS, H. R., MARCHWICKI, R. H., AND BINN, L. N., Intestinal infection of neonatal dogs and canine coronavirus 1-71: Studies by virologic, histologic, histochemical and immunofluorescent techniques, *Am. J. Vet. Res.* **27**:247–256 (1976).

138a. KIM, H. W., ARROBIO, J. O., BRANDT, C. D., JEFFRIES, B. C., PYLES, G., REID, J. L., CHANOCK, R. M., AND PARROTT, R. H., Epidemiology of respiratory syncytial virus infection in Washington, D.C. I. Importance of the virus in different respiratory tract disease syndromes and temporal distribution of infection, *Am. J. Epidemiol.* **98**:216–225 (1973).

139. KIM, H. W., BRANDT, C. D., KAPIKIAN, A. Z., WYATT, R. G., ARROBIO, J. O., RODRIGUEZ, W. J., CHANOCK, R. M., AND, PARROTT, R. H., Human reovirus-like agent (HRVLA) infection: Occurrence in adult contacts of pediatric patients with gastroenteritis, *J. Am. Med. Assoc.* **237**:404–407 (1977).

140. KOJIMA, S., FUKUMI, H., KUSAMA, H., YAMAMOTO, S., SUZUKI, S., UCHIDA, T., ISHIMARAU, T., OKA, T., KURETANI, K., OHMURA, K., NISHIKAWA, F., FUJIMOTO, J., FUJITA, K., NAKANO, A., AND SUNAKAWA, S., Studies on the causative agent of the infectious diarrhea: Records of the experiments on human volunteers, *Jpn. Med. J.* **1**:467–476 (1948).

141. KONNO, T., SUZUKI, H., IMAI, A., AND ISHIDA, N., Reovirus-like agent in acute epidemic gastroenteritis in Japanese infants: Fecal shedding and serologic response, *J. Infect. Dis.* **135**:259–266 (1977).

142. KONNO, T., SUZUKI, H., IMAI, A., KUTSUZAWA, T., ISHIDA, N., KATSUSHIMA, N., SAKAMOTO, M., KITAOKA, S., TSUBOI, R., AND ADACHI, M., A long term survey of rotavirus infection in Japanese children with acute gastroenteritis, *J. Infect. Dis.* **138**:569–576 (1978).

143. KONNO, T., SUZUKI, H., KUTSUZAWA, T., IMAI, A., KATSUSHIMA, M., SAKAMOTO, M., AND KITAOKA, S., Human rotavirus and intussuception, *N. Engl. J. Med.* **297**:945 (1977).

144. KURTZ, J. B., AND LEE, T. W., Astrovirus gastroenteritis age distribution of antibody, *Med. Microbiol. Immun.* **166**:227–230 (1978).

145. KURTZ, J. B., LEE, T. W., CRAIG, J. W., AND REED, S. E., Astrovirus infection in volunteers, *J. Med. Virol.* **3**:221–230 (1979).

146. KURTZ, J. B., LEE, T. W., AND PICKERING D., Astrovirus associated gastroenteritis in a children's ward, *J. Clin. Pathol.* **30**:948–952, (1977).

147. LAMBETH, L., AND MITCHELL, J. D., Transmission of human gastroenteritis virus to a monkey (abstract), *Aust. Paediatr. J.* **11**:127–128 (1975).

147a. LAPORTE, J., AND BOBULESCO, P., Growth of human

and canine enteric coronaviruses in a highly susceptible cell line: HRT 18, *Perspect. Virol.* **11**:189–193 (1981).

148. Lecce, J. G., King, M. W., and Mock, R., Reovirus-like agent associated with fatal diarrhea in neonatal pigs, *Infect. Immun.* **14**:816–825 (1976).

149. Levine, M. M., and Edelman, R., Acute diarrheal infections in infants. I. Epidemiology, treatment and prospects for immunoprophylaxis, *Hosp. Pract.* **14**:89–100 (1979).

150. Levy, A. G., Widerlite, L., Schwartz, C. J., Dolin, R., Blacklow, N. R., Gardner, J., Kimberg, D. V., and Trier, J. S., Jejunal adenylate cyclase activity in human subjects during viral gastroenteritis, *Gastroenterology* **70**:321–325 (1976).

151. Light, J. S., and Hodes, H. L., Studies on epidemic diarrhea of the newborn: Isolation of a filtrable agent causing diarrhea in calves, *Am. J. Public Health* **33**:1451–1454 (1943).

152. Madeley, C. R., Comparison of the features of astroviruses and caliciviruses, *J. Infect. Dis.* **139**:519–523 (1979).

153. Madeley, C. R., and Cosgrove, B. P., Caliciviruses in man, *Lancet* **1**:199–200 (1976).

154. Madeley, C. R., and Cosgrove, B. P., 28 nm particles in faeces in infantile gastroenteritis, *Lancet* **2**:451–452 (1975).

155. Madeley, C. R., and Cosgrove, B. P., Viruses in infantile gastroenteritis, *Lancet* **2**:124 (1975).

156. Madeley, C. R., Cosgrove, B. P., Bell, E. J., and Fallon, R. J., Stool viruses in babies in Glasgow. I. Hospital admissions with diarrhea, *J. Hyg. (Cambridge)*. **78**:261–273 (1977).

157. Maiya, P. P., Pereira, S. M., Mathan, M., Bhat, P., Albert, M. J., and Baker, J. J., Aetiology of acute gastroenteritis in infancy and early childhood in southern India, *Arch. Dis. Child.* **52**:482–485 (1977).

158. Malherbe, H. H., and Strickland-Cholmley, M., Simian viruse SA-11 and the related "O" agent, *Arch. Gesamte Virusforsch.* **22**:235–245 (1967).

159. Martin, M. L., Palmer, E. L., and Middleton, P. J., Ulstrastructure of infantile gastroenteritis virus, *Virology* **68**:146–153 (1975).

160. Mata, L., Rotavirus diarrhea in Costa Rica (abstract), 4th International Congress for Virology, The Hague, p. 469, 1978.

161. Mata, L. J., Urrutia, J. J., and Gordon, J. E., Diseases and disabilities, in: *The Children of Santa Maria Cauque: A Prospective Field Study of Health and Growth*, by L. J. Mata, pp. 254–292, The MIT Press, Cambridge, Massachusetts, and London, 1978.

162. Matsuno, S., Inouye, S., and Kono, R., Antigenic relationship between human and bovine rotaviruses as determined by neutralization, immune adherence

hemagglutination and complement-fixation tests, *Infect. Immun.* **17**:661–662 (1977).

163. Matsuno, S., Inouye, S., and Kono, R., Plaque assay of neonatal calf diarrhea virus and the neutralizing antibody in human sera, *J. Clin. Microbiol.* **5**:1–4 (1977).

164. Matsuno, S., and Nagayoshi, S., Quantitative estimation of infantile gastroenteritis virus antigens in stools by immune adherence hemagglutination test, *J. Clin. Microbiol.* **7**:310–311 (1978).

165. Matthews, R. E. F., The classification and nomenclature of viruses: Summary of results of meetings of the international committee on taxonomy of viruses in the Hague, September 1978, *Intervirology* **11**:133–135 (1979).

166. Mavromichalis, J., Evans, N., McNeish, A. S., Bryden, A. S., Davies, H. A., and Flewett, T. H., Intestinal damage in rotavirus and adenovirus gastroenteritis assessed by D-xylose malabsorption, *Arch. Dis. Child.* **52**:589–591 (1977).

167. McNulty, M. S., Allan, G. M., and Stuart, J. C., Rotavirus infection in avian species, *Vet. Rec.* **103**:319–320 (1978).

168. McNulty, M. S., Pearson, G. R., McFerran, J. B., Collins, D. S., and Allan, G. M., A reovirus like agent (rotavirus) associated with diarrhea in neonatal pigs, *Vet. Microbiol.* **1**:55–63 (1976).

168a. McSwiggan, D. A., Cubitt, D., and Moore, W., Calicivirus associated with winter disease, *Lancet* **2**:1215 (1978).

169. Mebus, C. A., Kono, M., Underdahl, N. R., and Twiehaus, M. J., Cell culture propagation of neonatal calf diarrhea (scours) virus, *Can. Vet. J.* **12**:69–72 (1971).

170. Mebus, C. A., Stair, E. L., Rhodes, M. B., and Twiehaus, M. J., Pathology of neonatal calf diarrhea induced by a coronavirus-like agent, *Vet. Pathol.* **10**:45 (1973).

171. Mebus, C. A., Torres-Medina, A., Twiehaus, M. J., and Bass, E. P., Immune response to orally administered calf reovirus-like agent and coronavirus vaccine, *Dev. Biol. Stand.* **33**:346–403 (1976).

172. Mebus, C. A., Wyatt, R. G., and Kapikian, A. Z., Intestinal lesions induced in gnotobiotic calves by the virus of human infantile gastroenteritis, *Vet. Pathol.* **14**:273–282 (1977).

173. Mebus, C. A., Wyatt, R. G., Sharpee, R. L., Sereno, M. M., Kalica, A. R., Kapikian, A. Z., and Twiehaus, M. J., Diarrhea in gnotobiotic calves caused by the reovirus-line agent of human infantile gastroenteritis, *Infect. Immun.* **14**:471–474 (1976).

174. Mebus, C. A., Underdahl, N. R., Rhodes, M. B., and Twiehaus, M. J., Calf diarrhea (scours): Reproduced with a virus from a field outbreak, *Univ. Nebraska Res. Bull.* **233**:1–16 (1969).

175. MEEROFF, J. C., SCHREIBER, D. S., TRIER, J. S., AND BLACKLOW, N. R., Abnormal gastric motor function in viral gastroenteritis, *Ann. Intern. Med.* **92**:370–373 (1980).

176. MEURMAN, O. H., AND LAINE, M. J., Rotavirus epidemic in adults, *N. Engl. J. Med.* **296**:1298–1299 (1977).

177. MIDDLETON, P. J., Analysis of the pattern of viral infection, in: Report of the 74th Ross Conference on Pediatric Research: Etiology, Pathology, and Treatment of Acute Gastroenteritis, Ponte Vedra Beach, Florida, March 20–22, 1977.

178. MIDDLETON, P. J., Pathogenesis of rotaviral infection, *J. Am. Vet. Med. Assoc.* **173**:544–546 (1978).

179. MIDDLETON, P. J., HOLDAWAY, M. D., PETRIC, M., SZYMANSKI, M. T., AND TAM, J. S., Solid-phase radioimmunoassay for the detection of rotavirus, *Infect. Immun.* **16**:439–444 (1977).

180. MIDDLETON, P. J., PETRIC, M., HEWITT, C. M., SZYMANSKI, M. T., AND TAM, J. S., Counter-immunoelectro-osmophoresis for the detection of infantile gastroenteritis virus (orbi-group) and antibody, *J. Clin. Pathol.* **29**:191–197 (1976).

181. MIDDLETON, P. J., PETRIC, M., AND SZYMANSKI, M. T., Propagation of infantile gastroenteritis virus (orbi-group) in conventional and germfree piglets, *Infect. Immun.* **12**:1276–1280 (1975).

182. MIDDLETON, P. J., SZYMANSKI, M. T., ABBOTT, G. D., BORTOLUSSI, R., AND HAMILTON, J. R., Orbivirus acute gastroenteritis of infancy, *Lancet* **1**:1241–1244 (1974).

183. MIDDLETON, P. J., SZYMANSKI, M. T., AND PETRIC, M., Viruses associated with acute gastroenteritis in young children, *Am. J. Dis. Child.* **131**:733–737 (1977).

184. MITCHELL, J. D., LAMBETH, L. A., SOSULA, L., MURPHY, A., AND ALBREY, M., Transmission of rotavirus gastroenteritis from children to a monkey, *Gut* **18**:156–160 (1977).

185. MORENS, D. M., ZWEIGHAFT, R. M., VERNON, T. M., GARY, G. W., ESLIEN, J. J., WOOD, B. T., HOLMAN, R. C., AND DOLIN, R., A waterbourne outbreak of gastroenteritis with secondary person-to-person spread association with a viral agent, *Lancet* **1**:964–966 (1979).

186. MORISHIMA, T., NAGAYOSHI, S., OZAKI, T., ISOMURA, S., AND SUZUKI, S., Immunofluorescence of human reovirus-like agent of infantile diarrhoea, *Lancet* **2**:695–696 (1976).

187. MUCH, D., AND ZAJAC, I., Purification and characterization of epizootic diarrhea of infant mice virus, *Infect. Immun.* **6**:1019–1024 (1972).

188. MURPHY, A. M., ALBREY, M. B., AND CREWE, E. B., Rotavirus infections of neonates, *Lancet* **2**:1149–1150 (1977).

189. MURPHY, A. M., GROHMANN, G. S., CHRISTOPHER, P. J., LOPEZ, W. A., AND MILLSOM, R. H., Oyster food poisoning, *Med. J. Aust.* **2**:439 (1978).

190. NALIN, D. R., LEVINE, M. M., MATA, L., DECESPEDES, C., VARGAS, W., LIZANO, C., LORIA, A. R., SIMHON, A., AND MOHS, E., Comparison of sucrose with glucose in oral therapy of infant diarrhea, *Lancet* **2**:277–279 (1978).

191. NEWMAN, J. F. E., BROWN, F., BRIDGER, J. D., AND WOODE, G. N., Characterization of a rotavirus, *Nature (London)* **258**:631–633 (1975).

192. OBIJESKI, J. F., PALMER, F. L., AND MARTIN, M. L., Biochemical characterization of infantile gastroenteritis virus (IGV), *J. Gen. Virol.* **34**:485–497 (1977).

193. OSHIRO, L. S., HALEY, C. E., ROBERTO, R. R., RIGGS, J. L., CROUGHAN, M., GREENBERG, H., AND KAPIKIAN, A., A 27 nm virus isolated during an outbreak of acute infectious nonbacterial gastroenteritis in a convalescent hospital: A possible new serotype *J. Infect. Dis.* **143**:791–795, 1981.

194. ORSTAVIK, I., FIGENSCHAU, K. J., HAUG, K. W., AND ULSTRUP, J. C., A reovirus-like agent (rotavirus) in gastroenteritis of children, *Scand. J. Infect. Dis.* **8**:1–5 (1976).

195. OSTRAVIK, I., HAUG, K. W., AND SOVDE, A., Rotavirus-associated gastroenteritis in two adults probably caused by virus reinfection, *Scand. J. Infect. Dis.* **8**:277–278 (1976).

196. PALMER, E. L., MARTIN, M. L., AND MURPHY, F. A., Morphology and stability of infantile gastroenteritis virus: Comparison with reovirus and bluetongue virus, *J. Gen. Virol.* **35**:403–414 (1977).

197. PARRINO, T. A., SCHREIBER, D. S., TRIER, J. S., KAPIKIAN, A. Z., AND BLACKLOW, N. R., Clinical immunity in acute gastroenteritis caused by the Norwalk agent, *N. Engl. J. Med.* **297**:86–89 (1977).

198. PARROTT, R. H., VARGOSKO, A. J., KIM, H. W., BELLANTI, J. A., AND CHANOCK, R. M., Myxovirus parainfluenza, *Am. J. Public Health* **52**:907–917 (1962).

199. PETERSON, M. W., SPENDLOVE, R. S., AND SMART, R. A., Detection of neonatal calf diarrhea virus, infant reovirus-like diarrhea virus and a coronavirus using the fluorescent virus precipitin test, *J. Clin. Microbiol.* **3**:376–377 (1976).

200. PETRIC, M., SZYMANSKI, M. T., AND MIDDLETON, P. J., Purification and preliminary characterization of infantile gastroenteritis virus (orbivirus group), *Intervirology* **5**:233–238 (1975).

201. PETRIC, M., TAM, J. S., AND MIDDLETON, P. J., Preliminary characterization of the nucleic acid of infantile gastroenteritis virus (orbivirus group), *Intervirology* **7**:176–180 (1976).

202. PORTNOY, B. L., CONKLIN, R. H., MENN, M., OLARTE, J., AND DUPONT, H. L., Reliable identification of reovirus-like agent in diarrheal stools, *J. Lab. Clin. Med.* **89**:560–563 (1977).

203. Public Health Service Laboratory (England), Rotavirus in rabbits, Communicable Disease Report 32 (1976).
204. Purdham, D. R., Purdham, P. A., Evans, N., and McNeish, A. S., Isolation of human rotavirus using human embryonic gut monolayers, *Lancet* **2**:977 (1975).
205. Reed, D. E., Daley, C. A., and Shave, H. J., Reovirus-like agent associated with neonatal diarrhea in pronghorn antelope, *J. Wildl. Dis.* **12**:488–491 (1976).
206. Reimann, H. A., Price, A. H., and Hodges, J. H., The cause of epidemic diarrhea, nausea and vomiting (viral dysentery?), *Proc. Soc. Exp. Biol. Med.* **59**:8–9 (1945).
207. Report of a WHO Scientific Working Group, Rotavirus and other viral diarrhoeas, *Bull. W.H.O.* **58**(2):183–198 (1980).
208. Retter, M., Middleton, P. J., Tam, J. S., and Petric, M., Enteric adenoviruses: Detection, implication and significance, *J. Clin. Microbiol.* **10**:574–578 (1979).
209. Ritchie, A. E., Deshmukh, D. R., Larsen, C. T., and Pomeroy, B. S., Electron microscopy of coronavirus-like particles characteristic of turkey bluecomb disease, *Avian Dis.* **17**:546–558 (1973).
210. Rodger, S. M., Craven, J. A., and William, I., Demonstration of reovirus-like particles in intestinal contents of piglets with diarrhea, *Aust. Vet. J.* **51**:536 (1975).
211. Rodger, S. M., Schnagl, R. D., and Holmes, I. H., Biochemical and biophysical characterization of diarrhea viruses of human and calf origin, *J. Virol.* **16**:1229–1235 (1975).
212. Rodger, S. M., Schnagl, R., and Holmes, I. H., Further biochemical characterization, including the detection of surface glucoproteins, of human, calf, and simian rotaviruses, *J. Virol.* **24**:91–98 (1977).
213. Rodriguez, W. J., Kim, H. W., Arrobio, J. O., Brandt, C. D., Chanock, R. M., Kapikian, A. Z., Wyatt, R. G., and Parrott, R. H., Clinical features of acute gastroenteritis associated with human reovirus-like agent in infants and young children, *J. Pediatr.* **91**:188–193 (1977).
214. Rodriguez, W. J., Kim, H. W., Brandt, C. D., Bise, B., Kapikian, A. Z., Chanock, R. M., Curlin, G., and Parrott, R. H., Incidence of pediatric rotavirus gastroenteritis resulting in admission to hospital in Washington, D.C. area, *Am. J. Dis. Child.* **134**:777–779 (1980).
215. Rodriguez, W. J., Kim, H. W., Brandt, C. D., Yolken, R. H., Arrobio, J. O., Kapikian, A. Z., and Chanock, R. M., Sequential enteric illnesses associated with different rotavirus serotypes, *Lancet* **2**:37 (1978).
216. Rodriguez, W. J., Kim, H. W., Brandt, C. D., Yolken, R. H., Richard, M., Arrobio, J. O., Schwartz, R. H., Kapikian, A. Z., Chanock, R. M., and Parrott, R. H., Common exposure outbreak of type 2 rotavirus gastroenteritis with high secondary attack rate within families, *J. Infect. Dis.* **140**:353–357 (1979).
217. Rohde, J. E., and Northrup, R. S., Taking science where the diarrhea is, in: *Acute Diarrhea in Childhood: Ciba Found. Symp. (new Ser.)* **42**:339–366 (1976).
218. Roseto, A., Lema, F., Sitbon, M., Cavalieri, F., Dianoux, L., and Peries, J., Detection of rotavirus in dogs, *Social Occupat. Med.* **7**:478 (1979).
219. Ryder, R. W., McGowan, J. E., Hatch, M. H., and Palmer, E. L., Reovirus-like agent as a cause of nosocomial diarrhea in infants, *J. Pediatr.* **90**:698–702 (1977).
220. Ryder, R. W., Sack, D. A., Kapikian, A. Z., McLaughlin, J. C., Chakraborty, J., Willis, J. G., Mizanur Rahman, A. S. M., and Merson, M. H., Entertotoxigenic *Escherichia coli* and reovirus-like agent in rural Bangladesh, *Lancet* **1**:659–663 (1976).
221. Sack, D. A., Chowdhury, A. M. A. K., Eusof, A., Ali, Md. A., Merson, M. H., Islam, S., Black, R. E., and Brown, K. H., A double blind comparison of sucrose with glucose electrolyte solution, *Lancet* **2**:280–283, (1978).
222. Sack, R. G., Human diarrheal disease caused by enterotoxigenic *Escherichia coli, Annu. Rev. Microbiol.* **29**:333–353 (1975).
223. Salmi, T. T., Arstila, P., and Koivikko, A., Central nervous system involvement in patients with rotavirus gastroenterititis, *Scand. J. Infect. Dis.* **10**:29–31 (1978).
223a. Sato, K., Inaba, Y., Shinozaki, T., Fujii, R., and Matumoto, M., Isolation of human rotavirus in cell cultures, *Arch. Virol.* **69**:155–160 (1981).
223b. Schaffer, F. L., Caliciviruses, in: *Comprehensive Virology, Vol. 14*, Plenum Press, New York and London, pp. 249–284, 1979.
224. Schaffer, F. L., and Soergel, M. E., Single major polypeptide of a calicivirus and characterization by polyacrylamide gel electrophoresis and stabilization of virions by cross-linking with dimethyl suberimidate, *J. Virol.* **19**:925–931 (1976).
225. Schnagl, R. D., and Holmes, I. H., Characteristics of the genome of human infantile enteritis (rotavirus) *J. Virol.* **19**:267–270 (1976).
226. Schnagl, R., Holmes, I. H., Moore, B., Lee, P., Dickinson-Jones, F., and Gust, I. D., An extensive rotavirus outbreak in aboriginal infants in Central Australia, *Med. J. Aust.* **1**:259–260 (1977).
227. Schoub, B. D., Koornof, J. H., Lecatsas, G., Prozesky, O. W., Freiman, I., Hartman, E., and Kassel, H., Viruses in acute summer gastroenteritis in black infants, *Lancet* **1**:1093–1094 (1975).
228. Schoub, B. D., Nel, J. D., Lecatsas, G., Greef, A.

S., Prozesky, O. W., Hay, I. T., and Prinsloo, J. G., Rotavirus as a cause of gastroenteritis in black South African infants, *South Afr. Med. J.* **50**:1124 (1976).

229. Schreiber, D. S., Blacklow, N. R., and Trier, J. S., The mucosal lesion of the proximal small intestine in acute infectious nonbacterial gastroenteritis, *N. Engl. J. Med.* **288**:1318–1323 (1973).

230. Schreiber, D. S., Blacklow, N. R., and Trier, J. S., The small intestinal lesion induced by Hawaii agent acute infectious nonbacterial gastroenteritis, *J. Infect. Dis.* **129**:705–708 (1974).

231. Scott, A. C., Luddington, J., Lucas, M., and Gilbert, F. R., Rotavirus in goats, *Vet. Rec.* **103**:145 (1978).

231. Sharpee, R., and Mebus, C. A., Rotaviruses (sic) of man and animals, *Lancet* **1**:639 (1975).

233. Shinozaki, T., Fujii, R., Sato, K., Takahashi, E., Ito, Y., and Inaba, Y., Hemagglutinin from human reovirus-like agent, *Lancet* **1**:878 (1978).

234. Simhon, A., and Mata, L., Anti-rotavirus antibody in human colostrum, *Lancet* **1**:39–40 (1978).

235. Snodgrass, D. R., Angus, K. W., and Gray, E. W., A rotavirus from kittens, *Vet. Rec.* **104**:222–223 (1979).

236. Snodgrass, D. R., and Gray, E. W., Detection and transmission of 30 nm virus particles (astroviruses) in faeces of lambs with diarrhea, *Arch. Virol.* **55**:287–291 (1977).

237. Snodgrass, D. R., Madeley, C. R., Wells, P. W., and Angus, K. W., Human rotavirus in lambs: Infection and passive protection, *Infect. Immun.* **16**:268–270 (1977).

238. Snodgrass, D. R., Smith, W., Gray, E. W., and Herring, J. A., A rotavirus in lambs with diarrhea, *Res. Vet. Sci.* **20**:113–114 (1976).

239. Snodgrass, D. R., and Wells, P. W., Rotavirus infection in lambs: Studies on passive protection, *Arch. Virol.* **52**:201–205 (1976).

240. Spence, L., Fauvel, M., Bouchard, S., Babiuk, L., and Saunders, J. R., Test for reovirus-like agent, *Lancet* **2**:322 (1975).

241. Spence, L., Fauvel, M., Petro, R., and Bloch, S., Comparison of counterimmunoelectrophoresis and electron microscopy for laboratory diagnosis of human reovirus-like agent-associated infantile gastroenteritis, *J. Clin. Microbiol.* **5**:248–249 (1977).

242. Spence, L., Fauvel, M., Petro, R., and Bloch, S., Hemagglutinin from rotavirus, *Lancet* **2**:1023 (1976).

243. Spendlove, R. S., Reoviridae: Rotavirus, in *Section H: Virology and Rickettsiology* (G. D. Hsuing and R. H. Green, sect. eds.), *Handbook Series in Clinical Laboratory Science* (D. Seligson, ed.-in-chief), pp. 251–265, CRC Press, West Palm Beach, Florida, 1978.

243a. Spratt, H. C., Park, M. I., Gomersall, M., Gill, P., and Pai, C. H., Nosocomial infantile gastroenteritis

associated with minirotavirus and calicivirus, *J. Pediatr.* **93**:922–926 (1978).

244. Stair, E. L., Rhodes, M. B., White, R. G., and Mebus, C. A., Neonatal calf diarrhea: Purification and electron microscopy of a coronavirus-like agent, *Am. J. Vet. Res.* **33**:1147–1156 (1972).

245. Steinhoff, M. C., Douglas, R. G., Jr., Greenberg, H. B., and Callahan, D. R., Bismuth subsalicylate therapy of viral gastroenteritis, *Gastroenterology* (in press).

246. Stintzing, G., Tufvesson, B., Habte, D., Back, E., Johnsson, T., and Wadstrom, T., Aetiology of acute diarrhoeal disease in infancy and childhood during the peak season Addis Ababa 1977: A preliminary report, *Ethiop. Med. J.* **15**:141–146 (1977).

247. Stuker, G., Oshiro, L., and Schmidt, N. H., Antigenic comparisons of two new rotaviruses from rhesus monkeys, *J. Clin. Microbiol.* **11**:202–203 (1980).

248. Suzuki, H., and Konno, T., Reovirus-like particles in jejunal mucosa of a Japanese infant with acute infectious non-bacterial gastroenteritis, *Tohoku J. Exp. Med.* **115**:119–211 (1975).

249. Suzuki, H., Konno, T., Kutsuzawa, T., Imai, A., Tazawa, F.; and Ishida, N., The occurrence of caliciviruses in infants with acute gastroenteritis, *J. Med. Virol.* **4**:321–326 (1979).

250. Szmuness, W., Dienstag, J. L., Purcell, R. H., Harle, E. J., Stevens, C. E., and Wong, D. C., Distribution of antibody to hepatitis A antigen in urban adult populations, *N. Engl. J. Med.* **295**:755–759 (1976).

251. Szmuness, W., Dienstag, J. L., Purcell, R. H., Stevens, C. E., Wong, D. C., Ikram, H., Bar-Shany, S., Beasley, R. P., Desmyter, J., and Gaon, J. A., The prevalence of antibody to hepatitis A antigen in various parts of the world: A pilot study, *Am. J. Epidemiol.* **106**:392–398 (1977).

252. Tallett, S., MacKenzie, C., Middleton, P., Kerzner, B., and Hamilton, R., Clinical, laboratory, and epidemiological features of a viral gastroenteritis in infants and children, *Pediatrics* **60**:217–222 (1977).

253. Tam, J. S., Szymanski, M. T., Middleton, P. J., and Petric, M., Studies on the particles of infantile gastroenteritis virus (orbivirus group), *Intervirology* **7**:181–191 (1976).

254. Theil, K. W., Bohl, E. H., and Agnes, A. G., Cell culture propagation of porcine rotavirus (reovirus-like agent), *Am. J. Vet. Res.* **28**:1765–1768 (1977).

255. Thornhill, T. S., Kalica, A. R., Wyatt, R. G., Kapikian, A. Z., and Chanock, R. M., Pattern of shedding of the Norwalk particle in stools during experimentally induced gastroenteritis in volunteers as determined by immune electron microscopy, *J. Infect. Dis.* **132**:28–34 (1975).

256. Thornhill, T. S., Wyatt, R. G., Kalica, A. R.,

DOLIN, R., CHANOCK, R. M., AND KAPIKIAN, A. Z., Detection by immune electron microscopy of 26–27 nm virus-like particles associated with two family outbreaks of gastroenteritis, *J. Infect. Dis.* **135**:20–27 (1977).

257. THOULESS, M. E., BRYDEN, A. S., AND FLEWETT, T. H., Rotavirus neutralization by human milk, *Br. Med. J.* **2**:1390 (1977).

258. THOULESS, M. E., BRYDEN, A. S., AND FLEWETT, T. H., Serotypes of human rotavirus, *Lancet* **1**:39 (1978).

259. THOULESS, M. E., BRYDEN, A. S., FLEWETT, T. H., WOODE, G. N., BRIDGER, J. C., SNODGRASS, G. R., AND HERRING, J. A., Serological relationships between rotaviruses from different species as studied by complement-fixation and neutralization, *Arch. Virol.* **53**:287–294 (1977).

260. TODD, D., AND MCNULTY, M. S., Biochemical studies on a reovirus-like agent (rotavirus) from lambs, *J. Virol.* **21**:1215–1218 (1977).

261. TORRES-MEDINA, A., WYATT, R. G., MEBUS, C. A., UNDERDAHL, N. R., AND KAPIKIAN, A. Z., Diarrhea in gnotobiotic piglets caused by the human reovirus-like agent of infantile gastroenteritis, *J. Infect. Dis.* **133**:22–27 (1976).

262. TORRES-MEDINA, A., WYATT, R. G., UNDERDAHL, N. R., AND KAPIKIAN, A. Z., Patterns of shedding of human reovirus-like agent in gnotobiotic newborn piglets with experimentally-induced diarrhea, *Intervirology* **7**:250–255 (1976).

263. TOTTERDELL, B. M., CHRYSTIE, I. L., AND BANATVALA, J. E., Rotavirus infections in a maternity unit, *Arch. Dis. Child.* **51**:924–928 (1976).

264. TUFVESSON, B., AND JOHNSSON, T., Immunoelectroosmophoresis for detection of reo-like virus: Methodology and comparison with electron microscopy, *Acta Pathol. Microbiol. Scand B* **84**:225–228 (1976).

265. TUFVESSON, B., AND JOHNSSON, T., Occurrence of reo-like viruses in young children with acute gastroenteritis, *Acta Pathol. Microbiol. Scand. B* **84**:22–28 (1976).

266. TUFVESSON, B., JOHNSON, T., AND PETERSON, B., Family infections by reo-like virus, *Scand. J. Infect. Dis.* **9**:257–261 (1977).

267. TZIPORI, S., Human rotavirus in young dogs, *Med. J. Austr.* **2**:922–923 (1977).

268. TZIPORI, S., CAPLE, I. W., AND BUTLER, R., Isolation of a rotavirus from deer, *Vet. Rec.* **99**:398 (1976).

269. URASAWA, S., TANIGUCHI, K., URASAWA, T., SAKURADA, N., KAWAMURA, S., AND AKATSUKA, K., Virus particle detected in an institutional outbreak of acute gastroenteritis, *Igaku no Ayumi* **109**(1):25–27 (1979).

270. VIERA DE TORRES, B., MAZZALI DE ILJA, R., AND ESPARZA, J., Epidemiological agents of rotavirus infection in hospitalized Venezuelan children with gastroenteritis, *Am. J. Trop. Med. Hyg.* **27**:567–572 (1978).

271. WALSH, J. A., AND WARREN, K. S., Selective primary health care and interim strategy for disease control in developing countries, *N. Engl. J. Med.* **301**:967–974 (1979).

272. WHORWELL, P. J., PHILLIPS, C. A., BEEKEN, W. L., LITTLE, P. K., AND ROESSNER, K. D., Isolation of reovirus-like virus agents from patients with Crohn's disease, *Lancet* **1**:1169–1171 (1977).

273. WIDERLITE, L., TRIER, J. S., BLACKLOW, N. R., AND SCHREIBER, D. S., Structure of the gastric mucosa in acute infectious nonbacterial gastroenteritis, *Gastroenterology* **68**:425–430 (1975).

274. WILLIAMS, T., BOURKE, P., AND GURWITH, M., Program abstracts, 15th Interscience Conference on Antimicrobial Agents and Chemotherapy, Washington, D.C. (Abstr 234), p. 232, 1975.

275. WOODE, G. N., AND BRIDGER, J. C., Isolation of small viruses resembling astroviruses and caliciviruses from acute enteritis of calves, *J. Med. Microbiol.* **11**:441–452 (1978).

276. WOODE, G. N., BRIDGER, J. C., HALL, G., AND DENNIS, M. J., The isolation of a reovirus-like agent associated with diarrhea in colostrum-deprived calves in Great Britain, *Res. Vet. Sci.* **16**:102–105 (1974).

277. WOODE, G. N., BRIDGER, J., HALL, G. A., JONES, J. M., AND JACKSON, G., The isolation of reoviruslike agents (rotavirus) from acute gastroenteritis of piglets, *J. Med. Microbiol.* **9**:203–209 (1976).

278. WOODE, G. N., BRIDGER, J. C., JONES, J. M., FLEWETT, T. H., BRYDEN, A. S., DAVIES, H. A., AND WHITE, G. B. B., Morphological and antigenic relationships between viruses (rotaviruses) from acute gastroenteritis of children, calves, piglets, mice, and foals, *Infect. Immun.* **14**:804–810 (1976).

279. WOODE, G. N., JONES, J., AND BRIDGER, J., Levels of colostral antibodies against neonatal calf diarrhoea virus, *Vet. Rec.* **97**:148–149 (1975).

280. WORLD HEALTH ORGANIZATION, Mortality due to diarrheal diseases in the world *Weekly Epidemiol. Rec.* **48**:409–416 (1973).

281. WYATT, R. G., Unpublished studies.

282. WYATT, R. G., DOLIN, R., BLACKLOW, N. R., DUPONT, H. L., BUSCHO, R. F., THORNHILL, T. S., KAPIKIAN, A. Z., AND CHANOCK, R. M., Comparison of three agents of acute infectious nonbacterial gastroenteritis by cross-challenge in volunteers, *J. Infect. Dis.* **129**:709–714 (1974).

283. WYATT, R. G., GILL, V. W., SERENO, M. M., KALICA, A. R., VAN KIRK, D. H., CHANOCK, R. M., AND KAPIKIAN, A. Z., Probable *in vitro* cultivation of human reovirus-like agent of infantile diarrhea, *Lancet* **1**:98 (1976).

284. WYATT, R. G., GREENBERG, H. B., DALGARD, D. W., ALLEN, W. P., SLY, D. L., THORNHILL, T. S., CHANOCK, R. M., AND KAPIKIAN, A. Z., Experimental infection of chimpanzees with the Norwalk agent of

epidemic viral gastroenteritis, *J. Med. Virol.* **2**:89–96 1978.

285. WYATT, R. G., JAMES, W. D., BOHL, E. H., THEIL, K. W., SAIF, L. J., KALICA, A. R., GREENBERG, H. B., KAPIKIAN, A. Z., AND CHANOCK, R. M., Human rotavirus type 2: Cultivation *in vitro, Science* **207**:189–191 (1980).

286. WYATT, R. G., KALICA, A. R., MEBUS, C. A., KIM, H. W., LONDON, W. T., CHANOCK, R. M., AND KAPIKIAN, A. Z., Reovirus-like agents (rotaviruses) associated with diarrheal illness in animals and man, *Perspect. Virol.* **10**:121–145 (1978).

287. WYATT, R. G., AND KAPIKIAN, A. Z., Viral agents associated with acute gastroenteritis in humans, *Am. J. Clin. Nutr.* **30**:1857–1870 (1977).

288. WYATT, R. G., KAPIKIAN, A. Z., THORNHILL, T. S., SERENO, M. M., KIM, H. W., AND CHANOCK, R. M., *In vitro* cultivation in human fetal intestinal organ culture of a reovirus-like agent associated with nonbacterial gastroenteritis in infants and children, *J. Infect. Dis.* **130**:523–528 (1974).

289. WYATT, R. G., MEBUS, C. A., YOLKEN, R. H., KALICA, A. R., JAMES, H. D., JR., KAPIKIAN, A. Z., AND CHANOCK, R. M., Rotaviral immunity in gnotobiotic calves: Heterologous resistance to human virus induced by bovine virus, *Science* **203**:548–550 (1979).

290. WYATT, R. G., SLY, D. L., LONDON, W. T., PALMER, A. E., KALICA, A. R., VAN KIRK, D. H., CHANOCK, R. M., AND KAPIKIAN, A. Z., Induction of diarrhea in colostrum-deprived newborn rhesus monkeys with the human reovirus-like agent of infantile gastroenteritis, *Arch. Viol.* **50**:17–27 (1976).

291. WYATT, R. G., YOLKEN, R. H., URRUTIA, J. J., MATA, L., GREENBERG, H. B., CHANOCK, R. M., AND KAPIKIAN, A. Z., Diarrhea associated with rotavirus in rural Guatemala: A longitudinal study of 24 infants and young children, *Am. J. Trop. Med. Hyg.* **28**:325–328 (1979).

292. YAMAMOTO, A., ZENNYGOGI, H., YANAGITA, K., AND KATO, S., Research into the causative agent of epidemic gastroenteritis which prevailed in Japan in 1948, *Jpn. Med. J.* **1**:379–384 (1948).

293. YOLKEN, R. H., BARBOUR, B., WYATT, R. G., KALICA, A. R., KAPIKIAN, A. Z., AND CHONICK, R. M., Enzyme-linked immunosorbent assay (ELISA) for identification of rotaviruses from different animal species, *Science* **201**:259–262 (1978).

294. YOLKEN, R. H., KIM, H. W., CLEM, T., WYATT, R. G., KALICA, A. R., CHANOCK, R. M., AND KAPIKIAN, A. Z., Enzyme linked immunosorbent assay (ELISA) for detection of human reovirus-like agent of infantile gastroenteritis, *Lancet* **2**:263–267 (1977).

295. YOLKEN, R. H., WYATT, R. G., MATA, L., URRUTIA, J. J., GARCIA, B., CHANOCK, R. M., AND KAPIKIAN, A. Z., Secretory antibody directed against rotavirus in human milk—measurement by means of enzyme linked immunosorbent assay, *J. Pediatr.* **93**:916–921 (1978).

296. YOLKEN, R. H., AND STOPA, P. J., Analysis of nonspecific reactions in enzyme-linked immunosorbent assay testing for human rotavirus, *J. Clin. Microbiol.* **10**:703–707 (1979).

297. YOLKEN, R. H., AND STOPA, P. J., Enzyme-linked fluorescence assay: Ultrasensitive solid-phase assay for detection of human rotavirus, *J. Clin. Microbiol.* **10**:317–321 (1979).

298. YOLKEN, R. H., WYATT, R. G., BARBOUR, B. A., KIM, H. W., KAPIKIAN, A. Z., AND CHANOCK, R. M., Measurement of anti-rotavirus antibody by an enzyme-linked immunosorbent (ELISA) blocking assay, *J. Clin. Microbiol.* **8**:283–287 (1978).

299. YOLKEN, R. H., WYATT, R. G., KALICA, A. R., KIM, H. W., BRANDT, C. D., PARROTT, R. H., KAPIKIAN, A. Z., AND CHANOCK, M. R., Use of a free viral immunofluorescence assay to detect human reovirus-like agent in human stools, *Infect. Immun.* **16**:467–470 (1977).

300. YOLKEN, R. H., WYATT, R. G., AND KAPIKIAN, A. Z., ELISA for rotavirus, *Lancet* **2**:818 (1977).

301. YOLKEN, R. H., WYATT, R. G., KIM, H. W., KAPIKIAN, A. Z., AND CHANOCK, R. M., Immunological response to infection with human reovirus-like agent: Measurement of anti-human reovirus-like agent immunoglobulin G and M levels by the method of enzyme-linked immunosorbent assay, *Infect. Immun.* **19**:540–546 (1978).

302. YOLKEN, R. H., WYATT, R. G., ZISSIS, G. P., BRANDT, C. D., RODRIGUEZ, W. J., KIM, H. W., PARROTT, R. H., URRUTIA, J. J., MATA, L., GREENBERG, H. B., KAPIKIAN, A. Z., AND CHANOCK, R. M., Epidemiology of human rotavirus types 1 and 2 as studied by enzyme-linked immunosorbent assay, *N. Engl. J. Med.* **299**:1156–1161 (1978).

302a. ZAHORSKY, J., Hyperemesis hiemis or the winter vomiting disease, *Arch. Pediatr.* **46**:391–395 (1929).

303. ZISSIS, G., AND LAMBERT, J. P., Different serotypes of human rotaviruses, *Lancet* **1**:38–39 (1978).

304. ZISSIS, G., LAMBERT, J. P., AND DE KEGEL, D., Routine diagnosis of human rotavirus in stools, *J. Clin. Pathol.* **31**:175–178 (1978).

305. ZISSIS, G., LAMBERT, J. P., FONTEYNE, J., AND DE KEGEL, D., Child–mother transmission of rotavirus, *Lancet* **1**:96 (1976).

12. Suggested Reading

BRANDT, C. D., KIM, H. W., YOLKEN, R. H., KAPIKIAN, A. S., ARROBIO, J. O., RODRIGUEZ, W. J., WYATT, R. G., CHANOCK, R. M., AND PARROTT, R. H., Comparative epidemiology of two rotavirus serotypes and other viral agents associated with pediatric gastroenteritis, *Am. J. Epidemiol.* **110**:243–254 (1979).

EDELMAN, R., AND LEVINE, M. M., Acute diarrheal infections in infants. II. Bacterial and viral causes, *Hosp. Pract.* **15**:97–104 (1980).

GREENBERG, H. B., WYATT, R. G., KALICA, A. R., YOLKEN, R. H., BLACK, R., KAPIKIAN, A. Z., AND CHANOCK, R. M., New insights in viral gastroenteritis, *Perspect. Virology* **11**:163–187 (1981).

HOLMES, I. H., Viral gastroenteritis, *Prog. Med. Virol.* **25**:1–36 (1979).

KAPIKIAN, A. Z., WYATT, R. G., GREENBERG, H. B., KALICA, A. R., KIM, H. W., BRANDT, C. D., RODRIGUEZ, W. J., PARROTT, R. H., AND CHANOCK, R. M., Approaches to immunization of infants and young children against gastroenteritis due to rotaviruses, *Rev. Infect. Dis.* **2**:459–469 (1980).

KAPIKIAN, A. S., YOLKEN, R. H., GREENBERG, H. B., WYATT. R. G., KALICA, A. R., CHANOCK, R. M., AND KIM, H. W., Gastroenteritis viruses, in: *Diagnostic Procedures for Viral, Rickettsial, and Chlamydial Infections,* 5th ed. (E. H. LENNETTE AND N. J. SCHMIDT, eds.), pp. 927–995, American Public Health Association, Washington, D.C., 1979.

SPENDLOVE, R. S., Reoviridae: Rotavirus, in: *Section H: Virology and Rickettsiology* (G. D. HSUING AND R. H. GREEN, sect. eds.), *Handbook Series in Clinical Laboratory Science* (D. SELIGSON, ed.-in-chief), pp. 251–265, CRC Press, West Palm Beach, Florida, 1978.

YOLKEN, R. H., WYATT, R. G., ZISSIS, G. P., BRANDT, C. D., RODRIGUEZ, W. J., KIM, H. W., PARROTT, R. H., URRUTIA, J. J., MATA, L., GREENBERG, H. B., KAPIKIAN, A. Z., AND CHANOCK, R. M., Epidemiology of human rotavirus types 1 and 2 as studied by enzyme-linked immunosorbent assay, *N. Engl. J. Med.* **299**:1156–1161 (1978).

Viral Hepatitis

Robert W. McCollum

1. Introduction

Evidence of acute inflammation of the liver may be observed in association with infections due to a number of different viruses, e.g., members of the herpesvirus group, yellow fever virus, coxsackieviruses, mumps virus, and a group of exotic viruses.[162] The term "viral hepatitis," however, is usually reserved for those infections due to one of at least three or more different and distinct agents collectively referred to as hepatitis viruses. These include the well-characterized hepatitis A virus (HAV) and hepatitis B virus (HBV), associated with, respectively, viral hepatitis type A (previously infectious hepatitis) and viral hepatitis type B (serum hepatitis), and the less well-defined non-A, non-B hepatitis virus(es). The clinical manifestations of these infections are sufficiently similar so that until recently, the differential diagnosis of the individual case rested almost entirely on epidemiological information or inference. Several specific serological tests are now available for diagnostic and epidemiological studies of both type A and type B infections. Diagnosis of non-A, non-B hepatitis is still based on exclusion rather than specific serological tests, but the rapid and sustained developments in hepatitis research during the past ten years give promise for early resolution of this remaining area of confusion.

Robert W. McCollum · Department of Epidemiology and Public Health, Yale University School of Medicine, New Haven, Connecticut.

2. Historical Background

The earliest descriptions of hepatitis (epidemic jaundice) are usually attributed to Hippocrates. More detailed observations were not recorded until the 17th and 18th centuries, when outbreaks of jaundice were noted particularly in association with military campaigns. For example, there were more than 70,000 cases of epidemic jaundice, presumed to be infectious (type A) hepatitis, during the Civil War. However, the infectious character of the disease was not recognized or widely accepted until the early part of the 20th century. Efforts to identify specific bacterial, leptospiral, and other possible etiological agents repeatedly met with total failure or spurious findings and ultimate lack of confirmation. By the beginning of World War II, however, sufficient evidence had been accumulated to support the probable existence of at least two distinct types of hepatitis, both of viral etiology but with apparently different epidemiological features. The military significance of hepatitis was given special emphasis by the recognition of a massive epidemic of over 40,000 cases of type B in association with yellow fever vaccine and repeated encounters with type A in Africa, the Mediterranean littoral, and other major areas of combat. These events stimulated an increase of research efforts, particularly in England and the United States, beginning in the early 1940s and continuing through the next decade. Repeated failures in attempts to find susceptible experimental animals or other laboratory methods for isolation and propagation of the etiological agents led to the initiation of controlled human-transmission studies that firmly established the basic etiological and epidemiological distinctions between type A (infectious) and type B (serum) hepatitis, the lack of cross-immunity, and the broad clinical spectrum of manifestations of infection.

After World War II, hepatitis, presumed to be mostly type B, followed in the wake of widespread civilian applications of developments in blood-banking technology and plasma fractionation that had been stimulated in large part by military medical needs. In addition, both sporadic cases and common-source outbreaks of hepatitis, presumed to be mostly type A, were recognized and reported with increasing frequency in many countries. The rising incidence appeared to be following a pattern previously noted in Scandinavian countries. This recognition of viral hepatitis as a major worldwide medical and public-health problem served as a continuing stimulus for research directed particularly at virological and serological methods for diagnosis and study. The rapidly developing tissue-culture technology of the 1950s disappointingly failed to provide the anticipated answers to long-standing questions about hepatitis viruses. However, limited human-transmission studies, particularly those of Krugman and his associates,[66] continued to add significantly to our knowledge of the natural behavior of viral hepatitis, including measures for its control and certain characteristics of the viruses. A landmark finding was the first clear demonstration of nonparenteral transmission of HBV.[67]

A new era in viral hepatitis research and understanding was opened with the discovery of Australia antigen [now designated hepatitis B surface antigen (HBsAg)] by Blumberg et al.[13,14] and the subsequent recognition by Prince[104] and others[42,96] of its specific relationship to type B viral hepatitis. This single discovery provided the essential key to many long-standing hepatitis riddles and served to initiate an intensive worldwide hepatitis research effort that still continues. Some of the early findings led almost immediately to significant specific control measures in relation to parenteral transmission of type B, particularly by blood transfusion, and to current field testing of specific vaccines.

The success with HBV also served to stimulate a renewed interest in pursuing the elusive HAV. Confirmation of earlier reports[30,79] of its propagation in marmosets, its identification by immune electron microscopy (IEM),[38] and the development of sero-

logical methods for measuring specific antibodies[86,108,109] rapidly opened the way for definitive studies of HAV infections and epidemiology. A more recent report of its adaptation to cell cultures[107] has provided a basis for optimism concerning future vaccine development.

With the capability of specific serological diagnoses of both type A and type B, it soon became apparent that a residue of illnesses characteristic of viral hepatitis must be due to other agents. These are now collectively referred to as non-A, non-B viruses and are believed to consist of at least two distinct members awaiting definitive characterization and designation.

3. Methodology Involved in Epidemiological Analysis

3.1. Mortality

Both HAV and HBV (and presumably non-A, non-B) infections generally have low clinical manifestation rates and relatively low case-fatality rates, so that mortality ascribed to hepatitis viruses is a poor indicator of disease incidence or overall infection rates. Furthermore, the special features that attend a higher mortality, such as older age, concomitant disease, and immunosuppression, make death rates unrepresentative of the usual epidemiological features. Also, there are problems in differential diagnosis and proper assignment to the rubrics provided under the International Classification of Disease.

3.2. Morbidity

Although some designation for viral hepatitis is included in the lists of notifiable diseases for most countries, type A and type B are still not officially reported separately in the majority. Even in those that provide for this distinction, the figures are available for only a few years at most, and their reliability is likely to be relatively poor. Only about one third of the countries report cases by age and sex. Indeed, overall reporting of viral hepatitis from the public-health viewpoint is so widely variable in both practice and efficiency that strict comparisons of data from different geographic areas or political units are likely to be unrewarding or even misleading.

While the limitations of both morbidity and mortality reporting are widely recognized, various patterns and trends can be discerned that are probably fair and reasonable indicators of the overall collective behavior of hepatitis. Data derived from hospital-discharge diagnoses or from intensive surveys of limited population groups may provide useful information and answers to specific questions, but they are unlikely to be representative of the hepatitis problem in general. Increasing availability and use of specific serological tests for diagnostic and epidemiological studies will provide a more reliable basis for reporting and comparative purposes.

3.3. Serological Surveys

Following the general acceptance of two major forms of hepatitis due to distinct viruses and the existence of unrecognized carriers, research in the 1940s included efforts to devise serological tests even in the absence of known viral antigens. In retrospect, it now appears that several investigators may have observed hepatitis-B-specific antigen–antibody reactions that were not successfully established by confirmatory studies. Others pursued the use of various biochemical tests of liver function, serum enzyme assays, as hepatitis markers for both diagnostic and epidemiological purposes, including blood-donor screening and transmission studies. Single-sample surveys rarely provided much helpful epidemiological information or insight, but serial determinations of enzyme levels have proved to be valuable for the intensive study of small populations exposed to infection with any type of hepatitis virus. Currently, such continued surveillance serves to identify non-A, non-B hepatitis following transfusion and among patients and staff members of dialysis units.

3.3.1. Background. The discovery in serum of the 20-nm Australia antigen particles by Blumberg et al.[13] and recognition of their specific relationship to type B hepatitis[104] provided the first basis for seroepidemiological studies of viral hepatitis. It also offered the first clues leading to the identification of the HBV itself, a 42-nm double-shelled spherical structure described by Dane et al.[29] in 1970. The core and surface were found to be antigenically distinct,[4] with "Australia" antigen particles appearing to represent excess production of free surface components. Within the next few years, serological studies revealed a common surface antigen (a) and an increasingly complex variety of antigenic subdeterminants. Those that are primarily associated with the surface component and are apparently coded for by the virus genome (d,y; r, w[1,2,3,4]) may serve as useful markers for epidemiological implications and investigations. Others (e,[1,2,3] and Δ) have both prognostic and epidemiological significance. Depending on their specific purposes, serological surveys may involve single or multiple antigenic or antibody measurements, or both, many of which are not routinely available

To date, there appears to be only one serotype of HAV with no recognized antigenic subdeterminants. Since circulating viral antigens cannot be readily detected except in limited infectivity studies, serological surveys are restricted to the measurement of antibodies.

Although infectivity and cross-challenge experiments in animals have demonstrated some diversity among agents derived from cases of non-A, non-B hepatitis, the current lack of well-documented viruses or tests for specific antibodies precludes serological surveys.

3.3.2. Terminology of Viral Hepatitis. In an attempt to bring some order into the complexity of terminology of the hepatitis viruses, antigens, and antibodies, the Committee on Viral Hepatitis of the National Research Council–National Academy of Sciences suggested a system of nomenclature and abbreviations in 1974.[27] This has subsequently been modified and extended in the report on an Expert Committee of the World Health Organization,[161] on which the following outline is based:

Hepatitis A: A disease due to infection with hepatitis A virus.

HAV	Hepatitis A virus; a small virus in the range of 25–28 nm possessing cubic symmetry.
anti-HAV	Antibody to hepatitis A virus.

Hepatitis B: A disease due to infection with hepatitis B virus.

HBV	Hepatitis B virus; a 42-nm double-shelled virus, originally known as the Dane particle.
HBsAg	Hepatitis B surface antigen; the hepatitis B antigen found on the surface of the virus and on the accompanying unattached spherical (22-nm) and tubular

particles, originally known as Australia antigen. At least eight distinct subtypes of HBsAg are recognized. Their alphabetical designations, if given, are indicated following a slash (/), e.g., HBsAg/adr.

HBcAg   Hepatitis B core antigen; the hepatitis B antigen found within the core of the virus.

HBeAg   The e antigen that is closely associated with hepatitis B infection.

anti-HBs   Antibody to hepatitis B surface antigen.

anti-HBc   Antibody to hepatitis B core antigen.

anti-HBe   Antibody to the e antigen.

Chronic carriers: Subjects in whom HBsAg has been found to circulate for more than 6 months.

Non-A, non-B hepatitis: A form of hepatitis that is not due to infection with HAV, HBV, or other known human viruses (such as Epstein–Barr virus and cytomegalovirus) that may cause hepatitis as part of a generalized infection.

The etiological agent or agents of this disease are unknown.

3.4. Laboratory Methods

A variety of biochemical tests that are indicative of hepatocellular damage with varying degrees of specificity are routinely used as the basis for both the diagnosis and the clinical management of viral hepatitis. With the exception of well-defined instances of common-source or limited-contact spread, these tests have not proved to be useful for epidemiological studies.

The quest for feasible methods for routine laboratory isolation and propagation of human hepatitis viruses is still far from being satisfactorily resolved. Certain species of marmosets are susceptible to infection with HAV, and chimpanzees are readily infected with HAV, HBV, and some non-A, non-B agents. However, the scarcity and expense of marmosets and chimpanzees impose severe restrictions on their availability and use. The recent adaptation of one marmoset-passaged strain of HAV to two different cell-culture systems[107] and unconfirmed reports of the direct isolation of HAV from human fecal specimens offer hope for this to become a routine viral diagnostic method. The cultivation of an HBsAg- (but not HBV-)producing continuous cell

line derived from a human hepatocellular carcinoma[76] has led to a renewed search for normal or malignant cell cultures susceptible to infection with HBV.

Both diagnostic and epidemiological studies of hepatitis are still dominated by serological methods related to HBV, although there have been significant developments in methods related to the detection of anti-HAV. Commercial reagents for both are becoming increasingly available and practical, but because of their wide array and their cost, most clinical and research laboratories will have to be selective.

3.4.1. Viral Hepatitis A. Following the detection of HAV in fecal extracts and their partial purification, it became possible to detect serum anti-HAV by IEM.[33] Subsequently, using viral antigen derived from the livers of marmosets, the far less cumbersome complement-fixation (CF) test[109] and the more sensitive immune adherence hemagglutination assay (IAHA)[86] were introduced. Even more sensitive radioimmunoassay (RIA)[110] and enzyme-linked immunosorbent assay (ELISA)[80] techniques have been developed. Comparisons and details of these methods have been reviewed by Dienstag *et al.*[35] Most RIA and ELISA tests detect both IgG and IgM and become positive at the onset of disease. IAHA tests appear to detect mostly IgM, so that the results become positive somewhat later in the course of infection. Such comparative results can be helpful for differential diagnosis in the acute phase of illness even when only a single serum sample is available. An IgM-specific RIA test system[18] should serve the same purpose.

3.4.2. Viral Hepatitis B. There are numerous methods readily and routinely available for the detection and measurement of HBsAg and anti-HBs. HBsAg was first detected by a method using agar-gel immunodiffusion (AGD). Although considered to be a relatively insensitive method as compared to techniques developed subsequently, AGD is still the only method that provides the high degree of specificity needed for reference purposes and for the identity of new HBsAg subtypes. A variety of tests employing techniques of counterelectrophoresis (CEP) or CF were found to be more sensitive than AGD and are still used in many settings for diagnosis and screening. However, they are being rapidly replaced by more sensitive red-cell agglutination (RCA) tests employing antibody-coated stabilized human or fowl[22] erythrocytes and RIA methods utilizing ^{125}I-labeled anti-HBs.[74,157] Reagents for both RCA and RIA tests are commercially available. While RIA is the more sensitive and objective method of the two, it requires expensive equipment and the reagents have a relatively short shelf life. The most recent test entry, also commercially available, is the ELISA.[160] It has a relatively long shelf life and involves no radioactivity. Its sensitivity appears to compare favorably with that of RIA.

AGD, CEP, and CF methods may also be used to detect anti-HBs, but they are all relatively insensitive and are no longer recommended for diagnostic or survey purposes. The more commonly used and commercially available tests are passive hemagglutination (PHA)[156] using HBsAg-coated erythrocytes, RIA,[101] and radioimmunoprecipitation (RIP).[71] RIA is perhaps the most sensitive test, but PHA offers the quantitative advantage of an endpoint titration result.

Antigentic subtypes of HBsAg were first demonstrated using AGD. This method is still the only one that can provide the fine degree of discrimination needed to distinguish the full range of recognized variants.[73] The necessary reference reagents for such studies are severely limited in quantity and distribution. However, reagents for determining the major subtypes (d,y; w,r) by RIA are available commercially. The determination of subtype-specific anti-HBs is currently impractical for clinical or epidemiological studies.

There are no routine methods for measuring circulating free HBcAg. Its detection after detergent treatment of serum as well as detection of specific DNA polymerase[60] are indicative directly of circulating HBV and indirectly of active viral replication in the hepatocytes and of infectivity. However, measurement of anti-HBc may provide the same information. Since anti-HBc appears before anti-HBs, it may serve as a marker of recent infection.[55] Several tests[41] for anti-HBc have been developed, but they are not yet widely used. IAHA, RIA, and RIP tests appear to be highly sensitive, but only the RIA reagents are now commercially available.

Originally identified by immunodiffusion, HBeAg and its antibody (anti-HBe) are now detected by more sensitive RIA techniques.[84] However, this method does not currently provide for detection of

the specific subcategories of e, i.e., e_1, e_2, and e_3, which are still differentiated only by AGD.

3.4.3. Non-A, Non-B Viral Hepatitis. At present, there are no specific laboratory tests for diagnostic or epidemiological studies of non-A, non-B hepatitis, since the designation is still derived only by exclusion of type A and type B hepatitis. There have been a number of reports of the isolation and experimental transmission of one or more agents associated with such cases. These and similar initial reports of serological tests for non-A, non-B antigens and antibodies[120,144,148,154] and immune complexes[34] remain to be critically compared and independently confirmed. However, the rapid progress to date and the intense interest in clarification of this problem provide encouragement for its resolution in the near future.

4. Biological Characteristics of the Human Hepatitis Viruses

Until 1970, relatively little was known about the characterization of human hepatitis viruses. On the basis of epidemiological observations and limited "inactivation" attempts carried out as part of human-transmission studies or limited control measures, both HAV and HBV had long been assumed to be unusually hardy agents, highly resistant to chlorination, disinfectants, heat, and ultraviolet irradiation, especially in the presence of serum proteins. During the decade of the 1970s, great strides were made in defining the morphological, antigenic, physiochemical, and biological characteristics of the hepatitis agents, but their precise classification among viruses is still unsettled.

4.1. Hepatitis A Virus

The animal-host range of HAV was thought to be restricted to man until 1961, when Hillis[53] reported an unusual outbreak of hepatitis, probably type A, among handlers of newly imported chimpanzees. Since then, similar episodes have been noted in relation to several other nonhuman primates presumably infected subsequent to capture. Little is known about the possible transmission or maintenance of HAV among nonhuman primates under natural conditions, but it is doubtful that such potential reservoirs are of importance in human infections. All experimental attempts to infect such animals had met with apparent failure until 1967, when Deinhardt et al.[30] reported the successful isolation and serial transmission of HAV in marmosets, findings subsequently confirmed and extended by others.[79] Although chimpanzees and other nonhuman primates may serve as experimental hosts, marmosets (*Saguinus* spp. and *Callithrix jacchus*) have continued to be the laboratory animals of choice. Nonhuman-primate responses to HAV infection tend to be mild, but are readily detected by serial biochemical or histopathological studies, or both. More recently, multiplication of marmoset-adapted HAV has been demonstrated in both human and simian cell cultures[107] without cytopathogenic effect. Prolonged or sustained serial passage has proved difficult. On the combined bases of human, marmoset, and cell-culture studies to date, it appears that HAV is an enterovirus with the following characteristics: 28-nm diameter, cubic symmetry, unenveloped, with a density of $1.34 \ g/cm^3$, a single-stranded RNA, and four polypeptides. It is stable for many years at $-20°C$ and is only partially inactivated at $60°C$ for 1 hr, but completely inactivated at $100°C$ for 5 min. Although it can withstand ether treatment (20%, 24 hr) and a pH of 3.0, it is inactivated by formalin (1:4000 at $37°C$ for 72 hr) and chlorine (1 mg/liter for 30 min). Comparative studies of HAV from different epidemiological and geographic sources have been too limited to permit definitive statements about antigenic or biological variations, but to date, no clear evidence of heterogeneity has been documented.

4.2. Hepatitis B Virus

Man appears to be the only natural host for HBV, with an experimental-host range that is limited to the higher primates. In the latter, infections tend to be mild and are usually detectable only on the basis of biochemical, serological, or histopathological examinations. Like man, chimpanzees may become long-term healthy carriers. Although they serve as important and reliable experimental hosts, their expense and limited availability severely restrict their use. No known tissue-culture system supports HBV replication.

Shortly after the discovery and confirmation of the diagnostic relationship between "Australia antigen" and type B hepatitis, Dane et al.[29] described the electron-micrographic appearance of an associated 42-nm double-shelled particle that is now accepted as the complete virion. Its classification among viruses appears to be unique, although an almost identical but distinct agent has been found in association with hepatitis in woodchucks.[130] The 27-nm inner core component, containing double-stranded DNA and a specific DNA polymerase as well as a specific antigen (HBcAg), is produced in the nuclei of hepatocytes. The outer coat is produced in the cytoplasm. It contains the surface antigen (HBsAg), which appears to be identical with that noted on the original Australia particles. These probably represent production of excess coat material released as spheres of variable size (17–25 nm) or elongated tubules. Some circulating coat material also appears as partially or completely empty shells. It has been suggested that such DNA-deficient structures may act as interfering particles.[59]

There do not appear to be demonstrable variants of HBcAg. In contrast, the antigenic complexity of HBsAg subtypes is still under investigation. In addition to a common group-specific antigen, a, there are at least two independent "allelic" sets of antigens, designated as d and y[72] and w and r,[8] yielding four major genotypes (adw, adr, ayw, ayr) that breed true. Several additional subtypes, as well as some hybrids, have been defined within this system.[93] A host of other reported determinants (q, x, f, t, n, j, s) presumed to be related to HBsAg have not been fully characterized or confirmed.[73]

In 1972, Magnius and Espmark[77] described a soluble antigen–antibody system (HBeAg/anti-HBe) found to be associated only with HBsAg-positive sera. Subsequent studies[142,158] have delineated three distinct specificities, HBeAg/1, /2, and /3, which may be found alone or in combination. The origin of HBeAg is still unclear, but it appears together with HBsAg early in HBV infection, disappears with clearance of HBsAg, and is followed by anti-HBe. In chronic HBs antigenemia, HBeAg may persist or be superseded by anti-HBe. Takekoshi et al.[145] suggested that one form of HBeAg originates from HBV core particles and that another form is associated with IgG.

4.3. Non-A, Non-B Hepatitis Viruses

Epidemiological and serological studies have pointed to the probability that there are more than two (HAV, HBV) human hepatitis viruses.[28,49,91,152] In addition, experimental chimpanzee-transmission studies have provided evidence to suggest at least two distinct non-A, non-B agents[7,143] with different incubation periods. Recent reports based on electron-micrographic studies of serum or hepatocytes[15,119] offer a variety of morphological observations with no clear agreement. However, lack of conformity may not be surprising in view of the expected multiplicity of agents. Infection with Epstein–Barr virus, cytomegalovirus, and a number of other well-characterized viruses may involve the liver sufficiently to cause hepatitis. However, such specific viruses are usually excluded from the non-A, non-B designation.

5. Descriptive Epidemiology

Until a few years ago, it was generally accepted that viral hepatitis type A was far more common than type B, that it was usually spread by the fecal–oral route while type B was limited to parenteral transmission, and that almost all sporadic cases were likely to be type A. On this basis, officially reported incidence figures were assumed to

be sufficiently weighted with type A to be representative of the distribution and epidemiological behavior of this type. In light of more recent studies based on the use of specific serological tests, these old concepts have been subjected to reconsideration. They are still subject to further revision as such tests become more widely used for diagnostic and epidemiological studies. These problems are illustrated by the United States experience based on reports to the Center for Disease Control. Figure 1 reveals that the total rates per 100,000 varied from 10 to 40 in the years 1952–1965, with peaks in 1954 and 1963. The basis for reporting cases as hepatitis A from 1966 on rests only on the clinical and epidemiological features and not on any laboratory test, except for exclusion in some of those in which HBsAg was demonstrable. Recent knowledge of non-A, non-B hepatitis suggests that some cases were probably included in the hepatitis A category, as well as some cases of HBV transmitted by nonparenteral routes. Given these limitations, it can be stated that viral hepatitis as a whole is one of the five most frequently reported diseases in the United States, but that the number of cases reported in 1978 was the lowest since 1968. The frequency of re-

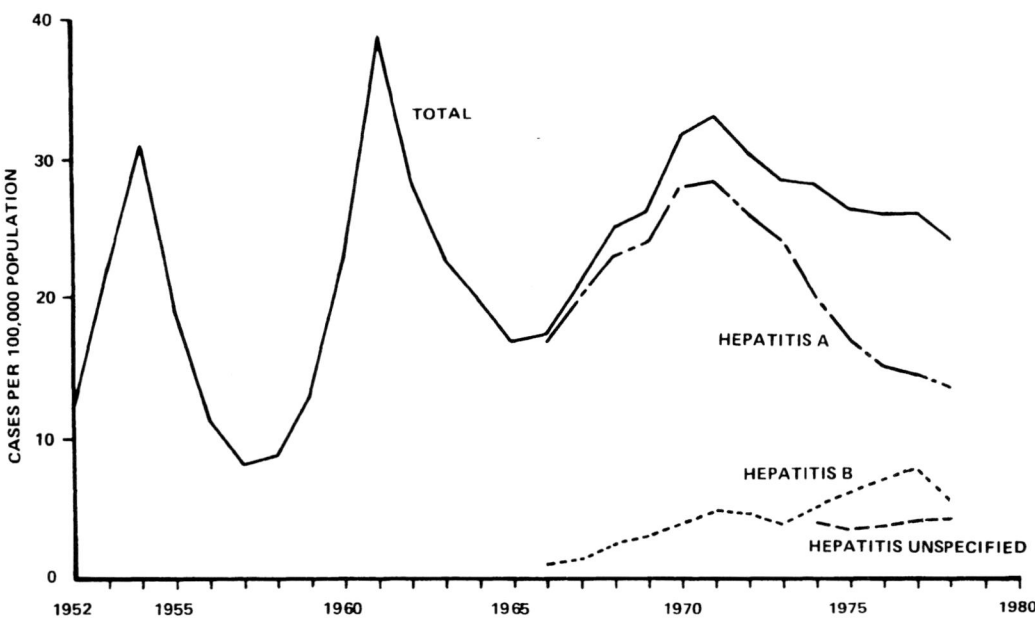

Fig. 1. Annual reported yearly viral hepatitis incidence rates in the U.S. (per 100,000 population) for 1952–1978, for hepatitis A and B 1966–1978, and unspecified 1974–78

ported cases designated as HAV has also decreased markedly since reaching a peak in 1971. A much clearer picture should emerge when the newer diagnostic tests for HAV can be used for routine diagnosis.

Reported annual figures of overall hepatitis incidence from other parts of the world vary from less than 10 per 100,000 in some, mostly tropical, countries, in which reporting is probably poor, to greater than 200 per 100,000 in several other countries (especially eastern Europe) where special reporting systems have been in effect for some 25–30 years. Incomplete and inaccurate reporting practices are unlikely to be corrected on a worldwide basis in the near future. At the moment, it is impossible to state with any degree of certainty, on the basis of either official reports or selected surveys, what the true proportionate distribution among A, B, and non-A, non-B is in most countries.

5.1. Viral Hepatitis A

Viral hepatitis A has long been considered to represent a secondary manifestation of an enteric infection spread primarily by the fecal–oral route. Most well-delineated epidemics, both large and small, can be accounted for by this mode of transmission, related either to close personal contact or to common-source food or water contamination. However, the majority of cases reported as type A do not fit neatly into this epidemic pattern, and such sporadic cases are frequently assumed to be linked to anicteric or unrecognized asymptomatic infections.

5.1.1. Geographic Distribution. HAV is believed to have a worldwide distribution. This assumption, previously based on clinical diagnoses, has been confirmed in each location included in comparative anti-HAV serological surveys.[39,122,133] Reported rates of disease vary considerably from country to country. In some, this may represent a reflection of age-related infection rates rather than relative overall levels of infection. In others, it may reflect true major differences in levels of endemicity and risk of infection. In some regions, Scandinavia and northern Europe and some parts of Japan, for example, it appears that currently, most HAV infections represent importations.[39,87] Rural and urban differences in hepatitis rates have been noted in Europe and the United States.[75] Within the United

States, there are marked geographic differences in reported rates of hepatitis A for recent years, with the lowest in the New England states, increasing to the south and west to the highest in the Mountain and Pacific states.[23]

The *prevalence* of HAV antibodies can now be measured by new and sensitive tests. Preliminary serological surveys indicate a pattern similar to that of other enteroviruses: worldwide distribution and early acquisition of antibody in developing countries. Frosner *et al.*[39] have compared the frequency of HAV antibody by age in seven European countries. Antibody was acquired earliest in Greece and latest in Sweden. The total antibody prevalence was highest in Greece (82%) and lowest in Norway (17%) and Sweden (13%). In population groups in five Pacific islands, a high frequency of anti-HAV antibody was found in each, ranging from 79.9 to 95.2% prevalence,[46] and the majority of infections were apparently acquired in the first decade of life. Similar surveys of other populations should soon be available.

5.1.2. Temporal Patterns. Hepatitis A infections occur sporadically and in epidemic clusters throughout the year in both tropical and temperate climates. In the latter regions, an autumn–winter seasonal peak has been observed, largely related to the younger age groups,[137] as well as a longer 6–7 to 10-year cycle or periodicity of incidence. Both these cyclical patterns were regular features of reported hepatitis occurrence in the United States between 1952 and 1970. Since then, seasonal variation has essentially disappeared, and annual incidence appears to be in a long, steady decline (Fig. 1). In Denmark, where peak incidence rates of over 500 per 100,000 were observed in the mid-1940s, a similar decline in hepatitis began in 1955 and proceeded to the point of virtual disappearance over the next two decades.

5.1.3. Age and Sex. Although nonimmune persons of all age groups are susceptible, hepatitis A has long been considered to be predominantly an infection of children, with the highest reported rates among preschool and school-age groups and the lowest among older adults, a presumably highly immune group. The major fluctuations between epidemic and nonepidemic years have been noted to occur in these younger age groups,[75] whereas rates among the older age groups tended to remain relatively unchanged from year to year. These patterns have continued to change in the United States during recent years and are now subject to clearer definition on the basis of specific diagnostic classification. It is likely that the earlier shift in reported peak age of incidence, particularly among males, to the 15 to 24-year age group, can be accounted for largely by type B, not type A, infections associated with illicit drug use.[45] While this age group continued to have the highest rates from 1972 to 1976, it was equaled by the 25 to 29-year age group in 1977.[24] A survey of antibodies against HAV in serum samples from New York,[25] Melbourne,[47] and several European countries[39] reveals age-related difference in this acquisition.

There is no convincing evidence that a sex differential exists for HAV infections, but reported sex-specific rates are usually slightly higher for males than for females, especially in the older age groups. In common-source epidemics, age and sex patterns will vary widely according to the composition of the population exposed. For example, raw-shellfish-associated epidemics occur almost entirely among adults, and particularly males, reflecting the age and sex distribution of this eating preference.

5.1.4. Occupation. There are no specific occupational associations except for handlers of certain recently imported primates in zoos or laboratories,[52] health professionals (including hospital personnel[21] and staff members of institutions for retarded children), government officials, military personnel, and missionaries[26] assigned to highly endemic areas.

5.2. Viral Hepatitis B

For a quarter of a century, from the mid-1940s until the late 1960s, HBV was widely presumed to be totally dependent on parenteral routes of transmission with limited distribution patterns determined largely by modern medical practices and procedures, except for cases associated with tattooing[123] and with shared equipment in illicit drug use.[127] Epidemics as such were unknown outside these restrictive bounds. With the discovery of HBsAg, its clear association with HBV infection, and the widespread application of rapidly improving and more sensitive methods for its detection, the epidemiological behavior of HBV has been subjected to a thorough and continuing reinvestigation and revision. Reported cases of hepatitis B for the United States are shown in Fig. 1. Current rates are in the range

of 0.4–0.6 per 100,000 and appear to be leveling off after a rise that can be attributed in part to increased illicit drug use and life styles of the late 1960s and 1970s, but also to better diagnosis and the recognition that HBV can be transmitted by nonparenteral routes.

5.2.1. Geographic Distribution. On the basis of extensive serological surveys for HBsAg and anti-HBs, HBV is now known to have penetrated and persisted throughout the world, even among remote and insular populations. Antigen-carrier (prevalence) rates vary widely among populations of otherwise presumably healthy subjects. Rates are higher in tropical zones (up to 20% or greater) than in most temperate areas (<0.1%). Such frequencies tend to correlate with overall HBV activity as indicated by age-specific prevalence rates for anti-HBs. Differences in the geographic distribution of certain HBsAg subtypes have been described[83] and may prove helpful in epidemiological determination of sources or movement of infection.[90] Since hepatitis B has been reported separately in only a few countries for a relatively short period, official rates are generally unavailable for comparisons over time or between countries. Within the United States, reported morbidity rates over the past few years have indicated "significant" geographic differences, with New England having the lowest and the Pacific States the highest,[23] the latter being sustained on a monthly basis over a 2-year period.

5.2.2. Temporal Distribution. There has never been any evidence to suggest, or any reason to suspect, a seasonal preference for HBV transmission or its clinical manifestations. Indeed, the recently observed flattening of seasonal peaks previously observed in overall viral hepatitis reporting in the United States has been attributed to an increasing proportion of type B infections. No long-term cycles in the temporal distribution of type B infection have been observed or suspected. However, there was a relatively steady rise in reported cases of type B in the United States from 1966 to 1977 in parallel with the increasing problem of illicit parenteral drug use and improved diagnostic capabilities. From 1977 to 1979, the 4-week periodic reporting of hepatitis B remained relatively fixed at rates between 0.4 and 0.6 per 100,000 population.[24]

5.2.3. Age and Sex. Nonimmune persons of all ages are susceptible to infection with HBV, but the recognized and reported disease is largely one of adults. In general, there is a slight to moderate excess of males among reported cases and among carriers. Sex differences in HBV infection rates among male and female homosexuals are striking. The excessively high rates among gay men[136] as compared with lesbians can probably be attributed to numbers of partners and types of sexual practices, rather than to sex alone.

Peak rates in the United States from 1972 to 1979 were regularly observed in the 15 to 29-year age group. However, such rates do not reflect true age patterns of infection, which may be more readily deduced from serum antibody surveys. These indicate an age- and socioeconomic-associated pattern of antibody acquisition, perhaps related to nonparenteral transmission. In some populations, infection rates among young children are so high that almost universal immunity is reached prior to adulthood.[46] The preponderance of adult cases is probably a combined reflection of increased clinical recognition (more severe host response) and perhaps a greater likelihood of parenteral infection. In any event, hepatitis B is no longer considered to be largely an adult infection. HBsAg carrier rates, however, have been observed to increase directly with age up to a late adult peak in all populations studied, but with a decline among older age groups,[135,138] suggesting the possibility that the carrier state is of self-limited duration in some persons.

5.2.4. Race. There is at present insufficient evidence for making distinctions concerning susceptibility of epidemiological behavior of HBV on the basis of race alone. Such variations as have been observed among different racial or ethnic groups may be attributed largely to environmental or other factors. Studies revealing marked variations in antigen-prevalence rates among blood donors of different ethnic groups in New York point to the likelihood that factors other than socioeconomic ones are significant determinants.[135] There has been considerable controversy over the role of genetic factors in relation to HBV infection, clinical response, and development of the carrier state since Blumberg first proposed a genetic hypothesis for his observed distribution of Australia antigen (HBsAg) among insular populations. The question, still far from settled, is a subject of continued study.[156] More recently, attention has been directed to searches for associations between specific HLA types and various outcomes of HBV infection, but the results

have been largely inconclusive and lacking in agreement.

5.2.5. Occupation. Increased risks of hepatitis related to occupation have been found among health professionals, hospital and other (especially staff members of hemodialysis units); among laboratory workers handling blood; among certain institutional employees (e.g., caretakers of mentally retarded); and recently among commercial processors of human plasma.[21,50,103,146] In most of these instances, it has been presumed that the increased risk represents largely an increased exposure to contaminated blood and blood products, with infection occurring by accidental inoculation or possibly by aerosol or oral routes. Serological surveys of anti-HBs among practicing United States physicians and dentists were conducted in the mid-1970s and revealed prevalence rates far in excess of those among blood donors matched for age and sex.[124] Rates increased with age and with years of practice. They were higher among Oriental (43%) than among white (16%) physicians, higher among surgeons and pathologists than among other specialty groups, and lowest among nonclinicians.[23] Another occupational group found to have a high prevalence of anti-HBs in some studies is prostitutes.[98]

5.2.6. Special Settings and Associations. During the late 1960s and early 1970s, members of the "hippie" culture and drug-using groups ran a high risk of hepatitis, probably A as well as B and non-A, non-B types. Not uncommonly, individual subjects suffered multiple episodes of jaundice. It was generally assumed that the risk was largely associated with the sharing of equipment for parenteral drug use, but the life style and communal living arrangements often adopted by such subjects fostered other mechanisms of transmission as well. There is now abundant evidence that HBV infection is readily transmitted by nonparenteral means in situations providing intimate or close personal contact, although the exact modes and mechanisms of transmission are not clearly defined or readily demonstrated. HBV has been found to be endemic in large institutions for mentally retarded, where antigen-carrier and antibody-prevalence rates are extremely high.[71] Secondary infection rates among household contacts of index hepatitis B cases and antigen carriers are also high, although clinical manifestations are relatively infrequent as compared to observations for type A in similar settings.[89,134,151] Risk of infection is highest among spouses and sexual partners.[64,112] Rates (up to 14% per year among susceptibles) among male homosexuals are among the highest recorded.[141] Extremely high carrier and illness rates have been observed among both patients and staff of hemodialysis units. These have been explained on the basis of a combination of factors including risk associated with blood usage, apparatus design, and sterilization methods and with immunological deficits among patients related to their basic illnesses or induced artificially for medical or organ-transplantation reasons.[78,125]

Both antigen- and antibody-prevalence studies among different populations have continued to support the original expectations that the prevalence rates are higher (and rise at earlier ages) among the lower socioeconomic groups in patterns consonant with those observed for other common infectious diseases in which crowding and lack of sanitation contribute to spread. Nutrition *per se* has not been studied carefully in relation to either infection or illness patterns.

5.3. Non-A, Non-B Viral Hepatitis

Until more definitive methods are available for segregating the components of this collective diagnostic category, specific statements concerning epidemiological features are difficult to interpret. It is presumed that agents belonging to the non-A, non-B category are as broadly distributed geographically as are HAV and HBV. No temporal patterns (seasonal or long-term trends) can be discerned from available data. Age and sex patterns have not been defined. On the basis of what probably represents selected reporting, certain groups are at particular risk of non-A, non-B infections. These include transfusion and blood-product recipients and dialysis patients and staff as well as other health professionals. In these respects, it would appear that at least one component of the non-A, non-B category shares epidemiological characteristics of HBV.

6. Mechanisms and Routes of Transmission

6.1. Viral Hepatitis A

Of the earliest recognized distinguishing features between type A and type B viral hepatitis, mechanisms and routes of transmission appeared to be among the most specific. On the basis of prior epidemiological observations and controlled transmission studies in the early 1940s, type A seemed to behave in a fashion typical of known enteric diseases, i.e., transmission by the fecal–oral route by way of contaminated food and water or by direct closer personal contact. Numerous small and large epidemics have been well documented as due to contamination of various foods, usually uncooked, or water, including individual wells, streams, or community supplies. Not uncommonly, secondary epidemic waves occur due to spread by close contact, particularly within households. The largest water-borne epidemic reported was one that occurred in New Delhi[85] when a temporary diversion in the course of the river resulted in massive sewage contamination of the water supply. More than 30,000 cases of hepatitis followed the event after an appropriate incubation period despite increased chlorination sufficient to inactivate most known pathogens. Although the outbreak was presumed at the time to be hepatitis A, the setting and age patterns of the cases served to cast doubt about the etiology. More recently, an outbreak of hepatitis that caused cancellation of most of a college football team's entire fall schedule was traced to a contaminated water line at the practice field.[88] A number of reports have suggested some relationship between hepatitis rates and community drinking water sources and treatment. A detailed study of one state with good reporting practices has failed to confirm such an association.[10]

That the fecal–oral route may not be exclusive has been suggested by findings related to a food-borne epidemic among Navy flight personnel who had consumed potato salad prepared with mayonnaise presumably contaminated with urine by a disturbed mess hall worker with anicteric hepatitis.[57]

Various levels of endemicity and epidemicity of hepatitis A have been commonly observed in institutional settings, especially those providing care for the mentally subnormal, in which personal hygiene and environmental sanitation problems cannot be adequately monitored and controlled. Since the infection is usually mild and anicteric in young children, the problem may be apparent only among susceptible adult employees. In addition to the fecal–oral route, parenteral transmission can occur, since there is a viremia during the latter half of the incubation period and the early acute phase of illness, an interval roughly paralleling fecal excretion of infective virus.[71] However, parenteral transmission is generally thought to be of little or no importance in the spread of HAV. Since the advent of specific serological tests for HAV, there has been no evidence in support of the existence of prolonged or chronic carrier states for hepatitis A infections. However, subjects with anicteric and asymptomatic infections are assumed to be as effective in virus excretion and transmission as are those with icterus.

It has frequently been proposed that HAV might be spread by the respiratory route,[56] but there is as yet no convincing experimental and little suggestive epidemiological evidence[2] to support this as an important mechanism of spread.

No biological vectors are known for HAV. During the past two decades, a number of well-studied shellfish-associated outbreaks of hepatitis[114,115] have clearly pointed to oysters and clams harvested from sewage-contaminated waters as effective HAV filters and as vehicles for transmission when eaten raw. Perhaps the most widely publicized such epidemic was the one recognized in New Jersey in 1961, which resulted in cases scattered over a wide area and led to the closing of Raritan Bay for clam-harvesting. However, there is no evidence to suggest that shellfish act as biological hosts or reservoirs for either HAV or HBV.

6.2. Viral Hepatitis B

The early experimental human hepatitis-transmission studies of the 1940s that clearly defined two distinct etiological agents also led to an epidemiological misunderstanding that prevailed for more than 20 years, i.e., the concept that HBV was transmitted only via the blood and was infective exclusively by the parenteral route. For these reasons, the perpetuation of hepatitis B was felt to be largely dependent on therapeutic and preventive health measures involving needles and syringes, blood, and blood products. Beginning in the 1930s, hepatitis was recognized as a risk associated with the use of pooled human convalescent serum to prevent diseases such as measles[105] and mumps.[12] The largest recorded epidemic occurred in 1942, when more than 45,000 United States military personnel developed hepatitis B following inoculation with live attenuated yellow fever virus vaccine that contained "normal" human serum as a stabilizer.[100]

The risk of hepatitis transmission in association with the transmission of whole blood or pooled human plasma, first recognized during World War II, became a major postwar civilian problem with the increasing therapeutic and prophylactic use of blood and blood products. A number of plasma protein fractions, particularly fibrinogen, and antihemophilic factor were found to carry a high frequency of HBV contamination and a high risk of infection.

Transmission has also been associated with a variety of medical, surgical, and dental instruments contaminated with blood or serum and inadequately cleansed and sterilized between uses. Aside from medical procedures, parenteral transmission has been associated with tattoo needles and injection equipment shared among illicit-drug users. Indeed, the latter mode of transmission may have accounted for a major share of recognized type B infections during the past decade in many countries.

The failure to demonstrate nonparenteral transmission of HBV in the volunteer studies of the 1940s was probably due in large part to the lack of sufficiently sensitive biochemical and specific serological tests for the detection of anicteric infections. Methods for measuring serum levels of transaminase, which are extremely sensitive indicators of hepatocellular damage, had been developed and carefully evaluated by the mid-1960s, when Krugman et al.[67] attempted oral transmission of HBV by feeding serum already known to be infective by the parenteral route. None of the resulting infections would have been recognized without the benefit of serial serum enzyme determinations over a period of several months. In a later study, testing of the same serum specimens for the presence of HBsAg provided additional evidence.[42] Subsequently, the demonstration of HBsAg in association with sporadic and contact cases of hepatitis clearly unrelated to possible parenteral transmission pointed to the need to seek further evidence in support of specific nonparenteral routes. Family clustering of infections related to acute cases and asymptomatic carriers of HBsAg[121,140] suggests the importance of the household setting without specifically defining the mechanism or route of transmission. Particularly high infection rates have been observed among all age groups in Swedish families who adopted HBsAg-carrier children from Asia.[92] There are many published claims and some contradictions concerning the presence or absence of HBsAg (and, by infer- ence, HBV) in urine, feces, saliva, and other body secretions,[51,150,153] all of which may be contami- nated to some degree with blood at one time or another. However, the mere presence of detectable antigen does not necessarily serve as a certain marker of infectivity.

The epidemiological evidence for fecal–oral trans- mission of HBV has never been convincing. The question now appears to have been settled by a careful study of samples collected from acute hep- atitis B cases and chronic antigen carriers (asymp- tomatic and postnecrotic cirrhosis). While the pres- ence of HBsAg was consistently demonstrated in the saliva, it was never found in the patient's feces,[37] even following ingestion of antigen-posi- tive serum or its direct mixture and incubation with normal feces. The latter finding is consistent with the presence of HBsAg "inhibitors" in human feces and intestinal mucosa as postulated by Piazza *et al.*[102]

The probability of sexual or venereal transmission of HBV has been a subject of intense interest and observation. Although it is generally agreed that susceptible sexual partners of acute and chronic HBsAg carriers are at high risk of infection, routes or mechanisms of transmission are not yet clearly defined for either heterosexual or homosexual re- lationships.[136] Reports of HBsAg in saliva, in semen,[51] in vaginal secretions, and in menstrual blood[82] of carriers provided fertile grounds for speculation. Subsequently, experimental transmis- sion of HBsAg-positive semen and saliva has been demonstrated in nonhuman primates.[6,9]

Perinatal transmission of HBV has been studied intensively since the advent of HBsAg testing. Chil- dren born of women who developed evidence of acute hepatitis B during the last trimester or within the early postpartum period run a high risk of neon- atal infection.[116] Infants born of asymptomatic HBsAg-*carrier* mothers in the United States and Eu- rope carry a relatively low risk of HBV infection (less than 10%), but extremely high rates (40–50%) have been observed in Taiwan and Japan. High levels of maternal antigenemia,[128] the presence of HBeAg,[40,95] and antigen-positive older siblings have all been found to be associated with the in- creased risk. Usually, these infants develop a per- sistent antigenemia with or without evidence of chronic hepatitis. Their ultimate fate and infectivity

remain to be determined, but it has been speculated that they play an important role in the maintenance of high levels of HBV endemicity in many areas. Rarely, neonatal infections result in an acute, fatal outcome.

6.2.1. Vectors and Reservoirs. No nonhuman natural reservoirs of HBV have been defined, al- though it is possible that infectious cycles may occur among chimpanzees and perhaps other lower pri- mates. A distinct, but closely related, virus has been discovered in association with hepatitis and hepa- tomas in woodchucks.[131] As far as is known, it does not infect men, nor have related viruses been found among other species in nature.

It has long been suspected that mosquitoes and other bloodsucking insects might act as parenteral transmitters of HBV. A number of investigators have reported demonstrating HBsAg in pools of wild-caught mosquitos in both tropical and tem- perate regions,[19,32,97] but such findings may be a reflection of the number of human antigen carriers serving blood meals at a given time and place. Ar- tificial mosquito-feeding experiments have so far provided no evidence in support of biological trans- mission, i.e., antigen persistence or replication, but this would not rule out the possibility of mechanical transmission in the course of interrupted and con- secutive feedings. HBsAg has also been demon- strated in bedbugs collected in Senegal[159] and South Africa,[58] but the possible role of the bedbug in transmission is still speculative.

6.3. Non-A, Non-B Viral Hepatitis

Transmission patterns of at least one, and pos- sibly more, of the non-A, non-B agents resemble those of HBV. Most cases of posttransfusion hep- atitis are now classified as non-A, non-B, as are most of those associated with plasma fractions and many of the episodes of hepatitis among the renal-dialysis patients and staff members. In addition to such ep- idemiological observations, experimental transmis- sion studies have provided evidence for the pres- ence of the agent(s) in blood[7,143] and plasma products[28] and for the existence of persistent car- riers.[7] However, a fair proportion of sporadic cases of non-A, non-B hepatitis do not have a history com- patible with parenteral transmission.

There is also the possibility that one or more of the non-A, non-B agents may resemble HAV in transmission patterns, i.e., fecal–oral. Relatively few institutional or food- or water-borne epidemics have been studied adequately since the recent advent of serological tests for HAV antibodies. A large water-borne epidemic in Kashmir has recently been attributed to a non-A, non-B agent.[62]

7. Pathogenesis and Immunity

7.1. Viral Hepatitis A

In the limited controlled-transmission studies of HAV carried out in the 1940s and 1950s,[71,155] it was demonstrated that fecal excretion of infective virus began approximately two thirds of the way in the incubation period, i.e., from about the 25th day after oral infection in one series. The specific cells or tissue sites of this early viral replication are still unknown. It may be suspected that the primary site of infection is in the intestine or some other nonhepatic site, since there is no clinical or biochemical evidence of hepatocellular damage at that early stage of infection. Discovery of the specific virus and the development of animal models and sensitive serological tests for both antigen and antibody have confirmed and extended these earlier studies. Peak infectivity probably occurs before the elevation of serum enzyme levels and onset of symptoms. Virus excretion subsides rapidly as the transaminase rises to peak levels and anti-HAV IgM appears.[17,36]

IgG begins to rise shortly thereafter and persists as the IgM falls over the next 3–6 months. The temporal association of these events suggests that the pathogenesis of liver damage may be due to an immune mechanism rather than simply hepatocyte destruction by virus replication. Circulating antigen–antibody complexes specific for HAV have not been demonstrated, nor have extrahepatic manifestations of infections suggested their presence in specific tissue sites. To date, there have been no reports of studies demonstrating cell-mediated immunity in hepatitis A.

Application of recently developed serological methods has provided for rapid advancement of knowledge concerning specific HAV antibodies. Previously, their existence was assumed on the basis of apparently solid immunity to experimental reinfection[48,67] and the protection afforded by even very small doses of pooled human immune serum globulin (γ-globulin).[129] Their specificity and protective efficacy are now well demonstrated. The suggestion has been made that there may be strains of varying degrees of virulence, but so far, there is no evidence of a multiplicity of either specific antigens or subtypes of HAV.

7.2. Viral Hepatitis B

The primary site of replication of HBV is unknown. The regular early appearance in the serum of large quantities of HBsAg, long before any biochemical or other evidence of hepatocellular damage, would suggest that the site might well be some cells other than hepatocytes or that these cells are relatively undamaged by the viral replication process. Studies of experimentally infected chimpanzees have revealed evidence of HBV core components in hepatocytes only 2 weeks after parenteral infection. Humoral immune responses are readily demonstrable in virtually all HBV infections. The appearance of anti-HBc[54,70] in close association with liver dysfunction (during the period of HBs antigenemia and long before detectable anti-HBs appears) suggests the possibility of an immune mechanism in the production of hepatocellular damage. It does not appear to play a role in resolution of the infection. The continued presence of anti-HBc in association with HBsAg and the absence of anti-HBs is believed to be indicative of persistent infection of hepatocytes and of infectivity.[32,55] Evidence strongly supports the view that immunological factors play a major role in determining the clinical response and outcome of HBV infections. Although the mechanism for persistence of antigenemia, particularly in the absence of apparent hepatic damage, is still far from fully explained, defects in cell-mediated immunity or other forms of immunodeficiency, or both, are likely to be significant factors.

Extrahepatic symptoms and lesions are not uncommon in association with HBV infection. A transient "serum sickness" syndrome may appear well in advance of hepatic symptoms,[5] in relation to circulating antigen–antibody complexes. Such complexes have also been demonstrated in association with vascular lesions of HBsAg-serum-positive cases of polyarteritis nodosa[43] and nephrosis or glomerulonephritis.[20]

Most HBV infections result in the development of specific antibodies (anti-HBs) against HBsAg as the antigenemia disappears. These antibodies presumably persist for life, usually at detectable levels. The observation that anti-HBs antibodies are strongly associated with immunity to reinfection has led to the development and trial of noninfectious purified HBsAg as an active immunizing agent.

7.3. Non-A, Non-B Viral Hepatitis

On the basis of histopathology, the hepatic changes associated with non-A, non-B hepatitis viruses cannot be readily distinguished from those identified with HAV and HBV infections. Presumably, each of these viruses replicates in the hepatocytes, and presumably, some immunological component plays a role in the tissue damage. The prolonged, sometimes intermittent and chronic, pattern of many non-A, non-B infections may be related to immune factors. Until specific non-A, non-B viruses are identified, both the early and late effects of such mechanisms can only be matters of speculation. However, it would seem safe to assume that infection with each virus results in specific long-term immunity to reinfection.

8. Patterns of Host Response

The diagnosis of acute hepatitis rested primarily on the occurrence of jaundice until the 1940s, when the first controlled human-transmission studies and extensive application of biochemical and histological methods confirmed the common occurrence of anicteric and asymptomatic infections. Since the latter are still ordinarily unrecognized and undiagnosed as viral hepatitis, their frequency and relative epidemiological importance remain matters for speculation.

The spectrum of acute clinical manifestations of infection appears to be similar for both type A and type B, and presumably for non-A, non-B. It ranges from mild to fatal, the distribution according to severity being dependent on a number of host factors, as yet only partially defined, and possibly on variations in virulence of the agents. The vast majority of symptomatic infections due to either virus will be followed by complete recovery. A small proportion will continue into one or another form of unresolved chronic liver disease. A much smaller proportion of acute infections will result in massive hepatic necrosis, coma, and death. In the past, it has been widely accepted that HBV infections tend to be more severe than those due to HAV. With the advent of accurate diagnostic tests, this belief has been upheld.

Fulminant or fatal outcomes of acute HAV are very rare, even among patients sufficiently ill to require hospitalization. Chronic or permanent liver disease directly attributable to HAV also appears to be infrequent.

Most HBV infections are also mild and proceed to complete recovery and immunity. Fatal acute infections are uncommon but more frequent than noted with HAV. Between 5 and 10% of hospitalized adult patients develop chronic antigenemia, but it is a more common outcome in very young infants (perinatal infection) and patients with immune deficiencies. Such carriers may remain asymptomatic or proceed to develop chronic active hepatitis or cirrhosis and in some instances progress to primary hepatocellular carcinoma.

While the clinical spectrum of non-A, non-B infections probably resembles that of A and B, anicteric infections are frequent among posttransfusion cases, and persistence of elevated enzyme levels is common and frequently associated with biopsy evidence of chronic active hepatitis.[111]

8.1. Clinical Features

Fever, malaise, fatigue, headache, anorexia, nausea, vomiting, and abdominal pain are common and usual features of variable severity associated with acute hepatitis of either type. However, when large numbers of cases have been well documented and grouped as either type A or type B for comparison, useful differentiating characteristics are frequently noted. The onset of type A is likely to be relatively more abrupt and febrile than that for type B, in which it tends to be more insidious with low or absent fever. The onset of hepatitis B not uncommonly follows a serum-sickness-like prodrome of urticaria, pruritis, or arthritis, or some combination thereof. The total duration of illness varies widely from a few weeks to a few months, with type B tending to be more prolonged. Some infections with HBV, and presumably also non-A, non-B viruses, progress to chronic liver damage with persistent, recurrent symptoms, eventually leading to posthepatitis cirrhosis. Those cases due to HBV, especially with persistence of antigenemia or very high titers of anti-HBc (both indicative of continuing active infection), may progress to the development of primary hepatocellular carcinoma with a fatal outcome.

8.2. Primary Hepatocellular Carcinoma

Primary hepatocellular carcinoma (hepatoma or PHC) is a relatively rare tumor in the United States and western Europe (2–3% of all cancers), but it represents an extremely common cancer (20–40%) and a frequent cause of death (20–100/100,000) in parts of Africa, Mozambique, Southeast Asia, and the Mediterranean littoral. It has long been known that there is a close relationship between the development of PHC and a preexisting cirrhosis of the posthepatitis type. Early suspicion of the possible etiological role of hepatitis viruses could not be assessed until specific serological tests for HBV infection became available. In early HBsAg serological surveys, high carrier rates were found in regions of high PHC mortality rates.[131,149] Rather marked variations have been observed in different regions of the same country, e.g., Greece and Mozambique.[61] More detailed studies within these areas revealed that the frequency of antigenemia and other markers of HBV infection was much higher in PHC patients (up to 85%) than in controls (up to 35%). In areas of low PHC mortality, such as the United States, the prevalence of HBsAg was lower among both patients (25%) and controls (0.3%), but the risk of PHC among carriers *per se* is thought to be of the same magnitude in all areas. However, not all patients with PHC have serological evidence of current or past HBV infection. HBsAg and HBcAg have been demonstrated in "normal" hepatocytes adjacent to areas of PHC,[118] but the specific manner in which HBV is involved in PHC is unclear. Early, perhaps perinatal, infection leading to chronic antigenemia appears to be an important feature, especially in Africa and Asia. Genetic, ethnic,[147] and environmentally related factors (malnutrition, aflatoxin, parasitic infections) may also play important roles in the pathogenesis of PHC. Prospective studies in high-risk populations should help ascertain the sequence and relationships of these suspected contributory factors, particularly the clear demonstration that HBV infection and chronic antigenemia precede any evidence of PHC. Among 115 cirrhosis patients followed for almost 5 years in Japan, 23% of those with HBsAg developed PHC, as compared with only 5.9% of those without HBsAg.[94] If HBV infection is an essential factor in most cases of PHC, widespread use of vaccine eventually should markedly reduce morbidity and mortality due to PHC.

Numerous attempts to culture cells from PHC have failed, but a few have yielded lines with appropriate characteristics. One of these[76] has consistently produced small quantities of HBsAg *in vitro* and, when transplanted to nude athymic mice,[31] *in vivo*. The HBV-related virus associated with woodchuck hepatitis does appear to be regularly associated with the PHC observed in these animals. Detailed studies of the pathogenesis of these tumors may lead to a clearer understanding of the human counterpart.

8.3. Laboratory Diagnosis

In addition to these clinical differences, certain laboratory tests may be helpful in differentiating between type A and type B hepatitis. The general patterns of serum transaminase, e.g., steepness of rise and duration, differ in consonance with the abrupt (type A) and insidious (type B) patterns of onset of symptoms. Serum thymol turbidity is elevated consistently and early in both icteric and anicteric infections with HAV. It usually remains normal in anicteric HBV infections.

The most useful and specific laboratory methods for differential diagnosis during the acute phase are sensitive serological tests for IgM-specific anti-HAV[16] and for HBsAg (and possibly anti-HBc). Later, a demonstrable rise in IgG anti-HAV or the disappearance of HBsAg (possibly with conversion to anti-HBs) may be accepted as diagnostic. Lacking any of these serology indicators, the presumptive diagnosis of non-A, non-B hepatitis may be made.

9. Control and Prevention

There is currently no approved vaccine for the prevention of either type A or type B hepatitis. However, recent developments would suggest that agents for active immunization against both may become available in the near future.

A formalin-inactivated HAV vaccine prepared from infected marmoset liver has been demonstrated to be effective in stimulating protective antibodies in marmosets subsequently challenged with active HAV.[106] This provides a sound experimental basis for pursuing a similar development with tissue-culture-adapted HAV.

Following the observations of Krugman *et al.*[69] that inoculation of heat-treated serum containing HBsAg would stimulate production of protective anti-HBs, several highly purified, inactivated HBsAg vaccines have been prepared. Three of these are currently under various stages of field testing.[81,141] All have been derived from plasma of human carriers and found to be immunogenic but noninfective for chimpanzees. It is anticipated that if they are proven to be protective under conditions of natural exposure to HBV infection, a licensed product will be available in the reasonably near future. Another potential vaccine source for the various antigens of HBV is through cloning in *Escherichia coli*. Initial experimental successes in this approach have been summarized and extended in a recent report.[99]

Until specific agents are identified for non-A, non-B, there is no basis for vaccine development.

9.1. Viral Hepatitis A

Since transmission of HAV is associated primarily with close personal contact and fecal contamination of food or water, those measures of personal hygiene and environmental sanitation that apply to control of other enteric infections are generally effective in limiting the spread of infection. The identification of common-source outbreaks will often lead to recognition of the vehicle of transmission, but usually too late for the institution of corrective measures to be beneficial except as they may be effective in preventing similar outbreaks in the future.

Pooled human immune serum globulin (ISG) as a 16% solution in a dose of 0.01–0.10 ml/kg body weight is highly effective in preventing or attenuating HAV infection among contacts of cases and among persons regularly exposed to or preparing to enter known endemic settings,[65] e.g., institutional employees, military and other travelers, or long-term visitors to recognized areas of high risk. The smaller dose is appropriate and effective when given during the early incubation period. The larger amounts are usually given in anticipation of risk of infection, the total single dose being proportional to the expected duration of risk (e.g., 1.0–2.0 ml/month for adults). In instances of more extended continuing exposure, injections may be repeated two or three times at intervals of 4–6 months. A primary aim in the use of ISG under such circumstances is that infection and active immunity will develop under the cover of this temporary passive protection.

9.2. Viral Hepatitis B

From the earliest recognition of blood as a vehicle for transmission of hepatitis B, three main approaches to control have been pursued: (1) the development of methods for the routine physical and/or chemical treatment of all blood, plasma, and pooled plasma protein fractions that would render them noninfective without diminishing or altering their therapeutic effectiveness; (2) the development of tests to identify carriers and/or infected blood in order to reduce the risk of transmission; and (3) the use of pooled human ISG for passive immunization of those at risk (or mixed directly with blood prior to transfusion in order to "neutralize" the virus *in vitro*).

The first of these approaches produced encouraging results from time to time, but no proven, practical, readily applicable methods were forthcoming after more than two decades of effort. Until the discovery of HBsAg and its widespread use in blood-donor-screening procedures, little progress was made in the second approach. Although markedly differing degrees of risk were found among different donor populations, particularly "commercial" or paid donors vs. volunteer or family donors,[3] relatively little heed was paid to the observation for almost two decades. This association has been confirmed and extended to include non-A, non-B posttransfusion hepatitis as well.[117] Since the introduction of Federal regulations in the United States mandating the testing of all donor blood for HBsAg and the subsequent introduction of extremely sensitive screening methods such as RIA,[74] the complete elimination of transfusion-associated hepatitis B has almost become a realistic goal. Pretesting and the use of only HBsAg-negative units for the preparation of pooled plasma fractions or for other specialized blood components should further reduce the risk of HBV transmission in therapeutic and prophylactic medical procedures to near zero.

Results of numerous prospective and variably controlled studies of the value of pooled human ISG in the prevention of viral hepatitis B have been characterized by inconsistency, perhaps at least partially explained by variations in infecting dose and in specific antibody content of the different globulin preparations tested. In a limited series of direct HBV parenteral-challenge studies, Krugman et al.[68] found a specific globulin preparation containing a high level of anti-HBs to be about 70% effective. Soulier et al.[126] also reported protection afforded by specific hepatitis B immune globulin (HBIG) given to 27 subjects during the first week after exposure to HBsAg-positive blood (19 after transfusion, 8 after accidental inoculation).

These observations have led to a number of controlled trials of HBIG, some in comparison with ISG of varying anti-HBs content. The findings and their interpretations have been subject to considerable controversy. Those completed prior to 1978 have been discussed and critically assessed by Grady.[44] HBIG has been licensed in the United States. Its use is recommended *only* for persons exposed to accidental HBV infection by injection, splashing, or oral ingestion of HBsAg-containing material. The suggested dose is 5 ml as soon as possible after exposure and again 1 month later. For chronic exposure to potential infection, e.g., dialysis-unit patients and staff, spouses or sexual partners or carriers, subjects in endemic institutional settings, it may be more efficacious to consider the regular (every 3–5 months) use of ISG, which currently contains respectable levels of anti-HBs. This recommendation is based on the results of several studies that have provided evidence of the efficacy of passive immunization under conditions of presumed nonparenteral transmission of HBV. A large-scale controlled study of United States military personnel in Korea, an area of high hepatitis incidence, indicated that a 5-ml dose of "standard" globulin provided significant protection for 6 months against both type B and non-B.[1] Szmuness et al.[139] compared the protective effect of standard and a special HBIG in a prospective study of children newly admitted to three institutions in which HBV was known to be endemic. Both appeared to be about equally, but far from completely, protective. No chronic antigen carriers were observed among the globulin recipients as compared to unimmunized children, among whom this outcome was common.

Another area of controversy in the efficacy of both ISG and HBIG is that of preventing infection among infants of HBsAg-carrier mothers. The long-term results of several trials have been far from successful,[11] but a much more intensive approach has been claimed to be effective.[113]

9.3. Non-A, Non-B Viral Hepatitis

A single report indicates that commercial immunoglobulin or a preparation with high levels of anti-HBs given preoperatively may reduce the incidence of posttransfusion non-A, non-B hepatitis among cardiac surgery patients receiving large amounts of blood.[63]

10. Unresolved Problems

Despite rapid and continuing progress in our total understanding of viral hepatitis during the past several years, many questions remain unresolved. The seemingly endless search for susceptible experimental animals has finally led to positive answers for type A, type B, and some non-A, non-B viruses, but the answers are less than totally satisfactory because of the relative scarcity of both chimpanzees and marmosets. It now appears doubtful that less exotic or more readily available species will be found to be equally acceptable substitutes. However, the woodchuck and its own brand of HBV-like virus may provide an excellent animal model system, particularly for studies related to the development of hepatoma in chronic carriers. Identification of feasible cell-culture systems for the regular isolation and propagation of all hepatitis viruses still represents a major challenge for both diagnostic and epidemiological studies as well as approaches to further development of routine serological reagents and ultimately vaccines, either inactivated or live attenuated strains. Readily available and reliable virus isolation and serological methods are needed to fill in large gaps in our epidemiological understanding of hepatitis and especially to clarify the meaning and importance of several suggested nonparenteral mechanisms of transmission of HBV.

In addition to the more practical considerations of their usefulness in diagnostic and epidemiological studies, it is becoming more and more apparent that immune responses are likely to play significant roles in the pathogenesis of viral hepatitis. Immune complexes involving HBsAg have also been demonstrated in association with certain nonhepatic diseases, e.g., polyarteritis nodosa, glomerulonephritis, and nephrosis, but their etiological significance and temporal relationship are not yet resolved. Still far from satisfactorily answered are the roles of immunodeficiency and immunosuppression in the development of persistent HBsAg—and presumably HBV—carriers as well as non-A, non-B chronic infections.

11. References

1. A Cooperative Study, Prophylactic gamma globulin for prevention of endemic hepatitis: Effects of U.S, gamma globulin upon the incidence of viral hepatitis and other infectious diseases in U.S. soldiers abroad, *Arch. Intern. Med.* **128**:723–738 (1971).
2. AACH, R. D., EVANS, J., AND LOSEE, J., An epidemic of infectious hepatitis possibly due to airborne transmission, *Am. J. Epidemiol.* **87**:99–109 (1968).
3. ALLEN, J. G., AND SAYMAN, W. H., Serum hepatitis from transfusions of blood, *J. Am. Med. Assoc.* **180**:1079–1085 (1962).
4. ALMEIDA, J., RUBENSTEIN, D., AND STOTT, E. J., New antigen–antibody system in Australia-antigen-positive hepatitis, *Lancet* **2**:1225–1227 (1971).
5. ALPERT, E., ISSELBACHER, K. J., AND SCHUR, P. H., The pathogenesis of arthritis associated with viral hepatitis, *N. Engl. J. Med.* **285**:185–189 (1971).
6. ALTER, H. J., PURCELL, R. H., AND GERIN, J. L., Transmission of hepatitis B to chimpanzees by hepatitis B surface antigen positive saliva and semen, *Infect. Immun.* **16**:928–933 (1977).
7. ALTER, H. J., PURCELL, R. H., HOLLAND, P. V., AND POPPER, H., Transmissible agent in non-A, non-B hepatitis, *Lancet* **1**:459–463 (1978).
8. BANCROFT, W., MUNDON, F., AND RUSSELL, P., Detection of additional antigenic determinants of hepatitis B antigen, *J. Immunol.* **109**:842–848 (1972).
9. BANCROFT, W. H., SNITBHAN, R., SCOTT, R., TINGPALAPONG, M., WATSON, W. T., TANTICHAROENYOS, P., KARWACKI, J. J., AND SRIMARUT, S., Transmission of hepatitis B virus to gibbons by exposure to human saliva containing hepatitis B surface antigen, *J. Infect. Dis.* **135**:79–85 (1977).
10. BATIK, O., CRAUN, G. F., TUTHILL, R. W., AND KRAEMER, D. F., An epidemiologic study of the relationship between hepatitis A and water supply characteristics and treatment, *Am. J. Public Health* **70**:167–178 (1980).
11. BEASLEY, R. P., AND STEVENS, C. E., Vertical transmission of HBV and interruption with globulin, in: *Viral Hepatitis* (G. N. VYAS, S. N. COHEN, AND R. SCHMID, (eds.), pp. 333–345, Franklin Institute Press, Philadelphia, 1978.
12. BEESON, P. B., CHESNEY, G., AND McFARLAN, A. M., Hepatitis following injection of mumps convalescent plasma, *Lancet* **1**:814–815 (1974).
13. BLUMBERG, B. S., ALTER, H. J., AND VISNICH, S., A "new" antigen in leukemia sera, *J. Am. Med. Assoc.* **191**:541–546 (1965).
14. BLUMBERG, B. S., GERSTLEY, B. J. S., HUNGERFORD, D. A., LONDON, W. T., AND SUTNICK, A. I., A serum antigen (Australia antigen) in Down's syndrome, leukemia and hepatitis, *Ann. Intern. Med.* **66**:924–931 (1967).
15. BRADLEY, D. W., COOK, E. H., MAYNARD, J. E., McCAUSTLAND, K. A., EBERT, J. W., DOLANA, G. H., PETZEL, R. A., KANTOR, R. J., HEILBRUNN, A., FIELDS, H. A., AND MURPHY, B. L., Experimental infection of chimpanzees with antihemophilic (Factor VIII) materials: Recovery of virus-like particles associated with non-A, non-B hepatitis, *J. Med. Virol.* **3**:253–269 (1979).
16. BRADLEY, D. W., FIELDS, H. A., McCAUSTLAND, K. A., MAYNARD, J. E., DECKER, R. H., WHITTINGTON, R., AND OVERBY, L. R., Serodiagnosis of viral hepatitis A by a modified competitive binding radioimmunoassay for immunoglobulin M and hepatitis A virus, *J. Clin. Microbiol.* **9**:120–127 (1979).
17. BRADLEY, D. W., GREVELLE, C. R., COOK, E. H., FIELDS, R. M., AND MAYNARD, J. E., Cyclic excretion of hepatitis A virus in experimentally infected chimpanzees: Biophysical characterization of the associated HAV particles, *J. Med. Virol.* **1**:133–138 (1977).
18. BRADLEY, D. W., MAYNARD, J. E., HINDMAN, S. H., HORNBECK, C. L., FIELDS, H. A., McCAUSTLAND, K. A., AND COOK, E. H., Serodiagnosis of viral hepatitis A: Detection of acute phase immunoglobulin M antihepatitis A virus by radioimmunoassay, *J. Clin. Microbiol.* **5**:521–530 (1977).
19. BROTMAN, B., PRINCE, A., AND GODFREY, H., Role of arthropods in transmission of hepatitis B virus in the tropics, *Lancet* **1**:1305–1308 (1973).
20. BRZOSKO, W., KRAWCZYNSKI, K., NAZAREWICZ, T., MORZYCKA, M., AND NOWOSLAWSKI, A., Glomerulonephritis associated with hepatitis B surface antigen immune complexes in children, *Lancet* **2**:477–481 (1974).
21. BYRNE, E. B., Viral hepatitis: An occupational hazard of medical personnel: Experience of the Yale-New Haven Hospital, 1952–1965, *J. Am. Med. Assoc.* **195**:362–364 (1966).
22. CAYZER, I., DANE, D. S., CAMERON, C. H., AND DENNING, J. V., A rapid haemagglutination test for hepatitis-B antigen, *Lancet* **1**:947–949 (1974).

23. CENTER FOR DISEASE CONTROL, Hepatitis Surveillance Report No. 43 (1979).

24. CENTER FOR DISEASE CONTROL, Hepatitis Surveillance Report No. 44 (1979).

25. CHERUBIN, C. E., NAIR, S. R., DIENSTAG, J. L., PURCELL, R. H., AND SZMUNESS, W., Antibody to hepatitis A and B in children in New York City, *Pediatrics* **61**:781–783 (1978).

26. CLINE, A. L., MOSLEY, J. W., AND SCOVEL, F. G., Viral hepatitis among American missionaries abroad: A preliminary study, *J. Am. Med. Assoc.* **199**:551–553 (1967).

27. COMMITTEE ON VIRAL HEPATITIS OF NRC-NAS, Nomenclature of antigens associated with viral hepatitis type B, *Morbid. Mortal. Weekly Rep.* **23**:29 (Jan. 26, 1974).

28. CRASKE, J., SPOONER, R. J. D., AND VANDERVELDE, E. M., Evidence for existence of at least two types of factor-VIII-associated non-B transfusion hepatitis, *Lancet* **2**:1051–1052 (1978).

29. DANE, D. S., CAMERON, C. H., AND BRIGGS, M., Virus-like particles in serum of patients with Australia-antigen-associated hepatitis, *Lancet* **1**:695–698 (1970).

30. DEINHARDT, F., HOLMES, A. W., CAPPS, R. B., AND POPPER, H., Studies on the transmission of human viral hepatitis to marmoset monkeys. I. Transmission of disease, serial passage and description of liver lesions, *J. Exp. Med.* **125**:673–687 (1967).

31. DESMYTER, J., RAY, M. B., BRADBURNE, A. F., AND ALEXANDER, J. J., Human HBsAg-positive hepatoma in nude athymic mice, in: *Viral Hepatitis* (G. N. VYAS, S. N. COHEN, AND R. SCHMID, eds.), pp. 459–460, Franklin Institute Press, Philadelphia, 1978.

32. DICK, S. J., TAMBURRO, C. H., AND LEEVY, C. M., Hepatitis B antigen in urban-caught mosquitoes, *J. Am. Med. Assoc.* **229**:1627–1629 (1974).

33. DIENSTAG, J. L., ALLING, D. W., AND PURCELL, R. H., Quantitation of antibody to hepatitis A antigen by immune electron microscopy, *Infect. Immun.* **13**:1209–1213 (1976).

34. DIENSTAG, J. L., BHAN, A. K., ALTER, H. J., FEINSTONE, S. M., AND PURCELL, R. H., Circulating immune complexes in non-A, non-B hepatitis, *Lancet* **1**:1265–1267 (1979).

35. DIENSTAG, J. L., MATHIESON, L. R., AND PURCELL, R. H., Test methods and animal models for HAV infection, in: *Viral Hepatitis* (G. N. VYAS, S, N. COHEN, AND R. SCHMID, eds.), pp. 13–29, Franklin Institute Press, Philadelphia, 1978.

36. DUERMEYER, W., WIELAARD, F., AND VAN DER VEEN, J., A new principle for the detection of specific IgM antibodies applied in an ELISA for hepatitis A, *J. Med. Virol.* **4**:25–32 (1979).

37. FEINMAN, S. V., BERRIS, B., REBANE, A., SINCLAIR, J. C., WILSON, S., AND WROBEL, D., Failure to detect hepatitis B surface antigen (HBsAg) in feces of HBsAg positive persons, *J. Infect. Dis.* **140**:407–410 (1979).

38. FEINSTONE, S. M., KAPIKIAN, A. Z., AND PURCELL, R. H., Hepatitis A: Detection by immune electron microscopy of a virus-like antigen associated with acute illness, *Science* **182**:1026–1028 (1973).

39. FROSNER, G. G., PAPAEVANGELOU, G., BUTLER, R., IWARSON, S., LINDHOLM, A., COUROUCE-PAUTY, A., HAAS, H., AND DEINHARDT, F., Antibody against hepatitis A in seven European countries. I. Comparison of prevalence data in different age groups, *Am. J. Epidemiol.* **110**:63–69 (1979).

40. GERETY, R. J., AND SCHWEITZER, I. L., Viral hepatitis type B during pregnancy, the neonatal period and infancy, *J. Pediatr.* **90**:368–374 (1977).

41. GERETY, R. J., TABOR, E., HOOFNAGLE, J. H., MITCHELL, F. D., AND BARKER, L. F., Tests for HBV associated antigens and antibodies, in: *Viral Hepatitis* (G. N. VYAS, S. N. COHEN, AND R. SCHMID, eds.), pp. 121–138, Franklin Institute Press, Philadelphia, 1978.

42. GILES, J. P., McCOLLUM, R. W., BERNDSTON, L. W., JR., AND KRUGMAN, S., Viral hepatitis: Relationship of Australia/SH antigen to the Willowbrook MS-2 strain, *N. Engl. J. Med.* **281**:119–121 (1969).

43. GOCKE, D. J., HSU, K., MORGAN, C., BOMBARDIERI, S., LOCKSHIN, M., AND CHRISTIAN, C. L., Association between polyarteritis and Australia antigen, *Lancet* **2**:1149–1153 (1970).

44. GRADY, G. F., Viral hepatitis; Passive prophylaxis with globulins—state of the art in 1978, in: *Viral Hepatitis* (G. N. VYAS, S. N. COHEN, AND R. SCHMID, eds.), pp. 467–476, Franklin Institute Press, Philadelphia, 1978.

45. GREGG, M. B., The changing epidemiology of viral hepatitis in the United States, *Am. J. Dis. Child.* **123**:350–354 (1972).

46. GUST, I. D., LEHMANN, N. I., AND DIMITRAKAKIS, M., A seroepidemiologic study of infections with HAV and HBV in five Pacific islands, *Am. J. Epidemiol.* **110**:237–242 (1979).

47. GUST, I. D., LEHMANN, N. I., LUCAS, C. R., FERRIS, A. A., AND LOCARNINI, S. A., Studies of the epidemiology of hepatitis A in Melbourne, in: *Viral Hepatitis* (G. N. VYAS, S. N. COHEN, AND R. SCHMID, eds.), pp. 105–112, Franklin Institute Press, Philadelphia, 1978.

48. HAVENS, W. P., JR., Immunity in experimentally induced infectious hepatitis, *J. Exp. Med.* **84**:403–406 (1946).

49. HAVENS, W. P., JR., Viral hepatitis: Multiple attacks in a narcotic addict, *Ann. Intern. Med.* **44**:199–203 (1956).

50. HAYASHI, S., NAKAMURA, R. M., AND GIORGI, E., Problems of prevention and detection of hepatitis in personnel of hospital hemodialysis units, *J. Occup. Med.* **13**:388–392 (1971).

51. HEATHCOTE, J., CAMERON, C. H., AND DANE, D. S., Hepatitis B antigen in saliva and semen, *Lancet* **1**:71–75 (1974).

52. Hepatitis Surveillance Report: Sub-human primate-associated hepatitis, Center for Disease Control, U.S. Department of Health, Education and Welfare, Atlanta, No. 34, pp. 10–14, (September 1971).

53. HILLIS, W. D., An outbreak of infectious hepatitis among chimpanzee handlers at a United States Air Force Base, *Am. J. Hyg.* **73**:316–328 (1961).

54. HOOFNAGLE, J. H., GERETY, R. J., AND BARKER, L. F., Antibody to hepatitis-B virus core in man, *Lancet* **2**:869–873 (1973).

55. HOOFNAGLE, J. H., GERETY, R. J., NI, L. Y., AND BARKER, L. F., Antibody to hepatitis B core antigen: A sensitive indicator of hepatitis B virus replication, *N. Engl. J. Med.* **290**:1336–1340 (1974).

56. IPSEN, J., DONOVAN, W. R., AND JAMES, G., Sociologic factors in the spread of epidemic hepatitis in a rural school district, *J. Hyg.* **50**:457–470 (1952).

57. JOSEPH, R. P., MILLAR, J. D., HENDERSON, D. A., NAUMANN, R. D., BAGLEY, C. S., SCHLANG, H. A., AND SHAW, G. A., An outbreak of hepatitis traced to food contamination, *N. Engl. J. Med.* **273**:188–194 (1965).

58. JUPP, P. G., PROZESKY, A. W., McELLIGOT, S. E., AND VAN WYCK, L. O. S., Infection of common bedbug (*Cimex lectularius* L.) with hepatitis B virus in South Africa, *S. Afr. Med. J.* **53**:598–600 (1978).

59. KAPLAN, P. M., FORD, E. C., PURCELL, R. H., AND GERIN, J. L., Demonstration of subpopulations of Dane particles, *J. Virol.* **17**:885–893 (1976).

60. KAPLAN, P. M., GREENMAN, R. L., GERIN, J. L., PURCELL, R. H., AND ROBINSON, W. S., DNA polymerase associated with human hepatitis B antigen, *J. Virol.* **12**:995–1005 (1973).

61. KEW, M. C., Hepatoma and the HBV, in: *Viral Hepatitis* (G. N. VYAS, S. N. COHEN, AND R. SCHMID, eds.), pp. 439–450, Franklin Institute Press, Philadelphia, 1978.

62. KHUROO, M. S., Study of an epidemic of non-A, non-B hepatitis: Possibility of another human hepatitis virus distinct from post-transfusion non-A, non-B type, *Am. J. Med.* **68**:818–824 (1980).

63. KNODELL, R. G., CONRAD, M. E., GINSBURG, A. L., BELL, C. J., AND FLANNERY, E. P., Efficacy of prophylactic gamma-globulin in preventing non-A, non-B post-transfusion hepatitis, *Lancet* **1**:557–561 (1976).

64. KOFF, R. S., SLAVIN, M. S., CONNELLY, L. J. D., POSEN, D. R., Contagiousness of acute hepatitis B: Secondary attack rates in household contacts, *Gastroenterology* **72**:297–300 (1977).

65. KRUGMAN, S., The clinical use of gamma globulin, *N. Engl. J. Med.* **269**:195–201 (1963).

66. KRUGMAN, S., AND GILES, J. P., Viral hepatitis, *J. Am. Med. Assoc.* **212**:1019–1029 (1970).

67. KRUGMAN, S., GILES, J. P., AND HAMMOND, J., Infectious hepatitis: Evidence for two distinctive clinical, epidemiological and immunological types of infection, *J. Am. Med. Assoc.* **200**:365–373 (1967).

68. KRUGMAN, S., GILES, J. P., AND HAMMOND, J., Viral hepatitis type B (Ms-2 strain): Prevention with specific hepatitis B immune serum globulin, *J. Am. Med. Assoc.* **218**:1665–1670 (1971).

69. KRUGMAN, S., GILES, J. P., AND HAMMOND, J., Viral hepatitis Type B (MS-2 strain): Studies on active immunization, *J. Am. Med. Assoc.* **217**:41–45 (1971).

70. KRUGMAN, S., HOOFNAGLE, J. H., GERETY, R. J., KAPLAN, P. M., AND GERIN, J. L., Viral hepatitis, type B: DNA polymerase activity and antibody to hepatitis B core antigen, *N. Engl. J. Med.* **290**:1331–1335 (1974).

71. KRUGMAN, S., WARD, R., AND GILES, J. P.: The natural history of infectious hepatitis, *Am. J. Med.* **32**:717–728 (1962).

71a. LANDER, J. M., ALTER, H. J., AND PURCELL, R. H., Frequency of antibody to hepatitis associated antigen as measured by a new radioimmunoassay technique, *J. Immunol.* **106**:1166–1171 (1871).

72. LEBOUVIER, G. L., The heterogeneity of Australia antigen, *J. Infect. Dis.* **123**:671–675 (1971).

73. LEBOUVIER, G., AND WILLIAMS, A., Serotypes of hepatitis B antigen (HBsAg): The problem of "new" determinants, as exemplified by "t," *Am. J. Med. Sci.* **270**:165–171 (1975).

74. LING, C. M., AND OVERBY, L. R., Prevalence of hepatitis B virus antigen as revealed by direct radioimmune assay with ^{125}I-antibody, *J. Immunol.* **109**:834–841 (1972).

75. LOBEL, H. O., AND McCOLLUM, R. W., Some observations on the ecology of infectious hepatitis, *Bull. WHO* **32**:675–682 (1965).

76. MACNAB, G. M., ALEXANDER, J. J., LECACSAS, G., BEY, E. M., AND URBANOWICZ, J. M., Hepatitis B surface antigen produced by a human hepatoma cell line, *Br. J. Cancer* **34**:509–515 (1976).

77. MAGNIUS, L. O., AND ESPMARK, J. A., New specificities in Australia antigen positive sera distinct from the LeBouvier determinants, *J. Immunol.* **109**:1017–1021 (1972).

78. MARMION, B. P., AND TONKIN, R. W., Control of hepatitis in dialysis units, *Br. Med. Bull.* **28**:169–179 (1972).

79. MASCOLI, C., ITTENSOHN, O., VILLAREJOS, V., ARGUEDAS, J., PROVOST, P., AND HILLEMAN, M.: Recovery of hepatitis agents in the marmoset from human cases occurring in Costa Rica, *Proc. Soc. Exp. Biol. Med.* **142**:276–282 (1973).

80. MATHIESEN, L. R., FEINSTONE, S. M., WONG, D. C., SKINHOJ, P., AND PURCELL, R. H., Enzyme-linked immunoabsorbent assay for detection of hepatitis A antigen in stool and antibody to hepatitis A antigen in

sera: Comparison with solid-phase radioimmunoassay, immune electron microscopy, and immune adherence hemagglutination assay, *J. Clin. Microbiol.* **7**:184–193 (1978).

81. MAUPAS, P., GOUDEAU, A., COURSAGET, P., DRUCKER, J., AND BAGROS, P., Hepatitis B vaccine: Efficacy in high risk settings, a two year study, *Intervirology* **10**:196–208 (1978).

82. MAZZUR, S., Menstrual blood as a vehicle of Australia antigen transmission, *Lancet* **1**:749–751 (1975).

83. MAZZUR, S., BURGERT, S., AND BLUMBERG, B. S., Geographical distribution of Australia antigen determinants d, y, and w, *Nature (London)* **247**:38–40 (1974).

84. MCAULIFFE, V. J., AND PURCELL, R. H., Current status of tests for HBeAg and anti-HBe, in: *Viral Hepatitis* (G. N. VYAS, S. N. COHEN, AND R. SCHMID, eds.), pp. 161–191, Franklin Institute Press, Philadelphia, 1978.

85. MELNICK, J. L., A water-borne urban epidemic of hepatitis, in: *Hepatitis Frontiers* (F. W. HARTMAN, ed.), pp. 211–225, Little Brown, Boston, 1957.

86. MILLER, W. J., PROVOST, P. J., MCALEER, W. J., ITTENSOHN, O. L., VILLAREJOS, V. M., AND HILLEMAN, M. R., Specific immune adherence assay for human hepatitis A antibody: Application to diagnostic and epidemiologic investigations (38783), *Proc. Soc. Exp. Biol. Med.* **149**:254–261 (1975).

87. MORITSUGU, Y., TOMOYUKI, T., AND SHIKATA, T., A preliminary serologic survey of hepatitis A virus infection in Japan, *Jpn. J. Med. Sci. Biol.* **31**:325–338 (1978).

88. MORSE, L. J., BRYAN, J. A., HURLEY, J. P., MURPHY, J. F., O'BRIEN, T. F., AND WACKER, W. E., The Holy Cross College football team hepatitis outbreak, *J. Am. Med. Assoc.* **219**:706–798 (1972).

89. MOSLEY, J. W., The epidemiology of viral hepatitis: An overview, *Am. J. Med. Sic.* **270**:253–270 (1975).

90. MOSLEY, J. W., EDWARDS, V. M., MEIHAUS, J. E., AND REDEKER, A. G., Subdeterminants d and y of hepatitis B antigen as epidemiologic markers, *Am. J. Epidemiol.* **95**:529–535 (1972).

91. MOSLEY, J. W., REDEKER, A. G., FEINSTONE, S. M., AND PURCELL, R. H., Multiple hepatitis viruses in multiple attacks of acute viral hepatitis, *N. Engl. J. Med.* **296**:75–78 (1977).

92. NORDENFELT, E., AND DALQUIST, E., HBsAg positive adopted children as a cause of intrafamilial spread of hepatitis B, *Scand. J. Infect. Dis.* **10**:161–163 (1978).

93. NORDENFELT, E., AND LEBOUVIER, G., Hepatitis B antigen with both d and y subspecificities on the same particle, *Intervirology* **2**:65–74 (1973).

94. OBATA, H., HAYASHI, N., MOTOIKE, Y., HISAMITSU, J., OKUDA, H., KOBAYASHI, S., AND NISHIOKA, K., A prospective study on the development of hepatocellular carcinoma from liver cirrhosis with persistent hepatitis B infection, *Int. J. Cancer* **25**:741–747 (1980).

95. OKADA, K., KAMIYAMA, I., INOMATA, M., MITSUNOBU, I., MIYAKAWA, Y., AND MAYUMI, M.: e antigen and anti-e in the serum of asymptomatic carrier mothers as indicators of positive and negative transmission of hepatitis B virus to their infants, *N. Engl. J. Med.* **294**:746–749 (1976).

96. OKOCHI, K., AND MURAKAMI, S., Observations on Australia antigen in Japanese, *Vox Sang.* **15**:374–385 (1968).

97. PAPAEVANGELOU, G., AND KOUREA-KREMASTINOU, T., Role of mosquitoes in transmission of hepatitis B virus infection, *J. Infect. Dis.* **130**:78–80 (1974).

98. PAPAEVANGELOU, G., TRICHOPOULOS, D., KREMASTINOU, T., AND PAPOUTSAKIS, G., Prevalence of hepatitis B antigen and antibody in prostitutes, *Br. Med. J.* **2**:256–258 (1974).

99. PASEK, M., GOTO, T., GILBERT, W., ZINK, B., SCHALLER, H., MACKAY, P., LEADBETTER, G., AND MURRAY, K., Hepatitis B virus genes and their expression in *E. coli*, *Nature (London)* **282**:575–579 (1979).

100. PAUL, J. R., AND GARDNER, H. T., "Viral hepatitis": Preventive medicine in World War II, *Communicable Dis.* **5**:411–462 (1960).

101. PETERSON, M. R., BARKER, L. F., AND SHADE, D. S., Detection of antibody to hepatitis-associated antigen in hemophilia patients and in voluntary blood donors, *Vox Sang.* **24**:66–75 (1973).

102. PIAZZA, M., DISTASIO, G., MAIO, G., AND MARZANO, L., Hepatitis B antigen inhibitor in human feces and intestinal mucosa, *Br. Med. J.* **2**:334–337 (1973).

103. POLAKOFF, S., Decrease in the incidence of hepatitis in dialysis units associated with prevention programme, *Br. Med. J.* **4**:751–754 (1974).

104. PRINCE, A. M., An antigen detected in the blood during the incubation period of serum hepatitis, *Proc. Natl. Acad. Sci. U.S.A.* **60**:814–821 (1968).

105. PROPERT, S. A., Hepatitis after prophylactic serum, *Br. Med. J.* **2**:677–678 (1938).

106. PROVOST, P. J., AND HILLEMAN, M. R., An inactivated hepatitis A virus vaccine prepared from infected marmoset liver, *Proc. Soc. Exp. Biol. Med.* **159**:201–203 (1978).

107. PROVOST, P. J., AND HILLEMAN, M. R., Propagation of human hepatitis A virus in cell culture *in vitro*, *Proc. Soc. Exp. Biol. Med.* **160**:213–221 (1979).

108. PROVOST, P. J., ITTENSOHN, O. L., VILLAREJOS, V. M., ARGUEDAS, J., HILLEMAN, M. R., Etiologic relationship of marmoset-propagated CR326 hepatitis A virus to hepatitis in man, *Proc. Soc. Exp. Biol. Med.* **142**:1257–1267 (1973).

109. PROVOST, P. J., ITTENSOHN, O. L., VILLAREJOS, V. M., AND HILLEMAN, M. R., A specific complement-fixation test for human hepatitis A employing CR326 virus antigen: Diagnosis and epidemiology (38669), *Proc. Soc. Exp. Biol. Med.* **148**:962–969 (1975).

110. Purcell, R. H., Wong, D. C., Moritsugu, Y., Dienstag, J. L., Routenberg, J. A., and Boggs, J. D., A microtiter solid-phase radioimmunoassay for hepatitis A antigen and antibody, *J. Immunol.* **116**:349–356 (1976).

111. Rakala, J., and Redeker, A. G., Long term follow-up after HBsAg negative hepatitis, *Gastroenterology* **72**:902–909 (1977).

112. Redeker, A., Mosley, J., Gocke, D., McKee, A., and Pollack, W., Hepatitis B immune globulin as a prophylactic measure for spouses exposed to acute type B hepatitis, *N. Engl. J. Med.* **293**:1055–1059 (1975).

113. Reesink, H. W., Reesink-Brongers, E. E., Lafeber-Schut, B. M. T., Kalshoven-Benschop, J., and Brummelhuis, H. G. J., Prevention of chronic HBsAg carrier state in infants of HBsAg-positive mothers by hepatitis B immunoglobulin, *Lancet* **2**:436–437 (1979).

114. Roos, B., Hepatitepidemi spridd genom ostron, *Svenska Lakert* **53**:989–1003 (1956).

115. Ruddy, S., Johnson, R., Mosley, J., Atwater, J., Rossetti, M., and Hart, J., An epidemic of clam-associated hepatitis, *J. Am. Med. Assoc.* **208**:649–655 (1969).

116. Schweitzer, I. L., Mosley, J. W., Ashcavai, M., Edwards, V. M., and Overby, L. B., Factors influencing neonatal infection by hepatitis B virus, *Gastroenterology* **65**:277–283 (1973).

117. Seef, L. B., Zimmerman, H. W., Wright, E. C., and McCollum, R. W., VA Cooperative study of post-transfusion hepatitis, 1969–1974: Incidence and characteristics of hepatitis and responsible risk factors, *Am. J. Med. Sci.* **270**:355–362 (1975).

118. Shikata, T.: Primary liver carcinoma and liver cirrhosis, in: *Hepatocellular Carcinoma* (K. Okunda and R. L. Peters, eds.), pp. 53–71, John Wiley, New York, 1976.

119. Shimizu, Y. K., Feinstone, S. M., Purcell, R. H., Alter, H. J., and London, W. T., non-A, non-b hepatitis: Ultrastructural evidence for two agents in experimentally infected chimpanzees, *Science* **205**:197–200 (1979).

120. Shirachi, R., Shiraishi, H., Tateda, A., Kikuchi, K., and Ishida, N., Hepatitis "C" antigen in non-A, non-B post-transfusion hepatitis, *Lancet* **2**:853–856 (1978).

121. Singleton, J. W., Kohler, P. F., and Merrill, D., Infectivity risk of household contact with chronic carriers of hepatitis B antigen, *Gastroenterology* **64**:172 (1973).

122. Skinhøj, P., Mikkelsen, F., and Hollinger, F. B., Hepatitis A in Greenland: Importance of specific antibody testing in epidemiologic surveillance, *Am. J. Epidemiol.* **105**:140–147 (1977).

123. Smith, B. F., Occurrence of hepatitis in recently tatooed service personnel, *J. Am. Med. Assoc.* **144**:1074–1076 (1950).

124. Smith, J. L., Maynard J., Berquist, K. R., Doto, I. L., Webster, H. M., and Sheller, M. J., Comparative risk of hepatitis B among physicians and dentists, *J. Infect. Dis.* **133**:705–706 (1976).

125. Snydman, D. R., Bregman, D., and Bryan, J. A., Hemodialysis-associated hepatitis in the United States, 1974, *J. Infect. Dis.* **135**:687–691 (1977).

126. Soulier, J. P., Blatix, C., Courouce, A. M., Bensamon, P., Amouch, P., and Drouet, J., Prevention of virus B hepatitis (SH hepatitis), *Am. J. Dis. Child.* **123**:429–435 (1972).

127. Steigman, F., Human, S., and Goldbloom, R., Infectious hepatitis (homologous serum type) in drug addicts, *Gastroenterology* **15**:642–645 (1950).

128. Stevens, C., Beasley, P., Tsui, J., and Lee, W., Vertical transmission of hepatitis B antigen in Taiwan, *N. Engl. J. Med.* **292**:771–774 (1975).

129. Stokes, J. Jr., and Neefe, J. R., The prevention and attenuation of infectious hepatitis by gamma globulin, *J. Am. Med. Assoc.* **127**:144–145 (1945).

130. Summers, J., Smolec, J. M., and Snyder, R., A virus similar to human hepatitis B virus associated with hepatitis and hepatoma in woodchucks, *Proc. Natl. Acad. Sci. U.S.A.* **75**:4533–4537 (1978).

131. Szmuness, W., Hepatocellular carcinoma and the hepatitis B virus: Evidence for a causal association, *Prog. Med. Virol.* **24**:40–49 (1978).

132. Szmuness, W., Large scale efficacy trials of hepatitis B vaccines in the USA: Baseline data and protocols, *J. Med. Virol.* **4**:327–40 (1979).

133. Szmuness, W., Dienstag, J. L., Purcell, R. H., Stevens, C. E., Wong, D. C., Ikram, H., Bar-Shany, S., Beasley, R. P., Desmyter, J., and Gaon, J. A., The prevalence of antibody to hepatitis A antigen in various parts of the world: A pilot study, *Am. J. Epidemiol.* **106**:392–398 (1977).

134. Szmuness, W., Harley, E. J., and Prince, A. M., Intrafamilial spread of asymptomatic hepatitis B, *Am. J. Med. Sci.* **270**:293–304 (1975).

135. Szmuness, W., Hirsch, R. L., Prince, A. M., Levine, R. W., Harley, E. J., and Ikram, H., Hepatitis B surface antigen in blood donors: Further observations, *J. Infect. Dis.* **131**:111–117 (1975).

136. Szmuness, W., Much, I., Prince, A., Hoofnagle, J., Cherubin, C., Harley, E., and Block, G., On the role of sexual behavior in the spread of hepatitis B infection, *Ann. Intern. Med.* **83**:489–495 (1975).

137. Szmuness, W., and Prince, A. M., Epidemiologic patterns of viral hepatitis in Eastern Europe in the light of recent findings concerning the serum hepatitis antigen, *J. Infect. Dis.* **123**:200–212 (1971).

138. Szmuness, W., Prince, A. M., Brotman, B., and Hirsch, R. L., Hepatitis B antigen and antibody in blood donors: An epidemiologic study, *J. Infect. Dis.* **127**:17–25 (1973).

139. Szmuness, W., Prince, A., Goodman, M., Ehrich, C., Pick, R., and Ansari, M., Hepatitis B immune serum

globulin in prevention of nonparenterally transmitted hepatitis B, *N. Engl. J. Med.* **290**:701–706 (1974).

140. SZMUNESS, W., PRINCE, A., HIRSCH, R., AND BROTMAN, B., Familial clustering of hepatitis B infection, *N. Engl. J. Med.* **289**:1162–1166 (1973).

141. SZMUNESS, W., STEVENS, C. E., HARLEY, E. J., ZANG, E. A., OLESZKO, W. R., WILLIAM, E. C., SADOVSKY, R., MORRISON, J. M., AND KELLNER, A., Hepatitis B vaccine demonstration of efficacy in a controlled clinical trial in a high risk population, *N. Engl. J. Med.* **303**:833–841 (1980).

142. TABOR, E., GERETY, R. J., AND BARKER, L. F., Detection of e antigen during acute and chronic hepatitis B virus infections in chimpanzees, *J. Infect. Dis.* **136**:541–547 (1977).

143. TABOR, E., GERETY, R. J., DRUCKER, J. A., SEEF, L. B., HOOFNAGLE, J. H., JACKSON, D. R., APRIL, M., BARKER, L. F., AND PINEDA-TAMONDONG, G., Transmission of non-A, non-B hepatitis from man to chimpanzee, *Lancet* **1**:463–466 (1978).

144. TABOR, E., SEEF, L. B., AND GERETY, R., Lack of susceptibility of marmosets to human non-A, non-B hepatitis, *J. Infect. Dis.* **140**:794–797 (1979).

145. TAKEKOSHI, Y., TANAKA, M., MIYAKAWA, Y., HIROSHI, Y., TAKEKOSHI, K., AND MAYUMI, M., Free "small" and IgG-associated "large" hepatitis B e antigen in the serum and glomerular capillary walls of two patients with membranous glomerulonephritis, *N. Engl. J. Med.* **300**:814–819 (1979).

146. TAYLOR, J. S., SHMUNES, E., AND HOLMES, A. W., Hepatitis B in plasma fractionation workers, *J. Am. Med. Assoc.* **230**:850–853 (1974).

147. TONG, M. J., WEINER, J. M., ASHCAVAI, M. W., REDEKER, A. G., COMPARINI, S., AND VYAS, G. N.: A comparative study of hepatitis B viral markers in the family members of Asian and non-Asian patients with hepatitis B surface antigen-positive hepatocellular carcinoma and with chronic hepatitis B infection, *J. Infect. Dis.* **140**:506–512 (1979).

148. TREPO, C. G., VITVITSKI, L., HANTZ, O., AND PRINCE, A. M., Detection in serum of a precipitating antigen antibody system supposedly associated with non-A non-B hepatitis, *Infection* **7**:209 (1979).

149. TRICHOPOULOS, D., GERETY, R. J., SPARROS, L., TABOR, E., XIROUCHAKI, E., MUNOZ, N., AND LINSELL, C. A., Hepatitis B and primary hepatocellular carcinoma in a European population, *Lancet* **2**:1217–1219 (1978).

150. TRIPATZIS, I., Australia antigen in urine and feces, *Am. J. Dis. Child.* **123**:401–404 (1972).

151. VILLAREJOS, V., GUTIERREZ, A., AND PELON, W., Identification of a type b hepatitis epidemic in Costa Rica, *Am. J. Epidemiol.* **96**:372–378 (1972).

152. VILLAREJOS, V. M., PROVOST, P. J., ITTENSOHN, O. L., McLEAN, A. A., AND HILLEMAN, M. R., Seroepide-

miologic investigations of human hepatitis caused by A, B and a possible third virus, *Proc. Soc. Exp. Biol. Med.* **152**:524–528 (1976).

153. VILLAREJOS, V. M., VISONA, K. A., GUTIERREZ, A., AND RODRIGUEZ, A., Role of saliva, urine and feces in the transmission of type B hepatitis, *N. Engl. J. Med.* **291**:1375–1378 (1974).

154. VITVITSKI, L., PRINCE, A. M., TREPO, C., AND BROTMAN, B., Detection of virus-associated antigen in serum and liver of patients with non-A/non-B hepatitis, *Lancet* **2**:1263–1267 (1979).

155. VOEGT, H., Zur Aetiologie der Hepatitis Epidemica, *Muench. Med. Wochenschr.* **89**:76–79 (1942).

156. VYAS, G. N., AND SHULMAN, N. R., Hemagglutination assay for antigen and antibody associated with viral hepatitis, *Science* **170**:332–333 (1970).

157. WALSH, J. H., YALOW, R., AND BERSON, S. D., Detection of Australia antigen and antibody by means of radioimmunoassay techniques, *J. Infect. Dis.* **121**:550–554 (1970).

158. WILLIAMS, A., AND LEBOUVIER, G., Heterogeneity and thermo-lability of "e," *Bibl. Haematol.* **42**:71–75 (1976).

159. WILLS, W., LAROUGE, B., LONDON, W. J., MILLMAN, I., WERNER, B. G., OGSTON, W., POURTAGHVA, M., DIALLO, S., AND BLUMBERG, B. S., Hepatitis B virus in bedbugs (*Cimex hemipterus*) from Senegal, *Lancet* **2**:217–219 (1977).

160. WOLTERS, G., KUIJPERS, L. P. C., KOCAKI, J., AND SCHUURS, H. W. M., Enzyme-linked immunoabsorbent assay for hepatitis B surface antigen, *J. Infect. Dis.* **136**:S311–S317 (1877).

161. WORLD HEALTH ORGANIZATION EXPERT COMMITTEE, Advances in viral hepatitis, *Tech. Rep. Ser.*, No. 602, WHO, Geneva (1977).

162. ZUCKERMAN, A. J., AND SIMPSON, D. I. H.: Exotic virus infections of the liver, in: *Progress in Liver Diseases*, Vol. VI (H. POPPER, AND F. SCHAFFNER, eds.), pp. 425–538, Grune and Stratton, New York, 1979.

12. Suggested Reading

ALTER, H. J., Hepatitis B, *Semin. in Liver Dis.* **1**:1–87, (1981).

KOFF, R. S., *Viral Hepatitis*, John Wiley & Sons, New York, 1978.

KRUGMAN, S. AND GOCKE, D. J. *Viral Hepatitis*, W. B. Saunders, Philadelphia, 1978.

SZMUNESS, W., ALTER, H. J. AND MAYNARD, J. E., eds. *Viral Hepatitis*. The Franklin Institute Press, Philadelphia, 1982, in press.

WHO EXPERT COMMITTEE. Advances in Viral Hepatitis, *Tech. Rep. Ser.* No. 602. WHO, Geneva, (1977).

CHAPTER 13

Herpes Simplex Viruses 1 and 2

André J. Nahmias and William E. Josey

1. Introduction and Social Aspects

Herpes simplex viruses (HSVs) are among the most common infectious agents of man. There are two distinct serotypes (HSV-1 and HSV-2), and they usually have different modes of transmission. HSV-1 is transmitted chiefly via a nongenital route, whereas HSV-2 is most often transmitted venereally or from a mother's genital infection to the newborn. The mode of spread of each of the two virus types is reflected by its relative prevalence at different ages and by its pattern of clinical distribution within the host. Thus, HSV-1 infections occur most frequently during childhood and usually affect body sites above the waist. HSV-2 infections, on the other hand, occur most often during adolescence and young adulthood and involve body sites below the waist, primarily the genitals. Most infections in newborns are also caused by HSV-2.

Although infections in persons without prior exposure to either virus (primary infections) may often be subclinical, they tend to be more severe than infections that occur in persons previously exposed to HSV-1 or HSV-2 or both. The clinical manifestations of either virus may also be more severe in certain types of hosts, e.g., the newborn or immunocompromised patient, and with involvement of certain sites, e.g., the central nervous system.[60]

Although not ubiquitous in all populations studied, infection with these viruses represents a socially significant problem for which no effective vaccine is yet available. HSV-2 infection is becoming appreciated as a common venereal disease in several countries, and more cases of neonatal HSV infections with fatal or severe sequelae are being recognized. HSV infections of the central nervous system are also often fatal or debilitating, and ocular infections may endanger normal vision. Recurrent HSV infections are very common and are often physically and psychologically distressing. With the greater usage of immunosuppressive and cytotoxic drugs, iatrogenic HSV infections of varying clinical severity are more commonly recognized. Because of incompleteness of information, the total impact of the relationship of HSVs to human cancers, abortions, birth defects, and chronic neurological diseases cannot be ascertained at present.

2. Evolutionary and Historical Background

HSVs belong to a family of DNA viruses that includes more than 60 other viruses affecting a wide

André J. Nahmias · Department of Pediatrics
William E. Josey · Department of Gynecology and Obstetrics, Emory University School of Medicine, Atlanta, Georgia.

range of species from fungi to man.[62] The other human viruses are cytomegalovirus (CMV), varicella–zoster virus (VZV), and Epstein–Barr virus (EBV). All these viruses have the capacity to persist in their natural host, either in neural cells, e.g., HSV and VZV, or in nonneural cells, e.g., CMV and EBV. The high prevalence in primitive societies of antibodies to the human herpesviruses, in contrast to the low prevalence of antibodies to other nonpersistent viruses,[10] emphasizes the survival advantage conveyed by viral persistence and suggests an early origin for viruses in the herpes family.

Many of the vertebrate herpesviruses have very similar clinicoepidemiological patterns, such as venereal transmission and the ability to cause encephalitis, keratitis, skin or genital lesions, and disseminated neonatal disease.[59] Despite the presence of common antigens among many of the herpesviruses and other common phenotypic expression, such as intranuclear inclusions in the infected cell, genetic similarities have been demonstrated with current technology primarily between HSV-1 and HSV-2. It therefore appears likely that one of these viruses evolved from the other; however, the origin of the HSVs from progenitors in lower species cannot be ruled out. Thus, the human viruses share common nucleotide sequences with the bovine mammilitis herpesvirus and common antigens with the B virus of macaques, which can produce an almost invariably fatal encephalitis in humans.

The term *herpes* (ερεπιυ, "to creep") has been used since the earliest epoch of Greek medicine to include spreading cutaneous lesions of varied etiology.[55] The "herpetic eruptions which appear about the mouth at the crisis of simple fevers" were first described around 100 A.D. by a Roman physician, Herodotus. About 1600 years later, herpes of the genital tract in both men and women was first reported by a French physician, Astruc. By the 19th century, the generally accepted use of the term *herpes* was restricted to certain diseases associated with vesicular eruptions; by the latter part of that century, a further distinction was made on the basis of cytopathological differences between infections of the pox and herpes groups. In the early part of the 20th century, herpes zoster was differentiated on clinical and epidemiological grounds from "herpes febrilis" and "herpes genitalis." This distinction was further supported by the studies of Grüter and other European workers who showed that specimens obtained from zoster lesions could not be transmitted to the rabbit cornea, in contrast to those obtained from the other two herpetic conditions. Around 1920, a German physician, Lipschütz, maintained that, although herpes febrilis and herpes genitalis were biologically related, they were etiologically different; however, this idea was not confirmed until recent years.

Over the next 40 years, the experimental host range of HSVs was widened to include other laboratory animals, chick embryos, and ultimately cell cultures. The clinical spectrum of HSV infections was augmented to include gingivostomatitis, encephalitis, meningitis, Kaposi's varicelliform eruption, and neonatal disease. It also became appreciated that HSV infections could recur in the presence of demonstrable levels of serum antibodies.

In the early 1960s, Schneweis[86] in West Germany and Plummer[72] in England found antigenic differences among HSV strains. By 1967, Nahmias and Dowdle[55] had demonstrated that the large majority of genital and newborn infections are caused by HSV-2 and that most nongenital infections are caused by HSV-1, relating these clinical findings with the usual mode of transmission of the two virus types. In more recent years, strain differences within each of the two HSV types have been demonstrated in their polypeptides and by restriction endonuclease analysis of their viral DNAs.[11–13,71] The application of modern biochemical and immunological technology, together with the broadening clinicopathological and epidemiological observations in more recent times, has thus provided new approaches to laboratory diagnosis, prevention, and therapy.[65]

3. Methodology Involved in Epidemiological Analysis

3.1. Mortality

HSV infections are not reported nationwide in the United States, other than the few fatal cases of HSV encephalitis (around 20 a year) that are reported to the Center for Disease Control (CDC).

Mortality from HSV infection occurs primarily in three types of hosts: newborns, older persons with encephalitis, and those who are compromised by immunological or skin defects or by severe malnutrition. The case-fatality rate is around 50% in infected newborns[63] and 70% in older persons with encephalitis.[47,111]

3.2. Morbidity

An attempt is being made in some European countries, such as Great Britain, to report genital herpes, primarily on the basis of clinical findings. Other than a recent effort by the CDC to obtain reports of cases of clinically diagnosed genital herpes in some venereal disease clinics,[15] and the few cases of HSV encephalitis reported every year to this agency, no official health records are available.

Any estimate of the true extent of HSV-1 and HSV-2 infections must take into consideration (1) the method of diagnosis; (2) the occurrence of inapparent infections, particularly of the mouth and urogenital areas; and (3) the facts that HSV-1 and HSV-2 can infect the same person at different times and even concomitantly and that HSV-1 or HSV-2 infection, or both, can be recurrent in the same person. It is therefore important to keep in mind the following possible circumstances in any one subject within a study population: (1) no evidence of infection with either HSV-1 or HSV-2; (2) a primary HSV-1 or HSV-2 infection, but without recurrences with either virus; (3) a recurrent infection with one HSV type only; (4) a recurrent infection with one HSV type and a first infection with the other type; or (5) recurrent infections with both HSV-1 and HSV-2. The recent observation that a given subject may acquire an exogenous reinfection with a different strain of the same HSV type[11,12] has added further complexity to such distinctions.

Information on prevalence rates is derived from clinical, virological, and cythohistopathological observations and by serological surveys in various populations in different parts of the world.

3.2.1. Clinical Methods. Clinical surveys without laboratory support will be accurate to different degrees, particularly when the information is obtained retrospectively and based primarily on the patient's recollection. Nevertheless, surveys on the prevalence of cold sores or herpetic keratitis are likely to be more reliable than those on genital or intraoral infections. The reason is that inapparent infections in the two latter sites are common and clinically manifest infections are more easily mis-

diagnosed. Skin herpetic infections may also be confused clinically with other entities. Infections of other sites, such as the central nervous system, cervix, or urethra, as well as cases of eczema herpeticum, require laboratory aids for diagnosis.

3.2.2. Virological Methods. Several types of virological approaches have been employed.[36,101] One is to detect infectious virus or viral antigens in clinically suspect herpetic conditions. A second is to demonstrate infectious virus or viral antigens in clinically inapparent cases. The most recent has been to detect latent virus in the sensory or autonomic nervous system ganglia of human cadavers.[5,6,107] Many studies are now providing information on whether HSV-1 or HSV-2 was specifically involved and, more recently, whether strains within a type were similar or different.

3.2.3. Cytohistopathological Methods. Papanicolaou screening of cervicovaginal smears for cervical cancer has offered another approach to determine the relative frequency of genital herpes in different female populations, since cellular changes associated with herpesviruses can be demonstrated in such smears.[68] This method is about two thirds as sensitive as viral isolation and has been found to be highly specific for genital HSV infection. We do not believe it possible to differentiate HSV-2 and HSV-1 infections, or to distinguish between primary and recurrent infections, by cytological methods.

Histological examination of biopsy or autopsy specimens may be helpful in cases of neonatal infection, encephalitis, or disseminated HSV infections. However, it should be appreciated that other viral infections and some noninfectious conditions may also produce intranuclear inclusions.

3.3. Serological Surveys

Until relatively recently, most serological surveys employed methods that did not differentiate antibodies to HSV-1 and HSV-2. In addition, complement-fixation (CF) tests used in some studies are not as sensitive as neutralization assays to detect HSV antibodies.[97,101] In general, neutralizing antibodies tend to persist for longer periods than CF antibodies. The serological tests currently in use for differentiating HSV-1 and HSV-2 antibodies have many technological problems, due primarily to the presence of common antigens in the two viruses.[87,99] The difficulty is much less with primary HSV-1 or

HSV-2 infections that it is in the case of persons who have been infected with both virus types. Microadapted serological tests to differentiate HSV antibodies have been until recently too cumbercome or too nonspecific for the ready performance of very large serological surveys. However, the use of more type-specific reagents adapted to enzyme-linked immunosorbent assays (ELISAs) or radioimmuno assays (RIAs)[48,104] promises to be useful for such surveys. The detection of HSV-2 antibodies in children between the ages of 6 months and 10 years can be employed to provide evidence of a clinically undiagnosed HSV-2 perinatally acquired infection.

3.4. Laboratory Diagnosis

3.4.1. Virological Methods. Clinical specimens for virus isolation should be processed as rapidly as possible or frozen at −70°C until processed. It is better to keep the specimen for a few hours at 4°C icebox temperature than in the −15°C freezing compartment. The development of a transport medium (Leibovitz–Emory) has facilitated the shipment of clinical specimens, since the swab with which the specimen is obtained, when placed in this medium, can be stored and shipped at ambient temperature.[57]

Virus can be isolated readily in a number of tissue-culture systems, and an almost pathognomic cytopathic effect (CPE) can be detected as rapidly as in a bacterial culture (usually within 1–3 days). Specific identification of HSV and its antigenic types can then be obtained by neutralization, immunofluorescence (IF), or immunoperoxidase techniques.[36] The latter two techniques can be used for rapid identification and direct typing of HSV in clinical specimens, but are not as sensitive or specific as viral cultures.[36] IF tests are particularly helpful for the diagnosis of HSV in brain biopsies of patients with encephalitis.

Embryonated eggs and laboratory animals such as mice or rabbits can be used for initial isolation of HSV; however, these assays are more laborious than tissue-culture methods. HSV typing can also be done in embryonated eggs (HSV-2 produces larger pocks than HSV-1) or by differences in the ability of HSV-1 and HSV-2 to grow in certain tissue-culture cells or to produce plaques of different size.[55] However, serological typing methods are more fi-

nite than these biological assays, which could yield erroneous virus typing results, particularly if the virus has been passaged many times in the laboratory.

HSV can also be demonstrated in vesicular fluid, biopsy, or autopsy specimens by the use of electron-microscopic techniques that would reveal enveloped or nonenveloped virus particles. The morphological appearance of HSV by this technique cannot be distinguished from that of other herpesviruses, such as CMV or VZV.

More recently, it has been possible to demonstrate HSV in sensory or autonomic nervous system ganglia obtained from human cadavers.[5,6,106] Two methods have usually been employed. The first consists of placing the ganglion explants in culture and observing CPE in fibroblastic cells growing from supporting cells or after supernates of the ganglion cultures are transferred to susceptible tissue-culture cells. Another method is to cocultivate the ganglion cells with susceptible cells. With either method, infectious virus is usually detectable no earlier than 8 days and as long as 40 days after incubation of the ganglion cultures.

3.4.2. Morphological Aids. The intranuclear inclusions and multinucleated giant cells that are seen in Papanicolaou-stained smears of cells, fixed in 90% alcohol and obtained by scraping the base of herpetic vesicles or ulcers of the skin or mouth or by scraping the conjunctiva or cornea, are characteristic of herpesviruses, including HSV and VZV.[68] Only the multinucleated giant cells are usually apparent in Wright- or Giemsa-stained smears. In most instances, there is little difficulty in differentiating clinically between HSV and VZV infection. The inclusions in urinary cells may make it difficult, however, to distinguish HSV from CMV infection. Papanicolaou smears of the cervix are particularly helpful in detecting subclinical herpetic cervicitis in women.[68] Biopsy or autopsy material should be preferably fixed in Bouin's fixative rather than formalin in order to enhance the demonstration of the characteristic inclusions and giant cells.

3.4.3. Serological Tests and Assays of Cell-Mediated Immunity. Many serological assays can be used to demonstrate HSV antibodies, including neutralization, CF passive hemagglutination, complement-mediated cytolytic, indirect immunofluorescence (IIF), and ELISA.[36,101] The HSV antibody type (type 1 or 2 or both) can be determined by more specialized serological procedures, such as micro-neutralization, kinetic neutralization, multiplicity analysis, inhibition passive hemagglutination tests, or RIAs.[36,73,101] The adaptation of the latter test or ELISA to more type-specific antigens in currently under development.[48,104] A primary infection is suggested by the finding of a 4-fold or greater rise in titer between the acute and the convalescent serum, obtained 1 week or more later. Since such a titer rise may be observed with recurrent infections, particularly in patients with certain cancers or those receiving certain cytotoxic drugs, the distinction between primary and recurrent infection is occasionally difficult.

IF and radioimmunological methods have been developed recently to detect HSV antibodies in the IgM, IgG, and IgA classes of immunoglobulins.[36,101] Thus, IgM HSV antibodies can be used to diagnose neonatal herpes in patients with no characteristic findings in the eye, throat, or skin, Such IgM antibodies usually appear within 1–4 weeks after birth and persist for at least 6 months. The detection of IgM or IgA antibodies in the serum of older persons unfortunately cannot be used to differentiate a primary from a recurrent HSV infection, since such antibodies can occasionally be found when infection is recurrent.

In vitro assays for cell-mediated immunity to HSV are still in the research stage, but may be potentially useful in diagnosis or in the demonstration of persons more prone to HSV recurrences.[49,95] Positive skin tests of delayed hypersensitivity can be elicited with inactivated HSV preparations that correlate well with the presence of serum neutralization antibodies;[113] such HSV skin-test materials are not currently available clinically.

4. Biological Characteristics of Herpes Simplex Viruses 1 and 2

HSV consist of four major components—a centrally located core surrounded by three concentric structures: the capsid, the tegument, and the envelope. The core contains DNA coiled around proteins arranged in the form of a barbell. The icosahedral capsid contains 162 capsomeres and measures around 100 nm. Between the capsid and the envelope is the tegument, composed of fibrillous material. The envelope, derived from nuclear and occasionally other cell membranes, confers on the complete virus particle a diameter of 150–200 nm. The lipid composition of the envelope makes the virus particularly susceptible to ether and other lipid solvents.

The DNAs of HSV-1 and HSV-2 are linear, double-stranded molecules, with a molecular weight of approximately 100 million. About half the HSV-1 and HSV-2 DNA sequences are homologous. *In vitro*, it is possible to infect cells with "naked" DNA free of virus proteins and to demonstrate defective DNA in some strains of HSV, of possible relevance to the oncogenic potential of HSV. Recent studies on temperature-sensitive mutants and genetic recombination between HSV-1 and HSV-2 are allowing the development of genetic maps and the definition of genes responsible for specific viral functions.[82,85]

There are at least 49 proteins specified by the virus, of which about 33 are found in the virion. There are five glycoproteins (a, b, c, d, e) detectable on the membranes of infected cells.[99] Glycoprotein c of HSV-1 is type-specific and glycoprotein e has the interesting property of being an Fc receptor for IgG. The proteins on the envelope of the virus appear to be similar to those found on the membranes of infected cells, so that immune mechanisms could operate not only on the virus itself but also on cells infected by the virus. Antibodies alone, for instance, are most often incapable of inhibiting cell-to-cell spread of the virus. Together with complement, or with killer (K) lymphocytes, monocytes, or polymorphonuclear leukocytes of seronegative or seropositive subjects, antibodies can lyse HSV-infected cells *in vitro*.[95] Such mechanisms could be operative *in vivo*, since early lysis of infected cells can occur with some of these systems before new viral progeny is produced.

The different lability of HSV-1 and HSV-2 to high-temperature exposure (HSV-2 is more labile at 39°C than HSV-1) and their different susceptibility to certain antiviral agents may potentially affect pathogenesis and therapy. For instance, fever is well appreciated to reactivate HSV-1 recurrences, but may not be as effective in reactivating HSV-2. The viruses are also labile to low pH, so that they are infrequently recovered from the gastrointestinal tract. Although HSV may survive for some time in skin scabs from patients with eczema herpeticum, it is unlikely that either HSV-1 or HSV-2 would remain infectious for any duration outside the human body.

HSV-1 and HSV-2 have a wide *in vitro* and *in vivo* host spectrum, being capable of infecting large numbers of cell cultures of human or animal origin and a great number of experimental animals, from mice to monkeys. Variability in the *in vitro* and *in vivo* behavior of the two virus types, as well as of different strains within each type, however, can be demonstrated in some of these systems. In humans, either HSV type appears to be capable of infecting similar body sites, if it can be transmitted to those sites by external or internal spread. In the case of neurological involvement in older persons, it appears, however, that the increased chance of meningitis with HSV-2 and of encephalitis with HSV-1 may be related to differences in the mode of viral spread—HSV-2 via the blood to the meninges and HSV-1 neurogenically to the brain.

As noted earlier, all herpesviruses have the capacity to persist throughout the host's lifetime, providing this group of viruses a great survival advantage. In the case of HSV, it has been appreciated that recrudescences occur in subjects with circulating HSV antibodies. Although the possibility of low-level virus multiplication around the site of involvement cannot be completely ruled out as a possible mechanism for viral persistence, the best evidence at present favors latency of the virus in a noninfectious form in sensory and autonomic nervous system ganglia. This conclusion is supported by a great amount of experimental data in mice, rabbits, guinea pigs, and humans.[5,6,106] Although infectious virus cannot be demonstrated in the ganglia, with the use of special cultivation methods (noted in Section 3.4), infectious virus can be reactivated within several days or weeks. The various types of HSV–cell interactions (productive infection, latency, and transformation) are further detailed in Chapter 26.

5. Descriptive Epidemiology

The epidemiological characteristics of HSVs can be divided into those that reflect the overall infection rate, as determined by various clinical or laboratory surveys, and those that are related to particular clinical entities.

5.1. General Epidemiology

The major epidemiological determinants of HSV infections are age, socioeconomic level, and geographic area. In case of HSV-2 infections, the degree of sexual exposure is particularly important. The interdependency of these variables causes some overlap in the following discussion.

5.1.1. Incidence and Prevalence. A high *prevalence* rate of HSV infection has been found in virological or serological studies of healthy subjects. In 1953, Buddingh *et al.*[14] reported on the recovery of HSV from the mouths of 20% of asymptomatic children 7 months to 2 years of age, 9% of children 3–14 years of age, and 2.4% of adolescents and adults. This high isolation rate has been questioned, because the technique used at that time for identifying HSV was chorioallantoic-membrane inoculation, which might yield nonspecific lesions.[94] By use of tissue-culture methods, the isolation rate in asymptomatic children has been found by later workers to be around 1%[34,44] and that in adults to be between 0.75 and 5%.[30,46,94] In studies of adults with serum HSV antibodies, serial samplings indicated that HSV could be recovered from oral secretions in up to 50% in the absence of clinical lesions.[22,31] In a children's home, 32% of the children with serum HSV antibodies were found to shed oral virus periodically, and most were asymptomatic.[18]

The occurrence of recurrent labial herpes as determined by retrospective epidemiological studies is summarized in Table 1, and the variability noted will be discussed in appropriate sections below.

A study on 80 trigeminal ganglia obtained from cadavers of adults has revealed 55% to contain latent HSV-1.[5] Close to 20% of 21 sacral ganglia were found to contain latent HSV-2.[6] These rates are only slightly less than those expected from serological studies in similar population groups.

Virological studies of HSV-2 in pregnant women of lower socioeconomic status have revealed genital viral excretion rates of 1:75–250.[40,103] Rates of genital isolation of HSV-2 as high as 12% have been recorded in young prostitutes.[23] Intermittent asymptomatic genital excretion of HSV has been observed in women prospectively followed at rates of 8–14%.[1,19,77] The duration of virus shedding and the frequency of virus isolation from the cervix varied from woman to woman.[16] The prevalence of

Table 1. Occurrence of Recurrent Herpes Labialis as Determined by Retrospective Epidemiological Studies[a]

Population	Recurrent herpes labialis		Ref. no.
	Number studied	Positive (%)	
Students of health-care professions[b] Philadelphia, Pennsylvania	1788	38.2	92
Medical students	343	44.6	93
Hospital patients Philadelphia, Pennsylvania	242	31.5	
Students of health-care professions[b]			25
South America	1713	16.0	
Asia	950	17.6	
Africa	404	30.2	
Europe	2085	30.9	
Australia	552	33.0	
North America	4155	37.9	
Patients in a general practice North Wales, England	1855	45.8	32
Patients attending a cancer-prevention center Chicago, Illinois	423	41.1	c
School of dentistry in Michigan			
Students	731	16.3	114
Faculty	300	30.7	
Students and scientific workers			
Philadelphia, Pennsylvania	146	35.6	107
Kyoto, Japan	245	24.1	

[a] Adapted from Rawls and Campione-Piccardo.[81]
[b] Students of medicine, dentistry, veterinary medicine, dental hygiene, and nursing.
[c] I. D. Rotkin and co-workers, Unpublished observation (1975).

asymptomatic cervical herpetic infection detected by cytological methods[68] has varied from 0.03 to 6.9% depending on the population studied (see Section 5.2). In asymptomatic males attending a Veterans Administration hospital, HSV was isolated from the urethra, prostate, or epididymis of 15% of the study group.[17] These high rates of asymptomatic uro-genital HSV infections in males have not been found by other workers.[39,51]

Antibody surveys have also established a high prevalence of infection with HSV. While early surveys did not differentiate between HSV-1 and HSV-2 antibodies, they are consistent with HSV-antibody prevalence rates in adult populations of 50% to close to 100%, depending on socioeconomic status.[81,97,109] Later differential antibody surveys confirmed these observations and in addition indicated prevalence rates of 10–70% for HSV-2, depending on sexual activity and socioeconomic level.[56,78–81,98]

The incidence of HSV (presumably HSV-1) infections has been measured largely in children's institutions through repeated bleedings or viral isolations or both over time. In one 6-year study in a children's home, Cesario et al.[18] found that of the 70 initially seronegative children, 8, or 11.4%, experienced a primary infection while in the home, of whom 6 had an associated illness. In an earlier Australian study in a home for children, all under 3 years of age, Anderson and Hamilton[3] found that 29 of 43 seronegative children (67.4%) developed HSV antibodies over a 1-year period, of whom 20 had an associated illness.

5.1.2. Epidemic Behavior. Epidemics of diseases associated with HSV have not been described. This is in large part because HSV infections, unlike varicella, are very often asymptomatic. However, clusters of cases in various environments have been reported. Scott[88] and Juretic[41] have reviewed such clusters in families, in hospitals, and in various closed populations. At least 17 families have been described in which two or more family members were found to be infected over a short period of time. The source of the infection was ascribed to adults with recurrent labial infections or children with primary oral infections.

Hospital outbreaks of eczema herpeticum or of gingivostomatitis have been described in England and in Yugoslavia.[41,75] In the contact outbreak of eczema herpeticum, four patients developed the infection in succession within 8 days. In addition, some of the nurses caring for the patients developed herpetic lesions on their hands. In crowded pediatric wards housing 37 children below 2 years of age, 17 of the infants developed, over a 1-month period, manifest forms of HSV infections. All of the affected infants had gingivostomatitis, but in 3 cases, this was also associated with herpetic keratitis or skin involvement. Nosocomial transmission of HSV infection has also been noted in an intensive care unit and in a newborn nursery.[13,45]

Outbreaks of herpetic stomatitis have been described in orphanage nurseries and children's homes. Within a 1-month period, the attack rate of the clinically apparent primary infections was around 80%.[33,41] The attack rate in another institution for young infants over an 11-month period was found to be 56%[3] Although these studies would imply that HSV spreads very readily in closed populations, another report demonstrated that only 10% of susceptible children developed HSV infections over a 6-year period.[18]

Several clusters of an unusual form of cutaneous HSV ("herpes gladiatorum") have also been reported.[74,89,110] Person-to-person spread from the close body contact associated with wrestling or other sports, such as rugby, has been observed repeatedly. Underlying skin conditions or mat burns increase the susceptibility of the wrestlers to this type of skin infection.

5.1.3. Geographic Distribution.
HSV infections are worldwide, as attested by the finding of antibodies to both HSV types in sera from all over the world, including remote islands and isolated primitive populations. For example, studies of remote and primitive Indian tribes in Brazil have demonstrated that sera from nearly all the Tiriyo tribe have HSV neutralizing antibodies; this is in contrast to the low incidence or even absence of antibodies to respiratory-transmitted infections, such as influenza and measles.[10] This observation was extended in a subsequent study of nine tribes on the periphery of the Amazon Basin in which the proportion of sera positive for HSV antibodies was higher than in New Haven, Connecticut, and other urban areas of the United States for each age group.

In an international study of health-care-professional students,[25] variability in responses of prior history of herpes labialis was noted (Table 1). Students from South America and Asia appeared to be about half as likely to have experienced this recurrent herpetic infection as those from Europe, Australia, or North America. Lower rates of recurrent labial herpes and of recovery of latent virus from trigeminal ganglia were found in Japanese than in Americans.[107]

Surveys for HSV-2 antibodies in healthy women, made in pursuit of a relationship between this virus and cervical cancer, have revealed wide geographic and socioeconomic variations.[80,81] The prevalence of HSV-2 antibodies in sera from women over 40 years old has ranged from 9% in one United States community to 77% in Uganda.

5.1.4. Temporal Distribution.
One report indicates that herpetic skin infections are more common in the summertime.[24] A significant increase in the occurrence in the summer months of genital herpetic infections was also observed in a university-student population.[102] This was explained in part by the recent detachment of students from parental restraints. Otherwise, no clear-cut yearly or seasonal pattern of infection has been demonstrated for either HSV-1 or HSV-2. It is still possible that such variations in infection rate might occur and go unrecognized because of the need for laboratory-based studies to identify the infection.

5.1.5. Age.
Herpetic infections, most often due to HSV-2, occur in newborns as a consequence usually of maternal genital infection.[63] Thereafter, during childhood, primary HSV-1 infections are most common and are reflected clinically as herpetic gingivostomatitis, and less often as infections of the eyes, skin, and central nervous system. Nevertheless, initial HSV-1 infections can occur in adulthood primarily as oral or genital infections.[19,30] Recurrent herpes labialis tends to be less frequent in childhood and adolescence and to decrease in frequency in older adults.[32,91] There is some indication from our own experience[2] that recurrent asymptomatic genital herpes as detected cytologically is less frequent in women beyond 49 years of age. The rate of isolation of HSV-2 was also noted to be 12% in prostitutes under 19 years of age, whereas it was only 2.8% in prostitutes over 30 years of age.[23]

HSV-2 infections and their clinical manifestations occur mainly after 14 years of age, when venereal exposure becomes a mechanism of spread. Two seroepidemiological studies, conducted in lower socioeconomic populations,[56,78] demonstrated essentially similar age patterns in the distribution of HSV-1 and HSV-2 antibodies. There was a sharp rise of HSV-1 antibodies between the ages of 1 and 5 years, at which time approximately half the children already demonstrated such antibodies. The frequency of HSV-1 antibodies thereafter rose gradually to reach around 90% by adulthood. On the other hand,

HSV-2 antibodies were not detected until around 14 years of age and peaked to 20–35% by 35 years of age. By use of virological or cytological methods, the peak age for detecting genital HSV infections has been found to be between 20 and 29 years of age.[19,58,68,70]

5.1.6. Race. A higher frequency of HSV-1 and HSV-2 antibodies has been found in black populations than in white populations.[8,81,97] This most likely reflects socioeconomic levels and sexual activities, rather than any differences in susceptibility or host response.

5.1.7. Sex. A slightly higher frequency of labial herpes in females has been noted in two reports.[32,69] Otherwise, no sex differences have been noted, if exposure patterns are kept in mind.

5.1.8. Occupation. An occupational risk has been noted in three groups. The first group includes medical, nursing, or dental personnel, who are at higher risk of developing herpetic paronychia.[13,83] A second group is comprised of college wrestlers, who have been noted in several studies to have a propensity to acquire "herpes gladiatorum," a special form of skin herpes.[74,89,110] A third group includes prostitutes, who are at high risk of developing genital herpes. The most striking observations are the high prevalence rates of HSV-2 antibodies of close to 70% in prostitutes[23] and the low frequency of 3% in chaste women.[56]

5.1.9. Occurrence in Different Settings. HSV-1 is transmitted by personal contact, so that settings with close and prolonged exposure such as families, nurseries, and orphanges can result in a higher rate of infection. Reactivation of HSV-1 infections is seen on hospital wards in patients having a variety of febrile illnesses or various cancers or being treated with immunosuppressants, and on ski slopes after ultraviolet exposure.

HSV-2 infections occur most commonly in settings associated with sexual activity and sexual promiscuity. It is not uncommon to find HSV-2 infections in association with other venereal diseases.[19,40,61]

5.1.10. Socioeconomic Status. The higher frequency of HSV infections in lower socioeconomic groups was well established in earlier antibody surveys.[14,97] While these did not differentiate type 1 and type 2 antibodies, the conclusions seem valid. Similar findings for HSV-1 have been seen in more recent work; for HSV-2, the association between

socioeconomic level and sexual activity has made interpretation more difficult, but the evidence is in the same direction.[79,81] Among upper social classes, HSV-2 antibodies are acquired later, and up to 50% of young adults may lack antibodies to either HSV type; the pattern is similar to that observed with EBV and CMV antibodies in different socioeconomic groups (see Chapters 8 and 10).

5.1.11. Other Factors. Trigeminal neurectomy and fever are well known to reactivate HSV oral infections. Certain forms of immunosuppression, such as is administered for cancer patients or renal-, bone-marrow-, or heart-transplant recipients, also increase the frequency of reactivation of HSV infections,[4,49,53,76] which tend to be more severe or chronic. Severe malnutrition does not appear to alter susceptibility, instead increasing markedly the severity of a herpetic infection.[9] Recent immunogenetic studies point to a higher frequency of HLA-1 antigens in persons with frequent recurrences of herpes labialis than in the general population.[84] Similar studies in patients with recurrent ocular infections failed to demonstrate a correlation with any histocompatability type.[50,115]

Whether the types or strains of HSV may differ in their ability to spread or to establish latency is still unclear. There is, however, some indication of a greater frequency of recurrences with genital than with labial infections and with genital HSV-2 than with genital HSV-1 infections.[19,81]

5.2. Epidemiological Aspects of Specific Clinical Entities

5.2.1. Genital Infections. Surveys of genital herpetic infections have been conducted most commonly in venereal disease clinics. As far back as 1880, the rates were found to be 7% in women and 1% in men attending a VD clinic in Hamburg; approximately similar rates have been observed recently in VD clinics in the United States, England, and Sweden.[40,61] Data are lacking to establish with certainty that genital herpes has been on the rise in the past decade in such clinics, since the entity has only recently received increasing awareness and recognition. However, it is most likely that a true increase has been occurring in certain segments of the general population who have become more promiscuous in recent years. Recent studies in college students[42,102] indicate an increasing recognition of genital herpes as a prevalent sexually transmitted disease, the disease being in fact more frequently diagnosed than syphilis or gonorrhea. Barring such published results and testimonials of similar experiences in practitioners' practices, the ratio of genital herpes to gonorrhea in VD clinics has been 1 case of herpes to 2–10 of gonorrhea.[15,19,61] Such information might permit a rough estimate of the number of cases of genital herpes in the United States. Thus, with about 2 million cases of gonorrhea a year, one might expect around 200,000–1 million cases of genital herpes, of which approximately one quarter would be primary infections.

By use of cytological methods for the detection of genital HSV infections, rates have varied from 0.03 to 6.9%, depending on the population studied.[68] The highest rates were in women attending VD clinics and in prostitutes. Comparative studies by the same group of workers revealed the rate in indigent women to be 0.31% and in private patients to be 0.02%.[70] In two different hospitals for indigent patients, the rates were 3 times higher in pregnant women than in nonpregnant women.[67,70] The median age for the detection of genital herpes in our hospital was found to be 22 years.

5.2.2. Oral Infections. The most thorough study of primary herpetic oral infection was performed by Juretic in Yugoslavia.[41] This worker found that over a 10-year period, about 13% of 18,730 children attending outpatient clinics had clinical evidence of oral herpes. No cases were recorded in the first 6 months of life. The frequency distribution of the total number of cases over the succeeding age periods was as follows: 6-12 months, 12%; 1–2 years, 35%; 2–3 years, 23%; 4–5 years, 11%; 5–6 years, 8%. Thereafter, cases continued to be observed at low frequency. No significant sex differences or seasonal variations were observed. These age distributions correspond well with those noted in South Africa in the severely malnourished children with fatal disseminated HSV infections whose initial site of infection was intraoral.[9] It should also be reemphasized that symptomatic primary oral herpetic infections can occur in adolescence and adulthood and that the virus has been associated with about 10% of cases of pharyngitis in student populations.[27,30] Extrapolated to the United States population, these various studies suggest that about half a million cases of oral herpetic infections occur yearly.

5.2.3. Labial Herpes. A positive history of recurrent herpes labialis was recorded in 38% of 1800 students attending professional schools at the University of Pennsylvania.[92] Among the students susceptible to recurrences, new lesions occurred once a month in 5%, at intervals of 2–11 months in 34%, and once a year or less often in 61%. Recurrent herpes labialis was also noted to occur 3 times as frequently in a group of febrile patients as in a group of nonfebrile controls.[31] This study corroborated the older findings that up to half of patients treated with fever therapy experienced reactivation of a herpetic infection, mostly on the lips. The Perinatal Study of the National Institutes of Health found 1% of pregnant women to have labial herpes at some time during pregnancy. Another study in the United States indicates that about 1% of nursery personnel had recurrent labial herpes within any one week.[29] Estimates based on various studies suggest that about 100 million episodes of recurrent labial herpes occur yearly in the United States.

5.2.4. Herpetic Keratitis. About 5% of patients attending an ophthalmology clinic were noted to have herpetic ocular disease. Close to half the patients would be expected to have at least one recurrence of herpetic keratitis within a 2-year period.[38]

5.2.5. Herpes of the Skin. The prevalence rate of herpetic skin infections was found to be around 1% of 7495 persons over 7 years of age in the county of Skaraborg in Sweden.[35] This investigation, performed during a mass X-ray survey of the lungs, showed little variation in rates according to age or sex. Another Swedish study found that 2% of men and 2.5% of women attending a dermatology clinic in Gothenburg over a 6-year period had clinical evidence of HSV skin infection.[24]

5.2.6. Respiratory Infections. In a 6-year study involving 1293 students attending a health clinic, 142 (11%) with respiratory illnesses were found with oral HSV, while only 11 (1%) of asymptomatic students shed virus.[30] Most of the respiratory illnesses, primary pharyngotonsillitis, were associated with primary HSV infections. This study provided strong support for the much-debated issue of the role of HSV in causing respiratory illnesses.[22, 27,46,52,94]

5.2.7. Neurological Infections. According to limited reports from the CDC, HSV encephalitis is associated with a higher case-fatality rate than encephalitis caused by other viruses, other than rabies. Prospective studies in the United States and England indicate a 70% fatality rate.[47,111] The incidence has been estimated to be 1 case per $\frac{1}{2}$–1 million population—so that around 250–500 cases are likely to occur every year in the United States. No estimate is available on the incidence of the benign meningitis most often associated with HSV-2 genital infections.

5.2.8. Neonatal Herpes. In a recent review of neonatal herpetic infections,[63] we noted that the numbers of cases being reported were increasing over the past decade. This may reflect increased awareness of this entity, which has been found to occur in over 25 countries in the world. An alternative explanation is the coincidence of this increase with that possibly occurring with genital HSV infections. On the basis of the number of cases observed in two hospitals for indigent patients, an estimate of the minimum number of cases of neonatal herpes in the United States is 120 per year.[63]

6. Mechanisms and Routes of Transmission

There are no known animal vectors for the transmission of HSVs. Although a few cases of HSV-1 or HSV-2 laboratory-acquired infections have occurred, the major mode of spread appears to be by close personal contact. The source of virus is a person with a subclinical or clinically inapparent primary or recurrent infection. It is also possible for a person to autoinfect himself. Exogenous reinfection in humans with the same virus type has recently been documented.[11]

The incubation period for either primary HSV-1 or HSV-2 infection ranges from 2 to 20 days, with an average of around 6 days. The incubation period for HSV encephalitis has been more difficult to define, but appears to be longer. The duration of recovery of infectious virus is usually longer with a primary genital infection (mean around 14 days) than with a recurrent genital infection or herpes labialis (mean around 4 days).[19,100]

The major source of virus to the newborn is the mother's HSV-2 (and occasionally HSV-1) genital infection around the time of delivery.[63] The virus is acquired by an ascending infection, if membranes are ruptured, or on passage of the infant through the infected birth canal. Postnatal acquisition of the virus from a maternal infection has been observed. Infant-to-infant transmission in a nursery, presumably via handling by nursery personnel, has also been noted.[29,45] On the other hand, the acquisition of virus by the newborn from nursery personnel with a herpetic infection, such as cold sores, is poorly documented.

Detailed information on the mode of spread of many types of HSV-1 nongenital infections is not available. Cases have been observed in which virus spread occurred via kissing or from body contact associated with wrestling. Spread by saliva is likely to have been involved in the outbreaks of herpetic stomatitis in orphanage nurseries and children's homes noted earlier (Section 5.1.2). Such spread is more directly evidenced by the cases of herpetic paronychia in medical, nursing, or dental personnel who treat the infected oral cavities of patients or handle contaminated tracheal catheters. Spread via air droplets or via infected skin squames has not been well documented. HSV-1 appears to have varying degrees of communicability, as suggested by surveys in closed populations.[3,18,33,41] HSV-1 has been demonstrated on occasion to be transmitted by oral-genital or oral-anal contact, and autoinoculation of oral virus to the genitals or other body sites can occur.

The venereal transmission of genital HSV infection was postulated during the 19th and early 20th centuries. Thereafter, despite a few case reports substantiating such transmission, the venereal route of spread was not accepted generally, most likely as a result of the lack of appreciation of subclinical genital infections. The advent of HSV type differentiation has provided more conclusive evidence of venereal transmission. The risk of developing genital HSV in female contacts of males with penile herpes is around 60–80%,[58,79] although the risk has not been defined in terms of single exposure. The risk of males developing genital HSV from contact with infected female partners has not been systematically studied, although many such cases have been observed. It is still unclear whether males are infectious to their sexual contacts between episodes of clinically evident penile infections. Homosexual transmission between males has been reported, resulting in HSV-1 or HSV-2 perianal lesions.[21] Similar transmission in female homosexuals, although likely to occur, has not yet been described. The transmission of HSV-2 by oral-genital contact, causing intraoral HSV-2 infections, has also been observed.[19,21]

HSV-2 infections of genital sites may occasionally involve neighboring areas, such as the perineum, thighs, or buttocks, either by autoinoculation or by contact with infected partners. Recurrences in these sites can occur independent of, or together with, recurrences at genital sites. In addition, HSV-2 infections of the hands have been acquired by medical or nursing personnel from contact with infected patients.

7. Pathogenesis and Immunity

Primary HSV-1 or HSV-2 infections are often clinically inapparent in both children and older persons, partly because the more common primary sites of infection, such as the mouth or cervix, are not readily visible. Primary infections, when clinically manifest, tend to be more severe (fever, more extensive lesions of longer duration, constitutional signs, and local adenopathy) than in persons with prior antibodies to either HSV-1 or HSV-2 or both.

Primary HSV infections are particularly severe in certain types of patients, including severely malnourished children and those with associated measles, patients with severe burns or chronic skin disorders such as eczema, patients receiving immunosuppressive therapy, patients with cancers, particularly of the lymphohematopoietic organs, and children with certain forms of immune deficiency, such as the Wiskott–Aldrich syndrome.[49,53,64] In such patients, as in the newborn, the virus may disseminate to internal organs. The pathogenesis of primary HSV infection has been defined most thoroughly in severely malnourished children.[9] In such cases, as a result of the initial replication of virus at the portal of entry, there is a primary viremia resulting in involvement of certain susceptible organ sites. A secondary viremia then ensues, with further dissemination to visceral organs and more extensive damage. Thus, the clinical spectrum may differ, depending on which organ sites are involved and the amount of cellular damage in these organs.

In the noncompromised host, recovery of virus from the blood or peripheral leukocytes has been infrequent.[20] It is therefore not clear at present whether virus affects areas other than the local site and regional lymph nodes. However, the recovery of HSV-2 from peripheral-blood leukocytes and

from the cerebrospinal fluid of patients with meningitis suggests that blood dissemination may ocur more commonly than has been appreciated in the past.[20,96] Several human and experimental-animal observations suggest that HSV may spread neurogenically when encephalitis occurs in otherwise normal subjects. Viral spread from superficial areas of skin to deeper layers may be prevented by the meshwork of connective tissue fibers, because of size factors, and by the possible effects on connective-tissue acid mucopolysaccharides of the negative electrical charge on the virus.[54] The pathogenesis of the deeper ocular manifestations associated with HSV has been attributed either to direct viral involvement or to a hypersensitivity reaction.

The pathogenesis of the disseminated form of neonatal herpes appears to be similar to that of primary herpes in the severely malnourished child, although the brain is involved much more often in the newborn.[63] Direct neurogenic spread to the brain, and possibly to the retina, appears to occur also in newborns.

The immunology of HSV infection in humans and experimental animals has been extensively reviewed recently.[95] In persons with a primary HSV infection, humoral antibodies can usually be detected within 1–3 weeks by a variety of neutralization, CF, complement-mediated cytolysis, antibody-mediated mononuclear cell cytolysis, or passive hemagglutination tests. With special serological methods, it is also possible to demonstrate an early rise of IgM antibodies to HSV, followed by IgA and IgG antibodies. In the newborn, IgM antibodies to HSV can be detected within 1–4 weeks after birth and are present for 6 or more months.

In addition to the humoral responses, various assays of cellular immunity *in vitro* have demonstrated a cell-mediated response within 1–2 weeks after onset of infection in both man and experimental animals. Individuals with serum neutralization antibodies will usually also demonstrate a delayed-hypersensitivity skin-test response to HSV antigens.

It is yet unclear which of these humoral or cellular factors operate in curtailing the virus in a primary infection or in a newborn without transplacental antibodies. In experimental animals, it has been demonstrated that a depression of T lymphocytes, macrophages, or interferon leads to increased mortality. It has been noted that HSV multiplies better in the macrophages of newborn mice or humans than in those of adults. Since any virus circulating in the blood would be affected greatly by the ability of reticuloendothelial cells in the liver or other organs to inactivate the virus or allow its multiplication and further spread, it is likely that macrophages play a central role in neonatal HSV infection and probably also in primary HSV infections of older persons. More recently, natural killer (NK) cells have also been involved in the immunity of mice to HSV infection. Both newborn mice and humans appear to have low or absent NK-cell activity.

Although HSV-1 or HSV-2 infections in patients with prior HSV-1 or HSV-2 infections, or both, tend to be less severe clinically than primary infections, such infections in compromised hosts tend to be more extensive and chronic. HSV encephalitis, which was formerly believed to occur only in association with a primary infection, has now been documented in patients with prior HSV infection. Similarly, although newborns with transplacental HSV antibodies were originally believed to be protected from acquiring HSV infections, several cases of neonatal herpetic disease, including fatalities, have been recorded in such infants.

In recurrent HSV infections, all persons appear to possess neutralizing antibodies in varying titers, usually higher than in those persons without recurrences. The antibodies most often do not rise after a recurrence, and it appears that clinically apparent or inapparent recurrences might be necessary to maintain the neutralizing titer at constant levels in the serum. There are also persons with frequent herpetic recurrences who possess persistent levels of IgG, IgA, and IgM antibodies to HSV in their serum and who may demonstrate a significant boost in titers to antibodies in the various classes after a recurrence.

Persons with recurrences also demonstrate positive responses in a variety of *in vitro* cell-mediated assays. There are conflicting data regarding the correlation between depression of cell-mediated immunity, including such lymphokines as interferon or leukocyte-inhibitory factor, with increased predilection to HSV recurrences. The importance of cell-mediated mechanisms, however, is suggested by studies in immunocompromised persons, who tend to develop more frequent and more severe herpetic recurrences.

In vitro studies indicate that both nonspecific and specific mechanisms are involved in stopping the cell-to-cell spread of HSV, since neutralizing anti-bodies alone cannot usually prevent this type of viral spread. In addition, *in vitro* observations indicate that neutralizing antibodies are unable to inactivate large amounts of extracellular virus and may operate together with complement or with nonimmune mononuclear or phagocytic cells in lysing HSV-infected cells.

8. Patterns of Host Response

Table 2 presents our most recent findings on close to 2000 subjects in whom HSV-1 or HSV-2 or both have been isolated from a variety of body sites. The occurrence in some subjects of simultaneous infections of different sites by HSV-1 and HSV-2 can be noted in the Table. It is important to emphasize that although one HSV type is more likely to occur in any one body site, the other HSV type can occasionally infect similar sites.

8.1. Mouth and Respiratory and Gastrointestinal Tracts

The mouth is the most common site of primary HSV-1 infection. Children are most often affected, but oral infections may also occur in older persons. The spectrum of oral infections ranges in the noncompromised subjects from inapparent infection to severe gingivostomatitis with extensive ulcerations of the mouth, tongue, and gums, cervical adenopathy, and fever, sometimes necessitating hospitalization for fluid and electrolyte restoration. The patients may occasionally infect themselves at other body sites, such as the face, fingers, or genitals. In the newborn or compromised host, and infrequently in the apparently normal person, oral infection may extend to involve the larynx, esophagus, or lungs, and may disseminate to involve the liver and other visceral organs or the brain.

Because of the common presence of HSV in the mouths or asymptomatic subjects, it has been difficult to ascertain the etiological role of HSV in upper respiratory infections, such as rhinitis and pharyngotonsillitis, and the role of the virus as a cause of recurrent lesions inside the mouth. However, recent data suggest strongly that HSV is etiologically related to these clinical manifestations.[30,108]

The large majority of cases of oral herpetic infections are caused by HSV-1, but HSV-2 has also been found to cause such infections as a consequence of fellatio (Table 2).

Table 2. Clinical Spectrum of Infections Caused by Herpes Simplex Viruses 1 and 2 in Newborns and Older Persons and the Type Isolated from Different Sites and Clinical Conditions[a]

	Number of persons with HSV type		
	Type 1	Type 2	Total
I. Usually mild to moderately severe (persons over 1 month of age)			
A. Urogenital infections			
1. Females (cervix, vulva, vagina, urethra)	51 (8[b])	514 (5[c])	565
2. Males (penis, urethra)	11 (2[b])	333 (1[d], 2[c])	344
B. Nongenital infections			
1. Gingivostomatitis or asymptomatic (mouth)	197	5 (3[c])	202
2. Herpes labialis (lips)	125	1	126
3. Keratitis and/or conjunctivitis (cornea and/or conjunctiva)	50	1	51
4. Dermatitis	6	0	6
a. Skin above waist	110 (2[e])	8	118
b. Skin below waist	11 (3[b], 2[e])	118 (6[e], 2[f])	129
c. Hands or arms	25 (2[f])	21 (2[f], 3[e])	46
C. Latent infections: Trigeminal or thoractic ganglia	26 (1[g])	0	26
Sacral ganglia	0	5	5
II. Usually severe to fatal (persons over 1 month of age)			
A. Meningoencephalitis (brain, spinal cord, CSF)	176	5	181
B. Multiple sclerosis (brain)	0	1	1
C. Eczema herpeticum (skin, lungs)	14	1	15
D. Generalized disease (visceral organs)	3	1 (1[h])	4
III. Newborns—localized or generalized infection (skin, eyes, brain, CSF, visceral organs)	57 (7[i])	142 (31[i])	199
TOTALS:	862	1156	2018

[a] Typing is done by microneutralization or direct IF tests.
[b] Simultaneous isolation of similar HSV type from mouth.
[c] Simultaneous isolation of HSV-2 from cervix or vulva and HSV-1 from lip or mouth.
[d] Simultaneous isolation of HSV-2 from penile lesion and HSV-1 from eye.
[e] Simultaneous isolation of same HSV type from genitals.
[f] Laboratory- or hospital-acquired infection.
[g] Simultaneous isolation of HSV-2 from sacral ganglia.
[h] Isolated also from brain.
[i] Same HSV type isolated from mother's genital tract.

8.2. Lips

Labial herpes is the most common form of recrudescence with HSV-1. The lesions, which are single or multiple, may involve the mucocutaneous junction, at or around the same site with every recurrence. Occasionally, the herpetic lesions may affect both sides and may be accompanied by involvement of other body sites. The lips may also be infrequently involved during a primary infection. Extensive local spread or persistence of the lesions for long periods may occur in compromised persons. The natural history of labial herpes has recently been well detailed.[(100)]

8.3. Eyes

The spectrum of ocular involvement includes conjunctivitis, keratitis (superficial and stromal), cataracts, iridocyclitis, and panuveitis. Although the more superficial ocular lesions in children and adults are usually associated with HSV-1, a few cases of HSV-2 infection have been recognized. In the newborn, the ocular lesions may be caused by either HSV-1 or HSV-2. The ill effects of corticosteroids in ocular herpes are worth reemphasizing here.

8.4. Skin

HSV vesicles on the skin are usually localized, may assume a zosteriform distribution in some instances, and may result from either a primary or a recrudescent infection. In the compromised subject, the skin lesions may be more extensive and chronic. In persons with atopic eczema or with other dermatoses (e.g., Darier's disease), HSV infection can be more generalized and involve both affected and nonaffected areas of the underlying skin condition, resulting in Kaposi's varicelliform eruption or eczema herpeticum.[75] Occasional recurrences of this entity have been described, and mortality may ensue from viral dissemination to vital organs or from bacterial superinfection.

Traumatic herpes occurs in areas of skin abrasions, burns, or puncture wounds. Laboratory HSV-1 or HSV-2 infections have occasionally resulted from such skin breaks in the hand (Table 2). Herpetic paronychia occurring in medical, nursing, or dental personnel and the skin infections occurring in wrestlers—herpes gladiatorum—were cited earlier. HSV infection of severe burns may be fatal, since it may lead to pneumonia and viral involvement of other vital organs. HSV infections may also be associated on occasion with the allergic manifestations of erythema multiforme.[90]

In general, skin lesions below the waist (Table 2) are caused by HSV-2, often in association with genital infection, whereas skin lesions above the waist are caused by HSV-1, reflecting the different modes of acquisition of the two virus types. Herpetic lesions of the hand or fingers can result from infection with either virus type.

8.5. Urogenital Tract

The term "herpes progenitalis" should be discarded, since in women genital infections occur commonly in the cervix and in either symptomatic or asymptomatic males the virus may be cultured not only from the penis but also from the urethra, prostate, and seminal vesicles.[17,39,51] Although HSV has been implicated as an occasional cause of urethritis, prostatitis, and cystitis, its exact role in these diseases remains to be elucidated. Cerebrospinal fluid pleocytosis in the presence or absence of meningeal signs, radiculitis, and myelitis has been observed occasionally in association with genital herpetic infections.[19,20]

8.6. Nervous System

The neurological manifestations associated with HSV infection include encephalitis, meningitis, radiculitis, and myelitis.[20,66] The association of a particular neurological manifestation with HSV-1 or with HSV-2 appears to depend on (1) the host, i.e., whether newborn or older person, and whether compromised or uncompromised; and (2) the prevalence of a particular HSV type at various ages and in different socioeconomic groups. Since HSV-1 is the viral type that has been recovered in all but five cases of herpetic encephalitis (Table 2), the possibility exists that the two HSV types also differ in their ability to spread neurogenically or via the blood to the brain. Further study is needed to substantiate the role of HSV in chronic central nervous system disease, psychiatric disorders, and Bell's palsy.

8.7. Fetus and Newborn

A wide spectrum of clinical manifestations has been observed with HSV infections in the newborn, the spectrum appearing to be similar whether HSV-1 or HSV-2 is the causal agent.[63] The most severe form is the disseminated disease with involvement of the liver and other visceral organs, including frequently th brain. HSV encephalitis, which can occur without evidence of viral blood dissemination to visceral organs, is also associated with a poor prognosis. Localized involvement of the eyes, skin, or mouth, or of any two or all three, may occur. Although fatality is rare in such cases, some of the infants have been found with neurological or ocular sequelae, or both. In contrast to CMV infections, subclinical HSV infections of the newborn are very infrequent.

The association of maternal genital herpetic infection with abortions, stillbirths and premature delivery has been reported.[63] Even though the virus has been recovered from abortus material, the possibility exists that the fetus was contaminated on passage through the mother's infected genital tract, as exemplified by two of our recent cases. The role of HSV in congenital malformations, suggested by the finding in some cases of microcephaly or chorioretinitis soon after birth,[28] also awaits more conclusive evidence.

9. Control and Prevention

Although there are several potential methods that might be used in the control of HSV infections, most have little scientific validation. These can be grouped into (1) prevention of the initial infection in a given person and (2) reduction of the source of virus transmissible to others.

9.1. Prevention of the Initial Infection

9.1.1. Active Immunization. There are great, although not insurmountable, problems associated with the development of effective HSV vaccines. The potential oncogenicity of HSV imposes a restriction as to the type of immunogen that could be employed in humans. Attenuated or inactivated viruses would still contain the viral DNA genome, which might be oncogenic. Thus, until the oncogenic component of the viral DNA is identified and mutants free of this portion are produced, the only option available is to work with viral proteins free of DNA. Although cell-membrane preparations of infected cells could be employed, there is serious question as to the possible immunopathology that could ensue from their administration. Efforts have therefore been directed at preparing envelope glycoproteins free of viral DNA. Such vaccines have been shown to be immunogenic and protective in animal experiments and are currently being evaluated in humans.[37] Prospects and problems in the use of HSV vaccines for prevention of HSV infections have been discussed elsewhere,[26] and their potential value in relation to cervical cancer is discussed in Chapter 26.

9.1.2. Passive Immunization. It has been found

in experimental animals that HSV antibodies will prevent infection if administered prior to virus inoculation. The effect is negligible, however, if antibodies are administered one or more days after virus inoculation. Hyperimmune HSV globulin is currently being prepared for human trials.[7] The protection afforded by γ-globulin, which contains a relatively high titer of HSV antibodies, has been inconsistent in a very small number of newborns exposed to maternal genital HSV infections at delivery. Although newborns can become infected despite the presence in their serum of transplacentally transmitted antibodies, it has not been determined whether these failures represent the rule rather than the exception.

Other potentially beneficial approaches still requiring clinical evaluation for persons at special risk, such as newborns, include interferon.

9.1.3. Interruption of Transmission. An approach in this direction has been made toward protecting newborns from acquiring HSV from their mother's genital infection around the time of delivery. Although the risk of the infant's acquiring the infection under these circumstances is not fully established (around 40–50% in a relatively small number of cases), cesarean section performed prior to or within 4 hr of rupture of membranes appears to be more usually protective on the basis of current information. The monitoring of women with genital herpes and other methods to prevent neonatal herpes have been detailed recently.[43,105]

The use of condoms or vaginal jellies to prevent transmission of genital infections has not yet been evaluated. It might be advisable to abstain from sexual contact with partners with obvious lesions. Similarly, close contact with persons with nongenital lesions, on the lips or skin, might be avoided. The problem, however, is that many times the genital or nongenital infections are asymptomatic.

The use of gloves by medical or dental personnel when handling oral catheters or treating the mouths of patients might prevent acquisition of herpetic paronychia. Similarly, isolation of patients with severe herpetic involvement, such as patients with eczema herpeticum, might prevent transmission to other hospitalized patients or to attending personnel. It has not yet been determined whether hospital personnel with herpetic lesions, most usually cold sores, should abstain from patient care.

9.2. Reduction of the Source of Virus Transmissible to Others

There are two main approaches toward reducing the source of virus in one person that would be transmissible to his or her contacts. The first is to reduce the duration of the lesions in primary or recurrent infections and hence of transmissible virus. This approach requires some effective method of treatment, administered either topically or systemically.

The first effective antiviral agent was iododeoxyuridine for the treatment of herpetic keratitis, which did not, however, reduce the recurrence rate. Oother drugs, including adenine arabinoside (vidarabine), trifluorothymidine, and acyclovir, have also been found to be effective for the treatment of ocular herpes. Systemically administered vidarabine was also shown in controlled trials to reduce the mortality associated with herpes simplex encephalitis and with neonatal herpes.[111,112] Acyclovir, topically or systemically administered, is currently under evaluation for the treatment of various forms of mucocutaneous or severe herpetic infections. Although antiviral therapy may reduce the duration of viral excretion, particularly if effective in the prodromal phase, it still would not affect an asymptomatic source of viral spread.

The more effective approach would be to find some means to decrease the frequency of recurrences or to prevent them completely, since a recurrent infection is not only often clinically problematic but also an important source of virus to others. Two strategies could be employed here. One would be to find some way to maintain the virus in its latent state in the ganglia. The current availability of several animal models and of human ganglia cultures for latency studies permits experimentation with a variety of chemicals toward this goal. The other strategy would be to enhance immune responses so as to abort virus propagation at the mucocutaneous sites and hence curb transmissibility.

10. Unresolved Problems

10.1. Reporting

A system for national reporting of certain forms of HSV infections, such as ocular and neonatal infections, should be established, and reporting of HSV infections of the genital tract and nervous system should be improved.

10.2. Virological Aspects

These include (1) improving our knowledge of the molecular and genetic aspects of these viruses; (2) increasing application of newer methods to differentiate strains within each of the HSV types to clinicoepidemiological problems; (3) use of HSV proteins or antibodies that are type-specific for seroepidemiological studies; and (4) further understanding of the basic mechanisms involved in latency.

10.3. Host Factors

Information needs to be expanded on the genetic and immune factors that might be associated with the severity or the frequency of recurrences of HSV infection in certain persons.

10.4. Control and Prevention

Further evaluation in the laboratory and in humans of the various possible approaches listed in Section 9 is required.

ACKNOWLEDGMENTS

The research reported herein was supported by grants from the National Institutes of Health and the March of Dimes–Birth Defects Foundation.

11. References

1. ADAM, E., KAUFMAN, R. H., MIRKOVIC, R. R., AND MELNICK, J. L., Persistence of virus shedding in asymptomatic women after recovery from herpes genitalis, *Obstet. Gynecol.* **54:**171–173 (1979).
2. ADELUSI, B., NAIB, Z., MUTHER, J., AND NAHMIAS, A., Epidemiological studies relating genital herpes simplex virus (HSV) infection with cervical neoplasia—An update, in: *The Human Herpesviruses: An Interdisciplinary Perspective* (A. NAHMIAS, W. DOWDLE, AND R. SCHINAZI, eds.), p. 627, Elsevier/North-Holland, New York, 1981.

3. ANDERSON, S. G., AND HAMILTON, J., The epidemiology of primary herpes simplex infection, *Med. J. Aust.* **1**:308–311 (1949).

4. ASTON, D. L., COHEN, A., AND SPINDLER, M., Herpesvirus hominis infection in patients with certain myeloproliferative and lymphoproliverative disorders, *Br. Med. J.* **4**:462–465 (1972).

5. BARINGER, J. R., AND SWOVELAND, P., Recovery of herpes simplex virus from human trigeminal ganglions, *N. Engl. J. Med.* **288**:648–650 (1973).

6. BARINGER, J. R., Recovery of herpes simplex virus from human sacral ganglions, *N. Engl. J. Med.* **291**:828–830 (1974).

7. BARON, S., GEORGIADES, J., AND WORTHINGTON, M., Potential for postexposure prophylaxis of neonatal herpes using passive antibody, in: *The Human Herpesviruses: An Interdisciplinary Perspective* (A. NAHMIAS, W. DOWDLE, AND R. SCHINAZI, eds.), pp. 491–495, Elsevier/North-Holland, New York, 1981.

8. BECKER, W. B., The epidemiology of herpesvirus infection in three racial communities in Cape Town, *S. Afr. Med. J.***40**:109–111 (1966).

9. BECKER, W. B., KIPPS, A., AND McKENZIE, D., Disseminated herpes simplex virus infections: Its pathogenesis based on virological and pathological studies in 33 cases, *Am. J. Dis. Child.* **115**:1–8 (1968).

10. BLACK, F. L., Infectious diseases in primitive societies, *Science* **187**:515–518 (1975).

11. BUCHMAN, T., ROIZMAN, B., AND NAHMIAS, A., Demonstration of exogenous genital reinfection with herpes simplex virus type 2 by restriction endonuclease fingerprinting of viral DNA, *J. Infect. Dis.* **140**:195–304 (1979).

12. BUCHMAN, T. G., SIMPSON, T., NOSAL, C., ROIZMAN, B., AND NAHMIAS, A. J., The structure of herpes simplex virus DNA and its application to molecular epidemiology, *Ann. N. Y. Acad. Sci.* **354**:279–290 (1980).

13. BUCHMAN, T. G., ROIZMAN, B., ADAMS, G., AND STOVER, G. H., Restriction endonuclease fingerprinting of herpes simplex virus DNA: A novel epidemiological tool applied to a nosocomial outbreak, *J. Infect. Dis.* **138**:488–498 (1978).

14. BUDDINGH, G. J., SCHRUM, D. I., LANIER, J. C., AND GUIDRY, D. J., Studies of the natural history of herpes simplex infections, *Pediatrics* **11**:595–610 (1953).

15. CENTER FOR DISEASE CONTROL, Non-reported sexually transmitted diseases in the United States, *Morbid. Mortal. Weekly Rep.* **28**:61–63 (1979).

16. CENTIFANTO, Y. M., HILDEBRANDT, R. J., HELD, B., AND KAUFMAN, H. E., Relationship of herpes simplex genital infection and carcinoma of the cervix: Population studies, *Am. J. Obstet. Gynecol.* **110**:690–692 (1971).

17. CENTIFANTO, Y. M., DRYLIE, D. M., DEARDOURFF, S. L., AND KAUFMAN, H., Herpesvirus type 2 in the male genitourinary tract, *Science* **178**:318–319 (1972).

18. CESARIO, T. C., POLAND, J. D., AND WULFF, H., Six years experience with herpes simplex virus in a children's home, *Am. J. Epidemiol.* **90**:416–422 (1969).

19. COREY, L., HOLMES, K. K., BENEDETTI, J., AND CRITCHLOW, C., Clinical course of genital herpes: Implications for therapeutic trials, in: *The Human Herpes viruses: An Interdisciplinary Perspective* (A. NAHMIAS, W. DOWDLE, AND R. SCHINAZI, eds.), pp. 496–502, Elsevier/North-Holland, New York, 1981.

20. CRAIG, C. P., AND NAHMIAS, A., Different patterns of neurologic involvement with herpes simplex virus types 1 and 2: Isolation of herpes simplex virus type 2 from the buffy coat of two adults with meningitis, *J. Infect. Dis.* **127**:365–372 (1973).

21. DOLIN, R., GILL, F., AND NAHMIAS, A., Genital herpes simplex virus type 1 infection—Variability in modes of spread, *J. Am. Ven. Dis. Assoc.* **2**:13–16 (1975).

22. DOUGLAS, R. G., JR., AND COUCH, R. B., A prospective study of chronic herpes simplex virus infection and recurrent herpes labialis in humans, *J. Immunol.* **104**:289–295 (1970).

23. DUENAS, A., ADAM, E., MELNICK, J. L., AND RAWLS, W. E., Herpesvirus type 2 in a prostitute population, *Am. J. Epidemiol.* **95**:483–489 (1972).

24. EILARD, U., AND HELLGREN, L., Herpes simplex: A statistical and clinical investigation based on 669 patients, *Dermatologica* **130**:101–106 (1965).

25. EMBIL, J. A., STEPHENS, R. G., AND MANUEL, F. R., Prevalence of recurrent herpes labialis and aphthous ulcers among young adults on six continents, *Can. Med. Assoc. J.* **113**:627–630 (1975).

26. ENNIS, F., Prevention of herpes simplex virus infection, in: *The Human Herpesviruses: An Interdisciplinary Perspective* (A. NAHMIAS, W. DOWDLE, AND R. SCHINAZI, eds.), pp. 440–446, Elsevier/North-Holland, New York, 1981.

27. EVANS, A. S., AND DICK, E. C., Acute pharyngitis and tonsillitis in University of Wisconsin students, *J. Am. Med. Assoc.* **190**:699–708 (1964).

28. FLORMAN, A. L., GERSHON, A. A., BLACKETT, P. R., AND NAHMIAS, A. J., Intrauterine infection with herpes simplex virus: Resultant congenital malformation, *J. Am. Med. Assoc.* **225**:129–132 (1973).

29. FRANCIS, D. P., HERRMANN, K. L., AND MacMAHON, J. R., Nosocomial and maternally acquired herpesvirus hominis infections: A report of four fatal cases in neonates, *Am. J. Dis. Child.* **129**(8):889–893 (1975).

30. GLEZEN, W. P., FERNALD, G. W., AND LOHR, J. A., Acute respiratory disease of university students with special reference to the etiologic role of herpesvirus hominis, *Am. J. Epidemiol.* **101**:111–121 (1975).

31. GREENBERG, M. S., BRIGHTMAN, V. J., AND SHIP, I. I., Clinical and laboratory differenitation of recurrent intraoral herpes simplex virus infections following fever, *J. Dent. Res.* **48**:385–391 (1969).

32. GROUT, P., AND BARBER, V. E., Cold sores—An epidemiological survey, *J. R. Coll. Gen. Pract.* **26:**428–434 (1976).

33. HALE, B. D., RENDTORFF, R. C., WALKER, L. C., AND ROBERTS, A. N., Epidemic herpetic stomatitis in an orphanage nursery, *J. Am. Med. Assoc.* **183:**1068–1072 (1963).

34. HAYNES, R. E., AZIMI, P. H., AND CRAMBLETT, H. G., Fatal herpesvirus hominis (herpes simplex virus) infections in children—Clinical, pathologic and virologic characteristics, *J. Am. Med. Assoc.* **206:**312–319 (1968).

35. HELLGREN, L., The prevalence of some skin diseases and joint diseases in total populations in different areas of Sweden, *Proc. North. Dermatol. Soc.,* 155–162 (1962).

36. HERRMANN, K. AND STEWART, J., Diagnosis of herpes simplex virus type 1 and 2 infections, in: *The Human Herpesviruses: An Interdisciplinary Perspective* (A. NAHMIAS, W. DOWDLE, AND R. SCHINAZI, eds.), pp. 343–350, Elsevier/North-Holland, New York, 1981.

37. HILLEMAN, M., LARSON, V. M., LEHMAN, E. D., SALERNO, R. A., CONARD, P. G., AND McLEAN, A. A., Subunit herpes simplex 2 vaccine, in: *The Human Herpesviruses: An Interdisciplinary Perspective* (A. NAHMIAS, W. DOWDLE, AND R. SCHINAZI, eds.), pp. 503–506, Elsevier/North-Holland, New York, 1981.

38. HOWARD, G. M., AND KAUFMAN, H. E., Herpes simplex keratitis, *Arch. Ophthalmol.* **67:**373–387 (1962).

39. JEANSSON, S., AND MOLIN, L., On the occurrence of genital herpes simplex virus infection: Clinical and virological findings and relation to gonorrhoea, *Acta Derm.-Venereol.* **54:**479–485 (1974).

40. JOSEY, W. E., NAHMIAS, A. J., AND NAIB, Z. M., The epidemiology of type 2 (genital) herpes simplex virus infection, *Obstet. Gynecol. Surv. Suppl.* **27:**295–302 (1972).

41. JURETIC, M., Natural history of herpetic infection, *Helv. Paediatr. Acta* **21:**356–368 (1966).

42. KALINYAK, J. E., FLEAGLE, G., AND DOCHERTY, J. J., Incidence and distribution of herpes simplex virus types 1 and 2 from genital lesions in college women, *J. Med. Virol.* **1:**173–181 (1977).

43. KIBRICK, S., Herpes simplex infections at term, *J. Am. Med. Assoc.* **243:**157–160 (1979).

44. KLOENE, W., BANG, F. B., CHAKRABORTY, S. M., COOPER, M. R., KULEMANN, H., OTA, M., AND SHAH, K. V., A two-year respiratory virus survey in four villages in West Bengal, India, *Am. J. Epidemiol.* **92:**307–320 (1970).

45. LINNEMANN, C. C., JR., BUCHMAN, T. G., LIGHT, I. J., BALLARD, J. L., AND ROIZMAN, B., Transmission of herpes-simplex virus type 1 in a nursery for the newborn: Identification of viral isolates by DNA fingerprinting, *Lancet* **1:**964–966 (1978).

46. LINDGREN, K. M., DOUGLAS, R. G., JR., AND COUCH, R. B., Significance of herpesvirus hominis in respiratory secretions of man, *N. Engl. J. Med.* **278:**517–523 (1968).

47. LONGSON, M., Herpes encephalitis, in: *Clinical Virology* (E. HEALTH, ed.), pp. 73–86, Pittman Medical, London, 1979.

48. MATSON, D. O., ADAM, E., MELNICK, J. L., AND DREESMAN, G. R., Prevalence of antibodies to herpes simplex virus (HSV) measured with a type-specific radioimmunoassay in cervical neoplasia—Case control studies, in: *The Human Herpesviruses: An Interdisciplinary Perspective* (A. NAHMIAS, W. DOWDLE, AND R. SCHINAZI, eds.), p. 628, Elsevier/North-Holland, New York, 1981.

49. MERIGAN, T., Immunosuppression and herpesviruses, in: *The Human Herpesviruses: An Interdisciplinary Perspective* (A. NAHMIAS, W. DOWDLE, AND R. SCHINZAI, eds.), pp. 309–316, Elsevier/North-Holland, New York, 1981.

50. MEYERS-ELLIOTT, R. H., ELLIOT, J. H., MAXWELL, W. A., PETIT, T. H., O'DAY, D. M., TERASAKI, P. I., AND BERNOCO, D., HLA antigens in herpes stromal keratitis, *Am. J. Ophthalmol.* **89:**54–57 (1980).

51. MORRISSEAU, P. M., PHILLIPS, C. A., AND LEADBETTER, G. W., JR., Viral prostatitis, *J. Urol.* **103:**767–769 (1970).

52. MUFSON, M. A., WEBB, P. A., AND KENNEDY, H., Etiology of upper respiratory tract illnesses among civilian adults, *J. Am. Med. Assoc.* **195:**1–7 (1966).

53. MULLER, S. A., HERRMANN, E. C., JR., AND WINKELMANN, R. K., Herpes simplex infections in hematologic malignancies, *Am. J. Med.* **52:**102–114 (1972).

54. NAHMIAS, A. J., AND KIBRICK, S., Inhibitory effect of heparin on herpes simplex virus, *J. Bacteriol.* **87:**1060–1066 (1964).

55. NAHMIAS, A. J., AND DOWDLE, W. R., Antigenic and biologic differences in herpesvirus hominis, *Prog. Med. Virol.* **10:**110–159 (1968).

56. NAHMIAS, A. J., JOSEY, W. E., NAIB, Z. M., LUCE, C., AND DUFFEY, C., Antibodies to herpesvirus hominis types 1 and 2 in humans. I. Patients with genital herpetic infection, *Am. J. Epidemiol.* **91:**539–546 (1970).

57. NAHMIAS, A., WICKLIFFE, C., PIPKIN, J., LEIBOVITZ, A., AND HUTTON, R., Transport media for herpes simplex virus types 1 and 2, *Appl. Microbiol.* **22:**451–454 (1971).

58. NAHMIAS, A. J., DOWDLE, W. R., NAIB, Z. M., JOSEY, W. E., McCLONE, D., AND DOMESCIK, G., Genital infection with type 2 herpesvirus hominis—A commonly occurring venereal disease, *Br. J. Vener. Dis.* **45:**294–298 (1969).

59. NAHMIAS, A. J., Herpesviruses from fish to man—A search for pathobiologic unity, *Pathobiol. Annu.* **2:**153–182 (1972).

60. NAHMIAS, A. J., AND ROIZMAN, B., Infection with

herpes simplex viruses 1 and 2, *N. Engl. J. Med.* **289**:667–674, 719–725, 781–789 (1973).

61. NAHMIAS, A. J., VON REYN, C. F., JOSEY, W. E., NAIB, Z. M., AND HUTTON, R., Genital herpes simplex virus infection and gonorrhoea—Association and analogies, *Br. J. Vener. Dis.* **49**:306–309 (1973).

62. NAHMIAS, A. J., The evolution (evovirology) of herpesviruses, in: *Viruses: Evolution and Cancer* (E. KURSTAK AND K. MARAMOROSCH, eds.), pp. 605–624, Academic Press, New York, 1974.

63. NAHMIAS, A., AND VISINTINE, A., Herpes simplex, in: *Infectious Diseases of the Fetus and Newborn Infant* (J. REMINGTON AND J. KLEIN, eds.), pp. 156–190, W. B. Saunders, Philadelphia, 1976.

64. NAHMIAS, A., AND NORRILD, B., Herpes simplex viruses 1 and 2—Basic and clinical aspects, *Dis.-Mon.* **25**(10):5–49 (1979).

65. NAHMIAS, A. J., DOWDLE, W. R., AND SCHINAZI, R. (eds.), *The Human Herpesviruses: An Interdisciplinary Perspective*, Elsevier/North-Holland, New York, 1981, 721 pp.

66. NAHMIAS, A., AND WHITLEY, R., Herpes simplex virus encephalitis in pediatrics, *Pediatrics in Review* **2**:259–266 (1981).

67. NAIB, Z.M., NAHMIAS, A. J., JOSEY, W. E., AND KRAMER, J., Genital herpetic infection: Association with cervical dysplasia and carcinoma, *Cancer* **23**:940–945 (1969).

68. NAIB, Z. M., NAHMIAS, A. J., JOSEY, W. E., AND ZAKI, S. A., Relation of cytohistopathology of genital herpesvirus infection to cervical anaplasia, *Cancer Res.* **33**:1452–1463 (1973).

69. NELSON, H. G., Epidemic cold sore, *Ir. Med. J.* **68**:527–534 (1975).

70. NG, A. B., REAGAN, J. W., AND YEN, S. S., Herpes genitalis—Clinical and cytopathologic experience with 256 patients, *Obstet. Gynecol.* **36**:645–651 (1970).

71. PEREIRA, L., CASSAI, E., HONESS, R., ROIZMAN, B., TERNI, M., AND NAHMIAS, A., Variability in the structural polypeptides of herpes simplex virus strains: Potential application in molecular epidemiology, *Infect. Immun.* **13**:211–220 (1976).

72. PLUMMER, G., Serological comparison of the herpesviruses, *Br. J. Exp. Pathol.* **45**:135–141 (1964).

73. PLUMMER, G., A review of the identification and titration of antibodies to herpes simplex viruses type 1 and type 2 in human sera, *Cancer Res.* **33**:1469–1476 (1973).

74. PORTER, P. S., AND BAUGHMAN, R. D., Epidemiology of herpes simplex among wrestlers, *J. Am. Med. Assoc.* **194**:998–1000 (1965).

75. PUGH, R. C. B., DUDGEON, J. A., AND BODIAN, M., Kaposi's varicelliform eruption (eczema herpeticum) with typical and atypical visceral necrosis, *J. Pathol.*

Bacteriol. **69**:67–80 (1955).

76. RAND, K. H., POLLARD, R. B., AND MERIGAN, T. C., Increased pulmonary superinfections in cardiac-transplant patients undergoing primary cytomegalovirus infection, *N. Engl. J. Med.* **298**:951–953 (1978).

77. RATTRAY, M. C., COREY, L., REEVES, W. C., VONTVER, L. A., AND HOLMES, K. K., Recurrent genital herpes among women: Symptomatic v. asymptomatic viral shedding, *Br. J. Vener. Dis.* **54**:262–265 (1978).

78. RAWLS, W. E., IWAMOTO, K., ADAM, E., AND MELNICK, J. L., Measurement of antibodies to herpesvirus types 1 and 2 in human sera, *J. Immunol.* **112**:728–736 (1974).

79. RAWLS, W. E., GARDNER, H. L., FLANDERS, R. W., LOWRY, S. P., KAUFMAN, R. H., AND MELNICK, J. L., Genital herpes in two social groups, *Am. J. Obstet. Gynecol.* **110**:682–689 (1971).

80. RAWLS, W. E., ADAM, E., AND MELNICK, J. L., Geographical variation in the association of antibodies to herpesvirus type 2 and carcinoma of the cervix, in: *Oncogenesis and Herpesviruses* (P. M. BIGGS, G. DE THE, AND L. N. PAYNE, eds.), pp. 424–427, Scientific Publication No. 2, International Agency for Research on Cancer, Lyon, 1972.

81. RAWLS, W. E., AND CAMPIONE-PICCARDO, J., Epidemiology of herpes simplex virus type 1 and type 2, in: *The Human Herpesviruses: An Interdisciplinary Perspective* (A. NAHMIAS, W. DOWDLE, AND R. SCHINAZI, eds.), pp. 137–152, Elsevier/North-Holland, New York, 1981.

82. ROIZMAN, B. R., The structure and isomerization of herpes simplex virus genomes, *Cell* **16**:481–494 (1979).

83. ROSATO, F. E., ROSATO, E. F., AND PLOTKIN, S. A., Herpetic paronychia—An occupational hazard of medical personnel, *N. Engl. J. Med.* **283**:804–805 (1970).

84. RUSSELL, A. S., AND SCHLANT, J., HLA transplantation antigens in subjects susceptible to recrudescent herpes labialis, *Tissue Antigens* **6**:257–261 (1975).

85. SCHAFFER, P., Molecular genetics of herpes simplex viruses, in: *The Human Herpesviruses: An Interdisciplinary Perspective* (A. NAHMIAS, W. DOWDLE, AND R. SCHINAZI, eds.), pp. 55–62, Elsevier/North-Holland, New York, 1981.

86. SCHNEWEIS, K. E., Serologische Untersuchungen zur Typendifferenzierung des *Herpesvirus hominis*, *Z. Immunitaetsforsch. Exp. Ther.* **124**:24–48 (1962).

87. SCHNEWEIS, K. E., AND NAHMIAS, A. J., Antigens of herpes simplex virus types 1 and 2—Immunodiffusion and inhibition passive hemagglutination studies, *Z. Immunitaetsforsch. Exp. Klin. Immunol.* **141**:471–487 (1971).

88. SCOTT, T. F. McN., Epidemiology of herpetic infections, *Am. J. Ophthalmol.* **43**:134–146 (1957).

89. SELLING, B., AND KIBRICK, S., An outbreak of herpes simplex among wrestlers (herpes gladiatorum), *N. Engl. J. Med.* **270**:979–982 (1964).

90. SHELLEY, W. B., Herpes simplex virus as a cause of erythema multiforme, *J. Am.Med. Assoc.* **201**:153–156 (1967).

91. SHIP, I. I., MILLER, M. F., AND RAM, C., A retrospective study of recurrent herpes labialis (RHL) in a professional population 1958–1971, *Oral Surg.* **44**:723–730 (1977).

92. SHIP, I. I., MORRIS, A. L., DUROCHER, R. T., AND BURKET, L. W., Recurrent aphthous ulcerations and recurrent herpes labialis in a professional school student population. I. Experience, *Oral Surg.* **13**:1191–1202 (1960).

93. SHIP, I. I., BRIGHTMAN, V. J., AND LASTER, L. L., The patient with recurrent aphthous ulcers and the patient with recurrent herpes labialis: A study of two population samples, *J. Am. Dent. Assoc.* **75**:645–654 (1967).

94. SHERIDAN, P. J., AND HERRMANN, E. C., JR., Intraoral lesions of adults associated with herpes simplex virus, *Oral Surg.* **32**:390–397 (1971).

95. SHORE, S., AND NAHMIAS, A., Immunology of herpes simplex virus infection, in: *Immunology of Human Infection*, Part II (A. NAHMIAS AND R. O'REILLY, eds.), pp. 21–72, Plenum Press, New York, 1981.

96. SKOLDENBERG, B., JEANSSON, S., AND WOLONTIS, S., Herpes simplex virus type 2 and acute aseptic meningitis: Clinical features of cases with isolation of herpes simplex virus from cerebrospinal fluids, *Scand. J. Infect. Dis.* **7**:227–232 (1975).

97. SMITH, I. W., PEUTHERER, J. F., AND MACCALLUM, F. O., The incidence of herpesvirus hominis antibody in the population, *J. Hyg.* **65**:395–408 (1967).

98. SMITH, I. W., ADAM, E., MELNICK, J. L., AND RAWLS, W. E., Use of the ^{51}Cr release test to demonstrate patterns of antibody response in humans to herpesvirus types 1 and 2, *J. Immunol.* **109**:554–564 (1972).

99. SPEAR, P. G., Composition and organization of herpesvirus virions and properties of some of the structural proteins, in: *The Oncogenic Herpesviruses* (F. RAPP, ed.), pp. 53–84, CRC Press, Boca Raton, Florida, 1980.

100. SPRUANCE, S. L., OVERALL, J. C., JR., KERN, E. R., KRUEGER, G. C., PLIAM, V., AND MILLER, W., The natural history of recurrent herpes simplex labialis: Implications for antiviral therapy, *N. Engl. J. Med.* **297**:69–75 (1977).

101. STEWART, J., AND NAHMIAS, A., Laboratory diagnosis of herpes simplex viruses, in: *Laboratory Diagnosis of Sexually Transmitted Diseases* A.P.H.A. (in press).

102. SUMAYA, C. V., MARX, J., AND ULLIS, F., Genital infection with herpes simplex virus in a university student population, *Sex. Transm. Dis.* **7**:16–20 (1980).

103. TEJANI, N., KLEIN, S. W., AND KAPLAN, M. Subclinical herpes simplex genitalis infections in the perinatal period, *Am. J. Obstet. Gynecol.* **135**:547 (1979).

104. VESTERGAARD, B. F., AND JENSEN, O., Diagnosis and typing of herpes simplex virus in clinical specimens by the enzyme-linked immunosorbent assay (ELISA), in: *The Human Herpesviruses: An Interdisciplinary Perspective* (A. NAHMIAS, W. DOWDLE, AND R. SCHINAZI, eds.), pp. 391–394, Elsevier/North-Holland, New York, 1981.

105. VISINTINE, A. M., NAHMIAS, A. J., AND JOSEY, W. E., Genital herpes, *Perinatal Care* **2**(9):32–41 (1978).

106. WARREN, K. G., BROWN, S. M., WROBLEWSKA, Z., GILDEN, D., KOPROWSKI, H., AND SUBAK-SHARPE, J., Isolation of latent herpes simplex virus from the superior cervical and vagus ganglions of human beings, *N. Engl. J. Med.* **298**:1068–1069 (1978).

107. WARREN, K. G., WROBLEWSKA, Z., OKABE, H., BROWN, S. M., GILDEN, D. H., KOPROWSKI, H., RORKE, L. B., SUBAK-SHARPE, J., AND YONEZAWA, T., Virology and histopathology of the trigeminal ganglia of Americans and Japanese, *Can. J. Neurol. Sci.* **5**:425–430 (1978).

108. WEATHERS, D. R., AND GRIFFIN, J. W., Intraoral ulcerations of recurrent herpes simplex and recurrent aphthae: Two distinct clinical entities, *J. Am. Dent. Assoc.* **81**:81–87 (1970).

109. WENTWORTH, B. B., AND ALEXANDER, E. R., Seroepidemiology of infections due to members of the herpesvirus group, *Am. J. Epidemiol.* **94**:496–507 (1971).

110. WHEELER, C. E., JR., AND CABANISS, W. H., JR., Epidemic cutaneous herpes simplex in wrestlers (herpes gladiatorum), *J. Am. Med. Assoc.* **194**:993–997 (1965).

111. WHITLEY, R. J., SOONG, S. J., DOLIN, R., GALASO, G. J., CHIEN, L. T., ALFORD, C. A., JR., AND THE NIAID COLLABORATIVE GROUP, Adenine arabinoside therapy of biopsy-proved herpes simplex encephalitis, *N. Engl. J. Med.* **297**:289–292 (1977).

112. WHITLEY, R. J., NAHMIAS, A. J., SOONG, S. J., VISINTINE, A., CONNOR, J. D., YEAGER, A., ALFORD, C. A., AND THE COLLABORATIVE STUDY GROUP, Vidarabine therapy of neonatal herpes simplex virus infection, *Pediatrics* **66**:495–500 (1980).

113. YAMAMOTO, Y., A re-evaluation of the skin test of herpes simplex virus, *Jpn. J. Microbiol.* **10**:67–77 (1966).

114. YOUNG, S. K., ROWE, N. H., AND BUCHANAN, R. A., A clinical study for the control of facial mucocutaneous herpes virus infections. I. Characterization of natural history in a professional school population, *Oral Surg.* **41**:498–507 (1976).

115. ZIMMERMAN, T. J., MCNEIL, J. T., RICHMAN, A., KAUFMAN, H. E., AND WALTMAN, S., HLA types and recurrent corneal herpes simplex infection, *Invest. Ophthalmol.* **16**:756–757 (1977).

12. Suggested Readings

JURETIC, M., *Herpetic Infections of Man*, University Press of New England, Hanover, New Hampshire, 1980.

KAPLAN, A. S. (ed.), *The Herpesviruses*, Academic Press, New York, 1973.

NAHMIAS, A., DOWDLE, R., AND SCHINAZI, R. (eds.), *The Human Herpesviruses: An Interdisciplinary Perspective*, Elsevier/North-Holland, New York, 1981.

RAPP, F. (ed.), *Oncogenic Herpesviruses*, Vol. 1 and 2, CRC Press, Boca Raton, Florida, 1980.

CHAPTER 14

Influenza Viruses

Fred M. Davenport

1. Introduction

Epidemic influenza remains the last great uncontrolled plague of mankind. Epidemics of influenza A and influenza B recur with monotonous frequency, and each quietly but relentlessly exacts its death toll. Periodically, worldwide pandemics levy larger and more conspicuous liens. Vaccines developed for control of influenza have been shown to be highly effective when applied to selected segments of the general population, but to date they have not been employed on a scale large enough to determine whether their use can interrupt nationwide epidemic spread. The primary strategy for partial containment of influenza has been to concentrate effort on prevention of lethal outcomes by vaccination of persons known to be at high risk. However, intensified efforts in education of the medical profession and the public concerning the importance of immunization against influenza and development of mechanisms for overcoming chronic vaccine shortages and maldistributions will be required in order to achieve a significant degree of control.[64]

Vaccine efficacy is conditioned by closeness of fit of vaccine-induced antibody to the surface antigens of influenza viruses, i.e., hemagglutinin and neur-

aminidase. Type A and B viruses are antigenically distinct. However, within type, both surface antigens exhibit differences that confer identity and similarities that indicate lineage. In succeeding epidemic years, variation of each occurs independently. When changes appear to take place gradually and are of such an extent that sharing of antigenic components is as readily discernible as are differences, the process is referred to as *antigenic drift*. At long intervals, abrupt changes occur, yielding variants so antigenically unique that serological relationships to strains formerly prevalent are difficult to recognize. This event is referred to an *antigenic shift*. Recognition of shifting among the hemagglutinins and neuraminidases of type A viruses has permitted definition of subtypes or families of strains. Nomenclature of the subtypes has evolved over time. Common synonyms for currently recognized prototypes are swine, A/swine/31, A/swine/Iowa/31 (Hsw1N1); PR8, A_0/PR/8/34, A/PR/8/34 (H0N1); FM1, A_1/FM/1/47, A/FM/1/47 (H1N1); A_2/Singapore/1/57, A/Singapore/1/57 (H2N2); A/Hong Kong/1/68 (H3N2). The term *A prime* has been used with reference to A_1 strains and the term *Asian* with reference to A_2 isolates. For completeness, strain designations identify serotype, host of origin, geographic origin, strain number, year of isolation, and, in parentheses, numerical indices of the antigenic character of viral hemagglutinin (H) and neuraminidase (N) subtype. Unless otherwise specified, the host of origin is man. Type B strains undergo antigenic drift, but to date have not exhibited antigenic shift.

Fred M. Davenport · Department of Epidemiology, School of Public Health, University of Michigan, Ann Arbor, Michigan.

2. Historical Background

In chronological surveys of influenza, Hirsch[55] and Thomson and Thomson[112] list 299 epidemics occurring between 1173 and 1875, an incidence of one outbreak every 2.4 years. Differences in extent and severity of episodes were clearly recognized. Some exhibited a low attack rate and limited distribution. Others, such as the first pandemic (recorded in 1580), struck much of the globe with a high incidence. Epidemics and pandemics were encountered more frequently in the 18th and 19th century than in preceding centuries. That difference is thought to be due to changes in size and distribution of the world's population and to changes in travel and commerce, rather than to changes in viruses or in fashions of reporting. East-to-west spread of pandemics was repeatedly documented, although progression in the opposite direction was less commonly observed. Clinical and epidemiological descriptions of influenza have remained remarkably similar over this period, lending credence to the authenticity of the chronicle.

In recent years, results of seroepidemiological studies have permitted reconstruction of part of the historical antigenic experience of mankind. Such a reconstruction is possible because of the major antigens of the strains of first infection of childhood impress an indelible orientation on the antibody-forming mechanism so that throughout life, on subsequent exposure to related strains, the level of primary antibody is reinforced. Persistence of antibody response to strains of first infection has been called "the doctrine of original antigenic sin."[45] Since, as will be seen, the initial antigenic experience of different cohorts of the population is sharply different, one can obtain a serological recapitulation of a population's past experience with the different antigens of influenza viruses by determining currently the pattern of age distribution of antibody oriented to different prototype strains.[27]

The serological evidence obtained by use of this technique identifies a period of prior prevalence of A/Equi/2/63-like viruses believed to have taken place between 1874 and 1889.[28] The great pandemic of 1889–1890 has been related to the first appearance of A_2 Asianlike strains that were succeeded in turn by the first appearance of Hong-Kong-like viruses in 1902.[24,31,52,72–76,84,118] The latter strains persisted in epidemic prevalance until swinelike strains evolved

as the virus responsible for the record-breaking pandemic of 1918.[2,27,66,77,97,102] Swinelike strains remained in epidemic prevalence until 1928, when type A_0 strains emerged.[26]

The modern annals of influenza have been compiled by mapping of viral prevalences and characterization of the antigenic composition of isolates. The virus of swine influenza was isolated in ferrets by Shope[101] in 1931. In 1933, Smith et al.[105] reported isolation of a virus from human cases occurring in England. Francis[40] and Burnet[6] confirmed their findings in the next outbreaks experienced in the New World and in Australia. On comparison of the early isolates of influenza A_0, it became clear that they were not identical antigenically, and minor antigenic variations continued to be observed during the remainder of the period of prevalence of A_0 subtype strains.[71]

This period was abruptly terminated when what later became known as A prime strains first appeared in Australia during the winter of 1946. By the succeeding winter in the northern hemisphere (1947), A prime strains had become the dominant prevailing form.[49] They constituted a major antigenic shift away from the set of antigens that had characterized their predecessors, and as time went on exhibited minor antigenic changes within the set that came to be recognized as those defining the A_1 subtype.[69] In 1957, strains of A_2 or Asian subtype of influenza viruses first appeared in the Kweichow Province of central China and emerged from the mainland via Hong Kong.[67,80] Antigenically, these strains were also only remotely related to their predecessors. As they became the dominant prevailing form in this and succeeding years, minor antigenic changes in the composition of the isolates of subsequent epidemics were observed. In 1968, from an unknown source in China, Hong Kong was again the scene of emergence of a new subtype of strains, and antigenic variation within this new subtype has occurred since.[10,95]

From the epidemiological events and serological findings, a general pattern of behavior of influenza A viruses has emerged. At intervals of 10–15 years, a different family or subtype of strains appears from an unknown source and site, usually resulting in the occurrence of a pandemic characterized by high attack rates and rapid spread in a population relatively devoid of antibodies to the major antigens of the emergent virus. In subsequent years, lesser outbreaks occur through recurrence of strains of the same subtype. These appear to undergo minor antigenic change or drift as antibody levels oriented to the set of antigens that characterize that subtype become progressively built up in the population. At saturation levels, a major antigenic shift occurs, and the sequence of events is repeated. Recycling of major antigenic viral components seems to have occurred as the resurgence in 1957 of Asian antigens once dominant in the virus involved in the pandemic of 1889–1890 and as the resurgence in 1968 of the Hong Kong antigens formerly emphasized in strains prevalent in 1902. Recycling of the 1918 pandemic swine antigens occurred in the United States in 1976, but despite the relative absence of swine antibodies in persons less than 55 years of age, the A/New Jersey/8/76 swinelike strains exhibited epidemic behavior only at Fort Dix, New Jersey.[8a] In 1977, recycling of A prime antigens in isolates of classic epidemic behavior occurred when A/USSR/90/77 (H1N1) viruses became prevalent. These last two recycling events had been predicted.[32a,54a] The reconstructed succession of strains is summarized in Table 1. Other reconstructions have been proposed by Masurel and Marine.[73,75,76]

Type B influenza virus was first isolated in 1940 by Francis,[42] who also demonstrated serologically that a related virus had been involved in the epidemic of 1936. Antigenic drift among strains isolated in subsequent years has been widely recognized, but the degree of change has not yet been great enough to permit recognition and designation of distinct subtypes.[96] The frequency of epidemics is less than that for influenza A, and severe pandemics have not been recognized.

A virus isolated by Taylor[111] in 1947 from a patient suspected to have influenza was found to be unrelated antigenically to type A or B viruses. In 1950, Francis et al.[47] isolated an identical virus from another suspect case. Principally because the virus could be implicated as the etiological agent involved in an institutional outbreak of influenza and because a high frequency of antibody was noted in the general population, the authors used the designation "type C influenza virus" in reporting their observations. Since that time, sporadic cases and local small outbreaks have been identified in various countries. Recent findings suggest that antigenic change among type C strains has occurred over time, but in this instance, too, the degree of change does not warrant separation into subtypes.[18]

However, the validity of the designation "influenza C" has been questioned. Hirst[56] demonstrated that the erythrocyte receptor of type C virus was qualitatively different from that of type A and B viruses. Melnick[79] cites structural differences, suggesting the need for taxonomic separation of type C from true influenza viruses. Kendal[63] was unable to detect neuraminidase on type C virus, yet that enzyme constitutes an important surface component of A and B strains. It seems not unlikely that influenza C virus will be reclassified.

Table 1. Hypothetical and Factual Summary of Periods of Prior Prevalence of Influenza A Viruses of Epidemiological Importance in Man

Virus	Antigen subtype	Prevalence
Equi/2/Miami/63-like	(H eq 2 N eq 2)	1874–1889[a]
A/Japan/305/57-like	(H2N2)	1890–1901[a]
A/Hong Kong/68-like	(H3N2)	1902–1917[a]
A/Swine/1973/31-like	(Hsw1 N1)	1918–1928[a]
A/PR/8/34	(H0N1)	1929[a] (1933–1943[b])
A/FM/1/47	(H1N1)	1947–1957[b]
A/Japan/305/57	(H2N2)	1957–1968[b]
A/Hong Kong/68	(H3N2)	1968[b]–1978[b]
A/New Jersey/8/76	(Hsw1 N1)	1976[b]
A/USSR/90/77	(H1N1)	1977[b]–

[a] Serological recapitulation   [b] Virus isolation.

3. Epidemiological Methodology

3.1. Mortality Data

William Farr introduced the concept of "excess mortality" in describing the epidemic that swept through London in 1847. He defined it as the number of deaths observed over and above the number of expected for the particular season and place where the epidemic occurred, and found that these excess deaths were ascribed not only to influenza but also to pneumonia, bronchitis, other respiratory diseases, and many nonrespiratory diseases as well. Excess total mortality still provides the most accurate measure of the impact of an influenza epidemic on a population. However, during mild or moderate epidemics, the total number of excess deaths may exceed the expected number only slightly, and the statistical procedures required to evaluate their significance become complex. The most sensitive index for measuring severity and extent of influenza epidemics is the record of excess deaths due to influenza and pneumonia.[69]

For monitoring current epidemics in the United States, weekly reports on the total number of deaths and deaths due to influenza–pneumonia are received by the Center for Disease Control (CDC), Atlanta, Georgia, via postcards sent from the Vital Statistics Offices of 121 large cities the populations of which comprise about one third of the total United States population. Deaths are listed by place of occurence and include those persons whose residence may have been elsewhere. Since reports consist of a count of death certificates filed each week, the tabulation may include some deaths that occurred in preceding weeks. Notorious lags in reporting accompany holidays. Pneumonia and influenza deaths for each city and region and an expected number for the country as a whole are published in Table IV of the *Morbidity and Mortality Weekly Report* (MMWR). Because of fatal outcome follows the onset of illness by a variable period and because it takes time for reports to get to local officials, perception of excess mortality occurs between 3 and 5 weeks after clinical disease is noted to be widespread.[7,39]

In addition to the tabulation, charts of pneumonia–influenza deaths are prepared by plotting the weekly number of reported deaths in relation to a curve of expectancy calculated to identify an epidemic threshold that takes into account seasonal variation and long-term trends.[99] Charts are constructed with data received from all 121 cities and from each of nine geographic subdivisions of the United States. By inspection of the latter, information on timing and relative impact of the epidemic in different regions may be obtained. Despite limitations in accuracy of reporting, these data provide the best readily available evidence on extent and severity of an epidemic in the country as a whole. Findings are published promptly in the MMWR and are summarized at least annually in the *Influenza–Respiratory Disease Surveillance Report* of the CDC.

Until recently, data on excess mortality comparable to those developed for the United States were available only from England and Wales and from Canada. Since 1970, however, the World Health Organization (WHO) has conducted a collaborative study on use of excess mortality from respiratory disease as a method for assessing the impact of influenza epidemics on 13 countries selected to encompass different climates and geographic distributions. Seasonal mortality curves with expected limits have been constructed by computers using data supplied by each country for the preceding 5–10 years. Charts are drawn to different scales to facilitate immediate comparison of influenza activity in reporting countries, irrespective of large variation in the numbers of events reported. The system provides a week-to-week record of deaths from acute respiratory disease in countries where weekly returns are available and a retrospective analysis of the disease pattern in collaborating countries. As in earlier studies, excess mortality from respiratory disease was found more useful in epidemiological studies than excess total deaths.[3] The WHO collaborative study will be continued for a number of years. It is hoped that systematic collection of data in epidemic and nonepidemic periods will provide a firm basis for numerical estimation of the intensity of different epidemics of influenza occurrring in these countries and these climates. Such information will contribute greatly to knowledge of the global impact of influenza and will point up the existence of regional and temporal differences.

3.2. Morbidity Data

Morbidity data are not reported regularly or systematically. During the influenza season, the CDC may conduct periodic telephone surveys with state epidemiologists in all 50 states. Information is requested on school and industrial absenteeism and on closed schools or colleges. While influenza is not a nationally reportable disease, 25 states currently report cases of influenza or influenzalike disease to CDC and publish them in their own state morbidity reports. Since 1972, additional information has been sought on the level of emergency-room visits to large community hospitals in major cities and on the findings in 60 cooperating virus-diagnostic laboratories; 44 states participate in the expanded program on a weekly basis. The data provide a rapid general assessment of influenza activity throughout the United States and are epitomized at appropriate intervals in the MMWR and CDC Surveillance Bulletins.

For the past 12 years, the National Health Survey has collected data on occurrence of influenzalike illness experienced in 800 households interviewed each week. The data can be used to provide a crude retrospective estimate of the overall attack rate experienced during epidemic years as measured against the self-reported background of diagnoses during nonepidemic years.[100]

Mass media provide timely news on occurrence of influenza outbreaks, but lack of uniformity of data collection precludes accurate analysis. All in all, the information available on morbidity due to influenza is highly unsatisfactory and unreliable unless carefully designed special studies are conducted.

3.3. Serological Surveys

The determination of influenza-antibody patterns in population groups was begun as early as 1935, shortly after the discovery of the virus. These early studies employed the neutralization test, which is cumbersome and expensive for mass application. The hemagglutination-inhibition (HI) test is now most commonly used. It is economical, reflects long-lasting antibody, has high strain specificity, and is adaptable to the microtiter system for testing. The complement-fixation (CF) test is group-specific as commonly employed and because it reflects antibody of shorter duration can be used to identify more recent outbreaks. Antibody to neuraminidase has now been introduced into population surveys to yield additional data on protection levels of immunity. The neutralization test has the highest strain specificity and is employed for special studies.

As previously described, serological surveys have proven useful for developing information about the antigenic composition of strains of influenza A prevalent before 1933. Serological surveillance of the incidence of influenza A and influenza B in defined populations has had limited use, but the findings have made important contributions to our knowledge of the epidemiology of influenza. In 1957, the fact that sera of persons less than 70 years of age were devoid of Asian antibody provided a unique opportunity to obtain serological age-specific infection rates, to compare them with age-specific clinical attack rates, and to follow the first and second waves of the epidemic curve as depicted by excess pneumonia–influenza deaths.[54,116] The results of these studies are presented in Section 5.

Serological sampling has also proved useful for rapid identification of the serotype of influenza virus causing an outbreak. Specimens are drawn at a given time from convalescents and from subjects of the same age who are in the early acute phase of illness. For each group of subjects, geometric mean antibody titers are then ascertained with type A and B strains. If, for example, the outbreak is caused by type A virus, geometric mean type B antibody levels in both sets of sera should be approximately equivalent, while type A geometric mean antibody titers of convalescents will be higher. A conventional Student's t test of mean log titers will establish the significance of any difference noted. As few as ten sera in each set will frequently suffice to establish etiology.[8] In interpandemic periods, prospective serological studies have also been used to ascertain total influenza clinical/subclinical ratios.[37a,37b]

3.4. Laboratory Methods

3.4.1. Isolation. The isolation of influenza virus early in the course of an epidemic is important in order to identify and characterize the antigenic composition of the prevailing strain. Throat swabs or garglings are obtained from patients within the first 3 or 4 days of onset of fever. Usually, no more than a dozen specimens are needed to determine the cause of an outbreak. Inoculation of primary rhesus-monkey-kidney-cell cultures and of 10- to 11-day-old embryonated eggs is recommended because influenza B strains are more readily isolated in monkey-kidney cells, while eggs are often more sensitive for isolation of influenza A viruses. In practice, however, most laboratories rely on one or the other culture system, accepting the possibility that the yield of isolates may be reduced thereby. Reports on isolation of influenza C strains have specified 7-day-old eggs. For successful egg inoculation, the amniotic route is required. Egg harvests are tested for hemagglutination with guinea pig or human type O erythrocytes and with chicken erythrocytes. Tissue-culture tubes are tested for hemadsorption with guinea pig cells, and, if positive, the supernate of companion tubes can be tested for hemagglutination.

Identification of isolates as type A or B strains is readily accomplished by CF using standardized reagents. Type C antisera should be used only if the isolate exhibits the unique cellular affinity characteristic of such strains, i.e., capacity to agglutinate chicken cells at 4°C but not at room temperature and inability to agglutinate guinea pig cells at either temperature. HI tests are also used for identification of isolates. Here, it is important to effect the removal of nonspecific inhibitors from test antisera by treatment with receptor-destroying enzyme (RDE) or trypsin and potassium periodate. Hemadsorption inhibition may be employed if culture tubes fail to yield an adequate titer of hemagglutinin. Test antisera should be prepared using the most recently isolated type A and B strains available.[30,32]

By use of a battery of sera prepared against present and earlier prototype isolates, one can establish by cross-HI or strain-specific CF tests a quantitative expression of the antigenic relationships of current strains to their predecessors. The principal antibody being measured in such tests is that directed against viral hemagglutinin. Viral neuraminidase, the minor surface antigen, is at times responsible for detectable low-level cross-reactions, but these can be eliminated by use of monospecific antisera. For completeness, the antigenic characteristics of both surface antigens should be established.[35]

3.4.2. Serological Tests. Serodiagnosis of influenza is most commonly employed in large-scale epidemiological studies. Paired sera drawn 2–3 weeks apart are used. The CF and HI tests are approximately equal in sensitivity, but use of either alone may result in missing as much as 15% of infections. Therefore, paired negative sera should be tested by the other technique. Use of "soluble" CF antigen will often, but not always, distinguish between antibody response to vaccination and that due to infection, since a rise in antibody level above $1/8$ is un-

common following vaccination. A single-radial-diffusion test has been developed that may prove to be well suited for field investigations, but to date experience is limited.[94]

4. Biological Characteristics of the Virus

Influenza virions are spherical particles 80–120 nm in diameter. The surface contains 500–1000 spikelike structures embedded in a lipid bilayer associated with an internal membrane derived from matrix (M) protein. Spikes are of two morphologically distinguishable types. One contains viral hemagglutinin (HA) protein responsible for attachment to mucoprotein cell receptors. The HA protein is a glycoprotein consisting of two polypeptides—HA1 and HA2—held together by disulfide bonds. HA1 is located at the free end of the spike and accounts for antigenic specificity of the hemagglutinins of different strains. The other spike contains viral neuraminidase (NA) responsible for release of virus from the host-cell surface following replication. The ratio is at least $2:1$.[98] The NA is also a glycoprotein and consists of one or two kinds of polypeptides joined in a tetramere. Mucoprotein cell receptors are cleaved by viral enzyme, yielding sialic acid. Antigenic variation of NA occurs, but it is less marked than that of HA. Antigenic distinction of spikes is conferred by differences in their amino acid composition, which is most elegantly reflected by differences in peptide maps of the appropriate components of different strains. The spikes, lipid, and internal protein membrane comprise the viral envelope that encloses the twisted and coiled nucleocapsid composed of nucleoprotein (NP) subunits associated with single-stranded RNA. The genome is segmented into eight pieces of unequal size, each of which codes for a particular viral polypeptide. Segmentation of RNA into components capable of rearrangement favors flexibility of genetic expression. The RNA segments of different strains may exhibit different mobilities in polyacrylamide-gel electrophoresis, permitting identification of gene donors in recombination (reassortment) experiments and providing information about the source of influenza viruses infecting man and animals.[88a] Polymerase activity has been related to three internal nonglycosylated proteins (P1, P2, P3).[65,90a] The

Table 2. Polypeptides of Influenza Virus

Designation	Molecular weight	Function	Approximate number of molecules per virus particle	Assignment to structural and antigenic components of virus	RNA segment code[a]
P1	81,000–94,000	Unknown	50	Minor, internal nonglycosylated proteins; unknown antigenic specificity; possibly associated with polymerase activity	RNA 2
P2					RNA 3
P3					RNA 1
NA	60,000	Neuraminidase	100–200	Surface glycoprotein; morphologically knob + fiber; antigenically variable, subtype specificity	RNA 6
NP	53,000	Nucleocapsid subunit	1000	Internal, nonglycosylated protein associated with RNA to form helical nucleocapsid; type-specific; antigenically stable	RNA 5
HA1[b]	58,000	Hemagglutinin components	1000	Surface glycoproteins; morphologically rods with triangular cross-section; heavy (HA1) and light (HA2) polypeptide chains linked by disulfide bonds; antigenically variable, subtype specificity	RNA 4
HA2[b]	28,000				
MP	25,000	Major, matrix, or membrane protein	3000	Major internal nonglycosylated protein; antigenically stable, type-specific; associated with inner surface of lipid layer of envelope	RNA 7
NS1	23,000	Unknown	—	Nonstructural virus coded proteins; synthesized in cytoplasm and migrate to nucleus of infected cells	RNA 8
NS2	11,000	Unknown	—		

[a] Ranked by rate of migration in polyacrylamide-gel electrophoresis.
[b] Hemagglutinin is synthesized as a single polypeptide of molecular weight 80,000 that is cleaved to HA1 and HA2 during virus maturation.

function of (an)other internal protein(s) (NS1, NS2) is completely unknown. Viral lipid is host-derived. Table 2 summarizes current information on eight virus-specific proteins (adapted from Schild[108a]).

5. Descriptive Epidemiology

5.1. Incidence and Prevalence Data

5.1.1. Mortality and Morbidity. By use of excess mortality due to influenza and pneumonia as an index,[69] Collins[12] compiled an impressive record of influenza-associated mortality extending from 1887 through 1956 (Fig. 1). Over the period of reporting, the intervals and sites have changed. After decades of quiescence, the pandemic of 1889–1890 erupted unexpectedly. The death toll of 1891–1892 was even greater, and high, sharp peaks of excess mortality recurred as "trailer" epidemics through 1908. Relative quiescence again ensued until 1915, when moderately severe epidemics reappeared. These failed to be predictive of the catastrophic pandemic of 1918–1919, in which globally over 20 million lives were lost. Subsequently, moderately severe outbreaks recurred through the early 1940s, but thereafter excess mortality declined conspicuously.

Another way of presenting the available data is

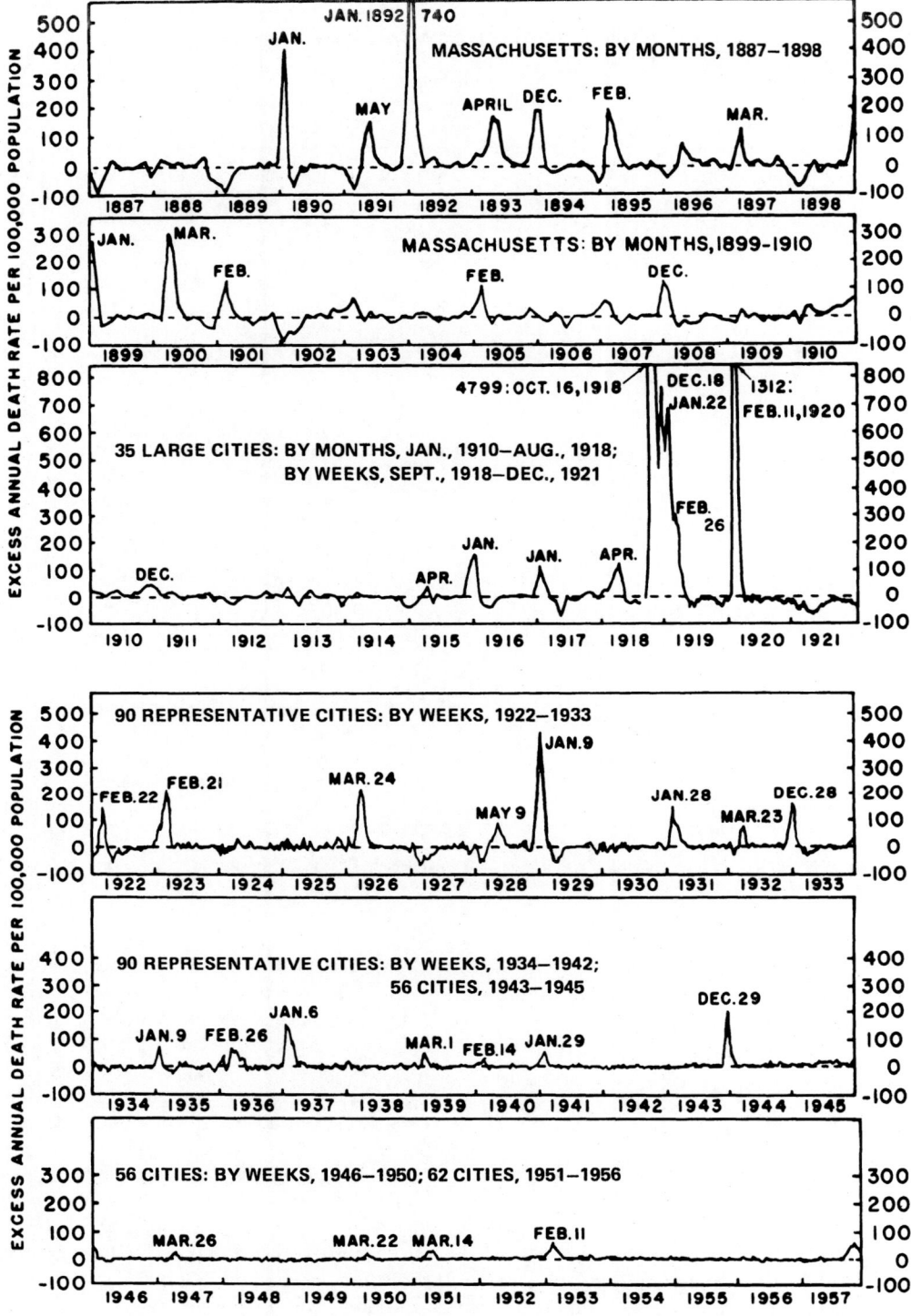

Fig. 1. Excess annual death rate in Massachusetts and in representative United States cities, 1887–1956.

in terms of bar graphs of total excess deaths and of excess pneumonia–influenza death rates observed during epidemic periods. Figure 2 summarizes information accumulated since 1934, a period wherein the identity of the causal viruses is known.[7] In the past 44 years, 22 epidemics of influenza A and 9 of influenza B were associated with excess mortality. The influenza B epidemic of 1976 was not (Fig. 2). Influenza B is clearly less frequent and less lethal than influenza A. Nevertheless, the impact of the 1936 epidemic of influenza B was outstanding, and there is no reason to believe that such a visitation might not recur. Over the entire period of record, 58 epidemics occurred in the 89 years elapsed since 1887.

The occurrence of excess deaths from influenza and pneumonia above the expected baseline is shown in Fig. 3 for 121 cities for 1975–1978 and for nine regions of the United States for 1977–1978. The influenza A epidemics of 1976 and 1978 are readily discernible. In the latter, excess mortality was most marked in the East North Central, East South Central, Middle Atlantic, Pacific, and South Atlantic sectors.[9,9a] These regional differences cannot be accounted for at present, except in general terms of unmeasurable differences in exposure and resistance of the populations involved.

5.1.2. High-Risk Categories. Detailed analysis of mortality data by criteria that describe the kinds of persons most likely to suffer a fatal outcome has led to identification of certain "high-risk groups," i.e., persons classified as being at increased risk of death during the course of an influenza epidemic.[19] From these findings and from clinical and laboratory data on influenza-associated deaths,[37] the Surgeon General's Advisory Committee on Influenza (USPHS) initiated in 1962 the policy that special emphasis should be given to protecting such persons in campaigns for better control of influenza.[15] They can readily be identified as (1) persons of all ages who suffer from chronic debilitating disease, e.g., chronic cardiovascular, pulmonary, renal, or metabolic disorders, in particular, patients with (a) rheumatic heart disease, especially those with mitral stenosis, (b) other cardiovascular disorders such as arteriosclerotic heart disease and hypertension, especially those with evidence of frank or incipient cardiac insufficiency, (c) chronic bronchopulmonary disease, e.g., chronic asthma, chronic bronchitis, bronchiectasis, pulmonary fibrosis, pulmonary emphysema, and pulmonary tuberculosis, (d) diabetes

mellitus, and (e) Addison's disease; (2) pregnant women; and (3) persons in older age groups, those over 45 and particularly those over 65 years of age. Subsequent advisory committees have deleted the category of pregnancy, since excess mortality in pregnancy, while apparent in epidemics occurring through 1931, was not discernible in less severe epidemics encountered in later years. The present system of registration and coding of deaths would preclude establishing such an association without special study, since an influenza–pneumonia death is coded as due to influenza and pneumonia regardless of whether pregnancy was noted or not.[37]

5.1.3. Incidence. Current usage tends to restrict the term *pandemic influenza* to episodes of spread of a known or presumed major antigenic variant in a population relatively devoid of antibody oriented to the novel strain. The literature on the incidence of influenza is enormous and in part contradictory. Discrepancies may be due in part to variability in criteria used for reporting and in part to actual differences in the experience of the several populations because of disparities in innate or acquired characteristics or in relative exposures. The statements that follow are believed to represent the average expectancy.

Data accumulated by household surveys in 1889–1890, 1918, 1957, and 1968 indicate that an incidence of 20–40% can be anticipated during the first wave of a new pandemic. Subsequent events cannot be summarized so simply. For unknown reasons, second waves at a short interval have been observed in certain pandemics and not in others. The rate of decline of intensity of epidemics during revisitations of strains of the same general antigenic character is also somewhat variable and irregular, as many be inferred by inspection of mortality curves in Figs. 1 and 2. Toward the end of the period of prevalence of some major variants, incidence may ultimately decline to as little as 2–5%.

5.2. Epidemic Behavior

Dissemination of influenza occurs in several forms. Infection may smolder in a population without clinical recognition, being manifest only by a 5–10% rate of titer increase discernible in serum samples collected to span interepidemic periods.[34] Introductions of novel serotypes of virus, as occurred in 1957 and 1968, may be followed by several months of sporadic, widely scattered, small outbreaks of

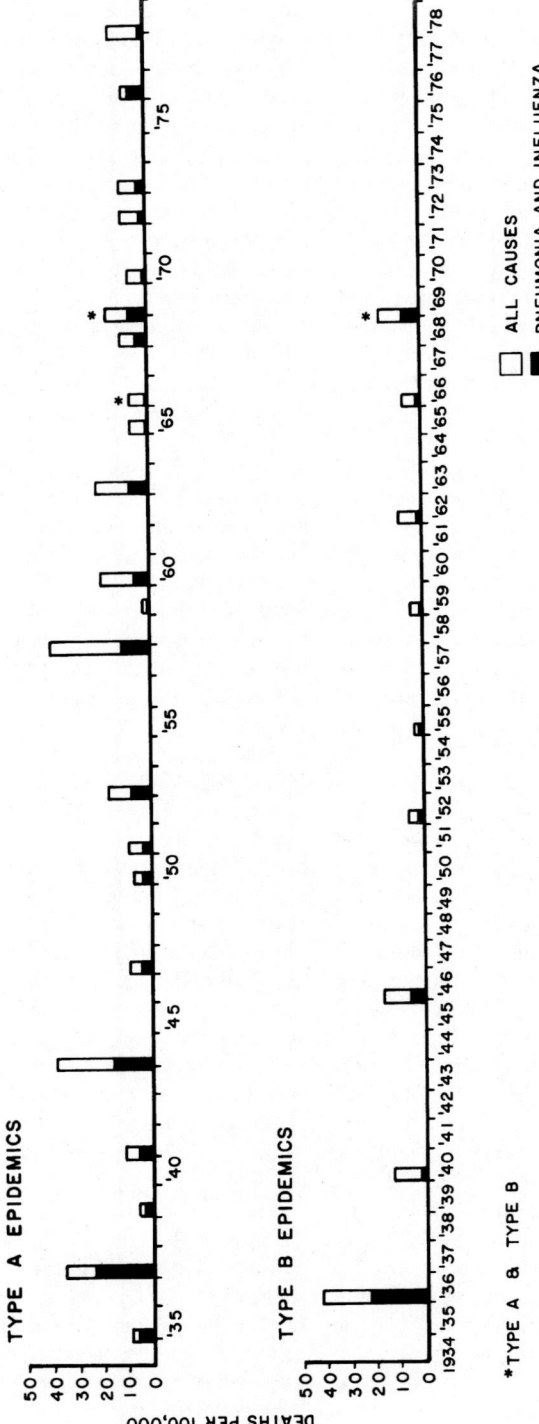

Fig. 2. Pneumonia–influenza death rates by month and excess mortality during epidemic periods, United States, 1934–1978. From Epidemiology Program, Center for Disease Control.

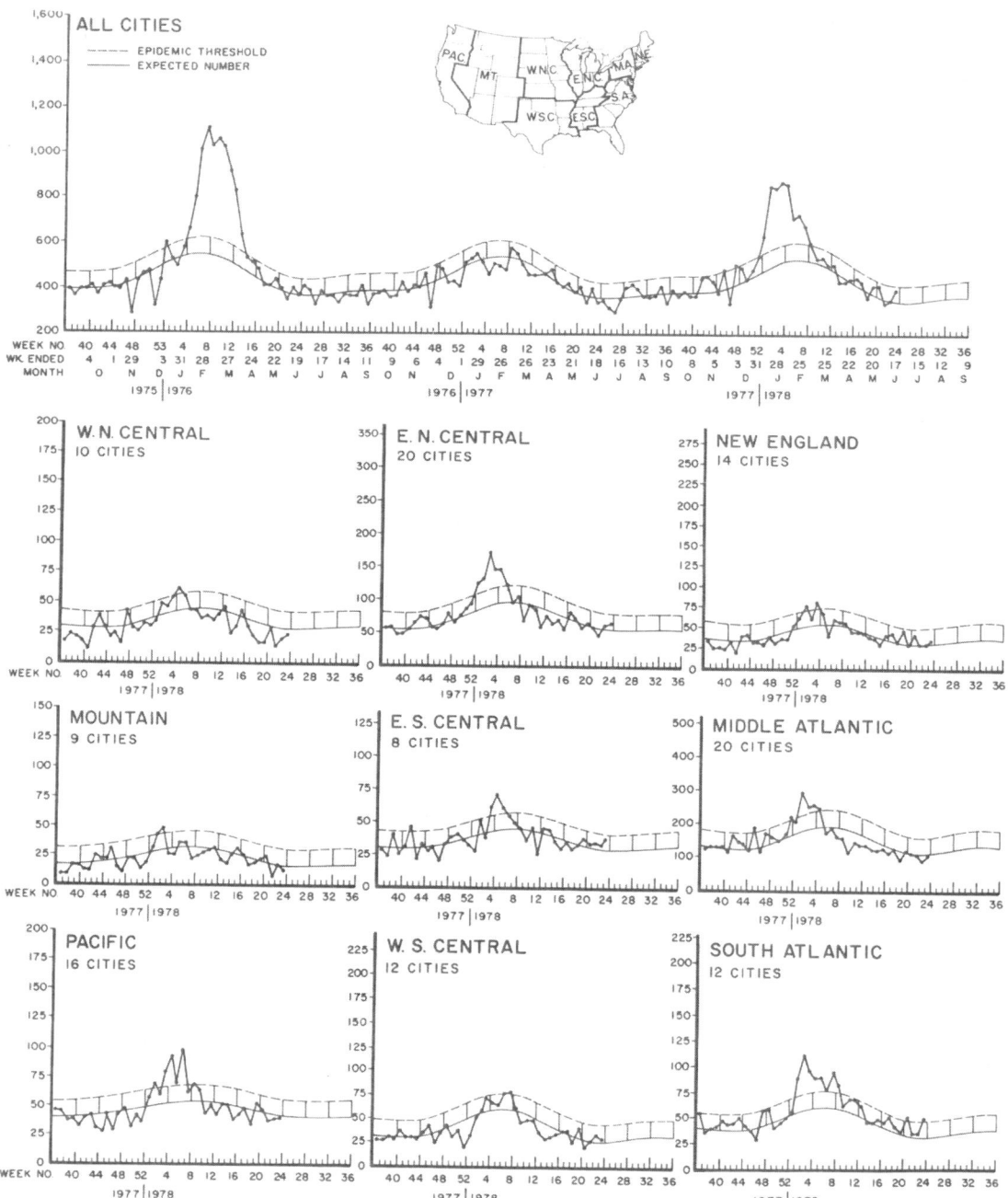

Fig. 3. Pneumonia–influenza deaths in 121 United States cities.

characteristic disease, indicating that widespread seeding of a country has preceded the subsequent epidemic explosion.[67] At other times, prior seeding is not detected and sharp outbreaks promptly follow importation with rapid but irregular spread over a region.

Once an outbreak begins, the epidemic behavior of influenza in any given locale is quite characteristic. Early cases are obscured by the background of noninfluenzal disease. Suddenly, the observer is confronted with an upsurge of patients exhibiting a precipitous onset of illness with fever, chills, aches, hacking nonproductive cough, and prostration, despite the absence of prominent physical findings in the respiratory tract. Uncomplicated recovery begins after 3–7 days of illness. The attack rate is high. The peak of the epidemic curve for areas of metropolitan size is often reached in 3–4 weeks, while the epidemic course may be essentially complete in an additional 3–4 weeks. This time scale is compressed for smaller geographic areas and expanded for larger ones. The clinical severity of disease, the high rate, and the steepness of the ascending limb of the epidemic curve are unique features of influenza that account for the fact that epidemic influenza remains the one respiratory disease of modern times capable of closing schools and factories and embarrassing or disrupting essential community services.

5.3. Geographic Distribution

Most epidemic strains of influenza A and influenza B extend globally. The origin of pandemics remains obscure. Earlier literature suggests that Turkestan or eastern Russia was an endemic source for westward spread of the major epidemics of man. The pandemic of 1889–1890 possibly arose in China. The severe pandemic strain of 1918 appeared first near the French battlefields in August, although there had been widespread scattered episodes during the preceding year. The source of emergence of influenza A_0 strains on or about 1928 is unknown. A_1 strains were isolated in Australia in the winter of 1946 before their introduction to North America early in 1947 followed by widespread extension in Europe during 1949. The 1957 Asian pandemic had its origin in Kweichow Province, China, and, after extending widely, broke out at Hong Kong shortly thereafter. The 1968 pandemic of Hong Kong influ-

enza erupted via the same city, presumably from the Chinese mainland. Focal outbreaks of swine influenza in man occurred in the United States in 1976, but contrary to early expectations, progressive widespread dissimination failed to occur. In May of 1977, H1N1 subtype strains first reappeared in China, and spread slowly there during the summer months. Explosive outbreaks were encountered in the U.S.S.R. and Hong Kong in November. Global spread then followed. The 1977 prototype virus is designated A/USSR/90/77 (H1N1). Contrary to prior experience, the occurrence of this antigenic shift was not followed by prompt displacement of H3N2 viruses. It is evident that the behavior of influenza continues to be surprising. Nevertheless, the accumulated record indicates that it is prudent to expect and to prepare for the occurrence of a severe pandemic of influenza every 10–15 years, followed by trailing epidemics of lesser intensity caused by minor antigenic variants of that pandemic subtype until the next major antigenic shift initiates another characteristic sequence.

5.4. Temporal Distribution

Major outbreaks of influenza A tend to recur at intervals of 2–3 years and of influenza B at intervals of 4–7 years. Either or both serotypes may exhibit yearly endemicity.[20] In the temperate zones, epidemics commonly occur during the period from early autumn to late spring, but there have been instances wherein they begin or extend during the warm seasons. In the tropics, epidemics tend to cluster in the rainy season, but pandemic influenza may be experienced at other times when invasion occurs from the northern or southern hemisphere. Influenza C has been recognized in sporadic cases or in small institutional outbreaks among children. The majority of type C infections are submerged in the viral smog that accompanies the early years of life.

5.5. Age

The highest incidence in a primary epidemic of influenza A is generally encountered in the 5- to 14-year-old group, frequently 5–9. A decline occurs to about 20–25 years, followed by a moderate but distinct rise to about age 30–35, the years of heaviest household exposure to school-aged children. Thereafter, the attack rate tends to decline slowly and somewhat progressively, bottoming out at about 10%. In secondary and subsequent waves, the highest age-specific attack rate tends to shift to older cohorts, reflecting persistence of acquired resistance in the age group most heavily involved at the first visitation as well as the apparent capacity of the virus to pick off the vulnerables spared during the first wave. Figure 4 illustrates these patterns with data collected from Tecumseh, Michigan, in 1957 and 1960.[54] The curve shown for 1957 is that of the first wave of Asian influenza, while the curve for 1960 reflects the third exposure of the population. The overall attack rate in the first wave of 1957 was 23.0% and in 1960 it was 17.3%, yet the age group in which the median case occurred in 1957 was 10–14, while in 1960 it was 30–34. Since the likelihood of fatal outcome increases with age, the findings help to explain why the case-fatality rate may rise in certain secondary epidemics. It is noteworthy that antigenic composition of the 1960 virus was virtually indistinguishable from that of 1957, and that the interval between the second wave of 1958 and the 1960 outbreak was less than 24 months. It seems likely that both factors may have contributed heavily to persistence of immunity in 1960 of those young people involved in the first two waves of Asian influenza. One would expect that the occurrence of a longer interval between outbreaks and the advent of viruses exhibting a marked antigenic drift

would tend to restore the curve of age incidence toward that seen in primary invasion. In 1977–1978, the incidence of A/USSR/90/77 (H1N1)-related influenza was largely confined to persons under 24 years of age, a cohort composed principally of H1N1-antibody-negative persons.

The data with respect to incidence and age distribution of influenza B are fewer. In 1937, an attack rate of 30–40% was noted in several communities in California.[41] The age–incidence curve was not unlike that seen in primary influenza A outbreaks.

Solov'ev in an extensive review of influenza morbidity, presents limited data indicating that age distribution of cases of influenza B is not dissimilar to that of influenza A.[119] In a comparison of the age distribution of pneumonia cases notified in Glasgow during the epidemic of influenza A in 1950–1951 and of influenza B in 1952, some excess of cases was noted in the 0–5 and 60+ year age groups during the A outbreak, but on the whole the curves were remarkably similar.[1] The results of several surveys carried out in the United States in 1961–1962 emphasized the high attack rate of influenza B in school-aged children, with a progressive slow decline after age 20.[14] In a small survey conducted in 1966, the decline after age 20 was described as more abrupt.[13] In 1974 and again in 1977, attack rates encountered in light epidemics of influenza B were high in affected schools, while industrial absenteeism was not noticeably increased. The picture that

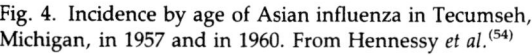
Fig. 4. Incidence by age of Asian influenza in Tecumseh, Michigan, in 1957 and in 1960. From Hennessy et al.[54]

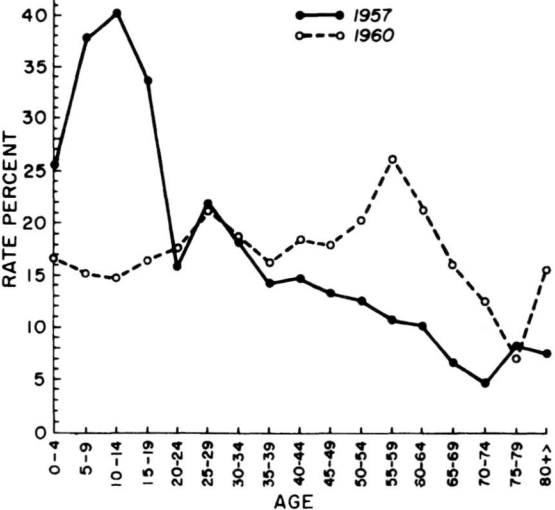

emerges from the scant data available is that the fatality rate drops abruptly and is maintained at low levels until age 35. From age 35 to age 60 a slow rise occurs, but at age 60, the slope of the curve rises abruptly and dramatically. In 1918, a high mortality occurred in the 20- to 40-year age group, especially males, converting the usual U-shaped respiratory mortality curve to a distinctive W-shaped one.[44] This change has been cited as a characteristic of "pandemic" influenza and has been interpreted to indicate that the virus of the 1918 pandemic was more pneumotropic and therefore more virulent than strains encountered before or since. However, the change is also conceived to be the result of excess physiological or environmental stresses contributing to pneumonia, rather than a selective viral effect.[46] The data cited on the age distribution of influenza-associated deaths relate largely to those associated with influenza A or with influenza of unknown etiology. As seen in Figs. 1 and 2, the mortality associated with influenza B is less pronounced, a finding consistent with the impression that the attack rate of influenza B in adults is lower than that of influenza A. The magnitude of the death toll varies enormously from epidemic to epidemic and from place to place. At present, there is no objective way to measure, either in the field or in the laboratory, the virulence of a strain of influenza virus. If influenza–pneumonia deaths are counted, important contributing factors are probably type and distribution of bacterial pathogens prevalent in different populations. In recent years, these factors are almost never under surveillance. Age composition of different populations is obviously another important variable. So too is the proportion of the population already handicapped by chronic disease, a circumstance of special importance when total excess mortality is being tabulated, since, as is evident from Fig. 2, the bulk of excess mortality encountered in influenza epidemics is attributed on death certificates to other causes. Conditions that indirectly influence magnitude of the attack rate, such as crowding, effects of climate on behavior, and history of past experience with influenza, also influence total impact as judged by mortality.

5.6. Other Factors

Presumably, the natural susceptibility of both sexes to influenza is equal. Nevertheless, in one attack rate of influenza B can simulate that of influenza A, but in general the incidence is lower, especially in adults. In either disease, an important component of the lowered incidence found in adults is, as in the case of other respiratory infections contracted in childhood, that of acquired immunity. The relative sparing of adults by influenza B is also consonant with the lesser degree of antigenic drifting that has been observed among type B strains.

The high incidence in school-aged children is undoubtedly related to the fact that schools provide an environment extremely favorable for transmission of respiratory pathogens. Daily assembly of a large mass of susceptibles who are intermittently partitioned in different classrooms with closed ventilation systems provides ideal tinder for conflagration once the spark of infection is introduced. In 1957, the opening of schools was promptly followed by an epidemic upsurge of Asian influenza after a summer of seeding of virus dispersed by focal outbreaks. In Japan, the epidemic peaked first in May while schools were in session, abated in July as vacations began, but peaked again after schools were reopened in September.[51] The ordinary seasonal incidence of influenza in temperate and tropical zones seems in large part due to climatic factors that determine their customary school schedules. The effects of crowding are also discernible in institutions other than schools. High attack rates on shipboard have been repeatedly observed, and epidemic dispersions through offices, industries, college dormitories, hospitals, and other institutions are familiar occurences. However, the possible effect of seasonal climatic changes on physiological host resistance or on survivorship of the virus in transit between hosts cannot be dismissed. It is known that influenza virus remains infectious for a longer time in cold, moist atmospheres. No convincing evidence for differences in attack rates in rural vs. urban communities exists, although instances of escape by isolated communities have been recorded.

As mentioned earlier, mortality is conditioned not only by the presence of chronic debilitating disease but also by age. The curve of age distribution of influenza–pneumonia deaths emphasizes the vulnerability of subjects at the extremes of the span of life. After the first year of life, the case-study, the attack rate was found to be higher in women than in men if the household contained children and adolescents. On the other hand, men exhibited a higher rate than women in households in which there were no subjects under 20 years of age. The findings were attributed to differences in exposures, women being more prone to acquire infection from their children and men from contacts outside the home.[54] Natural susceptibility of all races is apparently equal. Attack rates in different racial components of a population may be conditioned by population density, access to medical services, or prior exposures. Differences in attack rates in various socioeconomic groups probably reflect the effects of crowding. It has been shown that the attack rate in households increases as size of the household increases.[54] Occupational data have not been collected systematically in this country. In the U.S.S.R., the highest level of morbidity is observed in those branches of industry wherein contact between people in the course of production is greatest.[119] In the United States, incidence in pandemics is said to be high among doctors, nurses, and schoolteachers and their involvement to occur early in the course of an outbreak.

6. Transmission

At the height of illness, respiratory secretions commonly contain 1 million or more infectious viral particles per milliliter. One 50% human infectious dose is comprised of as few as 320 50% tissue-culture infectious doses when certain lines of virus are given to volunteers by nasal instillation.[17] Presumably, a tenth of that number, or fewer, would be required for infection if virus were aerosolized to yield droplets small enough to reach the alveoli, i.e., 1–5 μm. Clearly, the large amount of virus available for distribution from patients and the relatively small amount needed to bring down susceptibles are factors that help to explain the ready and rapid spread of influenza observed on the ascending limb of the epidemic curve. In nature, virus is easily transmitted by direct contact, by large-droplet infection, or by articles freshly contaminated by discharges from the noses and throats of infected persons. Further, true airborne transmission via droplet nuclei undoubtedly occurs in enclosed spaces, as evidenced by findings with sentinel animals[48,93] or by measures that promote air sterilization.[78] Unfortunately, precise information is lacking concerning the relative

importance of any of the mechanisms of transmission known to be involved.

7. Pathogenesis and Immunity

7.1. Pathogenesis

A more detailed description of the author's views on pathogenesis and immunity has been published previously.[21] Briefly, it is postulated that virus lodges first in the upper respiratory tract as a result of inhalation of infected droplets discharged into the air during talking, sneezing, and coughing. The viral hemagglutinin makes a specific combination with the complementary molecular configuration of heat-stable mucoproteins detectable as α inhibitors in respiratory secretions. Viral neuraminidase then rapidly lowers the viscosity of surface mucus, converting this material to a watery fluid and simultaneously laying bare cell surface receptors. Liquefaction of mucus prevents viral extrusion by ciliary action and promotes spread of virus to dependent portions of the respiratory tract. Next, penetration of virus in vacuoles or by intake of RNA from particles disrupted at the surface initiates viral reproduction. Finally, release of newly synthesized virus is facilitated by neuraminidase activity, and a new cycle of adsorption, penetration, synthesis, and release is begun. By analogy to observations in ferrets and mice, peak pulmonary virus titers in man are probably reached within 24 hr, remain at their fastigium for an additional 48 hr, and then at 72 hr decline almost as abruptly as they rose. The decline is accompanied, at least in mice, by the development of high levels of interferon in pulmonary tissue.[58] The incubation period in volunteer studies may be as short as 24 hr. Under conditions of natural exposure in isolated communities, 48 hr is a common interval between contact with a single source and development of symptomatic cases.

The early stage release of virus from infected cells is not accompanied by visible manifestations of cell injury. Later, necrosis and desquamation of respiratory epithelium occur, which may extend to the basement membrane. Intracellular spaces are distended with edema fluid and hemorrhagic extravasation. Cellular exudate is scanty. The nasopharynx, trachea, bronchi, and bronchioles are involved to a variable extent in different cases. Injury and reaction to it are focally distributed in both lungs. In fatal cases, degree and extent of pathological change increase distally. In the special case of influenza virus pneumonia, fixed alveolar cells show cytopathic changes accompanied by necrosis, capillary thrombosis, capillary hemorrhage, and focal leukocytic exudate. In some cases, hyaline membranes are seen. Pneumonia is most commonly due to superimposed bacterial infection, with the majority of fatal cases being associated with coagulase-positive staphylococci. Recovery is marked by epithelial hyperplasia and regeneration effected by proliferation from the basal-cell layers.[83]

Probably distribution of virus is generally limited to the respiratory tract. Attempts to demonstrate viremia in antibody-free natural cases proved negative in 1957.[81] However, isolation of virus from the blood of volunteers has been reported once.[107] In addition, virus—presumably blood-borne—has been found in the urine of children.[117] Finally, Oseasohn et al.[88] reported isolation of virus from extrapulmonary tissues obtained at autopsy from a few patients with fatal Asian influenza. Baron and Isaacs[4] failed to find interferon in extracts prepared with lungs of patients who died of influenza virus pneumonia. This circumstance would favor survival of virus and foster dissemination by leukocytes.[21]

7.2. Immunity

Resistance to influenza infection is a complex phenomenon. Human respiratory secretions contain a nonspecific humoral factor called β inhibitor. This heat-labile proteinaceous substance is capable of inactivating in vitro the infectivity of low concentrations of influenza viruses.[11] Francis[43] demonstrated in 1941 that nasal secretions contain specific neutralizing antibody and that plasma antibody can diffuse across mucous membranes to appear in respiratory secretions. The ratio of serum to nasal neutralizing activity was found to be about 10:1. Administration of inactivated vaccine subcutaneously was followed by enhanced nasal antibody titer levels.[43] Fazekas de St. Groth and Donnelley[38] showed that the best correlate with protection was the antibody titer of respiratory secretions rather than of serum. Kasel et al.[62] demonstrated that 11 S IgA secretory antibody levels were enhanced by administration of inactivated vaccines either by the nasopharyngeal route or subcutaneously, although ti-

ters tended to be higher after direct application. In volunteer studies, Couch et al.[16] found that the presence of serum antibody alone was associated with a reduction in the frequency of infection. When both serum and nasal secretion antibody were present, a still further reduction in frequency of infection occurred. The sole subject who possessed nasal secretion antibody but no serum antibody became infected, possibly because the distribution of nasal antibody tends to be restricted to the site of vaccine application.[115] Protection against natural disease by respiratory application of vaccine via aerosol has given irregular results.[114] At present, the common view is that secretory antibody constitutes the first line of natural defense, and the role of serum antibody is called into play when the inflammatory response results in diffusion of 7 S IgA and plasma constituents of 19 S IgM to areas of viral invasion. In man, the protective effect of serum antibody on the lung may be as important as that seen in ferrets.

The duration of immunity following natural infection is not known exactly. The results of community studies in Tecumseh demonstrate that resistance to Asian influenza was present 2 years, after the original assault.[54] Fry[50] found that immunity against Asian influenza lasted at least 4 years. Pickles et al.[89] came to the same conclusion with respect to previous experience with influenza A. During a 3-year period, Hall et al.[53] observed only a 2 and a 12% serological reinfection rate against influenza A and influenza B, respectively, in Seattle Virus Watch families. The prevailing view is that postinfection immunity measured by failure to exhibit disease lasts for several years after a previous attack, although subclinical reinfection probably occurs after a much shorter interval. However, under conditions of heavy exposure, clinical recurrence did affect a significant proportion of children after an interval as short as 2 years. The narrow specificity and rapid decline in antibody response of children would correlate with a less durable immunity.[103]

8. Patterns of Host Response

8.1. Clinical Features

The consequences of infection with influenza viruses extend from a totally asymptomatic state to fatal outcome despite heroic therapeutic efforts. Estimates of subclinical infection rates derived from clinical and serological studies indicate that for every febrile patient exhibiting symptoms compatible with influenza, there is another subject who denies illness or has at best a trivial experience self-diagnosed as a common cold.[54,92] Despite the range of symptoms in individual patients, clinical descriptions of influenza remain remarkably constant from year to year and observer to observer. This seeming paradox probably relates to the fact that physicians tend to reserve the clinical diagnosis of influenza for classic cases and diagnostic specimens are usually not processed for minor illnesses. The spectrum of clinical response is described in meticulous detail elsewhere.[46,108] The patient most likely to be recognized clinically as suffering influenza is one who 1–4 days after exposure (average 48 hr) experiences an abrupt onset with chills, fever, headache, malaise, backache, and nasal symptoms of sneezing and mild discharge. Hacking nonproductive cough is characteristic. At first, except for cough, the severity of constitutional symptoms far outweighs in importance to the patient the severity of respiratory symptoms. In the next 24 hr, fever reaches a substantial plateau and respiratory symptoms become more prominent. Obstructed nostrils, hoarseness, dry or sore throat, and substernal soreness may be pronounced, and troublesome cough persists. Retroorbital aching and photophobia are less common complaints. Anorexia, nausea, or vomiting may accompany fever, but diarrhea is not characteristic. Gastrointestinal symptoms are more common in children. Fever persists on the average for 3 days and may exhibit a diphasic course. Physical signs are few and not pathognomonic. Watery eyes, flushed face, and reddening of nasopharyngeal membranes are frequent findings. The chest is generally clear except for sibilant coarse rales heard best over larger bronchi in about one third of patients. When the patient experiences prostration, as is frequently the case, an apathetic appearance is characteristic. The leukocyte count generally is normal, but about one third of patients exhibit leukopenia with a relative increase in lymphocytes. Convalescence ordinarily begins on or about the 4th day, and most patients are back to full activity within 7–10 days. However, many experience prolonged lassitude or sense of debility and persistent cough. The clinical picture in children ordinarily tends to be milder and difficult to recognize. Croup and bron-

chiolitis may precipitate hospitalization, but the true incidence of these manifestations is unknown.

The most dreaded complication of influenza is pneumonia. Pneumonia should be suspected if fever persists beyond the 4th or 5th day or recurs abruptly after convalescence appears to have begun. It has been estimated that 80% of the pneumonias represent secondary bacterial infection. The clinical picture, physical findings, and laboratory data are markedly influenced by the type of bacterial invader, with staphylococci being the most lethal. Pure viral pneumonia may acccount for up to 20–25% of influenza-associated pneumonias, and it may be suspected when pneumonia is observed to occur in synchrony with influenza rather than after an interval. In viral pneumonia, few bacteria are seen on smear, and no significant pathogens are obtained on culture. Sputum is scant but bloody. Cyanosis and tachypnea are extreme, yet despite evidence of poor air exchange, pulmonary findings are diffuse rather than lobar. Rheumatic heart disease with mitral stenosis or insufficiency or both has been identified as an important predisposing factor. Bacterial pneumonias are more commonly seen in subjects bearing the additional diagnosis of chronic pulmonary disease, chronic cardiac disease, or pregnancy. Reye's syndrome, a rare acute highly fatal complication of influenza involving liver and brain by metabolic pathways, occurs mainly in children following attacks of influenza A or B.[8b,88b]

8.2. Diagnosis

The clinical diagnosis of influenza presents little problem in severe cases during epidemic or pandemic periods. The consistency of the clinical aspects from outbreak, the large numbers of persons presenting with similar features, and the tendency of influenza viruses to predominate over other causes of respiratory morbidity during such periods make the diagnosis easy and quite reliable. In sporadic and isolated cases, these clinical signs and symptoms are not characteristic enough to permit bedside recognition of influenza virus as the cause. Many other viruses can produce acute upper respiratory disease with similar findings. Reliance must be placed on laboratory diagnosis. This is based on isolation of the virus from the nasopharynx, or the demonstration of an antibody rise between acute and convalescent specimens, or both. These techniques are outlined in Section 3.4.

9. Control Measures

Prevention of the nationwide spread of influenza has never been accomplished. The task is formidable but theoretically not impossible. Sufficient epidemiological data are available to direct immunization concepts. It seems likely that an essential requirement for effective control would be vaccination of school-aged children, since at all times the attack rate in this cohort remains high and the role of this cohort in transmission important.[61] The demonstration that vaccination of schoolchildren confers a significant degree of protection on the rest of the community recommends adoption of this practice.[82] The development of nonreactogenic vaccines favors this approach.[25] However, extensive educational efforts would be required before large-scale vaccination of schoolchildren could be accomplished. It is estimated that in the United States, 60 million doses would be required for coverage of this cohort.

Vaccination of schoolchildren would not be expected to offer complete protection for persons at high risk of death during influenza epidemics, and for direct protection of these persons, an additional 40 million doses would be needed. At best, only about 25% of high-risk persons receive influenza virus vaccine, even in years of high promotional activity. This low level of coverage is conditioned by recurrent vaccine shortages and, more important, by perceptions of the public and of physicians concerning risk of influenza and the merits of vaccination.[91] Hence, it is not surprising that the use of influenza virus vaccine in this country has failed to effect a discernible decrease in the number of influenza-associated deaths.[68] More effective educational programs for vaccine utilization in high-risk subjects are clearly needed.

A large amount of the vaccine available in any given year is used in industry because many industrial physicians are convinced that vaccination minimizes economic loss due to absenteeism-related production setbacks.[90] Expansion of the volume used in this sector could probably be carried out quite efficiently, because industry provides a suitable milieu for vaccination campaigns. The potential savings are enormous. For example, Fox and Kilbourne reported Kavet's estimates that the indirect costs (loss of earnings and production deficits) of the 1968–1969 epidemic of Hong Kong influenza totaled $3,242,926,000.[39]

Use of vaccine for protection of strategic community services is recommended in years of anticipated high incidence. Doctors, nurses, schoolteachers, firemen, policmen, transportation workers, and others have been identified as appropriate priority groups. It is believed that use of vaccine for this purpose is sporadic and not well supported. Somewhere between 20 and 50 million doses of vaccine would be needed to protect against economic losses and for defense of strategic services.

As coverage of more and more of the population is extended, at some point the condition would be reached where the effects of herd immunity would become contributory. At present, there are no data that permit prediction of the level of coverage required to gain that advantage. Nevertheless, it is clear that the number of schoolchildren, high-risk persons, industrial employees, and employees in strategic community services sums to about 75% of our population, a level once—but no longer—believed capable of containing the spread of measles virus. The maximal amount of influenza virus vaccine previously produced in the United States without Federal subsidy was about 50 million doses.[87] The usual annual interpandemic volume is about 20 million doses. In 1976, under a Federal program to immunize against the potential threat of pandemic swine influenza, about 156 million doses were produced and almost 43 million doses administered by late February 1977. Coverage of those 18 years old or older was 32% and of those 65 or older, 43%. Delays in initiating vaccine production, failure of swine influenza to become pandemic, and a moratorium on vaccine use extending from December 16, 1976, through February 8, 1977, were factors that contributed to rates of coverage lower than those anticipated.

In view of recurrent shortages of influenza vaccines, the Surgeon General's Advisory Committee on Influenza first made the recommendation in 1962 that priority in use of vaccine be given to prevention of deaths in high-risk groups. This reecommendation has been retained by subsequent groups advisory to the United States Public Health Service, and was widely adopted abroad. However, implementation of the recommendation remains unsatisfactory due to failure to develop effective procedures for augmenting vaccine supplies and directing their distribution and utilization.[33]

This failure is distressing because the record of vaccine effectiveness demonstrates that in most years, a high degree of protection follows its use. For example, in seven vaccine trials carried out by the Commission on Influenza in the period 1943–1969, the range of protection was 80–90% effectiveness. In an additional five trials, the protection level was about 70%. Clearly, vaccination confers an important benefit to the recipient. This subject has been reviewed in detail elsewhere.[22,23,46,108,110]

Current influenza vaccines are associated with few side effects. Redness and induration at the site of injection of 1–2 days' duration may occur in less than one third of vaccinees. Fever, malaise, and myalgia starting 6–12 hr after vaccintion and lasting 1–2 days occur infrequently. This systemic reaction is more common in children and is readily controlled by aspirin at all ages. Guillian–Barré syndrome was associated with the anti-swine influenza campaign carried out in the United States in 1976. An attack rate of 10 cases per million persons vaccinated was observed in the first 10 weeks following vaccination, an incidence 5–6 times higher than that of unvaccinated persons. Allergy to eggs is a contraindication to administration of influenza virus vaccines due to the possibility of inducing hypersensitivity reactions.[9b]

Live influenza virus vaccines have been used extensively in the U.S.S.R. with results comparable to those achieved in other countries with killed vaccines. Francis and Maassab[46] have provided the most complete discussion of the Russian experience. Live virus vaccines are under active investigation in Great Britain and in the United States.[5,29,36,37,57,70, 85,86,103,104,113] Theoretically, their use might produce a superior degree of local immunity. Since they do not require concentration in order to attain an antibody-stimulating dose, the supply of vaccine rapidly available might be markedly enhanced. However, there are difficulties in regularly producing a sufficiently attenuated yet antigenic strain. Optimistically, genetic studies designed to identify the viral components responsible for virulence and techniques suitable for analysis of the viral genome may provide the information essential for reliable selection of vaccine candidate strains.[113a]

Until recently, it could be said that vaccination provided the sole proven means for prevention of influenza. At present, brief mention must be made of two other approaches. Solov'ev[106] describes the use of exogenous interferon for protection, but widespread application of the procedure described seems impractical. Amantadine hydrochloride has been found effective for prevention of Asian influenza, but is ineffective against influenza B. The therapeutic benefit of amantadine is at best slight. The expense and duration of drug administration militate against its widespread application, but consideration of use seems justified for high-risk persons exposed without vaccine protection, especially as household contacts.[59]

10. Unresolved Problems

At this time, the most striking of unresolved problems in the study of influenza relate to the questions of where the virus comes from and where it goes between epidemics and pandemics. There are data to support the concept that between epidemics, virus continues to be transmitted at a low frequency without causing recognized influenza and without reaching a level of virus shedding sufficient to permit virus isolation.[34,39,53] Presumably, antigenic drift occurs during this relatively quiescent phase. Pandemic strains have been postulated to erupt from animal or avian reservoirs, to arise by recombination of strains derived from human and subhuman sources, or to reappear when their nucleic acids have been reactivated by unknown forces acting on their reservoir in the human host.[32a,39,109] Conceivably, recycling of antigens involved in strains of prior pandemics and sharing of antigens among strains isolated from different species could come about, not be recent genetic interaction, but by genetic limitations imposed by the requirement that surface components of mutants must form a functioning limiting viral membrane.[31]

In contrast to the plethora of ideas relating to evolution of pandemic strains, there is a dearth of ideas relevant to the astonishing phenomenon that once a new subtype of viruses emerges, members of the old subtype generally cease to circulate, even though, susceptibles remain available in the population.

A satisfactory answer to these unresolved problems must explain disappearances as well as appearances. Intriguing though these questions are, there is no assurance that their solution will result in better control of influenza. To that end, the immediate objective is to enhance immunization capabilities.[64]

11. References

1. ANDERSON, T., GRIST, N. R., LANDSMAN, J. B., LAIDLAW, S. I. A., AND WEIR, I. B. L., An epidemic of influenza due to virus B, *Br. Med. J.* **1**:7–11 (1953).
2. ANDREWES, C. H., LAIDLAW, P. P., AND SMITH, W., Influenza: Observations on the antibody content of human sera, *Br. J. Exp. Pathol.* **16**:566–582 (1935).
3. ASSAAD, F., COCKBURN, W. C., AND SUNDARESAN, T. K., Use of excess mortality from respiratory diseases in the study of influenza, *Bull. WHO* **49**:219–233 (1973).
4. BARON, S., AND ISAACS, A., Absence of interferon in lungs from fatal cases of pneumonia, *Br. Med. J.* **1**:18–20 (1962).
5. BEARE, A. S., Methods of obtaining viruses suitable for live influenza vaccines and their potential efficacy in man, in: *Proceedings of the Symposium on Live Influenza Vaccine*, pp. 21–29, Yugoslav Academy of Sciences and Arts, Zagreb, 1971.
6. BURNET, F. M., Influenza virus isolated from an Australian epidemic, *Med. J. Aust.* **2**:651–653 (1935).
7. CENTER FOR DISEASE CONTROL, *Influenza—Respiratory Disease Surveillance*, Report No. 88, p. 8, January 1973.
8. CENTER FOR DISEASE CONTROL, *Influenza—Respiratory Disease Surveillance*, Report No. 89, p. 22, February 1974.
8a. CENTER FOR DISEASE CONTROL, *Influenza—Respiratory Disease Surveillance*, Report No. 91, pp. 27–30, July 1977.
8b. CENTER FOR DISEASE CONTROL, *Influenza—Respiratory Disease Surveillance*, Report No. 91, p. 2, July 1977.
9. CENTER FOR DISEASE CONTROL, *Morbid. Mortal. Weekly Rep.* **27**(13):114 (March 31, 1978).
9a. CENTER FOR DISEASE CONTROL, *Morbid. Mortal. Weekly Rep.* **27**(47):473 (Nov. 24, 1978).
9b. CENTER FOR DISEASE CONTROL, *Morbid. Mortal. Weekly Rep.* **27**(27):285–292 (Aug. 11, 1978).
10. CHANG, W. K., National influenza experience in Hong Kong, *Bull. WHO* **41**:349–351 (1968).
11. CHU, C. M., The action of normal mouse serum on influenza virus, *J. Gen. Microbiol.* **5**:739–757 (1951).
12. COLLINS, S. D., *Influenza in the United States 1887–1956*, Public Health Monograph No. 48, Government Printing Office, Washington, D.C., 1957.

13. COMMUNICABLE DISEASE CENTER, *Influenza—Respiratory Disease Surveillance*, Report No. 82, p. 6, June 30, 1966.
14. COMMUNICABLE DISEASE CENTER, *Influenza Surveillance*, Report No. 72, p. 10, May 31, 1962.
15. COMMUNICABLE DISEASE CENTER, *Influenza Surveillance*, Report No. 72, Supplement, May 31, 1962.
16. COUCH, R. B., DOUGLAS, R. G., ROSSEN, R., AND KASEL, J. A., Role of secretory antibody in influenza, in: *The Secretory Immunologic System* (D. H. DAYTON, JR., P. A. SMALL, JR., R. M. CHANOCK, H. E. KAUFMAN, AND T. B. TOMASI, eds.), pp. 93–112, National Institute of Child Health and Development, Government Printing Office, Washington, D.C., 1969.
17. COUCH, R. B., KASEL, J. A., GERIN, J. L., SCHULMAN, J. L., AND KILBOURNE, E. D., Induction of partial immunity to influenza by a neuraminidase-specific vaccine, *J. Infect. Dis.* **129**:411–420 (1974).
18. CZEKALOWSKI, J. W., AND PRASAD, A. K., Studies on influenza virus. I. Antigenic variation in influenza virus type C, *Arch. Gesamte Virusforsch.* **42**:215–227 (1973).
19. DAUER, C. C., AND SERFLING, R. E., Mortality from influenza 1957–1958 and 1959–1960, International Conference on Asian Influenza, *Am. Rev. Respir. Dis.* **83**(2): Part 2, 15–26 (1961).
20. DAVENPORT, F. M., Recent advances in prevention of influenza by vaccination, *Mod. Med.* **26**:115–122 (1958).
21. DAVENPORT, F. M., Pathogenesis of influenza, Conference on Airborn Infection, *Bacteriol. Rev.* **25**:294–300 (1961).
22. DAVENPORT, F. M., Killed influenza virus vaccines: Present status, suggested use, desirable developments, in: *Proceedings: International Conference on the Application of Vaccines Agaist Viral, Rickettsial and Bacterial Diseases of Man*, Pan American Health Organization—World Health Organization, Washington, D.C., December 14–18, 1970, pp. 85–95, PAHO Scientific Publication No. 226, 1971.
23. DAVENPORT, F. M., Control of influenza, Symposium on Influenza, *Med. J. Aust. Spec. Suppl.* **1**:33–38 (1973).
24. DAVENPORT, F. M., AND HENNESSY, A. V., The clinical epidemiology of Asian influenza, *Ann. Intern. Med.* **49**:493–501 (1958).
25. DAVENPORT, F. M., HENNESSY, A. V., BRANDON, F. M., WEBSTER, R. G., BARRETT, C. D., AND LEASE, G. O., Comparisons of serologic and febrile responses in humans to vaccination with influenza A viruses or their hemagglutinins, *J. Lab. Clin. Med.* **63**:5–13 (1964).
26. DAVENPORT, F. M., HENNESSY, A. V., DRESCHER, J., MULDER, J., AND FRANCIS, T., JR., Further observations on the relevance of serologic recapitulations of

human infection with influenza virus, *J. Exp. Med.* **120**:1087–1097 (1964).

27. DAVENPORT, F. M., HENNESSY, A. V., AND FRANCIS, T., JR., Epidemiologic and immunologic significance of age distribution of antibody to antigenic variants of influenza virus, *J. Exp. Med.* **98**:641–656 (1953).

28. DAVENPORT, F. M., HENNESSY, A. V., AND MINUSE, E., Further observations on the significance of A/Equine-2/63 antibodies in man, *J. Exp. Med.* **126**:1049–1061 (1967).

29. DAVENPORT, F. M., HENNESSY, A. V., MINUSE, E., MAASSAB, H. F., ANDERSON, G. R., MITCHELL, J. R., HEFFELFINGER, J. C., AND BARRETT, C. D., JR., Pilot studies on mono- and bivalent live attenuated influenza virus vaccines, in: *Proceedings of the Symposium on Live Influenza Vaccine*, pp. 105–113, Yugoslav Academy of Sciences and Arts, Zagreb, 1971.

30. DAVENPORT, F. M., AND MINUSE, E., Influenza viruses, in: *Diagnostic Procedures for Viral and Rickettsial Diseases*, 3rd ed. (E. H. LENNETTE AND N. J. SCHMIDT, eds.), pp. 455–469, American Public Health Association, New York, 1964.

31. DAVENPORT, F. M., MINUSE, E., HENNESSY, A. V., AND FRANCIS, T., JR., Interpretations of influenza antibody patterns of man, *Bull. WHO* **41**:453–460 (1969).

32. DAVENPORT, F. M., AND MONTO, A. S., Practical considerations in the diagnosis of myxovirus infections, *Am. J. Clin. Pathol.* **57**:777–782 (1972).

32a. DAVENPORT, F. M., Reflections on the epidemiology of myxovirus infections, *Med. Microbiol. Immunol.* **164**:69–76 (1977).

33. DAVIS, D. J., Problems of allocation and distribution of influenza vaccines, International Conference on Asian Influenza, *Am. Rev. Respir. Dis.* **83**(2): Part 2, 168–170 (1961).

34. DINGLE, J. H., BADGER, G. F., AND JORDAN, W. S., JR., *Illness in the Home*, p. 174, The Press of Western Reserve University, Cleveland, 1964.

35. DOWDLE, W. R., COLEMAN, M. T., HALL, E. C., AND KNEZ, V., Properties of the Hong Kong influenza virus. 2. Antigenic relationship of the Hong Kong virus hemagglutinin to that of other human influenza A viruses, *Bull. WHO* **41**:419–424, (1969).

36. EDWARDS, E. A., MAMMEN, R. E., ROSENBAUM, M. J., PECKINPAUGH, R. O., MITCHELL, J. R., MAASSAB, H. F., MINUSE, E., HENNESSY, A. V., AND DAVENPORT, F. M., Live influenza vaccine studies in human volunteers, in: *International Symposium on Influenza Vaccines for Men and Horses*, London, 1972 (F. T. PERKINS, London, AND R. H. REGAMEY, Geneva, eds.), pp. 289–294, 39th Symp., Ser. Immunobiol. Standard., Vol. 20, 1973.

37. EICKHOFF, T. C., SHERMAN, I. L., AND SERFLING, R. E., Observations on excess mortality associated with

epidemic influenza, *J. Am. Med. Assoc.* **176**:104–110 (1961).

37a. EVANS, A. S., NIEDERMAN, J. C., AND SAWYER, R. N., WITH THE TECHNICAL ASSISTANCE OF WANAT, J., CENABRE, L., SHEPARD, K., AND RICHARDS, V., Prospective studies of a group of Yale University freshmen. II. Occurrence of acute respiratory infections and rubella, *J. Infect. Dis.* **123**:271–278 (1971).

37b. EVANS, A. S., Serologic studies of acute respiratory infections in military personnel, *Yale J. Biol. Med.* **48**:201–209 (1975).

38. FAZEKAS DE ST. GROTH, S., AND DONNELLY, M., The protective value of active immunization, *Aust. J. Exp. Biol. Med. Sci.* **28**:61–75 (1950).

39. FOX, J. P., AND KILBOURNE, E. D., Epidemiology of influenza, Summary of Influenza Workshop IV, *J. Infect. Dis.* **128**:361–386 (1973).

40. FRANCIS, T., JR., Transmission of influenza by a filterable virus, *Science* **80**:457–459 (1934).

41. FRANCIS, T., JR., Epidemiological studies in influenza, *Am. J. Public Health* **27**:211–225 (1937).

42. FRANCIS, T., JR., A new type of virus from epidemic influenza, *Science* **92**:405–408 (1940).

43. FRANCIS, T., JR., Factors conditioning resistance to epidemic influenza, *Harvey Lect. Ser.* **37**:69–99 (1941).

44. FRANCIS, T., JR., Influenza: The newe acquayantance, *Ann. Intern. Med.* **39**:203–221 (1953).

45. FRANCIS, T., JR., On the doctrine of original antigenic sin, *Proc. Am. Philos. Soc.* **104**:572–578 (1960).

46. FRANCIS, T., JR., AND MAASSAB, H. F., Influenza viruses, in: *Viral and Rickettsial Infections of Man*, 4th ed. (F. L. HORSFALL, JR., AND I. TAMM, eds.), pp. 689–740, Lippincott, Philadelphia, 1965.

47. FRANCIS, T., JR., QUILLIGAN, J. J., JR., AND MINUSE, E., Identification of another epidemic respiratory disease, *Science* **112**:495–497 (1950).

48. FRANCIS, T., JR., SALK, J. E., PEARSON., H. E., AND BROWN, P. N., Protective effect of vaccination against induced influenza A, *J. Clin. Invest.* **24**:536–546 (1945).

49. FRANCIS, T., JR., SALK, J. E., AND QUILLIGAN, J. J., JR., Experience with vaccination against influenza in the spring of 1947, *Am. J. Public Health* **37**:1013–1016 (1947).

50. FRY, J., 1961 influenza pattern, *Br. Med. J.* **I**:745–746 (1961).

51. FUKUMI, H., Summary report on the Asian influenza epidemic in Japan 1957, *Bull. WHO* **20**:187–198 (1959).

52. FUKUMI, H., Interpretation of influenza antibody patterns in man, *Bull. WHO* **41**:469–473 (1969).

53. HALL, C. E., COONEY, M. K., AND FOX, J. P., The Seattle virus watch, *Am. J. Epidemiol.* **98**:365–380 (1973).

54. HENNESSY, A. V., DAVENPORT, F. M., HORTON, R. J.

M., NAPIER, J. A., AND FRANCIS, T., JR., Asian influenza: Occurrence and recurrence, a community and family study, *Mil. Med.* **129**:38–50 (1964).

54a. HENNESSY, A. V., DAVENPORT, F. M., AND FRANCIS, T., JR., Studies on antibodies to strains of influenza virus in persons of different ages in sera collected in a post epidemic period, *J. Immunol.* **75**:401–409 (1955).

55. HIRSCH, A., *Handbook of Geographical and Historical Pathology*, Vol. 1, pp. 7–17; translated from the second German edition by CHARLES CREIGHTON, New Sydenham Society, London, 1883.

56. HIRST, G. K., The relationship of the receptors of a new strain of virus to those of the mumps-NDV-influenza group, *J. Exp. Med.* **91**:177–184 (1950).

57. HOBSON, D., BEARE, A. S., AND GARDNER, A. W., Haemagglutination-inhibiting serum antibody titres as an index of the response of volunteers to intranasal infection with live attenuated strains of influenza virus, in: *Proceedings of the Symposium on Live Influenza Vaccine*, pp. 73–84, Yugoslav Academy of Sciences and Arts, Zagreb, 1971.

58. ISAACS, A., AND HITCHCOCK, G., Role of interferon in recovery from virus infections, *Lancet* **2**:69–71 (1960).

59. JACKSON, G. G., STANLEY, E. D., AND MULDOON, R. L., Prospects for the control of viral diseases with chemical substances, *PAHO Sci. Publ.* **226**:588–601 (1970).

60. JENSEN, K. E., AND FRANCIS, T., JR., The antigenic composition of influenza virus measured by antibody-absorption, *J. Exp. Med.* **98**:619–639 (1953).

61. JORDON, W. S., JR., DENNY, F. W., JR., BADGER, G. F., CURTIN, C., DINGLE, J. H., OSEASOHN, G., AND STEVENS, D. A., A study of illness in a group of Cleveland families. XVII. Occurrence of Asian influenza, *Am. J. Hyg.* **68**:190–212 (1958).

62. KASEL, J. A., HORNE, E. B., FULK, R. V., TOGO, Y., HUBER, M., AND HORNICK, R. B., Antibody responses in nasal secretions and serum of elderly persons following local or parenteral administration of inactivated influenza virus vaccine, *J. Immunol.* **102**:555–562 (1969).

63. KENDAL, A. P., A new receptor destroying enzyme in influenza C, in: *Symposium on Neuraminidase, Behring Institute Mitteilungen*, Vol. 55, pp. 18–34, Marburg, 1974.

64. KILBOURNE, E. D., CHANOCK, R. M. CHOPPIN, P. W., DAVENPORT, F. M., FOX., J. P., GREGG, M. B., JACKSON, G. G., AND PARKMAN, P. D., Influenza vaccines—Summary of Influenza Workshop V, *J. Infect. Dis.* **129**:750–771 (1974).

65. KILBOURNE, E. D., CHOPPIN, P. W., SCHULZE, I. T., SCHOLTISSEK, C., AND BUCHER, D. L., Summary of Workshop I, *J. Infect. Dis.* **125**:447–455 (1972).

66. LAIDLAW, P. P., Epidemic influenza: A virus disease, *Lancet* **1**:1118–1124 (1935).

67. LANGMUIR, A. D., Epidemiology of Asian influenza, *Am. Rev. Respir. Dis.* **83**(2): Part 2, 2–9 (1961).

68. LANGMUIR, A. D., HENDERSON, D. A., AND SERFLING, R. E., The epidemiological basis for control of influenza, *Am. J. Public Health* **54**:563–571 (1964).

69. LANGMUIR, A. D., AND HOUSWORTH, J., A critical evaluation of influenza surveillance, *Bull. WHO* **41**:393–398 (1969).

70. MACKENZIE, J. S., The use of temperature-sensitive mutants in live virus vaccines, in: *Proceedings of the Symposium on Live Influenza Vaccine*, pp. 35–41, Yugoslav Academy of Sciences and Arts, Zagreb, 1971.

71. MAGILL, T. P., AND FRANCIS, T., JR., Antigenic differences in strains of human influenza virus, *Proc. Soc. Exp. Biol. Med.* **35**:463–466 (1936).

72. MARINE, W. M., AND WORKMAN, W. M., Hong Kong influenza immunologic recapitulation, *Am. J. Epidemiol.* **901**:406–415 (1969).

73. MARINE, W. M., WORKMAN, W. M., AND WEBSTER, R. G., Immunological interrelationships of Hong Kong, Asian and Equi-2 influenza viruses in man, *Bull. WHO* **41**:475–482 (1969).

74. MASUREL, W. M., Relation between Hong Kong virus and former A₂ isolates and the A/Equi/2 virus in human sera collected before 1957, *Lancet* **1**:907–910 (1969).

75. MASUREL, N., Serological characteristics of a "new" serotype of influenza A virus: The Hong Kong strain, *Bull. WHO* **41**:461–468 (1969).

76. MASUREL, N., AND MARINE, W. M., Recycling of Asian and Hong Kong influenza A virus hemagglutinins in man, *Am. J. Epidemiol.* **97**:44–49 (1973).

77. MASUREL, N., AND MULDER, J., Studies on the content of haemagglutinin-inhibiting antibody for swine influenza virus, *A. Verk. Inst. Prev. Geneesk.* **52**:1 (1962).

78. MCLEAN, R. L., General discussion, International Conference on Asian Influenza, *Am. Rev. Respir. Dis.* **83**(2): Part 2, 36–38 (1961).

79. MELNICK, J. L., Classification and nomenclature of animal viruses 1971, *Prog. Med. Virol.* **13**:462–484 (1971).

80. MEYER, H. M., JR, HILLEMAN, M. R., MIESSE, M. L., CRAWFORD, I. P., AND BANKHEAD, A. S., New antigenic variant in Far East influenza epidemic, 1957, *Proc. Soc. Exp. Biol. Med.* **95**:609–616 (1957).

81. MINUSE, E., WILLIS, P. W., III, AND DAVENPORT, F. M., An attempt to demonstrate viremia in cases of Asian influenza, *J. Lab. Clin. Med.* **59**:1016–1019 (1962).

82. MONTO, A. S., DAVENPORT, F. M., NAPIER, J. A., AND FRANCIS, T., JR., Effect of vaccination of a school-age population upon the course of an A2 Hong Kong influenza epidemic, *Bull. WHO* **41**:537–542 (1969).

83. MULDER, J., AND HERS, J. F. P., *Influenza*, pp. 9–204, Wolters-Noordhoff, Groningen, The Netherlands, 1972.

84. MULDER, J., AND MASUREL, N., Pre-epidemic antibody against the 1957 strain of Asiatic influenza in the serum of older persons living in the Netherlands, *Lancet* **1**:810–814 (1958).

85. MURPHY, B. R., CHALHUB, E. G., NUSINOFF, S. R., AND CHANOCK, R. M., Temperature-sensitive mutants of influenza virus. II. Attenuation of *ts* recombinants for man, *J. Infect. Dis.* **126**:170–178 (1972).

86. MURPHY, B. R., CHALHUB, E. G., NUSINOFF, S. R., KASEL, J., AND CHANOCK, R. M., Attenuation of *ts* recombinants for man. III. Further characterization of *ts*-1 (E) influenza A recombinant (H_3N_2) virus in man, *J. Infect. Dis.* **128**:479–487 (1973).

87. MURRAY, R., Production and testing in the USA of influenza virus vaccine made from the Hong Kong variant in 1968–69, *Bull. WHO* **41**:495–496 (1969).

88. OSEASOHN, R., ADELSON, L., AND KAJI, M., Clinicopathologic study of thirty-three fatal cases of Asian influenza, *N. Engl. J. Med.* **260**:509–518 (1959).

88a. PALESE, P., AND RITCHEY, M. B., Polyacrylamide gel electrophoresis of the RNA's of new influenza virus strains: An epidemiological tool, in: *International Symposium on Influenza Immunization (II)*, Geneva, 1977 (F. T. PERKINS AND R. H. REGAMEY, Geneva, eds.), pp. 411–415, *Dev. Biol. Standard.*, Vol. 39, S. Karger, Basel, 1977.

88b. PARTIN, J. C., SCHUBERT, W., PARTIN, J. S., JACOBS, R., AND SAALFELD, K., Isolation of influenza virus from liver and muscle biopsy specimens from a surviving case of Reye's syndrome, *Lancet* **1**:599–602 (1976).

89. PICKLES, W. N., BURNET, F. M., AND MCARTHUR, N., Epidemic respiratory infection in a rural population with special reference to the influenza A epidemics of 1933, 1936–7 and 1943–4, *J. Hyg.* **45**:469–479 (1947).

90. PLUMMER, N., Essential industry and its role in an influenza epidemic, International Conference on Asian Influenza, *Am. Rev. Respir. Dis.* **83**(2): Part 2, 211–214 (1961).

90a. PONS, M. W., A reexamination of influenza single- and double-stranded RNA's by gel electrophoresis, *Virology* **69**:789–792 (1976).

91. ROSENSTOCK, I. M., Public acceptance of influenza vaccination programs, International Conference on Asian Influenza, *Am. Rev. Respir. Dis.* **83**(2): Part 2, 171–174 (1961).

92. SALK, J. E., MENKE, W. J., AND FRANCIS, T., JR., A clinical, epidemiological and immunological evaluation of vaccination against epidemic influenza, *Am. J. Public Health* **42**:57–93 (1945).

93. SALK, J. E., PEARSON, H. E., BROWN, P. N., AND FRAN-

CIS, T., JR., Protective effect of vaccination against induced influenza B, *J. Clin. Invest.* **24**:547–553 (1945).

94. SCHILD, G. C., HENRY-AYMARD, M., AND PEREIRA, H. G., A quantitative, single-radial-diffusion test for immunological studies with influenza virus, *J. Gen. Virol.* **16**:231–236 (1972).

95. SCHILD, G. C., HENRY-AYMARD, M., PEREIRA, M. S., CHAKRAVERTY, P., DOWDLE, W., COLEMAN, M., AND CHANG, W. K., Antigenic variation in current human type A influenza viruses: Antigenic characteristics of the variants and their geographic distribution, *Bull. WHO* **48**:269–278 (1973).

96. SCHILD, G. C., PEREIRA, M. S., CHAKRAVERTY, P., COLEMAN, M. T., DOWDLE, W. R., AND CHANG, W. K., Antigenic variants of influenza B virus, *Br. Med. J.* **4**:127–131 (1973).

97. SCHILD, G. C., AND STUART-HARRIS, C. H., Serologic epidemiological studies with influenza A viruses, *J. Hyg.* **63**:479–490 (1965).

98. SCHULZE, I. T., The structure of influenza virus: A model based on the morphology and composition of subviral particles, *Virology* **47**:181–196 (1972).

99. SERFLING, R. E., Methods for current statistical analysis of excess pneumonia–influenza deaths, *Public Health Rep.* **78**:494–506 (1963).

100. SHARRAR, R. G., National influenza experience in the U.S.A.; 1968–69, *Bull. WHO* **41**:361–366 (1969).

101. SHOPE, R. E., Swine influenza. III. Filtration experiments and etiology, *J. Exp. Med.* **54**:373–385 (1931).

102. SHOPE, R. E., The incidence of neutralizing antibodies for swine influenza virus on the sera of human beings of different ages, *J. Exp. Med.* **63**:669–684 (1936).

103. SIGEL, M. M., KITTS, A. W., LIGHT, A. B., AND HENLE, W., The recurrence of influenza A prime in a boarding school after 2 years, *J. Immunol.* **64**:33–38 (1950).

104. SLEPUSHKIN, A. N., SCHILD, G. C., BEARE, A. S., CHINN, S., FREESTONE, D., HALL, T., AND TYRRELL, D. A. J., Antineuraminidase antibody and resistance to vaccination with live influenza A2 Hong Kong vaccines, in: *Proceedings of the Symposium on Live Influenza Vaccine*, pp. 85–92, Yugoslav Academy of Sciences and Arts, Zagreb, 1971.

105. SMITH, W., ANDREWES, C. H., AND LAIDLAW, P. P., A virus obtained from influenza patients, *Lancet* **2**:66–68 (1933).

106. SOLOV'EV, V. D., The results of controlled observations on the prophylaxis of influenza with interferon, *Bull. WHO* **41**:683–688 (1969).

107. STANLEY, E. D., AND JACKSON, G. G., Viremia in Asian influenza, *Trans. Assoc. Am. Physicians* **79**:376–387 (1966).

108. STUART-HARRIS, C. H., *Influenza and Other Virus In-*

fections of the Respiratory Tract, pp. 8–21, Williams and Wilkins, Baltimore, 1965.

108a. STUART-HARRIS, SIR C. H., AND SCHILD, G. C., *Influenza: The Viruses and the Disease*, p. 27, Publishing Sciences Group, Littleton, Massachusetts, 1976.

109. STUART-HARRIS, SIR C. H., Pandemic influenza: An unresolved problem in prevention, *J. Infect. Dis.* **122**:108–115 (1970).

110. STUART-HARRIS, SIR C. H., Control of influenza, lack of knowledge versus lack of application of knowledge, *Arch. Environ. Health* **21**:276–284 (1970).

111. TAYLOR, R. M., A further note on 1233 ("influenza C") virus, *Arch. Gesamte Virusforsch.* **4**:485–500 (1951).

112. THOMSON, D., AND THOMSON, R., Influenza, *Ann. Pickett-Thomson Res. Lab.* **9**:4 (1933).

113. TYRRELL, D. A. J., AND BEARE, A. S., Live influenza virus vaccines: An interim report, *Pan Am. Health Organ. Sci. Publ.* **226**:96–100 (1971).

113a. TYRRELL, D. A. J., Using the genetics of influenza virus to make live attenuated vaccines, *Lancet* **1**:196–197 (1978).

114. WALDMAN, R. H., BOND, J. O., LEVITT, L. P., HARTWIG, E. C., PRATHER, E. C., BARATTA, R. L., NEILL, J. S., AND SMALL, P. A., JR., An evaluation of influenza immunization: Influence of route of administration and vaccine strain, *Bull. WHO* **41**:543–548 (1969).

115. WALDMAN, R. H., SMALL, P. A., JR., AND ROWE, D. S., Utilization of the secretory immunologic system for protection against disease, in: *The Secretory Immunologic System* (D. H. DAYTON, JR., P. A. SMALL, JR., R. M. CHANOCK, H. E. KAUFMAN, AND T. B. TOMASI, eds.), pp. 129–147, National Institute of Child Health and Development, Government Printing Office, Washington, D.C., 1969.

116. WIDELOCK, D., KLEIN, S., PEIZER, L. R., AND SIMONOVIC, O., A laboratory analysis of 1957–1958 influenza outbreak in New York City. II. A seroepidemiological study, *Am. J. Public Health* **49**:847–856 (1959).

117. ZAKSTELSKAYA, L. Y., Recovery of the virus from the urine of patients with epidemic influenza, *Gupp: OKUDR Trans. Ob'jed. Sess. Inst. AMN SSSR, Moscow*, 72 (1953).

118. ZAKSTELSKAJA, L. Y., EVSTIGNEEVA, N. A., ISACHENKO, V. A., SHENDEROVITCH, S. P., AND EFIMOVA, V. A., Influenza in the USSR: New antigenic variant A2/ Hong Kong/1/68 and its possible precursors, *Am. J. Epidemiol.* **90**:400–405 (1969).

119. ZHDANOV, V. M., SOLOV'EV, V. D., AND EPSHTEIN, F. G., *The Study of Influenza: Epidemiology*, pp. 648–732, Russian Scientific Translation Program, Division of General Medical Sciences, National Institutes of Health, Bethesda, Maryland, 1960.

12. Suggested Reading

FOX, J. P., AND KILBOURNE, E. D., Epidemiology of influenza, Summary of Influenza Workshop IV, *J. Infect. Dis.* **128**:361–386 (1973).

FRANCIS, T., JR., AND MAASSAB, H. F., Influenza viruses in: *Viral and Rickettsial Infections of Man*, 4th ed. (F. L. HORSFALL, JR., AND I. TAMM, eds.), pp. 689–740, Lippincott, Philadelphia, 1965.

HOYLE, L., *The Influenza Viruses*, Springer-Verlag, New york, 1968.

KILBOURNE, E. D., *The Influenza Viruses and Influenza*, Academic Press, New York, 1975.

STUART-HARRIS, SIR C. H., AND SCHILD, G. C., *Influenza: The Viruses and the Disease*, Publishing Sciences Group, Littleton, Massachusetts, 1976.

BEVERIDGE, W. D., *Influenza: The Last Great Plague*, Prodest, New york, 1977.

CROSBY, A. W., JR., *Epidemic and Peace, 1918*, Greenwood Press, Westport, Connecticut, 1976.

CHAPTER 15

Measles

Francis L. Black

1. Introduction

In 1948, Kenneth Maxcy[69] wrote in a chapter on epidemiology, "The simplest of all infectious diseases is measles." That was before the virus had been isolated or any serological test had become available. Several complicating situations have been found in the intervening years, but they are rare, and Maxcy's statement is true now, more than 30 years later, as it was then. This relative simplicity makes measles an ideal model for the study of infectious-disease epidemiology. Babbott and Gordon[5] reviewed our knowledge of measles epidemiology as of 1954. Much has been clarified since.

Measles is a relatively distinct disease both clinically and etiologically. The confusion that has sometimes occurred between measles and other exanthems, especially rubella and scarlatina, can usually be avoided except in sporadic atypical cases. A macular exanthem is the most prominent sign of measles in the Caucasian race, but the enanthem, referred to as Koplik spots, is more specifically characteristic. Respiratory-tract involvement that peaks with the onset of rash, but that may be complicated by secondary invaders, probably causes most of the mortality. The central nervous system is regularly involved to a minor degree, and frank encephalitis, which is usually immunologically mediated, occasionally follows as a delayed manifestation of the disease. Mortality is low when the underlying health is good, but it may reach 10% or more in unfavorable circumstances, and worldwide it is estimated[41] that measles accounted for 1% of all deaths in a typical prevaccine year.

2. Historical Background

The writings of Abu Becr,[1] known by his hometown name of Rhazes, provide our earliest description of measles. Rhazes lived in the 10th century, but he quoted other authors on measles from as far back as Al Yehudi, who lived in the 7th century.* Rhazes looked on measles as a relatively severe disease and considered it "more to be dreaded than smallpox." It is curious, then, that measles had not been described earlier; smallpox had been accurately described by Galen in the 2nd century A.D.

Hasbah, the Arabic word for measles, which Rhazes used, seems to be reasonably specific, although other exanthems were doubtless confused. This word carries much the same connotation as the English word "eruption." The precision of this name in Arabic is in contrast to classic Greek, which had no specific word, and Latin, which came to use the descriptive terms *rubeola* and *morbilla* only during the Middle Ages. The Teutonic languages have a common root word, *mazer*, which became *Masern*

Francis L. Black · Department of Epidemiology and Public Health, Yale University School of Medicine, New Haven, Connecticut.

* Some confusion has appeared in recent literature through the fact that the 1st century after the Hegira has been mistaken for the 1st century of the Christian era in dating Al Yehudi's life.

in German and *mislingar* in Icelandic, as well as "measles" in English. The divergence of the Teutonic words suggests considerable antiquity for the original recognition of the disease in northern Europe.

Measles requires a human population of several hundred thousand persons if it is to find a sufficient supply of new susceptibles to permit continuance of the virus.[20] Populations of this size did not exist prior to development of the Middle Eastern river-valley civilizations. Therefore, measles, as we now know it, must have arisen since that time, possibly by adaptation of rinderpest or canine distemper virus to man. This puts the appearance of the disease after 2500 B.C. The linguistic evidence suggests that it was much later than that. There were massive epidemics in the Roman Empire starting in 165 and in 251 A.D. and two similar epidemics in China in 162 and 310. McNeill[71] suggests that each of these represented virgin-soil outbreaks of smallpox and measles. Historical records suggest that smallpox came first in the West and measles first in the East.

Rhazes recognized the seasonal nature of measles epidemics, but seems not to have considered the disease infectious. Rather, he believed it a necessary part of growing up. Sydenham,[100] the first to describe measles in northern Europe, appears to have considered it infectious, but the first clear demonstration of this may be attributed to Home,[56] who, in 1758, attempted a procedure with measles analogous to variation with smallpox.

In 1846, Peter Panum went to the Faroe Islands to give help during a measles epidemic. While there, he carried out an extraordinarily fruitful investigation that led him to conclude that the source of this disease was solely through contagion. He was also able to define the 14-day incubation period and to show that infection conveyed lifetime immunity.[86] Hirsch[55] then built on Panum's work to reach the conclusion that an epidemic persisted "so long as there are found susceptible individuals affording the poison a soil adapted to its reproduction, whilst it perishes if there be no ground to reproduce itself." A very modern concept of the epidemic cycle involving input of new births and output of immunes to maintain a fluctuating population of susceptibles within stable limits was formulated by Hamer[52] in 1906.

Work on the epidemiology of measles continued in the 20th century because this was obviously a good model for the development of epidemic theory, but there were more false starts than constructive discoveries, and the picture became quite confused until 1954. In that year, Enders and Peebles[40] isolated the virus and demonstrated immune reactions by neutralization and complement-fixation tests. The serological tests proved to be of immense value in delineating the epidemiology of natural measles. The isolated virus was attenuated to provide a vaccine the use of which fundamentally changed the epidemiological pattern of this disease wherever it has been extensively used. These products of Enders's and Peebles's work are part of our modern understanding of this disease and will be described in subsequent sections.

3. Methodology Involved in Epidemiological Analysis

3.1. Sources of Mortality Data

Measles mortality rates are tabulated in the *World Health Statistics Annual* WHO, Geneva, and by various national vital statistics publications as, for instance, the Vital and Health Statistics published by the National Center for Disease Control (CDC) of the United States. Mortality rates are affected by intercurrent problems such as malnutrition and the age at which measles is contracted, so they do not give an accurate picture of measles incidence. Sometimes, however, where case reporting is very poor, mortality data may offer a better picture of changes in incidence within one political jurisdiction than those available from reported cases.

3.2. Sources of Morbidity Data

The reporting of measles cases to public-health authorities is mandatory in most sociologically advanced countries. However, measles is so commonly regarded as a routine part of childhood that reporting is notoriously incomplete. National statistics for the United States before 1967 probably included only 10–15% of the actual cases. Recognition of infection has also been inhibited by modification by γ-globulin injection in the prevaccine years and by atypical measles in inadequately immunized persons more recently. Confusion with other exanthems is also a problem in interepidemic periods, when measles cases are few. At these times, falsely diagnosed cases may make up a significant proportion of the total. On the basis of serological studies[23] and observations made during acute epidemics,[34] we may reasonably assume that except in extremely isolated populations, essentially everyone contracts measles unless vaccinated. On the other hand, the number of persons who experience measles more than once is very small—much less than 1%. Because of the inevitability of measles, the effectiveness of reporting may be estimated, over longer periods of time, by determining the ratio between reported cases and number of births (minus infant deaths). The efficiency of reporting may be quite variable. For instance, in the United States, reporting of cases in schoolchildren during the school year is usually more complete than reporting during the summer or reporting of cases in preschool children. Nevertheless, reporting is usually sufficiently consistent in any one administrative area that epidemics are well defined and major differences in age distribution are clearly discernible.

Figures on reported cases for the 19th century are available from a few European cities,[95] but, for the most part, reporting was initiated only near the beginning of the 20th century, when quarantine was in vogue for the control of infectious diseases. Prior to that time, there are numerous descriptions of epidemics of measles but little information on routine incidence. Currently, measles is a reportable disease in many countries, and the WHO *Weekly Epidemiologic Reports* tabulate these data. In the United States, the *Morbidity and Mortality Weekly Reports* of the CDC provide a current tabulation of reported cases.

3.3. Serological Surveys

Serological methods have been of immense value in confirming and sharpening the precision of the reported incidence of measles and in deciphering patterns of incidence where there has been no reporting. Several tests are available: complement fixation (CF), neutralization, hemagglutination-inhibition (HI), and hemolysis-inhibition.[21] All give similar results with serum from normal persons (Fig. 1). Antibodies are not found in persons unexposed to the virus except for maternal antibodies during the first year of life. CF titers in immune persons are only slightly less stable over extended periods of time than titers measured by other methods. Hemolysis-inhibition titers may be slightly elevated relative to titers obtained by other tests in certain specific diseases.[81] Hemolysin-inhibition titers are

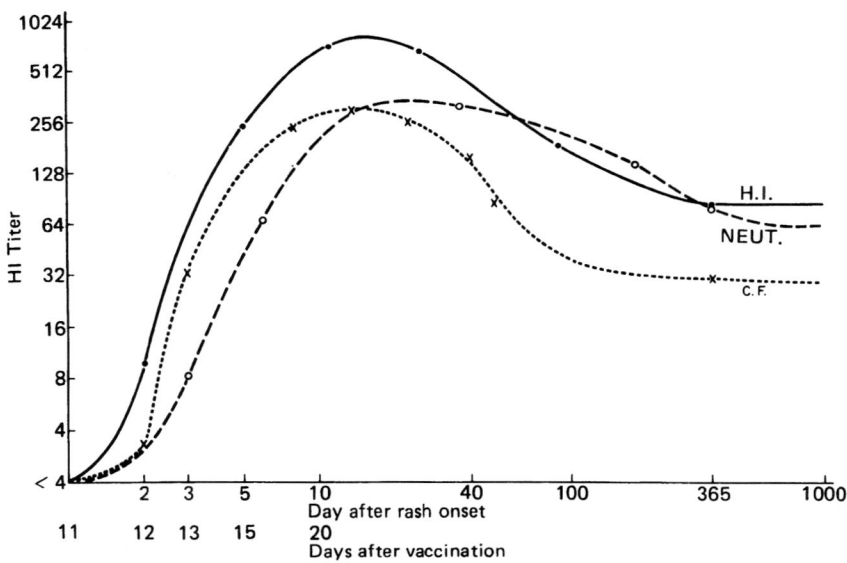

Fig. 1. Measles-antibody titers in serum relative to time after infection with vaccine (HI) or wild virus (neutralization and CF).

also relatively low in sera from persons immunized by killed virus vaccine.[82] The HI test is the most generally useful in epidemiological work because the test is sensitive, the titers are stable, and the procedure is not time-consuming.

The serological reactions to measles are remarkably specific, being unmodified by any other known human infection. Wherever these antibodies have been found, there has always been a history of measles activity in the community, and persons with demonstrable antibody are resistant to infection with wild or attenuated virus. Cross-reactions do occur with canine distemper and with rinderpest, but humans exposed to these viruses do not become naturally infected.

Antibody titers induced by measles infection are unusually stable.[23] There may be a slow decline in titer, but this is scarcely more than that attributable to the generalized reduction in antibody titer associated with aging. Measles-antibody titers in nearly everyone who has had the disease remain readily detectable for life (Fig. 1). Whether this antibody titer stability indicates persistence of latent virus remains unknown.

3.4. Laboratory Methods

Technical details of laboratory methods have been published elsewhere.[21,59] The HI test is the only test that has unusual features. For this test, sera must be treated with kaolin, or the γ-globulin must be separated by ammonium sulfate precipitation, to free it of nonspecific inhibitors. Old World monkey erythrocytes must be used for the test; red cells from the genus *Cercopithecus* are usually preferred. Antibody to these cells is removed from serum by extraction with packed erythrocytes. Untreated infected tissue culture fluid may be used as antigen, but treatment by ether and detergent or ultrasonics increases the hemagglutinin titer. The virus has no neuraminidase, and the test may be carried out at 37°C with less trouble from nonspecific reactions than at lower temperatures.

Virus isolation is always difficult and seldom necessary in the diagnosis of ordinary measles. It may, however, be important in establishing the relationship of measles virus to other less common diseases. For this, it is usually necessary to cocultivate cells from the diseased tissue with a recipient culture. A wide variety of primary, serial, and established

human and Old World monkey-cell cultures have been successfully used as the recipient culture. An important consideration is that it may be necessary to keep the culture under observation for several weeks, and a stable, low-acid-producing line as VERO may facilitate recognition of cytopathic effects.

IgG and IgM appear simultaneously and in comparable titers in the normal response, but IgM titers normally fall to undetectable levels within 60 days. Any persistence of IgM much beyond this period can be considered abnormal. Because IgM levels rarely exceed those of IgG, simple inactivation of one does not permit its identification. Physical separation of the two species by differential centrifugation, or sequential inactivation of both, is usually necessary.

4. Biological Characteristics of the Virus

Measles virus is morphologically a member of the paramyxovirus group, but it lacks neuraminidase and its hemagglutinin reacts with cells of Old World monkeys only. Curiously, human and chimpanzee erythrocytes are not agglutinated. The virus has a large single-stranded RNA genome and synthesizes shorter complementary RNAs during replication. The fact that the measles virus genome is comprised of a single molecule provides a partial explanation for the fact that strain variation is not observed. The covalent links between cistrons would make recombination much more complicated than in influenza virus with its multisegmented genome. The virion carries at least six different polypetides the size and structure of which are quite similar to those of the proteins of other Paramyxoviridae.[51]

Measles virus is labile. Half the infectivity is lost every 2 hr at 37°C even in favorable medium. It is inactivated by pH below 5, by proteolytic enzymes, and by strong light. It does not survive drying on a surface except when lyophilized.[18] These properties mean that it has a short survival time on contaminated fomites. The acid sensitivity also means that it does not infect through the stomach or lower alimentary tract and is not disseminated in the feces. However, the virus survives drying in microdroplets in the air relatively well.[58] In a droplet, the virus would not be mechanically crushed by surface tension, as it is in the last stage of drying on a flat surface. It is thus able to spread effectively as an aerosol.

5. Descriptive Epidemiology

5.1. Incidence

Wherever measles vaccine has been extensively used, measles epidemic patterns have been profoundly altered. Prior to the introduction of vaccine, reported measles cases in the United States numbered about 400,000 per annum, or slightly less than 10% of the number of infants entering the population. In localities where measles reporting received close attention, however, the number of reported cases was about half the number of births, and direct questioning of parents raised this to 80% or more. Even this is a low estimate because serological tests indicated that by age 18, at least 98% of the population had had experience with measles antigen. In fact, it appears, therefore, that in the United States, as in all but the most isolated corners of the world, the true incidence of measles was essentially equal to the number of surviving children.

Since the vaccine was introduced, the number of reported cases in the United States has fallen to about one tenth the former value (Fig. 2). We are left uncertain, however, whether this means that

the number of cases has been reduced to 10% or to 1% of the natural incidence. If there were no change in reporting efficiency, then only a 90% reduction in measles could be claimed, but if reporting has improved with reduction in total number of cases, the effect of vaccination may be as much as a 99% reduction in incidence. With cases occurring less frequently, each case generates more interest, and, coupled with intensified surveillance efforts, much better reporting is likely to result. On the other hand, most measles is occurring in persons who were not vaccinated, and these are the persons least likely to receive medical attention.

5.2. Epidemic Behavior

In populous parts of the world where the vaccine has not been extensively used, measles causes epidemics every 2–5 years, and each epidemic lasts 3–4 months. A few cases are usually reported each week in any very large population even when the epidemic cycle is at a low point. In economically advanced countries, measles epidemics are closely tied to the school year, building to a peak in the late spring and ceasing abruptly after the summer recess has begun. This pattern, however, is only slightly different from that which prevailed in the same countries before schooling became generally available. Sydenham[100] describes an epidemic that reached its peak in London in late March of 1670,

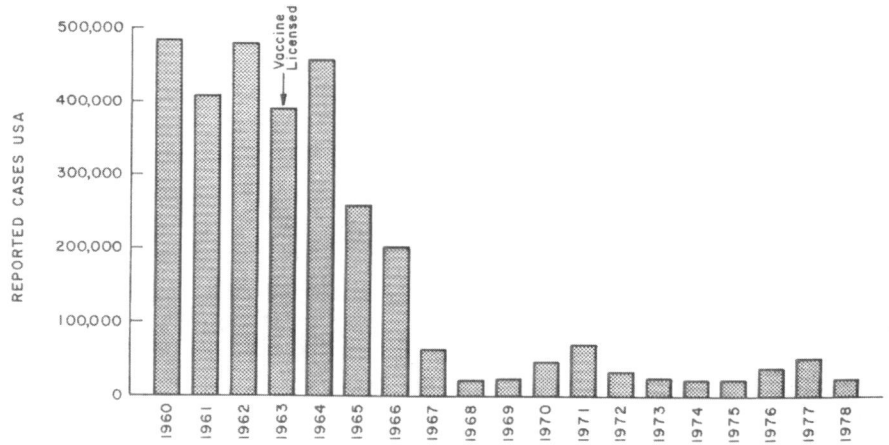

Fig. 2. Measles incidence in the United States as reported by the Center for Disease Control U.S.P.H.S. for the years 1960 to 1978.

and Schutz[95] provided data to demonstrate that March was the month of peak incidence in Hamburg in the early 19th century.

Much work has been done to devise mathematical formulas that will describe the sequence of measles epidemics and identify the parameters that control their course. With minor modifications, these formulas, developed from data on measles incidence, describe the epidemic pattern of any acute infectious disease. In the case of measles, one may start with the two premises that (1) all persons are equally susceptible initially and (2) when a susceptible is infected, he remains infectious for a limited period and then, through death or acquired immunity, withdraws from any further participation in the epidemic cycle. Following the pioneering work of Hamer [52] and Soper,[98] Bailey,[6] Bartlett,[7–9] and others have used measles as a model for definition of the parameters that control cyclical epidemics and for development of mathematical formulas to predict their course.

It is evident that over a short period of time, the number of people infected will be dependent on the number susceptible, as well as on the number who are already infected and capable of spreading the disease. The number susceptible is continuously modified by new births in the community and by removal of susceptibles through infection. Since the number infected in one round depends on the number infected in the previous round, it is relatively easy to develop formulas that will predict a cyclical oscillation in the epidemic pattern, as in Fig. 3A. The epidemic waves in these simple models, however, are always subject to damping and gradually approach a steady state. To get a more accurate picture of the way epidemics come and go, it is necessary to recognize the role played by chance.

When an epidemic is in the ebb phase, the number of cases may be quite small and the number of new contacts highly variable. Using computer technology, Bartlett[7] selected values for the number of new cases in each round randomly from pools of possible numbers. Epidemic curves based on this model show a remarkable resemblance to actual measles epidemic curves (Fig. 3B,C). Bartlett's equation has been used to predict that measles endemicity would exhibit breaks in continuity in any community with an average of fewer than 100 cases per week. Actual observations[8,9] are in agreement with this; an average of 80 cases in North America and of over 106 in England was required for continuity. In island populations where introductions are fewer and breaks in continuity more obvious, the critical value was between 260 and 320.[20]

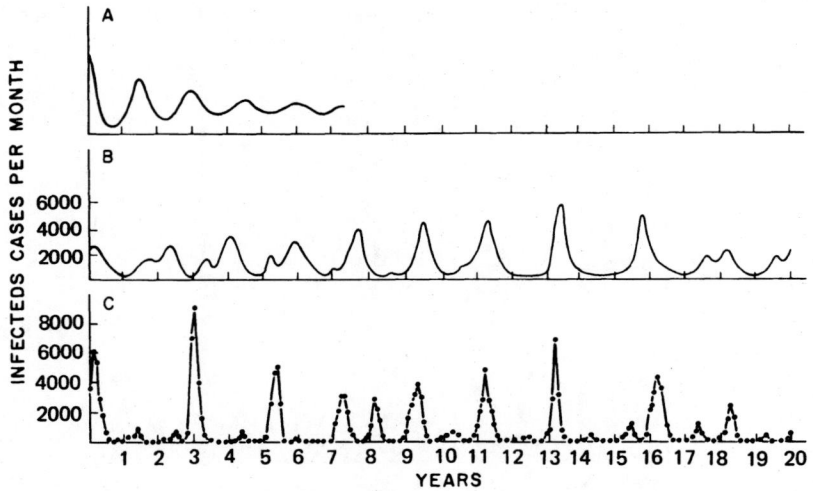

Fig. 3. Actual and model measles epidemic curves. (A) Curve derived from the deterministic model; (B) curve derived from the stochastic model; (C) actual curve for Baltimore, Maryland, 1900–1920. Curves are redrawn to a common scale from the work of Bartlett,[7] Griffiths,[49] and Hedrick.[53]

The equation also predicts that the average interval between epidemics will become shorter with increasing community size. This, too, confirms field observations. Griffiths [49] has used the formula to predict that vaccination of half the susceptibles in a community will have only a minor effect on the peak measles incidence during an epidemic, but will result in increased intervals between epidemics.

Even this model does not take into account a number of factors that modify natural outbreaks, such as the effect of uneven distribution of persons within a community, seasonal variations in habits and virus stability, and the fact that the disease is not transmissible during the early part of the incubation period. If these added factors can be incorporated into the formula, we may be better able to predict the course measles incidence will follow in the present situation of extensive but incomplete vaccination programs.

5.3. Geographic Distribution

Measles occurs regularly in every land, except in very remote and isolated areas. Strains of virus from different countries are indistinguishable, and antibody in sera from diverse populations shows the same specificity. Nevertheless, the epidemic patterns, average age at the time of infection, and the mortality vary considerably from one area to another (Fig. 4).

The average number of infective persons in a community will bear a constant relationship to the community size, if indeed all members are eventually infected. However, there may be differences from one community to another in proportion of persons infected at specific ages and proportion of the whole community susceptible to infection. In a North American city, young children spend much time isolated at home, but when they enter school, the number of contacts rises greatly. Most measles (prior to vaccination campaigns) occurs in the elementary school grades in these communities. Overall, up to 15% of the total population is susceptible. On the other hand, in less developed countries, young susceptible and infected children are commonly carried about by their mothers in the course of their daily chores, greatly increasing the number of contacts. Most measles occurs in children under 4 years of age, and the proportion of the total population susceptible may be less than 5%. When the

number of close contacts is raised to a very high level, as in military recruits, epidemics of measles have occurred where less than 2% were susceptible.

A characteristic of the epidemic curve noted by Hamer [52] is that it has momentum. The more intense the peak of the epidemic, the farther the epidemic will proceed below the equilibrium state before it subsides. In isolated communities, where introductions of measles are few, a large number of susceptibles accumulate in the interepidemic period. This may lead to a very intense epidemic peak, and before the epidemic subsides, nearly every susceptible person in the community will become infected. When measles was first introduced to Greenland in 1951, all but 5 persons in a susceptible population of more than 4000 were infected within 6 weeks. [34]

Another factor that affects the number of persons infected by each index case is simple population density. In Greenland, the population was confined to a few coastal towns, making the probability of contact high. If, however, the population is dispersed, the probability of virus transmission is reduced. This effect may be observed by comparing the duration of epidemics in various islands of comparable population but different area (Fig. 5).

5.4. Temporal Distribution

DeJong and Winkler [58] found that measles virus was most stable when the relative humidity was below 40%. There was a second optimum about 80% humidity. The favorable effect of dry air on virus would enhance spread in dry heated homes in the northern winter, as well as in the hot dry season of Rhazes' Persia [1] or modern Sahelian Africa, [75] and thus explain the relatively high incidence of measles during these seasons. However, it may equally well be that humans tend to congregate most in these inclement seasons and that the more important effect of climate is indirect, through its effect on human habits.

5.5. Age

Maternal antibody usually confers solid protection to infants against measles for 6 months, and the disease may be modified by marginal levels of maternal antibody remaining into the first part of

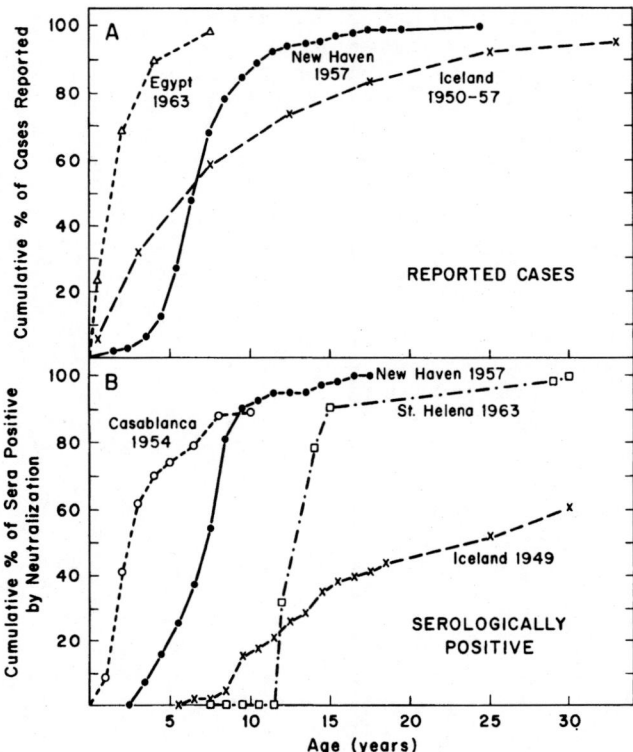

Fig. 4. Cumulative reported age-specific measles incidence (A) and age-specific percentage positive by serological test (B) in developed, underdeveloped, thinly populated, and isolated areas. Egypt and Casablanca are typical of the pattern observed in populous underdeveloped areas. New Haven is characteristic of developed countries. In Iceland, the population is relatively dispersed. St. Helena is representative of an isolated population, which last experienced a measles epidemic 12–13 years prior to the time the sera were collected. The two methods of determining the age-specific attack rate give similar results, except that in Iceland a significant part of the population escaped measles altogether and the proportion immune did not reach more than 60% even in the older age brackets.

the second year. Beyond this period, all ages seem to be equally susceptible to infection, and the age at which measles is most commonly contracted depends again on human habits rather than on the nature of the virus. In developed countries, children are commonly grouped into progressively larger units as they enter school and move through upper school into universities or the military. With extensive vaccine use, the number susceptible has been reduced to the point where continuity of transmission is not maintained in the small groups of young children, although it is maintained in the large groups. This has caused a pronounced shift in the age-specific attack rates.

Measles mortality is highest in the very young and very old. This may be demonstrated with data from England and France collected by Celers[30] or with data from two virgin-soil epidemics in the Arctic, where all ages were infected (Fig. 6). It is not always possible to dissociate direct effects of measles virus from the effect of secondary bacterial invaders in determining this mortality, but in the 1951

Greenland epidemic, a third of the deaths occurred in the period before the appearance of rash, when secondary infections probably had little effect, and these early deaths were distributed by age in the same manner as the total. Contrary to popular opinion, young adults were not more severely affected than children in the Arctic epidemics.

5.6. Sex

No difference has been noted between the sexes in either the incidence or the severity of measles. Antibody titers in women, however, are marginally higher than in men.

5.7. Race

It is commonly believed that measles is a more severe disease in races that have had limited prior experience with it. For example, popular theory has it that Polynesians and American Indians are more

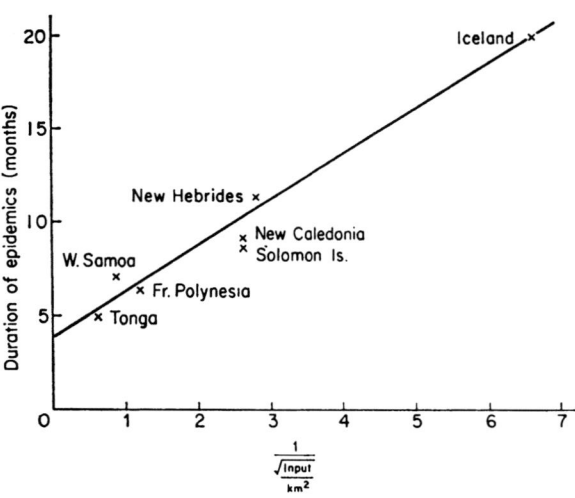

Fig. 5. Relationship between average duration of measles epidemics and dispersion of population in areas with about 2000–4000 new susceptible children per year. The abscissa plot of the inverse root of the number of new susceptibles introduced annually per square kilometer represents the mean distance between new susceptible persons.

severely affected than the Caucasian, Mongolian, and Negro races. This assumption has been based on the very high mortality that occurred during measles epidemics when the virus first reached these communities. In fact, however, it is based on very few data: specific numbers are nowhere available for measles deaths in any virgin-soil epidemic prior to 1951.

Severe breakdown of the social organization may occur during virgin-soil epidemics because so large a part of the whole population is affected at one time, and this disruption may have greatly increased

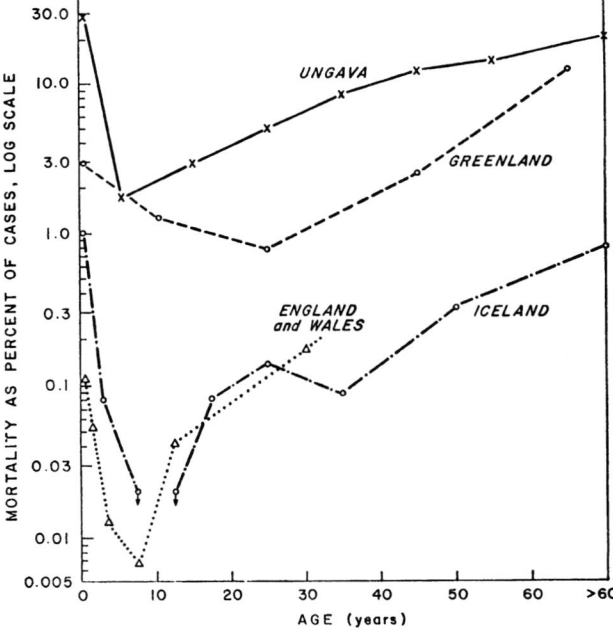

Fig. 6. Measles age-specific mortality rates in endemic and virgin-soil areas. (× —— ×) Ungava[89]; (O – – – O) Greenland[34]; (O – · – · O) Iceland[66]; (△ . . . . △) England and Wales.[30]

the mortality resulting from a moderate primary disease. Furthermore, high measles mortality is not limited to inexperienced peoples, but also occurs in parts of West Africa and Central America and occurred in Victorian Britain, where the disease had long been known (Table 1).

Since 1951, data have become available from several virgin-soil epidemics. These figures indicate that in the absence of medical assistance, the mortality was very high indeed, but that emergency medical aid could reduce the death rate considerably. Where, as in Greenland, there was a well-organized medical service, the mortality was less than 1%. Even this rate, however, is high relative to that in developed areas with good medical services, where measles mortality is usually about 0.02%. It is difficult to determine what part of the effect of medical care works on the primary measles infection and what part on secondary invaders. In the best-

characterized Greenland epidemic, deaths occurred before onset of rash in 0.6% of the cases. These deaths were presumably due directly to the virus, and they would have to be reduced to attain the lower mortality rates observed elsewhere.

Measles vaccine virus causes a mild form of disease with all the primary symptoms of natural measles but in reduced frequency and reduced severity. It therefore provides a model with which host response to measles virus may be tested under controlled conditions. Reactions to vaccine in Micronesians, who had not been exposed to natural measles for 20–30 years, were not significantly different from reactions in other races.[28] However, in four Amazon tribes that showed no serological evidence of ever having had experience with measles, the vaccine produced an average maximum fever 0.5°C higher than that which had been observed in several cosmopolitan populations.[22,104] This difference in

Table 1. Measles Mortality Rate

Place	Year	Number of cases[a]	Mortality (%)	Ref. no.	Medical care available
Endemic measles					
Glasgow, Scotland	1908	22,000	4.8	32	
Chile	1960	93,625	2.3	91	
Rural Guatemala	1960–1963	206	6.8	46	
Upper Volta	1963–1964	5,701	2.9	75	
England and Wales	1961	764,000	0.020	4	
Epidemic measles					
Caucasian					
Faroe Islands	1846	6,000	1.3	86	
Iceland	1882	5,500	4.5	55	
Iceland	1947–1956	21,091	0.12	66	
Oceanic					
Hawaii	1848	150,000	27	50	
Fiji	1873	115,000	26	37	
Samoa	1911	36,000	7.4	55	
Warburton Range, Australia	1961	206	3.0	101	
Amerindians					
Yagan, Argentina	1884	NA	50	27	−
Julianahaab, Greenland	1951	4,320	1.8	34	+
Ungava, Canada	1952	900	7.0	89	−
Baffin Island, Canada	1952	900	2.0	89	+
Xingu, Brazil	1954	298	27	83	−
Xingu, Brazil	1954	356	9.6	83	+
Jacobshaven, Greenland	1959	1,178	0.3	11	+
Several towns, Greenland	1962	10,722	0.5	12	+
Yanomama, Venezuela	1968	170	18	80	+

[a] NA = Not available.

Table 2. Social Characteristics Relative to Measles History[a]

	Number	Number of siblings	Residential neighborhood[b]	Father's education[c]
Positive history	388	2.75	3.54	11.0
Negative history	168	1.98	2.31	12.5

[a] Children in the first school grade in New Haven, Connecticut, 1962, with serologically confirmed histories.
[b] Rated on the 6-point scale of Myers[77]: 1 the most and 6 the least favored.
[c] Average years of schooling.

febrile response may not seem large but is the same as that achieved by giving γ-globulin with the less attenuated (Edmonston) vaccine strains. The Indian tribes live under conditions that are very different from those of the comparison groups, and it is by no means clear that the differences in the reactions are attributable to race. Malnutrition is believed to be the cause of the severe reactions in Africa,[75] but the Indian tribes were well nourished as indicated by body weight, by hair root diameter, and by tabulation of available foodstuffs.

At this time, it seems probable that racial differences in response to measles do exist, but that these differences are only a partial explanation of the high mortality rates that have been observed in isolated populations.

5.8. Occupation

As has been observed in Section 5.2, occupations and institutions do not ordinarily affect the nearly 100% incidence rate ultimately observed with measles. They do affect the age at which measles is usually contracted and the rapidity of its spread by isolating or congregating susceptible individuals.

5.9. Social Setting

Family size and circumstance exert a clear influence on the age at which measles is contracted.[42] The several factors represented in Table 2 all showed significant correlation with measles history. However, these differences are of rather modest magnitude in comparison to the effects of the same factors in other infections. In the first school grade, most of the observed differences are attributable to incidence of infection during the preschool years. Within a few years of entering school, nearly all these children will have contracted measles regardless of family setting.

Gathering large numbers of recruits together increases the opportunities for measles transmission, both by congregating them and by continually introducing new susceptibles. Measles epidemics were a major problem in the Civil War, significant in World War I, minor in World War II, and of little consequence in United States armed forces since that time (Table 3). These changes seem to reflect changes in the rural–urban distribution and in school-district size, which have reduced the number of persons growing up in very small communities, rather than any change in the military. The changes in national social structure have resulted in a highly immune population at the time of induction. For example, in 1962, at least 98.8% of the entering United States recruit population had antibody. Nevertheless, 0.1% of the military population developed measles annually.[19]

5.10. Socioeconomic Status

Socioeconomic status is related to many of the other factors described above and hence often shows a correlation to age at which measles infec-

Table 3. Measles Rates in United States Armed Forces

	Cases per 1000 man-years	Deaths
Civil War	32.2	2.0
Spanish-American War	26.1	0.32
World War I	23.8	0.57
World War II	4.7	0.004
Vietnam War, 1966	0.9	—

tion occurs. This correlation, however, is weak when compared to the effects observed with many other virus infections. The weakness of the association seems to be characteristic of viruses spread by the respiratory route, which is little affected by standard hygienic practices.

5.11. Nutrition

It is generally believed that malnutrition may increase the severity of measles substantially, but controlled tests of this correlation are almost impossible to obtain. Scrimshaw *et al.*[96] noted that measles mortality in young children living in one Guatemalan village was reduced from 1 to 0.3% per annum when the children were offered a protein-rich dietary supplement. The rate stayed near 0.7% in a control village not offered the supplement. However, since only 27% of the children who had the extra protein available to them actually took it regularly, it would appear that the observed change was not entirely due to the food supplement. Morley[76] noted a clinical correlation between severe measles and kwashiorkor in West Africa and by means of a mail poll found that severe measles was more common in areas where kwashiorkor was relatively frequent.

6. Transmission

Proof that the transmission of measles is an unusually efficient process lies in the evidence, presented above, that it spreads very rapidly and reduces the susceptible proportion of a population to extremely low levels. The chief mechanism of transmission is clearly via aerosol. The fact that the most infectious stage of the disease is associated with sneezing and coughing doubtless increases the amount of virus put into suspension.

Measles virus grows in tissues throughout the body, but the mucosal cells of the respiratory tract are the main source of disseminated virus. Infected cells are not rapidly killed, but continue to release virus for several days. Adjacent cells are often fused into syncytia, and these may slough off. Whether inside sloughed cells or free, the virus is delivered directly to the respiratory and urinary excretions in a form that is readily put into aerosol. Virus excretion from the respiratory tract is reduced promptly on development of antibodies, a process that is synchronous with appearance of the rash, but the urine remains infectious a few days longer.[48] How often urine is the source of infection is not clear, but the possibility of infection via the urine a few days after appearance of rash must be recognized. Experiments with vaccine virus suggest that the lower respiratory tract is the most susceptible portal of entry. Vaccine virus did not infect when dropped in the eye or when swabbed on the buccal mucosa.[24] On the other hand, vaccine virus dropped into the nose infected half the recipients and, given as an aerosol fine enough to reach the lower respiratory tract, infected nearly 100%.[63] It is uncertain whether the more virulent wild virus used by Papp[86a] infected the conjunctiva more efficiently than the vaccine strain or whether the virus she administered drained through the lacrimal duct into the respiratory tract.

The fact that aerosols are important in measles transmission does not mean that other mechanisms are not operative. The lability of the virus, however, would make indirect mechanisms inefficient. There is no significant vector of measles virus and no animal reservoir. Old World primates may be infected naturally or experimentally, but they usually get a mild disease.[26] Animals caught in the wild are free of measles antibody unless they have lived in proximity to humans or have been held in cages with large numbers of other animals.[16] Unlike the situation with yellow fever, the monkey does not serve to maintain measles endemicity.

7. Pathogenesis and Immunity

Although commonly classed as an exanthem, measles involves many body tissues. The lymphatic and mucosal epithelial cells are most prominently involved during the period when virus is multiplying.

Infection with measles virus is followed by an incubation period that usually lasts 10–12 days. This incubation period is longer in older persons, and in adults may last as long as 3 weeks. Failure to recognize the extended period in older persons has sometimes invalidated quarantine precautions.[34] Administration of virus by injection, whether wild virus strains as used by Home[56] or vaccine virus as in current immunization practice, shortens the incubation period by 2 or 3 days. Differences in the size of the infecting dose also have an effect on the duration of this period,[70] but it is doubtful that large inocula are commonly encountered in nature.

The only evidence of disease during the incubation period is a decreasing leukocyte count, especially eosinophils and lymphocytes.[14,25] Berg and Rosenthal[15] showed that the virus is capable of growing in leukocytes. It is possible that this leukopenia is a direct result of virus action.

With the onset of the prodromal period, virus appears in the tears, nasal secretions, throat, and urine. Little is known of the sequence and relative titer of virus in these fluids. Isolation of virus from natural sources has never been an easy procedure because of the narrow tissue specificity of wild virus and the fact that the early stages of disease are difficult to identify. The virus is doubtless widespread in the body during the prodrome; it may be isolated from the blood at this time, and giant cells have been found in the lymph nodes, tonsils, and appendix. Neutrophil counts decline, lymphocyte counts remain depressed, and eosinophils practically disappear during this period. Hypersensitivity reactions to a wide variety of antigens are suppressed during the prodromal period. This effect may be nearly complete for a few days before and after onset of rash. Normal reactions to dermal antigens return slowly, with some anergy being demonstrable for about 1 month.[54] It is tempting to attribute this anergy to the destruction of lymphocytes; measles virus has been shown to grow in vitro in both T- and B-like lymphocyte cell lines,[44] but T cells uniquely exhibit surface binding sites of measles virus.[103] As discussed in the next section, the electroencephalogram may indicate brain involvement during the prodromal period.

Koplik spots appear on the oral membranes and sometimes on other mucosal surfaces toward the end of the prodromal period. These seem to be a direct manifestation of virus pathology, and cells in the spots have been shown to contain virus nucleocapsid.[99]

With the appearance of rash, both IgG and IgM antibodies become detectable by neutralization or HI tests. IgM antibody titers do not greatly exceed the IgG even in the early stages. Peak IgM titers are

reached at about 10 days after rash, and they become undetectable again by about 30 days.[94] IgG titers reach a peak at about 30 days, fall 2- to 4-fold during the ensuing 6 months, and then remain very nearly stationary for life. Little is known of IgA antibody or cellular responses. Both are part of the immune response to measles,[13,102] and it seems probable that they play important roles in natural protection. Even though circulating globulins passively administered will confer protection, it cannot be assumed that circulating antibody titer gives an adequate picture of measles immunity. Cellular immunity is probably involved in eliminating foci of infected cells.

Free virus is quickly cleared from the blood with the appearance of antibody, but remains detectable in the leukocytes for 1 or 2 days longer. Lymphocyte and eosinophil counts return to the normal range quickly. The neutrophils remain depressed for a day or two and then recover their numbers gradually.

Like the Koplik spots, cells in the macules of the rash contain nucleocapsidlike structures.[99] The two lesions show similar pathological changes except that there are more inflammatory cells in the skin lesions. It seems probable that Koplik spots and rash are basically similar but that under the skin the lesions are not visible until an immunological reaction with virus antigen on the surface of the cells of the capillary endothelium causes dilation and extravasation. The synchrony between the appearance of rash and of circulating measles antibody is striking (Fig. 7) and suggestive of an etiological relationship. However, it is quite possible that cellular immunity, too, appears at this time and that it, rather than antibody, causes the rash.

Once infectious measles virus is cleared from the body, within a few days of the rash, it does not reappear. No instance has been reported where new cases of measles have been attributed to contact with persons who had had measles in the past. Nevertheless, the presence of measles virus antigens and recoverable virus in the brains of patients with subacute sclerosing panencephalitis (SSPE) indicates that the virus may occasionaly persist in the body for long periods. The stability of antibody titers throughout life further suggests that a continuing source of antigenic stimulation is the rule, not the exception.

The lifelong immunity that follows natural mea-

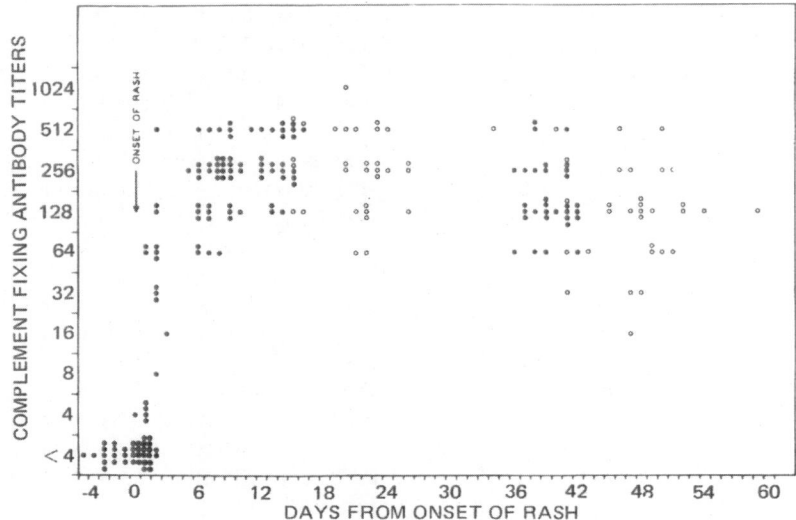

Fig. 7. Measles CF antibody titers in Greenlanders relative to the time of onset of measles rash. Data from Bech.[10]

sles infecton is unusually effective. While secondary cases occur, they are extremely rare and difficult to document. Only the persistent encephalitic infection SSPE represents a well-documented form of measles activity in an immune person. The attenuated vaccines more often fail to provide lasting immunity, especially when they are inhibited by passively acquired γ-globulin, but even they are more than 90% effective for periods of 10 years or more. The extraordinary effectiveness of this immunity suggests that it is not solely dependent on any one element of the immune response. Certainly, passively acquired IgG protects either infants or exposed persons quite effectively in the absence of any cellular immunity. Even killed vaccines, which induce no antihemolysin,[82] confer temporary protection. On the other hand, agammaglobulinemic children usually develop immunity to measles, and the cell-associated system has been found responsive in immune persons with low specific immune globulin levels.[92] In view of the ability of measles virus to spread in tissue culture in the presence of specific IgG, it seems probable that complement-mediated, or T-cell-mediated, lysis of infected cells is needed to eliminate an established infection, but perhaps either, in the absence of the other, can provide protection.

8. Patterns of Host Response

The usual pattern of host response to infection with measles has been described in Section 7. There are also certain rarer and more serious forms the disease may take.

8.1. Clinical Features of Unusual Forms

8.1.1. Atypical Measles in Partially Immunized Persons. Atypical reactions were first noted in persons who had received killed measles vaccine and been exposed to live virus more than a few months later.[43] Although deaths have not been reported as a result of this syndrome, those who have come to medical attention have been more seriously ill than characteristic of their age group with measles. In this syndrome, the rash usually begins on the distal extremities and progresses centripetally. Like the usual measles rash, it is maculopapular, but it is more likely to become petechial or hemorrhagic. The syndrome frequently includes pneumonia and severe myalgia and other pain. Children sensitized by killed vaccine may exhibit a local reaction of pain and swelling at the site of injection of live vaccine. Such revaccination with live vaccine does not, however, eliminate the possibility of a subsequent atypical response to infection with wild virus.[62] Similar atypical reactions have been observed after live virus vaccination, but rarely, relative to the number of vaccine recipients.[33,106]

8.1.2. Encephalitis. The incidence of measles encephalitis is about 1 in 2000 measles cases in the more developed countries of the world, when the denominator is corrected for underreporting of uncomplicated cases. Geographic variations in this rate are not of sufficient magnitude to be visible against the varied background of different reporting efficiencies. Increasing age is accompanied by an increasing proportion of measles patients affected by encephalitis, and encephalitis occurs 2 or 3 times as frequently with measles in children over 10 as in those under 5.[47] Onset may be from 1 to 15 days after appearance of rash, but there is a rather sharp peak frequency on the 6th day.

Abnormal electroencephalograms have been reported in most acute-stage measles cases[45] and in all prodromal stage cases[85] examined in one report. However, the virus has very seldom been isolated from encephalitic brain, and then only by cocultivation with other cells.[74] The timing and pathology of measles encephalitis suggest that immunological reactions may be responsible for many of the symptoms.[61] Direct virus involvement of the central nervous system may occur more frequently in preencephalitic phases of the disease, but, if it does, it causes little distinctive symptomatology. In this, the virus behaves in the brain as it does in the skin. In the brain, however, the most serious symptoms are usually further delayed until some time after the rash. This has given rise to the hypothesis that immunological damage may be related to autoimmunity, generated during the virus infection, against normally sequestered brain antigens.

A high proportion of children with measles encephalitis are left with sequelae, and there is some evidence that even neurological involvement too mild to be diagnosed as encephalitis may leave residua in many children.[42,85]

8.1.3. Subacute Sclerosing Panencephalitis. SSPE is a rare, slow, neurological disease, usually seen in school-age children, that is accompanied by high measles antibody titers in blood and spinal fluid. Measles IgM antibody, commonly demonstrable in the serum, is suggestive of a suppressor-T-cell defect. Children suffering from SSPE usually give a history of measles infection some years previously, 50% before the 2nd birthday. Reported cases in the

United States show a concentration in boys from rural parts of the southeastern states.[39] The geographic disproportion may, however, be an artifact of survey procedures.

A virus can often be isolated from affected tissue by cocultivation of brain cells with a cell line that is competent to replicate measles.[57] These SSPE strains frequently differ from ordinary measles virus in host specificity, but there has been no consistent pattern to these differences. Several SSPE strains have been compared to a measles strain with respect to antigenicity, and no differences were found. Payne and Baublis[88] reported that five SSPE strains were all neutralized less effectively than one measles strain regardless of whether SSPE or measles antiserum was used in the test, but they could isolate an SSPE-like strain from their measles stock after a single selective passage in the presence of antiserum.

It is difficult to reconcile the idea of a distinct SSPE agent with the epidemiology of the disease. The antigenic similarity probably means that infection with either SSPE or measles virus would confer immunity to the other. This means the SSPE agent could move only in those few persons who have no history of measles. If distribution of SSPE virus were this restricted, the cases would probably be more distinctly clustered in time and space than they are.

Rather, each SSPE strain may represent a separate variant of measles virus. The question, then, is whether the variants arise during the primary period of measles infection and determine the neurological involvement or whether they appear only secondarily as a result of selective pressures in the immune host, or even during the protracted and selective manipulations that are required to rescue the virus from nervous tissue. In any case, the development of SSPE strains might be attributable to host-related factors—immunological deficiency that allowed modified virus to persist or a physiological anomaly that allowed virus to penetrate the nervous system. The fact that most SSPE follows measles at a very early age implies that host factors are important. A more detailed presentation of SSPE is given in Chapter 27.

8.2. Diagnosis

8.2.1. Clinical. In the absence of modifying factors, such as γ-globulin prophylaxis or vaccines, the majority of measles infections follow a typical course that is quite distinctive. Koplik spots are particularly useful because they appear early and are not seen in other exanthems. The prodromal period is longer and associated with more fever than the rubella prodrome. Catarrhal symptoms are more prominent than in roseola or scarlatina. The rash is more macular than that of scarlatina, and unlike the case with roseola, fever persists with rash. The pattern of lymphadenopathy is not distinctive as with rubella or scarlatina.

In compilation of measles statistics, the reliability of positive case reports is higher than that for most other infectious disease. Problems may occur when vaccine use has reduced the number of new measles infections to a low level and atypical cases make up a large part of the remainder, but failure to report typical cases represents a greater problem.

8.2.2. Laboratory. Diagnosis by virus isolation is difficult, but serological techniques are useful. Appearance of humoral antibody is sufficiently rapid and regular that paired specimens collected during the first week of rash will show a significant increase in titer even when collected only a few days apart. Reexposure of immune persons to the virus does not usually produce a boost in titer, and no serologically related virus is known to infect man. Laboratory-confirmed diagnoses have very high reliability, and this fact makes measles an ideal model for the study of detailed points in infectious-disease epidemiology.

9. Control and Prevention

Quarantine has been tried and has proven futile in the prevention of measles, except as a temporary expedient in small isolated populations when used to gain time until vaccine can be administered.

A killed vaccine against measles was found effective in conferring temporary protection, but a hypersensitive state sometimes followed this immunization, in which infection with either wild or attenuated live measles virus caused unusual and possibly serious disease.[43] This vaccine has been withdrawn, but recent studies[31,62] show that some people who had received this vaccine remain sensitized to the virus more than 10 years later. Sensitivity seemed to be correlated with exaggerated lymphocyte responsiveness.

Early forms of the live attenuated vaccine caused considerable reaction,[60] and there was reluctance to use them, especially in mass campaigns. γ-Globulin was commonly given in a separate site at the same time as the early vaccine virus strains to reduce the reaction. This procedure has now been almost entirely replaced by use of newer "further attenuated" vaccine strains that cause a reaction comparable to typhoid vaccine.[64] Little or no virus is excreted by vaccinees, and secondary spread to contacts is not a mechanism that increases vaccine coverage as the live poliovirus vaccine. The vaccine can be safely and effectively administered in combination with other vaccine viruses such as rubella, mumps, yellow fever, and smallpox. As shown in Fig. 2, these vaccines have been eminently successful in reducing measles incidence to a low level. Some cases continue, however. The small peaks of higher incidence in 1971 and 1977 seem to be related to a slackening in the vaccination campaigns, and their reversal was associated with renewed efforts to attain full coverage. Cases in recent years have occurred in progressively older age groups, as can be seen by comparing recent age incidence[73] with prevaccine data.[17] With less measles around, the chances of a susceptible person's postponing the disease are increased, but also, in our society, older children and adults associate in larger groups than the young, further increasing their chance of infection.

It is clear that the continuing cases of measles are occurring not only in unvaccinated persons but also in some persons who have been vaccinated. In a 1970 measles epidemic in St. Louis, Cherry et al.[33] reported that 44% of 10,000 cases occurred in persons with a history of vaccination, and this proportion has been higher in subsequent epidemics where more of the population had been previously immunized.[90,97] It is still not altogether clear what proportion of the disease in vaccinees is due to initial failure of the vaccine to immunize and what proportion to waning immunity. There is substantial evidence that in the United States, failures in children vaccinated before 12 months of age and also shortly after their first birthday are relatively common,[3,97] and Yeager et al.[106] believe that vaccine failure accounts for most disease in vaccinees. The report of Deseda-Tous et al.[38] that persons who respond poorly to their first immunization fail to maintain high antibody titers after revaccination is disturbing. It may be that these represent a preexisting group who would always make low titers, but it may also be that early faulty immunization inhibits the later response.

Whether waning immunity also contributes significantly to measles in vaccinated persons is the subject of divergent opinion. The British Measles Sub-committee[72] found no evidence of waning protection 12 years after vaccination with Schwarz strain in a study of 5000 children. There has been limited evidence in the United States and Canada of more measles in persons vaccinated earlier,[90,106] but patterns have been erratic, and differences in vaccination procedure may have played a role. Antibody titers in vaccinees living in open communities have not declined significantly (65,67) over extended periods, but Krugman[65] reported a steady decline over 15 years in antibody titers in one institutionalized group. Brown et al.[29] presented evidence of an irregular decline in titer over 5 years in an isolated island population, but we found no decline over 8 years in isolated forest populations.[68] Krugman attributes the difference in antibody stability in his open and institutionalized populations to the effect of reexposure in the open community, but in view of the present high average age of measles infection, it seems unlikely that reexposure has occurred with regularity, and inevitably there are other differences between institutionalized and healthy children. It is clear that measles-vaccine-induced immunity is more stable than vaccinia-induced smallpox immunity, and at this time there has been no strong call for general revaccination.

Distribution of measles vaccine is hampered by the fact that it must be delayed until the child has reached an age when visits to the pediatric clinic are less frequent and the mother may have become less concerned about preventive care. This is particularly true in the poorer elements of our society, where other concerns are more pressing and medical care often entails long delays in a waiting room. As we have seen, herd immunity has postponed the age at which the unvaccinated acquire the disease, but it has not protected them. Continued efforts to publicize the need and simplify the process are required to counter this difficulty.

Different countries differ greatly in recommendations for measles immunization. At the time of writing, the CDC recommendation for the United States is vaccination with live vaccine "about 15 months of age." After exposure to measles has occurred, measles immune globulin (0.1 ml per pound body weight) may be used if no more than 6 days have elapsed, but this must be followed by vaccination no less than 3 months later.

10. Unresolved Problems

10.1. Vaccine Distribution in Developing Countries

Many developing countries are now organizing mass programs for measles vaccination. It is in these areas that mortality rates are highest and the need greatest. Much of the mortality, however, occurs very early in life, even before the first birthday, making the problem particularly difficult. Conventional advice would be to vaccinate twice, once at 6–9 months of age and once at 15 months, thus protecting both those who lose maternal antibody early and those who lose it late. However, this is an expensive vaccine, and health officials in many countries are hard pressed to find the funds for a single dose. A recent influential study by a WHO team in Kenya[105] showed that children living in Nairobi responded to vaccine at a younger age than children who have been studied heretofore in the developed countries. It recommends vaccination at 7–8 months of age to prevent as much mortality as possible.

This proposal raises a number of problems. First, until we know the reason for the difference, we don't know where the recommendation applies. Is the earlier response due to rapid metabolism of maternal antibody in the malnourished child? Is it due to low original maternal titers perhaps due in turn to the mother's having had measles at an early age? Or is it a genetically determined character? Early vaccination may prevent the greatest number of deaths because so many of these occur in the very young patient, but it will inevitably leave a substantial proportion of the vaccinees unprotected. This will tend to discredit the vaccine and make cooperation by the mothers less enthusiastic. It will also provide fuel for a continuing high level of endemicity and continued threat to the young infant. If, on the other hand, vaccine were distributed with the goal of immunizing the greatest proportion of the recipients, a successful campaign would raise the average age of attack and might protect the infant indirectly. Until a basis for generalization is found, these questions will have to be answered by each country arbitrarily.

10.2. Eradication

The recent success attained in eradicating smallpox prompts a new look at the possibility of eradicating measles. Like smallpox, measles appears to have no effective nonhuman reservoir. As we have seen, the measles vaccine has its imperfections, but it is probably at least as effective as the smallpox vaccine, which offers only medium-term durability. Nathanson et al.[79] have pointed out that because measles needs a large population for its maintenance, it probably cannot persist long in remote corners of the world and that a campaign patterned on the smallpox campaign, concentrated on limiting the spread of recognized outbreaks, would probably be successful in the United States.

In the United States, Federal authorities have promised a campaign to achieve eradication by 1982. Initial efforts to achieve this goal, however, have not followed the pattern that succeeded with smallpox, but have concentrated on immunizing children who reach school age without immunity.

Measles appears to be rather more infectious than smallpox and spreads more rapidly, but on the other hand, the virus is not known to persist in dried particulates matter and thus lacks this temporary reservoir. The main difference, however, may be the stage of the battle. The smallpox-eradication campaign was undertaken only after the disease had been eliminated from much of the world and greatly reduced in the rest by a long-term program of attrition. Until the disease is better controlled in the rest of the world, reintroductions would be frequent. Until the questions raised in Section 10.1 are answered, it seems unlikely that the disease can also be eliminated from developing countries.

10.3. Measles and Multiple Sclerosis

A third unsolved problem is the relationship of measles to multiple sclerosis (MS). Adams and Imagawa[2] noted that the average measles antibody titer in serum from MS patients was 1.4 times higher than in controls. This difference is small, but it has been confirmed in many subsequent studies. It also appears in persons with HLA antigens A3 and B7,[87] two types that occur in MS patients with unusual frequency. This suggests a possible confounding factor, but even more striking than the serum data, measles antibody was present in the CSF of 70% of the patients and none of the controls. At first, it seemed possible that the CSF antibody represented material that had leaked nonspecifically from the serum as a result of disease-induced damage, but Salmi et al.[93] have shown that whereas the titer of nonspecifically transferred antibodies in the CSF was usually 1/320th or less of the serum titer, measles titers in the CSF might be 1/10th the serum titer. Other studies[35,102] show that lymphocyte migration is not inhibited by measles antigen to the same extent with cells from MS patients as with cells from controls. This effect, however, could not be confirmed by thymidine-uptake techniques, and it is not altogether specific to measles antigen.[84] Attempts to isolate a virus from the brain have yielded no consistent result.

Epidemiological data indicate that some event occurring in the second decade of life initiates a process that leads to MS, usually a decade or more later. This triggering event may be infection with measles virus or with the related canine distemper virus or with some other virus,[36,78] but in any event, many genetic and environmental factors influence the outcome, and no one virus appears to be uniquely essential to the process.

11. References

1. ABU BECR, M., *A Discourse on the Smallpox and Measles* (trans. R. Mead), J. Brindley, London, 1748.
2. ADAMS, J. M., AND IMAGAWA, D. T., Measles antibodies in multiple sclerosis, *Proc. Soc. Exp. Biol. Med.* **111:**562–566 (1962).
3. ALBRECHT, P., ENNIS, F. H., SALTZMEN, E. J., AND KRUGMAN, S., Persistence of maternal antibody beyond twelve months: Mechanisms of measles vaccine failure, *J. Pediatr.* **91:**766–767 (1977).
4. BABBOTT, F. L., GALBRAITH, N. S., McDONALD, J. C., SHAW, A., AND ZUCKERMAN, A. J., Deaths from measles in England and Wales in 1961, *Mon. Bull. Minist. Health Public Health Lab. Serv.* **22:**167–175 (1963).
5. BABBOTT, F. L., AND GORDON, J. E., Modern measles, *Am. J. Med. Sci.* **228:**334–361 (1954).
6. BAILEY, N. T. J., *The Mathematical Theory of Epidemics*, Griffin, London, 1957.

7. Bartlett, M. S., Deterministic and stochastic models for recurrent epidemics, *Third Berkeley Symp. Math. Stat. Prob.* **4**:81–109 (1956).

8. Bartlett, M. S., Measles periodicity and community size, *J. R. Stat. Soc. Ser. A* **120**:40–70 (1957).

9. Bartlett, M. S., The critical community size for measles in the United States, *J. R. Stat. Soc. Ser. A* **123**:37–44 (1960).

10. Bech, V., Studies on the development of complement fixing antibodies in measles patients, *J. Immunol.* **83**:267–275 (1959).

11. Bech, V., Measles epidemics in Greenland, *Am. J. Dis. Child.* **103**:252–253 (1962).

12. Bech, V., The measles epidemic in Greenland, *Arch. Gesamte Virusforsch.* **16**:53–56 (1965).

13. Bellanti, J. A., Sanga, R. L., Klutinis, B., Brandt, B., and Artenstein, M. S., Antibody responses in serum and nasal secretion of children immunized with inactivated and attenuated measles virus vaccines, *N. Engl. J. Med.* **280**:628–633 (1969).

14. Benjamin, B., and Ward, S. M., Leukocyte response to measles, *Am. J. Dis. Child.* **44**:921–963 (1932).

15. Berg, R. B., and Rosenthal, M. S., Propagation of measles virus in suspensions of human and monkey leukocytes, *Proc. Soc. Exp. Biol. Med.* **106**:581–585 (1961).

16. Bhatt, P. N., Brandt, C. D., Weiss, R. A., Fox, J. P., and Shaffer, M. F., Viral infections of monkeys in their natural habitat in southern India, *Am. J. Trop. Med. Hyg.* **15**:561–566 (1966).

17. Black, F. L., Serological epidemiology in measles, *Yale J. Biol. Med.* **32**:44–50 (1959).

18. Black, F. L., Growth and stability of measles virus, *Virology* **7**:184–192 (1959).

19. Black, F. L., A nationwide survey of United States military recruits, 1962. III. Measles and mumps antibodies, *Am J. Hyg.* **80**:304–307 (1964).

20. Black, F. L., Measles endemicity in insular populations: Critical community size and its evolutionary implication, *Theor. Biol.* **11**:207–211 (1965).

21. Black, F. L., Measles, in: *Manual of Clinical Microbiology*, 2nd ed. (E. H. Lennette and J. P. Truant, eds.), American Society of Microbiology, Bethesda, Maryland, 1974.

22. Black, F. L., Hierholzer, W., Woodall, J. P., and Pinheiro, F., Intensified reactions to measles vaccine in unexposed populations of American Indians *J. Infect. Dis.* **124**:306–317 (1971).

23. Black, F. L., and Rosen, L., Patterns of measles antibodies in residents of Tahiti and their stability in the absence of re-exposure, *J. Immunol.* **88**:725–731 (1962).

24. Black, F. L., and Sheridan, S. R., Studies on attenuated measles-virus vaccine. IV. Administration of vaccine by several routes, *N. Engl. J. Med.* **263**:166–170 (1960).

25. Black, F. L., and Sheridan, S. R., Blood leukocyte response to live measles vaccine, *Am. J. Dis. Child.* **113**:301–304 (1967).

26. Blake, F. C., and Trask, J. D., Studies on measles. II. Symptomatology and pathology in monkeys experimentally infected, *J. Exp. Med.* **33**:413–422 (1921).

27. Bridges, E. L., *Uttermost Part of the Earth*, Dutton, New York, 1949.

28. Brown, P., Basright, M., and Gajdusek, D. C., Response to live attenuated measles vaccine in susceptible island populations in Micronesia, *Am. J. Epidemiol.* **82**:115–122 (1965).

29. Brown, P. D., Gajdusek, C., and Tsai, T., Persistence of measles antibody in the absence of circulating natural virus five years after immunization of a virgin population with Edmonston B vaccine, *Am. J. Epidemiol.* **90**:514–518 (1969).

30. Celers, J., Problèmes de santé publique posés par la rougeole dans les pay favorisés, *Arch. Gesamte Virusforsch.* **16**:5–18 (1965).

31. Center for Disease Control, Atypical measles—California 1974–1975, *Morbid. Mortal. Weekly Rep.* **25**:245–246 (1976).

32. Chalmers, A. K., *The Health of Glasgow 1818–1925*, Bell and Bain, Glasgow, 1930.

33. Cherry, J. D., Feigin, R. D., Lobes, L. A., Jr., Hinthorn, D. R., Shackleford, P. G., Shirley, R. H., Lins, R. D., and Choi, S. C., Urban measles in the vaccine era: A clinical, epidemiologic and serologic study, *J. Pediatr.* **81**:217–230 (1972).

34. Christensen, P. E., Henning, S., Bang, H. O., Andersen, V., Jordal, B., and Jensen, O., An epidemic of measles in southern Greenland, 1951: Measles in virgin soil. II. The epidemic proper, *Acta Med. Scand.* **144**:430–449 (1952).

35. Ciongoli, A. K., Platz, P., Dupont, B., Svejgaard, A., Fog, T., and Jerslid, C., Lack of antigen response to myxoviruses in multiple sclerosis, *Lancet* **2**:1147 (1973).

36. Cook, S. D., Dowling, P. D., and Russell, W. C., Multiple sclerosis and canine distemper, *Lancet* **1**:605–606 (1978).

37. Corney, B. G., The behavior of certain epidemic diseases in natives of Polynesia with especial reference to the Fiji Islands, *Trans. Epidemiol. Soc. London (N. Ser.)* **3**:76–95 (1884).

38. Deseda-Tous, J., Cherry, J. D., Spencer, M. J., Williver, R. C., Boyer, K. M., Dudley, J. P., Zahradnik, J. M., Krause, P. J., and Walbergh, E. W., Measles revaccination, persistence and degree of antibody titer by type of immune response, *Am. J. Dis. Child.* **132**:287–290 (1978).

39. Detels, R., Brody, J. A., McNew, J., and Edgar, A. H., Further epidemiological studies of sub-acute sclerosing panencephalitis, *Lancet* **2**:11–14 (1973).

40. ENDERS, J. F., AND PEEBLES, T. C., Propagation in tissue cultures of cytopathogenic agents from patients with measles, *Proc. Soc. Exp. Biol. Med.* **86:**277–286 (1954).

41. FENNER, F., *The Impact of Civilization on the Biology of Man* (S. V. BOYDEN, ed.), University of Toronto Press, Toronto, 1970.

42. FOX, J. P., BLACK, F. L., AND KOGON, A., Measles and readiness for reading and learning. V. Evaluative comparison of the studies and overall conclusions, *Am. J. Epidemiol.* **88:**168–175 (1969).

43. FULGINITI, V. A., ELLER, J. J., DOWNIE, A. W., AND KEMPE, C. H., Altered reactivity to measles virus: Atypical measles in children previously immunized with inactivated measles virus vaccines, *J. Am. Med. Assoc.* **202:**1075–1080 (1967).

44. GALLAGHER, M., AND FLANAGAN, T. D., Growth of measles in continuous lymphoid cell lines, *Fed. Proc. Fed. Am. Soc. Exp. Biol.* **34:**948 (1975).

45. GIBBS, F. A., GIBBS, E. L., CARPENTER, P. R., AND SPIES, H. W., Electroencephalographic abnormality in "uncomplicated" childhood diseases, *J. Am. Med. Assoc.* **171:**1050–1055 (1959).

46. GORDON, J. E., JANSSEN, A. A. J., AND ASCOLI, W., Measles in rural Guatemala, *J. Pediatr.* **66:**779–786 (1965).

47. GREENBERG, M., PELLITTERI, O., AND EISENSTEIN, D., T., Measles encephalitis. 1. Prophylactic effect of gamma globulin, *J. Pediatr.* **46:**642–647 (1955).

48. GRESSER, I., AND KATZ, S. L., Isolation of measles virus from urine, *N. Engl. J. Med.* **263:**452–454 (1960).

49. GRIFFITHS, D. A., The effect of measles vaccination on the incidence of measles in the community, *J. R. Stat. Soc. Ser. A* **136:**441–449 (1973).

50. GULICK, L. H., On the climate, diseases and materia medica of the Sandwich (Hawaiian) Islands, *N. Y. J. Med.* **14:**169–211 (1855).

51. HALL, W. W., AND MARTIN, S. J., The structural proteins of measles virus, in: *Negative Strand Viruses* (B. W. J. MAHY AND R. D. BARRY, eds.), pp. 89–103, Academic Press, London, 1975.

52. HAMER, W. H., The Milroy lectures on epidemic disease in England—The evidence of variability and persistency of type, *Lancet* **1:**733–739 (1906).

53. HEDRICK, A. W., Monthly estimates of the child population susceptible to measles 1900–1931, *Am. J. Hyg.* **17:**613–636 (1933).

54. HELMS, S., AND HELMS, P., Tuberculin sensitivity during measles, *Acta Tuberc. Scand.* **35:**166–171 (1956).

55. HIRSCH, A., *Handbook of Geographical and Historical Pathology,* Vol. 1, pp. 154–170, New Sydenham Society, London, 1883.

56. HOME, F., *Medical Facts and Experiments,* A. Millar, London, 1759.

57. HORTA-BARBOSA, L., FUCCILO, D. A., HAMILTON, R.,

TRAUB, R., LEY, A., AND SEVER, J. L., Some characteristics of SSPE measles virus, *Proc. Soc. Exp. Biol. Med.* **134:**17–21 (1970).

58. DEJONG, J. G., AND WINKLER, K. O., Survival of measles virus in air, *Nature (London)* **201:**1054–1055 (1964).

59. KATZ, S. L., AND ENDERS, J. F., Measles virus, in: *Diagnostic Procedures for Viral and Rickettsial Infections,* 4th ed. (E. H. LENNETTE AND N. J. SCHMIDT, eds.), pp. 504–528, American Public Health Association, New York, 1969.

60. KATZ, S. L., KEMPE, C. H., BLACK, F. L., LEPOW, M. L., KRUGMAN, S., HAGGERTY, R. J., AND ENDERS, J. F., Studies on an attenuated measles-virus vaccine. VIII. General summary and evaluation of the results of vaccination, *N. Engl. J. Med.* **273:**180–184 (1960).

61. KOPROWSKI, H., The role of hyperergy in measles encephalitis, *Am. J. Dis. Child.* **103:**273–278 (1962).

62. KRAUSE, P. J., CHERRY, J. D., NAIDITCH, M. J., DESADÁ-TOUS, J., AND WALBERGH, E. W., Revaccination of previous recipients of killed measles vaccine: Clinical and immunological studies, *J. Pediatr.* **93:**565–571 (1978).

63. KRESS, S., SCHLUEDERBERG, A. E., HORNICK, R. B., MORSE, L. J., COLE, J. L., SLATER, E. A., AND MCCRUMB, F. R., Studies with live attenuated measles-virus vaccine. II. Clinical and immunological response of children in an open community, *Am. J. Dis. Child.* **101:**701–707 (1961).

64. KRUGMAN, S., GILES, J. P., JACOBS, A. M., AND FRIEDMAN, H., Studies with a further attenuated live measles-virus vaccine, *Pediatrics* **66:**471–488 (1965).

65. KRUGMAN, S., Present status of measles and rubella immunization in the United States: A medical progress report, *J. Pediatr.* **90:**1–12 (1977).

66. Landlaekni, Heilbrigdisskyslur (Public Health in Iceland, Rikisprentsmidjan Gutenberg, Reykjavik, 1941–1950.

67. LEPOW, M. L., AND NANKERVIS, G. A., Eight-year serological evaluation of Edmonston live measles vaccine, *J. Pediatr.* **75:**407–411 (1969).

68. LIAN, J.-F., Quantitative approach to measles humoral immunity, Ph.D. Dissertation, Yale University, 1979.

69. MAXCY, K. F., Principles and methods of epidemiology, in: *Viral and Rickettsial Infections of Man* (T. M. RIVERS, ed.), pp. 128–146, Lippincott, Philadelphia, 1948.

70. MCCRUMB, F. R., KRESS, S., SAUNDERS, E., SNYDER, M. J., AND SCHLUEDERBERG, A. E., Studies with live attenuated measles vaccine. I. Clinical and immunological responses in institutionalized children, *Am. J. Dis. Child.* **101:**689–700 (1961).

71. MCNEILL, W. H., *Plagues and Peoples: A Natural History of Infectious Diseases,* Doubleday, New York, 1976.

72. MEASLES SUB-COMMITTE: COMMITTEE ON DEVELOPMENT

OF VACCINES AND IMMUNIZATION PROCEDURES, Clinical trial of live measles vaccine given alone and live vaccine preceded by killed vaccine, *Lancet* **2**:571–575 (1977).

73. Measles—United States, first 36 weeks, 1977–1978, *Morbid. Mortal. Weekly Rep.* **27**:235–237 (1978).

74. TER MEULEN, V., MÜLLER, D., KÄCKELL, Y., KATZ, M., AND MAYERMANN, R., Isolation of infectious measles virus in measles encephalitis, *Lancet* **2**:1172–1175 (1972).

75. MEYER, H. M., Mass vaccination against measles in Upper Volta, *Arch. Gesamte Virusforsch.* **16**:243–245 (1965).

76. MORLEY, D., The severe measles of West Africa, *Proc. R. Soc. Med.* **57**:846–849 (1969).

77. MYERS, J. M., Assimilation to the ecological and social systems of a community, *Am. Sociol. Rev.* **15**:367–370 (1950).

78. NATHANSON, N., AND MILLER, A., Epidemiology of multiple sclerosis: Critique of the evidence for a viral etiology, *Am. J. Epidemiol.* **107**:451–461 (1978).

79. NATHANSON, N., YORKE, J. A., PIANIGIANI, G., AND MARTIN, J., Requirements for perpetuation and eradication of viruses in populations, in: *Persistent Viruses* (J. D. STEVENS, G. J. TODARO, AND C. F. FOY, eds.), pp. 75–100, Academic Press, New York, 1978.

80. NEEL, J. V., CENTERWALL, W. R., CHAGNON, N. A., AND CASEY, H. L., Notes on the effects of measles in virgin-soil population of South American Indians, *Am. J. Epidemiol.* **91**:418–429 (1970).

81. NORRBY, E., Viral antibodies in multiple sclerosis, *Prog. Med. Virol.* **24**:1–39 (1978).

82. . NORRBY, E., ENDERS-RUCKLE, G., AND TER MEULEN, V., Differences in the appearance of antibodies to structural components of measles virus after immunization with inactivated and live virus, *J. Infect. Dis.* **132**:262–269 (1975).

83. NUTELS, N., Medical problems of newly contacted Indian groups, *Pan. Am. Health Organ. Sci. Publ.* **165**:68–76 (1968).

84. OFFNER, H., AMMITZBOLL, T., CLAUSEN, J., FOG, F., HYLLESTED, K., AND EINSTEIN, E., Immune response of lymphocytes from patients with multiple sclerosis to phytohemagglutinin, basic protein myelin and measles antigens, *Acta. Neurol. Scand.* **50**:373–381 (1974).

85. PAMPIGLIONE, G., Prodromal phase of measles: Some neurophysiological studies, *Br. Med. J.* **2**:1296–1300 (1964).

86. PANUM, P. L., *Observations Made During the Epidemic of Measles on the Faroe Islands in the Year 1846*, American Publishing Association, New York, 1940.

86a. PAPP, K., Experiences prouvant que a voie d'infection de la rougeole est la contamination de la muguese conjontivale, *Rev. d'Immunol.* **20**:27–36 (1956).

87. PATY, D. W., FURESZ, J., BOUCHER, W., RAND, C. G., AND STILLER, C. R., Measles antibodies as related to HLA types in multiple sclerosis, *Neurology* **20**:651–655 (1976).

88. PAYNE, F. E., AND BAUBLIS, J. V., Decreased reactivity of SSPE strains of measles virus with antibody, *J. Infect. Dis.* **127**:505–511 (1973).

89. PEART, A. F. W., AND NAGLER, F. P., Measles in the Canadian Arctic 1952, *Can. J. Public Health* **45**:146–157 (1954).

90. RAWLS, W. E., RAWLS, M. L., AND CHERNESKY, M. H., Analysis of a measles epidemic: Possible role of vaccine failures, *Can. Med. Assoc. J.* **113**:941–944 (1975).

91. RISTORI, C., BOCCARDO, H., BORGOÑO, J. M., AND ARMIJO, R., Medical importance of measles in Chile, *Am. J. Dis. Child.* **103**:236–241 (1962).

92. RUCKDESCHEL, J. C., GRAZIANO, K. D., AND MARDINEY, M. R., JR., Additional evidence that the cell-associated immune system is the primary host defense against measles, *Cell. Immunol.* **17**:11–18 (1975).

93. SALMI, A. A., NORRBY, E., AND PANELIUS, M., Identification of different measles virus-specific antibodies in the serum and cerebro-spinal fluid from patients with sub-acute sclerosing panencephalitis and multiple sclerosis, *Infect. Immun.* **6**:248–254 (1972).

94. SCHLUEDERBERG, A. E., Immune globulins in human viral infections, *Nature (London)* **205**:1232–1233 (1965).

95. SCHUTZ, F., *Die Epidemiologie der Masern*, Gustav Fisher, Jena, 1925.

96. SCRIMSHAW, N. S., SOLOMON, J. B., BRUCH, H. A., AND GORDON, J. E., Studies of diarrheal disease in Central America. VIII. Measles, diarrhea and nutritional deficiency in Guatemala, *Am. J. Trop. Med.* **15**:625–631 (1966).

97. SHASBY, D. M., SHOPE, T. C., DOWNS, H., HERRMANN, K. L., AND POLKOWSKI, J., Epidemic measles in a highly vaccinated population, *N. Engl. J. Med.* **296**:585–589 (1977).

98. SOPER, H. E., The interpretation of periodicity in disease prevalence, *J. R. Stat. Soc. Ser. A* **92**:34–61 (1929).

99. SURINGA, D. W. R., BANK, L. J., AND ACKERMAN, A. B., Role of measles in skin lesions and Koplik spots, *N. Engl. J. Med.* **283**:1139–1142 (1970).

100. SYDENHAM, T., *The Works of Thomas Sydenham*, Vol. 2, pp. 250–251, Sydenham Society, London, 1922.

101. TOOTH, J. S. H., AND LEWIS, I. C., Measles epidemic in a primitive isolated community, *Med. J. Aust.* **1**:182–186 (1963).

102. UTERMOHLEN, V., AND ZABRISKIE, J. B., A suppression of cellular immunity in patients with multiple sclerosis, *J. Exp. Med.* **138**:1591–1596 (1973).

103. VALDIMARSSON, H., AGNARSDOTTIR, G., AND LACH-

MANN, P. J., Measles virus receptor on human T lymphocytes, *Nature (London)* **225:**554–556 (1975).

104. VIEIRA, J. P. B., JR., Vacinacão dos indios Surui contrâ o sarapo, *Rev. Assoc. Med. Brazil* **16:**183–186 (1968).

105. WORLD HEALTH ORGANIZATION, Measles immunity in the first year after birth and the optimum age for vaccination in Kenyan children, *WHO Bull.* **55:**21–31 (1977).

106. YEAGER, A. S., DAVIS, J. H., ROSS, L. A., AND HARVEY, B. S., Measles immunization successes and failures, *J. Am. Med. Assoc.* **237:**347–351 (1977).

Mumps

Harry A. Feldman

1. Introduction

Mumps is an acute communicable disease of children and young adults caused by a single strain of a myxovirus. Epidemiologically, mumps has played an important role in armies during mobilization, resulting in widespread morbidity. In addition to producing the well-known syndrome of parotitis, it also is a common cause of meningoencephalitis; additional manifestations include orchitis, pancreatitis, mastitis, and oophoritis.

2. Historical Background

An outbreak of what was probably mumps or epidemic parotitis was described by Hippocrates in the 5th century B. C. as an illness accompanied by swelling near the ear and painful enlargement of the testes, either unilaterally or bilaterally. Hamilton in 1790 not only emphasized the importance of orchitis as a manifestation of the disease, but also thought that some patients had symptoms related to the central nervous system. The latter was recognized early in the present century.

But until relatively recently, mumps was viewed primarily as an illness that affected armies during times of mobilization. Its history has been summarized as follows[79]:

Harry A. Feldman · Department of Preventive Medicine, State University of New York, Upstate Medical Center, Syracuse, New York.

Knowledge of mumps has developed within 3 periods. The first was concerned chiefly with the study of frank epidemics, and established both the communicability of the condition and its wide distribution. Hirsch's collection of some 150 epidemics, occurring between 1714 and 1859, showed the disease to be prevalent from Iceland to Egypt, and from Alaska to Polynesia. Accumulated evidence from outbreaks in the first half of the 19th century demonstrated another epidemiologic feature of mumps, its predilection for prisons, orphanages, boarding schools, garrisons, and ships. The second general advance was concerned with better definition of the clinical features of mumps, credit for which goes in large part to a brilliant line of French army surgeons. The third era was initiated with the production of mumps experimentally and the recognition of the specific infectious agent.

Gordon and Heeren,[56] in a review of the epidemiology of mumps in anticipation of America's becoming involved in World War II, quoted Haven Emerson that in World War I, mumps was the most important cause of days lost from active duty in the American army in France. Stokes [133] found that the annual hospital admission rate was 55.8/1000 average strength in World War I, exceeded only by influenza and gonorrhea. Blacks were affected 2.7 times more than white recruits. While the peak rate was 75.5 in 1918, it was only 6.9 in World War II (1943).

In their landmark report of the successful transmission of mumps from patients to rhesus monkeys in 1934, Johnson and Goodpasture[79] clearly demonstrated that mumps was caused by a filtrable virus present in saliva. With the development of specific serological techniques, it soon became evident that mumps was a generalized disease with a proclivity for glandular tissues such as the parotids, ovaries, testes, and pancreas, but on occasion the central nervous system, myocardium, and kidneys. Furthermore, 30–40% of people were found to be immune, apparently as the result of asymptomatic infections. When coupled with underreporting (only about 12% are recorded), the gathering of precise epidemiological data becomes very difficult.

Cultivation of mumps virus in the developing chick embryo was described by Habel[60] in 1945, and an experimental vaccine produced in 1946[61] was used in humans in 1951.[62] A live mumps virus vaccine has been used in Russia since the early 1960s.[129] Successful trials of a live attenuated mumps virus vaccine in the United States by Weibel et al. [146] led to its licensure in December 1967.

3. The Agent

Myxovirus parotiditis, the cause of epidemic parotitis, is a member of the group that includes the influenza, parainfluenza, and Newcastle disease viruses. It is an RNA virus with a nucleoprotein core [soluble (S) antigen] surrounded by a lipid-containing outer membrane that is susceptible to ether and chloroform. The outer surface contains a neuraminidase and a hemagglutinin [viral (V) antigen] and induces protective antibodies. There is only one serotype. Readily destroyed by heat, the virus is also inactivated by 0.2% formalin, ultraviolet light, and other agents.

Mumps virus is found only in man, but has been adapted to monkeys, chick embryos, and tissue cultures. Newcastle disease and parainfluenza viruses, but not influenza, produced antibodies that cross-react with mumps virus. Antibodies to the various components of mumps virus appear at different rates and time intervals. Those to the S antigen are apparent by the 7th day after the onset of illness and reach their peak within about 2 weeks. Antibodies to the V antigen appear somewhat slower, requiring 2–3 weeks for detection and another week or two for maximum titers, but are detectable for longer periods than are those induced by the S antigen. Antibodies for the S antigen are measurable by complement fixation (CF) and do not seem to relate to protection. Several varieties of antibodies—

CF, hemagglutination-inhibition (HI), and neutralizaton (N)—are induced by the V antigen and are indicative of immunity. Delayed hypersensitivity with positive skin reactions also develops in those who have had mumps or have received either inactivated or live virus vaccines.

Immunity follows both clinically apparent and inapparent infections. Second infections can occur, but their rate is unknown and their clinical expression and complications are infrequent.

4. Methodology Involved in Epidemiological Analysis

4.1. Sources of Data

In view of the frequency with which clinically asymptomatic and undiagnosed cases of mumps occur and the fact that most cases are not reported, all epidemiological data are somewhat suspect. It comes as no surprise that much of the information on incidence, prevalence, complications, and fatalities is drawn from military sources, where epidemics have been almost a tradition. These will be dealt with in subsequent sections.

In recent years, the source of the most useful data has been the Epidemiology Program of the Centers for Disease Control (CDC), which instituted a mumps surveillance program in January 1968 when, coincidentally with the licensing of attenuated live virus mumps vaccine, mumps was reinstated as a notifiable disease. First put on the notifiable list in 1922, it had been removed in 1950, although some states had continued, with variable effectiveness, their own reporting systems. The fourth and latest such report (July 1974–December 1976) was issued in July 1978.[30] Mumps is recorded in the *Morbidity and Mortality Weekly Reports* (MMWR), which are published by the CDC and summarized annually.

All incidence and prevalence data err on the low side for several reasons: at least some reported cases of aseptic meningitis and encephalitis are related to mumps, subclinical cases of mumps are frequent, and under-reporting is common. Aside from the CDC data, many individual local and state health departments continue to provide information for their areas. Other useful information has been provided from military experiences, especially those in World War I and World War II.[56,57,89,104]

4.2. Serological Surveys

A number of serological surveys utilizing the method(s) available at a particular time have been reported. For these purposes, CF, HI, and N techniques, as well as skin tests, were employed.[17,18,43,70,74,82,97,99,114]

4.3. Laboratory Methods

Henle[68] reviewed the laboratory procedures available for the study of patients and populations for mumps.

4.3.1. Virus Isolation. The virus was first transmitted to monkeys by Johnson and Goodpasture,[79] but Habel[60] adapted it to developing chick embryos from infected monkey parotid tissue and found both CF and skin-test antigens to be produced. Henle and McDougall[72] transmitted the virus directly to chick embryos with spinal fluid from a human patient. Later, Levens and Enders[96] demonstrated hemagglutinins in the amniotic fluids of such infected eggs. Virus has been isolated from saliva, blood, spinal fluid, and parotids, but this is not often attempted, since several effective serological techniques are available.

4.3.2. Neutralization (N). N antibodies have been detected in serum–virus mixtures inoculated into embryonated eggs or tissue cultures. The latter generally are used, with the end points being cytopathic effect (CPE), hemadsorption, or interference. Titers as low as 1:2 are accepted as indicative of specific immunity.

4.3.3. Hemolysis-in-Gel. Recently, a new hemolysis-in-gel test was described[58] that is said to correlate well with the N system. It is simpler and can be performed more rapidly than N, but further evaluation is required before this new test can be placed in perspective.

4.3.4. Complement Fixation (CF). Two antigens are used for CF,[68] each supplying somewhat different information. Antibodies to soluble (S) antigen appear early, while those to viral (V) antigen appear in convalescence and persist for many years. Thus, a positive test with S antigen and a negative test with V antigen indicate an early stage of infection, whereas the reverse suggests convalescence or later.

4.3.5. Skin Test. The antigen for the skin test, originally produced from mumps-infected monkey parotid, is usually made from infected chick embryos. It is difficult to standardize, but generally contains a defined amount of hemagglutinating antigen (HA) or CF antigen. Reactions are of the delayed type. A minimum of 10 mm of erythema is usually required for a "positive," but some authors insist on a larger area. Positive reactions are assumed to indicate immunity, but variable results have been reported. Skin tests probably do not induce primary antibody responses, but do initiate a secondary response. Possibly useful for the study of cell-mediated immunity, mumps-virus skin tests are no longer recommended for the estimation of resistance to infection.

4.3.6. Hemagglutination Inhibition (HI). Levens and Enders[96] found allantoic fluid from infected chick embryos to agglutinate fowl erythrocytes that were inhibited by both human and monkey convalescent sera. This reaction, similar in all respects to that produced by influenza viruses, has been evaluated by several investigators and correlates quite well with CF tests. A variety of red cells can be used and antibodies seem to persist, but clear end points are sometimes difficult to achieve.

5. Descriptive Epidemiology

5.1. Incidence and Prevalence

In the United States during 1977, 21,436 cases of mumps were reported,[31] as opposed to 38,492 during the preceding year and 59,647 the year before that. The cases reported to the CDC in 1977 represented a disease incidence of 8.5 per 100,000, the lowest in the history of mumps surveillance. The rates of reported cases of mumps, by year, in the United States from 1922 to 1976 are depicted in Fig. 1.[30] The largest number of cases since 1960 was recorded in 1964, with 212,932 and a rate of approximately 84 per 100,000. Since the licensing of mumps vaccine in December 1967, there has been a steady decrease annually in reported cases to well below 50,000. The reason for this is not entirely certain, but the fact that in the 5 years preceding vaccine introduction no year had fewer than 114,000 reported cases strongly suggests that the decrease is probably associated with vaccine utilization.

The incidence of mumps encephalitis, mumps aseptic meningitis, and mumps deaths is compared in Fig. 2[30] with the incidence of reported mumps

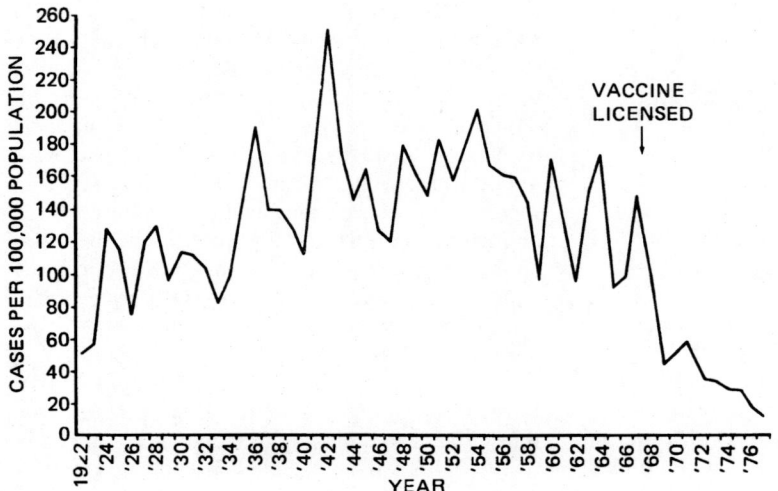

Fig. 1. Reported cases of mumps, United States, 1922–1976. From the CDC.[30]

for the years 1960–1976. Decreases in all four categories are self-evident.

As mentioned in Section 4.1, the reported cases of mumps fall far short of their actual number. Such underreporting results, in part, from the necessity for patients to first seek care by physicians, which may not be done in mild cases. These physicians must not only make the proper diagnosis but also report it to the health department. Furthermore, even if all clinical cases were recognized and reported, the total would be grossly underestimated because of the predominance of mild and subclinical cases. An example of the magnitude of such errors is illustrated by a seroepidemiological study of 126

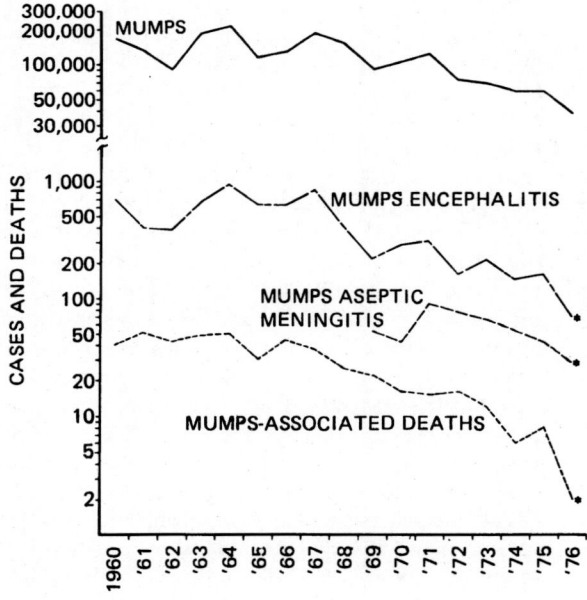

Fig. 2. Reported cases of mumps, mumps encephalitis, mumps aseptic meningitis, and mumps-associated deaths, by year, United States, 1960–1976. From the CDC.[30]

cases and 233 contacts in Florida.[97] From this experience, it was estimated that the yearly incidence rate was 19.5 per 1000, or about 10 times the national surveillance figure based on reported cases alone. Of the 126 cases identified, only 27% visited a physician and only 6% were actually reported. In addition to the clinical cases, serological tests revealed that 25% of the family contacts had had inapparent infections. From 14 to 46% of family contacts develop secondary clinical cases, the rate varying with the age of the contact. No serological evidence of reinfection was found in reexposed adults by the CF or HI tests.

5.2. Survey Data

Several types of population surveys have been carried out to determine the patterns of susceptibility and immunity within a community. These have used questionnaire and interview data, skin tests, and various laboratory determinations of mumps antibody (CF, HI, and N).

Questionnaire data were used by Harris et al.[65] to define the incidence of mumps among various members of the health profession and general university faculty members. By age, highest attack rates occurred in the 20- to 29-year-old group, by profession among pediatricians; the lowest attack rates were in those over 50 years of age and among the general university faculty. An inverse relationship was found between the student's age and the frequency of mumps in the teacher. Household surveys conducted in Buffalo, New York, also by Harris et al.,[66] indicated that the peak incidence of cases was at 7 years and that 74% had experienced mumps by age 10. Some investigators feel that a history of mumps is not a reliable indicator of immunity.[82]

Using skin and CF tests, Henle et al.[70] carried out an early study of 1800 residents in the Philadelphia area. Among persons with a past history of mumps, 70–80% had positive skin or CF tests. While reactivity was not an absolute criterion, fewer than 2% of persons with CF or skin-test reactivity acquired mumps. Both tests were needed because they did not always agree. Variability among different lots of commercial skin-test antigens has been found in comparison studies with serum N tests.[19,122] Since skin-test results do not accurately reflect susceptibility or immunity, this procedure is no longer

recommended. The presence of N antibody is a reliable indicator of immunity, [19,20] but this should be measured before any skin test to avoid an anamnestic response.[122] The CF test has been a fairly good indicator of immunity to mumps.[82]

Antibody surveys of healthy populations have been widely employed to indicate the past experience of a community with mumps in terms of its remaining susceptibles (i.e., lacking antibody). The results of surveys employing various tests are summarized in Table 1. The first nationwide recruit study of Liao and Benenson[99] in 1951 revealed CF antibody levels of 1:8 or more in 54% of recruits tested. Clinical histories of mumps were provided by 70% (51% prior to age 10). Among the 29% who had no prior history of mumps, 39% had positive CF tests. In a second survey of 2400 United States recruits by Black[17] in 1962, 76% had HI antibody in the 1:10 dilution. In a study of 1385 Brazilian recruits by Niederman et al.[114] in 1964, 83% were positive in the 1:10 dilution.

Wide variations in antibody prevalence were found in serum collections from the WHO Serum Bank at Yale University. These retrospective tests were performed by Black and Houghton[18] and included Eskimos and subjects from Iceland, New Haven, Connecticut, and several islands. Overall, in the 5- to 9-year age group, the percentages with mumps antibody were: Point Barrow, 0%; Tahiti, 15%; Cape Verde Islands, 55%; Iceland, 79%, New Haven, Connecticut, 52%; and Bahamas, 74%. The lowest prevalence rates were found in Point Barrow, Alaska, where no one had antibody until age 15 or more. A good correlation was found between a history of mumps and a relatively high HI titer. The titers declined slowly, about 2-fold per decade. In another remote island off Alaska, St. Paul, a virgin-soil population was identified in which only 12% of the residents had neutralizing antibody, and on St. George only 7% were positive. This contrasts with United States medical students, of whom 88% had neutralizing antibody.[19]

Kenny et al.[84] more recently reported their mumps N antibody test results as determined among 3000 1- to 15-year-old Middle America children and 2221 United States children of similar ages. The results obtained among 1- to 3-year-olds and 4- to 6-year-olds are incorporated into Table 1. It will be noted that mumps immunity is acquired somewhat later than was that for measles in the prevaccine era.

Table 1. Results of Serological Surveys for Mumps Antibody

Type of population tested	Country	Year bled	Number tested	Test used	Titer "positive"	Immune (%)[a]	Ref. no.
Army recruits	United States	1951	2625	CF	1:8	54	99
Army recruits	United States	1962	2400	HI	1:10	76	17
Army recruits	United States	1962	2400	HI	1:20	47	17
Army recruits	Brazil	1964	1385	HI	1:10	83	114
Rural	Iceland	1962, 1965	384	HI	1:20	73	18
First grade	New Haven, Connecticut	1964, 1965	419	HI	1:20	52	18
Eskimos	Point Barrow, Alaska	1949	97	HI	1:20	14	18
Aleutian Islanders	St. Paul Island, Alaska	1968	195	N	1:4	12	102
Aleutian Islanders	St. George Island, Alaska	1963	57	CF	1:4	7	120
Medical students	United States	1971 (?)	59	N	1:2	88	19
1–3 years old	Dominican Republic	1971–1973	1033	N	1:4	16±	84
4–6 years old	Dominican Republic	1971–1973	725	N	1:4	60	84
1–3 years old	Honduras	1972	593	N	1:4	20	84
4–6 years old	Honduras	1972	69	N	1:4	35±	84
1–3 years old	Panama	1973	150	N	1:4	11	84
4–6 years old	Panama	1973	98	N	1:4	51	84
1–3 years old	United States	1970–1973	792	N	1:4	20	84
4–6 years old	United States	1970–1973	468	N	1:4	75	84

[a] Based on antibody tests rounded off to nearest whole number.

5.3. Epidemic Behavior and Contagiousness

The term "epidemic parotitis" reflects the capacity of mumps virus to cause outbreaks, even though it fails to indicate that infection is always generalized rather than localized to the parotid gland. Outbreaks of mumps occur periodically at intervals from 2–3 to 7 years. Local outbreaks are common wherever there are large aggregations of children and young adults in close contact. This includes military barracks, institutions, and boarding schools.

The contagiousness of mumps can be judged from outbreaks in virgin populations. Three isolated island groups off Alaska have been studied in this regard. On St. Lawrence and adjacent islands, where no prior outbreak of mumps was known, a mumps outbreak occurred in 1957. Of the 561 resident Eskimos, 65% had clinical mumps over a 6-month period. The clinical attack rates were highest in the 5-9 and 10-14 year age groups, in which the incidence was 86 and 87%, respectively, in two villages.[117] A second island outbreak in a virgin population occurred on St. George Island in 1965. No known exposure to mumps had been recorded since

1907, and 93% of 57 preepidemic sera obtained in 1963 lacked antibody.[120] During the outbreak, 56% of the 212 native residents had clinical mumps and 20% had subclinical infections, as revealed by serological tests. Again, the highest incidence of clinical mumps occurred in the 5–9 year (74%) and 10–14 year age groups (91%). The subclinical rates were 16 and 6%, respectively, in these age groups. In ten persons over age 60, who had been exposed in 1907 or before, there were no clinical cases, but six subclinical reinfections were identified. In a third island outbreak on St. Paul Island in 1967–1968, preillness sera indicated that 88% of residents were susceptible. A mumps vaccination program was promptly initiated in part of the population. Among the nonvaccinated persons lacking antibody, mumps subsequently infected 59%, and clinical mumps occurred in 35%. While a similar attack rate occurred in vaccinees, the vaccination may have prevented the exhaustion of the pool of susceptibles. These studies show a high contagiousness of mumps in susceptible populations similar to that of influenza and rubella in open and susceptible groups, but lower than that in measles and chicken pox.

5.4. Geographic Distribution

Except for very isolated island groups and remote villages, mumps occurs throughout the world. In the United States, variations in the incidence of reported cases occur from year to year within most states and from one region to another within a given year. Urban centers are capable of supporting the virus endemically with sporadic outbreaks in schools and other institutions, whereas the virus tends to die out in rural areas until enough susceptibles have accumulated. Some 80–90% of city residents may acquire mumps infection by age 16, whereas only 10–20% are infected by this age in relatively remote communities.[150] In a study of a large military outbreak in 1917–1918 involving over 1000 cases, only 15% occurred in soldiers from cities as opposed to 85% from rural areas.[150]

Gordon and Heeren[56] concluded that mumps is quite endemic within urban populations, but of somewhat irregular incidence. They thought that epidemics were unusual except among closely crowded populations, although some Scandinavian data suggested that increased prevalence occurred at approximately 7- to 8-year intervals.

5.5. Temporal Distribution

In the North Temperate zone, mumps seems to occur more often in the winter and spring than at other times of the year, especially the summer.

Cases may be seen in any month, but March and April have the greatest number of outbreaks (see Fig. 3). There are no seasonal increases in tropical areas.

5.6. Age

In the United States, more than 50% of reported cases occur in the 5–9 year age group and 90% in children 14 years old or less. Cases in adolescents and adults have a peak age distribution later than that of measles or rubella. The cumulative frequency by age is shown in Fig. 4.[28] In Massachusetts, Gordon and Heeren[56] reported almost 90% of reported cases to be in children under age 15 years. A household interview survey carried out in Buffalo, New York,[66] indicated that 10% of those less than 5 years of age and 33% of those 5–9 years had had mumps previously. The peak age of recorded cases was 7 years, but 74% were experienced by age 10 and only 5% after age 20. Cooney et al.[33] found in families that the virus was spread mostly by 2- to 5-year-olds. Illness occurred in 77% of infants and in 75% of those older than 9 years.

Encephalitis, as is true of mumps in general, is most common in the 5–9 year age group. Of 529 reported cases in the United States in 1973–1975,[30] 52% of the patients were age 5–9, 14% age 0–4, and 19% age 10–14. The remaining cases were scattered throughout all other age groups. A similar age distribution is seen in the 166 cases of mumps among

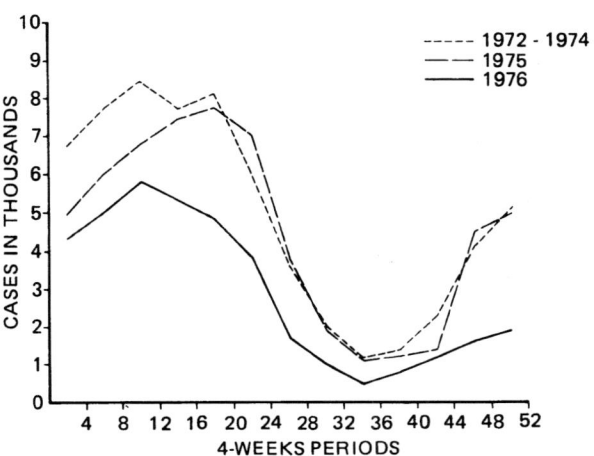

Fig. 3. Reported cases of mumps, by 4-week period, United States, 1972–1976. *Three-year average used for 1972–1974. From the CDC.[30]

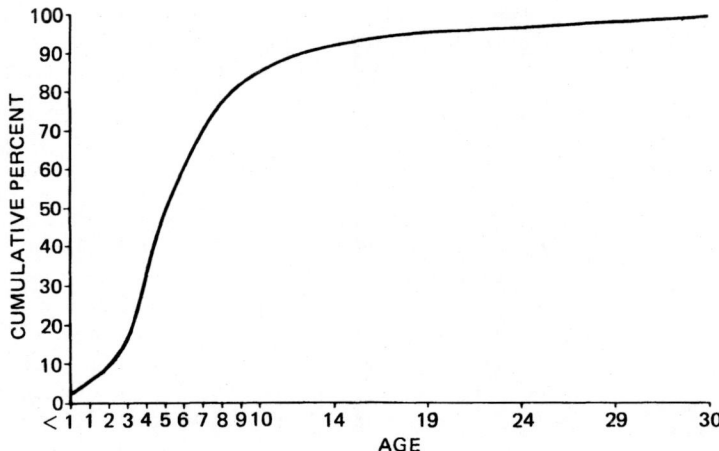

Fig. 4. Reported cases of mumps, cumulative percentage by age. From the CDC.[28]

the United States aseptic meningitides reported in 1975[25] and from Stockholm from 1955 to 1976.[16] Mumps-associated deaths in 200 cases from 1966 to 1975 were distributed by age as follows: 41% over age 40, 22% ages 5–9 years, and 19% ages 0–4 years.[30]

5.7. Sex

Males and females are affected with equal frequency, although one survey reported males to have a history of mumps more often than females.[66] Encephalitis has been reported 3–4 times more often in males, but deaths are equally divided between the sexes.[16,30] While the predominance of encephalitis in males is currently unexplainable, it has also been noted with paralytic poliomyelitis and bacterial meningitis.

5.8. Race and Occupation

Race *per se* appears to exert no effect, although blacks tend to have higher rates at an earlier age than whites.[66] Occupation also does not seem to play any role, except that susceptible adults who deal with young children are more likely to acquire infections.

5.9. Occurrence in Different Settings

Outbreaks are common in families, schools, institutions, and especially the military, where mumps can be a major cause of morbidity among recruit populations. Outbreaks may be persistent in the latter setting because of the continuing input of new recruits in contrast to the limited susceptibles available in elementary and secondary schools.

5.9.1. In the Family. As with so many other diseases, the young school-age child most often introduces mumps into the home, where it may spread to other susceptible siblings and adults. On the other hand, Cooney *et al.*[33] concluded that mumps virus ". . . is spread largely by 2–5 year-old children." In households with more than one child, the younger sibling acquires the disease at an earlier age.

5.9.2. In Military Personnel. Wesselhoeft and Walcott[150] reviewed mumps in the military and reported that the U.S. Army had had major epidemics during the Civil War and World War I, but not in the Spanish-American War. Mumps did not assume great prominence during World War II. Both the Army and Navy were affected during World War I, and epidemics were so severe that training and embarkation schedules sometimes were disrupted. From 1917 through 1919, there were 231,490 cases in the U.S. Army; there were 168,519 during 1918 alone, with 8020 men "noneffective" at any one time. The seasonal nature of mumps was illustrated by the occurrence of 70% of these cases in the winter and spring. The total noneffective days for the Army during World War I was 3,884,147, making mumps third in incidence after venereal disease and influenza.

Kneeland[89] has emphasized the lower incidence of mumps in the U.S. Army in World War II as compared with World War I: in World War I, there were 237,000 cases of mumps, but only 103,055 were reported during World War II from a much larger force. Others have made similar observations. Gordon and Kilham[57] analyzed these military experiences somewhat differently, but also concluded that the admission rate for mumps (U.S. Army) per 1000 strength was higher in World War I than in World War II, with a ratio of about 11:1. In Europe, the difference was almost 16 times greater. Nonetheless, mumps was more frequent than rubella, measles, meningococcal infections, diphtheria, and scarlet fever.

Mumps has been the most frequent communicable disease of childhood diagnosed in military personnel, but has had a very low mortality. It was estimated that the case-fatality rate during World War I was 0.08% when mumps represented the primary reason for hospital admission. Deaths generally were due to secondary infections such as pneumonia. During all of World War II, only five deaths were attributed to mumps in the entire U.S. Army. The average number of days lost from duty by a patient during World War II was 18. Since the disease was primarily one of recruits, it was relatively infrequent after they arrived overseas.[89]

McGuiness and Gall[104] summarized the U.S. Army's experience during 1943. They, like others, believed that mumps was not likely to repeat the World War I experience because of "the tremendous increase in travel during the past 25 years and the resultant decrease in isolation in rural areas, where many persons formerly reached adult life without exposure to the usual communicable diseases." In this report, they described an epidemic at Camp McCoy, Wisconsin, in which 1378 mumps patients were admitted to the station hospital between November 22, 1942, and June 23, 1943. The outbreak progressed at a fairly slow rate, but one company had 19% of its 194 members ill with mumps at some time during the 16 weeks between the first and last cases. The maximum number ill in any one week was 2.5%. This epidemic was unique for several reasons. It seemed to move slowly through the camp, which was not a recruit-training center. The peak incidence for the entire camp was late, occurring in the 17th week, at which time there were 194 cases. Because this was a wartime publication, no information as to strength or number of persons exposed was provided. One of the conclusions of the authors is that the men affected were predominantly those who came from the rural areas of the South and Southwest.

The prevalence of mumps antibody in military recruits has already been presented in Table 1.

5.9.3. In Hospitals and Institutions. Outbreaks also occur in hospitals and other institutions. Sparling[132] described such an episode in an Alaskan hospital in which an asymptomatic infection in a nurse was the probable source. Thus, mumps virus may be considered to be a potential, but relatively uncommon, cause of nosocomial disease.

5.10. Other Factors

Socioeconomic factors play little role in incidence except that the impoverished tend to live under more crowded conditions (if in cities) and thus acquire the infection at earlier ages. Additional factors that may play significant roles in other diseases, such as nutritional state and genetics, do not seem to be of any consequence in relation to mumps except for the usual increased risks for those who either have abnormal immunological systems or are being "immunosuppressed" for therapeutic purposes.

6. Mechanisms and Routes of Transmission

There are no known animal reservoirs or insect vectors of mumps virus. The route of transmission is by infected droplets containing live virus that is being secreted in the throat or from the salivary glands. Presumably, infection could be transmitted during mouth-to-mouth resuscitation. The period of infectiousness of mumps ranges from about 3 days prior to the onset of clinical mumps to about the 4th day of active disease. Transmission by persons with inapparent infections is also an important source of spread of mumps virus. "Reactivation" among the immunosuppressed has not been demonstrated. Evidence for transplacental transfer of virus is indecisive, but some is discussed in Sections 8.1 and 8.6. Long-term human carriers are unknown, so that a continuing source of both acutely infected persons and susceptible contacts is needed to maintain the virus in a community.

7. Pathogenesis and Immunity

The usual sources of mumps virus are saliva and respiratory secretions. The virus is acquired through the respiratory tract, following which the available evidence indicates there is local multiplication in both the upper respiratory tract and the regional lymph nodes. After an incubation period of 16–18 days, a viremia follows that persists for 3–5 days. During this stage, virus may be disseminated widely to the meninges and glands such as the salivary, testes, pancreas, ovaries, and sometimes thyroid and mammaries. Virus seems to be present in saliva for about 7–10 days (about one third before and about two thirds after the appearance of symptoms). It has been isolated from saliva, blood, urine, stool, and spinal fluid. Viruria is frequent, lasting about 10 days, sometimes longer, after the onset of symptoms. Whether urine serves as a means of transmission has not been established. About a week or more after the onset of parotitis, orchitis may occur in as many as one third of postpubertal males. Other complications may make their appearance at this time or, occasionally, seriatim.

Mumps is generally considered to be less contagious than measles or chicken pox, which may explain why so many children reach adulthood without having been immunized by naturally acquired virus. As many as one third of mumps infections are totally asymptomatic, but the reasons are unknown. One would anticipate that if this were because of the acquisition of naturally attenuated viruses, they would not be readily transmissible. Such does not seem to be the case. In symptomatic infections, the clinical severity varies greatly, and, in fact, even a rare death may occur.

Parotitis is unilateral in at least 25% of cases.[92] Estimates of the frequency of central nervous system involvement differ, depending greatly on the frequency with which spinal fluids were examined.

Kilham[85] first isolated mumps virus from the bloodstream, and also from milk.[87] The latter had been obtained at the beginning of lactation, 3 days after the delivery of an infant to a 23-year-old woman with parotitis of 2 days' duration. Two of her other children had had mumps during the preceding 3 weeks. The infant remained symptom-free, while the mother had an 8-fold rise in antibodies during the following 3 weeks. The baby never developed antibodies, but was not breast fed. Virus could not be isolated from the placenta. This virus, after egg passage, was inoculated into two lactating monkeys, one of which developed parotitis and a rise in antibodies. Virus was not isolated from its milk. Its infant failed to develop antibodies and never became ill. In the other, mumps virus appeared in the milk 6 days after inoculation and persisted for 9 days, but no parotid swelling, signs of breast infection, or fever was noted. There was a maternal rise in antibodies, but the infant developed none. Kilham concluded that the virus probably multiplies in the lactating breast.

Utz et al.[141] inoculated ultracentrifugates of urine from 13 mumps patients into monkey-kidney tissue cultures and obtained isolates 3 times as often as from simple urine dilutions. Isolations were made from all specimens as early as the 1st and up until the 14th day of illness. No patient had orchitis, and in 7 viruria could be detected after there was no longer clinical parotitis. Subsequently, Utz and Szwed[140] expanded these investigations to a larger group and demonstrated viruria not only often (80% of specimens collected during the first 5 days), but also as late as 15 days after the onset of illness. In another study,[139] they found that 15 of 20 young servicemen with mumps had viruria at some time, usually within the first 5 days of illness. Of 55 specimens, 12 were positive on the 11th through the 25th days; the 5 from patients with orchitis were all positive. Abnormal renal function was detected at some time in each person: 17 had abnormal creatinine clearances, 15 abnormal PSP excretion, 8 microscopic hematuria, and 4 proteinuria, and all had at least one abnormal Fishberg test. Generalized edema or hypertension or both were not detected in any, and all had negative cultures and normal renal function by the end of the study. It was concluded that renal involvement, when it occurs, is mild.

Virus has been found in saliva as long as 7 days before the appearance of parotitis[45] and for 3 days subsequently. Henle et al.[71] had earlier made a similar observation following the inoculation of egg-passage virus into volunteers.

Antibodies for mumps are transmitted across the placenta.[47,76] Since approximately 80% of adults have antibodies, most infants are immune for about 6 months. This can be detected by CF, HI, or N tests and probably accounts for the rarity of the clinical disease in young infants.

Interferon is produced during mumps infections, with the highest titers being detected within the first 3 days. Levels in saliva parallel those in serum,[144] and interferon has been reported in spinal fluid.

Second attacks of mumps are assumed to occur,[92] but their rate is unknown. One reason is that the substantial proportion of asymptomatic infections makes a prior history of mumps an unreliable indicator of past infection. Another reason is that parotitis may be caused by other agents. Nonetheless, Biedel[14] reported three cases of recurrent parotitis in persons known to have postvaccine, or infection-acquired, antibodies. In general, one attack, whether symptomatic or asymptomatic, may be assumed to induce lifelong immunity. Clinically expressed reinfections, if they do occur, probably account for fewer than 5% of all cases.

The value of fluorescent-antibody and other rapid diagnostic techniques in urine, saliva, spinal fluid, and other sources for evidence of mumps-virus infection requires exploration.

8. Patterns of Host Response

8.1. Common Clinical Features

Mumps-virus infections are generalized, but produce no symptoms in about one third of infected persons. The wide range of responses in those with clinical disease reflects the attraction of glandular and nerve tissue for the virus. The most common signs are fever and swelling of the parotid glands, either unilaterally or bilaterally. The sublingual and submaxillaries may also be involved. With these signs may appear simultaneously, or in any sequence, pancreatitis, oophoritis, mastitis, myocarditis, meningoencephalitis, cranial nerve involvement (especially the eighth nerve), and, in adult males, epididymo-orchitis. The occurrence of virus in urine and of abnormal renal function suggests that mumps virus produces an infection of the kidney. In some instances, parotitis may be absent and one or more of the other complications occur. Kilham,[86] for example, found 13 of 25 patients with mumps meningoencephalitis to have no clinical parotitis, and he was also able to isolate virus from cerebrospinal fluid as late as the 6th day of disease. Azimi et al.[7] described the case of an 11-year-old

male with meningoencephalitis in whom pleocytosis persisted for at least 102 days. Not infrequently, mumps virus has been found in the saliva in the absence of evident enlargement of the salivary glands.

Various complications are often reported as individual cases, so that their rates cannot be calculated. Rarely have attempts been made to estimate their incidence in closed or limited populations. All the studies performed in the Army during World War I and most during World War II were based on clinical findings without support from serological tests or the isolation of viruses. One study in which rates could be calculated is that of Philip et al.,[117] who investigated a virgin-soil epidemic of mumps among 561 Eskimos living on St. Lawrence Island in the Bering Sea (see Table 2). This outbreak was mentioned in Section 5.3. The villages were visited after the epidemic had begun, but 57 cases were available for examination. Members of each household were interviewed, and the records of the village nurse were reviewed. Orchitis was age-related, increasing sharply at puberty: the youngest patient was a boy of 9 and the oldest a man of 51. Of 205 males with clinical mumps, 52 had orchitis, 37% bilateral. Among 158 female patients, 15% had mastitis, which increased in incidence with puberty. The youngest was a girl of 12 and the oldest a woman of 61. Among the female patients 15 years of age or older, 31% had mastitis. In a few instances, there were swelling and tenderness over the thyroid area, and a few women had lower abdominal pain, suggestive of oophoritis. Stiffness of the neck was reported by 40 patients, sometimes with delirium, vomiting, and high fever, but all recovered. Of 4 deaths noted during the outbreak, 3 were apparently unrelated to mumps. The fourth death, 2 days after the appearance of parotitis, was a 10-month-old girl. Since no one was in attendance, the cause of her death could not be determined. Of additional interest were the women who were in the first trimester of pregnancy; 4 aborted. Of the 15 who were in their second or third trimester, none had either a stillbirth or a miscarriage. Of the 4 who aborted, 3 were among 8 women with clinical mumps. In contrast, only 1 of 12 women with inapparent mumps aborted. No congenital malformations were detected in the 17 infants whose mothers were exposed to mumps during pregnancy. Serological follow-up some 10 years later of 12 chil-

Table 2. Incidence of Infection and Clinical Disease in a Virgin-Soil Outbreak of Mumps in 561 Residents of St. Lawrence Island, Bering Sea[a]

	Feature	Number	%
1.	Mumps infection[b]	460[c]	82
2. a.	Males	300[c]	53
	With clinical mumps	205	68
	Without clinical mumps	95	32
b.	Females	261[c]	47
	With clinical mumps	158	61
	Without clinical mumps	103	40
c.	Both sexes	561	100
	With clinical mumps	363[c]	65
	Without clinical mumps	198[c]	35
	Total infection rate[d]	—	85
3.	Clinical mumps	363[c]	65
a.	With salivary gland swelling	344	95
b.	With stiffness of neck	40	11
c.	With scrotal swelling (males)	52	25
d.	With swelling of breasts (females)	24	15

[a] Data derived from Philip et al.[117]   [b] Based on serological data.   [c] Of total population of 561.   [d] An additional 3% had disease without antibodies.

dren whose mothers had mumps during pregnancy revealed the absence of N antibody, but the presence of positive skin tests, in many children.[1] This suggests the possibility that infection *in utero* fails to induce humoral antibodies but does activate cell-mediated responses.

8.2. Involvement of the Central Nervous System

Mumps can cause aseptic meningitis, meningoencephalitis, and encephalitis. It is one of the most important causes of these syndromes in the United States. Of 824 cases of aseptic meningitis in military personnel in the period 1941–1952, Adair et al.[2] found 12% associated with mumps virus. Among 1,085,084 mumps cases reported to the CDC from 1966 to 1976, there were 3,464 cases (0.3%) of encephalitis.[30] Other data from 407 cases in Cleveland revealed a relationship to mumps in 7.8%,[95] and from 511 cases in Los Angeles, an association in 8.2%.[93] Altered encephalograms are uncommon during mumps parotitis,[54] suggesting that the meninges, rather than the brain, are the more common site of involvement.

Epidemiological and clinical investigations of mumps meningoencephalitis have been made by a number of investigators.[6,80,98,106,134] In Toronto, mumps accounted for 8.7% of 43 patients diagnosed as having meningoencephalitis in 1963.[106] Boys are more commonly affected than girls, the ratio being 3:1. Parotitis may be absent in 25–50% of patients with this syndrome. Similar experiences have been reported from Stockholm.[15]

Mumps is the most common cause of viral encephalitis in the United States. It accounted for 36% of the cases reported to the CDC in 1967, 20% in 1971, and 13% in 1972.[29] Most patients recover without sequelae. Of 11 surviving patients from an outbreak in Guam in 1947–1948, 8 were without sequelae when examined 10 years later.[118] The remaining 3 were without complaints, but minimal neurological changes were detected. Isolated cases of encephalitis have been reported.[37,38,127] The CDC recorded 63 deaths from 1963 through 1972.[29] The Guillain–Barré syndrome[53,108] and a variety of rare central nervous system complications have been described.[10,11,13,35,64,80,105,107,127,137]

Deafness is an important residual complication of mumps infection and may occur unattended by meningitis or encephalitis.[119,143] An important recent report described the first isolation of mumps virus from perilymph.[21] Some hearing loss was found in 4.4% of 298 mumps patients in a military epidemic in Finland who were evaluated audiometrically,[143] an incidence rate of about 1 per 200,000 persons. In the United States, this would be equivalent to 1100 cases annually.

8.3. Involvement of the Heart

As it does in other acute infections. myocarditis may occur during mumps.[40,94,121,136] Some investigators have suggested that intrauterine infection may lead to endocardial fibroelastosis.[41,52,115,123,124,126,142] The relationship to the latter syndrome has been based on correlations among the syndrome, positive mumps skin tests, circulating antibody, and a history of maternal exposure to mumps. The evidence is conflicting, and additional data are required before the issue can be settled.

8.4. Orchitis and Sterility

Since orchitis frequently occurs during mumps, there has been a great deal of interest in whether or not this results in residual difficulties such as sterility. At least half of orchitis cases resolve completely, and most are unilateral.[92] The follow-ups of World War I and II cases failed to demonstrate impotence and sterility to be important consequences of mumps infection. By history, orchitis occurred in 4.9% of 2000 males aged 14–43, and among those over 13 years of age, the frequency increased to 19%.[148] The disease was unilateral in two thirds and bilateral in one third. Atrophy occurred in one third of the orchitis cases. Sperm counts for 49 males with histories of mumps orchitis and for 91 without such histories revealed little difference.[149] Only one instance of aspermia was identified among those who had a history of mumps and none in controls.[149] Testicular atrophy did not appear to be an important factor in sperm production qualitatively or quantitatively. These studies suggest that mumps is not an important cause of sterility in the male population. About 30 cases of neoplasm of the testes have been reported following the atrophy of mumps orchitis.[12,83] No increase in genitourinary-tract malformations was noted among the offspring of fathers who had had mumps orchitis.[12] One case of breast cancer 36 years after atrophic mumps orchitis has also been recorded.[113]

8.5. Mumps and Diabetes

While some isolated instances of diabetes have occurred in children following mumps infection,[34,48,75,81,88,103,109] a causal relationship has yet to be demonstrated. A speculative, preliminary report from Erie County, New York, considers juvenile diabetes and mumps to have similar periodicities, with the former separated from the latter by time.[135] This is based on clinical diagnoses with no supporting laboratory data. Furthermore, this study is based on diabetics, and there is no comparative control group. Higher antibody levels to coxsackieviruses, especially type B4, have been found in insulin-dependent diabetics of 3 months' duration or more than in control groups.[49] There was a seasonal pattern consistent with coxsackievirus B4 infections, but not with other viruses.[50] These results were not confirmed in a subsequent study.[73] Madden et al.,[100] in a well-matched study of pregnant women, found the frequencies of mumps, various coxsackievirus B, and respiratory syncytial virus antibodies not to differ significantly between diabetic and nondiabetic participants. The relationship of mumps and coxsackievirus infections to diabetes is thus contradictory and inconclusive. Its solution requires proper prospective studies, including supportive isolation or serological data or both.

8.6. Other Complications

A variety of other acute and delayed complications have been reported following mumps infection. These include arthritis in adults.[5,24,55,131,138] An arthritis incidence of 0.44% was noted among 1334 patients during an outbreak in Paris in 1923–1924.[24] Viruria is common in mumps infection, and this may be accompanied by abnormal renal-function tests,[140] and rarely by nephritis,[4,78,101,111] which may be fatal.[4,78] Hematological complications are rare, but include a leukemoid reaction[51] and paroxysmal cold hemoglobinuria.[32] No evidence of a relationship to leukemia was found in children of mothers who had mumps during pregnancy.[3] Holowach et al.[77] described a case of congenital chorioretinitis in a 6-month-old infant whose mother had been infected by mumps in the latter part of her first trimester. These authors concluded on review of the literature that mumps infection at this stage could affect the fetus. In a prospective study of 19 mumps infections among 4930 pregnant women,[90] no evidence of any fetal abnormalities or of endocardial fibroelastosis was found.

The possible relationship of mumps and other viruses to multiple sclerosis has been studied. No differences in skin reactivity to viral antigens were found in 20 patients compared to controls.[125] Of 43 patients with multiple sclerosis tested, immunoglobulin M (IgM) mumps-specific antibody was present in the sera of two patients and measles-specific IgM in 4 patients. None of the serum samples from 43 patients with other neurological diseases or from 43 healthy controls contained mumps IgM antibody, but 1 of the former had measles IgM antibody.[110] The significance of these findings is not clear, but one explanation is that persistent IgM antibody may reflect persistence of the virus.

9. Control and Prevention

Since mumps was long viewed as a disease primarily of childhood, often inapparent, usually mild, and leaving only infrequent, inconsequential complications, mumps vaccine understandably failed to induce great enthusiasm for a general immunization program. The one exception perhaps was the military, where mumps has always seemed to produce problems, especially in times of general mobilization. Yet the various complications—such as orchitis with testicular atrophy, central nervous system involvement with permanent damage especially to the eighth nerve, myocarditis of clinical significance, potential teratogenesis, pancreatitis, and perhaps a relationship with the onset if not the induction of diabetes—led some to believe that its control by vaccine was warranted. Enders et al.[42] foresaw this early and reported in 1946 that the mumps virus that he had adapted to the monkey, when passed continuously in chick embryos, lost its virulence for the monkey and probably for man. After 25 passages, no parotitis was produced in the monkey, but immunity followed the apparently subclinical infection. CF and HI antibodies were induced when the virus was sprayed into the mouth and throat, but immunity followed irregularly. In one experiment, there was a suggestion that single-egg-passage virus (less attenuated) might do better.

Henle et al.[69] used formalin-inactivated mumps virus as a vaccine and gave this to a number of children. N antibodies were formed following multiple doses, and there was evidence of clinical protection, although the occurrence of subclinical disease was not altered. Deinhardt and Shramek[36] reviewed this problem extensively and stated that immunization was a worthwhile goal but that killed antigens were inadequate inducers of long-range protection. They felt that attenuated vaccines should be the objective, and, in fact, one was already being tested at that time.

Penttinen et al.[116] related the experiences of the Finnish military forces, in which inactivated mumps vaccine (formalin-treated allantoic fluid) has been used routinely since 1960. Among some 200,000 servicemen who had received two injections of vaccine following induction, the only reactions encountered were small and localized. The seroconversion rate by CF varied between 73 and 92%, depending on the year. From 1955 to 1959, prior to vaccine, the rate for mumps in these forces was 31 per 1000, whereas from 1961 to 1966 it was 1.9 per 1000, or a reduction of 94%. Until immunization was put into routine effect, the military was contributing about 10% of all the cases reported in Finland. This, too, decreased 10fold with vaccine usage. Penttinen and co-workers also found that even with vaccine, mumps was most frequent in the first month of service, too early for adequate immunity to have developed. It was about twice as frequent in those from rural areas as in those from urban centers. Overall, orchitis was 25 times less frequent among the vaccinated than among the nonvaccinated. The authors also pointed out that during World War II, mumps occurred at the rate of 250–300 per 1000 men in the Finnish army.

Buynak and Hilleman[22] described the attenuated mumps virus vaccine licensed in the United States in December 1967 and made available for general use soon thereafter. Initiated in 1963, the virus is grown in both embryonated chicken eggs and tissue cultures of chick embryos. It stores well when it is lyophilized, and it is rehydrated just prior to use. Following clinical trials in thousands of susceptible children and adults, it was concluded that about 97% of children and about 93% of adults are converted from seronegative to seropositive by a single dose of the vaccine.[146] Protection from natural infection is of the order of 95%. In follow-up studies, the same group demonstrated that N antibodies persist for at least 9.5 years with concomitant protective immunity.[145] Ennis *et al.*,[44] in a careful study of this vaccine, found no clinical reactions as the result of its administration. While N, HI, and CF antibodies were formed, virus could not be isolated from the blood, urine, or saliva of its recipients. Antibody titers were somewhat lower than after natural infection, but 1 year later, N antibodies could still be detected.

Subsequently, Buynak *et al.*[23] demonstrated that mumps virus could be administered combined with live measles and rubella virus vaccines without altering the immunological responses to any. Smorodintsev *et al.*[130] did the same with their Russian vaccine strains and also believed the results to be as good as when each was used alone. The American trivalent vaccine was subsequently tested by Krugman *et al.*[91] in 40 susceptible infants and found to be well tolerated and to induce the usual immunological responses. Combined live measles and mumps vaccine was also tested by Weibel *et al.*[147] in children under 7 years of age, with a 99% response to the measles and 96% to the mumps antigens. Sinha and Carlson [128] administered triple vaccine to 150 mentally retarded children, with normally expected seroconversion rates. Balfour and Amren[9] administered combined rubella, measles, and mumps vaccine to 141 infants 11 months or older and found the usual responses to be expected in such a group. The use of such combination vaccines simplifies the problems of supply and administration considerably, as well as increases patient acceptance.

The Public Health Service Advisory Committee on Immunization Practices recommends[26] that live virus mumps vaccine be given to children after 12 months of age and to others known to be susceptible or who have not had mumps. Like other live virus vaccines, it should *not* be given during pregnancy, or to those who are immunodeficient, either congenitally or otherwise. The mumps skin test is not a reliable indicator of immunity and is no longer commercially available. Because the vaccine is derived from chick cells, those allergic to egg proteins should not be inoculated.

Cases that might represent complications of mumps immunization have been reported. Among these are one each of hemolytic–uremic syndrome,[39] possible deafness,[67] encephalopathy with convulsions,[46]

and one of the Guillain-Barré type following combined mumps–rubella vaccine.[59] The last began only 2 days after administration of live attenuated vaccine and was followed by complete recovery. From 1968 to 1976, 16 cases of central nervous system illness within 2 months of receiving live mumps vaccine were reported to the *Mumps Surveillance Reports* of the CDC.[30] No clustering was apparent, and so their relationship to the vaccine remains something of a mystery.

Yamauchi *et al.*[152] administered vaccine to five women (three susceptible and two immune) 7–10 days prior to the scheduled termination of their pregnancies with intraamniotically infused hypertonic saline. Mumps virus was recovered from the placentas of two of the three seronegative women, but not from fetal tissues. The suggestion was made that the vaccine be given with caution to postpubertal females.

Live mumps virus vaccine, like any other live virus vaccine, depresses lymphocyte function,[112] and may interfere with tuberculin reactions for at least 5 weeks. Vaccine induction of cell-mediated immunity is probable, but not proven.

Preparatory to the licensing of vaccine, mumps was again reinstituted as a notifiable disease. Listings of vaccine usage, complications, cases reported, and eradication programs are summarized in the *Mumps Surveillance Reports*. The latest[30] was issued in July 1978 and covers the period July 1974–December 1976. Recorded mumps incidence is now at the lowest level since its surveillance began. Further, the number of encephalitis cases reported annually since 1968 has been lower than in prior years, accounting in 1977 for only 1.1% of all viral encephalitides.[27] In children less than 15 years old, males have encephalitis 3 times more often than females, but this difference is not carried into adulthood. Deaths, too, have declined steadily since 1968. There is no sex predominance, but 38% are in persons over 40 years old.

For the years 1973–1976, the U.S. Immunization Survey found that in the population 1–9 years, the vaccination rate had increased from 33 to 49%.[30] From 1968 to 1976, 31 million doses of mumps-containing vaccine were distributed in the United States. As with other live virus vaccines, failure may be expected in about 5% of recipients. Complications, mostly involving the central nervous system, have been reported in 24 persons within 2 months

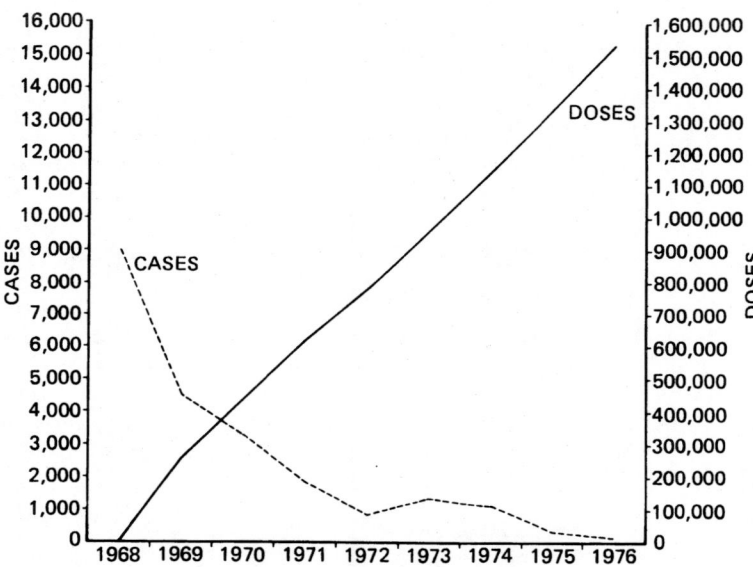

Fig. 5. Reported cases of mumps, and cumulative doses of mumps vaccine administered, Massachusetts, 1968–1976. From the CDC.[30]

of vaccination, but almost all have recovered fully. Some cases undoubtedly were caused by other agents. Surveillance for possible vaccine-related complications is continuing, but at this writing, the problem does not appear to be very significant.

Soon after mumps vaccine was licensed, the State of Massachusetts initiated the first full-scale immunization program early in 1969. During the first 2 years of the program, the concentration was on schoolchildren aged 5–14 years, but in 1971, the program was broadened to include preschool children. The most recent summary of cases reported in the State of Massachusetts (1968–1976) is illustrated in Fig. 5.[30] There was a remarkable drop in the number of reported cases coincident with the institution of the program. An increasing number of states continue to add mumps vaccine to the vaccines required for school admission.

Witte and Karchmer,[151] in a surveillance study meant to serve as a background for the use of vaccine, found that the incidence of mumps has no apparent cyclical pattern and varies markedly from year to year. It is most frequent, as has been noted, in the early school years. While cases are only slightly more prevalent in males than in females, encephalitis seems to occur excessively in males (some 70% of the total). Witte and Karchmer rightfully emphasize the importance of maintaining surveillance to determine the effectiveness and the best

possible utilization of vaccine and any complications that might result therefrom.

Bader,[8] Bjorvatn, and Skoldenberg,[15] and Harasek[63] have made good cases for the favorable cost-benefits to be anticipated from the widespread use of mumps vaccine in young children. Bader also feels confident that since mumps virus is wholly dependent on man, it may be possible to eliminate the disease entirely by the general use of vaccine in the pediatric population. The achievement of this eminently worthwhile goal seems possible now, in view of the increasing pressure to immunize all children for all preventable diseases, the availability of combined measles, mumps, and rubella vaccines, and the steadily widening requirement that such programs be completed as a prerequisite for school entry.

10. Unresolved Problems

That complete solutions for biological problems represent unachievable goals is generally accepted; mumps certainly is no exception. A long list of unresolved issues could be constructed rather readily, but much of it would serve little purpose now that an effective vaccine is available and in ever-increasing use.

Among the problems that seem most important at this time are:

1. Will live virus vaccine administered in childhood prevent mumps and its complications in adulthood, especially orchitis, partial or total deafness, central nervous system disease, and, possibly, fetal teratogenesis? These will require continuing surveillance based on sound epidemiological principles aided by specific laboratory procedures.
2. What is the meaning of reactivity to mumps skin-test antigen(s)? May this be acquired from infections other than with this virus? Does it have a role in any disease state, including endocardial fibroelastosis? Would purified antigens help to sort out the answers to these questions?
3. Do mumps-virus infections cause either juvenile- or adult-onset diabetes, or both? Can any such relationship be determined by other than prospective studies following natural or vaccine infections?
4. What are the roles of secretory IgA and cell-mediated immunity in the prevention or pathogenesis of mumps virus infections?
5. Is there a chronic degenerative central nervous system disease state induced by mumps virus, as has been demonstrated to follow some other viral infections (e.g., measles)?

11. References

1. Aase, J. M., Noren, G. R., Reddy, D. V., and St. Geme, J. W., Jr., Mumps-virus infection in pregnant women and the immunologic response of their offspring, N. Engl. J. Med. 286:1379–1382 (1972).
2. Adair, C. V., Gauld, R. L., and Smadel, J. E., Aseptic meningitis, a disease of diverse etiology: Clinical and etiologic studies on 854 cases, Ann. Intern. Med. 39:675–704 (1953).
3. Adelstein, A. M., and Donovan, J. W., Malignant disease in children whose mothers had chickenpox, mumps, or rubella in pregnancy, Br. Med. J. 4:629–631 (1972).
4. Anderson, D. M., and Hutchinson, D. N., Renal damage and virus infection, Br. Med. J. 3:680–681 (1968).
5. Appelbaum, E., Kohn, J., Steinman, R. E., and Shearn, M. A., Mumps arthritis, Arch. Intern. Med. 90:217–223 (1952).
6. Azimi, P. H., Cramblett, H. G., and Haynes, R. E., Mumps meningoencephalitis in children, J. Am. Med. Assoc. 207:509–512 (1969).
7. Azimi, P. H., Shaban, S., Hilty, M. D., and Haynes, R. E., Mumps meningoencephalitis: Prolonged abnormality of cerebrospinal fluid, J. Am. Med. Assoc. 234:1161–1162 (1975).
8. Bader, M., Mumps in Seattle–King County, Washington 1920–1976, Am. J. Public Health 67:1090–1091 (1977).
9. Balfour, H. H., Jr., and Amren, D. P., Rubella, measles and mumps antibodies following vaccination of children: A potential rubella problem, Am. J. Dis. Child. 132:573–577 (1978).
10. Balfour, H. H., Jr., Hable, K. A., Carlson, G. S., Isenberg, J. N., and Siem, R. A., Mumps associated with coma or exanthems: A clinical study including an instance of dual mumps and varicella infection, Clin. Pediatr. 11:88–92 (1972).
11. Beal, D. D., and Naunton, R. F., Mumps hearing loss: A case report, Laryngoscope 76:1786–1791 (1966).
12. Beard, C. M., Benson, R. C., Jr., Kelalis, P. P., Elveback, L. R., and Kurland, L. T., The incidence and outcome of mumps orchitis in Rochester, Minnesota, 1934 to 1974, Mayo Clin. Proc. 52:3–7 (1977).
13. Beardwell, A., Facial palsy due to the mumps virus, Br. J. Clin. Pract. 23:37–38 (1969).
14. Biedel, C. W., Recurrent mumps parotitis following natural infection and immunization, Am. J. Dis. Child. 132:678–680 (1978).
15. Bjorvatn, B., and Skoldenberg, B., Mumps and its complications in Stockholm, Br. Med. J. 1:788 (1978).
16. Bjorvatn, B., and Skoldenberg, B., Mumps, meningitis, and orchitis in Stockholm during 1955–1976: An epidemiological background for a vaccination policy, Lakartidningen 75:2295–2298 (1978).
17. Black, F. L., A nationwide serum survey of United States military recruits, 1962. III. Measles and mumps antibodies, Am. J. Hyg. 80:304–307 (1964).
18. Black, F. L., and Houghton, W. J., The significance of mumps hemagglutinin inhibition titers in normal populations, Am. J. Epidemiol. 85:101–107 (1967).
19. Brickman, A., and Brunell, P. A., Susceptibility of medical students to mumps: Comparison of serum neutralizing antibody and skin test, Pediatrics 48:447–450 (1972).
20. Brunell, P. A., Brickman, A., O'Hare, D., and Steinberg, S., Ineffectiveness of isolation of patients as a method of preventing the spread of mumps: Failure of the mumps skin-test antigen to predict immune status, N. Engl. J. Med. 279:1357–1361 (1968).
21. Bureau of Epidemiology (Ottawa), Isolation of mumps virus from perilymph in a case of sudden deafness—England, Can. Dis. Weekly Rep. 4-42:168 (October 1978).

22. Buynak, E. B., and Hilleman, M. R., Live attenuated mumps virus vaccine. 1. Vaccine development, *Proc. Soc. Exp. Biol. Med.* **123**:768–775 (1966).

23. Buynak, E. B., Weibel, R. E., Whitman, J. E. Jr., Stokes, J., Jr., and Hilleman, M. R., Combined live measles, mumps and rubella virus vaccines, *J. Am. Med. Assoc.* **207**:2259–2262 (1969).

24. Caranasos, G. J., and Felker, J. R., Mumps arthritis, *Arch. Intern. Med.* **119**:394–398 (1967).

25. Center for Disease Control, *Encephalitis Surveillance Rep., Annu. Summary 1975* (issued May 1977).

26. Center for Disease Control, *Morbid. Mortal. Weekly Rep.* **26**:393–394 (December 1977).

27. Center for Disease Control, *Morbid. Mortal. Weekly Rep.* **27**:379–381 (October 1978).

28. Center for Disease Control, *Mumps Surveillance, Report No. 2* (September 1972).

29. Center for Disease Control, *Mumps Surveillance, January 1972–June 1974* (issued October 1974).

30. Center for Disease Control, *Mumps Surveillance, July 1974–December 1976* (issued July 1978).

31. Center for Disease Control, Reported Morbidity and Mortality in the United States, *Morbid. Mortal. Weekly Rep., Annu. Summary 1977,* **26**(No. 53) (September 1978).

32. Colley, E. W., Paroxysmal cold haemoglobinuria after mumps, *Br. Med. J.* **1**:1552–1553 (1964).

33. Cooney, M. K., Fox, J. P., and Hall, C. E., The Seattle virus watch. VI. Observations of infections with and illness due to parainfluenza, mumps and respiratory syncytial viruses and *Mycoplasma pneumoniae, Am. J. Epidemiol.* **101**:532–551 (1975).

34. Dacou-Voutetakis, C., Constantinidis, M., Moschos, A., Vlachou, C., and Matsaniotis, N., Diabetes mellitus following mumps: Insulin reserve, *Am. J. Dis. Child.* **127**:890–891 (1974).

35. Davis, L. E., Harms, A. C., and Chin, T. D. Y., Transient cortical blindness and cerebellar ataxia associated with mumps, *Arch. Ophthalmol.* **85**:366–368 (1971).

36. Deinhardt, F., and Shramek, G. J., Immunization against mumps, in: *Prog. Med. Virol.* **11**:126–153 (1969).

37. Donohue, W. L., The pathology of mumps encephalitis: With report of a fatal case, *J. Pediatr.* **19**:42–52 (1941).

38. Donohue, W. L., Playfair, F. D., and Whitaker, L., Mumps encephalitis, *J. Pediatr.* **47**:395–412 (1955).

39. Dosik, H., and Tricarico, F., Haemolytic–uraemic syndrome following mumps vaccination, *Lancet* **1**:247 (1970).

40. Editorial, Mumps of the heart, *Br. Med. J.* **5481**:187–188 (1966).

41. Editorial, Mumps and the endocardium, *N. Engl. J. Med.* **275**:393 (1966).

42. Enders, J. F., Levens, J. H., Stokes, J., Jr., Maris, E.

P., and Berenberg, W., Attenuation of virulence with retention of antigenicity of mumps virus after passage in the embryonated egg, *J. Immunol.* **54**:283–291 (1946).

43. Ennis, F. A., Immunity to mumps in an institutional epidemic: Correlation of unsusceptibility to mumps with serum plaque neutralizing and hemagglutination-inhibiting antibodies, *J. Infect. Dis.* **119**:654–657 (1969).

44. Ennis, F. A., Douglas, R. D., Hopps, H. E., Meyer, H. M., Jr., Brown, E. R., Hobbins, T. E., and Biehusen, F. C., Clinical studies with virulent and attenuated mumps viruses, *Am. J. Epidemiol.* **89**:175–183 (1969).

45. Ennis, F. A., and Jackson, D., Isolation of virus during the incubation period of mumps infection, *J. Pediatr.* **72**:536–537 (1968).

46. *Epidemiological Bulletin,* Health and Welfare, Canada, **18**(1):10 (January 1974).

47. Florman, A. L., Schick, B., and Scalettar, H. E., Placental transmission of mumps and streptococcus MG antibodies, *Proc. Soc. Exp. Biol. Med.* **78**:126–128 (1951).

48. Freeman, A. G., Mumps followed by diabetes (letter to the editor), *Lancet* **2**:96 (1962).

49. Gamble, D. R., Kinsley, M. L., Fitzgerald, M. G., Bolton, R., and Taylor, K. W., Viral antibodies in diabetes mellitus, *Br. Med. J.* **3**:627–630 (1969).

50. Gamble, D. R., and Taylor, K. W., Seasonal incidence of diabetes mellitus, *Br. Med. J.* **3**:631–633 (1969).

51. Garcia, R., and Rasch, C. A., Leukemoid reaction to mumps virus, *N. Engl. J. Med.* **271**:251–252 (1964).

52. Gersony, W. M., Katz, S. L., and Nadas, A. S., Endocardial fibroelastosis and the mumps virus, *Pediatrics* **37**:430–434 (1966).

53. Ghosh, S., Guillain–Barré syndrome complicating mumps, *Lancet* **1**:895 (1967).

54. Gibbs, F. A., Gibbs, E. L., Spies, H. W., and Carpenter, P. R., Common types of childhood encephalitis: Electroencephalographic and clinical relationships, *Arch. Neurol.* **10**:1–11 (1964).

55. Gold, H. E., Boxerbaum, B., and Leslie, H. J., Jr., Mumps arthritis, *Am. J. Dis. Child.* **116**:547–548 (1968).

56. Gordon, J. E., and Heeren, R. H., The epidemiology of mumps, *Am. J. Med. Sci.* **200**:412–428 (1940).

57. Gordon, J. E., and Kilham, L., Ten years in the epidemiology of mumps, *Am. J. Med. Sci.* **218**:338–359 (1949).

58. Grillner, L., and Blomberg, J., Hemolysis-in-gel and neutralization tests for determination of antibodies to mumps virus, *J. Clin. Microbiol.* **4**:11–15 (1976).

59. Gunderman, J. R., Guillain–Barré syndrome: Occurrence following combined mumps–rubella vaccine, *Am. J. Dis. Child.* **125**:834–835 (1973).

60. HABEL, K., Cultivation of mumps virus in the developing chick embryo and its application to studies of immunity to mumps in man, *Public Health Rep.* **60:**201–212 (1945).

61. HABEL, K., Preparation of mumps vaccine and immunization of monkeys against experimental mumps infection, *Public Health Rep.* **61:**1655–1664 (1946).

62. HABEL, K., Vaccination of human beings against mumps; vaccine administered at the start of an epidemic. I. Incidence and severity of mumps in vaccinated and control groups, *Am. J. Hyg.* **54:**295–311 (1951).

63. HARASEK, V. B., Mumpsmeningitis und mumpsimpfung, *Wien. Klin. Wochenschr.* **90:**7–10 (1978).

64. HARBERT, F., AND YOUNG, I. M., Sudden deafness with complete recovery, *Arch. Otolaryngol.* **79:**459–471 (1964).

65. HARRIS, R. W., KEHRER, A. F., AND ISACSON, P., Relationship of occupation to risk of clinical mumps in adults, *Am. J. Epidemiol.* **89:**264–270 (1969).

66. HARRIS, R. W., TURNBEULL, C. D., ISACSON, P., KARSON, D. T., AND WINKELSTEIN, W., JR., Mumps in a northeast metropolitan community. I. Epidemiology of clinical mumps, *Am. J. Epidemiol.* **88:**224–233 (1968).

67. HEALY, C. E., Mumps vaccine and nerve deafness (letter to the editor), *Am. J. Dis. Child.* **123:**612 (1972).

68. HENLE, W., Mumps virus, in: *Diagnostic Procedures for Viral and Rickettsial Infections,* 4th ed. (E. H. LENNETTE AND N. J. SCHMIDT, eds.), pp. 457–482, American Public Health Association, New York, 1969.

69. HENLE, W., CRAWFORD, M. N., HENLE, G., TABIO, H. F., DEINHARDT, F., CHABAU, A. G., AND OLSHIN, I. J., Studies on the prevention of mumps. VII. Evaluation of dosage schedules for inactivated mumps vaccine, *J. Immunol.* **83:**17–28 (1959).

70. HENLE, G., HENLE, W., BURGOON, J. S., BASHE, W. J., JR., AND STOKES, J., JR., Studies on the prevention of mumps. I. The determination of susceptibility, *J. Immunol.* **66:**535–549 (1951).

71. HENLE, G., HENLE, W., WENDELL, K. K., and ROSENBERG, P., Isolation of mumps virus from human beings with induced apparent or inapparent infections, *J. Exp. Med.* **88:**223–232 (1948).

72. HENLE, G., AND McDOUGALL, C. L., Mumps meningoencephalitis: Isolation in chick embryos of virus from spinal fluid of a patient, *Proc. Soc. Exp. Biol. Med.* **66:**209–211 (1947).

73. HIERHOLZER, J. C., AND FARRIS, W. A., Follow-up of children infected in a coxsackievirus B-3 and B-4 outbreak: No evidence of diabetes mellitus, *J. Infect. Dis.* **129:**741–746 (1974).

74. HILDES, J. A., WILT, J. C., PARKER, W. L., STACKIW, W., AND DELAAT, A., Surveys of respiratory virus antibodies in an Arctic Indian population, *Can. Med. Assoc. J.* **93:**1015–1018 (1965).

75. HINDEN, E., Mumps followed by diabetes, *Lancet* **1:**1381 (1962).

76. HODES, D., AND BRUNELL, P. A., Mumps antibody: Placental transfer and disappearance during the first year of life, *Pediatrics* **45:**99–101 (1970).

77. HOLOWACH, J., THURSTON, D. L., AND BECKER, B., Congenital defects in infants following mumps during pregnancy: A review of the literature and a report of chorioretinitis due to fetal infection, *J. Pediatr.* **50:**689–694 (1957).

78. HUGHES, W. T., STEIGMAN, A. J., AND DELONG, H. F., Some implications of fatal nephritis associated with mumps, *Am. J. Dis. Child.* **111:**297–301 (1966).

79. JOHNSON, C. D., AND GOODPASTURE, E. W., An investigation of the etiology of mumps, *J. Exp. Med.* **59:**1–19 (1934).

80. JOHNSTONE, J. A., ROSS, C. A. C., AND DUNN, M., Meningitis and encephalitis associated with mumps infection: A 10-year survey, *Arch. Dis. Child.* **47:**647–651 (1972).

81. KAHANA, D., AND BERANT, M., Diabetes in an infant following inapparent mumps, *Clin. Pediatr.* **6:**124–125 (1967).

82. KALTER, S. S., AND PRIER, J. E., Immunity to mumps among physicians, *Am. J. Med. Sci.* **229:**161–164 (1955).

83. KAUFMAN, J. J., AND BRUCE, P. T., Testicular atrophy following mumps: A cause of testis tumour?, *Br. J. Urol.* **35:**65–69 (1963).

84. KENNY, M. T., JACKSON, J. E., MEDLER, E. M., MILLER, S. A., AND OSBORN, R., Age-related immunity to measles, mumps and rubella in Middle American and United States children, *Am. J. Epidemiol.* **103:**174–180 (1976).

85. KILHAM, L., Isolation of mumps virus from the blood of a patient, *Proc. Soc. Exp. Biol. Med.* **69:**99–100 (1948).

86. KILHAM, L., Mumps meningoencephalitis with and without parotitis, *Am. J. Dis. Child.* **78:** 324–333 (1949).

87. KILHAM, L., Mumps virus in human milk and in milk of infected monkey, *J. Am. Med. Assoc.* **146:**1231–1232 (1951).

88. KING, R. C., Mumps followed by diabetes (letter to the editor), *Lancet* **2:**1055 (1962).

89. KNEELAND, Y., JR., Mumps, in: *Internal Medicine in World War II,* Vol. II (J. B. COATES, JR., ed. in chief; W. P. HAVENS, JR., ed. for internal medicine), pp. 35–38, Office of the Surgeon General, Department of the Army, Washington, D.C., 1963.

90. KORONES, S. B., TODARO, J., ROANE, J. A., AND SEVER, J. L., Maternal virus infection after the first trimester of pregnancy and status of offspring to 4 years of age in a predominantly Negro population, *J. Pediatr.* **77:**245–251 (1970).

91. KRUGMAN, S., MURIEL, G., AND FONTANA, V. J., Combined live measles, mumps, rubella vaccine: Immu-

nological response, *Am. J. Dis. Child.* **121**:380–381 (1971).

92. KRUGMAN, S., WARD, R., AND KATZ, S. L. (eds.), Mumps (epidemic parotitis), in: *Infectious Diseases of Children*, pp. 181–193, C. V. Mosby, St. Louis, 1977.

93. LENNETTE, E. H., MAGOFFIN, R. L., AND KNOUF, E. G., Viral central nervous system disease, *J. Am. Med. Assoc.* **179**:687–695 (1962).

94. LEONIDAS, J. C., ATHANASIADES, T., AND ZOUMBOU-LAKIS, D., Mumps myocarditis: Case report, *J. Pediatr.* **68**:650–653 (1966).

95. LEPOW, M. L., CARVER, D. H., WRIGHT, H. T., JR., WOODS, W. A., AND ROBBINS, F. C., A clinical, epidemiologic and laboratory investigation of aseptic meningitis during the four-year period, 1955–58. I. Observations concerning etiology and epidemiology, *N. Engl. J. Med.* **266**:1181–1187 (1962).

96. LEVENS, J. H., AND ENDERS, J. F., The hemoagglutinative properties of amniotic fluid from embryonated eggs infected with mumps virus, *Science* **102**:117–120 (1945).

97. LEVITT, L. P., MAHONEY, D. H., JR., CASEY, H. L., AND BOND, J. O., Mumps in a general population: A seroepidemiologic study, *Am. J. Dis. Child.* **120**:134–138 (1970).

98. LEVITT, L. P., RICH, T. A., KINDE, S. W., LEWIS, A. L., GATES, E. H., AND BOND, J. O., Central nervous system mumps: A review of 64 cases, *Neurology* **20**:829–834 (1970).

99. LIAO, S. J., AND BENENSON, A. S., Immunity status of military recruits in 1951 in the United States. II. Results of mumps complement-fixation tests, *Am. J. Hyg.* **59**:273–281 (1954).

100. MADDEN, D. L., FUCCILLO, D. A., TRAUB, R. G., LEY, A. C., SEVER, J. L., AND BEADLE, E. L., Juvenile onset diabetes mellitus in pregnant women: Failure to associate with Coxsackie B1–6, mumps, or respiratory syncytial virus infections, *J. Pediatr.* **92**:959–960 (1978).

101. MASSON, A. M., AND NICKERSON, G. H., Mumps with nephritis, *Can. Med. Assoc. J.* **97**:866–867 (1967).

102. MAYNARD, J. E., SHRAMEK, G., NOBLE, G. R., DEINHARDT, F., AND CLARK, P., Use of attenuated live mumps virus vaccine during a "virgin soil" epidemic of mumps on St. Paul Island, Alaska, *Am. J. Epidemiol.* **92**:301–306 (1970).

103. MCCRAE, W. M., Diabetes mellitus following mumps, *Lancet* **1**:1300–1301 (1963).

104. MCGUINNESS, A. C., AND GALL, E. A., Mumps at Army camps in 1943, *War Med.* **5**:95–104 (1944).

105. MCKAIG, C. B., AND WOLTMAN, H. W., Neurologic complications of epidemic parotitis: Report of a case of parotitic myelitis, *Arch. Neurol. Psychiatry* **31**:794–808 (1934).

106. MCLEAN, D. M., BACH, R. D., LARKE, R. P. B., AND

McNAUGHTON, G. A., Mumps meningoencephalitis, Toronto, 1963, *Can. Med. Assoc. J.* **90**:458–462 (1964).

107. MEDNICK, J. P., AND LEONARDS, R., An unusual central nervous system complication of mumps, *Calif. Med.* **101**:42–43 (1964).

108. MELNICK, S. C., AND FLEWETT, T. H., Role of infection in the Guillain–Barré syndrome, *J. Neurol. Neurosurg. Psychiatry* **27**:395–407 (1964).

109. MESSARITAKIS, J., KARABULA, C., KATTAMIS, C., AND MATSANIOTIS, N., Diabetes following mumps in sibs, *Arch. Dis. Child.* **46**:561–562 (1971).

110. MILLAR, J. H. D., FRASER, K. B., HAIRE, M., CONNOLLY, J. H., SHIRODARIA, P. V., AND HADDEN, D. S. M., Immunoglobulin M specific for measles and mumps in multiple sclerosis, *Br. Med. J.* **2**:378–380 (1971).

111. MONTEIRO, G. E., AND LILLICRAP, C. A., Case of mumps nephritis, *Br. Med. J.* **4**:721–722 (1967).

112. MUNYER, T. P., MANGI, R. J., DOLAN, T., AND KANTOR, F. S., Depressed lymphocyte function after measles–mumps–rubella vaccination, *J. Infect. Dis.* **132**:75–78 (1975).

113. NICOLIS, G. L., SABETGHADAM, R., HSU, C. C. S., SOHVAL, A. R., AND GABRILOVE, J. L., Breast cancer after mumps orchitis, *J. Am. Med. Assoc.* **223**:1032–1033 (1973).

114. NIEDERMAN, J. C., HENDERSON, J. R., OPTON, E. M., BLACK, F. L., AND SKVRNOVA, K., A nationwide serum survey of Brazilian military recruits, 1964. II. Antibody patterns with arboviruses, polioviruses, measles and mumps, *Am. J. Epidemiol.* **86**:319–329 (1967).

115. NOREN, G. R., ADAMS, P., JR., AND ANDERSON, R. C., Positive skin reactivity to mumps virus antigen in endocardial fibroelastosis, *J. Pediatr.* **62**:604–606 (1963).

116. PENTTINEN, K., CANTELL, K., SOMER, P., AND POIKO-LAINEN, A., Mumps vaccination in the Finnish defense forces, *Am. J. Epidemiol.* **88**:234–244 (1968).

117. PHILIP, R. N., REINHARD, K. R., AND LACKMAN, D. B., Observations on a mumps epidemic in a "virgin" population, *Am. J. Hyg.* **69**:91–111 (1959).

118. PIEPER, S. J. L., JR., AND KURLAND, L. T., Sequelae of Japanese B and mumps encephalitis: Recent follow-up of patients affected in 1947–1948 epidemic on Guam, *Am. J. Trop. Med. Hyg.* **7**:481–490 (1958).

119. PRASAD, L. N., Complete bilateral deafness following mumps, *J. Laryngol.* **77**:809–811 (1963).

120. REED, D., BROWN, G., MERRICK, R., SEVER, J., AND FELTZ, E., A mumps epidemic on St. George Island, Alaska, *J. Am. Med. Assoc.* **199**:967–971 (1967).

121. ROBERTS, W. C., AND FOX, S. M., III, Mumps of the heart: Clinical and pathologic features, *Circulation* **32**:342–345 (1965).

122. ST. GEME, J. W., JR., Susceptibility of medical students to mumps: Dubious value of currently available skin test antigens (letter to the editor), *Pediatrics* **49**:314–315 (1972).

123. ST. GEME, J. W., JR., NOREN, G. R., AND ADAMS, P., JR., Proposed embryopathic relation between mumps virus and primary endocardial fibroelastosis, *N. Engl. J. Med.* **275:**339–347 (1966).

124. ST. GEME, J. W., JR., PERALTA, H., FARIAS, E., DAVIS, C. W. C., AND NOREN, G. R., Experimental gestational mumps virus infection and endocardial fibroelastosis, *Pediatrics* **48:**821–826 (1971).

125. SEVER, J. L., AND KURTZKE, J. F., Delayed dermal hypersensitivity to measles and mumps antigens among multiple sclerosis and control patients, *Neurology* **19:**113–115 (1969).

126. SHONE, J. D., ARMAS, S. M., MANNING, J. A., AND KEITH, J. D., The mumps antigen skin test in endocardial fibroelastosis, *Pediatrics* **37:**423–429 (1966).

127. SILVERMAN, A. C., Mumps complicated by a preceding myelitis, *N. Engl. J. Med.* **241:**262–266 (1949).

128. SINHA, S. K., AND CARLSON, S. D., Immune responses of mentally retarded subjects to measles, mumps and rubella vaccines, *Wisc. Med. J.* **74:**S75–S77 (1975).

129. SMORODINTSEV, A. A., LUZIANINA, T. Y., AND MIKUTSKAYA, B. A., Data on the efficiency of live mumps vaccine from chick embryo cell cultures, *Acta Virol.* **9:**240–247 (1965).

130. SMORODINTSEV, A. A., NASIBOV, M. N., AND JAKOVLEVA, N. V., Experience with live rubella virus vaccine combined with live vaccines against measles and mumps, *Bull. WHO* **42:**283–289 (1970).

131. SOLEM, J. H., Mumps arthritis without parotitis, *Scand. J. Infect. Dis.* **3:**173–175 (1971).

132. SPARLING, D., Transmission of mumps (letter to the editor), *N. Engl. J. Med.* **280:**276 (1969).

133. STOKES, J., JR., Mumps, in: *Preventive Medicine in World War II,* Vol. IV, *Communicable Diseases Transmitted Chiefly through Respiratory and Alimentary Tracts,* Prepared by The Historical Unit, U.S. Army Medical Service, pp. 135–140, U.S. Government Printing Office, Washington, D.C., 1960.

134. STRUSSBERG, S., WINTER, S., FRIEDMAN, A., BENDERLY, A., KAHANA, D., AND FREUNDLICH, E., Notes on mumps meningoencephalitis: Some features of 199 cases in children, *Clin. Pediatr.* **8:**373–374 (1969).

135. SULTZ, H. A., HART, B. A., ZIELEZNY, M., AND SCHLESINGER, E. R., Is mumps virus an etiologic factor in juvenile diabetes mellitus? Preliminary report, *J. Pediatr.* **86:**654–656 (1975).

136. THOMPSON W. M., JR., AND NOLAN, T. B., Atrioventricular dissociation associated with Adams–Stokes syndrome presumably due to mumps myocarditis, *J. Pediatr.* **68:**601–607 (1966).

137. TIMMONS, G. D., AND JOHNSON, K. P., Aqueductal stenosis and hydrocephalus after mumps encephalitis, *N. Engl. J. Med.* **283:**1505–1507 (1970).

138. TRACEY, J. P., AND RIGGENBACH, R. D., Mumps arthritis associated with positive latex fixation reaction, *South. Med. J.* **63:**1122, 1126 (1970).

139. UTZ, J. P., HOUK, V. N., AND ALLING, D. W., Clinical and laboratory studies of mumps. IV. Viruria and abnormal renal function, *N. Engl. J. Med.* **270:**1283–1286 (1964).

140. UTZ, J. P., AND SZWED, C. F., Mumps, III. Comparison of methods for detection of viruria, *Proc. Soc. Exp. Biol. Med.* **110:**841–844 (1962).

141. UTZ, J. P., SZWED, C. F., AND KASEL, J. A., Clinical and laboratory studies of mumps. II. Detection and duration of excretion of virus in urine, *Proc. Soc. Exp. Biol. Med.* **99:**259–261 (1958).

142. VOSBURGH, J. B., DIEHL, A. M., LIU, C., LAUER, R. M., AND FABIYI, A., Relationship of mumps to endocardial fibroelastosis: Complement-fixation, hemagglutination-inhibition and intradermal skin tests for mumps in children with and without endocardial fibroelastosis, *Am. J. Dis. Child.* **109:**69–73 (1965).

143. VUORI, M., LAHIKAINEN, E. A., AND PELTONEN, T., Perceptive deafness in connection with mumps: A study of 298 servicemen suffering from mumps, *Acta Oto-Laryngol.* **55:**231–236 (1962).

144. WADDELL, D. J., WILBUR, J. R., AND MERIGAN, T. C., Interferon production in human mumps infections, *Proc. Soc. Exp. Biol. Med.* **127:**320–324 (1968).

145. WEIBEL, R. E., BUYNAK, E. B., MCLEAN, A. A., AND HILLEMAN, M. R., Persistence of antibody after administration of monovalent and combined live attenuated measles, mumps, and rubella virus vaccines, *Pediatrics* **61:**5–11 (1978).

146. WEIBEL, R. E., STOKES, J., JR., BUYNAK, E. B., WHITMAN, J., AND HILLEMAN, M. R., Live attenuated mumps-virus vaccine. 3. Clinical and serologic aspects in a field evaluation, *N. Engl. J. Med.* **276:**245–251 (1967).

147. WEIBEL, R. E., VILLAREJOS, V. M., HERNANDEZ, C. G., STOKES, J., JR., BUYNAK, E. B., AND HILLEMAN, M. R., Combined live measles–mumps virus vaccine, *Arch. Dis. Child.* **48:**532–536 (1973).

148. WERNER, C. A., Mumps orchitis and testicular atrophy. I. Occurrence, *Ann. Intern. Med.* **32:**1066–1974 (1950).

149. WERNER, C. A., Mumps orchitis and testicular atrophy. II. A factor in male sterility, *Ann. Intern. Med.* **32:**1075–1086 (1950).

150. WESSELHOEFT, C., AND WALCOTT, C. F., Mumps as a military disease and its control, *War Med.* **2:**213–222 (1942).

151. WITTE, J. J., AND KARCHMER, A. W., Surveillance of mumps in the United States as background for use of vaccine, *Public Health Rep.* **83:**95–100 (1968).

152. YAMAUCHI, T., WILSON, C., AND ST., GEME, J. W., JR., Transmission of live, attenuated mumps virus to the human placenta, *N. Engl. J. Med.* **290:**710–712 (1974).

12. Suggested Reading

BEARD, C. M., BENSON, R. C., JR., KELALIS, P. P., ELVEBACK, L. R., AND KURLAND, L. T., The incidence and outcome of mumps orchitis in Rochester, Minnesota, 1934 to 1974, *Mayo Clin. Proc.* **52**:3–7 (1977).

UTZ, J. P., HOUK, V. N., AND ALLING, D. W., Clinical and laboratory studies of mumps. IV. Viruria and abnormal renal function, *N. Engl. J. Med.* **270**:1283–1286 (1964).

VUORI, M., LAHIKAINEN, E. A., AND PELTONEN, T., Perceptive deafness in connection with mumps: A study of 298 servicemen suffering from mumps, *Acta Oto-Laryngol.* **55**:231–236 (1962).

WEIBEL, R. E., VILLAREJOS, V. M., HERNANDEZ, C. G., STOKES, J., JR., BUYNAK, E. B., AND HILLEMAN, M. R., Combined live measles–mumps virus vaccine, *Arch. Dis. Child.* **48**:532–536 (1973).

CHAPTER 17

Parainfluenza Viruses

W. Paul Glezen, Frank A. Loda, and Floyd W. Denny

1. Introduction

The parainfluenza viruses are species of the genus *Paramyxovirus*, family Paramyxoviridae.[51a] They are exceeded only by respiratory syncytial virus (RSV) as important causes of lower respiratory disease in young children, and they commonly reinfect older children and adults to produce upper respiratory illnesses. There is considerable diversity in both epidemiological and clinical manifestations of infections due to the parainfluenza viruses. Parainfluenza virus type 1 (Para 1) is the principal cause of croup (laryngotracheobronchitis) in children, and parainfluenza virus type 3 (Para 3) is second only to RSV as a cause of pneumonia and bronchiolitis in infants less than 6 months of age. Parainfluenza virus type 2 (Para 2) resembles Para 1 in clinical manifestations, but serious illnesses occur less frequently; infections with parainfluenza virus type 4 (Para 4) are detected infrequently, and associated illnesses are usually inconsequential.

2. Historical Background

Chanock[9] reported the first isolation of parainfluenza virus from human sources in 1956 in Cin-cinnati; this virus, recovered from children with croup, was designated originally as the "croup-associated" (CA) virus. Two additional parainfluenza strains were identified in 1958 by their ability to adsorb guinea pig erythrocytes onto infected rhesus monkey kidney cells in culture.[11] Because these viruses, first designated "HA-1" and "HA-2," or hemadsorption 1 and 2, shared many biological properties with CA virus while being antigenically distinct, they were reclassified as parainfluenza viruses: Para 1 (HA-2), Para 2 (CA), and Para 3 (HA-1).[4] Type 4 was first isolated in 1960.[45] During the same period, these viruses were compared with isolates obtained from animals. The Sendai virus,[54] recovered from rodents, was found to share antigens with Para 1 and is classifed as a subtype of this strain.[16,17] In 1959, a hemadsorbing virus,[77] antigenically similar to Para 3 virus,[1] was recovered from cattle with "shipping fever." A simian virus, SV5,[42] has been shown to be related to Para 2 virus.[41,92]

3. Methodology Involved in Epidemiological Analysis

3.1. Sources of Mortality Data

Limited mortality data are available and consist of sporadic case reports[2,96]; the failure to identify more fatal cases may be a result of the lability of these viruses in postmortem specimens. Most deaths due to parainfluenza virus infections are probably

W. Paul Glezen · Department of and Microbiology Immunology, Baylor College of Medicine, Houston, Texas   Frank A. Loda and Floyd W. Denny · Department of Pediatrics, School of Medicine, University of North Carolina, Chapel Hill, North Carolina.

related to Para 3 virus infections in young infants, but even in this age group, mortality is not documented with sufficient frequency to allow a reasonable estimate of the mortality rate in the general population. Mortality data do not reflect the occurrence of these agents or the amount of morbidity that they cause.

3.2. Sources of Morbidity Data

Official morbidity reports do not include acute respiratory infections; furthermore, laboratory diagnosis is required to establish the diagnosis of a parainfluenza virus infection. Morbidity data, therefore, are based on special research studies of the etiology of respiratory disease in various communities around the world.

Standardized techniques have been employed by reliable investigators to provide some estimate of the impact of parainfluenza viruses as causes of acute respiratory disease in diverse populations. Most studies have been cross-sectional studies of the etiology of either illnesses of hospitalized patients or epidemics in closed populations. These studies provide a limited view of the total morbidity resulting from infections with these viruses. Five investigations of the etiology of acute respiratory disease conducted over extended periods of time and involving large populations merit special mention because of the broader perspective that they provide. These five studies in Washington, D.C.,[7,10] Chapel Hill, North Carolina,[26,28] Tecumseh, Michigan,[65] Seattle, Washington,[19] and Great Britain[15] have differed in methods of patient selection, types of illnesses surveyed, and ages of the subjects, but taken together, they constitute an extensive survey of respiratory illness over an extended time period in widely diverse geographic environments and socioeconomic groups. Numerous other studies have focused on the occurrence of respiratory illness in specialized population groups. Children seen on the wards and in the clinics of hospitals have been studied extensively both in North America and in Great Britain.[23,36,37,40,61,73,89,97] Studies of uncomplicated respiratory disease in insitutionalized children,[3,12,35,47] day-care groups,[57] and school-children[80] have contributed information about the spectrum of disease due to these agents. Mild illnesses occurring within families have been described in both the United States[29] and Great Britain.[5,38]

The role of parainfluenza viruses as etiological agents in respiratory illnesses of adults has also been investigated.[17a,18,25,31,34,64,68,83,93] These studies have reported sampling of patients with acute respiratory disease in hospitals, military services, university student-health services, and industrial medical facilities. The ability of parainfluenza viruses to infect volunteers has been demonstrated in studies in both the United States[48,76,81,86] and Great Britain.[85,87,88] There have also been studies of the role of respiratory pathogens including the parainfluenza viruses in asthmatic children[60] and in patients with chronic bronchitis.[82] Evidence of infections with paramyxoviruses has been obtained in all areas of the world[55,67,84,91] including tropical climates[6,52,66,71] and isolated communities,[8,59] except for the absence of Para 1 and 2 antibody in children in very remote Indian tribes in South America.[6a]

3.3. Serological Surveys

In an effort to delineate the importance of the parainfluenza viruses as etiological agents of respiratory disease, numerous serological studies have been conducted. Such serological surveys have frequently sought to determine whether the pattern of occurrences of parainfluenza virus infection is similar in special population groups to that reported elsewhere. Such studies have been useful in demonstrating the ubiquity of these agents and the relative similarity of age at acquisition of antibody in various areas of the world.[8,55,66,67,84] Many community studies have utilized both serological and isolation data, but have relied heavily on serological data to determine the frequency of infection within the population.[18,19,33,64,65] Care should be taken in the interpretation of studies that rely solely on the measurement of hemagglutination-inhibition (HI) or complement-fixation (CF) antibodies because cross-reactions are frequent among the paramyxovirus group, which includes mumps virus as well as the parainfluenza viruses.

3.4. Laboratory Methods

Most studies have utilized primary monkey-kidney tissue culture for isolation of parainfluenza viruses from clinical specimens; this is the most practical system for isolation, although human embryonic tissues may be used. Infection is usually detected by adding guinea pig erythrocytes, which will adsorb to infected tissue-culture cells. This property is useful for identification of isolates, which is accomplished by inhibition of hemadsorption with monospecific antisera raised in laboratory animals.[43] Rapid identification can be accomplished by use of fluorescent-tagged antisera for the major hemadsorbing viruses including Para 1, 2, and 3.[23] Antibody in serum and nasal secretions can be measured by neutralization (N), HI, and CF.[13] All the serological tests have been adapted to microtiter techniques.[95] The end point of titers of N antibodies to parainfluenza viruses can be detected by hemadsorption; Para 3 virus can be adapted readily to produce recognizable cytopathic effect in continuous cell lines, and the observation of cytopathology can also be used as an end point in N tests.

4. Biological Characteristics of the Virus That Affect the Epidemiological Pattern

The parainfluenza viruses are RNA-containing viruses consisting of a lipoprotein envelope with hemagglutinin spikes surrounding the nucleocapsid.[43] The viruses are ether-sensitive and acid-labile. They apparently are antigenically stable. Para 3 virus remains infectious in an aerosol for periods greater than 1 hr.[63] Studies have shown that 10% of virus particles aerosolized are infectious after 1 hr in 20% relative humidity. No systematic studies of the stability of other parinfluenza viruses in aerosol have been reported, but Para 1 virus has been isolated from air samples obtained in the vicinity of infected children.[62]

The biological characteristic of parainfluenza viruses that seems to be the most important determinant of their success as respiratory pathogens is their ability to replicate in the respiratory epithelium without deeper invasion. The virus is extruded from the cell membrane without immediately destroying the cell, which allows continued release of particles from a single cell.[43] Furthermore, Para 3 virus may infect the mucosa of infants in the presence of maternally derived circulating antibodies[10,23,28,69] and also frequently may reinfect older children who have circulating antibodies.[12] Excretion of virus may be prolonged up to 1 month or longer, even with the second or third infection.[30,56,57] Epidemiological evidence suggests that reinfected children are infectious for their contacts.[12]

The incubation period is short, and the virus spreads rapidly to a high percentage of persons in closed populations, which indicates that the virus possesses a high degree of infectiousness. Adult volunteers with preexisting antibody were infected with as little as 1500 median tissue-culture infectious doses ($TCID_{50}$).[88] More than half the volunteers infected with the virus developed signs and symptoms of an upper respiratory illness.

5. Descriptive Epidemiology

5.1. Incidence and Prevalence Data

5.1.1. Serological Surveys. Available evidence supports strongly the view that parainfluenza viruses are ubiquitous viruses that infect most persons during childhood. Serological surveys have uniformly demonstrated that 90–100% of children have antibodies to Para 3 virus by age 5 years.[8,33,66] Antibodies to Para 1 and 2 viruses do not develop as rapidly or as universally as do antibodies to Para 3 virus or RSV; however, 74% of the children over 5 years of age tested in Washington, D.C., possessed antibody against Para 1 virus and 59% possessed antibody against Para 2 virus.[72] Similar data have been obtained in serological surveys in a wide variety of geographical areas,[8,33,55,59,66,71] but not in remote tribes in South America.[6a]

5.1.2. Association of Para 1 and 2 Viruses with Illnesses. Studies of lower respiratory disease have shown the highest isolation rates of Para 1 and 2 viruses to be between 4 months and 5 years of age.[10,28] The rate for lower respiratory disease associated with Para 1 virus infections in Chapel Hill pediatric practice was 17 per 1000 children per year for children under 4 years of age.[26,28] Lower respiratory disease after that age was relatively uncommon.[68,83]

Studies of outbreaks of Para 1 and 2 viruses in day-care centers and in families suggest a high attack rate in young antibody-negative children. An outbreak of Para 1 virus infections in a residential home in Washington, D.C., resulted in the development of N antibody in 65% of the children without prior antibody.[12] In studies at the same home for children in Washington, D.C., 21 or 49 residents without antibody were infected during a Para 2 outbreak.[47] In two other outbreaks of Para 2 virus infection, one in a day-care center in Chapel Hill[57] and the other in a children's home in Kansas City, Kansas,[35] the infection rates were 79 and 65%, respectively, in antibody-negative children. Most illnesses in both studies were afebrile and involved the upper respiratory tract. These results suggest that Para 1 and 2 viruses are less effective than Para 3 virus in spreading through a susceptible population.[12]

5.1.3. Association of Para 3 Virus with Illnesses. Para 3 virus infections have been detected in all studies of hospitalized children with acute lower respiratory disease,[7,10,61,70,97] and this virus is now recognized to be second only to RSV as a cause of bronchiolitis and pneumonia in infants.[15,23,26,28,69] Few studies of open populations have had denominator data to allow calculation of attack rates. In Chapel Hill, studies of children with lower respiratory disease presenting to a pediatric practice from 1966 to 1971 showed that 15 children per 1000 per year were infected with Para 3 virus each year for the first 3 years of life.[26,28]

A small group of infants in Chapel Hill were followed longitudinally through the first 2 years of life, and 21 of 62 (34%) developed respiratory illnesses associated with Para 3 virus infection; 6 of the 21 had evidence of involvement of the lower respiratory tract.[25] Of 15 children infected during the first year of life, 4 were reinfected during the second year; 66% of the total had N antibodies at the end of 2 years, indicated that mild or inapparent infections occurred in a number equal to the number of those presenting with illness.

Studies in Seattle in a prepaid group health-care program have reported isolation rates of Para 3 virus considerably lower than those observed in the Chapel Hill pediatric practice, but in the patients with paired serum specimens, a high percentage showed antibody rises to this virus.[19]

In closed populations such as children's homes and nurseries, infections with Para 3 virus were frequent.[3,12] The investigations of Junior Village in Washington, D.C., showed that all infants without preexisting antibodies were infected and 90% of the children with N antibody titers between 1:8 and 1:32 were reinfected, while only one third of those with higher antibody levels were reinfected.[12] In contrast, the studies focused on school-age children[80] and young adults[18,34,64] have revealed a relatively low rate of isolation of parainfluenza viruses, although infections by these agents are well documented in adults.

5.1.4. Para 4 Virus Infections. Para 4 virus has not been isolated frequently, but serological surveys indicate that infection may be common.[24,49,87] Most of these infections are considered to be asymptomatic, but isolation of the virus may be missed in some ill children because of the technical problems in identifying the virus in tissue culture.[24]

5.2. Epidemic Behavior

5.2.1. Para 1 and 2 Viruses. The longest continuous observation of the epidemic behavior of Para 1 virus has been at the Children's Hospital of the District of Columbia. From the initiation of the studies in 1957 until 1961, the virus was endemic.[10] Beginning in 1962, sharp epidemics of Para 1 virus began to occur every 2 years in the autumn of even-numbered years.[7,10] A similar pattern was noted in Great Britain between 1962 and 1977.[15,58a] In Chapel Hill, epidemics of Para 1 virus have occurred every 2 years since 1964, synchronously with these other epidemics.[26] Epidemics of Para 1 virus occurring in the fall of even-numbered years after 1962 have been described in other reports as well.[36,37,40,61] Evidence suggests that the epidemic occurrence of Para 1 virus at these times was not limited to a few communities, but occurred over a wide geographic area. In contrast, in other longitudinal studies, including those in Tecumseh,[65] Para 1 virus occurred in the endemic pattern seen in Washington, D.C., prior to 1962. A more irregular pattern of epidemic occurrence was noted in Seattle, where Para 1 virus epidemics were associated with increased incidence of croup during the winters of 1966–1967, 1967–1968, and 1970–1971.[19] The evidence suggests that Para 1 virus can, at different times and at different places, assume different patterns of occurrence varying from an endemic pattern over several years to sharp epidemics associated with a marked increase in the incidence of croup. Continued surveillance over time in different areas will be necessary before a predominant pattern can be established, if indeed such a pattern does exist.

Para 2 virus would appear to be as nearly ubiquitous as Para 1 virus on the basis of serological surveys, but it is not associated as frequently with severe clinical disease as is Para 1 virus. Because many studies depend on the isolation of the agent from lower respiratory disease to establish the presence of the virus in the community, there is less information on the occurrence of Para 2 virus. The available data suggest that it occurs in a sporadic epidemic pattern, often disappearing from the community for fairly long periods of time. In Chapel Hill, Para 2 virus epidemics occurred in the fall of the odd-numbered years, the years in which Para 1 virus was absent from the population.[26] A similar pattern occurred in Washington, D.C.[7] In Great Britain[15] and in Tecumseh,[65] Para 2 virus tended to occur in well-defined, but somewhat erratic, epidemic patterns, while in the Seattle surveillance studies,[19] it was rarely identified. In surveillance studies of young children with minor respiratory illness, Para 2 virus has had a distinct epidemic pattern with high attack rates in small, defined populations.[35,47,57]

5.2.2. Para 3 Virus. Infections with Para 3 virus have been invariably endemic in nature, occurring in all seasons of the year.[7,26] Small outbreaks have been noted, but there has been no predictable periodicity in their occurrence. Most major respiratory viruses have caused relatively discrete epidemics, but outbreaks of Para 3 virus have occurred concurrently when other viruses were epidemic.[26] This virus has been prevalent in Chapel Hill during RSV influenza virus, or Para 1 virus epidemics.

The high reinfection rate of Para 3 virus allows it to spread in populations containing majorities of people with previous experience with the virus. Observations in Chapel Hill of families with a child under 2 years of age showed that Para 3 virus infected these infants regardless of family constellation, while RSV infections were more likely to occur in infants with an older sibling who might bring the virus into the home.[25] A latent state of infection in adults has been suggested,[30] and this could explain the ability of parents to transmit infection to their infants.

5.3. Geographic Distribution

Available evidence indicates that parainfluenza viruses are found throughout the world and in all areas cause illness in young children. There is remarkable similarity of serological and isolation data obtained from tropical,[6,66] temperate,[12,33,84] and arctic[59] climates. However, antibody to Para 1 was found in very few Tiriyo Indians in South America and in none under age 20; in the Xikrin tribe, there was no antibody under age 17. Para 2 antibody was present in Xikrin of all ages, but almost entirely absent in other tribes. This suggests that fresh in-

troductions of virus are needed in very remote tribes in which the population base is too small to sustain the infection.[6a]

5.4. Temporal Distribution

Parainfluenza viruses can be isolated in any month of the year, in both temperate[10,26] and tropical climates.[6,52,71] The most common time for the occurrence of epidemics of Para 1 virus has been during the fall months.[7,15,19,26,36]

A similar occurrence in the fall has been noted for Para 2 virus in studies in Chapel Hill[26] and Washington, D.C.,[7] while studies in Tecumseh[66] showed a peak occurrence of Para 2 virus in the winter.

Para 3 virus infections occur endemically throughout the year. During the first 7 years of studies at the Children's Hospital of the District of Columbia, infections with Para 3 virus were associated with respiratory illness in 70 of 81 months.[10] A similar endemicity was noted in studies in the Chapel Hill pediatric practice, where this virus was associated with lower respiratory illness in 63 of 91 months.[26]

5.5. Age Distribution

5.5.1. Para 1 and 2 Viruses. Maternal antibody apparently prevents severe disease in very young infants infected with either Para 1 or 2 virus. Data from studies of lower respiratory disease show few cases of severe disease in infants under 4 months of age.[6,15,19,23,28,97] After 4 months of age, there is a rise in the number of cases of croup and other lower respiratory diseases.[28] This high incidence continues until approximately age 6 years. After a child reaches school age, there is a much lower incidence of lower respiratory symptomatology, and lower respiratory illnesses in persons infected by Para 1 and 2 viruses are distinctly unusual in adolescents[26] and adults,[68,83] although they have been reported.[93]

Studies of milder illness have shown a similar age distribution. Infection and minor clinical illness have been demonstrated more frequently in younger children than in adolescents and adults.[5,29,65] Infections do occur in older persons,[15,18,34,38,64,65] most of which presumably represent recurrent infections in persons with antibody. The studies conducted in Tecumseh[65] showed serological evidence of frequent infections in young adults in the age groups who would be likely to be the parents of young children. In family studies, infection in adults occurred concurrently with illness in their children, but attack rates in adults were distinctly lower than those in younger family members.[5,29]

5.5.2. Para 3 Virus. Initial infections with Para 3 virus occur early in life. Several investigators have noted that, like RSV infections, Para 3 virus infections often occur in the first months of life when infants still possess circulating antibodies derived from their mothers.[10,15,23,28,69] In the studies of lower respiratory disease in the Chapel Hill pediatric group practice, the age-specific attack rate for Para 3 disease paralleled that of RSV.[28] The average annual attack rate for the period from 1966 to 1971 was 15 lower respiratory illnesses per 1000 children per year for children under 3 years of age.[26] After the first 3 years of life, the incidence of lower respiratory illnesses associated with this virus falls off considerably, but studies in other populations indicate that reinfections are common in older children and adults, but usually are not associated with evidence of lower tract involvement.[12,18,29,31,34]

5.6. Sex

The greater frequency of croup in males has long been recognized.[75] Studies in the Chapel Hill pediatric practice demonstrated infection rates for Para 1 virus of 1.8 lower respiratory illnesses per 100 boys compared to 1.1 per 100 girls.[28] This sex difference disappeared after age 6 years. A similar predominance of serious illness in young males has been noted in other studies of lower respiratory disease.[58] The available information suggests that rates of infection in young boys and girls are the same, but that the clinical manifestations of infection are more severe in boys.[26]

There were insufficient numbers of cases of Para 2 virus infections to analyze.

Para 3 virus had identical rates of lower respiratory illness in males and females.[26] The attack rates for lower respiratory illnesses due to Para 3 virus infections in the Chapel Hill pediatric practice were 12 and 11 per 1000 children per year for boys and girls under 6 years of age.

5.7. Race and Occupation

No differences in infection rates or in the consequences of infection with parainfluenza viruses have been noted in different racial or occupational groups.

5.8. Occurrence in Special Epidemiological Settings

The frequencies of infections with parainfluenza viruses are greater in studies of young children hospitalized with lower respiratory disease[69] or day-care facilities.[57] Infections associated with respiratory disease occur but are usually mild or inapparent in school-age children,[80] university students,[18,34] military recruits,[64,93] and adults.[29,31,38,68,83]

Nosocomial infections with respiratory viruses may occur readily if susceptible infants are not kept isolated from children with respiratory disease. Mufson et al.[70] reported infections with Para 3 virus in 18% of infants who were well or infected with some other respiratory pathogen at the time of admission to Cook County Children's Hospital.

5.9. Socioeconomic Status

There is some evidence to suggest that infants from low-income families are more likely to be hospitalized with bronchiolitis or pneumonia in the first months of life than are infants from middle-income families.[22] RSV and Para 3 virus are frequent etiological agents of these illnesses. There may be many factors involved in this situation. The decision to hospitalize an infant may be based on the social milieu in which the child lives and not necessarily on the severity of the presenting signs and symptoms; however, some evidence suggests that young infants in low-income familes do have more severe illnesses, and this may result from exposures to relatively large inocula at an earlier age.

Unlike the case with Para 3 virus, there does not appear to be any difference in severity of disease due to Para 1 and 2 viruses in children of different socioeconomic groups.[26]

6. Mechanisms and Route of Transmission

Transmission of parainfluenza viruses is by direct person-to-person contact or large-droplet spread. These viruses do not persist long in the environment, but Para 1 virus has been recovered from air samples collected in the vicinity of infected patients, and from 1 to 10% of Para 3 virus particles in aerosols may be viable after 1 hr.[63] Adult volunteers who have had prior natural infection have been reinfected experimentally by inoculation of the upper airway with a coarse aerosol or nasal drops or both.[48,88] The high rate of infection early in life coupled with the frequency of reinfection suggests that the virus spreads readily, that reinfected persons may be infectious, and that a relatively small inoculum is necessary to produce an infection.

There is little evidence of animal reservoirs for human disease and no evidence of vector spread. The Sendai virus is a rodent strain of Para 1 virus, but there is no evidence that it is related to disease in humans.[43] SV5, a simian virus related to Para 2 virus, has been reported to cause human infections on rare occasions[41,92]; reports of human infections must be reviewed critically because this virus often contaminates monkey-kidney tissue cultures.[42] A virus that is antigenically similar to human Para 3 virus has been isolated from several animals, but particularly cattle[77] and sheep.[39] Bovine Para 3 virus is at least one of the agents commonly associated with an economically important disease of cattle usually called "shipping fever,"[79] but there is no evidence of spread between cattle and man.

7. Pathogenesis and Immunity

7.1. Pathogenesis

Little is known about the pathogenesis of infections with Para 1 and 2 viruses. Pathological studies have noted the predilection for the marked inflammatory response of glottic tissues[96] that is evident from the serious clinical manifestation (croup) of infections with these viruses.

Because infection with Para 3 virus may occur early in life in the presence of maternal antibody, the possibility of an immunopathological process similar to that proposed for RSV disease must be considered. Gardner et al.[23] noted the similarity of the clinical manifestations of infections with these two viruses in early infancy and the need for learning more about the pathogenesis. Although it is well accepted that infection with Para 3 virus may occur in the presence of low levels of maternal antibody,

there is no direct evidence that maternal antibody will enhance the pathogenicity of the host–virus interaction. Experimental studies in hamsters have not demonstrated enhanced virulence in the presence of passive antibody.[27] In fact, the pulmonary infiltrations were less in animals with passive antibody than in those without; however, animals with primary infection occurring with passive antibody had significantly greater infiltrate at the time of reinfection. This suggests that passive antibody may dampen some part or parts of the immune response to the primary infection, which allows for development of more disease at the time of reinfection. Studies have demonstrated that the primary serum antibody response to infection is decreased by passive antibody, but it is unknown whether other parameters such as surface antibody production and cellular immune response are affected. Viremia has been reported both with primary infection[78] and with reinfection.[30,46] It is difficult to determine the consequences of this, because clinical and pathological evidence of infection has been noted only in the respiratory tract. Viremia with reinfection was reported to have occurred in the presence of circulating antibodies; more work is necessary to determine the factors inherent in these observations.

7.2. Immunity

Studies with Para 1 virus[81] and Para 2 virus[86] have revealed that immunity is better correlated with the presence of nasal antibody than with the level of serum antibody. The protective immune response to Para 3 virus infection in humans has not been established. Clinical studies have shown that the risk of reinfection is inversely related to the level of circulating antibodies,[12] but the relationship to surface antibody or cellular immunity is unknown. Although reinfection is common, the consequences of subsequent infections seem to be negligible. Lower respiratory involvement with reinfection is unusual , and mild upper respiratory symptoms are the rule.

Studies in calves infected with Para 3 virus indicate that maternal antibody derived from colostrum is protective.[20] Calves are usually protected for 10–23 weeks after birth if allowed to suckle. Inactivated vaccines injected parenterally have provided some protection against natural and experimental challenge, but attenuated viruses inoculated intranasally provide better protection.[32] There is some evidence that hyperimmunization of dams with inactivated vaccines to increase antibody titers in colostrum will decrease the morbidity of their offspring.[53]

In summary, studies of bovine disease and experimental infections of hamsters do not support the hypothesis that passive antibody may contribute to the pathogenesis of disease in early life. The data suggest that passively acquired antibody may provide at least partial protection.

8. Patterns of Host Response

8.1. Clinical Manifestations

Primary infections with parainfluenza viruses are usually symptomatic, but the clinical manifestations may range from an afebrile upper respiratory illness to severe and life-threatening lower respiratory disease (Table 1). The most characteristic and clinically important syndrome associated with infections with Para 1 and 2 viruses is croup or laryngotracheobronchitis. Para 1 virus was isolated from 20% of patients with croup in studies in the Chapel Hill pediatric practice.[28] Para 2 virus is much less frequently associated with croup than is Para 1 virus.[10,26] Mortality has been reported with both these agents, but is rare.[6,23,73,92] Studies in ambulatory populations suggest that most initial infections with Para 1 virus result in febrile upper respiratory illness, while initial infections with Para 2 virus result in somewhat less severe upper respiratory illnesses, with a high proportion being afebrile.[35,57] Reinfection with either of these agents is associated with upper respiratory symptoms indistinguishable from those due to other viruses.[29]

The clinical manifestations of infections with Para 3 virus are varied. In studies in the Chapel Hill pe-

diatric practice of children presenting with lower respiratory disease, the diagnosis varied with age[26]; infants under 1 year of age were likely to present with bronchiolitis or pneumonia, while children from 6 to 18 months might develop croup. Older children were usually diagnosed as having tracheobronchitis. In general, though, it should be stated that there was no consistent clinical presentation of Para 3 virus infection.

Prospective studies of children indicate that primary infection with Para 3 virus is usually symptomatic but often mild.[57] In children followed for the first 2 years of life, about one third of primary infections involved the lower respiratory tract, but only 5% of primary infections resulted in lower respiratory illnesses for which families sought medical care.[25] Frequency of reinfection—both symptomatic and asymptomatic—decreased with age (and experience with the virus). Reinfection was symptomatic among young children at Junior Village 20% of the time,[12] but this frequency is probably higher than that in open populations; the circumstances of living conditions in this nursery could have resulted in a greater inoculum than would occur ordinarily.

The incidence of reinfection in adult populations is difficult to determine because of the cross-reactions that may occur by serological testing—particularly if the HI or CF test is used. The viruses have been isolated rarely from asymptomatic adults.[25]

8.2. Diagnosis

Clinical diagnosis of the etiology of sporadic episodes of acute respiratory disease is difficult; however, infections with parainfluenza viruses may be suspected by combining the clinical manifestations with known epidemiological patterns.[26] As noted in Section 5.2.1, Para 1 virus infections have pro-

Table 1. Parainfluenza Viruses: Serotypes and Associated Clinical and Epidemiological Manifestations

Human serotype	Major clinical syndrome	Peak age (months)	Sex predominance	Periodicity[a]	Antigenically related animal strains
Para 1	Croup	6–24	Male	Epidemic (fall)	Sendai virus (rodents)
Para 2	Croup	6–24	Male	Epidemic (fall)	Simian virus 5 (SV5)
Para 3	Pneumonia and bronchiolitis	0–6	None	Endemic	Bovine Para 3 virus
Para 4	URI	Unknown	Unknown	Endemic	None

[a] Peak season in parentheses.

duced predictable epidemics of croup in the autumn of even-numbered years in widely scattered geographic areas observed for periods up to 10 years. Croup is most common in boys between 6 months and 3 years of age. With knowledge of the patterns of parainfluenza virus infections provided by regional laboratories, it may be possible to predict the occurrence of epidemics of Para 1 or 2 virus infections and thereby establish an estimate of the etiology of respiratory illnesses—particularly when they present with a major clinical manifestation such as croup.

Para 3 virus infections are much less predictable, but this etiology should be considered for infants less than 6 months of age with bronchiolitis or pneumonia occurring at times other than during RSV epidemics.[26] Although RSV-associated bronchiolitis has been more common in male infants, lower respiratory illnesses associated with Para 3 virus have had an even sex distribution.

Laboratory diagnosis is best accomplished by identification of virus in respiratory secretions or tissue because of cross-reactions that may be observed among parainfluenza viruses when employing serological tests. Cross-reactions appear to be less frequent with tests measuring N antibodies than with those for CF or HI antibodies. Methods for virus isolation and identification are described in Section 3.4. Identification of hemadsorbing viruses can be expedited by the use of immunofluorescent technique.[23] These viruses can be identified directly in infected epithelial cells shed in respiratory secretions collected from patients by aspiration or washings of the upper respiratory passages. The cells must be washed to separate them from mucus and fixed on slides in six "spots" that are then exposed to specific antisera. Usually, a battery of antisera to parainfluenza viruses and influenza A and B viruses are used along with preimmunization serum from the same animal host. After the slides are washed, fluorscein-tagged antiserum against the animal host globulin is used to counterstain the cells. This method may allow specific diagnosis within a few hours after the specimen is collected.

9. Control and Prevention Based on Epidemiological Data

As soon as the clinical importance of the parainfluenza viruses was demonstrated, efforts were begun to develop effective vaccines. Most early efforts involved the use of formalin-inactivated, parenterally administered vaccines grown in embryonated hens' eggs.[14,22,44,50] These preparations were given either as a monovalent preparation,[21] as a trivalent parainfluenza vaccine, or as a multivalent vaccine including other respiratory pathogens. Most preparations were aqueous suspensions, but one alum-adsorbed egg-grown Para 3 vaccine was tested.[21] One group employed a monkey-kidney-grown, formalin-killed, alum-precipitated parainfluenza vaccine given both as a trivalent parainfluenza vaccine and as a multivalent respiratory vaccine.[90] A high proportion of subjects developed serum antibody rises with parenterally administered, formalin-inactivated vaccines—particularly antibody-negative subjects. Antibody rises occurred in a smaller proportion of subjects with preexisting antibody, either passively acquired maternal antibody or antibody secondary to natural infection.[19] All studies uniformly failed to show evidence of protection even in subjects with good serum antibody responses. There was no evidence of more severe disease in the subjects given the trivalent aqueous parainfluenza vaccine, an important finding in view of the fact that infants given alum-precipitated RSV vaccine had more severe illness than expected when they were naturally infected.[50,50a]

The demonstration that protective immunity is more closely related to the level of secretory nasal antibody than to serum antibody,[81,86] and the actual worsening of disease seen with inactivated RSV vaccine, has led to a reevaluation of the use of parenteral respiratory vaccines. Efforts have focused on use of attenuated live vaccines given intranasally. Initial trials of a temperature-sensitive Para 1 mutant in animals were promising,[74] but an attenuated strain suitable for use in humans has not been developed. It has been shown that aerosol inoculation of an inactivated Para 2 vaccine will safely stimulate nasal secretory antibody in adults.[94] The effectiveness of this method of vaccine administration has not been tested further.

Epidemiological data suggest that the most important age group to immunize against Para 1 and 2 viruses is children over 4 months of age. This contrasts with Para 3 virus and RSV, which cause significant illness between 1 and 3 months of age and which would require immunization in early infancy.

For bovine Para 3 virus infections, both inactivated and attenuated vaccines administered parenterally and intranasally have been used in calves.[32] The results are not consistent, but it would appear that attenuated strains given intranasally are more effective. Evidence suggests that in calves, vaccine-induced antibody is associated with protection and does not cause more severe disease. However, until more is known about the pathogenesis of human parainfluenza disease, care must be exercised in the use of any vaccine—particularly in infants.

10. Unresolved Problems

The clinical spectrum of illness, age incidence, and ubiquity of parainfluenza virus infections have been demonstrated (Table 1). There remains some question about the epidemic patterns associated with Para 1 and 2 viruses that can be clarified by further observations over time. The most important needs at the present time are for more intense study of the pathogenesis of disease—especially that associated with Para 3 virus—and a better understanding of the total immune response to all parainfluenza viruses in order to facilitate the development of effective vaccines.

11. References

1. ABINANTI, R. R., CHANOCK, R. M., COOK, M. K., WONG, D., AND WARFIELD, M., Relationship of human and bovine strains of myxovirus parainfluenza 3, *Proc. Soc. Exp. Biol. Med.* **106**:466–469 (1961).
2. AHERNE, W., BIRD, T., COURT, S. D. M., GARDNER, P. S., AND McQUILLEN, J., Pathological changes in virus infections of the lower respiratory tract in children. *J. Clin. Pathol.* **23**:7–18 (1970).
3. AITKEN, C. J. D., MOFFAT, M. A. J., AND SUTHERLAND, J. A. W., Respiratory illness and viral infection in an Edinburgh nursery, *J. Hyg.* **65**:25–36 (1967).
4. ANDREWES, C. H., BANG, M. B., CHANOCK, R. M., AND ZHDANOV, B. M., Parainfluenza viruses 1, 2 and 3: Suggested names for recently described myxoviruses, *Virology* **8**:129–130 (May 1959).
5. BANATVALA, J. E., ANDERSON, T. B., AND REISS, B. B., Parainfluenza infections in the community, *Br. Med. J.* **1**:537–540 (February 1964).
6. BISNO, A. L., BARRATT, N. P., SWANSTON, W. H., AND SPENCE, L. P., An outbreak of acute respiratory disease in Trinidad associated with parainfluenza viruses, *Am. J. Epidemiol.* **91**:68 (1970).
6a. BLACK, F. L., HIERHOLZER, W. J., DE PINHEIRO, P. F.

7. EVANS, A. S., WOODHALL, J. P., OPTON, E. M., EMMONS, J. E., WEST, B. S., EDSALL, G., DOWNS, W. G., AND WALLACE, E. D., Evidence for persistence of infectious agents in isolated human populations, *Am. J. Epidemiol.* **100**:230–250 (1974).
7. BRANDT, C. D., KIM, H. W., CHANOCK, R. M., AND PARROTT, R. S., Parainfluenza virus epidemiology, *Pediatr. Res.* **8**:422 (1974).
8. BROWN, P. K., AND TAYLOR-ROBINSON, D., Respiratory virus antibodies in sera of persons living in isolated communities, *Bull. WHO* **34**:895–900 (1966).
9. CHANOCK, R. M., Association of a new type of cytopathogenic myxovirus with infantile croup, *J. Exp. Med.* **104**:555 (1956).
10. CHANOCK, R. M., AND PARROTT, R. H., Acute respiratory disease in infancy and childhood: Present understanding and prospects for prevention, *Pediatrics* **36**:21–39 (1965).
11. CHANOCK, R. M., PARROTT, R. H., COOK, K., ANDREWS, B. E., BELL, J. A., REICHELDERFER, T., KAPIKIAN, A. Z., MASTROTA, F. M., AND HUEBNER, R. J., Newly recognized myxoviruses from children with respiratory disease, *N. Engl. J. Med.* **258**:207 (1958).
12. CHANOCK, R. M., PARROTT, R. H., JOHNSON, K. M., KAPIKIAN, A. Z., AND BELL, J. A., Myxoviruses: Parainfluenza, *Am. Rev. Respir. Dis.* **88**:152 (1963).
13. CHANOCK, R. M., WONG, D. C., HUEBNER, R. J., AND BELL, J. A., Serologic response in individuals infected with parainfluenza viruses, *Am. J. Pub. Health* **50**:1858 (1960).
14. CHIN, J., MAGOFFIN, R. L. SHEARER, L. A., SCHIEBLE, J. H., AND LENNETTE, E. H., Field evaluation of a respiratory syncytial virus vaccine and a trivalent parainfluenza virus vaccine in a pediatric population, *Am. J. Epidemiol.* **89**: 449 (1969).
15. CLARKE, S. K. R., Parainfluenza virus infections, *Postgrad. Med. J.* **49**:792–797 (1973).
16. COOK, M. K., ANDREWS, B. E., FOX, H. H., TURNER, H. C., JAMES, W. D., AND CHANOCK, R. M., Antigenic relationships among the "newer" myxoviruses (parainfluenza), *Am. J. Hyg.* **69**:250–264 (1959).
17. COOK, M. K., AND CHANOCK, R. M., *In vivo* antigenic studies of parainfluenza viruses, *Am. J. Hyg.* **77**:150–159 (1963).
17a. EVANS, A. S., Infections with hemadsorption virus in University of Wisconsin students, *N. Engl. J. Med.* **263**:233–237 (1960).
18. EVANS, A. S., AND DICK, E. C., Acute pharyngitis and tonsillitis in University of Wisconsin students, *J. Am. Med. Assoc.* **190**:699 (1964).
19. FOY, H. M., COONEY, M. K., MALETZKY, A. J., AND GRAYSTON, J. T., Incidence and etiology of pneumonia, croup and bronchiolitis in preschool children belonging to a prepaid medical care group over a four-year period, *Am. J. Epidemiol.* **97**:80 (1973).

20. FRANK, G. H., AND MARSHALL, R. G., Parainfluenza 3 virus infection of cattle, *J. Am. Vet. Med. Assoc.* **163**:858–860 (1973).
21. FULGINITI, V. A., SIEBER, O. F., JOHN, T. J., ASKIN, P., AND UMLANT, H. J., JR., Parainfluenza virus immunization. II. The influence of age and maternal antibody upon successful immunization with an alum-adsorbed parainfluenza type 3 vaccine, *Pediatr. Res.* **1**:50–58 (1967).
22. FULGINITI, V. A., ELLER, J. J., SIEBER, O. F., JOYNER, J. W., MINAMITANI, M., AND MEIKLEJOHN, G., Respiratory virus immunization. I. A field trial of two inactivated respiratory virus vaccine: an aqueous trivalent parainfluenza virus vaccine and an alum-precipitated respiratory syncytial virus vaccine, *Am. J. Epidemiol.* **89**:435 (1969).
23. GARDNER, P. S., McQUILLIN, J., McGUCKIN, R., AND DITCHBURN, R. K., Observations on clinical and immunofluorescent diagnosis of parainfluenza virus infections, *Br. Med. J.* **2**:7–12 (1971).
24. GARDNER, S. D., The isolation of parainfluenza 4 subtypes A and B in England and serological studies of their prevalance, *J. Hyg.* **67**:545–550 (1969).
25. GLEZEN, W. P., Unpublished data.
26. GLEZEN, W. P., AND DENNY, F. W., Epidemiology of acute lower respiratory disease in children, *N. Engl. J. Med.* **288**:498–505 (1973).
27. GLEZEN, W. P., AND FERNALD, G. W., Effect of passive antibody on parainfluenza virus type 3 pneumonia in hamsters, *Infect. Immun.* **14**: 212 (1976).
28. GLEZEN, W. P., LODA, F. A., CLYDE, W. A., JR., SENIOR, R. J., SHEAFFER, C. I., CONLEY, W. G., AND DENNY, F. W., Epidemiologic patterns of acute lower respiratory disease of children in pediatric group practice, *J. Pediatr.* **78**:397 (1971).
29. GLEZEN, W. P., WULFF, H., LAMB, G. A., RAY, C. G., CHIN, T. D. Y., AND WENNER, H. A., Patterns of virus infections in families with acute respiratory illnesses, *Am. J. Epidemiol.* **86**:350 (1967).
30. GROSS, P. A., GREEN, R. H., AND CURNEN, M. C. M., Persistent infection with parainfluenza type 3 virus in man, *Am. Rev. Respir. Dis.* **108**:894–898 (1973).
31. GWALTNEY, J. M., JR., HENDLEY, J. O., SIMON, G., AND JORDAN, W. S., Rhinovirus infections in an industrial population. I. The occurrence of illness, *N. Engl. J. Med.* **275**:1261–1268 (1966).
32. GUTEKUNST, D. E., PATON, I. M., AND VOLANCE, F. J., Parainfluenza 3 vaccine in cattle: Comparative efficacy of intranasal and intramuscular routes, *J. Am. Vet. Med. Assoc.* **155**:1879–1885 (1969).
33. HALL, C. E., BRANDT, C. D., FROTHINGHAM, T. E., SPIGLAND, I., COONEY, M. K., AND FOX, J. P., The Virus Watch Program: A continuing surveillance of viral infections in metropolitan New York families. IX. A comparison of infections with several respiratory pathogens in New York and New Orleans families, *Am. J. Epidemiol.* **94**:367 (1971).
34. HAMRE, D., CONNELLY, A. P., AND PROCKNOW, J. J., Virologic studies of acute respiratory disease in young adults. IV. Virus isolations during four years of surveillance, *Am. J. Epidemiol.* **83**:238 (1966).
35. HARRIS, D. J., WULFF, H., RAY, C. G., POLAND, J. D., CHIN, T. D. Y., AND WENNER, H. A., Viruses and disease. II. An outbreak of parainfluenza type 2 in a children's home, *Am. J. Epidemiol.* **87**:419 (1968).
36. HERRMANN, E. C., AND, HABLE, K. A., Experiences in laboratory diagnosis of parainfluenza viruses in routine medical practice, *Mayo Clin. Proc.* **45**:177 (1970).
37. HOLZEL, A., PARKER, L., PATTERSON, W. H., CARTMEL, D., WHITE, L. L. R., PURDY, R., THOMPSON, K. M., AND TOBIN, J., Virus isolations from throats of children admitted to hospital with respiratory and other diseases, *Br. Med. J.* **1**:614 (1965).
38. HOPE-SIMPSON, R. E., AND HIGGINS, P. G., A respiratory virus study in Great Britain: Review and evaluation, *Prog. Med. Virol.* **11**:354 (1969).
39. HORE, D. E., STEVENSON, R. G., GILMOUR, N. J. L., VANTISIS, J. T., AND THOMPSON, D. A., Isolation of parainfluenza virus from the lungs and nasal passages of sheep showing respiratory disease, *J. Comp. Pathol.* **78**:259–265 (1968).
40. HORTSMANN, D. M., AND HSIUNG, G. D., Myxovirus infections and respiratory illnesses in children, *Clin. Pediatr.* **2**:378 (1963).
41. HSIUNG, G. D., ISACSON, P., AND TUCKER, G., Studies of parainfluenza viruses. II. Serologic interrelationships in humans, *Yale J. Biol. Med.* **35**:534–544 (1963).
42. HULL, R. N., MINNER, J. R., AND SMITH, J. W., New agents recovered from tissue cultures of monkey kidney cells, *Am. J. Hyg.* **63**:204–215 (1956).
43. JACKSON, G. G., AND MULDOON, R. L., Viruses causing common respiratory infections in man. II. Enteroviruses and paramyxoviruses, *J. Infect. Dis.* **128**:387–469 (1973).
44. JENSEN, K. E., PEELER, B. E., AND DULWORTH, W. G., Immunizations against parainfluenza infections, *J. Immunol.* **89**:216–226 (1962).
45. JOHNSON, K. M., CHANOCK, R. M., COOK, M. K., AND HUEBNER, R. J., Studies of a new human hemadsorption virus. I. Isolation, properties and characterization, *Am. J. Hyg.* **71**:81–92 (1960).
46. JOHNSON, D. P., AND GREEN, R. H., Viremia during parainfluenza type 3 virus infection of hamsters, *Proc. Soc. Exp. Biol. Med.* **144**:745–748 (1973).
47. KAPIKIAN, A. Z., BELL, J. A., MASTROTA, F. M., HUEBNER, R. J., WONG, D. C., AND CHANOCK, R. M., An outbreak of parainfluenza 2 (croup-associated) virus infection, *J. Am. Med. Assoc.* **183**:324 (1963).
48. KAPIKIAN, A. Z., CHANOCK, R. M., REICHELDERFER, T. E., WARD, T. G., HUEBNER, R. J., AND BELL, J. A.,

Inoculation of human volunteers with parainfluenza virus type 3, *J. Am. Med. Assoc.* **18**:537–541 (1961).

49. KILLGORE, G. E., AND DOWDLE, W. R., Antigenic characterization of parainfluenza 4A and 4B by the hemagglutination-inhibition test and distribution of HI antibody in human sera, *Am. J. Epidemiol.* **91**:308–316 (1970).

50. KIM, H. W., CANCHOLA, J. G., VARGOSKO, A. J., ARROBIO, J. O., DE MEIO, J. L., AND PARROTT, R. H., Immunogenicity of inactivated parainfluenza type 1, type 2, and type 3 vaccines in infants, *J. Am. Med. Assoc.* **196**:819 (1966).

50a. KIM, H. W., CANCHOLA, J. G., BRANDT, C. D., PYLES, G., CHANOCK, R. M., JENSEN, K., AND PARROTT, R. H., Respiratory syncytial virus disease in infants despite prior administration of antigenic inactivated vaccine, *Am. J. Epidemiol.* **89**:422–434 (1969).

51. KIM, H. W., VARGOSKO, E. J., CHANOCK, R. M., AND PARROTT, R. H., Parainfluenza 2 (CA) virus: Etiologic association with croup, *Pediatrics* **28**:614–621 (1961).

51a. KINGSBURY, D. W., BRATT, M. A., CHOPPIN, P. W., HANSON, R. P., HOSAKA, Y., TER MUELEN, V., NORRBY, E., PLOWRIGHT, W., ROTT, R., AND WUNNER, W. H., Paramyxoviridae, *Intervirology* **10**:137 (1978).

52. KLOENE, W., BANG, F. B., CHAKRABORTY, S. M., COOPER, M. R., KULEMANN, H., OTA, M., AND SHAH, K. V., A two-year respiratory virus survey in four villages in West Bengal, India, *Am. J. Epidemiol.* **92**:307 (1970).

53. KOLAR, J. R., JR., SHECHMEISTER, I. L., AND STRACK, L. E., Field experiments with formalin-killed-virus vaccine against infectious bovine rhinotracheitis, bovine viral diarrhea, and parainfluenza-3, *Am. J. Vet. Res.* **34**:1469–1471 (1973).

54. KUROYA, M., AND ISHIDA, N., Newborn virus pneumonitis (type Sendai). II. Isolation of a new virus possessing hemagglutinin activity, *Yokohoma Med. Bull.* **4**:217–233 (1953).

55. LAPLACA, M., AND MOSCOVICI, C., Distribution of parainfluenza antibodies in different groups of population, *J. Immunol.* **88**:72 (1962).

56. LODA, F. A., COLLIER, A. M., AND GLEZEN, W. P., Unpublished observations.

57. LODA, F. A., GLEZEN, W. P., AND CLYDE, W. A., Respiratory disease in group day care, *Pediatrics* **48**:428 (1972).

58. MALETZKY, A. J., COONEY, M. K., LUCE, R., KENNY, G. E., AND GRAYSTON, J. T., Epidemiology of viral and mycoplasmal agents associated with childhood lower respiratory illness in a civilian population, *J. Pediatr.* **78**:407–414 (1971).

58a. MARTIN, A. J., GARDNER, P. S., AND McQUILLIN, J., Epidemiology of respiratory viral infection among pediatric inpatients over a six-year period in northeast England, *Lancet* **2**:1035 (1978).

59. MAYNARD, J. E., FELTZ, E. T., WULFF, H., FORTUINE, R., POLAND, J. D., AND CHIN, T. D. Y., Surveillance of respiratory virus infections among Alaskan Eskimo children, *J. Am. Med. Assoc.* **200**:927 (1967).

60. McINTOSH, K., ELLIS, E. F., HOFFMAN, L. S., LYBASS, T. G., ELLER, J. J., AND FULGINITI, V. A., The association of viral and bacterial respiratory infections with exacerbations of wheezing in young asthmatic children, *J. Pediatr.* **82**:578 (1973).

61. McLEAN, D. M., BACH, R., LAVKE, R. P. B., AND McNAUGHTON, G. A., Myxoviruses associated with acute laryngotracheobronchitis in Toronto, 1962–1963, *Can. Med. Assoc. J.* **89**:1257 (1963).

62. McLEAN, D. M., BANNATYNE, R. M., AND GIBAN, K., Myxovirus dissemination by air, *Can. Med. Assoc. J.* **96**:1449 (1967).

63. MILLER, W. S., AND ARTENSTEIN, M. S., Aerosol stability of three acute respiratory disease viruses, *Proc. Soc. Exp. Biol. Med.* **125**:222–227 (1967).

64. MOGABGAB, W. J., Acute respiratory illnesses in university (1962–1966), military and industrial (1962–1963) populations, *Am. Rev. Respir. Dis.* **98**:359–379 (1968).

65. MONTO, A. A., The Tecumseh study of respiratory illness. V. Patterns of infection with the parainfluenza viruses, *Am. J. Epidemiol.* **97**:338–348 (1973).

66. MONTO, A. S., AND JOHNSON, K. M., Respiratory infections in the American tropics, *Am. J. Trop. Med. Hyg.* **17**:867–874 (1968).

67. MONOZENKO, M. A., BANYSHEVA, A. E., TEMOFEYEVA, G. A., BYSTOYAKAVA, L. V., AND KALINNIKOVA, O. N., Diagnostic value of the complement fixation reaction in viral respiratory infections of infants, *Acta Virol.* **7**:534–541 (1963).

68. MUFSON, M. A., CHANG, V., GILL, V., WOOD, S. C., ROMANSKY, M. J., AND CHANOCK, R. M., The role of viruses, mycoplasmas and bacteria in acute pneumonia in civilian adults, *Am. J. Epidemiol.* **86**:526 (1967).

69. MUFSON, M. A., KRAUSE, H. E., MOCEGA, H. E., AND DAWSON, F. W., Viruses, *Mycoplasma pneumoniae* and bacteria associated with lower respiratory tract disease among infants, *Am. J. Epidemiol.* **91**:192–202 (1970).

70. MUFSON, M. A., MOCEGA, H. E., AND KRAUSE, H. E., Acquisition of parainfluenza 3 virus infection by hospitalized children. I. Frequencies, rates, and temporal data, *J. Infect. Dis.* **128**:141–147 (1973).

71. OLSON, L. C., LEXOMBOON, U., SITHISARN, P., AND NOYES, H. E., The etiology of respiratory tract infections in a tropical country, *Am. J. Epidemiol.* **97**:34 (1973).

72. PARROTT, R. H., VARGOSKO, A. J., KIM, H. W., BELL, J. A., AND CHANOCK, R. M., III. Myxoviruses: Parainfluenza, *Am. J. Public Health* **52**:907–917 (1962).

73. PEREIRA, M. S., AND FISHER, O. D., An outbreak of acute laryngotracheobronchitis associated with parainfluenza 2 virus, *Lancet* **2**:790 (1960).

74. POTASH, L., LEES, R., GREENBERGER, J. L., HOYRUP, A., DENNEY, L. D., AND CHANOCK, R. M., A mutant of parainfluenza type 1 virus with decreased capacity for growth at 38°C and 39°C, *J. Infect. Dis.* **121**:640–647 (1970).

75. RABE, E. F., Infectious croup. II. "Virus" croup, *Pediatrics* **2**:415 (1948).

76. REICHELDERFER, T. E., CHANOCK, R. M., CRAIGHEAD, J. E., HUEBNER, R. J. WARD, T. J., TURNER, H. C., AND JAMES, W. D., Infection of human volunteers with type 2 hemadsorption virus, *Science,* **128**:779–780 (1958).

77. REISINGER, R. C., HEDDLESTON, K. L., AND MANTHEI, C. A., A myxovirus SF-4 associated with shipping fever of cattle, *J. Am. Vet. Med. Assoc.* **135**:147–152 (1959).

78. ROCCHI, G., ARANGRO-RUIZ, G., GIANNINI, V., JEMOLO, A. M., ANDREONI, G., AND ARCHETTI, I., Detection of viremia in acute respiratory disease of man, *Acta Virol.* **14**:405–407 (1970).

79. ROSNER, S. F., Bovine parainfluenza type 3 virus infection and pasteurellosis, *J. Am. Vet. Med. Assoc.* **159**:1375–1381 (1971).

80. SALIBA, G. S., GLEZEN, W. P., AND CHIN, T. D. Y., Etiologic studies of acute respiratory illness among children attending public schools, *Am. Rev. Respir. Dis.* **95**:592 (1967).

81. SMITH, C. B., PURCELL, R. H., BELLANTI, J. A., AND CHANOCK, R. M., Protective effect of antibody to parainfluenza type 1 virus, *N. Engl. J. Med.* **275**:1145 (1966).

82. STARK, J. D., HEATH, R. B., AND CURWEN, M. P. Infection with influenza and parainfluenza viruses in chronic bronchitis, *Thorax* **20**:124 (1965).

83. SULLIVAN, R. J., DOWDLE, W. R., MARINE, W. M., AND HIERHOLZER, J. C., Adult pneumonia in a general hospital, *Arch. Intern. Med.* **129**:935 (1972).

84. TAI, F.-H., AND CHING, C.-M., Antibody patterns of parainfluenza viruses in human populations on Taiwan, *Am. Rev. Respir. Dis.* **97**:941 (1968).

85. TAYLOR-ROBINSON, D., AND BYNOE, M. L., Parainfluenza 2 virus infections in adult volunteers, *J. Hyg.* **61**:407 (1963).

86. TREMONTI, L. P., LIN, J. S. L., AND JACKSON, G. C., Neutralizing activity in nasal secretions and serum in resistance of volunteers to parainfluenza virus type 2, *J. Immunol.* **101**:572 (1968).

87. TYRRELL, D. A. J., AND BYNOE, M. L., Studies on parainfluenza type 2 and 4 viruses obtained from patients with common colds, *Br. Med. J.* **1**:471 (1969).

88. TYRRELL, D. A. J., BYNOE, M. L., BIRKUM, K., PETERSEN, S., AND PEREIRA, M. S., Inoculation of human volunteers with parainfluenza viruses 1 and 3 (HA₂ and HA₁), *Br. Med. J.* **2**:909 (1959). *Med. J.* **2**:909 (1959).

89. VARGOSKO, A. J., CHANOCK, R. M., HUEBNER, R. J., LUCKEY, A. H., KIM, H. W., CUMMINGS, C., AND PARROTT, R. A., Association of type 2 hemadsorption (parainfluenza 1) virus and Asian influenza A virus with infectious croup, *N. Engl. J. Med.* **261**:1–9 (1959).

90. VELLA, P. P., WEIBEL, R. E., WOODHOUR, A. F., MASCOLI, C. C., LEAGUS, M. B., ITTENSOHN, O. L., STOKES, J., JR., AND HILLEMAN, M. R., Respiratory virus vaccines. VIII. Field evaluation of trivalent parainfluenza virus vaccine among preschool children in families, 1967–1968, *Am. Rev. Respir. Dis.* **99**:526 (1969).

91. VIHMA, L., Surveillance of acute viral respiratory diseases in children, *Acta Paediatr. Scand. Suppl.* **192**:1 (1969).

92. VON EULER, L. V., KANTOR, F. S., AND HSIUNG, G. D., Studies of parainfluenza viruses. I. Clinical, pathological and virological observations, *Yale J. Biol. Med.* **35**:523 (1963).

93. WENZEL, R. P., MCCORMICK, D. P., AND BEAM, W. E., JR., Parainfluenza pneumonia in adults, *J. Am. Med. Assoc.* **221**:294 (1972).

94. WIGLEY, F. M., FRUCHTMAN, M. H., AND WALDMAN, R. H., Aerosol immunization of humans with inactivated parainfluenza type 2 vaccine, *N. Engl. J. Med.* **283**:1250 (1970).

95. WULFF, H., SOEKEN, J., POLAND, J. D., AND CHIN, T. D. Y., A new micro-neutralization test for antibody determination and typing of parainfluenza and influenza viruses, *Proc. Soc. Exp. Biol. Med.* **125**:1045–1049 (1967).

96. ZINSERLING, A., Peculiarities of lesion in viral and mycoplasma infections of the respiratory tract, *Virchows Arch. A.* **356**:259–273 (1972).

97. ZOLLAR, L. M., KRAUSE, H. E., AND MUFSON, M. A., Microbiologic studies on young infants with lower respiratory tract disease, *Am. J. Dis. Child.* **126**:56 (1973).

12. Suggested Reading

CHANOCK, R. M., AND PARROTT, R. H., Acute respiratory disease in infancy and childhood: Present understanding and prospects for prevention, *Pediatrics* **36**:21–39 (1965).

CLARKE, S. K. R., Parainfluenza virus infections, *Postgrad. Med. J.* **49**:792–797 (1973).

GLEZEN, W. P., AND DENNY, F. W., Epidemiology of acute lower respiratory disease in children, *N. Engl. J. Med.* **288**:498–505 (1973).

JACKSON, G. G., AND MULDOON, R. L., Viruses causing common respiratory infections in man. II. Enteroviruses and paramyxoviruses, *J. Infect. Dis.* **128**:387–469 (1973).

MONTO, A. S., The Tecumseh study of respiratory illness. V. Patterns of infection with the parainfluenza viruses, *Am. J. Epidemiol.* **97**:338–348 (1973).

CHAPTER 18

Rabies

Robert E. Shope

1. Introduction

Rabies is an acute central nervous system (CNS) disease of man and domestic and wild animals that usually results in death. The disease follows infection with a virus that is bullet-shaped, has an envelope, and contains single-stranded RNA. In the classic pathogenesis, the virus gains entry by the bite of a rabid animal, usually a dog or cat but also a wild animal such as a bat, wolf, fox, skunk, raccoon, meerkat, or coyote. During an incubation period of from days to several months, the virus is believed to multiply in the muscle[42] at the site of entry and then to travel centripetally via nerves to the ganglia and to the CNS. Once the CNS is infected, overt disease appears in the form of fever, acute excitation, convulsions, excess lacrimation and salivation, insomnia, anxiety, difficulty in swallowing, and sometimes maniacal behavior. A form of the disease called "dumb rabies" is characterized by progressive lassitude, coma, and death. There is no cure for rabies, but prevention by cleansing of the wound, vaccination, and immune serum therapy is effective in many cases.

Laboratory animals may survive overt disease,[6] and there have now been at least three cases of survival in man.[9c,24,48b] There is thus reason for optimism that something can be done about rabies in man.

2. Historical Background

The pre-Mosaic Eshnunna Code from the 3rd millennium B.C. refers to death in man following dog bite.[61] Democritus in 500 B.C. and Aristotle in 322 B.C. recognized rabies in dogs and other domestic animals. Thus, it can be assumed that the disease existed in Asia, Europe, and perhaps Africa for centuries in a stable form. Periodic epizootics occurred in wild vertebrates; Johnson[28] cites wolf rabies in western Europe in 1271 and in the same region seven major epizootics in foxes from 1803 to 1925. After World War II, another epizootic in foxes swept through Europe from east to west at a rate of about 30 km each year, and the westward movement still continues. Domestic dog rabies probably stemmed from infection in wild vertebrates. The first recorded sizable dog rabies outbreak was in Italy in 1708, and England had epizootic rabies in 1734.

Rabies virus probably evolved in the Old World, perhaps Africa or Asia. Rabies was unknown in the New World until 1753, when dogs in the colony of Virginia were infected, and in South America until 1803, when it occurred in dogs in Peru. Thus, the virus was probably imported into the New World in the 18th century. The existence in Africa of at least five viruses serologically related to rabies[53,61a] (see Sections 5.3 and 10.2) supports the hypothesis of its African origin with the parallel evolution of several related viruses. Rabies virus has now become widely established in wildlife in the Americas including vampire bats in South and Central America[25] and insectivorous bats in North America.[10]

Robert E. Shope · Department of Epidemiology and Public Health, Yale University School of Medicine, New Haven, Connecticut.

The history of rabies has been documented by a long series of observations relating to prevention, treatment, and laboratory diagnosis. Celsius in A.D. 100 treated rabies by cautery, and Galen in A.D. 200, by amputation. Zuike, in 1804, first transmitted rabies to a normal dog by inoculation of infected saliva. This observation led to institution of dog control and muzzle laws that resulted in elimination of rabies from Denmark, Norway, and Sweden by 1826. In 1879, Galtier[22] first used the domestic rabbit as a laboratory host, enabling the classic experiments in which Pasteur et al.[47] developed virus attenuated for the dog but having a uniform (fixed) incubation period in the rabbit. Pasteur subsequently used this virus, grown in rabbit spinal cords and dried for varying periods, to give virus doses graded from noninfectious to fully infectious for immunization of dogs and man.[46] The first vaccine in man was given in 1885 to a 12-year-old boy, and, because of early success, no controlled clinical trial of vaccine effectiveness has ever been carried out.

In 1903, Negri[43] described intracytoplasmic inclusion bodies in neurons of man and other vertebrate animals, facilitating the early diagnosis of rabies. In 1908, Fermi developed the first chemically treated vaccine, and in 1919, Semple showed that phenol could inactivate rabies virus without destroying antigenicity. The Semple vaccine has been used in man extensively for 50 years. In 1935, rabies immune serum was shown to be effective postexposure in preventing disease,[55] and in 1949, a live virus vaccine using the Flury strain of egg-adapted virus was developed for use in dogs.[37] Both killed and live virus vaccines are effective in preventing rabies in domestic animals. Their widespread use in the United States, and the introduction of the Habel test for vaccine standardization, has resulted since 1960 in excellent control of rabies in dogs and consequently a marked decrease in numbers of cases in man.

3. Methodology Involved in Epidemiological Analysis

3.1. Sources of Mortality Data

Rabies in man is a specified notifiable disease in the United States, and reporting is generally required in other countries. United States statistics for man and animal are compiled from state health departments by the National Rabies Surveillance Program of the Center for Disease Control (CDC) and are published in the *Mobidity and Mortality Weekly Report*. The World Health Organization (WHO), through the Veterinary Public Health Section, collects data from national governments on deaths in man, numbers of persons exposed, and numbers of doses of rabies vaccine administered. These data are distributed annually to national governments.

Death rates, where rabies is looked for, accurately represent incidence rates of infection in man and probably in animals because the disease, for statistical purposes, can be regarded as 100% fatal. Animals that develop disease usually die, but it is not clearly established whether or not naturally infected animals can develop antibodies and recover from or escape disease. Mortality data can be reliable, provided the diagnosis is made accurately. Underreporting is common in some parts of the world. For instance, there were estimated to be 400–500 human deaths from rabies in Thailand in 1966, more than 10 times the officially reported number.[32]

3.2. Sources of Morbidity Data

There are at least three documented cases in man of recovery from rabies.[9c,24,48b] Exposures and potential exposures to bites of rabid animals, however, are documented indirectly in some countries by recording of the number of vaccine doses sold or used. These estimates are crude, but are useful to show trends.

3.3. Serological Surveys

Serological surveys in man[50] and domestic[1] and wild animals have been done by the neutralization (N) test in mice,[29] by the indirect fluorescent-antibody (FA) test,[39] and by the Ouchterlony agar-gel precipitin test.[1] Serological surveys are infrequently used in the study of rabies epidemiology; those surveys reported in the literature should be interpreted with caution. Naturally occurring substances in sera neutralize or react with rabies virus, and these substances cannot a priori be considered to be antibody unless they are also shown to be localized in the immunoglobulin (Ig) fractions of serum. Rabies often has a long incubation period during which humoral antibody may appear in an animal that is later destined to become rabid.[8] The presence of antibody in animal sera does not necessarily mean, therefore, that inapparent rabies infection has occurred, as claimed by some.[16] On the other hand, Bell and co-workers have reported abortive rabies in laboratory experiments with mice[7] and have reviewed the evidence for inapparent infection and antibody formation in animals.[6]

The interpretation of survey results in Africa may also be complicated by the potential existence of cross-reacting heterologous antibody to rabies-related viruses,[53,61a] although such antibody has not yet been found in nature.

Detection of antibody responses to vaccination may be important in evaluating vaccines and in assessing risk in high-exposure populations. The rabies fluorescent focus-inhibition test[33,39] gives a rapid, reliable determination. Rabies antibody prevents the formation in tissue culture of foci of infected cells as visualized under the fluorescence microscope. This technique is not yet in general use for serological surveys, but should be equally useful as the mouse N test and quicker and less expensive. At present, there is no simple, specific, and inexpensive antibody test in use for rabies serological surveys of large populations.

3.4. Laboratory Methods

Since other forms of encephalitis may be confused with rabies, it is essential that epidemiological studies be based on carefully documented laboratory confirmation of disease or death from rabies virus infection. Laboratory techniques have evolved for more than 100 years, and while successful variations are in use in many laboratories, the standard techniques approved by the WHO Expert Committee on Rabies[33] are recommended and widely used. Included are methods for collection, preparation, and shipping rabies specimens; this WHO source and a review by H. N. Johnson[28] have been used freely in the following description. Methods include examination of brains for Negri bodies, laboratory-animal inoculation, use of FA for detection of rabies virus infection, and specific virus identification by FA and N tests. For regulations governing shipment of potentially infectious specimens, the local public-health laboratory should be consulted.

Negri bodies are cytoplasmic inclusions seen under the light microscope. They contain rabies ribonucleoprotein, which accumulates in quantities large enough to stain by the Sellers, Giemsa, or Mann method and be visualized. The Ammon's horn is the portion of the brain usually examined by smear. Artifacts and inclusions produced by other viruses can be differentiated only after considerable experience. Nevertheless, histopathological examination offers a diagnosis as quickly as 30 min after the laboratory receives a specimen. For epidemiological studies, confirmation of Negri bodies by FA or by animal inoculation and serological identification should be attempted, since in some laboratories histopathological diagnosis misses 15–20% of rabies infections.[33]

The weanling mouse is highly susceptible to rabies infection by intracerebral inoculation. The time from inoculation to illness varies from 4 days to 3 weeks, but the presence of rabies antigen in mouse brain may sometimes be confirmed much earlier by FA or complement-fixation tests. The identity of the suspected rabies isolate should always be determined serologically, because animals may die of intercurrent infection or as a result of infection by other viruses in the original specimen. In Africa, the identity of the suspected rabies isolate should be confirmed by N test rather than by the FA technique, since African viruses related to rabies cross-react significantly in the FA test.[53]

The direct FA test uses a fluorescein dye conjugated to rabies immune globulin, which in turn is reacted with a smear from the brain of the presumed rabid animal or person. The antigen–antibody reaction is detected by observing fluorescence under light of the appropriate wavelength. The test is rapid and as reliable as animal inoculation when used by an experienced worker. It should not supplant animal inoculation unless the operator is skilled and maintains adequate controls.

Diagnosis can sometimes be made during life by FA tests of skin biopsies taken usually from the buccal mucosa or nape of the neck where nerve plexi are prominent.[9a,38b] In about half of rabies cases, corneal cells obtained by touch impressions are FA-positive during life.[9f,57b]

Recent reports[38a,57a] of the isolation of field strains from saliva and from brain of a variety of rabid animals by inoculation of either BHK-21, CER, or mouse neuroblastoma cells appear promising. At this time, however, the mouse is the method of choice for primary isolation of rabies virus until more experience with cell cultures has accrued.

4. Biological Characteristics of the Virus That Affect the Epidemiological Pattern

The biological characteristics of rabies virus have a very definite although incompletely understood effect on the epidemiological pattern, especially in wildlife.

Rabies in man is a dead-end disease; man does not usually transmit or maintain the infection cycle. Biological properties of the virus that affect the epidemiology must therefore be properties referable to the domestic animal or wildlife cycle. The incubation period is long—Debbie[15] cites ranges in animals from 10 to 209 days of the natural infection, and in man exceptionally as long as 3 years, with 4–10% 6 months or longer. The long incubation period in dogs is responsible for the ease of introduction of rabies into rabies-free areas. Because of the long incubation period in wildlife, smoldering epizootics allow time for new susceptible offspring to enter a population so that the virus continually has fertile ground for maintenance of the cycle. In Europe, the spread of fox rabies from east to west is gradual (30 km/yr), and this can be related to the approximate distance that young infected animals range during the long incubation period.

Two other biological properties—neurotropism and shedding from exocrine glands in dogs, cats, and wildlife—account for the unique mode of transmission via saliva following bites. As R. T. Johnson has written, "No other virus is so diabolically adapted to selective neuronal populations that it can drive the host in a fury to transmit the virus to another host animal."[31] Here, he refers to the selective relative localization of lesions to the limbic system and the transmission through bite via infected saliva.

Biological properties of the virus also undoubtedly account for some of the unexplained apparent contradictions in the epidemiology of rabies. For instance, data collected by the U.S. Public Health Service indicate that there is relative geographic compartmentalization of rabies to a single animal species.[26] Where rabies occurs in skunks (Califor-

nia, midwestern United States), there is little or no fox rabies; where rabies occurs in foxes (southeastern United States), there is a scarcity of skunk rabies; where raccoons are infected (Florida and Georgia), there is little infection in other wildlife populations. There appears to be a predilection of the virus of a given geographic area to one animal and even to a single species of that animal, as in Virginia, where infection of the gray fox was more common than infection of the red fox.[9b] Sikes[56] has given a plausible explanation for such compartmentalization: A strain of virus from a fox has biological properties such that (1) it requires 100 times less virus to infect a fox than a skunk and (2) if a fox is infected with a large dose, the fox develops a rapidly progressive disease and dies before the salivary glands have time to become infected. Thus, most of the foxes that transmit rabies have relatively low virus titers in the saliva—titers high enough to infect other foxes, but not skunks.

The epidemiology of rabies in bat caves may also be influenced by a little-understood biological property of rabies-virus strains of bats—a predilection for nasal mucosa.[12] The spread of these strains by the airborne route in bat caves may explain transmission of rabies virus to persons who entered Frio Cave, Texas, where the air was subsequently shown to contain rabies virus.[67] Recently, a bat isolate spread among foxes in an airborne epizootic in a laboratory building.[69]

5. Descriptive Epidemiology

5.1. Incidence

The number of human rabies cases in most areas is directly related to the prevalence of rabid dogs. In the United States, where dog rabies was controlled by a highly effective vaccination program and by leash laws, human rabies dropped from 33 cases reported in 1946 to 3 or fewer cases per year since 1962.[26] This striking decrease in human rabies is shown in Fig. 1. In other parts of the world where dog rabies is still prevalent, such as parts of South America, Africa, and Asia, human rabies still constitutes a major public-health problem. Concomitantly with the decrease in dog rabies has come a decrease in the reported cases of rabies in domestic animals and an increase in reported cases in wild

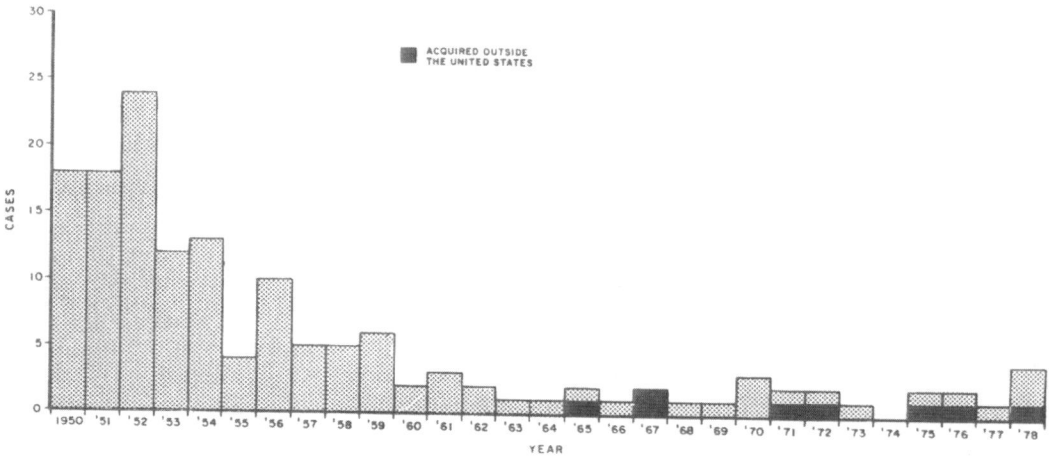

Fig. 1. Reported cases of rabies in humans by year, United States, 1950–1978.

animals (Fig. 2). The increase in rabies of wild animals may reflect better recognition.

In some parts of Africa, because of an unusual virus biotype that produces paralytic or dumb rabies in dogs rather than the furious type, the dogs do not transmit frequently to man. This type of rabies is referred to as *Oulou Fato*.

Where dog rabies is controlled, the incidence in man relates almost entirely to exposure to wildlife. In the United States between 1946 and 1950, nearly all the 94 human rabies cases were traced to rabid dogs and cats. Between 1951 and 1970, dog- and cat-transmitted rabies virtually disappeared; skunks were responsible for 10 rabies deaths in man between 1951 and 1970, foxes 6, and bats 7.[68] Skunks commonly live near man and have been sold as household pets. One study of 69 skunks sold as pets showed that 80 of 366 persons in contact with the pet skunks were bitten, and 15 of these people received postexposure rabies prophylaxis.[23]

During 1977, 3182 rabid animals were reported in the United States and areas under its jurisdiction[9d]; the percentage distribution in Puerto Rico and 47 states was as follows: skunks, 51%; bats, 20%; rac-

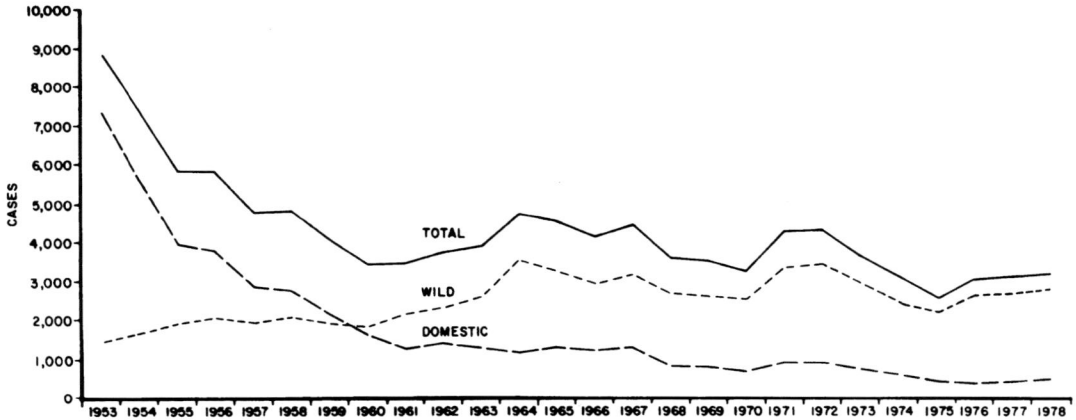

Fig. 2. Reported cases of rabies in wild and domestic animals by year, United States, 1953–1978.

coons, 9%; cattle, 6%; dogs, 4%; foxes, 4%; cats, 3%; and others, 3%.

A minority of persons bitten by a rabid animal become infected, and it is also possible that one can be infected without developing disease. Factors that influence the initiation of infection and the incubation period are those that influence the dose of virus transmitted, such as the titer of virus in saliva and whether the bite was through clothing. In addition, the threshold of infection (the titer needed to initiate infection) varies with the host species and with the individual strain of virus.[56] If the skin is broken at the time of exposure, infection is much more likely to occur.

Detection of serological positive reactions in apparently normal animals and persons[1,8,50] has been reported on rare occasions, but the reactive substances have not usually been shown to be in the Ig fraction of sera, and thus the validity of these results is in doubt.

5.2. Epidemic Behavior

Rabies epidemics are of two types: (1) cases resulting from a single rabid animal biting several people in series and (2) cases resulting from geographically localized increase of rabies in a domestic or wild animal population, the infection spilling over into the human population.

The first type of epidemic is well illustrated by the now famous episode in 1954 in which a rabid wolf in Iran attacked 29 persons, inflicting severe head wounds.[5] This afforded the first opportunity to test the efficacy of rabies immune serum as an adjunct to vaccine postexposure treatment.

The dynamics of the second type of epidemics are poorly understood. Epizootics in wild animals have historically swept over large areas,[28] infecting people where contact with wild animals occurred. The distribution of the epizootics did not necessarily conform to that of susceptible animal populations, and their cessation was not related to public-health control measures as far as is known. Areas of infection appear to be limited in part by topography such as bodies of water and mountain ranges.[9b] The behavioral and mobility patterns of the animal species, its eating and biting habits, the availability of vegetation and meat sources, and the stress of inclement weather or extending foraging practices undoubtedly affect the incidence and spread of ra-

bies in nature, but the interplay and separate importance of these factors have not been carefully evaluated.

5.3. Geographic Distribution

The distribution of rabies in man is directly related to its distribution in wild and domestic animals. In the United States, rabies occurs in bats in all 48 contiguous states. Skunks, foxes, raccoons, and several less frequently infected animals serve as reservoirs of infection in different parts of the country. In Alaska, the arctic fox is the reservoir, transmitting to sled dogs, wolves, and coyotes.

In South and Central America, dog and cattle rabies is widespread. Vampire bats are an important reservoir; it is likely that nearly a million cattle die each year of vampire-bat-transmitted rabies in Latin America, and losses are estimated at $250,000,000 annually.[60] The mongoose is also a reservoir of rabies in Puerto Rico, Cuba, and Grenada, although not in Trinidad.

In Southeast Asia, dog rabies is highly enzootic except in Japan, Taiwan, and Okinawa, where rabies does not occur. Wild animals in some parts of Southeast Asia such as the Philippine Islands are apparently not infected with rabies virus despite high infection rates in domestic dogs. This lack of a wildlife reservoir has led some to propose that eradication of rabies in the Philippines, which has the highest attack rate of human rabies in the world, is feasible.[2a]

Eastern and central Europe are currently involved in a major outbreak of fox rabies that has now spread into Switzerland and France. North Africa has enzootic dog rabies, and in sub-Saharan Africa, the jackal, the yellow mongoose, the cape polecat, the weasel, and the civet cat, in addition to the dog, are known to be rabid.[28]

There are five viruses serologically related to rabies that can be distinguished in the laboratory. These viruses occur in sub-Saharan Africa. They include Lagos bat, Mokola, and kotonkan viruses in Nigeria; Obodhiang virus in Sudan; and Duvenhage virus in South Africa. Kemp et al.[35] have postulated that antibody to a rabies-related virus in the cattle population of West Africa could account for the rarity of observed rabies in cattle in that region.[35]

Several areas are free of rabies either because of their island status or because of strict quarantine and dog control. These include Australia, New Zealand, Japan, Hawaii, the British Isles, and much of Scandinavia.

5.4. Temporal Distribution

Rabies occurs throughout the year. However, peak numbers of rabid animals in the United States are found in the spring or, in some areas, in the winter. This seasonality is preceded by dispersal of young susceptible animals and coincides with the breeding season.[8,9b] Human exposures are common in the summer, and this may relate to the period in which people enjoy peak outdoor activity.

5.5. Age, Sex, Race, Occupation, Socioeconomic, Nutritional, and Genetic Factors

Rabies occurs more commonly in children than in adults. This may be a result of increased susceptibility in the young, but is more fully explained by the greater contact of children with dogs and wildlife, the uninhibited curiosity of children, and their inability to evade a rabid animal. By the same token, male children are more likely to be exposed than female children. There do not appear to be racial, genetic, nutritional, or socioeconomic differences in susceptibility to rabies virus. Members of certain occupations such as veterinarians, laboratory workers, and persons living in developing tropical areas are at higher risk of rabies exposure.

6. Mechanisms and Route of Transmission

Rabies is transmitted by the bite of rabid animals. Intact skin protects against virus entry,[28] although infection may occur through small cuts and scratches or by way of mucous membranes. The chances of infection are believed to be less if the bite occurs through clothing. Virus appears in the saliva of dogs and other animals in most cases only shortly before disease is evident and not before infection of the brain. Fekadu,[20] however, has reported in dogs what must be a rare exception: five animals survived from 9 to 39 months after first isolation of rabies virus from their saliva. While one dog died of rabies and another of pneumonia, three were still alive and apparently well for at least 2 years. Rabies virus was isolated repeatedly from these animals. Bell[6] has suggested that some rabies strains in Africa are attenuated with "accommodation between host and virus."

The offspring of one of these dogs developed rabies, and the possibility of transplacental or milk-borne infection must be entertained. Transplacental transmission in a naturally infected cow has been reported.[40]

Oral transmission through ingestion of rabies-contaminated meat has been amply demonstrated in experimental animals,[21,58] and Charles Darwin, in *The Voyage of the Beagle*, described possible cases of rabies in men in Peru after they consumed the meat of a rabid bullock.[13] The oral route of infection might explain natural transmission to carnivores that frequently eat sick or dead rabid animals.

Airborne transmission of rabies has been shown experimentally in the laboratory,[67] and by an elegant experiment by Constantine,[11] who showed infection of foxes and coyotes to occur when they were placed in a tightly meshed wire cage in bat-occupied Frio Cave, near Uvalde, Texas. This seems to explain how rabies occurred in two men who entered Frio Cave in 1956 and 1958.[27] In 1977, a laboratory worker who was exposed to aerosolized rabies virus subsequently developed rabies.[9c]

Transmission by apparently healthy animal carriers or by the oral, milk-borne, and airborne routes must be considered unusual and relatively unimportant from the point of view of human infection or the transmission of rabies by dogs and cats. Strong evidence indicating that dog and cat bites are the important route in human rabies is the near elimination of human rabies in the United States by effective vaccination of pets and by leash laws.

Cattle rabies in Latin America remains the major economic rabies problem in the New World. This disease is transmitted primarily by vampire bats, which maintain the infection in the bat population as a closed cycle with approximately 1% of normal-appearing vampire bats infected at any time.[10] The bats probably maintain the cycle by biting each other; the transmission of bat rabies to cattle and occasionally to man occurs secondary to natural feeding and does not necessitate the bats' being furious or sick. Bats reportedly[48] have virus in their saliva for more than 3 months after infection, but the mechanism by which the bat remains infected and without disease, while other animals regularly become sick following infection, is not well understood.

In 1978, a case of surgical transmission of rabies occurred in a woman who received a corneal transplant from a man who died of rabies.[26a] In addition, physicians and veterinarians have inadvertently transmitted rabies virus by needle, giving improperly inactivated vaccine to man [45] or incompletely attenuated vaccine to dogs.[48a]

7. Pathogenesis and Immunity

Naturally occurring (street) rabies virus buds from the endothelial reticulum in the cytoplasm of the neuron and not, as in some other viral infections of the CNS, from the plasma membrane.[41] Cell structure remains intact, and in 14.6% of the brains examined in one study of human cases, inflammation was absent.[17]

Until recently, it was believed that the virus failed to multiply at the site of introduction. There was no rise in virus titer demonstrable in muscle tissue[7] and antigen could not be visualized at the inoculation site.[30] However, Murphy et al.[42] have now shown by the FA technique that antigen is present in muscle cells of hamsters at 36 hr postinoculation. This is before antigen is demonstrable by fluorescence methods in other parts of the body, including the CNS.

Rabies virus spreads via the axoplasm centripetally along peripheral nerves to ganglia or to the CNS. Experiments in mice show that amputation of the inoculated limb prevents spread of infection and saves the animal. In mice infected with street virus, amputation done as long as 18 days after inoculation still permits animal survival.[4] Virus multiplication occurs next in the ganglia serving the nerves from the inoculation site.

The CNS is invaded, and rapid spread occurs by either nerve pathways, cerebrospinal fluid (CSF), or both. Within hours, the virus becomes detectable throughout the CNS and later in virtually all organs of the body. Viremia at this stage has been detected but is a rare event and is of too low a titer to have epidemiological significance.

The salivary glands of most rabid animals become infected during the period before onset of signs. Dogs, cats, and skunks shed virus in saliva 1–3 days before disease appears, and in some animals, the titer of virus in salivary glands considerably exceeds that in brain.[52] Virus is also found in the respiratory tract, the kidneys, and the milk of infected animals, but these sites are not usually implicated in the spread of rabies to man.

The widespread distribution of rabies antigen in man just prior to the onset of disease has been the basis of tests for early diagnosis. For example, FA methods to detect antigen in skin biopsies, buccal mucosa, and corneal tissue may sometimes yield a positive diagnosis before clinical disease develops. However, a negative test does not rule out rabies infection.

Antibody may be found in serum at the onset of illness. N antibody appears in high titer in the brain and CSF of infected individuals[7] and is considered a reliable indication of a CNS infection. There is no doubt that humoral antibody prolongs the incubation period of rabies infection, as demonstrated by passive immunization in experimental animals.[4] The question has been asked, however, whether the immune reaction may in some instances be detrimental and actually contribute to the pathogenesis of clinical disease.[38] Monkeys that were inoculated with relatively poor antibody-inducing vaccines following exposure to rabies virus died earlier than rabies-infected animals not given vaccine.[57] Tignor et al.[62] have demonstrated in mice that immunosuppression induced by drugs and by thymectomy and irradiation can prolong the incubation period in experimentally infected animals and that administration of antibody can induce an early death associated with inflammatory lesions of the neurons in rabies-infected animals. This suggests that clinical rabies may involve an immunopathological mechanism of disease.

8. Patterns of Host Response

8.1 Clinical Features

Rabies is often cited in epidemiological teaching as the classic example of an infection that is universally fatal and in which no inapparent-to-apparent ratio exists. There are, however, many anecdotal reports and some clear evidence disputing this, as reviewed by Bell.[6] Bats have been reported to have long-term inapparent infection accompanied by virus shedding[48]; foxes may survive experimental infection and develop rabies antibody and resistance to challenge[56]; and normal-appearing dogs have been reported to shed virus in saliva for as long as 2 years.[2,20,63] In addition to inapparent infections, abortive infections also occur; three well-established cases of survival with recovery in man have been reported.[9c,24,48b]

It is not known where or in what form the virus resides during at least part of the incubation period. If the clinical disease, rabies, has an immunological basis (i.e., antigen–antibody reaction), instead of being the consequence of a direct lytic effect of the virus, then the long period between exposure and disease in dogs, man, and other animals might represent an inapparent infection with a delayed immunological response, rather than a long incubation period in the traditional sense. Admittedly, there are other rational explanations for the long incubation period,[4] but if delayed immunological response exists, there could be many unrecognized infections of this type, especially among the many people who, although bitten by proved rabid animals, never become ill. The regular employment of rabies vaccine in man following exposure does not permit differentiation of humoral antibody to vaccine from humoral antibody to natural infection. Thus, inapparent infections could go undetected.

Rabies is a neurotropic illness, and the signs relate to neurological functions. A prodromal stage lasting 2–4 days includes moderate fever, malaise, loss of appetite, headache, and nausea. Presenting symptoms include hyperexcitability, and pain and tightness in the chest; aerophobia (spasms of the pharyngeal muscles elicited by fanning the face) is a useful sign to confirm the diagnosis.[66a] There may be pain or other abnormal sensation at the site of the original wound; unusual sensitivity to light, noise, or sensory stimulation may follow; and increased muscle tension and tics are common. The sympathetic nervous system is often involved in the form of increased sweating, salivation, or lacrimation. Excitement manifested both by maniacal behavior, anxiety, and painful muscle contractions in spasms (often precipitated by swallowing and called "hydrophobia") and by paralytic signs may be seen during different stages of the disease. Ascending paralysis, especially in bat-transmitted rabies, has been described. Death after 2–6 days may be secondary to respiratory or cardiac failure and is often

signaled by a convulsion. The patient is usually alert throughout most of the illness.

8.2. Diagnosis

The differential diagnosis includes poliomyelitis, tetanus, herpes encephalitis, arboviral encephalitis, tularemia, and (in Africa) the rabies-related viruses Mokola and Duvenhage, which cause CNS disease in man. The diagnosis during life may be established by FA staining of corneal impressions, mucosal scrapings, skin biopsy, or brain biopsy. A rise in antibody titer may be diagnostic if the patient has not received vaccine or serum treatment. After death, the demonstration of Negri bodies, isolation of virus in mice, or the finding of specific antigen in brain or other tissues by the FA technique reliably makes the diagnosis. In animals, the use of FA examination of the brain has permitted early diagnosis; suckling mice are also highly susceptible to infection, but may take up to 3 weeks to develop disease, thus delaying diagnosis. The nearest public-health laboratory should be consulted about the collection and shipment of specimens as well as the management of the exposed person.

9. Control and Prevention

9.1. Epidemiological Methods

Effective control of human rabies in the United States and much of Europe was achieved by dog and cat measures that included leash laws, licensing of dogs, and administration of killed or live attenuated vaccines.

The spread of rabies into susceptible areas such as Great Britain, Scandinavia, Australia, New Zealand, Hawaii, and Taiwan is prevented by vaccination and strict quarantine of imported animals prior to or on entry into the country. Since the incubation period of rabies may be 6 months or longer, animals must have continued surveillance even after the quarantine, and care must be taken that exposure to a rabid animal does not occur in the quarantine facility.

It is not possible to eradicate rabies in the New World, Africa, or much of Asia and Europe where wildlife reservoirs occur. Depopulation of infected wildlife populations serves to control rabies temporarily and is justified where potentially rabid animals are frequently in contact with people, i.e., around campsites and garbage dumps. However, depopulation by vacating of previously occupied territory also allows more of the young vigorous animals to grow up and thrive. These same young animals are highly susceptible, and unless the control measures are enforced to the point of marked population reduction, depopulation is not successful.

An alternative suggestion that has been successful experimentally is vaccination of wildlife using oral vaccines contained in animal bait.[3] This appears to be a feasible procedure, but the safety to nontarget animals of infected bait distributed in the environment has not yet been established.

Of the insectivorous bats submitted for rabies diagnosis in the United States, it is common to find

10% or more positive.[17a,64] Bats may cohabit houses and may become a serious public-health hazard and, equally important, a severe psychological threat to a family. The commonly implicated bat is the big brown bat, which is controlled by application of DDT as a dust or less effectively as a 6% spray. The treatment is followed by structural improvements to prevent reentry of bats into the home.[64] Permits to use DDT are issued only after state authorities receive approval from the CDC.

9.2. Immunization Concepts and Practice

The management of susceptible persons following exposure is outlined in Tables 1 and 2 according to recommendations of the CDC.[9e] Effective prevention of infection is achieved by thorough cleansing of the wound immediately after the bite. Soap and

Table 1. Rabies Postexposure Prophylaxis Guide—March 1980[a]

The following recommendations are only a guide. In applying them, take into account the animal species involved, the circumstances of the bite or other exposure, the vaccination status of the animal, and the presence of rabies in the region. *Local or state public-health officials should be consulted if questions arise about the need for rabies prophylaxis.*

Animal species	Condition of animal at time of attack	Treatment of exposed person[b]
Domestic		
Dog and cat	Healthy and available for 10 days of observation	None, unless animal develops rabies[c]
	Rabid or suspected rabid	RIG[d] and HDCV[e]
	Unknown (escaped)	Consult public health officials. If treatment is indicated, give RIG[d] and HDCV.[c]
Wild		
Skunk, bat, fox, coyote, raccoon, bobcat, and other carnivores	Regard as rabid unless proven negative by laboratory tests.[f]	RIG[d] and HDCV[e]
Other		
Livestock, rodents, and lagomorphs (rabbits and hares)	Consider individually. Local and state public-health officials should be consulted on questions about the need for rabies prophylaxis. Bites of squirrels, hamsters, guinea pigs, gerbils, chipmunks, rats, mice, other rodents, rabbits, and hares almost never call for antirabies prophylaxis.	

[a] From the CDC.[9e]

[b] *All bites and wounds should immediately be thoroughly cleansed with soap and water.* If antirabies treatment is indicated, both rabies immune globulin (RIG[d]) and human diploid-cell rabies vaccine (HDCV[e]) should be given as soon as possible, *regardless* of the interval from exposure.

[c] During the usual holding period of 10 days, begin treatment with RIG[d] and vaccine (preferably with HDCV[e]) at first sign of rabies in a dog or cat that has bitten someone. The symptomatic animal should be killed immediately and tested.

[d] If RIG is not available, use antirabies serum, equine (ARS). Do not use more than the recommended dosage.

[e] If HDCV is not available, use duck-embryo vaccine (DEV). Local reactions to vaccines are common and do not contraindicate continuing treatment. Discontinue vaccine if fluorescent-antibody (FA) tests of the animal are negative.

[f] The animal should be killed and tested as soon as possible. Holding for observation is not recommended.

Table 2. Rabies Immunization Regiments—March 1980[a]

Rabies vaccine	Number of 1-ml doses	Route of administration	Intervals between doses	If no antibody response to primary series, give[b]:
Preexposure: Preexposure rabies, prophylaxis for persons with special risks of exposure to rabies, such as animal-care and control personnel and selected laboratory workers, consists of immunization with either human diploid-cell rabies vaccine (HDCV) or duck-embryo vaccine (DEV), according to the following schedule.				
HDCV	3	Intramuscular	1 week between 1st and 2nd; 2–3 weeks between 2nd and 3rd[c]	1 booster dose[c]
DEV	3	Subcutaneous	1 month between 1st and 2nd; 6–7 months between 2nd and 3rd[c]	2 booster doses, 1 week apart[c]
	or		or	
	4		1 week between 1st, 2nd, and 3rd; 3 months between 3rd and 4th[c]	
Postexposure: Postexposure rabies prophylaxis for persons exposed to rabies consists of the immediate, through cleansing of all wounds with soap and water, administration of rabies immune globulin (RIG) or, if RIG is not available, antirabies serum, equine (ARS), and the initiation of either HDCV or DEV, according to the following schedule.[d]				
HDCV	5[e]	Intramuscular	Doses to be given on days 0, 3, 7, 14, and 28[c]	1 additional booster dose[c]
DEV	23	Subcutaneous	21 daily doses followed by a booster on day 31 and another on day 41[c]	3 doses of HDCV at weekly intervals[c]
			or	
			2 daily doses in the first 7 days, followed by 7 daily doses; then 1 booster on day 24, and another on day 34[c]	

[a] From the CDC.[(9e)]
[b] If no antibody response is documented after the recommended additional booster dose(s), consult the state health department or the CDC.
[c] Serum for rabies antibody testing should be collected 2–3 weeks after the last dose.
[d] The postexposure regimen is greatly modified for someone with previously demonstrated rabies antibody (see reference 9e for details).
[e] The WHO recommends a 6th dose 90 days after the 1st dose.

water is an excellent preventative in experimental rabies exposures.[(14)] Quarternary ammonium compounds and rabies immune serum are equally effective. Saline, however, is not recommended; substances that actually bind or neutralize the virus or physically destroy receptor sites appear to be required for preventing infection.

Human immune globulin is now commercially available in the United States (Hyperab,® Cutter Laboratories, Berkeley, California) and should be administered intramuscularly in a dose of 20 IU/kg, with one half the dose being infiltrated around the wound. Alternatively, where horse serum is substituted for human globulin, it should be given at 40 IU/kg. Appropriate tests for sensitivity to horse serum should be carried out before administration.

Inactivated vaccines are administered immediately after serum therapy. Nervous-tissue vaccines are used successfully in much of the world; in the United States, human diploid-cell vaccine (HDCV) became available in 1980 and is administered according to the schedule in Table 2. Prior to 1980, duck-embryo vaccine (DEV) was used almost exclusively because of the low rate of neurological complications following its use.

Preexposure vaccination (Table 2) is recommended for people who because of their profession or avocation are at high risk. These include veterinarians, hunters, campers, laboratory workers, and persons (especially children) living in areas of the world where dog and cat rabies is not controlled. Serum should be tested for rabies antibody 2–3 weeks after the last inoculation. Testing can be arranged through state health departments. Booster doses should be given at least every 2 years unless antibody titer remains satisfactory. When an immunized person who has developed antibody is exposed to rabies, the person should be revaccinated with HDCV immediately and 3 days later, or with DEV in 5 daily doses plus a booster dose 20 days after the fifth daily injection. Immune globulin should not be given.

There are risks involved in the use of both vaccine and immune horse serum. Actual transmission of rabies virus through an inadvertent failure to inactivate the vaccine properly has occurred,[36] and demyelinating disease and both local and generalized allergic reactions following DEV and nervous-tissue vaccines are reported.[49] With nervous-tissue vaccines, it is estimated that from 1:600 to 1:8000 persons develop neurological complications and 1:35,000 die. With DEV, 1:25,000 are reported to have neurological complications and 1:225,000 die.[49] The DEV, while safer, does not induce N antibody as well as nervous-tissue vaccines or as well as the new HDCV that is available and widely used with rabies immune globulin in Europe and Asia,[4a] and that in 1980 was licensed in the United States. Serum sickness and severe skin reactions (avoidable by using human rabies immune globulin) have been recorded in 16.3% of persons given antiserum prepared in horses.[34] Because of these risks and the expense of postexposure treatment, it is important to establish that the biting animal was or was not rabid. If laboratory tests are negative, or if the biting animal is of a species that can reasonably be judged not to carry rabies, or if rabies is known to be absent from that community or country, then treatment should not be given; New York City and Philadelphia changed their health codes in 1975 to discourage rabies treatment of persons bitten by cats and dogs, since rabies had not been reported in dogs and cats for more than 20 years in these cities.

While immune serum in conjunction with vaccination is believed to be highly effective in prevention following exposure, the risk of horse serum must be carefully weighed against the risk of developing rabies.

10. Unresolved Problems

10.1. Epizootiology of Wildlife Rabies

Wildlife rabies constitutes the major reservoir and the source of most exposures of man in the United States and much of Europe today. Populations of foxes, skunks, raccoons, coyotes, and bats are infected, often in apparently compartmentalized epizootics, i.e., without very much transmission between different populations. Studies of the incidence of rabies in these populations, the means by which the virus is transmitted among animals, the incubation periods and the prevalence of transplacental infection, the occurrence of abortive infection and of carrier states, and the frequency and duration of shedding of virus in the saliva are all needed. A special situation may exist in Czechoslovakia and other parts of Europe, where rabies in rodents has been reported in a cycle separate from that in foxes.[59] More information is needed to understand this cycle and its possible implications as a permanent reservoir should rabies in foxes be controlled eventually in neighboring regions.

10.2. Rabies-Related Viruses

There are five viruses serologically related to rabies but easily distinguished by their antigenic properties: (1) Lagos bat, isolated from *Eidolon helvum* in Lagos, Nigeria[9]; (2) Mokola, from *Crocidura* spp. shrews in Ibadan, Nigeria[54]; (3) Duvenhage, from brain of a man bitten on the lip by a bat, in South Africa[61a]; (4) kotonkan, from *Culicoides* midges in Ibadan, Nigeria[35]; and (5) Obodhiang, from *Mansonia uniformis* mosquitos in Sudan.[51] These viruses appear to be limited in their geographic distribution to regions of Africa and limited in their host range to specific animals or insects. Duvenhage infects man in South Africa, and alert physicians in Nigeria have diagnosed two cases of Mokola virus infection in children—one a fatal poliomyelitislike illness[19] and the other a nonfatal one with febrile convulsions.[18] Important questions remain to be answered: Are rabies-related viruses limited to Africa? How often is man infected? How are these viruses transmitted in nature, and how are they transmitted to man? What is the role of arthropods in their natural cycles? Will rabies vaccines prevent Duvenhage and Mokola virus infections in man?

10.3. Vaccines

The further development of inexpensive, safe, potent vaccines for man that could be given in a shorter regimen is needed throughout the world. A new HDCV[66] is effective postexposure when given in conjunction with rabies antibody[4a] and represents an important advance. This vaccine, however, is still too expensive for use in many areas of the world. The observation that effective vaccines also induce interferon[4,65] has suggested that interferon might be effective as adjunct to postexposure administration of commerical vaccines. Both exogenous and endogenous interferon should be tried.

Oral vaccines for wildlife and for feral dogs and cats have been developed experimentally.[3] There is a need for continued research on oral vaccines to increase their potency, stability, and field-delivery facility and to test and ensure their safety to nontarget animals in the field.

Many developing countries where rabies exists also lack adequate diagnostic facilities, vaccine programs for domestic animals, effective surveillance, and the means of producing their own vaccine and sera. Standardization of potency and of safety of these materials on an international basis is required.

10.4. Pathogenesis and Virulence

If it were possible to understand the pathogenesis of rabies, one might interrupt the infection process by chemical or immunological means. Clearly, no treatment or cure for the disease is now in sight. However in laboratory animals, the incubation period can be prolonged by immunosuppression,[62] and induction of antibody in both rabies-infected animals[57] and man[44] is sometimes associated with death earlier than expected. Careful studies are needed to assess the role of interferon, defective-interfering virus, temperature-sensitive virus, complement, cell-mediated immunity, and humoral immunity in the pathogenesis of rabies.

Neither do we understand what changes occur in rabies virus when it becomes fixed or attenuated. Perhaps if it were possible to find or to derive a strain of virus that was immunogenic and at the same time was not neurotropic, a live virus vaccine for man could be developed. Solid advances have been made recently: it has been shown that the diploid-cell killed vaccine can be effective, that inter-

feron is a promising adjunct to vaccine, and that tissue culture can be useful for isolation of field strains. Perhaps it is not too much to expect that research on pathogenesis and virulence may eventually lead to control and treatment of rabies.

11. References

1. AFSHAR, A., AND BAHMANYAR, M., A contribution to the detection of inapparent rabies in stray dogs, *Vet. Rec.* **91**:562–565 (1972).
2. ANDRAL, L., AND SERIE, C., Etudes experimentales sur la rage in Ethiopie, *Ann. Inst. Pasteur* **93**:475–488 (1957).
2a. ARAMBULO, P. V., III, BERAN, G. W., ESCUDERO, S. H., II, AND STEELE, J. H., Rabies in the Republic of the Philippines: With notes on its field control and possible eradication, *Acta Med. Philipp.* **10**:20–37 (1974).
3. BAER, G. M., ABELSETH, M. K., AND DEBBIE, J. G., Oral vaccination of foxes against rabies, *Am. J. Epidemiol.* **93**:487–490 (1971).
4. BAER, G. M., AND CLEARY, W. F., A model in mice for the pathogenesis and treatment of rabies, *J. Infect. Dis.* **125**:520–527 (1972).
4a. BAHMANYAR, M., FAYZ, A., NOUR-SALEHI, S., MOHAMMADI, M., AND KOPROWSKI, H., Successful protection of humans exposed to rabies infection, *J. Am. Med. Assoc.* **236**:2751–2754 (1976).
5. BALTAZARD, M., AND BAHMANYAR, M., Essai pratique du serum antirabique chez les mordus par loups enrages, *Bull. WHO* **13**:747–772 (1955).
6. BELL, J. F., Latency and abortive rabies, in: *The Natural History of Rabies*, Vol. 1 (G. M. BAER, ed.), pp. 331–354, Academic Press, New York, 1975.
7. BELL, J. F., LODMELL, D. L., MOORE, G. J., AND RAYMOND, G. H., Brain neutralization in rabies virus to distinguish recovered animals from previously vaccinated animals, *J. Immunol.* **97**:747–753 (1966).
8. BIGLER, W. J., MCLEAN, R. G., AND TREVINO, H. A., Epizootiologic aspects of raccoon rabies in Florida, *Am. J. Epidemiol.* **93**:326–335 (1973).
9. BOULGER, L. R., AND PORTERFIELD, J. S., Isolation of a virus from Nigerian fruit bats, *Trans. R. Soc. Trop. Med. Hyg.* **52**:421–424 (1958).
9a. BRYCESON, A. D. M., GREENWOOD, B. M., AND WARREL, D. A., Demonstration during life of rabies antigen in humans, *J. Infect. Dis.* **131**:71–74 (1975).
9b. CAREY, A. B., GILFS, R. H., JR., AND MCLEAN, R. G., The landscape epidemiology of rabies in Virginia, *Am. J. Trop. Med. Hyg.* **27**:573–580 (1978).
9c. CENTER FOR DISEASE CONTROL, *Rabies Surveillance January–June 1977* (issued February 1978).

9d. CENTER FOR DISEASE CONTROL, *Morbidity and Mortality Weekly Report* **27**:499–500 (1978).

9e. CENTER FOR DISEASE CONTROL, *Morbidity and Mortality Weekly Report* **29**:265–280 (1980).

9f. CIFUENTES, E., CALDERON, E., AND BIJLENGA, G., Rabies in a child diagnosed by a new intra-vitam method: The cornea test, *J. Trop. Med. Hyg.* **74**:23–25 (1971).

10. CONSTANTINE, D. G., Bat rabies: Current knowledge and future research, in: *Rabies* (Y. NAGANO AND F. M. DAVENPORT, eds.), pp. 253–262, University of Tokyo Press, Tokyo, 1971.

11. CONSTANTINE, D. G., Rabies transmission by non-bite route, *Public Health Rep.* **77**:287–289 (1962).

12. CONSTANTINE, D. G., EMMONS, R. W., AND WOODIE, J. D., Rabies virus in nasal mucosa of naturally infected bats, *Science* **175**:1255–1256 (1972).

13. DARWIN, C., Cited in BELL, J. F., AND MOORE, G. J., Susceptibility of Carnivora to rabies virus administered orally, *Am. J. Epidemiol.* **93**:176–182 (1971).

14. DEAN, D. J., BAER, G. M., AND THOMPSON, W. R., Studies on the local treatment of rabies-infected wounds, *Bull. WHO* **28**:277–486 (1963).

15. DEBBIE, J. G., Rabies, *Prog. Med. Virol.* **18**:241–256 (1974).

16. DOEGE, T. C., AND NORTHROP, R. L., Evidence for inapparent rabies infection, *Lancet* **2**:826–829 (1974).

17. DUPONT, J. R., AND EARLE, K. M., Human rabies encephalitis: A study of forty-nine fatal cases with a review of the literature, *Neurology* **15**:1024–1034 (1965).

17a. EVANS, A. S., Rabies in Wisconsin, *Wisc. Med. J.* **62**:329–333 (1963).

18. FAMILUSI, J. B., AND MOORE, D. L., Isolation of rabies-related virus from the cerebrospinal fluid of a child with aseptic meningitis, *Afr. J. Med. Sci.* **3**:93–96 (1972).

19. FAMILUSI, J. B., OSUNKOYA, B. O., MOORE, D. L., KEMP, G. E., AND FABIYI, A., A fatal human infection with Mokola virus, *Am. J. Trop. Med. Hyg.* **21**:959–963 (1972).

20. FEKADU, M., Atypical rabies in dogs in Ethiopia, *Ethiopian Med. J.* **10**:79–86 (1972).

21. FISCHMAN, H. R., AND WARD, F. E., III, Oral transmission of rabies virus in experimental animals, *Am. J. Epidemiol.* **88**:132–138 (1968).

22. GALTIER, V., Etudes sur la rage, *C. R. Acad. Sci.* **89**:444–446 (1879).

23. HATTWICK, M. A. W., MARCUSE, E. K., BRITT, M. R., ZEHMER, R. B., CURRIER, R. W., II, AND ELLEDGE, W. N., Skunk rabies: The risk to man—or never trust a skunk, *Am. J. Public Health* **63**:1080–1084 (1973).

24. HATTWICK, M. A. W., WEIS, T. T., STECHSCHULTE, J., BAER, G. M., AND GREGG, M. B., Recovery from rabies: A case report, *Ann. Intern. Med.* **76**:931–942 (1972).

25. HAUPT, H., AND REHAAG, H., Durch Fledermäuse ver-

breitete seuchenhafte Tollwut unter Viehbeständen in Santa Catharina (Süd-Brasilien), *Z. Infectionskr. Haustiers* **22**:76–88, 104–127 (1921).

26. HELD, J. R., TIERKEL, E. S., AND STEELE, J. H., Rabies in man and animals in the United States, 1946–65, *Public Health Rep.* **82**:1009–1018 (1967).

26a. HOUFF, S. A., BURTON, R. C., WILSON, R. W., HENSON, T. E., LONDON, W. T., BAER, G. M., ANDERSON, L. J., WINKLER, W. G., MADDEN, D. L., AND SEVER, J. L., Human-to-human transmission of rabies virus by corneal transplant, *N. Engl. J. Med.* **300**:603–604 (1979).

27. HUMPHREY, G. L., KEMP, G. E., AND WOOD, E. G., A fatal case of rabies in a woman bitten by an insectivorous bat, *Public Health Rep.* **75**:317–325 (1960).

28. JOHNSON, H. N., Rabies, in: *Viral and Rickettsial Infections of Man* (T. M. RIVERS, ed.), pp. 267–299, J. B. Lippincott, Philadelphia, 1952.

29. JOHNSON, H. N., The serum-virus neutralization test, in: *Laboratory Techniques in Rabies,* 2nd ed., Vol. 23, pp. 81–84, WHO Monograph Series, 1966.

30. JOHNSON, R. T., Experimental rabies: Studies of cellular vulnerability and pathogenesis using fluorescent antibody staining, *J. Neuropathol. Exp. Neurol.* **24**:662–674 (1965).

31. JOHNSON, R. T., The pathogenesis of experimental rabies, in: *Rabies* (Y. NAGANO AND F. M. DAVENPORT, eds.), pp. 59–75, University of Tokyo Press, Tokyo, 1970.

32. KAPLAN, M. M., Epidemiology of rabies, *Nature (London)* **221**:421–425 (1969).

33. KAPLAN, M., AND KOPROWSKI, H. (eds.), *Laboratory Techniques in Rabies,* World Health Organization, Geneva, 1973, 367 pp.

34. KARLINER, J. S., AND BELAVAL, G. S., Incidence of reactions following administration of anti rabies serum, *J. Am. Med. Assoc.* **193**:359–362 (1965).

35. KEMP, G. E., LEE, V. H., MOORE, D. L., SHOPE, R. E., CAUSEY, O. R., AND MURPHY, F. A., Kotonkan, a new rhabdovirus related to Mokola of the rabies serogroup, *Am. J. Epidemiol.* **98**:43–49 (1973).

36. KOPROWSKI, H., Vaccines against rabies: Present and future, in: *First International Conference on Vaccines Against Viral and Rickettsial Diseases of Man,* p. 488, Scientific Publication No. 147, Pan American Health Organization, Washington, D.C., 1967.

37. KOPROWSKI, H., AND BLACK, J., Studies on chick embryo adapted rabies virus. III. Duration of immunity in vaccinated dogs, *Proc. Soc. Exp. Biol. Med.* **80**:410–415 (1952).

38. KOPROWSKI, H., AND COX, H. R., Studies on chick embryo adapted rabies virus. I. Culture characteristics and pathogenicity, *J. Immunol.* **60**:533–554 (1948).

38a. LARGHI, O. P., NEBEL, A. E., LAZARO, L., AND SAVY, V. L., Sensitivity of BHK-21 cells supplemented with diethylaminoethyldextran for detection of street rabies virus in saliva samples, *J. Clin. Microbiol.* 1:243–245 (1975).

38b. LARGHI, O. P., GONZALEZ, L. E., AND HELD, J. R., Evaluation of the corneal test as a laboratory method for rabies diagnosis, *Appl. Microbiol.* 25:187–189 (1973).

39. LENNETTE, E. H., AND EMMONS, R. W., The laboratory diagnosis of rabies: Review and perspective, in: *Rabies* (Y. NAGANO AND F. M. DAVENPORT, eds.), pp. 77–90, University of Tokyo Press, Tokyo, 1970.

40. MARTELL, D. M. A., MONTES, F. C., AND ALCOCER, B. R., Transplacental transmission of bovine rabies after natural infection, *J. Infect. Dis.* 127:291–293 (1973).

41. MIYAMOTO, K., AND MATSUMOTO, S., Comparative studies between pathogenesis of street and fixed rabies infection, *J. Exp. Med.* 125:447–456 (1967).

42. MURPHY, F. M., BAUER, S. P., HARRISON, A. K., AND WINN, W. C., JR., Comparative pathogenesis of rabies-like viruses, *Lab. Invest.* 28:361–376 (1973).

43. NEGRI, A., Beitrag zum Studium der Aetiologie der Tollwuth, *Z. Hyg. Infektionskr.* 43:507–528 (1903).

44. PAN AMERICAN HEALTH ORGANIZATION, Epidemiological surveillance of rabies for the Americas, Centro Panamericano de Zoonosis, September (1976).

45. PARA, M., An outbreak of post-vaccinal rabies (rage de laboratoire) in Fortaleza, Brazil, in 1960: Residual fixed virus as the etiological agent, *Bull. WHO* 33:177–182 (1965).

46. PASTEUR, L., Méthode pour prévenir la rage après morsure, *C. R. Acad. Sci.* 101:765–772 (1885).

47. PASTEUR, L., CHAMBERLAND, C., AND ROUX, E., Nouvelle communication sur la rage, *C. R. Acad. Sci.* 98:457–464 (1884).

48. PAWAN, J. L., Rabies in the vampire bat of Trinidad, with special reference to the clinical course and the latency of infection, *Ann. Trop. Med. Parasitol.* 30:401–422 (1936).

48a. PEDERSEN, N. C., EMMONS, R. W., SELCER, R., WOODIE, J. D., HOLLIDAY, T. A., AND WEISS, M., Rabies vaccine virus infection in three dogs, *J. Am. Vet. Med. Assoc.* 172:1092–1096 (1978).

48b. PORRAS, C., BARBOZA, J. J., FUENZALIDA, E., ADAROS, L. H., DIAZ, A. M. O., AND FURST, J., Recovery from rabies in man, *Ann. Intern. Med.* 85:44–48 (1976).

49. RUBIN, R. H., GREGG, M. B., AND SIKES, R. K., Rabies in citizens of the United States, 1963–1968: Epidemiology, treatment, and complications of treatment, *J. Infect. Dis.* 120:268–273 (1969).

50. RUEGSEGGER, J. M., BLACK, J., AND SHARPLESS, G. R., Primary antirabies immunization in man with HEP virus vaccine, *Am. J. Public Health* 51:706–714 (1961).

51. SCHMIDT, J. R., WILLIAMS, M. C., LULE, M., MIVULE, A., AND MUJOMBA, E., Viruses isolated from mosquitoes collected in the southern Sudan and western Ethiopia, *East Afr. Virus Res. Inst. Rep.* 15:24–25 (1965).

52. SCHNEIDER, L., Spread of virus from the central nervous system, in: *The Natural History of Rabies*, Vol. 1 (G. M. BAER, ed.), pp. 273–301, Academic Press, New York, 1975.

53. SHOPE, R. E., Rabies virus antigenic relationships, in: *The Natural History of Rabies*, Vol. 1 (G. M. BAER, ed.), pp. 141–152, Academic Press, New York, 1975.

54. SHOPE, R. E., MURPHY, F. A., HARRISON, A. K., CAUSEY, O. R., KEMP, G. E., SIMPSON, D. I. H., AND MOORE, D. L., Two African viruses serologically and morphologically related to rabies virus, *J. Virol.* 6:690–692 (1970).

55. SHORTT, H. E., McGUIRE, J. P., BROOKS, A. G., AND STEPHENS, E. D., Antirabies immunization: Probable lines of progress in improvement of methods, *Indian J. Med. Res.* 22:537 (1935).

56. SIKES, R. K., Pathogenesis of rabies in wildlife. I. Comparative effect of varying doses of rabies virus inoculated into foxes and skunks, *Am. J. Vet. Res.* 23:1041–1047 (1962).

57. SIKES, R. K., CLEARY, W. F., KOPROWSKI, H., WIKTOR, T. J., AND KAPLAN, M. M., Effective protection of monkeys against death from street virus by postexposure administration of tissue-culture rabies vaccine, *Bull. WHO* 45:1–11 (1971).

57a. SMITH, A. L., TIGNOR, G. H., EMMONS, R. W., AND WOODIE, J. D., Isolation of field rabies virus strains in CER and murine neuroblastoma cell cultures, *Intervirology* 9:359–361 (1978).

57b. SMITH, W. B., BLENDEN, D. C., AND FUH, R. H., Diagnosis of rabies by immunofluorescent staining of frozen sections of skin, *J. Am. Vet. Med. Assoc.* 161:1495–1501 (1972).

58. SOAVE, O. A., Transmission of rabies to mice by ingestion of infected tissue, *Am. J. Vet. Res.* 27:44–46 (1966).

59. SODJA, I., LIM, D., AND MATOUCH, O., Isolation of rabies-like virus from murine rodents, *J. Hyg. Epidemiol. Microbiol. Immunol.* 15:229–230 (1971).

60. STEELE, J. H., International aspects of veterinary medicine and its relation to health, nutrition and human welfare, *Mil. Med.* 131:765–778 (1966).

61. TIERKEL, E. S., Historical review of rabies in Asia, in: *Rabies* (Y. NAGANO AND F. M. DAVENPORT, eds.), pp. 3–9, University of Tokyo Press, Tokyo, 1971.

61a. TIGNOR, G. H., MURPHY, F. A., CLARK, H. F., SHOPE, R. E., MADORE, P., BAUER, S. P., BUCKLEY, S. M., AND MEREDITH, C. D., Duvenhage virus: Morphological, biochemical, histopathological and antigenic relationship to the rabies serogroup, *J. Gen. Virol.* 37:595–611 (1977).

62. TIGNOR, G. H., SHOPE, R. E., GERSHON, R. K., AND WAKSMAN, B. H., Immunopathologic aspects of in-

fection with Lagos bat virus of the rabies serogroup, *J. Immunol.* **112**:260–265 (1974).

63. VEERARAGHAVAN, N., GAJANANA, A., RANGSAMI, R., OONNUNNI, P. T., SARASWATHI, K. C., DEVARAJ, R., AND HALLAN, K. M., Studies on the salivary excretion of rabies virus by the dog from Surandai, in: *Coonoor Scientific Report*, p. 66, Pasteur Institute of Southern India, Coonoor, Tamilnadu, India, 1969.

64. WELLS, L. F., JR., AND GIRARD, K. F., Bats, rabies and DDT, *N. Engl. J. Med.* **297**:390–392 (1977).

65. WIKTOR, T. J., POSTIC, B., HO, M., AND KOPROWSKI, H., Role of interferon induction in the protective activity of rabies vaccine, *J. Infect. Dis.* **126**:408–418 (1972).

66. WIKTOR, T. J., SOKOL, F., KUWERT, E., AND KOPROWSKI, H., Immunogenicity of concentrated and purified rabies vaccine of tissue culture origin, *Proc. Soc. Exp. Biol. Med.* **131**:799–805 (1969).

66a. WILSON, J. M., HETTIARACHI, J., AND WIJESURIYA, L. M., Presenting features and diagnosis of rabies, *Lancet* **2**:1139–1140 (1975).

67. WINKLER, W. G., Airborne rabies virus isolation, *Bull. Wildl. Dis. Assoc.* **4**:37–40 (1968).

68. WINKLER, W. G., Rabies in the United States, 1951–1970, *J. Infect. Dis.* **125**:674–675 (1972).

69. WINKLER, W. G., BAKER, E. F., AND HOPKINS, C. C., An outbreak of non-bite transmitted rabies in a laboratory animal colony, *Am. J. Epidemiol.* **95**:267–277 (1972).

12. Suggested Reading

BAER, G. M. (ed.), *The Natural History of Rabies*, Vol. 1, 454 pp., and Vol. 2, 408 pp., Academic Press, New York, 1975.

JOHNSON, H. N., Rabies virus, in: *Viral and Rickettsial Infections of Man* (F. L. HORSFALL, JR., AND I. TAMM, eds.), pp. 814–840, J. B. Lippincott, Philadelphia, 1965.

KAPLAN, M., AND KOPROWSKI, H. (eds.), *Laboratory Techniques in Rabies*, World Health Organization, Geneva, 1973, 367 pp.

NAGANO, Y., AND DAVENPORT, F. M., eds., *Rabies*, University of Tokyo Pres., Tokyo, 1971, 406 pp.

CHAPTER 19

Respiratory Syncytial Virus

Robert M. Chanock, Hyun Wha Kim, Carl D. Brandt, and Robert H. Parrott

1. Introduction and Historical Background

Respiratory syncytial virus (RSV) was first isolated from a chimpanzee with common-cold-like illness.[77] Shortly thereafter, the virus was recovered from young children with severe lower respiratory tract disease in Baltimore.[16,21] Since its initial isolation from infants with respiratory disease almost 23 years ago, RSV has emerged as the major lower respiratory tract pathogen of infancy and early childhood throughout the world.[3,18,19,29,36,39,60,69,70,98,100] It is now clear that in all geographic areas, RSV is the major cause of bronchiolitis and pneumonia in infants and young children. RSV presents a special challenge to the epidemiologist, since this virus exhibits a pattern of infection and disease unlike that of any of the other known respiratory tract viral pathogens. Unanswered are many pressing questions concerning the pathogenesis of serious life-threatening disease of the lower respiratory tract produced by this virus during early infancy. A safe, effective vaccine for prevention of serious, pediatric RSV illness is not available at this time. However, studies now in progress offer some hope that ultimately it should be possible to develop effective immunoprophylaxis for RSV bronchiolitis and pneumonia.

RSV is a medium-sized (120–200 nm) enveloped virus that contains a lipoprotein coat and an RNA genome.[6,57,79,80] The virus matures at the limiting membrane of the infected cell.[57,80] Its internal component consists of ribonucleoprotein (RNP), which exhibits helical symmetry, while its outer envelope is studded with glycoprotein, spikelike projections.[56,106] Although there is some controversy concerning the dimensions of the inner RNP helix, it appears to have a diameter of 13 nm.[6,56,106] It is thus intermediate in size between the helix of the orthomyxoviruses (9 nm) and that of the paramyxoviruses (18 nm).[101] For this reason, it has been suggested that RSV and the pneumonia virus of mice, which also has a 13-nm inner helix, may comprise a group of enveloped RNA viruses distinct from the orthomyxoviruses (the influenza viruses) and the paramyxoviruses (parainfluenza viruses, mumps virus, Newcastle disease virus, and measles, rinderpest, and distemper viruses).[6,101]

Robert M. Chanock, Hyun Wha Kim, Carl D. Brandt, and Robert H. Parrott · Laboratory of Infectious Diseases, National Institute of Allergy and Infectious Diseases, National Institutes of Health, Bethesda, Maryland; Children's Hospital National Medical Center of Washington, D.C.; and George Washington University School of Medicine and Health Sciences, Department of Child Health and Development, Washington, D.C.

2. Methodology Involved in Epidemiological Analysis

2.1. Sources of Mortality Data

Limited information is available concerning the importance of RSV in fatal respiratory disease; however, from the serious nature of RSV bronchiolitis and pneumonia of infancy, there is reason to suspect that the virus is a major cause of fatal respiratory tract disease during the first year of life. This view is supported by two reports from Britain concerning 46 infants and children who died with lower respiratory tract disease; 36 of the patients were less than 1 year of age. RSV was isolated from 13 of the patients postmortem.[24,33] In another study in Great Britain, RSV was recovered from 3 of 12 infants who died with lower respiratory tract disease.[53] One of these infants had bilateral hydronephrosis and another Down's syndrome, and these conditions were thought to contribute to the fatal outcome of their disease. RSV or viral antigens have been detected postmortem in the lungs of a varying proportion of infants with the sudden infant death syndrome (SIDS).[9,24,88] This suggests that the virus may play a role in this important cause of infant mortality; however, the magnitude of its contribution to SIDS remains to be determined.

2.2. Sources of Morbidity Data

Although the importance of RSV in fatal respiratory tract disease in early life, or in any age group for that matter, has not been defined clearly, there is abundant evidence that suggests that this virus is a major cause of serious life-threatening disease of the lower respiratory tract during early life. The data that suggest that causality come from cross-sectional studies of pediatric patients admitted to the hospital with a diagnosis of bronchiolitis, pneumonia, bronchitis, or croup.

Estimates of the contribution of RSV to pediatric respiratory disease generally represent an undervaluation of the role of this agent. For example, human heteroploid-cell cultures commonly used for the recovery of RSV frequently exhibit marked variation of sensitivity to the agent; at times, such cell cultures may be completely resistant to RSV.[99] Another factor that should be considered in assessing the impact of RSV in pediatric respiratory disease is the inefficiency of the complement-fixation (CF), neutralization (N), and enzyme-linked immunosorbent assay (ELISA) techniques for the detection of serological evidence of infection in young infants.[18,83,90–92] This poses a special difficulty, since it is the young infant who is at greatest risk of developing RSV disease serious enough to require admission to the hospital.

The behavior of RSV in pediatric populations throughout the world has been discerned primarily from the pattern of serious respiratory disease produced by this virus. Although surveillance of seriously ill infants and children can serve as a barometer of the virus in the community, this type of study cannot, in itself, yield an estimate of the incidence of infection, the type and severity of clinical syndromes produced, or the risk of serious illness during infection. Such information, however, has been obtained from prospective studies of families, children in a day-care center, or residents of a semi-closed nursery.[44,49,58,76]

2.3. Serological Surveys

Serological surveys have been performed using the CF and N techniques. The former method is relatively less sensitive than the latter, especially if the plaque-reduction technique is used to measure N antibody. In most studies, N antibody has been assayed by the roller-tube culture N technique, which is less sensitive than the plaque-reduction technique.[22a] Nonetheless, in the first seroepidemiological survey performed, the former technique was sufficiently sensitive to show that the proportion of subjects with serum N antibody to RSV increased rapidly with age and reached 80% by 4 years of age in the Baltimore area.[16] In later studies using this technique, it was found that all adults tested possessed serum N antibody, and the level of antibody was significantly higher than that detected in the serum of seropositive children.[55] Finally, newborn infants were shown to possess the same level of serum N antibody as their mothers.[2] In later studies, the plaque-reduction technique was employed for seroepidemiological purposes, since it was shown to be approximately 10 times more sensitive for measurement of antibody than the roller-tube culture N method. In a recent study, each of a group of infants 1–5 months of age was found to possess serum N antibody when measured by the plaque-reduction technique; in addition, the majority of infants who were 6–7 months of age also possessed such neutralizing activity in their serum.[82] These infants were born after the last epidemic of RSV and presumably had not been infected with the virus. The mean titer of antibody decreased with age, dropping approximately 2-fold per month. This suggested that the antibody measured was passively acquired from the mother.

In summary, serological surveys using techniques of varying sensitivity have shown that all adults possess serum N antibody, as do infants at the time of birth. Antibody found in the serum of newborn infants represents passively acquired antibody; this antibody has a half-life of approximately 1 month and cannot be detected after 6–7 months of age unless the infant has been infected with RSV.

2.4. Laboratory Methods

RSV is very labile, and for this reason reliance on virus-isolation data often results in an underestimate of the importance of the agent in the population under study. For optimum results, secretions from the respiratory tract should be inoculated directly at the bedside into roller-tube cell cultures of known sensitivity to RSV. Freezing and thawing of respiratory tract secretions or nasopharyngeal washings often result in a significant decrease in titer of virus as well as failure to recover virus from such specimens.[3] Most investigators have used one of a series of heteroploid human cell lines for recovery of RSV, and it would appear that there are a number of such cell lines that are reasonably effective for this purpose. Among those used most extensively are the HEp-2 and Bristol HeLa cells. It cannot be overemphasized that cell cultures used for the recovery of RSV must be constantly monitored and tested for their sensitivity to RSV, in terms of both development of characteristic syncytial cytopathic effects during infection and capacity to detect small quantities of virus.

3. Biological Characteristics of the Virus That Affect the Epidemiological Pattern

There is no information that would link various biological properties of RSV with its unusual epidemiological behavior. Its lability does not seem to limit its spread in a susceptible population.

Antigenic variation among RSV viruses has been recognized in tests with convalescent sera obtained from RSV-infected ferrets.[22a] However, these differences were not evident when tests were performed with convalescent sera from young infants with RSV bronchiolitis. Thus, the major epidemiological patterns of RSV and the occurrence of reinfection are not dependent on antigenic variation as with the influenza A viruses.

Persistent infection in tissue culture can be initiated with certain temperature-sensitive mutants of RSV without recourse to reverse transcription of viral RNA to complementary DNA.[87] Nevertheless, the occurrence of a chronic carrier state has not been demonstrated in man. The capacity of the virus to reinfect and reinstitute pharyngeal carriage is probably a major mechanism of survival and spread. Although the relative importance of primary infection vs. reinfection as a source of virus in the community has not been studied formally, it is likely that the latter predominates.

4. Descriptive Epidemiology

4.1. Incidence and Prevalence Data

4.1.1. Risk of Infection and Reinfection. On the basis of serological surveys, infection with RSV appears to be a common occurrence during the first few years of life. In a study performed in Baltimore shortly after isolation of the first human strains of RSV, it was found that 48% of children possessed serum N antibody for the virus by 2 years of age and 77% by 3 years of age.[16] In a study employing the more sensitive plaque-reduction method, it was found that approximately half the infants who lived through one RSV epidemic in the Washington, D.C., area were infected during this period.[82] Furthermore, almost all children who had lived through two successive RSV epidemics were infected, as indicated by the presence of N antibody in their serum. Thus, the risk of infection for previously uninfected infants and young children is extremely high. In a recent prospective study in Houston, 22 of 42 infants were infected by their first birthday, and 19 of the remaining 20 children underwent primary infection by their second birthday.[37] When one considers the overall impact of RSV in pediatric respiratory disease throughout the world, it is likely that initial RSV infection also occurs early in life in most geographic areas.

Reinfection appears to be a relatively frequent event and was documented in 18 of 22 children during their second year of life in the Houston longitudinal study.[37] A similar frequency of reinfection was observed for young children in a day-care center.[49] In this population, 98% of seronegative infants and young children were infected with RSV, while during two succeeding exposures to the virus, the frequency of reinfection was 74 and 65%, respectively. In a recent longitudinal study, RSV infection was detected in 45% of 36 families studied during one epidemic period.[44] It is of interest that 9 of 21 persons 17–45 years of age became infected when virus was introduced into the family. This observation supports the view that reinfection is a common event even in adults.

In summary, it appears that most people become infected with RSV early in life, and few escape attack by this virus during infancy or early childhood. Further, reinfection occurs with appreciable frequency in older children and young adults and probably plays a major role in the spread of virus to the young infant, who is the target host for serious disease. It is highly unlikely that infants with serious RSV disease are the usual source of infection for other young infants.

In surveys of serum from adults, it was shown that 33–99% of subjects possessed CF antibody for RSV.[23,48,54] The presence of such antibody in serum is most likely a reflection of the frequent occurrence of reinfection, rather than long-term persistence of antibody following a limited, superficial infection of the respiratory tract.

4.1.2. Risk of Serious Bronchiolitis or Pneumonia during Infancy.

The risk of RSV illness serious enough to require admission of the affected person to the hospital has been estimated by three groups of investigators. First, in a study spanning 11 consecutive yearly RSV epidemics in the Washington, D.C., area, it was estimated that 1 in 200 infants (0–12 months) developed RSV bronchiolitis or pneumonia or both requiring hospitalization.[60] Second, during a collaborative study in the United Kingdom involving ten centers, the estimate for all infants was 1 in 120, while in highly industrialized areas, the estimate was 1 in 70.[29] For all infants 1–3 months of age, the estimate was 1 in 55, while in

industrial areas, it was 1 in 40. Third, during a prospective study in Houston, 2 of 98 infants were hospitalized during the first half year of life for RSV lower respiratory tract disease.[37]

Of course, the toll of RSV in infancy is considerably higher, since for every hospital admission for RSV bronchiolotis or pneumonia, there are many infants who develop respiratory disease that is almost as serious as that seen in the infants admitted to the hospital. At the other end of the spectrum is upper respiratory illness that may not be severe enough for the mother to bring her affected infant or young child to the outpatient clinic of the hospital or to a physician's office.

4.1.3. Risk of Pneumonia and Febrile Disease.

Of 90 institutionalized infants and young children, 40% developed pneumonia over a 4-week period during an outbreak of RSV infection that occurred in a welfare nursery in Washington, D.C.[58] An additional 53% of the nursery residents developed a febrile illness. The relationship of the virus to illness was determined by cross-sectional analysis in which the illness attack rate during a 5-day period bracketing initial virus isolation (test period) among infants and children who were RSV-positive was compared with the attack rate during the same 5-day period among children who were RSV-negative. This type of analysis indicated a significant association of virus with febrile illness and with pneumonia. The cross-sectional analysis, however, did not adjust for attributes such as age, sex, race, and duration of residence in the nursery, some of which might influence the occurrence of illness. Therefore, a horizontal analysis was made comparing the febrile-illness experiences of those children from whom RSV was isolated with the febrile experiences of the same children 2 weeks before and 2 weeks after a 5-day period (test period) bracketing initial virus isolation. This type of horizontal analysis indicated that the children who were RSV-positive experienced an onset of febrile respiratory disease 3 times more often than the expected number of febrile episodes ($p = 0.001$). This finding indicated a striking association between the recovery of RSV and the onset of a febrile illness in the children involved in the nursery outbreak. In a second outbreak of RSV infection that occurred in the same nursery 6 years later, only 10% of infants and young children developed pneumonia.[59] There is no obvious reason (or reasons) for this difference in response at this time. It should be emphasized that in both outbreaks, the population consisted of a mixture of infants and children, of whom some were probably completely susceptible to both infection and disease, while others had experienced several RSV infections previously and undoubtedly had developed some resistance to this virus.

An outbreak of RSV that occurred in a nursery in Taiwan also provided significant information about the pathogenic potential of RSV.[67] The outbreak involved 15 normal infants ranging between $7\frac{1}{2}$ and 12 months of age. The clinical attack rate was 100%; each of the infants developed symptoms of respiratory disease, and 13 of the 15 developed a febrile response that exceeded 38°C. A similar experience was recorded during an outbreak of RSV infection in a home for infants in Stockholm.[97] Thus, it appears that infection with RSV has a high degree of clinical penetrance and that most infections that occur in infancy and early childhood lead to the development of signs and symptoms of respiratory tract disease, and in most instances an associated febrile response occurs. Most adults undergoing reinfection also develop acute respiratory tract disease, but fever is less common than observed in infants and children.[44]

4.1.4. Role of RSV in Different Clinical Syndromes. In a 13-year surveillance of infants and young children admitted to the Children's Hospital of D.C. with lower respiratory tract disease, RSV infection was detected in 43% admitted with the diagnosis of bronchiolitis and in 25% of patients with pneumonia.[60] RSV infection was detected less often in the syndromes of bronchitis (10.6%) and croup (9.8%). In contrast, RSV infection was detected in only 5.4% of infants and children seen in the clinic or admitted to the hospital for nonrespiratory illness during this interval. The findings that emerged from this study of approximately 5000 infants and children with lower respiratory tract disease are representative of observations made by others during the past 21 years. Thus, it is clear that RSV is the major cause of bronchiolitis of early infancy. In addition, the virus is a major cause of pneumonia during the first few years of life.

4.2. Epidemic Behavior

One of the most remarkable features of the epidemiology of RSV is the consistent pattern of infection and disease. Other respiratory viruses cause epidemics at irregular intervals or exhibit a mixed endemic–epidemic pattern, but RSV is the only respiratory viral pathogen that produces a sizable epidemic every year in large urban centers.[20,82] This pattern has been observed wherever RSV has been studied. In the temperate areas of the world, RSV epidemics have occurred primarily in the late fall, winter, or spring, but never during the summer. In Washington, D.C., over an interval of 13 years, RSV was most active during the period from January to April and virtually absent from the community during August and September.[60] Large annual variations in the impact of RSV on the pediatric population of the Washington, D.C., area were not observed over this 13-year period. During 11 consecutive epidemics studied intensively, the number and proportion of infants and children admitted to the Children's Hospital of D.C. for RSV lower respiratory tract disease did not vary more than 2.7-fold.[60] Also remarkable was the consistency with which RSV produced the same clinical pattern of respiratory tract disease, especially bronchiolitis and pneumonia, year after year. These illnesses were barometers of RSV infection in the community; when the virus was at its epidemic peak, hospitalization for bronchiolitis and pneumonia in infants and young children soared.[60] A similar temporal association of RSV infection and serious lower respiratory illness in infants was also documented in Scotland.[39]

More than 15,000 infants and young children were studied for RSV infection during 11 consecutive outbreaks in the Washington, D.C., area. Data obtained at monthly intervals during the outbreaks were combined to plot a composite epidemic curve, which showed a normal distribution.[8] Of more than 1000 respiratory-disease patients who yielded an RSV isolate during the composite outbreak, 40% shed virus during the peak epidemic month and 82% shed virus during the period encompassing the peak month and the month preceding and following it; this indicated the sharpness of the yearly epidemics of the virus in the Washington, D.C., area. During the peak month of the composite epidemic, RSV was recovered from 46% of all inpatients hospitalized with bronchiolitis, from 34% of all patients hospitalized with any type of respiratory disease, and from 32% of patients with respiratory disease who were seen as outpatients in the hospital. Control subjects who were free of respiratory disease rarely yielded RSV (less than 1%). As indicated by virus recovery or the development of serum CF antibody, or both, 70% of bronchiolitis patients and 56% of all respiratory-disease inpatients exhibited evidence of RSV infection during the peak epidemic month. A similar epidemic wave was seen in males compared to females and in black compared to nonblack children.

4.3. Geographic Distribution

RSV has emerged as the major pediatric respiratory tract pathogen wherever appropriate studies have been performed to detect infection. Furthermore, the epidemic pattern of disease just described for the Washington, D.C., area appears to be characteristic of the behavior of this virus in large urban centers throughout the world. Serological surveys of subjects from remote isolated populations have in each instance revealed evidence of prior RSV infection (R. M. Chanock, unpublished studies).

4.4. Temporal Distribution

In the United States and other temperate areas, RSV epidemics occur in the late fall, winter, or spring, but not during the summer.[60,78] The virus is rarely isolated during August or September. In Washington, D.C., outbreak peaks were observed to occur in six different calendar months over a period of 13 years.[8,60] The outbreak peak occurred as late as June and as early as December. Each RSV epidemic lasted approximately 5 months.[60] In Chicago, the peaks of three successive outbreaks were separated by an interval of 55–58 weeks.[78] A fourth outbreak occurred after a shorter interval of 39 weeks, and this was followed by a fifth outbreak in which the interval between peaks was prolonged to 62 weeks. Analysis of 13 successive outbreaks that occurred in Washington, D.C. suggested that the interval between successive peaks was alternately long (13–16 months) and then short (7–12 months), resulting in an outbreak later in the respiratory season the next year.[60]

In one semitropical area (Trinidad), RSV was found to exhibit a temporal pattern different from that characteristic of temperate regions. Over a 3-year period of surveillance, RSV epidemics occurred in Trinidad during the rainy season that extended from June through December.[96] The Trinidad epidemics started in June 1964, September 1965, and August 1966.

4.5. Age

In a large cross-sectional study of RSV infection in pediatric patients admitted to the hospital, the peak incidence of RSV bronchiolitis and pneumonia was observed at 2 months of age.[82] Thereafter, the incidence of these diseases decreased with increasing age, more rapidly for bronchiolitis than for pneumonia. Except for the first month of life, the incidence curve of RSV bronchiolitis exhibited a marked downward slope, so that by 10–12 months of age, few infants were admitted to the hospital with this diagnosis. During the first month, the incidence of RSV bronchiolitis was approximately one third that observed during the second month, the period of peak occurrence of the disease. Although RSV pneumonia occurred most often at 2 months of age, the incidence of this disease decreased rather slowly with increasing age. It was not unusual for the virus to cause pneumonia in older children. It should be emphasized that the age distribution of the most serious RSV disease, i.e., bronchiolitis, is unique among viral infections of man. RSV is the only virus that preferentially produces severe disease and has its maximum impact during the first few months of life.[17,82]

In the various age groups investigated in the Tecumseh, Michigan, seroepidemiological study, a serological response to RSV occurred most frequently in school-age children 5–9 years old.[76] The rate of infection (which presumably was reinfection) fell rapidly with increasing age during childhood and then more slowly among adults. In children 5–9 years of age, approximately 20% underwent infection during yearly epidemics of RSV in the community. Of children 10–14 years of age, 17% appeared to have been infected, whereas the estimate for young people 15–19 years of age was 10%.

In a prospective study that extended over one RSV epidemic season in Rochester, New York, it was observed that the rate of infection did not vary appreciably with age except during infancy.[44] Infection was monitored by virus isolation, which is generally a more sensitive indicator of reinfection than serology. Infection was detected in 16 of the 36 families under surveillance. In familes into which the virus was introduced, approximately 40% of family members 1–45 years of age became infected, while the rate was higher for infants—62%. In these families, it appeared that children were primarily responsible for introducing virus into the home.

4.6. Sex

Severe RSV disease that requires hospitalization occurs approximately 30% more often among male infants than among female infants.[82]

4.7. Race

In a study of 13 consecutive epidemics in the Washington, D.C. area, the proportion of nonblack patients with various forms of lower respiratory disease associated with RSV infection was somewhat higher than that of black patients.[82] A plot of all hospitalized respiratory disease patients indicated that in every age category, black patients yielded RSV slightly less often than nonblack patients; however, the age pattern of RSV bronchiolitis was the same for both groups of patients. The nonblack patients were in most instances from the suburbs of the Washington, D.C., area, whereas the black patients tended to come from the poorer areas of the District of Columbia immediately surrounding the Children's Hospital.

4.8. Occupation

We have no information about any relationship of RSV infection to occupation.

4.9. Occurrence in Different Settings

Differences in the spread of RSV within different families were noted in a seroepidemiological study performed in Tecumseh, Michigan.[76] As the number of members in the family increased from three to six persons, there was an increase in the proportion of families in which one or more members were infected with RSV. This apparently was a reflection of the additional opportunity for introduction of infection into a larger family. The increased number of persons at risk in larger families also resulted in more multiple infections within the family once the virus was introduced. In the Tecumseh study, only 5.5% of persons in families with three members were infected with RSV, whereas the proportion increased to 16.3% in families that had six members. Data from this study support the view that the virus is most often introduced into the family unit by a school-aged child.

4.10. Socioeconomic Status

Data from a study in North Carolina suggested that serious RSV disease occurred more frequently in infants of low socioeconomic status from a rural area than in infants of higher socioeconomic status living in an urban center.[36] In this situation, socioeconomic factors may have influenced the risk of infection during early infancy, and this in turn influenced the pattern of disease. It is likely that delay of primary infection past the age of vulnerability (i.e., the first 6 months of life) increases the probability that disease will be mild rather than severe. Observations made during the multicenter study in the United Kingdom also indicated that the incidence of serious RSV illness during infancy varied significantly in relation to social class. The incidence was 12-fold higher among infants from the lowest social class compared to those of the highest class.[29]

4.11. Other Factors

We have no information concerning other factors.

5. Mechanisms and Routes of Transmission

RSV infection appears to be transmitted from person to person through respiratory secretions. Small-particle aerosol does not seem to be important. There is evidence that suggests that coarse particles and direct contamination by secretions represent the most common modes for spread of virus.[42,45]

A virus that is similar antigenically and biologically to RSV has been recovered from cattle with respiratory disease in Europe, Asia, and the United States.[51,52,81] The bovine strains appear to be related antigenically to the human strains, but the ability of bovine strains to infect man and of human strains to infect cows has not been ascertained as yet.

6. Pathogenesis and Immunity

From information obtained during outbreaks in closed populations, it was estimated that the incubation period from exposure to development of fever and signs of RSV lower respiratory disease was approximately 4–5 days.[58,97] When adults were experimentally infected with RSV, the incubation period averaged 5 days, and illness lasted an average of 5½ days.[55,65]

The behavior of RSV in young infants provides an opportunity to assess the protective effect of serum antibody for this agent in the absence of any potential effect of local respiratory tract immunity. During the first 6 months of life, the young infant possesses maternally derived serum antibody, whereas local antibody, which is not transferred passively from the mother, is presumably not present. The observation that serious RSV disease occurs most often during this period when infants possess passively transferred serum antibody clearly indicates that such N antibody (presumably IgG) does not provide effective protection against the most serious effects of the virus. The high frequency with which RSV infection occurs in young infants also indicates that serum antibody does not provide effective resistance to infection. In one study, infants who developed severe RSV disease did not differ significantly from their age-matched nonill cohorts with respect to serum N antibody.[82] Thus, acute-phase sera of young infants admitted to the hospital with RSV bronchiolitis or pneumonia contained moderate to high levels of N antibody as measured by the plaque-reduction technique.[82] The age pattern of antibody in the acute-phase sera of patients with RSV bronchiolitis or pneumonia was similar to that of infants without respiratory tract disease, and the level of antibody was inversely related to age, suggesting that this antibody was derived passively from the mother. In another study, almost all young infants, 3 months or younger, had N antibodies in their serum when admitted to the hospital for RSV disease.[37]

Additional evidence that serum N antibody does not provide effective protection was obtained during the study of an RSV outbreak that occurred in a semiclosed nursery the residents of which ranged in age from 6 to 65 months.[58] Preoutbreak serum specimens were available from 85 of the nursery residents, and these specimens were assayed for N antibody by the plaque-reduction technique. The occurrence of pneumonia was not related to the level of preexisting serum N antibody in this population. It should be emphasized, however, that in most instances the pneumonia illnesses that occurred in these older infants and young children were not severe. Although the mothers' passive

contribution of RSV IgG antibodies does not appear to protect her infant, there is recent evidence that immune factors in colostrum and milk may provide some protection.[25] The proportion of infants hospitalized for RSV disease who were breast fed was only one fourth that of age-matched controls. The nature, extent, and duration of this type of passive immunity remain to be determined.

Older children and adults usually develop less serious illness during reinfection with RSV than do young infants undergoing primary infection. In the Chapel Hill longitudinal day-care study, there was a steady reduction in the occurrence of lower respiratory tract illness, middle ear disease, and fever during second and third infections with RSV.[49] Since serum N antibody does not appear to be protective, other mechanisms of resistance are probably involved. Systemic cell-mediated immunity (CMI) does not appear to play a significant role in resistance, since an inactivated RSV vaccine that stimulated a heightened CMI response (as measured by lymphocyte transformation *in vitro*) did not provide resistance to either RSV infection or the development of disease.[64] These considerations led to an examination of local respiratory tract immune mechanisms in an attempt to explain resistance to RSV. A series of studies were performed in adult volunteers to evaluate the properties and effects of local respiratory-tract antibody to RSV. Initially, antibody in nasal secretions of adults was characterized and shown to be predominantly of the 11 S, IgA variety.[74,75] Each of the 104 adults tested possessed such RSV-specific, secretory antibody, and levels varied over a wide range. In addition, experimentally infected adults were shown to develop neutralizing activity in their nasal secretions during convalescence.[75] In two recent studies, it was shown that the majority of young infants developed RSV-specific IgA antibodies in their nasal secretions following RSV disease.[31,73] These antibodies, which were detectable by immunofluorescence, did not possess demonstrable neutralizing activity and hence appeared to have low avidity.[73] Nonetheless, this type of response indicated that the respiratory-tract secretory-antibody system operates early in life.

The significance of local antibody was investigated in a volunteer study, in which subjects were challenged intranasally with 500 plaque-forming units (PFU) of RSV.[75] Eight men had a low level of prechallenge nasal-secretion neutralizing activity, while the other eight subjects had a high level, and there was no overlap in level of antibody between the two groups. Each of the volunteers possessed a moderately high level of serum N antibody. Following challenge, each of the men in the two groups shed virus, and the temporal pattern of virus shedding was the same for men in either group. However, when the virus content of the nasopharyngeal washings was estimated by the plaque technique, it was found that men in the low-nasal-antibody group shed large quantities of virus (up to 10^5 PFU/ml of nasaopharyngeal washing), whereas the washings from the high-antibody group contained very little virus. The difference was related to nasal antibody and not serum antibody, since the two groups differed primarily in their level of prechallenge nasal antibody. Following infection, none of the high-nasal-antibody men developed a serum N, serum CF, or nasal-secretion N antibody response. In contrast, six of the eight low-nasal-antibody group developed a rise in one or more of these antibodies. The findings from this study indicate that the level of preexisting local antibody did not influence susceptibility to infection; however, the level of this antibody had a marked effect on the level of virus replication and secondarily on the immune response to infection. This interpretation supports the thesis that resistance to RSV disease is a function of the local respiratory-tract secretory-antibody system.

One can only speculate about the capacity of RSV to evade the host's defense mechanisms and to reinfect with relatively high frequency. RSV characteristically induces syncytium formation in tissue culture. This type of virus–host cell interaction may lessen the protective role of local immune defenses, since syncytium formation permits recruitment of uninfected cells into the disease process under conditions that minimize the effectiveness of antibody in halting extension of infection and tissue damage.

Although the pathogenesis of RSV disease in early infancy is not understood, there are several observations that suggest that immunological factors play a role. The level of serum N antibody by age during infancy resembles the age distribution of RSV bronchiolitis except during the first month. This similarity has prompted the suggestion that serum antibody might participate in an immunopathological reaction with RSV antigens in the lungs and that this reaction might contribute to the development

and severity of bronchiolitis.[17] Any hypothesis that attempts to explain the pathogenesis of serious RSV disease in early life, however, must take into account the intrinsic pathogenic potential of the virus itself. For example, in several well-studied nursery outbreaks, RSV was found to cause pneumonia in children who lacked detectable serum N antibody. If immunological factors are important in lower respiratory tract disease, they must act to enhance the basic pathogenic effects of the virus.

The level of N antibody by age in the sera of normal infants and in the acute-phase sera of infants with RSV bronchiolitis and pneumonia was reexamined recently using the plaque-reduction N technique.[82] Each of the control infants 1–5 months of age possessed serum N antibody, as did the majority of control infants 6–7 months of age. These infants were born after the last epidemic of RSV and presumably had not been infected with the virus. In addition, the mean titer of antibody decreased with age, suggesting that the antibody measured was passively acquired from the mother. The antibody pattern of infants with RSV bronchiolitis or pneumonia resembled that of the control group; however, a larger proportion of the respiratory-disease patients lacked detectable serum antibody at 5–7 months of age. Failure to detect acute-phase serum antibody in some patients with RSV bronchiolitis at 5–7 months of age casts some doubt on the essential role of serum antibody in the pathogenesis of RSV bronchiolitis. Furthermore, no relationship was observed between the severity of RSV illness and the titer of CF antibody in acute-phase serum.[11] Although the significance of serum antibody in the pathogenesis of disease may not be clear at this time, it is evident, nonetheless, that high levels of this type of antibody during the first 3–4 months of life do not protect the young infant from bronchiolitis or pneumonia caused by RSV.

Other findings make it difficult to dismiss completely the possibility that immunopathological factors play an important role in RSV bronchiolitis. There was a strong suggestion that an inactivated RSV vaccine, prepared in monkey-kidney tissue culture, potentiated the response of vaccinees to RSV infection through an immunological mechanism.[22,28,59,63] This vaccine was found to be highly antigenic, stimulating high levels of serum plaque-reduction antibody and a heightened systemic CMI response in young infants.[59,64] In several field trials, a significant proportion of young children who received the inactivated RSV vaccine during infancy developed severe bronchiolitis when they subsequently underwent natural RSV infection at an age when RSV bronchiolitis rarely occurs.[59,63] It is possible, of course, that the pathogenesis of infantile bronchiolitis is different from that of vaccine-associated bronchiolitis. But this seems unlikely in view of the marked similarity of clinical course and progression of these conditions.

Possibly an age-related nonimmunologically determined factor could be responsible for the unusual pattern of RSV illness in early infancy. This would mean that the age–disease–antibody relationships that exist are merely fortuitous. The simplest nonimmunological explanation for the unusual predilection for RSV disease in early infancy is that the air pathways at this time are smaller and more easily obstructed than later in life. This anatomical factor may contribute to the occurrence of RSV disease in the first months of life and could explain in part the observation that the frequency of bronchiolitis during primary RSV infection decreases with increasing age.[49] But it should be emphasized that the majority of RSV vaccinees who developed severe obstructive pulmonary disease were older than the usual unvaccinated infant with bronchiolitis. More than two thirds of non-vaccine-associated RSV disease in the community occurs in infants in the first half year of life, whereas 63% of the vaccinees who exhibited altered reactivity to RSV developed obstructive disease (bronchiolitis) after 6 months of age.[63] The development of severe, typical, obstructive RSV bronchiolitic disease by the older vaccinees makes it unlikely that the size of the air pathways is the only determinant in the unusual age pattern of RSV illness.

In the early studies of RSV infection in young infants, as well as in more recent studies, it was observed that the serum antibody response of young infants to this virus was impaired.[18,83,92] Also, the local secretory IgA antibodies produced in response to RSV infection during infancy appear to be relatively ineffective in neutralizing this virus.[73] A delayed, decreased, or inefficient immunological response to infection could contribute to the increased severity of RSV disease during infancy. Recent studies of parainfluenza 1 virus and vesicular stomatitis virus in mice have shown the occurrence of an early immunological response in the lungs that

developed several days before antibody was detected in serum.[7] If this type of early pulmonary immunological response plays a role in the resolution of infection, which is likely, a delay, decrease, or defect in the response could lead to a more serious type of disease. One factor that might contribute to such an impaired response is immunological suppression produced by maternally derived serum antibody. This type of immunological suppression is known to affect the development of serum antibody, but it is not known whether local respiratory-tract secretory antibody can be suppressed in a similar manner. The possible role of impaired immunological response due to immunological immaturity or immunosuppression or both should be kept in mind and evaluated in future studies of RSV disease of infancy.

There is one observation that is difficult to explain on the basis of serum-antibody-induced immunopathology or an impaired immunological response mechanism. This concerns the relative sparing of 1-month-old infants from RSV bronchiolitis. RSV bronchiolitis occurs approximately one third as often among infants 1 month of age as during the time of peak occurrence at 2 months of age.[82]. Furthermore, young neonates (under 3 weeks of age) who undergo nosocomial infection with RSV have less lower respiratory tract disease than older infants.[47] The basis for this early resistance to RSV disease is not understood. If either or both of the two immunological mechanisms are important in the pathogenesis of RSV disease, one would anticipate a very high (or the highest) incidence of disease during the first month of life, and this is not the case.

Another hypothesis that has been offered to explain the pathogenesis of RSV bronchiolitis envisions the essential process in this disease as an allergic reaction.[32] According to this hypothesis, the first exposure to RSV during infancy results in a silent, but sensitizing, infection. Subsequently, disease occurs during a second infection when the virus induces an allergic, IgE-mediated reaction in the sensitized host. In contrast, RSV pneumonia is postulated not to require a prior sensitizing RSV infection. The question of one vs. two infections in RSV bronchiolitis is not merely of academic interest, since efforts to immunize infants with live attenuated virus have begun and are being continued with the expectation that protection rather than sensitization will result.[61,62,105] The evidence that the sensitization hypothesis is correct is based on the study of autopsy material from infants with bronchiolitis or pneumonia. The lungs of the infants with bronchiolitis contained small quantities of virus and RSV immunofluorescent antigen, whereas the lungs of young infants who died of pneumonia contained large amounts of virus and immunofluorescent antigen.[32]

The sensitization hypothesis was recently evaluated by analyzing a composite RSV outbreak constructed from data obtained during 11 consecutive outbreaks in the Washington, D.C., area.[8] If the sensitization hypothesis were correct, one would expect that during an RSV epidemic, the incidence of RSV bronchiolitis would increase more slowly and peak later than other respiratory-disease syndromes caused by the virus, such as pneumonia. In other words, a period of time would be required for young infants born after the last yearly RSV epidemic to undergo their first RSV infection, and this should produce a shift in the time frame of RSV bronchiolitis. In addition, early in an RSV epidemic, bronchiolitis patients would be especially likely to be 6 months of age or older, because young infants would not have been born in time to experience a previous infection. At the epidemic peak, RSV bronchiolitis patients should be younger than such patients seen prior to the epidemic peak. Finally, with increasing age, relatively more infants and young children should be hospitalized with RSV bronchiolitis than with RSV pneumonia. None of the expectations was confirmed by analysis of the composite RSV epidemic; the age pattern of RSV bronchiolitis remained the same throughout the epidemic.[8] Furthermore, the majority of young infants with bronchiolitis who are less than 6 months of age exhibit a slow antibody response or a very poor antibody response that is more characteristic of a primary than of a secondary immunological reaction.[18,83,91,92] Thus, there was no support for the sensitization hypothesis from the analysis of RSV epidemics or from a study of the immunological response of young infants to this virus.

In addition, Polmar et al.[84] and L. Senterfit and H. W. Kim (unpublished observations, 1974) found normal levels of serum IgE in infants during the acute stage of RSV bronchiolitis. If an allergic reaction were involved in pathogenesis of RSV bronchiolitis, one would expect a proportion of infants with the disease to have an elevated level of serum IgE. This expectation is based on the observation that many patients with extrinsic (allergic) asthma have an elevated level of serum IgE.[5,35,66] Cortisone, which is highly effective in allergic asthma, does not appear to affect the course of infantile bronchiolitis.[68] Finally, a recent evaluation of 35 children who had RSV bronchiolitis 8 years earlier during infancy suggested that this disease and childhood asthma were not closely related.[94] Nevertheless, exercise–induced bronchial reactivity of the children with a history of RSV infantile bronchiolitis was significantly greater than that of control children.[94]

Recently, two additional hypotheses have been suggested to explain the unusual pathogenesis of RSV lower respiratory tract disease. First, infants with RSV bronchiolitis were observed to develop a greater systemic CMI response (as measured by lymphocyte transformation in vitro) than infants who had pneumonia or an upper respiratory illness associated with their RSV infection.[93,102] It was suggested that an altered CMI response might affect peripheral-airway reactivity. The observation that the inactivated RSV vaccine stimulated a heightened systemic CMI response is compatible with this suggestion, since these vaccinees developed severe bronchiolitis with high frequency during RSV infection.[64]

Second, infants with RSV lower respiratory tract disease were observed to develop a very poor local interferon response.[43,71] In contrast, other pediatric patients with influenza A or parainfluenza type 1 virus illness developed an interferon response with higher frequency.[43,71] Failure to stimulate an adequate interferon response may contribute to the severity of RSV disease in early life.

7. Patterns of Host Response

7.1. Symptoms

The effect of RSV on the host ranges from inapparent infection to severe respiratory tract disease such as bronchiolitis or pneumonia. Response to infection is influenced by age and immunological status. Bronchiolitis and pneumonia caused by RSV occur in most instances during the first year of life. Initially in an RSV infection in infancy and early childhood, there are involvement and inflammation of the mucous membranes of the nose and throat. Paranasal and eustachian tube obstruction and otitis media occur commonly. In a significant proportion of infections in early infancy, and in a minority of instances in later life, there is an extension of the inflammatory process in the trachea, the bronchioles, and the parenchyma of the lung. In young infants, there is a tendency for necrotizing bronchiolitis and pneumonia to develop, and apnea may occur in a significant proportion of such illnesses.[10] Bronchiolar obstruction results in focal areas of atelectasis or emphysema. The clinical picture may be dominated by obstructive bronchiolitis or pneumonitis or a combination of the two patterns. Inflammation and edema of the larynx may occur, but this condition is less frequently observed than bronchiolitis or pneumonia. Older children or adults who undergo reinfection with RSV often develop mild upper respiratory tract illness indistinguishable from that produced by the multitude of other viruses that cause the common cold. However, more serious disease involving the lower respiratory tract may occur and require bed rest.[26,46] This type of febrile response resembling influenza in severity occurs more commonly than previously appreciated and is associated with an increase in total respiratory resistance and altered airway reactivity to carbachol challenge that lasts at least 8 weeks.[46]

It has been suggested that exacerbation of chronic bronchitis and emphysema in adults is frequently associated with reinfection with RSV.[14,95] Recent studies have failed to yield evidence that would support this view. However, exacerbations of wheezing in asthmatic children are often associated with RSV infection.[72]

In fatal illnesses in young infants caused by RSV, the most prominent change is necrotizing or interstitial pneumonitis, peribronchiolar lymphocytic infiltration, necrosis of tracheobronchiolar epithelium, atelectasis, and emphysema.[1,33,53] Cytoplasmic inclusions may be present in infected areas of the lungs.

7.2. Diagnosis

Diagnosis of RSV infection can be made by virus isolation, detection of antigen in exfoliated cells by immunofluorescence, demonstration of a rise in serum antibody during convalescence, or some combination of these techniques. Examination of exfoliated cells from the respiratory tract by immunofluorescence provides a highly efficient method for the diagnosis of RSV infection.[30,38] Virus is present in the nasal and pharyngeal secretions of infected persons and can be isolated with greatest efficiency when specimens are inoculated directly into cell culture without prior freezing.[40,41] It is possible, however, to isolate a large proportion of strains from frozen specimens when veal infusion broth with 0.5% bovine albumin is used as the collecting medium. Human heteroploid-cell cultures (e.g., HeLa, HEp-2) represent the most sensitive host system for recovery of naturally occurring virus. Characteristic syncytial cytopathic changes usually develop 3–10 days after inoculation of clinical specimens containing RSV. Since sublines of HeLa and HEp-2 cells differ considerably in sensitivity to RSV, it is essential that cultures of a sensitive cell line be used in virus-isolation attempts.[99] Human embryonic kidney and human diploid fibroblast cultures can also be used for virus isolation, but these are generally less sensitive than the heteroploid cell cultures described above. Except in early infancy, the CF, ELISA, and tissue-culture N techniques are relatively efficient serological procedures for diagnosis of RSV infection. Infants, less than 7 months of age develop N, CF and ELISA antibodies less often following RSV infection than do older persons.[18,83,91,92] In addition, a greater concentration of antigen is required for detection of CF antibody during early life.[83] In young infants, infection is most accurately determined by virus isolation or by immunofluorescence.

8. Control and Prevention

It is unlikely that an effective, inactivated RSV vaccine can be developed for prevention of serious disease in early life. First, the unusual age distribution of RSV bronchiolitis and pneumonia makes it difficult to consider the use of an inactivated vaccine. If a vaccine is to have a major impact on RSV bronchiolitis and pneumonia, it must be capable of stimulating effective host resistance in the first month of life, since the peak incidence of disease occurs during the second month of life. Second, a highly antigenic, formalin-inactivated vaccine was tested in older infants and was found to be ineffective in terms of preventing both infection and disease.[22,28,59,63]

The inactivated vaccine was prepared in African green monkey kidney (AGMK) tissue culture, and virus was concentrated by centrifugation and by adsorption to alum. This vaccine stimulated high levels of serum antibody in seronegative infants.[59] In addition, the vaccine induced a heightened systemic CMI response.[64] Unfortunately, the vaccine did not confer protection against subsequent infection caused by RSV. Thus, when RSV was prevalent in the community following the period of immunization, the frequency of infection among RSV vaccinees was not remarkably different from that of age-matched subjects who received a tissue-culture-grown type 1 parainfluenza vaccine or an egg-grown trivalent parainfluenza virus vaccine.[22,28,63] More striking than the failure of the vaccine to protect against the virus was the unexpected response to infection exhibited by the vaccinees. In one vaccine trial, 9 (60%) of 15 vaccinees, 6–23 months of age, developed pneumonia or bronchiolitis or both; in 5 instances, disease was severe enough to require hospitalization.[59] In contrast, only 4 (8%) of 47 unvaccinated controls developed pneumonia, and none of these children required admission to the hospital. This difference in response indicated that the vaccine had induced an altered, exaggerated reactivity to infection. Definite evidence of such an altered response to infection was not seen among older vaccinees, who were 24–65 months of age. In another study, 78% of RSV vaccinees required hospitalization when infected subsequently with the virus under natural conditions; hospitalization was necessary because of serious obstructive lower respiratory tract disease.[63] In contrast, only 5% of parainfluenza vaccinees who became infected with RSV-developed illness of similar severity. In fact, the illness experienced by the RSV vaccinees was more severe than that seen in younger, unvaccinated hospitalized patients from the community. The parainfluenza type 1 vaccine used in the comparison group was prepared in AGMK tissue cultures in a manner identical to that of the RSV vaccine; in fact, the two vaccines were prepared by the same pharmaceutical manufacturer. Since the parainfluenza vaccinees did not exhibit an exaggerated response to RSV infection, it was unlikely that a monkey-kidney antigen was responsible for the altered reactivity associated with the RSV vaccine. Instead, it appeared that a component of the RSV itself was responsible for the potentiation of disease by the vaccine.

The difficulties encountered with the formalin-inactivated RSV vaccine parallel in several respects the problems associated with formalin-inactivated measles virus vaccine. The latter vaccine stimulated serum HI antibodies, but vaccinees lost their resistance to infection after several years. Furthermore, many vaccinees developed an altered, more severe form of disease when infected with measles virus. These adverse effects have been attributed to a selective action of formalin upon the surface glycoproteins of measles virus.[79a] Antigenicity of the fusion glycoprotein is destroyed by formalin, whereas the hemagglutinin glycoprotein, responsible for attachment of virus to the cell surface, is unaffected.[79a] The potentiating effect of the inactivated measles vaccine as well as its failure to stimulate durable protection is now ascribed to failure of the vaccine to induce immunity to the viral fusion glycoprotein. A similar type of incomplete immunity may explain the failure and adverse effects of the inactivated RSV vaccine. RSV appears to possess a surface protein that is involved in penetration of virus into the cell and in fusion of infected cells with uninfected cells to form syncytia.[4a] It should be possible to determine whether formalin selectively destroys antigenicity of the putative RSV fusion protein once methods are available for measuring specific antibodies to this protein.

Naturally acquired RSV infection appears to confer a definite degree of protection against illness caused by the virus. This observation coupled with the ineffectiveness of serum antibody suggests that local defense mechanisms in the respiratory tract play a major role in resistance to illness caused by RSV. For this reason, an attenuated strain of RSV that could infect the respiratory tract and induce resistance without producing significant illness has been sought.[15] In the initial attempts to develop an attenuated vaccine, a low-temperature-adapted strain of RSV was produced in the laboratory, and this strain was found to produce a silent infection in infants and young children who had been infected with RSV previously.[27] However, mild lower respiratory tract disease developed when the potential vaccine strain was given to young infants who lacked prior experience with RSV. These findings indicated that a measurable degree of attenuation had been achieved by low-temperature adaptation, but the residual virulence of the low-temperature-adapted strain made it unacceptable for use in young infants, the group for whom an RSV vaccine is most urgently needed.

Encouraged by partial success with the low-temperature RSV strain, other candidate vaccine strains that might offer the possibility of greater attenuation were developed. The most promising of the candidate strains was the temperature-sensitive (ts) mutant designated ts-1, which was induced by the chemical mutagen 5-fluorouridine.[34] This strain was chosen for clinical trial on the basis of its behavior in vitro in tissue culture and in vivo in the hamster.[34,104] This mutant did not produce plaques, i.e., did not initiate foci of infection in tissue culture, at or above 37°C, unlike wild-type virus, which produced plaques without restriction at 39°C.[34] In the hamster, infection with the mutant was limited to the cooler upper respiratory tract, where the temperature was 32–34°C, and virus was not found in the lungs, where the temperature was 37°C.[104] The temperature-sensitive characteristics of this mutant were stable following growth in cell culture and in hamsters; i.e., there was no evidence of reversion to the wild phenotype.[104] When administered into the nasopharynx, the mutant infected adult volunteers, did not produce disease, and induced resistance to subsequent challenge with virulent wild-type virus.[103] Finally, the mutant appeared to be genetically stable in adults in that isolates obtained from the volunteers retained their ts property. When tested in young children, · the ts mutant was acceptably attenuated. The mutant induced mild rhinitis in infants who had no prior experience with RSV, but this was considered to be an acceptable price to pay for protection against serious RSV disease of the lower respiratory tract.[61,105] However, one of the young infants developed a mild otitis media following rhinitis, and this was thought to be an unacceptable property of the ts-1 strain. In addition, a proportion of infants and young children experimentally infected with the ts-1 mutant shed virus that appeared to be altered genetically in that it was able to produce plaques at 37, 38, or 39°C, temperatures that were restrictive for the ts-1 mutant.[50] The emergence of genetically altered virus with wild-type temperature sensitivity was not associated with any signs or symptoms of lower respiratory tract disease.[61] Nonetheless, this pattern of genetic alteration offered some cause for concern. Although the ts-1 mutant may not be the definitive RSV vaccine strain, the initial studies were helpful in providing a frame of reference for evaluation of other mutants of this virus. In these studies, a sharper definition of the properties required for an acceptable vaccine strain was developed, and it was shown that an attenuated strain could infect and induce an antibody response in young infants without attendant lower respiratory tract disease. Infants who were experimentally infected with the ts-1 mutant did not exhibit an altered, exaggerated response to infection when they were subsequently reinfected with naturally occurring virus 1–2 years later (H. W. Kim, unpublished findings, 1978). Current efforts are directed at the production of temperature-sensitive mutants of RSV that are more restricted in their growth in the upper respiratory tract.[4,89]

Recently, workers at the Merck Institute for Therapeutic Research reported another approach to the immunoprophylaxis of RSV disease. It was shown that parenteral administration of live, wild-type RSV, grown in human diploid cells, induced the development of serum N antibody in young seronegative children without causing signs or symptoms of disease. Importantly, this vaccine did not appear to induce a state of altered reactivity to RSV, as had been observed previously with the inactivated RSV vaccine.[12,13]

A more detailed study of parenteral immunization with live RSV indicated that intramuscular (IM) inoculation of 10^2–10^4 PFU of virus induced complete resistance in both the upper and lower portions of the respiratory tract of the cotton rat.[85,86] Virus was not recovered from the local site of inoculation after 5 min and was never detected in the respiratory tract of IM inoculated rats. Attempts to detect viral antigens at the site of inoculation using indirect immunofluorescence were unsuccessful. However, inactivation of infectivity of three different strains of RSV by ultraviolet light markedly reduced or completely ablated antigenicity and protective efficacy by the IM route. This suggests that these viruses underwent limited replication, perhaps restricted to an abortive cycle, at the local site of inoculation. Finally, an immunosuppressive effect of passive maternally derived immunity was observed. Only

50% of weanling rats possessing passive maternal serum antibody were successfully immunized by IM vaccination with live virus.

An immunosuppressive effect of maternally transmitted antibody was also observed by the Merck group in that none of 15 seropositive infants 2–6 months of age developed a seroresponse when given virus parenterally.[12] In a recent double blind field trial, the Merck vaccine failed to protect seronegative or seropositive children against RSV disease.[4b]

9. Unresolved Problems

The major unresolved problem in our understanding of RSV concerns the mechanism whereby the virus produces its most frequent and most severe disease manifestations during the first few months of life. The role and relative importance of age, immunological immaturity, immunosuppression, and immunopathology in serious RSV lower respiratory disease of early infancy must be assessed in a more definitive manner than in past studies. Greater insight in these areas is required before the final strategy for prevention or therapy of RSV disease can be planned.

In addition, we need a more complete understanding of the manner in which RSV evades the host's defense mechanisms and reinfects the same person with appreciable frequency over a period of years. Greater comprehension in this area may allow us to manipulate the host's defenses so that the reinfection can be diminished and the quantity of virus available for infection of susceptible infants can be decreased significantly.

10. References

1. ADAMS, J. M., IMAGAWA, D. T., AND ZIKE, K., Relationship of pneumonitis in infants to respiratory syncytial virus, *Lancet* **81**:502–506 (1961).
2. BEEM, M., EGERER, R., AND ANDERSON, J., Respiratory syncytial virus neutralizing antibodies in persons residing in Chicago, Illinois, *Pediatrics* **34**:761–770 (1964).
3. BEEM, M., WRIGHT, F. H., HAMRE, D., EGERER, R., AND OEHME, M., Association of the chimpanzee coryza agent with acute respiratory disease in children, *N. Engl. J. Med.* **263**:523–530 (1960).
4. BELSHE, R. B., RICHARDSON, L. S., LONDON, W. T., SLY, D. L., CAMARGO, E., PREVAR, D. A., AND CHANOCK, R. M., Evaluation of five temperature-sensitive mutants of respiratory syncytial virus in primates. II. Genetic analysis of virus recovered during infection, *J. Med. Virol.* **3**:101–110 (1978).
4a. BELSHE, R. B., RICHARDSON, L. S., SCHNITZER, T. J., PREVAR, D. A., CAMARGO, E., AND CHANOCK, R. M., Further characterization of the complementation group B temperature-sensitive mutant of respiratory syncytial virus, *J. Virol.* **24**:8–12 (1977).
4b. BELSHE, R. B., VAN VORIS, L. P., AND MUFSON, M. A., Results of a field trial with parenterally administered live respiratory syncytial virus vaccine, *Clinical Res.* **27**:4, 650a (1979).
5. BERG, T., AND JOHANSSON, S. G. O., IgE concentrations in children with atopic diseases, *Ann. Allergy* **36**:219–232 (1969).
6. BERTHIAUME, L., JONCAS, J., AND PAVILANIS, V., Comparative structure, morphogenesis and biological characteristics of the respiratory syncytial (RS) virus and the pneumonia virus of mice, *Arch. Gesamte Virusforsch.* **45**:39–51 (1974).
7. BLANDFORD, C., AND HEATH, R. B., Studies on the immune response and pathogenesis of Sendai virus infection of mice. I. The fate of viral antigens, *Immunology* **22**(4):637–650 (1972).
8. BRANDT, C. D., KIM, H. W., ARROBIO, J. O., JEFFRIES, B. C., WOOD, S. C., CHANOCK, R. M., AND PARROTT, R. H., Epidemiology of respiratory syncytial virus infection in Washington, D.C. III. Composite analysis of eleven consecutive yearly epidemics, *Am. J. Epidemiol.* **98**:355–364 (1973).
9. BRANDT, C. D., PARROTT, R. H., PATRICK, J. R., KIM, H. W., ARROBIO, J. O., CHANDRA, R., JEFFRIES, B. C., AND CHANOCK, R. M., Epidemiology—SIDS and viral respiratory disease in metropolitan Washington D.C., in: *S.I.D.S. Proceedings of the Francis E. Camps International Symposium on Sudden and Unexpected Death in Infancy* (R. R. ROBINSON, ed.), pp. 117–129, Canadian Foundation for the Study of Infant Death, 1974.
10. BRUHN, F. W., MOKROHISKY, S. T., AND MCINTOSH, K., Apnea associated with respiratory syncytial virus infection in young infants, *J. Pediatr.* **90**:382–386 (1977).
11. BRUHN, F. W., AND YEAGER, A. S., Respiratory syncytial virus in early infancy, *Am. J. Dis. Child.* **131**:145–148 (1977).
12. BUYNAK, E. B., WEIBEL, R. E., MCLEAN, A. A., AND HILLEMAN, M. R., Live respiratory syncytial virus vaccine administered parenterally, *Proc. Soc. Exp. Biol. Med.* **157**:636–642 (1978).

13. BUYNAK, E. B., WEIBEL, R. E., CARLSON, A. J., MCLEAN, A. A., AND HILLEMAN, M. R., Further investigations of live respiratory syncytial virus vaccine administered parenterally, *Proc. Soc. Exp. Biol. Med.* **160**:272–277 (1979).

14. CARILLI, A. D., GOHD, R. S., AND GORDON, W., A virologic study of chronic bronchitis, *N. Engl. J. Med.* **270**:123–127 (1964).

15. CHANOCK, R. M., Prospects for control of acute viral and mycoplasmal respiratory tract disease by vaccination, *Science* **169**:248–256 (1970).

16. CHANOCK, R. M., AND FINBERG, L., Recovery from infants with respiratory illness of a virus related to chimpanzee coryza agent (CCA). II. Epidemiological aspects of infection in infants and young children, *Am. J. Hyg.* **66**:291–300 (1957).

17. CHANOCK, R. M., KAPIKIAN, A. Z., MILLS, J., KIM, H. W., AND PARROTT, R. H., Influence of immunological factors in respiratory syncytial virus disease, *Arch. Environ. Health* **21**:347–356 (1970).

18. CHANOCK, R. M., KIM, H. W., VARGOSKO, A. J., DELEVA, A., JOHNSON, K. M., CUMMING, C., AND PARROTT, R. H., Respiratory syncytial virus. I. Virus recovery and other observations during 1960 outbreak of bronchiolitis, pneumonia, and minor respiratory diseases in children, *J. Am. Med. Assoc.* **176**:647–653 (1961).

19. CHANOCK, R. M., AND PARROTT, R. H., Acute respiratory disease in infancy and childhood: Present understanding and prospects for prevention, *Pediatrics* **36**:21–39 (1965).

20. CHANOCK, R. M., PARROTT, R. H., JOHNSON, K. M., MUFSON, M. A., AND KNIGHT, V., Biology and ecology of two major lower respiratory tract pathogens—RS virus and Eaton PPLO, in: *Perspectives in Virology* (M. POLLARD, ed.), pp. 257–281, Burgess, Minneapolis, 1963.

21. CHANOCK, R. M., ROIZMAN, B., AND MYERS, R., Recovery from infants with respiratory illness of a virus related to chimpanzee coryza agent. I. Isolation, properties and characterization, *Am. J. Hyg.* **66**:281–290 (1957).

22. CHIN, J., MAGOFFIN, R. L., SHEARER, L. A., SCHIEBLE, J. H., AND LENNETE, E. H., Field evaluation of a respiratory syncytial virus vaccine and a trivalent parainfluenza virus vaccine in a pediatric population, *Am. J. Epidemiol.* **89**:449–463 (1969).

22a. COATES, H. V., ALLING, D. W., AND CHANOCK R. M., An antigenic analysis of respiratory syncytial virus isolates by a plaque reduction neutralization test, *Am. J. Epidemiol.* **89**:299–313 (1966).

23. DOGGETT, J. E., Antibodies to respiratory syncytial virus in human sera from different regions of the world, *Bull. WHO* **32**:849–853 (1965).

24. DOWNHAM, M. A. P. S., GARDNER, P. S., MCQUILLIN, J., AND FERRIS, J. A. J., Role of respiratory viruses in childhood mortality, *Br. Med. J.* **1**:235–239 (1975).

25. DOWNHAM, M. A. P. S., SCOTT, R., SIMS, D. G., WEBB, J. K. G., AND GARDNER, P. S., Breast-feeding protects against respiratory syncytial virus infections, *Br. Med. J.* **2**:274–276 (1976).

26. FRANSEN, H., STERNER, G., FORSGREN, M., HEIGL, Z., WOLONTIS, S., SVEDMYR, A., AND TUNEVALL, G., Acute lower respiratory illness in elderly patients with respiratory syncytial virus infection, *Acta Med. Scand.* **182**:323–330 (1967).

27. FRIEDEWALD, W. T., FORSYTH, B. R., SMITH, C. B., GHARPURE, M. S., AND CHANOCK, R. M., Low-temperature-grown RS virus in adult volunteers, *J. Am. Med. Assoc.* **204**:690–694 (1968).

28. FULGINITI, V. A., ELLER, J. J., SIEBER, O. F., JOYNER, J. W., MINAMITANI, M., AND MEIKLEJOHN, G., Respiratory virus immunization. I. A field trial of two inactivated respiratory virus vaccines: An aqueous trivalent parainfluenza virus vaccine and an alum-precipitated respiratory syncytial virus vaccine, *Am. J. Epidemiol.* **89**:435–448 (1969).

29. GARDNER, P. S., Respiratory syncytial virus infection: Admissions to hospital in industrial, urban, and rural areas: Report to the Medical Research Council subcommittee on Respiratory Syncytial Virus Vaccines, *Br. Med. J* **2**:796–798 (1978).

30. GARDNER, P. S., AND MCQUILLIN, J., Application of immunofluorescent antibody technique in rapid diagnosis of respiratory syncytial virus infection, *Br. Med. J.* **3**:340–343 (1968).

31. GARDNER, P. S., AND MCQUILLIN, J., The coating of respiratory syncytial (RS) virus-infected cells in the respiratory tract by immunoglobulins, *J. Med. Virol.* **2**:165–173 (1978).

32. GARDNER, P. S., MCQUILLIN, J., AND COURT, S. D. M., Speculation on pathogenesis in death from respiratory syncytial virus infection, *Br. Med. J.* **1**:327–330 (1970).

33. GARDNER, P. S., TURK, D. C., AHERNE, W. A., BIRD, T., HOLDAWAY, M. D., AND COURT, S. D. M., Deaths associated with respiratory tract infection in childhood, *Br. Med. J.* **4**:316–320 (1967).

34. GHARPURE, M. A., WRIGHT, P. F., AND CHANOCK, R. M., Temperature-sensitive mutant of respiratory syncytial virus, *J. Virol.* **3**:414–421 (1969).

35. GLEICH, G. J., AVERBECK, A. K., AND SWEDLUNG, H. A., Measurement of IgE in normal and allergic serum by radioimmunoassay, *J. Lab. Clin. Med.* **77**:690–698 (1971).

36. GLEZEN, W. P., AND DENNY, F. W., Epidemiology of acute lower respiratory disease in children, *N. Engl. J. Med.* **288**:498–505 (1973).

37. GLEZEN, W. P., TABER, L. H., PAREDES, A., ALLISON, J. E., AND FRANK, A. L., Pathogenesis of respiratory syncytial (RS) virus bronchiolitis in infants, *Pediatr. Res.* **12**:492 (1978).

38. GRAY, K. G., MACFARLANE, D. E., AND SOMERVILLE, R. G., Direct immunofluorescent identification of respiratory syncytial virus in throat swabs from children with respiratory illness, *Lancet* **1**:446–448 (1968).

39. GRIST, N. R., ROSS, C. A. C., AND STOTT, E. J., Influenza, respiratory syncytial virus, and pneumonia in Glasgow 1962–1965, *Br. Med. J.* **1**:456–457 (1967).

40. HALL, C. B., DOUGLAS, R. G., JR., AND GEIMAN, J. M., Quantitative shedding patterns of respiratory syncytial virus in infants, *J. Infect. Dis.* **132**:151–156 (1975).

41. HALL, C. B., DOUGLAS, R. G., JR., AND GEIMAN, J. M., Respiratory syncytial virus infections in infants: Quantitation and duration of shedding, *J. Pediatr.* **89**:11–15 (1976).

42. HALL, C. B., DOUGLAS, R. G., JR, GEIMAN, J. M., AND MESSNER, M. K., Nosocomial respiratory syncytial virus infections, *N. Engl. J. Med.* **293**:1343–1346 (1975).

43. HALL, C. B., DOUGLAS, R. G., JR., SIMONS, R. L., AND GEIMAN, B. S., Interferon production in children with respiratory syncytial, influenza and parainfluenza virus infections, *J. Pediatr.* **98**:23–32 (1978).

44. HALL, C. B., GEIMAN, J. M., BIGGAR, R., KOTOK, D. I., HOGAN, P. M., AND DOUGLAS, R. G., JR., Respiratory syncytial virus infections within families, *N. Engl. J. Med.* **294**:414–419 (1976).

45. HALL, C. B., GEIMAN, J. M., DOUGLAS, R. G., JR., AND MEAGHER, M. P., Control of nosocomial respiratory syncytial viral infections, *Pediatrics* **62**:728–732 (1978).

46. HALL, W. J., HALL, C. B., AND SPEERS, D. M., Respiratory syncytial virus infection in adults: Clinical, virologic, and serial pulmonary function studies, *Ann. Intern. Med.* **88**:203–205 (1978).

47. HALL, C. B., KOPELMAN, A. E., DOUGLAS, R. G., JR., GEIMAN, J. M., AND MEAGHER, M. P., Neonatal respiratory syncytial virus infection, *N. Engl. J. Med.* **300**:393–396 (1979).

48. HAMBLING, M. H., A survey of antibodies to respiratory syncytial virus in the population, *Br. Med. J.* **1**:1223–1225 (1964).

49. HENDERSON, F. W., COLLIER, A. M., CLYDE, W. A., AND DENNY, F. W., Respiratory syncytial virus infection, reinfection and immunity: A prospective longitudinal study in young children, *N. Engl. J. Med.* **300**:530–535 (1979).

50. HODES, D. S., KIM, H. W., PARROTT, R. H., CAMARGO, E., AND CHANOCK, R. M., Genetic alteration in a temperature-sensitive mutant of respiratory syncytial virus after replication *in vivo*, *Proc. Soc. Exp. Biol. Med.* **145**:1158–1164 (1974).

51. INABA, Y., TANAKA, Y., SATO, K., OMORI, T., AND MATUMOTO, M., Bovine respiratory syncytial virus: Studies on an outbreak in Japan, 1968–1969, *Jpn. J. Microbiol.* **16**:373–383 (1972).

52. JACOBS, J. W., AND EDGINGTON, N., Isolation of respiratory syncytial virus from cattle in Britain, *Vet. Rec.* **87**:694 (1971).

53. JACOBS, J. W., PEACOCK, D. B., CORNER, B. D., CAUL, E. O., AND CLARKE, S. K. R., Respiratory syncytial and other viruses associated with respiratory disease in infants, *Lancet* **1**:871–876 (1971).

54. JENNINGS, R., Adenovirus, parainfluenza virus and respiratory syncytial virus antibodies in the sera of Jamaicans, *J. Hyg.* **70**:523–529 (1972).

55. JOHNSON, K. M., CHANOCK, R. M., RIFKIND, D., KRAVETZ, H. M., AND KNIGHT, V., Respiratory syncytial virus. IV. Correlation on virus shedding, serologic response, and illness in adult volunteers, *J. Am. Med. Assoc.* **176**:663–667 (1961).

56. JONCAS, J., BERTHIAUME, L., AND PAVILANIS, V., The structure of the respiratory syncytial virus, *Virology* **38**:493–496 (1969).

57. KALICA, A. R., WRIGHT, P. F., HETRICK, F. M., AND CHANOCK, R. M., Electron microscopic studies of respiratory syncytial temperature-sensitivie mutants, *Arch. Gesamte Virusforsch.* **41**:248–258 (1973).

58. KAPIKIAN, A. Z., BELL, J. A., MASTROTA, F. M., JOHNSON, K. M., HUEBNER, R. J., AND CHANOCK, R. M., An outbreak of febrile illness and pneumonia associated with respiratory syncytial virus infection, *Am. J. Hyg.* **74**:234–248 (1961).

59. KAPIKIAN, A. Z., MITCHELL, R. H., CHANOCK, R. M., SHVEDOFF, R. A., AND STEWART, C. E., An epidemiologic study of altered clinical reactivity to respiratory syncytial (RS) virus infection in children previously vaccinated with an inactivated RS virus vaccine, *Am. J. Epidemiol* **89**:405–421 (1969).

60. KIM, H. W., ARROBIO, J. O., BRANDT, C. D., JEFFRIES, B. C., PYLES, G., REID, J. L., CHANOCK, R. M., AND PARROTT, R. H., Epidemiology of respiratory syncytial virus in Washington, D.C. I. Importance of the virus in different respiratory tract disease syndromes and temporal distribution of infection, *Am. J. Epidemiol.* **98**:216–225 (1973).

61. KIM, H. W., ARROBIO. J. O., BRANDT, C. D., WRIGHT, P., HODES, D., CHANOCK, R. M., AND PARROTT, R. H., Safety and antigenicity of temperature-sensitive (*ts*) mutant respiratory syncytial (RS) virus in infants and children, *Pediatrics* **52**:56–63 (1973).

62. KIM, H. W., ARROBIO, J. O., PYLES, G., BRANDT, C. D., CAMARGO, E., CHANOCK, R. M., AND PARROTT, R. H., Clinical and immunological response of infants and children to administration of low temperature adapted respiratory syncytial virus, *Pediatrics* **48**:745–755 (1971).

63. KIM, H. W., CANCHOLA, J. G., BRANDT, C. D., PYLES,

G., CHANOCK, R. M., JENSEN, K., AND PARROTT, R. H., Respiratory syncytial virus disease in infants despite prior administration of antigenic inactivated vaccine, *Am. J. Epidemiol.* **89:**422–434 (1969).

64. KIM, H. W., LEIKIN, S. L., ARROBIO, J. O., BRANDT, C. D., CHANOCK, R. M., AND PARROTT, R. H., Cell-mediated immunity to respiratory syncytial virus induced by inactivated vaccine or by infection, *Pediatr. Res.* **10:**75–78 (1976).

65. KRAVETZ, H. M., KNIGHT, V., CHANOCK, R. M., MORRIS, A. J., JOHNSON, K. M., RIFKIND, D., AND UTZ, J. P., Respiratory syncytial virus. III. Production of illness and clinical observations in adult volunteers, *J. Am Med. Assoc.* **176:**657–663 (1961).

66. KUMAR, L., NEWCOMB, R. W., ISHIZAKA, K., MIDDLETON, E., AND HORNBROOK, M. M., IgE levels in sera of children with asthma, *Pediatrics* **47:**848–856 (1971).

67. LEE, C., FUNK, G. A., CHEN, S., AND HUANG, T., An outbreak of respiratory syncytial virus infection in an infant nursery, *J. Formosan Med. Assoc.* **72:**39–46 (1973).

68. LEER, H. W., BLOOMFIELD, N. J., GREEN, J. L., HEIMLICH, E. M., HYDE, J. S., MOFFET, H. L., YOUNG, G. A., AND BARRON, B. A., Corticosteroid treatment in bronchiolitis, *Am. J. Dis. Child.* **117:**495–503 (1969).

69. LODA, F. A., CLYDE, W. A., GLEZEN, W. P., SENIOR, R. J., SHEAFFER, C. I., AND DENNY, F. W., Studies on the role of viruses, bacteria and *M. pneumoniae* as causes of lower respiratory tract infections in children, *J. Pediatr.* **72:**161–176 (1968).

70. MARTIN, A. J., GARDNER, P. S., AND McQUILLIN, J., Epidemiology of respiratory viral infection among pediatric inpatients over a six-year period in Northeast England, *Lancet* **2:**1035–1038 (1978).

71. McINTOSH, K., Interferon in nasal secretions from infants with viral respiratory tract infections, *J. Pediatrics* **93:**33–36 (1978).

72. McINTOSH, K., ELLIS, E. F., HOFFMAN, L. S., LYBASS, T. G., ELLER, J. J., AND FULGINITI, V. A., The association of viral and bacterial respiratory infections with exacerabations of wheezing in young asthmatic children, *J. Pediatr.* **82:**578–590 (1973).

73. McINTOSH, K., MASTERS, H. B., ORR, I., CHAO, R. K., AND BARKIN, R. M., The immunologic response to infection with respiratory syncytial virus in infants, *J. Infect. Dis* **138:**24–32 (1978).

74. MILLS, J., KNOPF, H. L. S., VANKIRK, J., AND CHANOCK, R. M., Significance of local respiratory tract antibody to respiratory syncytial virus, in: *The Secretory Immunological System* (D. H. DAYTON, JR., P. A. SMALL, JR., R. M. CHANOCK, H. E. KAUFMAN, AND T. B. TOMASI, eds.), pp. 149–165, U.S. Government Printing Office, Washington, D.C., 1971.

75. MILLS, J., VANKIRK, J. E., WRIGHT, P. F., AND CHAN-

OCK, R. M., Experimental respiratory syncytial virus infection of adults, *J. Immunol.* **107:**123–130 (1971).

76. MONTO, A. S., AND LIM, S. K., The Tecumseh study of respiratory illness. III. Incidence and periodicity of respiratory syncytial virus and mycoplasma pneumonia infections, *Am. J. Epidemiol.* **94:**290–301 (1971).

77. MORRIS, J. A., BLOUNT, R. E., JR., AND SAVAGE, R. E., Recovery of cytopathogenic agent from chimpanzees with coryza, *Proc. Soc. Exp. Biol. Med.* **92:**544 (1956).

78. MUFSON, M. A., LEVINE, H. D., WASIL, R. E., MOCEGAGONZALEZ, H. E., AND KRAUSE, H. E., Epidemiology of respiratory syncytial virus infection among infants and children in Chicago, *Am. J. Epidemiol.* **98:**88–95 (1973).

79. NORRBY, E., Myxoviridae: Pseudomyxovirus—Respiratory syncytial (RS) virus, in: *Handbook Series in Clinical Laboratory Science* (D. SELIGSON, ed.), pp. 401–409, CRC Press, West Palm Beach, Florida, 1979.

79a. NORRBY, E., AND GOLLMAR, Y., Identification of measles virus-specific hemolysis-inhibiting antibodies separate from hemagglutination-inhibiting antibodies, *Infect. Immun.* **11:**231–239, (1975).

80. NORRBY, E., MARUSYK, H., AND ORVELL, C., Ultrastructural studies of the multiplication of RS (respiratory syncytial) virus, *Acta Pathol. Microbiol. Scand. Sect. B* **78:**268 (1970).

81. PACCAUD, M. R., AND JACQUIER, C., A respiratory syncytial virus of bovine origin, *Arch. Gesamte Virusforsch.* **30:**327–342 (1970).

82. PARROTT, R. H., KIM, H. W., ARROBIO, J. O., HODES, D. S., MURPHY, B. R., BRANDT, C. D., CAMARGO, E., AND CHANOCK, R. M., Epidemiology of respiratory syncytial virus infection in Washington, D.C. II. Infection and disease with respect to age, immunologic status, race and sex, *Am. J. Epidemiol.* **98:**289–300 (1973).

83. PARROTT, R. H., VARGOSKO, A. J., KIM, H. W., CUMMING, C., TURNER, J., HUEBNER, R. J., AND CHANOCK, R. M., Respiratory syncytial virus. II. Serologic studies over a 34-month period of children with bronchiolitis, pneumonia, and minor respiratory disease, *J. Am. Med. Assoc.* **176:**653–657 (1961).

84. POLMAR, S. H., ROBINSON, S. D., AND MINNEFOR, A. B., Immunoglobulin E in bronchiolitis, *Pediatrics* **50:**279–284 (1972).

85. PRINCE, G. A., JENSON, A. B., HORSWOOD, R. L., CAMARGO, E., AND CHANOCK, R. M., The pathogenesis of respiratory syncytial virus infection in cotton rats, *Am. J. Pathol.* **93:**771–783 (1978).

86. PRINCE, G. A., POTASH, L., HORSWOOD, R. L., CAMARGO, E., SUFFIN, S. C., JOHNSON, R. A., AND CHANOCK, R. M., Intramuscular inoculation of live respiratory syncytial virus induces immunity in cotton rats, *Infect. Immun.* **23:**723–728 (1979).

87. PRINGLE, C. R., SHIRODARIA, P. V., CASH, P., CHISWELL, D. J., AND MALLOY, P., Initiation and maintenance of persistent infection by respiratory syncytial virus, *J. Virol.* **23**:199–211 (1978).

88. RAVEN, C., MAVERAKIS, N. H., EVELAND, W. C., AND ACKERMAN, W. W., The sudden infant death syndrome: A possible hypersensitivity reaction determined by distribution of IgG in lungs, *J. Forensic Sci.* **23**:116–138 (1978).

89. RICHARDSON, L. S., BELSHE, R. B., LONDON, W. T., SLY, D. L., PREVAR, D. A., CAMARGO, E., AND CHANOCK, R. M., Evaluation of five temperature sensitive mutants of respiratory syncytial virus in primates. I. Viral shedding, immunologic response and associated illness, *J. Med. Virol.* **3**:91–100 (1978).

90. RICHARDSON, L. S., YOLKEN, R. H., BELSHE, R. B., CAMARGO, E., KIM, H. W., AND CHANOCK, R. M., Enzyme-linked immunosorbent assay for measurement of serological response to respiratory syncytial virus infection, *Infect. Immun.* **23**:660–664 (1978).

91. ROSS, C. A. C., PINKERTON, I. W., AND ASSAAD, F. A., Pathogenesis of respiratory syncytial virus diseases in infancy, *Arch. Dis. Child.* **46**:702–704 (1971).

92. ROSS, C. A. C., STOTT, E. J., McMICHAEL, S., AND CROWTHER, I. A., Problems of laboratory diagnosis or respiratory syncytial virus infection in childhood, *Arch. Gesamte Virusforsch.* **14**:553–562 (1964).

93. SCOTT, R., KAUL, A., CHIBA, Y., AND OGRA, P. L., Development of *in vitro* correlates of cell-mediated immunity to respiratory syncytial virus infection in humans, *J. Infect. Dis.* **137**:810–817 (1978).

94. SIMS, D. G., DOWNHAM, M. A. P. S., GARDNER, P. S., WEBB, J. K. G., AND WEIGHTMAN, D., Study of 8-year-old children with a history of respiratory syncytial virus bronchiolitis in infancy, *Br. Med. J.* **1**:11–14 (1978).

95. SOMMERVILLE, R. G., Respiratory syncytial virus in acute exacerbations of chronic bronchitis, *Lancet* **2**:1246–1248 (1963).

96. SPENCE, L., AND BARRATT, N., Respiratory syncytial virus associated with acute respiratory infections in Trinidadian patients, *Am. J. Epidemiol.* **88**:257–266 (1968).

97. STERNER, G., WOLONTIS, S., BLOTH, B., AND DeHEVESY, G., Respiratory syncytial virus: An outbreak of acute respiratory illnesses in home for infants, *Acta Paediatr. Scand.* **55**:273–279 (1966).

98. SUTO, T., YANO, N., IKEDA, M., MIYAMOTO, M., TAKAI, S., SHIGETA, S., HINUMA, Y., AND ISHIDA, N., Respiratory syncytial virus infection and its serologic epidemiology, *Am. J. Epidemiol.* **82**:211–224 (1965).

99. TYRRELL, D. A. J., Discovering and defining the etiology of acute respiratory disease, *Am. Rev. Respir. Dis.* **88**:77–84 (1963).

100. TYRRELL, D. A. J., A collaborative study of the aetiology of acute respiratory infections in Britain 1961–1964, *Br. Med. J.* **2**:319–326 (1965).

101. WATERSON, A. P., AND HOBSON, D., Relationship between respiratory syncytial virus and Newcastle disease—Parainfluenza group, *Br. Med. J.* **2**:1166–1167 (1962).

102. WELLIVER, R. C., KAUL, A., AND OGRA, P. L., Cell-mediated immune response to respiratory syncytial virus infection: Relationship to the development of reactive airway disease, *J. Pediatr.* **94**:370–375 (1979).

103. WRIGHT, P. F., MILLS, J., AND CHANOCK, R. M., Evaluation of a temperature-sensitive mutant of respiratory syncytial virus in adults, *J. Infect. Dis.* **124**:505–511 (1971).

104. WRIGHT, P. F., WOODEND, W. G., AND CHANOCK, R. M., Temperature-sensitive mutants of respiratory syncytial virus: *In vivo* studies in hamsters, *J. Infect. Dis.* **122**:501–512 (1970).

105. WRIGHT, P. F., SHINOVAKI, T., FLEET, W., SELL, S. H., THOMPSON, J., AND KARZON, D. T., Evaluation of live, attenuated respiratory syncytial virus vaccine instance, *J. Pediatr.* **88**:931–936 (1976).

106. ZAKSTELSKAYA, L. Y., AND SHENDERVOCH, S. F., On mechanisms of interference of respiratory syncytial virus by influenza A2 virus, *Vopr. Virusol.* **15**:552–555 (1970).

CHAPTER 20

Rhinoviruses

Jack M. Gwaltney, Jr.

1. Introduction

Rhinoviruses are the most important common cold viruses to be discovered. The name *rhinovirus* reflects the prominent nasal involvement seen in infections with these viruses. The large rhinovirus genus, which is a member of the picornavirus family, contains over 100 different antigenic types. The discovery of the rhinoviruses led to the realization that the common cold is an enormously complex syndrome. The number of antigenically distinct rhinoviruses is so large that man can be infected with a different rhinovirus each year and still not experience all the known types in a lifetime. Awareness of the complexity of the rhinovirus problem has discouraged work on the development of common-cold vaccines and stimulated interest in alternative approaches to control, such as chemoprophylaxis and environmental measures. Although rhinoviruses are the best studied of the common-cold viruses, major gaps still remain in knowledge of their epidemiological behavior. The fundamental question of the number of antigenic types in existence is unanswered, as is the related question of the possible occurrence of antigenic drift of serotypes.

Jack M. Gwaltney, Jr. · Department of Internal Medicine, University of Virginia School of Medicine, Charlottesville, Virginia.

2. Historical Background

Another member of the picornavirus family, poliovirus, is known to have caused disease in ancient times, so it is probable that rhinoviruses were in existence then also. Colds were a nuisance in early civilization; then, as now, many useless remedies were proposed for their treatment. In 400 B.C., Hippocrates noted that bleeding was a frequently used, although worthless, treatment for colds. In the 1st century, Pliny the Younger prescribed "kissing the hairy muzzle of a mouse" for colds. The first sound epidemiological knowledge about acute respiratory disease came with the observations that sea voyagers and the inhabitants of isolated communities were free of colds while not in contact with the outside world, but developed colds when such contact was reestablished. This led to the important conclusion that colds are contagious.

Direct evidence of the infectious nature of colds came in 1914 from the volunteer studies of Kruse,[97] who produced experimental colds in volunteers by intranasal inoculation of cell-free filtrates of nasal secretions from persons with colds. Similar experiments by Dochez *et al.*[38] in 1930 confirmed that colds could be transmitted by bacteria-free filtrates, suggesting that the responsible agents might be viruses. At the same time, epidemiological studies of acute respiratory disease in populations had been started. Van Loghem[168] measured the incidence of colds and observed their relationship to the seasons.

Frost and Gover[57] made the perceptive observation that common respiratory disease appearing during the months of high prevalence, September to March, was composed of a series of short epidemics of irregular sequences and magnitude. This suggested that colds were caused by a variety of different agents occurring in succession. In the 1940s and 1950s, long-term studies of colds in the home by Dingle et al.[36] yielded precise information on attack rates by age and the importance of the home as a site for transmission of respiratory infections. During the same period, a group at the Common Cold Research Unit at Salisbury, England, headed by Andrewes and later Tyrrell, was vigorously pursuing questions related to the etiology and epidemiology of colds.[1] Colds were successfully transmitted in volunteers using nasal secretions that were later shown to contain rhinoviruses. Attempts at the time to establish growth of the virus in artificial culture were unsuccessful.

Specific work on rhinoviruses began in 1956 when Pelon et al.[126] and Price,[135] working separately, reported the isolation of a new virus that was subsequently given the designation rhinovirus 1A. Within a few years, Ketler et al.,[93] using the highly sensitive human embryonic lung cells developed by Hayflick and Moorhead[74] and employing growth methods developed at the Salisbury Common Cold Unit,[167] isolated a number of different serological types, indicating that the rhinovirus group would not be small. Epidemiological studies conducted by Hamre and Procknow[70] during the same period established that rhinoviruses were responsible for a significant amount of acute respiratory disease. Specific rhinovirus infection rates and the finding of recurrent fall peaks of rhinovirus colds were reported from a longitudinal study by Gwaltney et al.[62] In further studies of rhinovirus epidemiology by Monto,[113] Dick et al.,[35] and Hendley et al.,[77] the importance of the family setting and of schoolchildren in particular in favoring rhinovirus transmission was demonstrated. Couch et al.[28] noted the surprisingly small amount of virus necessary to initiate experimental infections in volunteers. This group also provided important information on the pathogenesis[42] and immunology of rhinovirus infections.[143] In 1967, a collaborative program directed by Kapikian et al.[89] assigned numbers 1A–55 to the rhinovirus types then known. In 1971, a second phase of this program added types 56–89.[90]

Results of a third phase of the numbering program currently in progress indicate that approximately 20 more rhinovirus types will be added to the genus.[71]

3. Methodology Involved in Epidemiological Analysis

3.1. Surveillance and Sampling

Three longitudinal studies of rhinovirus epidemiology have provided data on rhinovirus attack rates. Surveillance of a population of young adults at an insurance company in Charlottesville, Virginia, was conducted by collecting illness data on symptom-record cards in conjunction with weekly personal contact by a nurse-epidemiologist.[62] This nurse also collected samples at the time of illness. In addition, samples were obtained weekly from asymptomatic persons in a randomly selected sample of the study population. In another study, families from representative segments of the population in Tecumseh, Michigan, were surveyed by weekly telephone contact with a single household respondent who provided illness information for the family.[119] In the third investigation, mothers of families with newborn infants in a group health cooperative in Seattle, Washington, recorded illness information on their families and were visited twice weekly for routine sampling.[55] In the latter two studies, specimens were collected during home visits by a nurse-epidemiologist when illness was reported to the study team by telephone.

3.2. Methods of Virus Isolation and Propagation

Cell culture is the standard method for rhinovirus isolation and propagation. Rhinoviruses grow best at temperatures of 33–34°C under conditions of motion[87] and will not grow in embryonated eggs or suckling mice. Most epidemiological studies have employed human embryonic lung cells, strains WI26 and WI38, or strains of human embryonic lung cells originated by the laboratory conducting the study. Rhinovirus cytopathic effect in WI38 cell culture is readily discernible, making this an easy system with which to work. The sensitivity of WI38 cells to rhinoviruses appears to be similar to that of the nasal mucosa of volunteers. Volunteer challenge experiments comparing rhinovirus median human and tissue culture infectious dose (HID_{50} and $TCID_{50}$) have shown 1 HID_{50} to be equivalent to 0.03–0.75 $TCID_{50}$.[39]

There are problems, however, with the use of human embryonic lung-cell cultures. The sensitivity to rhinovirus of cell strains of different origin may vary 100-fold or more, for poorly understood reasons.[8] Also, different lots of the same strain, such as WI38, may have unpredictable variations in rhinovirus sensitivity that are unexplained.[61] Interpretations of rhinovirus morbidity data must take these variations into account, since rates of rhinovirus-associated illness are directly related to the sensitivity of the cell cultures used.

Rhinoviruses will grow in other cell lines and strains derived from human and primate tissues, including rhesus monkey kidney, human embryonic kidney, and KB. The sensitivity of these cells for rhinoviruses tends to be less consistent than that of WI38 cells. A strain of HeLa cells with enhanced sensitivity to rhinoviruses has been developed and proven useful for propagation of antigen and for serological procedures.[23] These M-HeLa cells have been used to grow rhinovirus harvests with exceptionally high titers (10^9 PFU/ml)[25] and to prepare large quantities of antigen in suspension cultures.[162] Certain rhinovirus serotypes were recovered from original specimens with M-HeLa cells but not with human diploid-cell cultures.[27a,97b] All the first 55 numbered rhinovirus types have been plaqued using a method that employs HeLa cells and an agarose overlay containing medium with added magnesium and DEAE–dextran.[51]

The earlier division of rhinoviruses into H and M strains on the basis of growth in cells of human or monkey origin has been of limited epidemiological importance. M strains tend to grow better in cell culture, and thus were more easily recovered with the less sensitive systems used in earlier studies.[65] Consideration should be given to the greater ease of recovery of M strains when epidemiological data are being evaluated, since this variable could result in overestimation of the importance of M rhinoviruses. Recent work has shown that H strains can be adapted to grow in monkey-kidney cells, suggesting that the division into H and M strains is not based on major differences in the biological properties of rhinoviruses.[41]

Organ cultures of fetal human trachea and other ciliated epithelium have been used to isolate rhinoviruses that did not grow initially in cell culture.[82,166] Comparison of the sensitivity for rhinovirus isolation of standard cell culture and of organ culture has failed to show clear superiority of the organ-culture system;[79] both systems are necessary for optimal recovery of these viruses. Once isolated in organ culture, rhinoviruses can usually be adapted to cell culture. The organ-culture strains have been found to be types that have also been recovered in cell culture. Because of the limited supply of fetal material, it has not been possible to use organ-culture systems in large epidemiological studies.

Experimental infections with human rhinoviruses have been produced in chimpanzees[34] and gibbons,[133] but attempts to infect small laboratory animals have not been successful. Rhinoviruses have been isolated from cattle,[112] and respiratory viruses with characteristics similar to those of human rhinoviruses have been recovered from cats[30] and horses.[37]

3.3. Methods Used for Serological Surveys and Antibody Measurements

The multiplicity of rhinovirus types and their relative immunological specificity have prevented the general use of serological techniques for measuring infection rates. Serological study of infection rates is possible, however, when the types of rhinoviruses circulating in small populations, such as families, are known from viral cultures. Testing for the presence of rhinovirus antibody has been done with the neutralization (N) test, since this method was the only one available until recently. The N test has also been used to identify specific antigenic types of viruses and to measure antibody in human serum and nasal secretions.

In experimental rhinovirus infection, virus shedding was found to be more sensitive than antibody response as a means of detecting infection,[75] while in studies of natural infections, either procedure alone identified only about two-thirds of the diagnosed infections.[4] In family studies, 20–40% of total infections were detected only by serology in persons who had both tests performed.[35,77]

For typing rhinoviruses, hyperimmune rhinovirus antisera have been produced in a number of animal species, including rabbits, guinea pigs, calves, goats, and baboons. Some goat and calf antisera have contained cytotoxic substances that have caused difficulties in the interpretation of N test results.[23] The large number of rhinovirus serotypes has led to the use of antisera pools for serotype identification. An efficient method of antisera pooling is the combinatorial method.[92] Serological identifications of rhinoviruses in large epidemiological studies can be done with pooled antisera used in microneutralization systems.[59,96]

The accepted standard for serological identity of an unknown rhinovirus is neutralization of virus concentrations ranging from 10 to 300 $TCID_{50}$ by 20 units of antibody.[87] For measuring N antibody in human serum and nasal washings, it is necessary to use small doses of virus (3–30 $TCID_{50}$) for the test to have satisfactory sensitivity.[45] Somewhat more sensitive plaque-reduction methods of antibody measurement have been developed[161] but have not been used extensively as an epidemiological tool.

Complement-fixation (CF) tests with rhinoviruses have been reported[20,33] but have not been useful as a method of collecting morbidity data. Also, rhinoviruses have been found to agglutinate sheep erythrocytes,[155] although not all serological types show hemagglutination under the conditions of pH and temperature that were studied. A passive hemagglutination test for rhinovirus type 17 has been reported.[133a]

4. Characteristics of the Virus That Affect the Epidemiological Pattern

4.1. Physical and Biochemical Characteristics

Rhinoviruses have physical and biochemical properties that put them in the picornavirus family (Table 1).[12a,170] This family also includes enterovirus and calicivirus. While sharing basic properties with enteroviruses, such as size, shape, nucleic acid composition, and ether resistance, rhinoviruses differ in having a greater buoyant density and a susceptibility to inactivation by exposure to an acid environment.[144] The basis for acid lability remains unclear, although treatment with acid results in the loss from the virion of the smallest of the four size classes of rhinovirus polypeptides (VP1–4).[95] Rhinoviruses are structurally similar to enteroviruses.[105,106] Their gene and cleavage patterns have been found to be similar to those of

poliovirus.[103] Thus, the sum of evidence on the physical and biochemical nature of rhinoviruses suggests that they and enteroviruses are descended from a common ancestor. Similarity in physical nature of the two groups may help explain similarities in epidemiological behavior, i.e., increased prevalence in late summer and fall and possible spread by direct contact with infectious secretions.

4.2. Biological Characteristics

The biochemical basis for the optimal temperature range for rhinovirus growth is unknown, but this property may be of major epidemiological importance (Table 1). The mean temperature of nasal mucosa, 33–35°C, corresponds to the optimal temperature for rhinovirus replication. At 37°C, virus yields fall to 10–50% of optimum.[156,167] In natural infection in man, rhinovirus concentrations are higher in nasal secretions than in pharyngeal secretions, saliva, or secretions obtained by simulated coughs and sneezes.[78] Attempts to isolate rhinovirus from blood have not been successful,[42,47] nor does rhinovirus survive and replicate in the intestinal tract. Studies of rhinovirus survival in the gut suggest that the temperature of 37°C may be a decisive factor in inhibiting growth, although gastrointestinal secretions and transit time may also have adverse effects on virus survival.[17] On the basis of these observations, it is tempting to speculate that one reason for the different pathogenic and epidemiological behavior of enteroviruses and rhinoviruses is the difference in the optimal temperature for growth of the two groups of viruses.

Rhinovirus receptors are insensitive to neuraminidase but sensitive to proteolytic enzymes.[101a] Studies using HeLa cell cultures have shown that rhinoviruses can be separated into at least two different groups on the basis of attachment at receptor sites on the cell surface.[99]

4.3. Antigenic Characteristics

Rhinoviruses in their native state contain type-specific surface antigens (Table 1). On the basis of a collaborative program, they have been classified as serotypes 1–89 and subtype 1A.[88–90] Further work on rhinovirus numbering is nearing comple-

Table 1. Characteristics of Rhinovirus

Physical and biochemical	Biological
Size: 28–34 nm	Optimal temperature of growth 33–35°C and restriction of growth at 37°C
Shape: capsid with icosahedral symmetry with proposed structure of 60 copies each of four polypeptides (VP1–VP4)	Inability to survive and replicate in the intestinal tract
Nucleic acid: single-stranded RNA of $2.6 \pm 0.1 \times 10^6$ daltons (30% of total particle mass)	Survival on skin and environmental surfaces
Ether: resistant	Two or more receptor families for host cells
Acid: labile (pH 3–5)	
Virus synthesis and maturation in cytoplasm	

Antigenic

Native antigenicity: type-specific (D antigenicity)
One hundred or more numbered native antigenic types
Direct and indirect antigenic relationships between some native antigenic types demonstrable with hyperimmune sera
Altered antigenicity (by heat or urea): cross-reactive between types (C antigenicity)

tion, and approximately 20 more types will be added to the classification.[71] There are a large number of rhinovirus strains that have been recovered in epidemiological studies that are not neutralized by antisera to the numbered types.

The criterion for the selection of numbered prototype viruses was the absence of cross-neutralization with other prototype candidates using animal hyperimmune antiserum at dilutions of 1:2–20 in a standard N test. There was a virtual absence of cross-reactions with the antisera that were used in the numbering program. Recent work with high-titered hyperimmune antisera, discussed below, has disclosed antigenic relationships among some of the numbered types that were not discovered in the collaborative program. Despite these findings, which are discussed in the next paragraph, the large number of antigenically different types of rhinoviruses is undoubtedly an important characteristic of the group, influencing epidemiological behavior and accounting for the frequency of rhinovirus colds.

In an early study, antigenic relationships among different rhinovirus types were reported, using hyperimmune bovine antisera in N tests.[50] The bovine antisera were later recognized to contain anticellular antibody. When this antibody was removed, the antigenic cross-reactions largely disappeared.[22] More recently, potent monotypic animal antisera were

used to demonstrate both reciprocal and one-way cross-reactions among numbered rhinovirus types studied.[26,146a] The cross-reactions were usually minor. A number of these relationships were indirect and were demonstrable only by primary immunization with one rhinovirus type followed by immunization with a different but related type.

The importance of cross-reactions in immunity in man is currently unknown, and the results of work in this area are contradictory. N tests carried out with paired sera from patients have usually not shown significant cross-reactions following natural rhinovirus infections.[73] On the other hand, in a study of experimental infections in volunteers, heterotypic antibody responses were relatively common after infection with some types.[53]

The native antigenicity of rhinoviruses can be altered by experimental means. Treatment at pH 5 at 56°C or in 2 M urea produces virus particles that react in immunodiffusion and CF tests with heterologous types.[101,101a] When the virus is in this C-antigenic state, which results from a configurational change that exposes normally hidden determinants, it is unable to attach to cell receptors. This alteration in antigenicity, which also occurs after virus attachment to host cells, may be an important step in the initiation of infection,[100] but probably plays no role in immunity to infection.

5. Descriptive Epidemiology

5.1. Incidence and Prevalence of Infection

5.1.1. Age- and Sex-Specific Infection and Illness Rates.

Rhinovirus infections are the most common of the acute respiratory infections[24,65] and probably the most common of all acute infections of man. Infection rates based on virus isolations from routine specimens from family members in Seattle with and without symptoms were 0.59 per person-year (Table 2A). Rates in this population ranged from 1.21 in the 0–1 year age group to 0.20 in mothers; values were intermediate in children 2–9 years of age. Similar data collected from medical students in Chicago[69] and insurance company employees in Charlottesville[62,65] gave rhinovirus infection rates of 0.74 and 0.77 per person-year, respectively.

True rhinovirus infection rates are probably higher than reported, since currently available rhinovirus culture methods lack optimal sensitivity (see Section 3). The overall rhinovirus infection rates of 0.74 and 0.77 per person-year in Chicago and Charlottesville, respectively, are probably minimum values for the true incidence of rhinovirus infections in young adults. Adjustment of the Seattle rates for children to those measured for young adults in Chicago and Charlottesville gives projected rhinovirus infection rates in young children of up to 1.5 per person-year. Of particular interest was the slight increase in incidence of rhinovirus infections in young adults, 20–29 years old, in the Michigan population and the increased incidence in females in the 16–24 age group in the Charlottesville population. These findings may relate to the importance of young children in disseminating rhinovirus in the home, particularly to mothers. This is discussed in Section 5.2.1.

Rhinovirus illness rates have been measured in long-term studies of families and insurance company workers. In Tecumseh, Michigan, the rhinovirus illness rate for all ages was 0.29 per person-year.[120] Rates ranged from 0.58 for infants less than 1 year old to 0.14 for adults over the age of 50 (Table 2B). Rates declined proportionately with increasing age. Data collected from the insurance company population of young adults yielded a rhinovirus illness rate of 0.53.[62] Rates for males and females derived from this study were 0.51 and 0.55, respectively. The higher rate in females reflected a greater incidence of total colds in females and not an increased incidence of rhinovirus recovery from females, since the rhinovirus isolation percentages from males and females were not different. The reason for the differences in rhinovirus illness rates in these studies is not clear, but may relate to variables such as the methods of surveillance, criteria used in counting colds, and varying sensitivities of the cell cultures used for virus recovery.

5.1.2. Prevalence of Antibody and Geographic Distribution.

Studies of the prevalence of rhinovirus antibody support the conclusion that rhinovirus infections begin in early childhood and continue into adult life (Fig. 1). Antibody to the various rhinovirus types begins to appear at an early age and increases in prevalence throughout childhood and adolescence.[117,159,165] The prevalence of antibody reaches a peak in young adults (mean percentage positive: 50%), probably reflecting the effect of exposure to young children in the home.[72] Antibody prevalence then declines to a slightly lower level that persists throughout adulthood. Studies of antibody in sera collected serially from the same person show persistence of antibody at relatively stable levels for years.[159] The mechanisms by which rhinovirus serum antibody levels persist are unknown and could include inherent stability of antibody formed initially, or recurrent antigenic stimulation from infection with the same or related types, or both. The slight decrease in prevalence of antibody after the early adult peak (Fig. 1) suggests that a decline in antibody occurs when viral exposure is lessened. Limited work has also shown that artificially induced N antibody in nasal secretions may persist for at least 330 days following intranasal vaccination.[11]

Information is also available on the prevalence of serum N antibody in adults to each of the different serotypes, 1A–55. In the groups studied, antibody was present in all the types tested (Fig. 2).[72] The prevalence of antibody ranged from a low of approximately 10% to a high of approximately 80%, and there was no sharp dividing point between types associated with high and low antibody prevalence. It is of interest that types with high antibody prevalence tended to be M strains and types with low antibody prevalence were H strains.

Studies of rhinovirus-antibody prevalence in specimens from many different parts of the world have shown that rhinoviruses have a worldwide

Table 2A. Rhinovirus Infection Rates: Calculated from Surveillance and Sampling of All Persons—Well and Ill

Location	Age (yr)	Person-yr of observation	Infections per person-yr
Seattle Washington[24]	0–1	144	1.21
	2–5	135	0.54
	6–9	22	0.55
	Mothers	208	0.20
	All ages	510	0.59
Chicago, Illinois[69]	19–32	466	0.74[a]
Charlottesville, Virginia[62]	16–45	500	0.77[b]

[a] Rhinovirus isolation percentages for well and ill persons 1.5 and 25.4%, respectively; sampling interval of well persons 6 weeks; data collected over four periods of 9 months and adjusted to annual rates.
[b] Rhinovirus isolation percentages for well and ill persons 2.1 and 23.3%, respectively; sampling interval of well persons arbitrarily adjusted to 6 weeks; data collected over 1 year.

Table 2B. Rhinovirus Illness Rates: Calculated from Surveillance and Sampling of Persons with Colds

Location	Age (yr)	Person-yr of observation	Number of respiratory illnesses per person-yr	Number of rhinovirus illnesses per person-yr
Tecumseh, Michigan[120]	<1	726	6.1	0.58[a]
	1–4	3,516	5.2	0.50
	5–9	5,064	3.5	0.33
	10–19	6,228	2.5	0.24
	20–29	3,786	2.75	0.26
	30–49	8,394	2.0	0.19
	50+	1,716	1.45	0.14
	All ages:	29,430	3.0	0.29
Charlottesville, Virginia[62,65]	Males			
	16–24	240	2.2	0.51[b]
	25–34	204	2.1	0.50
	35–44	111	2.3	0.54
	45+	24	2.2	0.51
	All males:	579	2.2	0.51
	Females			
	16–24	477	2.6	0.60
	25–34	237	2.1	0.49
	34–44	84	2.1	0.49
	45+	24	1.3	0.31
	All females:	822	2.4	0.55
	All persons:	1,401	2.3	0.53

[a] All rates calculated using rhinovirus isolation percentage of 9.6%.
[b] All rates calculated using rhinovirus isolation percentage of 23.3% (observed: 22.9% in males, 23.6% in females).

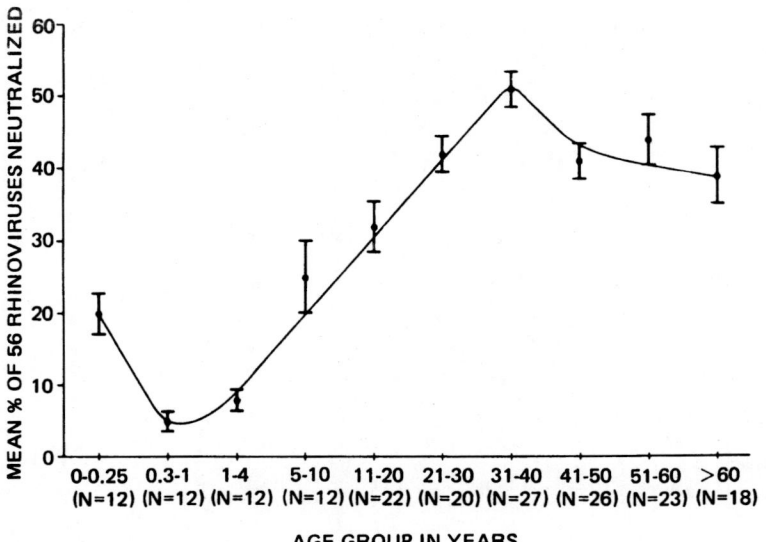

Fig. 1. Distribution of N antibody in human sera according to age. A total of 184 sera were tested at 1:4 dilutions vs. rhinovirus types 1A–55. The vertical brackets represent the S.E.M. With permission of Hamparian *et al.*[72]

distribution.[160] Broadly speaking, there were differences in prevalence of antibody among countries for any particular virus tested. Rhinovirus-antibody prevalence in tropical areas is equal to or greater than that in the temperate zone.

5.1.3. Seasonal Distribution of Infections. In an early epidemiological study of acute respiratory disease in which virological methods were not available, Frost and Gover[57] noted that "during the sea-

son of high prevalence, from September to March, inclusive, the incidence curve [for colds] in each locality exhibited a series of oscillations, constituting a succession of epidemics, each of several weeks' duration, rather irregular in sequence and magnitude, but clearly not attributable to mere chance fluctuation." The data from this study showed that one of the recurrent epidemic peaks of colds occurred in the early fall, usually in September. Later,

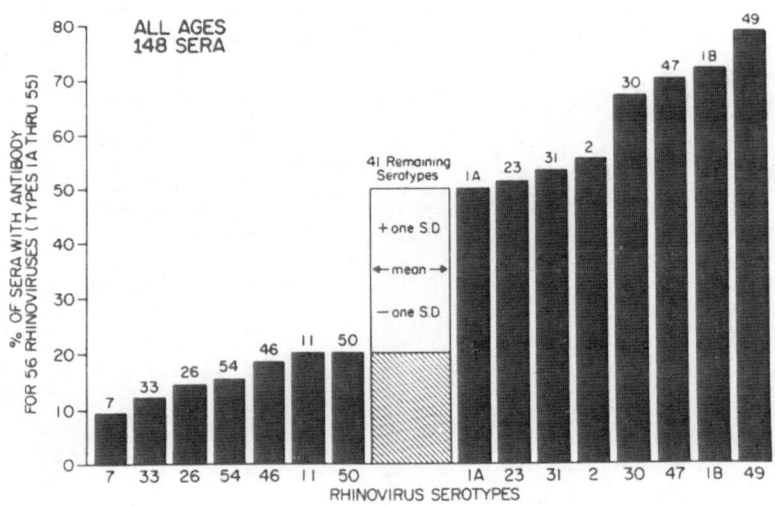

Fig. 2. Percentages of human sera with N antibody to rhinovirus types 1A–55. A total of 148 sera were tested at a 1:4 dilution. With permission of Hamparian *et al.*[72]

in the Cleveland family study of minor illness, a September peak of colds was a prominent feature of the seasonal pattern of illness, although no respiratory viruses could be associated with this period.[36] Studies using virus cultures have now shown that rhinoviruses account for a major part of this early fall outbreak of colds that annually initiates the respiratory-disease season (Fig. 3).[62,114] In adults with colds in the eastern United States, rhinovirus infection rates reached their highest annual point (3.5 illnesses/1000 per day, 1.28 per person-year) in September. At this time, rhinoviruses accounted for approximately 40% of all colds and greater than 90% of diagnosed colds. Rhinovirus infection rates fell and remained low (1–1.5/1000 per day) in the winter and early spring. A second peak of rhinovirus illness occurred in April and May. Although total respiratory rates were falling in the spring, rhinoviruses were associated with a substantial fraction of all colds during that time. Throughout the summer, rhinovirus infections continued to account for an important part of all colds, although respiratory illness rates reach their lowest point at this time.

In the tropics, the respiratory-disease season coincides with the rainy season, beginning in May and June and ending in November and December.[118] Most rhinovirus infections occur during the rainy season,[117] but more precise monitoring of the seasonal prevalence of rhinovirus colds has not been done. In arctic locations, where the respiratory-disease season coincides with cold weather as in temperature climates, rhinovirus outbreaks have been observed, but precise patterns have not been studied.[171]

Although there is a well-established correlation between the lowered temperatures during the fall, winter, and spring months and the increased occurrence of acute respiratory disease during that period,[83] there is no evidence to support a direct causal relationship between thermal cold and increased rates of infection. As to meterological effects that specifically influence rhinovirus infections, a thorough study of weather and colds showed that none of nine weather variables including temperature had a distribution remotely resembling the autumn (presumed rhinovirus) peak of colds.[98] This is in keeping with the observations from two long-term studies of rhinovirus infections in which prominent September peaks of rhinovirus colds were associated with mild seasonal fall weather and not with the more severe cold of winter that requires heating of homes and alterations in living patterns.[76,116] More direct evidence on this question comes from a volunteer study with rhinovirus type 15 in which exposure to thermal cold showed no adverse effect on susceptibility to experimental infection or severity of illness.[46]

The reason for seasonal variation in the incidence of colds remains a mystery. Speculations include the idea that cold weather, like rain in the tropics, leads to crowding indoors, thus providing better conditions for virus spread.[84] Also, school openings in the fall bring together into large groups a segment of the population highly susceptible to rhinoviruses and other respiratory viruses. There has also been speculation on the effect of weather changes on virus infectivity and host resistance. Changes in humidity have been shown to influence the survival of respiratory viruses,[9] and seasonal changes may

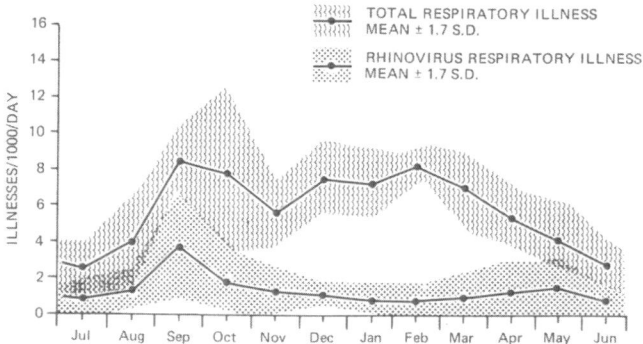

Fig. 3. Total and rhinovirus respiratory illness rates (±1.7 S.D.) in young adults. Data collected over a 7-year period (1963–1969). Adapted from Gwaltney et al.[62]

affect hormonal functions in man that influence susceptibility to infection.[164] In this regard, female volunteers were found to be more susceptible to experimental colds in the middle trimester than during other times in the menstrual cycle.[48]

5.1.4. Distribution of Serotypes. A tally of rhinovirus serotypes in the United States based on published studies revealed wide dispersal of most types throughout the country.[68] Of the first 55 numbered types, only type 5, a virus first isolated in England, had not been recovered in the United States. The serological survey cited earlier[72] showed antibody to type 5 virus in sera from United States populations. Thus, the conclusion that rhinovirus types are widely distributed throughout the United States and the world is supported by both virus isolation and serological data.

The current impression, based on longitudinal studies, is that multiple types circulate in a geographic area at any given time with no discernible pattern to their appearance or reappearance.[64,68] Over several years, some types were endemic, while others appeared only once or twice. It has been proposed, however, that certain rhinovirus types might possess a higher degree of infectivity than others, increasing their importance as a cause of colds and making them prime candidates for inclusion in vaccines.[115] Analysis of the frequency of isolation of the various rhinovirus types, however, does not show a sharp division between "common" and "uncommon" types. Also, types most commonly encountered in one study have not necessarily been the same as those in other studies. From the analysis of combined data from several studies, it was not possible to designate a particular year as a nationwide epidemic year for a particular type, nor was it possible to detect pathways of rhinovirus transmission by type across the country.[68]

One general pattern of serotype distribution has emerged that raises a basic question about the antigenic nature of rhinoviruses. Long-term studies have shown a gradual change with time in the overall distribution of serotypes in a given geographic location.[14,55a] Serotypes with lower numbers, which in general were discovered earlier, have been replaced by higher-numbered, "newer" types and strains that cannot be typed with available antisera. The reason for the shift in types is unknown; one possibility is that all of a very large number of stable antigenic types have not cycled through the loca-

tions where rhinovirus surveillance is in progress and so have not been discovered. Another possibility is that rhinoviruses are undergoing antigenic drift. If this is occurring with sufficient speed to result in marked changes in the already-numbered viruses, they could be mistaken for "new" types. Bearing on the second possibility are two studies showing antigenic differences between strains of the same types isolated several years apart.[146,157] In one instance, the newer strain had broader antigenicity than the prototype.

5.2. Occurrence in Different Settings

5.2.1. Family. One of the major sites of rhinovirus spread in civilian populations is the home.[35,77,113] The characteristic epidemiological pattern in this setting is for a schoolchild to introduce virus into the home, after which transmission occurs to other members of the family (Fig. 4). Secondary infections are most common in young children and mothers, but all members of the household including fathers, other adults working outside the home, and adolescents are affected. Intervals of 2–5 days are commonly seen between onsets of cases.

In one study, total respiratory illness rates were highest in preschool children.[77] Rates in housewives were similar to those in schoolchildren and were consistently higher than rates in adults working outside the home. During the height of the epidemic, the frequency of rhinovirus infection as determined by culture and serology was similar in all age groups. Later, in October, total illness rates were seen to decline in adults and older children, while young children continued to have frequent colds for which no etiology could be established. The presence of children in the home was associated with total respiratory illness infection rates for adults that were higher than for adults who did not have this exposure. At the height of a September peak of illness, rhinovirus respiratory illness rates for all family members, adults and children, were approximately 8/1000 per day (2.92 per person-year), calculated on the basis of rhinovirus causing 40% of fall colds.

In one family study, the rhinovirus attack rates for two epidemic types were 25 and 50%,[35] while the attack rate for type 16 in an outbreak in families in a small Alaskan community was nearly 70%.[171] In another study, the secondary attack rates for

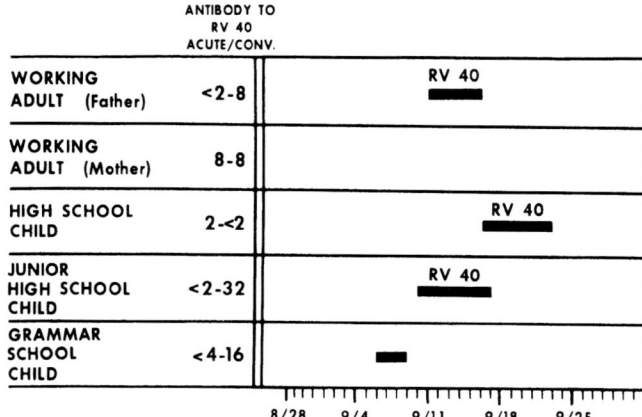

Fig. 4. A family outbreak of colds due to rhinovirus type 40. (■) Periods of symptomatic illness; (RV 40) positive virus culture. The diagnosis of rhinovirus infection in the index case (grammar-school child) was made by serology. Adapted from Hendley et al.[75]

members of families into which a rhinovirus had been introduced were inversely proportional to preexposure serum antibody levels: 71, 50, and 21% of persons with titers of ≤2, 4, and 8–32, respectively, were infected.[75,77] Based on the results of a study of colds in the tropics,[113] the secondary attack rate with type 39 was calculated to be 56% in antibody-free persons.[75]

5.2.2. **Schools.** A key study has shown that rhinoviruses spread efficiently among children in nursery school,[4] thus establishing transmission in school as an important step in rhinovirus dissemination in civilian populations. Spread of some types in the schoolroom was extensive, involving up to 77% of children. However, half the serotypes introduced into the groups showed no evidence of spread. The reason for the lack of spread of some types is unknown, but the authors concluded that it was not due to characteristics of the associated illness, patterns of virus shedding, or levels of immunity. Spread was most pronounced during March and April, a recognized time of increased prevalence of rhinovirus colds. The study unfortunately did not extend through the September peak of rhinovirus infections.

Rhinovirus activity has been observed in day-school groups at various grade levels[127] and in boarding-school, university, and medical-school populations.[66,69,91,111,132] Rhinoviruses are a prominent cause of morbidity in these groups, although information on their specific epidemiological behavior is not available. Presumably, spread in older children, adolescents, and young adults who are part of closed populations such as boarding schools oc-

curs among roommates, friends, members of athletic teams, and the like.

5.2.3. **Military.** Rhinoviruses account for a large amount of the morbidity associated with upper respiratory tract infections in military populations.[54,86,111] In a prospective study of Navy and Marine recruits, 90% of the men developed rhinovirus infection during a 28-day period in basic training, giving an attack rate for this period of 11.7 per person-year![141] Of these infections, 75% occurred within the first 2 weeks of training, and simultaneous or closely spaced infections with two different serotypes in the same man were common. The epidemiological behavior of the numbered rhinoviruses in military populations is generally similar to that in civilians, showing a constantly changing mosaic of different types.[121]

6. Mechanisms and Routes of Transmission

The exact mechanism by which rhinoviruses are passed from person to person is unknown. As discussed above, schoolchildren are the most important reservoir of the virus, and home and school are the places where spread most often occurs. In volunteer experiments, close personal contact appears to be necessary for virus to spread efficiently from an infected to a susceptible subject.[32,81b] These facts alone suggest that spread is most often by some type of short-range exposure to infectious secretions. Information on the various steps in the sequence of transmission is best evaluated in relation to the question of spread by direct manual contact with infectious secretions vs. spread by contact with virus in contaminated aerosols of large or small particle sizes.[66a]

Virus shedding, the first step in the sequence, occurs primarily from the nose. Under experimental conditions, the amount of rhinovirus in the nasopharyngeal washes of volunteers peaked (832 $TCID_{50}$/ml) on the 3rd day after inoculation and then fell to low levels that persisted for up to 2 weeks.[42] Some volunteers showed a different pattern of nasal shedding characterized by delayed onset and slow buildup over 7 days to relatively low maximum virus concentrations (41 $TCID_{50}$/ml). Comparisons of rhinovirus concentrations in respiratory secretions from subjects with natural colds have shown that the quantity of virus in nasal mucus tends to be 10- to 100-fold greater than in pharyngeal secretions.[78] Also, virus was present only 50% of the time in saliva, where it was found in low concentrations. In keeping with the relative scarcity of rhinovirus in saliva was the finding that virus was infrequently recovered from simulated coughs and sneezes.

The relatively poor yield of virus in saliva can be interpreted as evidence against spread through the air, since aerosols produced by coughing and sneezing are mainly of oral origin, coming primarily from the pool of saliva in the anterior part of the mouth.[7,85] On the other hand, the idea of nasal mucus as a direct source of transmissible virus is appealing because of the relatively high titers of virus in mucus and the great potential for people with colds to contaminate the environment, including fingers, with this substance. Rhinovirus has been recovered from the hands of 40–90% of adults with natural[78] and experimental[131] colds[32a,66b, 138a] and from 6 and 15% of selected objects in the environment of persons with experimental and natural colds, respectively.[66b,138a] Information obtained on the second step in transmission, virus survival in the environment, indicates that rhinovirus in concentrations found in nasal mucus survives regularly for up to 3 hr on skin and a variety of surfaces such as wood, plastic, steel, Formica, and hard fabrics.[78]

Evidence in favor of spread through the air comes from experiments in which biological tracers, the spores of *Bacillus mycoides*, were placed in the nose. These experiments showed that blowing the nose and especially sneezing could produce droplets containing the tracer that were small enough to remain airborne and yet in the size range (3–16 μm) that is likely to be trapped in the nose.[10] Rhinovirus survival in aerosol is enhanced by low temperature and high humidity.[81a]

Whatever the method of transfer, virus must reach an appropriate portal of entry to complete the sequence of events leading to successful spread. Under experimental conditions, small quantities of rhinovirus (the HID_{50} equivalent to 0.032–0.75 $TCID_{50}$) placed in the nose in coarse drops will efficiently initiate infection.[39] There is indirect evidence that similar small amounts of virus may initiate infection under natural conditions.[75] Experimental infections have been produced by the inhalation of rhinovirus aerosols with particle sizes in the true droplet nuclei range (0.3–2.5 μm) but require approximately 20-fold greater concentrations of virus than intranasal challenge. Thus, it appears that the nasal mucosa is more susceptible to rhinovirus than is the lower respiratory tract.[28] In this experiment, it was not possible to exclude the possibility that infection resulted from the fraction of the viral aerosol that was deposited in the nose rather than that reaching the lower respiratory tract. Experimental rhinovirus colds have also been produced by dropping small amounts of virus on the conjunctiva,[13,78] indicating that the eye may be another portal of entry for rhinovirus. In contrast, rhinovirus placed in the mouth does not readily initiate infection.[78] In related experiments in which infected and susceptible volunteers kissed under controlled conditions, oral contact was an inefficient method of causing spread.[131]

From the results of the work cited above, it appears that rhinovirus must reach the nasal or perhaps the conjunctival mucosa for efficient initiation of infection. Observations carried out on adults at medical conferences and in Sunday school show that normal behavior includes placing fingers into the nose or onto the conjunctiva with regularity.[78] Episodes in which finger contact with nasal and conjunctival mucosa occurred were measured on the average of 2 per 3 person-hr of observation. This type of behavior provides sufficient opportunity for accidental self-inoculation if the fingers are contaminated with virus. The alternative method of spread, transmission via airborne particles with deposition in the respiratory tract, is also feasible. The average adult is effectively exposed by inhalation to large amounts (approximately 10 liters/min) of air, thus,

Table 3. Postulates to Test a Hypothesis of Microbial Transmission

1. Infectious microorganism must be produced in infected host at proposed anatomical source.
2. It must be present in secretions or tissues that are shed from host by proposed route.
3. It must be present and survive in or on the appropriate environmental substance or object.
4. The contaminated environmental substance or object must reach the proposed portal of entry.
5. Interruption of transmission by the hypothesized route must prevent spread of infection.

small concentrations of virus in the air may be sufficient to transmit infection.

Direct evidence on the relative importance of these different methods of spread is limited to studies of experimental infections. In one study, airborne transmission of rhinovirus did not occur across a wire-mesh barrier from infected to susceptible volunteers in closed barracks.[39] In another, infected volunteers who engaged in singing and other activity designed to create infectious aerosols failed to spread rhinovirus to susceptible subjects confined in the same closed room.[32] The efficiencies of viral spread by three routes were compared in volunteers, and the hand-contact/self-inoculation route was decidedly more efficient.[66b] Of 15 volunteers, 11 were infected after hand-contact exposure, compared to 1 of 12 exposed at close range to respiratory secretions in air (large particle) and none of 10 exposed to infected persons residing across a wire barrier (small particle).

The sum of evidence, particularly the frequent finding of rhinovirus on the hands and its relative scarcity in secretions from simulated coughs and sneezes, suggests that manual contact with nasal mucus may be the more important mode of spread. It is possible, however, that more than one method contributes to rhinovirus dispersal under natural conditions. To find a more definite answer to the question, it will be necessary to satisfy several postulates, which include a requirement for proof that interruption of spread by the hypothesized route results in a reduction in natural infections (Table 3).[66a]

7. Pathogenesis

The acute stage of viral rhinitis is characterized by hyperemia and edema of the mucous membrane with exudation of serous and mucinous fluid.[140] The nasal cavities are narrowed by thickening of the membrane and engorgement of the turbinates. Histologically, there is marked edema of subepithelial connective tissue with sparse infiltration of neutrophils, lymphocytes, plasma cells, and eosinophils. The secretory activity of the mucus-secreting submucosal glands is increased.

Specific work on the gross and histotological findings in acute rhinovirus infections is limited. In one study, nasal biopsies were obtained by currettage from volunteers with experimental rhinovirus infection.[40] Fixed smears stained by the Papanicolaou technique showed no consistent changes associated with either infection or illness. Cellular pathology was also absent on microscopic examination of nasal-polyp organ cultures infected with rhinovirus.[67b] In contrast, scanning electron microscopy of bovine tracheal organ cultures infected with a bovine rhinovirus showed extrusion of degenerating ciliated and nonciliated cells and relatively smooth areas of denuded epithelium (Fig. 5).[137] If similar anatomical abnormalities occur in human rhinovirus infections, they could explain the depressions in nasal mucociliary flow rates that have been observed in volunteers with experimental infection.[145]

The mechanism by which rhinovirus produces rhinitis is unknown, but information on the correlation of peak virus titers and illness onsets suggests that an important mechanism may be direct cell injury secondary to the cycle of virus replication.[39,42] In experimental rhinovirus infection, virus may be recovered from nasopharyngeal wash in small amounts by 24 hr after inoculation. Virus concentrations then rise rapidly to peak values on days 2 and 3. Maximal virus shedding is followed within 24 hr by the release of large quantities of protein from the mucous membrane. The incubation period is usually 2–3 days, and the onset of illness is very closely related to the time of peak virus shedding. At this time, nasal-epithelial-cell biopsies are uniformly positive for virus; later, when lesser amounts

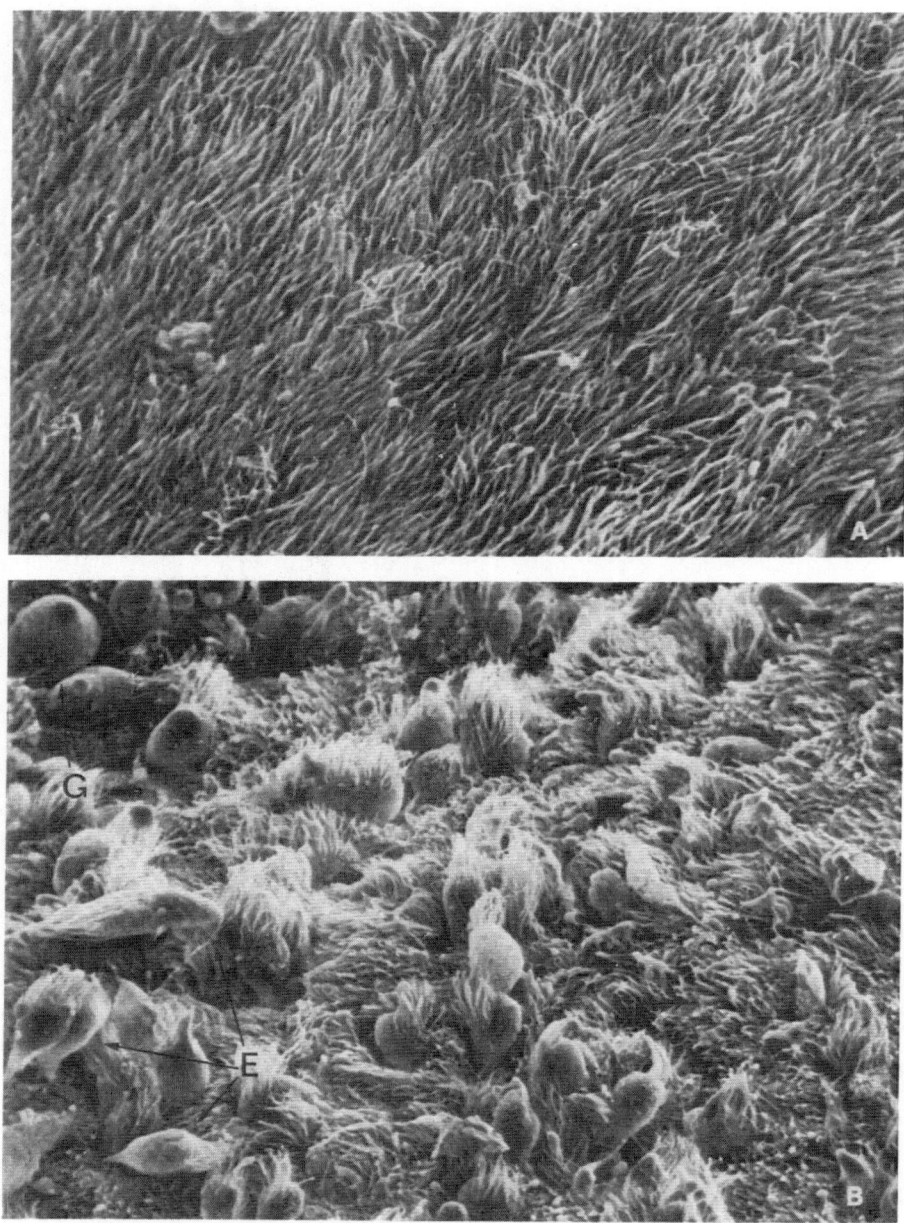

Fig. 5. Organ cultures of bovine tracheal epithelium. (A) Uninfected control culture. Field width 100 μm. (B) Culture infected with bovine rhinovirus, fixed 6 days after inoculation: (E) extruding ciliated cells; (G) extruding goblet cells. Field width 180 μm. Reprinted from Reed and Boyde [137] by permission of the authors and the Editor of the American Society for Microbiology.

of virus are shed, they are only occasionally positive.[39,40]

The anatomical limits of rhinovirus infection have not been determined. Comparisons of virus concentrations recovered from the nose, throat, saliva, coughs, and sneezes (discussed in Section 6) suggest that the major site of infection is usually in the nose. It is currently unknown whether virus recovered from the pharynx and saliva is produced in these sites or merely represents contamination with nasal secretions. In reports on children with wheezing[82b] and adults with chronic bronchitis or asthama,[97a] rhinovirus was recovered more often from sputum than from the nose or throat, suggesting that viral replication was occurring in the lower respiratory tract. However, there still remains no direct evidence on the question as might be obtained by transtracheal aspiration or long puncture.

There have been multiple reports of rhinovirus infection in patients, especially children, with disease of the lower respiratory tract.[21,31,58,130] The possibility cannot be excluded that concurrent infection with other viral or bacterial pathogens may have been present and caused the illness seen in some cases. The opinion of several workers in the field has been that rhinoviruses are not an important cause of viral pneumonia, croup, and bronchiolitis in children.[6,67,122,134,171] More recent studies have, however, implicated rhinovirus infection as an important precipitant of asthmatic attacks in children.[81,82a,b,102,109,109b] The mechanism for this is unknown, but a decrease in granulocytic β-adrenergic and H_2 histamine receptor responses has been observed in volunteers with peripheral-airway obstruction associated with experimental rhinovirus infection.[11a]

Rhinovirus infections have also been associated with periods of acute exacerbation in patients with chronic bronchitis.[49,104,153]

A decline in pulmonary function has been observed in patients with chronic obstructive pulmonary disease in association with rhinovirus infection.[152] However, the abnormalities have been mild and transient. Similar changes in pulmonary function have been seen in cigarette smokers[56] and healthy adults[5,18] with rhinovirus infection. The mechanisms by which rhinovirus infection might alter pulmonary function are unknown. Direct invasion of the lower respiratory tract by the virus is a possibility, but reflex mechanisms or secondary bacterial infection might also play a role. The hypothesis that rhinovirus invades the bronchopulmonary tree must be reconciled with the observation that rhinovirus grows relatively poorly at the core body temperature of 37°C.

8. Immunity

Work on the immunology of rhinovirus infections has focused on humoral immunity, particularly the role of antibody in respiratory secretions. No information is available on the role, if any, of cellular immunity in resistance to rhinovirus infection.

Serum N antibody titers rise in up to 75–80% of persons with natural or experimental rhinovirus colds[15,63,65,77]; once present, antibody in serum is well maintained.[159] The level of naturally acquired serum N antibody prior to natural or experimental challenge is inversely proportional to the subsequent infection rate. Under conditions of exposure to rhinovirus in the home, naturally acquired serum antibody at a level of 8 was associated with a sharp reduction in the infection rate, and serum antibody levels of ≥16 were associated with solid immunity.[77] With artificial challenge, it is possible to infect, although at a reduced rate, volunteers who have higher titers of naturally acquired serum antibody. In one study using relatively small challenge doses of virus (0.05–50 $TCID_{50}$), no infections occurred in volunteers with prechallenge titers of 64 or higher.[75] In other studies in which the infecting inocula contained more virus (17–10,000 $TCID_{50}$), infections were observed in volunteers with prechallenge titers of up to 512, presumably as a result of the overwhelming of normal immunity by an artificially large virus challenge.[19,123]

The findings cited above do not necessarily indicate that serum N antibody is the primary immune mechanism responsible for resistance to rhinovirus, since naturally acquired serum antibody is found in close association with antibody in nasal secretions.[123,129] The ratio of nasal-secretion to serum N antibody after recent infection (approximately 1:2) appears to be higher than that after remote infection (approximately 1:16), suggesting a decline in nasal-secretion antibody with time.[19] Actual measurements of nasal immunoglobulin concentrations have confirmed that significant falls in titers did occur over a 5-month period after infection.[81b]

Several attempts have been made to determine the relative importance and specific roles of serum and nasal-secretion antibody in protection against rhinovirus infection. Naturally acquired antibody in nasal-wash specimens and serum was associated with resistance to "infection" if present in sufficient titer before artificial challenge, but it did not appear to modify "illness" or virus shedding.[19] Because of the close association of naturally acquired antibody in serum and nasal secretions, the findings of this study did not answer the questions posed. Another approach to the problem was to administer inactivated rhinovirus vaccine by either the parenteral or the intranasal route to selectively elicit nasal-secretion or serum antibody or both. Vaccine given intranasally in large amounts led to the production of antibody in both serum and nasal secretions, while parenteral vaccination resulted primarily in serum-antibody production.[128,129] Intranasal challenge with rhinovirus at a later date resulted in the reduction of *illness* and virus shedding only in volunteers who received the intranasal vaccine.[11,128,129] In these studies, intranasal vaccination was not associated with a clear-cut reduction in *infection* rate determined by antibody response. Therefore, this work suggested that the primary effect of nasal antibody was to modify illness and reduce virus shedding. This conclusion is in conflict with that of the investigation cited above[19] and of other reports that have found that the major effect of humoral (serum) immunity was prevention of infection and not modification of illness.[42,75,77,123] Other studies have reported on finding an association between naturally acquired[63] and vaccine-induced[44] serum antibody and reduction of illness and, in the latter study, diminished virus shedding. Thus, currently available data from studies of the relative importance of nasal and serum antibody associated with immunity are not in complete agreement; further work is necessary to provide a clear understanding of this area.

′ Naturally acquired neutralizing activity against rhinovirus in serum has been found to sediment primarily in the 5–7 S region and to be associated with fractions containing immunoglobulin A (IgA) and IgG.[19,142] After recent experimentally induced rhinovirus infection or intranasal vaccination with inactivated rhinovirus vaccine, neutralizing activity has also been associated with 19 S IgM.[19,94,142]

Under normal conditions, nasal secretions contain 12 different identifiable proteins found in serum as well as 6 antigenic components not present in serum.[143] Secretory IgA, the most abundant protein in nasal secretions, is synthesized locally at sites adjacent to the mucosa and accounts for 30% or more of total protein in nasal secretions. Rhinovirus neutralizing activity in nasal secretions is associated primarily with IgA in 9–11 S fractions, although secretory IgA is not entirely homogeneous in its sedimentation characteristics, being found also in 7 and 19 S regions.[94] The symptomatic period of rhinovirus illness is associated with considerable transudation of serum proteins, including IgG, into nasal secretions.[12,143] After cessation of illness, the concentration of serum proteins in nasal secretions falls rapidly; at this time, the IgA concentration begins a progressive sustained increase. The IgA that appears during this period is not associated with an increase in specific neutralizing activity for the infecting virus. Specific N antibody first appears in nasal secretions and serum at approximately 2 weeks in volunteers lacking detectable antibody. Antibody concentrations increase most rapidly between the 3rd and 4th weeks, by which time virus shedding is completed. Volunteers with preexisting serum antibody may show rises in nasal antibody titers by as early as day 7. N antibody to rhinovirus has also been found in tears and parotid saliva, where it is associated with the IgA fraction.[47]

Because of the sequence of events described above, it is felt that recovery from rhinovirus infection and illness is not dependent on humoral immunity.[19] It has been shown that interferon is released into respiratory secretions during the course of experimental rhinovirus infection. This has led to the suggestion that in rhinovirus colds, as in other viral infections, interferon may have an important role in recovery.[16]

In one study, resistance to experimental rhinovirus infection was reported to occur as a result of recent infection with a heterologous rhinovirus type.[52] The mechanism for this, which is unknown, was not related to humoral immunity. However, in epidemiological studies of children[4,109a] and military recruits,[141] many instances of closely spaced rhinovirus infections have been seen, raising the question of how important this nonspecific resistance is in natural infection. Psychological factors may also play a role in susceptibility to infection or illness or both. In one interesting study, volunteers exposed to psychological stress before infection with rhinovirus had more severe illness than nonstressed controls.[163a]

9. Patterns of Host Response

9.1. Clinical Features

Rhinoviruses produce a typical common cold characterized by rhinorrhea, nasal obstruction, sneezing, pharyngeal discomfort, and cough. The median length of natural illness in young adults is 7 days, with peak symptomatology occurring on the 2nd and 3rd days of illness.[63] Symptoms last up to 2 weeks in one-fourth of cases and may be prolonged

to 1 month, although secondary bacterial infection may play a role when this occurs. The profile of rhinovirus illness can be distinguished from that of influenza by the relative severity of systemic complaints and cough that occur with influenza (Fig. 6). Rhinovirus colds differ from group A β-hemolytic streptococcal pharyngitis in having more nasal involvement and cough and less severe and prolonged pharyngeal discomfort. This information is unfortunately of limited value to the clinician. In the individual patient, it is impossible to distinguish, on clinical grounds, rhinovirus colds from those caused by other common respiratory viruses.

In children, rhinoviruses also produce the common cold syndrome.[6,139] Whether rhinoviruses

Fig. 6. Comparison of symptom profiles of rhinovirus colds (139 cases), type A₂ influenza (33 cases), and group A β-hemolytic streptococcal pharyngitis (17 cases). Adapted from Gwaltney et al.[63]

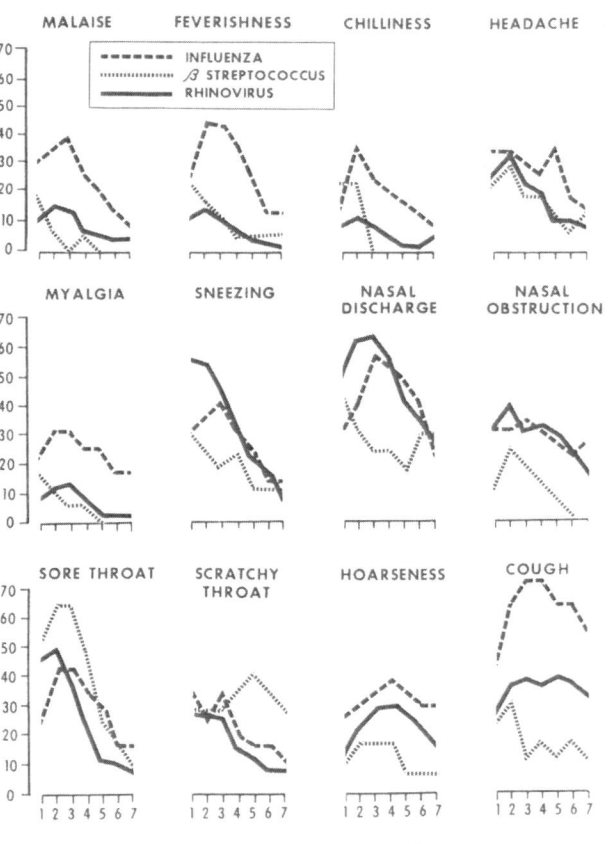

cause more serious disease in children, such as viral pneumonia, croup, and bronchiolitis, is still not clear. As discussed in Section 7, the prevailing opinion is that rhinoviruses, unlike parainfluenza viruses and respiratory syncytial virus, do not commonly cause these diseases.

Cough is a prominent feature of rhinovirus colds in patients of all ages, indicating that involvement of the lower respiratory tract of some type does occur. The frequency and duration of cough are markedly increased in cigarette smokers, particularly females, with rhinovirus colds.[63] Also, it has been reported that up to 40% of exacerbations in patients with chronic bronchitis may be associated with rhinovirus infections.[49,97a,104,153]

Rhinoviruses are among the respiratory viruses that precipitate asthmatic attacks in children.[81,102,109] They appear to play an especially important role in causing wheezing in older children.[82a,b,109] Multiple serotypes have been implicated.[109b] Also, asthmatic children have been found to experience a significantly greater number of viral respiratory infections, primarily due to rhinoviruses, than do nonasthmatic controls.[108] These recent findings are of interest in view of an earlier report that volunteers with a history of allergy have enhanced susceptibility to experimental colds.[84]

During acute rhinovirus illness in volunteers, there is a modest increase in circulating neutrophils.[15] Later in the infection, moderate elevations in the erythrocyte sedimentation rate may occur. The diagnosis of rhinovirus infection is best accomplished by isolation of the virus from nose-and-throat-swab or nasal-wash specimens. There is currently very limited availability of facilities for the laboratory diagnosis of rhinovirus infections in routine medical practice.[130]

9.2. Apparent/Inapparent Infection Ratios

Data based on virus isolations are available from several studies for calculating apparent/inapparent infection ratios for rhinoviruses. The results, which are in good agreement, indicate that the majority of rhinovirus infections are associated with symptomatic respiratory illness. The percentages of rhinovirus infections associated with illness were 63% in families,[93a] 88% in medical students,[69] 69% in insurance-company employees,[62] and 70–74% in military trainees.[86,121] Thus, the ratio of apparent to inapparent infections is approximately 3:1.

10. Control and Prevention

No methods for controlling or preventing rhinovirus infections are available at present. Studies with experimental monovalent rhinovirus vaccines given parenterally have met with only partial success. Rhinovirus antigens are inferior to poliovirus antigens for vaccine production. In volunteers, parenteral vaccination has been followed by reduction in illness and virus shedding but not infection.[2,44,123] It is difficult to evaluate studies of parenteral-vaccine efficacy under natural conditions because of the multiplicity of serotypes.[110,136]

The discovery of ever-increasing numbers of specific antigenic types has led to pessimism over the prospects of developing rhinovirus vaccines with practical value. However, there is still some hope that advances in immunology and vaccine development may eventually make it possible to use the antigenic relationships that have been found among some of the numbered rhinoviruses to develop useful vaccines.[55a,146a,154] In rabbits, potent monovalent rhinovirus antigens have been used successfully to stimulate heterotypic antibody responses to one or more different rhinovirus types.[27] Also, volunteers who received formalin-inactivated decavalent rhinovirus vaccines developed a limited number of antibody responses to heterologous antigens not present in the vaccines.[67a]

The problem of vaccine development is further complicated by the findings discussed in Section 8 that indicate an important role for secretory antibody in resistance to rhinovirus infection. Parenteral vaccination does not appear to be an efficient means of stimulating rhinovirus N antibody in nasal secretions, suggesting that immunization via the respiratory tract may be necessary for optimum protection. This has led to interest in the development of vaccines prepared with live attenuated strains of rhinovirus.[43]

Control of rhinovirus infection by chemoprophylaxis and chemotherapy have also been under investigation. In early work, rhinoviruses were found to be susceptible to 2-(α-hydroxybenzyl) benzimidazole and related compounds that have specific actions on virus replication.[147,158] Since then, a number of other compounds with activity against rhinoviruses *in vitro* have been discovered.[10a,60,138, 149,151,151a] Compounds with antirhinovirus activity that have been tested in humans have not been effective, however.[138,150,163] Interferon has also been shown to have activity against rhinoviruses,[14a] and several clinical trials with human leukocyte interferon or interferon-inducing agents have been conducted.[3a,47a,80,107,124,168a] A reduction in the severity of clinical illness has been observed in some of the studies, but drug administration prior to virus challenge appears necessary to achieve a beneficial effect.

In recent years, a controversy has arisen over the proposal that large doses of vitamin C be used for the prevention and treatment of common colds.[125] Early controlled trials of the effectiveness of 1 and 2 g per day of vitamin C in the prevention of natural colds showed an approximately 30% reduction of days of disability or morbidity among volunteers taking this compound.[3,29] There was no reduction in the total number of illnesses. In a similar study conducted more recently, the beneficial effects of vitamin C in ameliorating illness were considered, at most, small or equivocal.[90a] The frequency of illness was again not altered. Also, it was discovered that many subjects tasted the contents of the capsules that they were given and thus were able to guess correctly whether they were receiving vitamin C or placebo. These events have led the authors of two careful reviews of the question to conclude that no beneficial effects have been established for vitamin C in the prevention or treatment of natural colds.[19b,48a] Also, in other studies, 3 g per day of vitamin C did not prevent experimental rhinovirus infections in volunteers and produced at most an unimpressive reduction in the illness scores of prophylaxed subjects over those of controls.[148,169] A recommendation for the general prophylactic or therapeutic use of large doses of vitamin C for colds does not seem warranted.

Rhinovirus colds might also be controlled if ways are discovered to interrupt their spread from person to person. The development of environmental control measures is largely dependent on precise knowledge of the mechanism of rhinovirus spread. If accidental self-inoculation of the nose or eye with virus contaminating the fingers is of importance, then the simple expedients of avoiding finger contact with the nose and eyes and of hand-washing, particularly when a household member develops a cold, may be beneficial in reducing the risk of infection.[19a,172]

11. Unresolved Problems

A number of important questions concerning rhinoviruses remain unanswered. These include the number of virus serotypes and their antigenic stability, the extent of antigenic relatedness, the mechanisms by which rhinoviruses produce disease and stimulate host immunity, their mode of transmission, and finally the biochemical nature of the virus, particularly as it relates to the action of antivirals with potential clinical usefulness. The answers to these questions may have a direct effect on the success of solving the most important practical problem, which is the development of methods for rhinovirus control. The increasing awareness of the importance of rhinoviruses, not only as a major cause of the morbidity of common colds and their complications, but also as precipitants of more serious illness such as chronic bronchitis, asthma, and sinusitis, should stimulate an increasing effort to understand rhinovirus behavior.

12. References

1. Andrewes, C., in: *The Common Cold*, Norton, New York, 1965.
2. Andrewes, C., Tyrrell, D. A. J., Stones, P. B., Beale, A. J., Andrews, R. D., Edward, D. G., Goffe, A. P., Doggett, J. E., Homer, R. F., Crespi, R. S., and Clements, E. M. B., Prevention of colds by vaccination against a rhinovirus: A report by the scientific committee on common cold vaccines, *Br. Med. J.* **1:**1344 (1965).
3. Anderson, T. W., Reid, D. B. W., and Beaton, G. H., Vitamin C and the common cold: A double-blind trial, *Can. Med. Assoc. J.* **107:**503 (1972).
3a. Aoki, F. Y., Reed, S. E., Craig, J. W., Tyrrell, D. A. J., and Lees, L. J., Effect of a polynucleotide interferon inducer of fungal origin on experimental rhinovirus infection in humans, *J. Infect. Dis.* **137:**82–86, (1978).
4. Beem, M. O., Acute respiratory illness in nursery school children: A longitudinal study of the occurrence of illness and respiratory viruses, *Am. J. Epidemiol.* **90:**30 (1969).

5. BLAIR, H. T., GREENBERG, S. B., STEVENS, P. M., BI-
LUNOS, P. A., AND COUCH, R. B., Effects of rhinovirus
infection on pulmonary function of healthy human
volunteers, *Am. Rev. Respir. Dis.* **114**:95 (1976).

6. BLOOM, H. H., FORSYTH, B. R., JOHNSON, K. M., AND
CHANOCK, R. M., Relationship of rhinovirus infection to mild upper respiratory disease. 1. Results of
a survey in young adults and children, *J. Am. Med.
Assoc.* **186**:38 (1963).

7. BOURDILLON, R. B., AND LIDWELL, O. M., Sneezing
and the spread of infection, *Lancet* **2**:365 (1941).

8. BROWN, P. K., AND TYRRELL, D. A. J., Experiments
on the sensitivity of strains of human fibroblasts to
infection with rhinovirus, *Br. J. Exp. Pathol.* **45**:571
(1964).

9. BUCKLAND, F. E., AND TYRRELL, D. A. J., Loss of infectivity on drying various viruses, *Nature (London)*
195:1063 (1962).

10. BUCKLAND, F. E., AND TYRRELL, D. A. J., Experiments
on the spread of colds. 1. Laboratory studies on the
dispersal of nasal secretion. *J. Hyg.* **62**:365 (1964).

10a. BUCKNALL, R. A., SWALLOW, D. L., MOORES, H., AND
HARRAD, J., A novel substituted guanidine with high
activity *in vitro* against rhinovirus, *Nature (London)*
246:144–145, (1973).

11. BUSCHO, R. F., PERKINS, J. C., KNOPF, H. L. S., KA-
PIKIAN, A. Z., AND CHANOCK, R. M., Further characterization of the local respiratory tract antibody
response induced by intranasal instillation of inactivated rhinovirus 13 vaccine, *J. Immunol.* **108**:169
(1972).

11a. BUSH, R. K., BUSSE, W., FLAHERTY, D., WARSHAUER,
D., DICK, E. C., AND REED, C. E., Effects of experimental rhinovirus 16 infection on airways and leukocyte function in normal subjects, *J. Allergy Clin.
Immunol.* **61**:80 (1978).

12. BUTLER, W. T., WALDMANN, T. A., ROSSEN, R. D.,
DOUGLAS, R. G., JR., AND COUCH, R. B., Changes in
IgA and IgG concentrations in nasal secretions prior
to the appearance of antibody during viral respiratory infection in man, *J. Immunol.* **105**:584 (1970).

12a. BUTTERWORTH, B. E., GRUNERT, R. R., KORANT, B. D.,
LONBERG-HOLM, K., AND YIN, F. H., Replication of
rhinoviruses: Brief review, *Arch. Virol.* **51**:169 (1976).

13. BYNOE, M. L., HOBSON, D., HORNER, J., KIPPS, A.,
SCHILD, G. C., AND TYRRELL, D. A. J., Inoculation of
human volunteers with a strain of virus from a common cold, *Lancet* **1**:1194 (1961).

14. CALHOUN, A. M., JORDAN, W. S., JR, AND GWALTNEY,
J. M., JR., Rhinovirus infections in an industrial pop-
ulation. V. Change in distribution of serotypes, *Am.
J. Epidemiol.* **99**:58 (1974).

14a. CAME, P. E., SCHAFER, T. W., AND SILVER, G. H.,
Sensitivity of rhinoviruses to human leukocyte and
fibroblast interferons. *J. Infect. Dis.* **133**:A136 (1976).

15. CATE, T. R., COUCH, R. B., AND JOHNSON, K. M.,
Studies with rhinoviruses in volunteers: Production
of illness, effect of naturally acquired antibody, and
demonstration of a protective effect not associated
with serum antibody, *J. Clin. Invest.* **43**:56 (1964).

16. CATE, T. R., DOUGLAS, R. G., JR., AND COUCH, R. B.,
Interferon and resistance to upper respiratory virus
illness, *Proc. Soc. Exp. Biol. Med.* **131**:631 (1969).

17. CATE, T. R., DOUGLAS, R. G., JR., JOHNSON, K. M.,
COUCH, R. B., AND KNIGHT, V., Studies on the inability of rhinovirus to survive and replicate in the
intestinal tract of volunteers, *Proc. Soc. Exp. Biol.
Med.* **124**:1290 (1967).

18. CATE, T. R., ROBERTS, J. S., RUSS, M. A., AND PIERCE,
J. A., Effects of common colds on pulmonary function, *Am. Rev. Respir. Dis.* **108**:858 (1973).

19. CATE, T. R., ROSSEN, R. D., DOUGLAS, R. G., JR.,
BUTLER, W. T., AND COUCH, R. B., The role of nasal
secretion and serum antibody in the rhinovirus common cold, *Am. J. Epidemiol.* **84**:352 (1966).

19a. CATE, T. R., Self-control of the common cold?, *Ann.
Intern. Med.* **88**:569 (1978).

19b. CHALMERS, T. C., Effects of ascorbic acid on the common cold: An evaluation of the evidence, *Am. J. Med.*
58:532 (1975).

20. CHAPPLE, P. J., HEAD, B., AND, TYRRELL, D. A. J., A
complement fixing antigen from an M rhinovirus,
Arch. Gesamte Virusforsch. **21**:123 (1967).

21. CHERRY, J. D., DIDDAMS, J. A., AND DICK, E. C., Rhinovirus infections in hospitalized children: Provoc-
ative bacterial interrelationships, *Arch. Environ. Health*
14:390 (1967).

22. CONANT, R. M., AND HAMPARIAN V. V., Rhinoviruses: Basis for a numbering system. II. Serologic
characterization of prototype strains, *J. Immunol.*
100:114 (1968).

23. CONANT, R. M., SOMERSON, N. L., AND HAMPARIAN,
V. V., Rhinovirus: Basis for a numbering system. 1.
HeLa cell for propagation and serologic procedures,
J. Immunol. **100**:107 (1968).

24. COONEY, M. K., HALL, C. E., AND FOX, J. P., The
Seattle virus watch. III. Evaluation of isolation methods and summary of infections detected by virus
isolations, *Am. J. Epidemiol.* **96**:286 (1972).

25. COONEY, M. K., AND KENNY, G. E., Immunogenicity
of rhinoviruses, *Proc. Soc. Exp. Biol. Med.* **133**:645
(1969).

26. COONEY, M. K., KENNY, G. E., TAM, R., AND FOX, J.
P., Cross relationships among 37 rhinoviruses demonstrated by virus neutralization with potent monotypic rabbit antisera, *Infect. Immun.* **7**:335 (1973).

27. COONEY, M. K., AND WISE, J. A., Heterotypic stimulation of rhinovirus antibodies in rabbits, in: *Abstr.
Annu. Meet. Am. Soc. Microbiol.*, p. 114, May 6–11,
1973.

27a. COONEY, M. K., AND KENNY, G. E., Demonstration of dual rhinovirus infection in humans by isolation of different serotypes in human heteroploid (HeLa) and human diploid fibroblast cell cultures, *J. Clin. Microbiol.* **5**:202 (1977).

28. COUCH, R. B., CATE, T. R., DOUGLAS, R. G., JR., GERONE, P. J., AND KNIGHT, V., Effect of route of inoculation on experimental respiratory viral disease in volunteers and evidence for airborne transmission, *Bacteriol. Rev.* **30**:517 (1966).

29. COULEHAN, J. L., REISINGER, K. S., ROGERS, K. D., AND BRADLEY, D. W., Vitamin C prophylaxis in a boarding school, *N. Engl. J. Med.* **290**:6 (1974).

30. CRANDELL, R. A., A description of eight feline picornaviruses and an attempt to classify them, *Proc. Soc. Exp. Biol. Med.* **126**:240 (1967).

31. CRAIGHEAD, J. E., MEIER, M., AND COOLEY, M. H., Pulmonary infection due to rhinovirus type 13, *N. Engl. J. Med.* **281**:1403 (1969).

32. D'ALESSIO, D., DICK, C. R., AND DICK, E. C., Transmission of rhinovirus type 55 in human volunteers, in: *International Virology 2* (J. L. MELNICK, ed.), p. 115, S. Karger, Basel, 1972.

32a. D'ALESSIO, D. J., PETERSON, J. A., DICK, C. R., AND DICK, E. C., Transmission of experimental rhinovirus colds in volunteer married couples, *J. Infect. Dis.* **133**:28 (1976).

33. DANS, P. E., FORSYTH, B. R., AND, CHANOCK, R. M., Density of infectious virus and complement-fixing antigens of two rhinovirus strains, *J. Bacteriol.* **91**:1605 (1966).

34. DICK, E. C., Experimental infection of chimpanzees with human rhinovirus type 14 and 43, *Proc. Soc. Exp. Biol. Med.* **127**:1079 (1968).

35. DICK, E. C., BLUMER, C. R., AND EVANS, A. S., Epidemiology of infections with rhinovirus types 43 and 55 in a group of University of Wisconsin student families, *Am. J. Epidemiol.* **86**:386 (1967).

36. DINGLE, J. H., BADGER, G. F., AND JORDAN, W. S., JR., Patterns of illness, in: *Illness in the Home*, p. 19, Western Reserve University, Cleveland, 1964.

37. DITCHFIELD, W. J. B., Rhinoviruses and parainfluenza viruses of horses, *J. Am. Vet. Med. Assoc.* **155**:384 (1969).

38. DOCHEZ, A. R., SHIBLEY, G. S., AND MILLS, K. C., Studies in the common cold. IV. Experimental transmission of the common cold to anthropoid apes and human beings by means of a filtrable agent, *J. Exp. Med.* **52**:701 (1930).

39. DOUGLAS, R. G., JR., Pathogenesis of rhinovirus common colds in human volunteers, *Ann. Otol. Rhinol. Laryngol.* **79**:563 (1970).

40. DOUGLAS, R. G., JR., ALFORD, B. R., AND COUCH, R. B., Atraumatic nasal biopsy for studies of respiratory virus infection in volunteers, *Antimicrob. Agents Chemother.* **8**:340 (1968).

41. DOUGLAS, R. G., JR., CATE, T. R., AND COUCH, R. B., Growth and cytopathic effect of H type rhinoviruses in monkey kidney tissue culture, *Proc. Soc. Exp. Biol. Med.* **123**:238 (1966).

42. DOUGLAS, R. G., JR., CATE, T. R., GERONE, P. J., AND COUCH, R. B., Quantitative rhinovirus shedding patterns in volunteers, *Am. Rev. Respir. Dis.* **94**:159 (1966).

43. DOUGLAS, R. G., JR., AND COUCH, R. B., Attenuation of rhinovirus type 15 for humans, *Nature (London)* **223**:213 (1969).

44. DOUGLAS, R. G., JR., AND COUCH, R. B., Parenteral inactivated rhinovirus vaccine: Minimal protective effect, *Proc. Soc. Exp. Biol. Med.* **139**:899 (1972).

45. DOUGLAS, R. G., JR., FLEET, W. F., CATE, T. R., AND COUCH, R. B., Antibody to rhinovirus in human sera. I. Standardization of a neutralization test, *Proc. Soc. Exp. Biol. Med.* **127**:497 (1968).

46. DOUGLAS, R. G., JR., LINDGREN, K. M., AND COUCH, R. B., Exposure to cold environment and rhinovirus common cold: Failure to demonstrate effect, *N. Engl. J. Med.* **279**:743 (1968).

47. DOUGLAS, R. G., JR., ROSSEN, R. D., BUTLER, W. T., AND COUCH, R. B., Rhinovirus neutralizing antibody in tears, parotid saliva, nasal secretions and serum, *J. Immunol.* **99**:297 (1967).

47a. DOUGLAS, R. G., JR., AND BETTS, R. F., Effect of induced interferon in experimental rhinovirus infection in volunteers, *Infect. Immun.* **9**:506 (1974).

48. DOWLING, H. F., JACKSON, G. G., AND INOUYE, T., Transmission of the experimental common cold in volunteers. II. The effect of certain host factors upon susceptibility, *J. Lab. Clin. Med.* **50**:516 (1957).

48a. DYKES, M. H. M., AND MEIER, P., Ascorbic acid and the common cold: Evaluation of its efficacy and toxicity, *J. Am. Med. Assoc.* **231**:1073 (1975).

49. EADIE, M. B., STOTT, E. J., AND GRIST, N. R., Virological studies in chronic bronchitis, *Br. Med. J.* **2**:671 (1966).

50. FENTERS, J. D., GILLUM, S. S., HOLPER, J. C., AND MARQUIS, G. S., Serotypic relationships among rhinoviruses, *Am. J. Epidemiol.* **84**:10 (1966).

51. FIALA, M., Plaque formation by 55 rhinovirus serotypes, *Appl. Microbiol.* **16**:1445 (1968).

52. FLEET, W. F., COUCH, R. B., CATE, T. R., AND KNIGHT, V., Homologous and heterologous resistance to rhinovirus common cold, *Am. J. Epidemiol.* **82**:185 (1965).

53. FLEET, W. F., DOUGLAS, R. G., JR, CATE, T. R., AND COUCH, R. B., Antibody to rhinovirus in human sera. II. Heterotypic responses, *Proc. Soc. Exp. Biol. Med.* **127**:503 (1968).

54. FORSYTH, B. R., BLOOM, H. H., JOHNSON, K. M., AND

CHANOCK, R. M., Patterns of illness in rhinovirus infections of military personnel, *N. Engl. J. Med.* **269**:602 (1963).

55. Fox, J. P., HALL, C. E., COONEY, M. K., LUCE, R. E., AND KRONMAL, R. A., The Seattle virus watch. II. Objectives, study population and its observation, data processing and summary of illnesses, *Am. J. Epidemiol.* **96**:270 (1972).

55a. Fox, J. P., Is a rhinovirus vaccine possible?, *Am. J. Epidemiol.* **103**:345 (1976).

56. FRIDY, W. W., INGRAM, R. H., HIERHOLZER, J. C., AND COLEMAN, M. T., Airways function during mild viral respiratory illnesses: The effect of rhinovirus infection in cigarette smokers, *Ann. Intern. Med.* **80**:150 (1974).

57. FROST, W. H., AND GOVER, M., The incidence and time distribution of common colds in several groups kept under continuous observation, in: *Papers of Wade Hampton Frost, M.D.* (K. F. MAXCY, ed.), p. 359, Commonwealth Fund, New York, 1941.

58. GEORGE, R. B., AND MOGABGAB, W. J., Atypical pneumonia in young men with rhinovirus infections, *Ann. Intern. Med.* **71**:1073 (1969).

59. GWALTNEY, J. M., JR., Micro-neutralization test for identification of rhinovirus serotypes, *Proc. Soc. Exp. Biol. Med.* **122**:1137 (1966).

60. GWALTNEY, J. M., JR., Rhinovirus inhibition by 3-substituted triazinoindoles, *Proc. Soc. Exp. Biol. Med.* **133**:1148 (1970).

61. GWALTNEY, J. M., JR., AND EDMONDSON, W. P., JR., Etiology and Epidemiology of Acute Respiratory Disease, Annual Progress Report to the Commission on Acute Respiratory Disease of the Armed Forces Epidemiological Board, Contract No. DADA-49-007-MD-1000, September 15, 1968.

62. GWALTNEY, J. M., JR., HENDLEY, J. O., SIMON, G., AND JORDAN, W. S., JR., Rhinovirus infections in an industrial population. I. The occurrence of illness, *N. Engl. J. Med.* **275**:1261 (1966).

63. GWALTNEY, J. M., JR., HENDLEY, J. O., SIMON, G., AND JORDAN, W. S., JR., Rhinovirus infections in an industrial population. II. Characteristics of illness and antibody response, *J. Am. Med. Assoc.* **202**:494 (1967).

64. GWALTNEY, J. M., JR, HENDLEY, J. O., SIMON, G., AND JORDAN, W. S., JR., Rhinovirus infections in an industrial population. III. Number and prevalence of serotypes, *Am. J. Epidemiol.* **87**:158 (1968).

65. GWALTNEY, J. M., JR., AND JORDAN, W. S., JR., Rhinoviruses and respiratory disease, *Bacteriol. Rev.* **28**:409 (1964).

66. GWALTNEY, J. M., JR., AND JORDAN, W. S., JR., Rhinoviruses and respiratory illness in university students, *Am. Rev. Respir. Dis.* **93**:362 (1966).

66a. GWALTNEY, J. M., JR., AND HENDLEY, J. O., Rhino-

virus transmission: One if by air, two if by hand, *Am. J. Epidemiol.* **107**:357 (1978).

66b. GWALTNEY, J. M., JR., MOSKALSKI, P. B., AND HENDLEY, J. O., Hand-to-hand transmission of rhinovirus colds, *Ann. Intern. Med.* **88**:463 (1978).

67. GLEZEN, W. P., LODA, F. A., CLYDE, W. A., SENIOR, R. J., SHEAFFER, C. I., CONLEY, W. G., AND DENNY, F. W., Epidemiologic patterns of acute lower respiratory disease of children in a pediatric group practice, *J. Pediatr.* **78**:397 (1971).

67a. HAMORY, B. H., HAMPARIAN, V. V., CONANT, R. M., AND GWALTNEY, J. M., JR., Human responses to two decavalent rhinovirus vaccines, *J. Infect. Dis.* **132**:623 (1975).

67b. HAMORY, B. H., HENDLEY, J. O., AND GWALTNEY, J. M., JR., Rhinovirus growth in nasal polyp organ culture, *Proc. Soc. Exp. Biol. Med.* **155**:577 (1977).

68. HAMRE, D., Rhinoviruses in: *Monographs in Virology 1* (J. L. MELNICK, ed.) p. 52, S. Karger, Basel, 1968.

69. HAMRE, D., CONNELLY, A. P., JR., AND PROCKNOW, J. J., Virologic studies of acute respiratory disease in young adults. IV. Virus isolations during four years of surveillance, *Am. J. Epidemiol.* **83**:238 (1966).

70. HAMRE, D., AND PROCKNOW, J. J., Viruses isolated from natural common colds among young adult medical students, *Am. Rev. Respir. Dis.* **88**:277 (1963).

71. HAMPARIAN, V. V., Personal communication.

72. HAMPARIAN, V. V., CONANT, R. M., AND THOMAS, D. C., Rhinovirus Reference Laboratory, Annual Contract Progress Report to the National Institute of Allergy and Infectious Diseases, National Institutes of Health, Bethesda, Maryland, Contract No. 69-2062, December 1, 1969–November 30, 1970.

73. HAMPARIAN, V. V., LEAGUS, M. B., HILLEMAN, M. R., AND STOKES, J., JR., Epidemiologic investigations of rhinovirus infections, *Proc. Soc. Exp. Biol. Med.* **117**:469 (1964).

74. HAYFLICK, L., AND MOORHEAD, P. S., The serial cultivation of human diploid cell strains, *Exp. Cell Res.* **25**:585 (1961).

75. HENDLEY, J. O., EDMONDSON, W. P., JR, AND GWALTNEY, J. M., JR., Relation between naturally acquired immunity and infectivity of two rhinoviruses in volunteers, *J. Infect. Dis.* **125**:243 (1972).

76. HENDLEY, J. O., AND GWALTNEY, J. M., JR., Relation of the weather and respiratory illness: Resume of analysis to date, conclusions and prospects, Unpublished data.

77. HENDLEY, J. O., GWALTNEY, J. M., JR., AND JORDAN, W. S., JR., Rhinovirus infections in an industrial population. IV. Infections within families of employees during two fall peaks of respiratory illness, *Am. J. Epidemiol.* **89**:184 (1969).

78. HENDLEY, J. O., WENZEL, R. P., AND GWALTNEY, J.

M., Jr., Transmission of rhinovirus colds by self-inoculation, *N. Engl. J. Med.* **288**:1361 (1973).

79. Higgins, P. G., Ellis, E. M., and Woolley, D. A., A comparative study of standard methods and organ culture for the isolation of respiratory viruses, *J. Med. Microsc.* **2**:109 (1969).

80. Hill, D. A., Baron, S., Perkins, J. C., Worthington, M., Van Kirk, J. E., Mills, J., Kapikian, A. Z., and, Chanock, R. M., Evaluation of an interferon inducer in viral respiratory disease, *J. Am. Med. Assoc.* **219**:1179 (1972).

81. Hilleman, M. R., Reilly, C. M., Stokes, J., Jr., and Hamparian, V. V., Clinical epidemiologic findings in coryzavirus infections, *Am. Rev. Respir. Dis. Suppl.* **88**:274 (1963).

81a. Holmes, M. J., Deig, E. F., Williams, J. A., and Ehreshmann, D. W., Stability of airborne rhinovirus type 2 under atmospheric and physiological conditions, *Abstr. Annu. Meet. Am. Soc. Microbiol.* Q 18 (1976).

81b. Holmes, M. J., Reed, S. E., Stott, E. J., and Tyrrell, D. A. J., Studies of experimental rhinovirus type 2 infections in polar isolation and in England, *J. Hyg. (Cambridge)* **76**:379 (1976).

82. Hoorn, B., and, Tyrrell, D. A. J., On the growth of certain "newer" respiratory viruses in organ cultures, *Br. J. Exp. Pathol.* **46**:109 (1965).

82a. Horn, M. E. C., and Gregg, I., Role of viral infection and host factors in acute episodes of asthma and chronic bronchitis, *Chest* **63**:44S (1973).

82b. Horn, M. E. C., Reed, S. E., and Taylor, P., The role of viruses and bacteria in acute wheezy bronchitis in childhood: A study of sputum, *Arch. Dis. Child.* **54**:587 (1979).

83. Ipsen, J., Relationships of Acute Respiratory Disease to Measurements of Atmospheric Pollution and Local Meteorological Conditions, Final Report to the Department of Health, Education, and Welfare, Public Health Service, Bureau of State Services (October 5, 1960–March 30, 1964), Henry Phipps Institute, University of Pennsylvania, Contract No. PH 86-63-25, March 1965.

84. Jackson, G. G., Dowling, H. F., and Muldoon, R. L., Acute respiratory diseases of viral etiology. VII. Present concepts of the common cold, *Am. J. Public Health* **52**:940 (1962).

85. Jennison, M. W., Atomisation of mouth and nose secretions into the air as revealed by high speed photography, *Summ. Proc. Am. Assoc. Adv. Sci.* **17**:106 (1942).

86. Johnson, K. M., Bloom, H. H., Forsyth, B. R., and Chanock, R. M., Relationship of rhinovirus infection to mild upper respiratory disease. II. Epidemiologic observations in male military trainees, *Am. J. Epidemiol.* **81**:131 (1965).

87. Kapikian, A. Z., Rhinoviruses, in: *Diagnostic Procedures for Viral and Rickettsial Infections*, 4th ed. (E. H. Lennette and N. J. Schmidt, eds.), pp. 603–640, American Public Health Association, New York, 1969.

88. Kapikian, A. Z., Rhinoviruses, in: *Strains of Human Viruses* (M. Majer and S. A. Plotkin, eds.), S. Karger, Basel, 1972.

89. Kapikian, A. Z., Conant, R. M., Hamparian, V. V., Chanock, R. M., Chapple, P. J., Dick, E. C., Fenters, J. D., Gwaltney, J. M., Jr., Hamre, D., Hopler, J. C., Jordan, W. S., Jr., Lennette, E. H., Melnick, J. L., Mogabgab, W. J., Mufson, M. A., Phillips, C. A., Schieble, J. H., and Tyrrell, D. A. J., Rhinoviruses: A numbering system, *Nature (London)* **213**:761 (1967).

90. Kapikian, A. Z., Conant, R. M., Hamparian, V., V., Chanock, R. M., Dick, E. C., Gwaltney, J. M., Jr., Hamre, D., Jordan, W. S., Jr., Kenny, G. E., Lennette, E. H., Melnick, J. L., Mogabgab, W. J., Phillips, C. A., Schieble, J. H., Stott, E. J., and Tyrrell, D. A. J., A collaborative report: Rhinoviruses—extension of the numbering system, *Virology* **43**:524 (1971).

90a. Karlowski, T. R., Chalmers, T. C., Frenkel, L. D., Kapikian, A. Z., Lewis, T. L., and Lynch, J. M., Ascorbic acid for the common cold: A prophylactic and therapeutic trial, *J. Am. Med. Assoc.* **231**:1038 (1975).

91. Kendall, E. J. C., Bynoe, M. L., and Tyrrell, D. A. J., Virus isolations from common colds occurring in a residential school, *Br. Med. J.* **2**:82 (1962).

92. Kenny, G. E., Cooney, M. K., and Thompson, D. J., Analysis of serum pooling schemes for identification of large numbers of viruses, *Am. J. Epidemiol.* **91**:439 (1970).

93. Ketler, A., Hamparian, V. V., and Hilleman, M. R., Characterization and classification of ECHO 28–rhinovirus–coryzavirus agents, *Proc. Soc. Exp. Biol. Med.* **110**:821 (1962).

93a. Ketler, A., Hall, C. E., Fox, J. P., Elveback, L., and Cooney, M. K., The virus watch program: A continuing surveillance of viral infections in metropolitan New York families. VII. Rhinovirus infections: Observations of virus excretion, intrafamilial spread and clinical response, *Am. J. Epidemiol.* **90**:244 (1969).

94. Knopf, H. L. S., Perkins, J. C., Bertran, D. M., Kapikian, A. Z., and Chanock, R. M., Analysis of the neutralizing activity in nasal wash and serum following intranasal vaccination with inactivated type 13 rhinovirus, *J. Immunol.* **104**:566 (1970).

95. Korant, B. D., Lonberg-Holm, K., Noble, J., and Stasny, J. T., Naturally occurring and artificially

produced components of three rhinoviruses, *Virology* **48**:71 (1972).

96. KRIEL, R. L., WULFF, H., AND CHIN, T. D. Y., Microneutralization test for determination of rhinovirus and coxsackievirus A antibody in human diploid cells, *Appl. Micrbiol.* **17**:611 (1969).

97. KRUSE, W., Die Erregen von Husten und Schnupfen (The etiology of cough and nasal catarrh), *Munch. Med. Wochenschr.* **61**:1574 (1914).

97a. LAMBERT, H. P., AND, STERN, H., Infective factors in exacerbations of bronchitis and asthma, *Br. Med. J.* **3**:323 (1972).

97b. LEWIS, F. A., AND KENNETT, M. L., Comparison of rhinovirus-sensitive HeLa cells and human embryo fibroblasts for isolation of rhinoviruses from patients with respiratory disease, *J. Clin. Microbiol.* **3**:528 (1976).

98. LIDWELL, O. M., MORGAN, R. W., AND WILLIAMS, R. E. O., The epidemiology of the common cold. IV. The effect of weather, *J. Hyg. (Cambridge)* **63**:427 (1965).

99. LONBERG-HOLM, K., AND KORANT, B. D., Early interaction of rhinoviruses with host cells, *J. Virol.* **9**:29 (1972).

100. LONBERG-HOLM, K., AND NOBLE-HARVEY, J., Comparison of *in vitro* and cell-mediated alteration of a human rhinovirus and its inhibition by sodium dodecyl sulfate, *J. Virol.* **12**:19 (1973).

101. LONBERG-HOLM, K. AND YIN, F. H. Antigenic determinants of infective and inactivated human rhinoviruses type 2, *J. Virol.* **12**:114 (1973).

101a. LONBERG-HOLM, K., AND PHILIPSON, L., Molecular aspects of virus receptors and cell surfaces, in: *Cell Membranes and Viral Envelopes*, Vol. 2 (H. A. BLOUGH AND J. M. TIFFANY, eds.), pp. 789–848, Academic Press, New York, 1980.

102. MCINTOSH, K., ELLIS, E. F., HOFFMAN, L. S., LYBASS, T. G., ELLER, J. J, AND FULGINITI, V. A., The association of viral and bacterial respiratory infections with exacerbations of wheezing in young asthmatic children, *J. Pediatr.* **82**:578 (1973).

103. MCLEAN, C., AND RUECKERT, R. R., Picornaviral gene order: Comparison of a rhinovirus with a cardiovirus, *J. Virol.* **11**:341 (1973).

104. MCNAMARA, M. J., PHILLIPS, I. A., AND WILLIAMS, O. B., Viral and *Mycoplasma pneumoniae* infections in exacerbations of chronic lung disease, *Am. Rev. Respir. Dis.* **100**:19 (1969).

105. MEDAPPA, K. C., MCLEAN, C., AND RUECKERT, R. R., On the structure of rhinovirus 1A, *Virology* **44**:259 (1971).

106. MEDAPPA, K. C., AND RUECKERT, R. R., Binding of cesium ions to human rhinovirus-14 (R-14), in: *Abstr. Annu. Meet. Am. Soc. Microbiol.* p. 207, May 12–17, 1974.

107. MERIGAN, T. C., HALL, T. S., REED, S. E., AND TYRELL, D. A. J., Inhibition of respiratory virus infection by locally applied interferon, *Lancet* **1**:563 (1973).

108. MINOR, T. E., BAKER, J. W., DICK, E. C., DEMEO, A. N., OUELLETTE, J. J., COHEN, M., AND REED, C. E., Greater frequency of viral respiratory infections in asthmatic children as compared with their nonasthmatic siblings, *J. Pediatr.* **85**:472 (1974).

109. MINOR, T. E., DICK, E. C., DEMEO, A. N., OUELLETTE, J. J., COHEN, M., AND REED, C. E., Viruses as precipitants of asthmatic attacks in children, *J. Am. Med. Assoc.* **227**:292 (1974).

109a. MINOR, T. E., DICK, E. C., PETERSON, J. A., AND DOCHERTY, D. E., Failure of naturally acquired rhinovirus infections to produce temporal immunity to heterologous serotypes, *Infect. Immun.* **10**:1192 (1974).

109b. MINOR, T. E., DICK, E. C., BAKER, J. W., OUELLETTE, J. J., COHEN, M., AND REED, C. E., Rhinovirus and influenza type A infections as precipitants of asthma, *Am. Rev. Respir. Dis.* **113**:149 (1976).

110. MOGABGAB, W. J., Upper respiratory illness vaccines—Perspectives and trials, *Ann. Intern. Med.* **57**:526 (1962).

111. MOGABGAB, W. J., Acute respiratory illnesses in university (1962–1966), military and industrial (1962–1963) populations, *Am. Rev. Respir. Dis.* **98**:359 (1968).

112. MOHANTY, S. B., LILLIE, M. G., AND ALBERT, T. F., Experimental exposure of calves to a bovine rhinovirus, *Am. J. Vet. Res.* **30**:1105 (1969).

113. MONTO, A. S., A community study of respiratory infections in the tropics. III. Introduction and transmission of infections within families, *Am. J. Epidemiol.* **88**:69 (1968).

114. MONTO, A. S., AND CAVALLARO, J. J., The Tecumseh study of respiratory illness II. Patterns of occurrence of infection with respiratory pathogens, 1965–1969, *Am. J. Epidemiol.* **94**:280 (1971).

115. MONTO, A. S., AND CAVALLARO, J. J., The Tecumseh study of respiratory illness. IV. Prevalence of rhinovirus serotypes, 1966–1969, *Am. J. Epidemiol.* **96**:352 (1972).

116. MONTO, A. S., CAVALLARO, J. J., AND KELLER, J. B., Seasonal patterns of acute infection in Tecumseh, Mich., *Arch. Environ. Health* **21**:408 (1970).

117. MONTO, A. S., AND JOHNSON, K. M., A community study of respiratory infections in the tropics. II. The spread of six rhinovirus isolates within the community, *Am. J. Epidemiol.* **88**:55 (1968).

118. MONTO, A. S., AND JOHNSON, K. M., Respiratory infections in the American tropics, *Am. J. Trop. Med. Hug.* **17**:867 (1968).

119. MONTO, A. S., NAPIER, J. A., AND METZNER, H. L., The Tecumseh study of respiratory illness. I. Plan

of study and observations on syndromes of acute respiratory disease, *Am. J. Epidemiol.* **94**:269 (1971).

120. MONTO, A. S., AND ULLMAN, B. M., Acute respiratory illness in an American community: The Tecumseh study, *J. Am. Med. Assoc.* **227**:164 (1974).

121. MUFSON, M. A., BLOOM, H. H., FORSYTH, B. R., AND CHANOCK, R. M., Relationship of rhinovirus to mild upper respiratory disease. III. Further epidemiologic observations in military personnel, *Am. J. Epidemiol.* **83**:379 (1966).

122. MUFSON, M. A., KRAUSE, H. E., MOCEGA, H. E., AND DAWSON, F. W., Viruses, *Mycoplasma pneumoniae* and bacteria associated with lower respiratory tract disease among infants, *Am. J. Epidemiol.* **91**:192 (1970).

123. MUFSON, M. A., LUDWIG, W. M., JAMES, H. D., JR., GAULD, L. W., ROURKE, J. A., HOLPER, J. C., AND CHANOCK, R. M., Effect of neutralizing antibody on experimental rhinovirus infection, *J. Am. Med. Assoc.* **186**:578 (1963).

124. PANUSARN, C., STANLEY, E. D., DIRDA, V., RUBENIS, M., AND JACKSON, G. G., The prevention of illness from rhinovirus infection by a topical interferon inducer, *N. Engl. J. Med.* **291**:57 (1974).

125. PAULING, L. C., *Vitamin C and the Common Cold*, Freeman, San Francisco, 1970.

126. PELON, W., MOGABGAB, W. J., PHILLIPS, I. A., AND PIERCE, W. E., A cytopathogenic agent isolated from naval recruits with mild respiratory illness, *Proc. Soc. Exp. Biol. Med.* **94**:262 (1957).

127. PEREIRA, M. A., ANDREWS, B. E., AND GARDNER, S., D., A study on the virus aetiology of mild respiratory infections in the primary school child, *J. Hyg. (Cambridge)* **65**:475 (1967).

128. PERKINS, J. C., TUCKER, D. N., KNOPF, H. L. S., WENZEL, R. P., HORNICK, R. B., KAPIKIAN, A. Z., AND CHANOCK, R. M., Evidence for protective effect of an inactivated rhinovirus vaccine administered by the nasal route, *Am. J. Epidemiol.* **90**:319 (1969).

129. PERKINS, J. C., TUCKER, D. N., KNOPF, H. L. S., WENZEL, R. P., KAPIKIAN, A. Z., AND CHANOCK, R. M., Comparison of protective effect of neutralizing antibody in serum and nasal secretions in experimental rhinovirus type 13 illness, *Am. J. Epidemiol.* **90**:519 (1969).

130. PERSON, D. A., AND HERRMANN, E. C., JR., Experiences in laboratory diagnosis of rhinovirus infections in routine medical practice, *Mayo Clin. Proc.* **45**:517 (1970).

131. PETERSON, J. A., D'ALESSIO, D. J., AND DICK, E. C., Studies on the fialure of direct oral contact to transmit rhinovirus infection between human volunteers, in: *Abstr. Annu. Meet. Am. Soc. Microbiol.* p. 214, May 6–11, 1973.

132. PHILLIPS, C. A., MELNICK, J. L., AND GRIM, C. A., Rhinovirus infections in a student population: Iso-

lation of five new serotypes, *Am. J. Epidemiol.* **87**:447 (1968).

133. PINTO, C. A., AND HAFF, R. F., Experimental infection of gibbons with rhinovirus, *Nature (London)* **224**:1310 (1969).

133a. PONOMAREVA, T. I., LEVI, M. I., AND DREIZIN, R. S., A stable antibody-sensitized erythrocyte diagnostic preparation for detection of rhinovirus type 17 and its antibody, *Acta Virol.* **20**:232 (1976).

134. PORTNOY, B., ECKERT, H. L., AND SALVATORE, M. A., Rhinovirus infection in children with acute lower respiratory disease: Evidence against etiological importance, *Pediatrics* **35**:899 (1965).

135. PRICE, W. H., The isolation of a new virus associated with respiratory clinical disease in humans, *Proc. Natl. Acad. Sci. U.S.A.* **42**:892 (1956).

136. PRICE, W. H., Vaccine for the prevention in humans of cold-like symptoms associated with the JH virus, *Proc. Natl. Acad. Sci U.S.A.* **43**:790 (1957).

137. REED, S. E., AND BOYDE, A., Organ cultures of respiratory epithelium infected with rhinovirus or parainfluenza virus studies in a scanning electron microscope, *Infect. Immun.* **6**:68 (1972).

138. REED, S. E., AND BYNOE, M. L., The antiviral activity of isoquinoline drugs for rhinoviruses *in vitro* and *in vivo*, *J. Med. Microbiol.* **3**:346 (1970).

138a. REED, S. E., An investigation of the possible transmission of rhinovirus colds through indirect contact. *J. Hyg. (Cambridge)* **75**:249 (1975).

139. REILLY, C. M., HOCH, S. M., STOKES, J., McCLELLAND, L., HAMPARIAN, V. V., KETLER, A., AND HILLEMAN, M. R., Clinical and laboratory findings in cases of respiratory illness caused by coryzaviruses, *Ann. Intern. Med.* **57**:515 (1962).

140. ROBBINS, S. L., in: *Pathologic Basis of Disease*, p. 846, W. B. Saunders, Philadelphia, 1974.

141. ROSENBAUM, M. J., DE BERRY, P., SULLIVAN, E. J., PIERCE, W. E., MUELLER, R. E., AND PECKINPAUGH, R. O., Epidemiology of the common cold in military recruits with emphasis on infections by rhinovirus types 1A, 2, and two unclassified rhinoviruses, *Am. J. Epidemiol.* **93**:183 (1971).

142. ROSSEN, R. D., DOUGLAS, R. G., JR., CATE, T. R., COUCH, R. B., AND BUTLER, W. T., The sedimentation behavior of rhinovirus neutralizing activity in nasal secretion and serum following the rhinovirus common cold, *J. Immunol.* **97**:532 (1966).

143. ROSSEN, R. D., KASEL, J. A., AND COUCH, R. B., The secretory immune system: Its relation to respiratory viral infection, in: *Progress in Medical Virology* (J. L. MELNICK, ed.), pp. 194–238, S. Karger, Basel, 1971.

144. RUECKERT, R. R., Picornaviral architecture, in: *Comparative Virology*, pp. 225–306, Academic Press, New York, 1971.

145. SASAKI, Y., TOGO, Y., WAGNER, H. N., JR., HORNICK,

R. B., SCHWARTZ, A. R., AND PROCTOR, D. F., Mucociliary function during experimentally induced rhinovirus infection in man, *Ann. Otol.* **82**:203 (1973).

146. SCHIEBLE, J. H., LENNETTE, E. H., AND FOX, V. L., Antigenic variation of rhinovirus type 22, *Proc. Soc. Exp. Biol. Med.* **133**:329 (1970).

146a. SCHIEBLE, J. H., FOX, V. L., LESTER, F., AND LENNETTE, E. H., Rhinoviruses: An antigenic study of the prototype virus strains, *Proc. Soc. Exp. Biol. Med.* **147**:541 (1974).

147. SCHLEICHER, J. B., AQUINO, F., RUETER, A., RODERICK, W. R., AND APPELL, R. N., Antiviral activity in tissue culture systems of bis-benzimidazoles, potent inhibitors of rhinoviruses, *App. Microbiol.* **23**:113 (1972).

148. SCHWARTZ, A. R., TOGO, Y., HORNICK, R. B., TOMINAGA, S., AND GLECKMAN, R. A., Evaluation of the efficacy of ascorbic acid in prophylaxis of induced rhinovirus 44 infection in man, *J. Infect. Dis.* **128**:500 (1973).

149. SHANNON, W. M., ARNETT, G., AND SCHABEL, F. M., JR., 3-Deazauridine: Inhibition of ribonucleic acid virus-induced cytopathogenic effect *in vitro, Antimicrob. Agents Chemother.* **2**:159 (1972).

150. SHIPOWITZ, N. E., BOWER, R. R., SCHLEICHER, J. B., AQUINO, F., APPELL, R. N., AND RODERICK, W. R., Antiviral activity of a bis-benzimidazole against experimental rhinovirus infection in chimpanzees, *Appl. Microbiol.* **23**:117 (1972).

151. SIDWELL, R. W., HUFFMAN, J. H., KHARE, G. P., ALLEN, L. B., WITKOWSKI, J. T., AND ROBINS, R. K., Broad-spectrum antiviral activity of virazole: 1-β-D-ribofuranosyl-1,2,4-triazole-3-carboxamide, *Science* **177**:705 (1972).

151a. SIDWELL, R. W., HUFFMAN, J. H., ALLEN, L. B., MEYER, R. B., JR., SHUMAN, D. A., SIMON, L. N., AND ROBINS, R. K., *In vitro* antiviral activity of 6-substituted 9-β-D-ribofuranosylpurine-3',5'-cyclic phosphates, *Antimicrob. Agents Chemother.* **5**:652 (1974).

152. SMITH, C. B., KANNER, R. E., GOLDEN, C. A., KLAUBER, M. R., AND RENZETTI, A. D., Effect of viral infections on pulmonary function in patients with chronic obstructive pulmonary diseases (abstract), p. 11, 18th Interscience Conference on Antimicrobial Agents and Chemotherapy, 1978.

153. STENHOUSE, A. C., Rhinovirus infection in acute exacerbations of chronic bronchitis: A controlled prospective study, *Br. Med. J.* **3**:461 (1967).

154. STOTT, E. J., DRAPER, C., STONES, P. B., AND TYRRELL, D. A. J., Absence of heterologous antibody responses in human volunteers after rhinovirus vaccination, *Arch. Gesamte Virusforsch.* **28**:89 (1969).

155. STOTT, E. J., AND KILLINGTON, R. A., Haemagglutination by rhinoviruses, *Lancet* **1**:1369 (1972).

156. STOTT, E. J., AND KILLINGTON, R. A., Rhinoviruses, *Annu. Rev. Microbiol.* **26**:503 (1972).

157. STOTT, E. J., AND WALKER, M., Antigenic variation among strains of rhinovirus type 51, *Nature (London)* **224**:1311 (1969).

158. TAMM, I., AND CALIGUIRI, L. A., 2-(α-Hydroxybenzyl)-benzimidazole and related compounds, in: *The International Encyclopedia of Pharmacology and Therapeutics*, Section 61 (D. J. BAUER, ed.), Pergamon Press, New York, 1972.

159. TAYLOR-ROBINSON, D., Studies on some viruses (rhinoviruses) isolated from common colds, *Arch. Gesamte Virusforsch.* **13**:281 (1963).

160. TAYLOR-ROBINSON, D., Respiratory virus antibodies in human sera from different regions of the world, *Bull. WHO* **32**:833 (1965).

161. TAYLOR-ROBINSON, D., JOHNSON, K. M., BLOOM, H. H., PARROTT, R. H., MUFSON, M. A., AND CHANOCK, R. M., Rhinovirus neutralizing antibody responses and their measurement, *Am. J. Hyg.* **78**:285 (1963).

162. THOMAS, D. C., CONANT, R. M., AND HAMPARIAN, V. V., Rhinovirus replication in suspension cultures of HeLa cells, *Proc. Soc. Exp. Biol. Med.* **133**:62 (1970).

163. TOGO, Y., SCHWARTZ, A. R., AND HORNICK, R. B., Failure of a 3-substituted triazinoindole in the prevention of experimental human rhinovirus infection, *Chemotherapy* **18**:17 (1973).

163a. TOTMAN, R., REED, S. E., AND CRAIG, J. W., Cognitive dissonance, stress and virus-induced common colds, *J. Psychosom. Res.* **21**:55 (1977).

164. TROMP, S. W., Biometeorological effect on healthy man (physiological biometeorology), in: *Medical Biometeorology*, Part IV, pp. 279–280, Elsevier, New York, 1963.

165. TYRRELL, D. A. J., Rhinoviruses, in: *Virology Monographs 2* (S. GARD, C. HALLAUER, AND K. F. MYER, eds.), p. 67, Springer-Verlag, New York, 1968.

166. TYRRELL, D. A. J., BYNOE, M. L., AND HOORN, B., Cultivation of "difficult" viruses from patients with colds, *Br. Med. J.* **1**:606 (1968).

167. TYRRELL, D. A. J., SHEFF, M. D., AND PARSONS, R., Some virus isolations from common colds. III. Cytopathic effects in tissue cultures, *Lancet* **1**:239 (1960).

168. VAN LOGHEM, J. J., Epidemiologische bijdrage tot de kennis van de ziekten der ademhalingsorganen, *Ned. Tijdschr. Geneeskd.* **72**:666 (1928).

168a. WALDMAN, R. H., AND GANGULY, R., Effect of CP-20, 961, an interferon inducer, on upper respiratory tract infections due to rhinovirus type 21 in volunteers, *J. Infect. Dis.* **138**:531 (1978).

169. WALKER, G. H., BYNOE, M. L., AND TYRRELL, D. A. J., Trial of ascorbic acid in prevention of colds, *Br. Med. J.* **1**:603 (1967).

170. WILDY, P., Classification and nomenclature of viruses, in: *Monographs in Virology* (J. L. MELNICK, ed.), p. 56, S. Karger, Basel, 1971.

171. WULFF, H., NOBLE, G. R., MAYNARD, J. E., FELTZ, E.

T., POLAND, J. D., AND CHIN, T. D. Y., An outbreak of respiratory infection in children associated with rhinovirus types 16 and 29, *Am. J. Epidemiol.* **90:**304 (1969).

172. Leading Article, Spread of colds, *Br. Med. J.* **4:**123–124 (1973).

13. Suggested Reading

ANDREWES, C., in: *The Common Cold*, Norton, New York, 1965.

GWALTNEY. J. M., JR., AND JORDAN, W. S., JR., Rhinoviruses and respiratory disease, *Bacteriol. Rev.* **28:**409 (1964).

HAMRE, D. Rhinoviruses, in: *Monographs in Virology 1* (J. L. MELNICK, ed.), S. Karger, New York, 1968.

JACKSON, G. G., AND MULDOON, R. L., Viruses causing common respiratory infections in man, *J. Infect. Dis.* **127:**328 (1973).

STOTT, E. J., AND KILLINGTON, R. A., Rhinoviruses, *Annu. Rev. Microbiol.* **26:**503 (1972).

TYRRELL, D. A. J., AND CHANOCK, R. M., Rhinoviruses: A description, *Science* **141:**152 (1963).

CHAPTER 21

Rubella

Dorothy M. Horstmann

1. Introduction

Rubella (German measles) is a common contagious
disease with mild constitutional symptoms and a
generalized rash. In childhood, it is an inconsequential illness, but when it occurs during pregnancy, there is a significant risk of severe damage
to the fetus.

2. Historical Background

Despite its recognition as a clinical entity by German authors in the 18th century, rubella continued
to be regarded by most physicians as a mild form
of measles or a combination of measles and scarlet
fever until the late 19th century.[26] Finally, in 1881,
the International Congress of Medicine in London
gave official approval to its independent status. That
it is not generally called by its German name,
Rötheln, is due to Veale, a Scottish physician who
in 1866 published a paper in the *Edinburgh Medical
Journal* recommending a short and euphonius name
that could be easily pronounced, namely, *rubella*.[113]

The discovery that changed the concept of rubella
from an inconsequential disease of childhood to one
of great concern to the medical profession did not
come until 1941. In that year, Sir Norman Gregg,
an Australian ophthalmologist, reported that an
unusual number of newborns with congenital cataracts had suddenly appeared in Sydney and elsewhere in Australia and that in almost all cases the
mothers of the infants had experienced rubella in
the first trimester of pregnancy.[33] Gregg also noted
the presence of other ocular abnormalities in the
affected infants as well as a high incidence of cardiac
lesions. The medical community was slow to accept
his findings, and an editorial published in *The Lancet*
in 1944 questioned their validity.[20] But once the
way had been pointed out, confirmatory reports of
Gregg's remarkable discovery began to come in
from various parts of the world during the next decade.

At first, it was difficult to quantitate the potential
risk of fetal damage associated with maternal rubella
because most of the data came from retrospective
analyses of cases in which the patients had been
hospitalized. Estimates ranged as high as a 90% rate
of stillbirths or congenital anomalies when the disease occurred in the first 12 weeks of pregnancy. In
the 1950s, prospective studies in England,[77] the
United States,[103] and Sweden[76] permitted a more
accurate calculation of the risk of fetal damage. This
was found to be of the order of 15–20% at birth
when rubella occurred during the first trimester of
pregnancy. Subsequent prospective studies raised
the figure to 35% as hearing deficits and other late
anomalies were recognized.[57]

The viral nature of the infection had been postulated as early as 1914 by Hess[44] on the basis of
transmission studies in rhesus monkeys. This was
confirmed in 1938 by Hiro and Tasaka,[45] who produced rubella in children by inoculation of nasal

Dorothy M. Horstmann · Department of Epidemiology
and Public Health and Department of Pediatrics, Yale
University School of Medicine, New Haven, Connecticut.

washings, and in 1942 by Habel,[34] who also succeeded in infecting monkeys using nasal washings
and blood. In volunteer studies in the 1950s, Krugman and Ward[64] and Krugman et al.[65] showed
that viremia occurs in the preeruptive stage and
proved that the infection can occur without rash.

With the new prominence of rubella, increased
efforts were made in many laboratories to isolate
the etiological agent, but none met with success.
Following the introduction of practical tissue-culture methods in the late 1940s, renewed attempts
were made to cultivate rubella virus *in vitro*. Finally,
in 1962, this was accomplished. In that year, two
groups of investigators, Weller and Neva[116] at the
Harvard School of Publich Health and Parkman *et
al.*[86] at the Walter Reed Army Institute of Research,
simultaneously reported the growth of rubella virus
in cultured cells. This breakthrough was a landmark:
it made possible an accurate delineation of the clinical epidemiology of the disease, made available
tools to determine the behavior of the virus in population groups, and, most significantly, provided
the basis for the development of vaccines for the
control of congenital rubella. In the United States,
the $HPV_{77}DE_5$ strain of live attenuated rubella virus
vaccine developed by Meyer et al.[80] was licensed
in 1969, and the Cendehill strain[90] shortly thereafter; the RA 27/3 strain of Plotkin[89] was adopted
for use in several European countries at about the
same time (see Section 9.1). These vaccines have
been widely used during the past 10 years; their
impact on the rubella problem is currently being
assessed.

3. Methodology

3.1. Mortality Data

Since death from rubella is such a rare event,
mortality data are not of significance in understanding the epidemiology of the disease.

3.2. Morbidity Data

Rubella and congenital rubella became nationally
reportable in the United States in 1966, and in 1969,
the Center for Disease Control (CDC) established
the National Registry for Congenital Rubella Syndrome.[11] Before 1966, information on the incidence

of the acquired disease came from the 27 states in
which reporting had been mandatory for many
years. Official statistics tell far less than half the
story, however. The reasons for this are several: (1)
the disease is usually so mild that medical care may
not be sought; (2) the clinical syndrome is not highly
specific, and sporadic cases therefore frequently go
unrecognized and undiagnosed; and (3) the reporting of even diagnosed cases by physicians is poor,
as is true for other notifiable conditions, particularly
mild diseases like rubella that do not seem to have
great public-health importance. These factors result
in the reporting of only about one in five or one in
ten clinical cases. In addition—and most significant—for every frank case there are one or more
completely inapparent infections, which in epidemiological terms are as important as the clinically
manifest ones.

3.3. Serological Surveys

Surveys of healthy population groups, primarily
using the hemagglutination-inhibition (HI) test,
have been of major importance in mapping the epidemiology of rubella and documenting differences
in its behavior in various parts of the world and
under various circumstances. The HI test is specific
and simple and can be adapted to microtiter testing
of large numbers of sera; since it measures an antibody that is long-lasting, it is highly suitable for
survey purposes. Several other tests including immunodiffusion, radioimmunoassay (RIA), hemolysin in gel, and the enzyme-linked immunosorbent
assay (ELISA) are also satisfactory for such use.

3.4. Laboratory Methods

3.4.1. Virus Isolation. Unadapted rubella virus
does not produce significant cytopathic effect (CPE)
in cells in tissue culture. Because of this, the most
commonly employed technique for isolation of the
agent makes use of viral interference as an indicator[86]: blood or throat swabs (or other materials to
be tested) are inoculated onto monolayer primary
African green monkey kidney (GMK) tissue cultures, and after 9–12 days, the cultures are challenged with a virus that normally induces cytopathic
changes and destroys the cell sheet. If rubella virus
is present, it interferes with the challenge virus, and

no CPE develops. A second passage is often required before the interference effect can be detected. The first passage may be performed in some other sensitive cell system such as VERO, a GMK continuous line, but passage into primary GMK cultures is necessary for demonstration of interference.

Growth of rubella virus in tissue culture can also be detected by measuring the production of hemagglutinin[73,95] or of complement-fixation (CF) antigens[94] and by immunofluorescence techniques.[119]

3.4.2. Serological Tests. There are a number of serological methods available for the measurement of antibodies to rubella virus. The most commonly used is HI,[73,74,107] and less frequently CF[101]; others include neutralization, (N),[87] precipitin,[10a,67,68] immunodiffusion,[30a,96] indirect fluorescent-antibody (IFA),[8] platelet-aggregation (PA),[112] hemadsorption-inhibition (HADI),[88] RIA,[107] hemolysis in gel,[106b] and the ELISA[113a] tests. All are highly specific. The one selected depends in large measure on the nature of the clinical situation and the purpose for which testing is being done. For screening large numbers of sera, immunodiffusion and hemolysis-in-gel tests are simple and inexpensive. ELISA and RIA have also been recommended for this purpose.

However, there has been more experience with the HI test both for diagnosis and for antibody surveys, and it is still the one used by most laboratories. The test has been standardized and is reproducible when nonspecific inhibitors, present in all human sera, are adequately removed. The most reliable methods for doing so are treatment with heparin–manganese chloride or with dextran sulfate.[73,74] Absence of antibody as measured by an HI titer of less than 1:8 correlates well with susceptibility to infection. The titers of more than 90% of antibody-positive sera from naturally infected persons fall between 1:16 and 1:256. Levels of 1:1024 or higher suggest incomplete removal of inhibitors; in such instances, the test should be repeated after careful retreatment of the original serum to remove inhibitors. A very low titer—i.e., 1:8—probably indicates an antibody-positive serum if the result is reproducible. However, since it is not certain how protective such a low level is, it is preferable to consider a titer of 1:8 as indicating lack of immunity.

Elevated rubella HI antibody levels of 1:256 or higher have been observed in 15–30% of patients with diseases characterized by disturbed immune mechanisms, such as sarcoidosis,[9a] systemic lupus erythematosus,[93b] and chronic active hepatitis.[109a] The mechanisms involved in this response are unclear.

As in viral infections generally, neutralizing antibodies to rubella virus are considered to be most closely correlated with protective immunity. Two basic tissue-culture methods for their detection are available, the indirect interference test,[87] and direct tests employing virus adapted to a cell line such as SIRC[69] or VERO,[97a] in which the end point is read by neutralization of CPE. Both types of tests are slower, more expensive, and more cumbersome than the HI test. In general, the results of rubella HI and N tests parallel one another, but there is evidence that persons with HI but no detectable N antibody are subject to reinfection, and when this occurs in pregnancy, the fetus may be involved.[20a,27a] The HI-positive, N-negative antibody profile occurs more frequently in vaccinated persons than in those who acquired infection naturally.[97a]

Among other serological methods available, the CF test is useful in establishing the current nature of an infection, for CF antibodies appear later than HI or N antibodies; thus, significant rises in titer between paired sera can be demonstrated by CF when the first specimen has been collected too late in the course to show a significant increase in titer by HI test. Since CF antibody tends to disappear in many persons over a period of years, it is not suitable for use in serological surveys.

Detection of rubella-specific immunoglobulin M (IgM) antibody, present transiently following primary infection, is also a means of identifying recent or current experience with the virus.[2a,35,62a] The test is useful in determining whether rubella antibody present in a newborn infant is of maternal origin or represents a response to endogenous infection, since IgM molecules (unlike IgG) are not transferred across the placenta.

4. Biological Characteristics of the Virus

Rubella is an ether-sensitive RNA virus, readily inactivated by a variety of chemical agents, by a pH below 6.8 or above 8.1, and by ultraviolet irradiation. It is unstable at room temperature and at 37 and 56°C, and is best preserved at −60°C or below.

In thin sections of infected tissue-culture cells examined in the electron microscope, the virus appears as spherical particles measuring 50–70 nm in diameter with 30-nm electron-dense cores; the virions can be seen budding into intracellular vesicles or directly from the marginal membrane.[82] Released virus is covered with projections 5–6 nm in length[46] that cause the particles to hemagglutinate certain fowl red blood cells and human O cells.[83a,36,107]

Not only is the morphological picture of rubella similar to that of alphaviruses (group A arboviruses), but also there are other similarities. The rubella nucleocapsid core sediments at 150 S and contains a single strand of infectious RNA that sediments at about 40 S.[55,98] Instability of the core has thwarted definitive studies of its structure. The rubella virion has been reported to contain from three to eight structural proteins, the three major ones being two glycoproteins and a nonglycosylated core protein.[55,75,110]

The taxonomic position of rubella virus is with the togaviruses, because it is an RNA virus with an envelope (toga). There appears to be only one antigenic type, and no cross-reactions with alphaviruses or other members of the togavirus group have been found.[79] Differences in the biological behavior of different strains have been demonstrated, however; these include capacity to induce interferon *in vitro*,[4] and transmissibility to rabbit fetuses.[62]

5. Descriptive Epidemiology

5.1. Incidence and Prevalence

The incidence of rubella infection depends on the periodicity of the epidemic cycle, the degree of exposure within a group or community, and the number of susceptible persons at risk—i.e., lacking antibody.

Prospective serological studies of children in institutions have shown that virtually 100% of susceptibles living in cottages in which rubella occurs become infected as secondary and tertiary waves occur.[53] The situation is analogous to spread in families[29] and in military installations,[52,70] where close contact also results in a similar high degree of communicability. Among susceptible college students, a somewhat lower infection rate (64%) has been recorded.[24]

Data on the incidence of reported rubella cases in ten selected areas of the United States are shown in Fig. 1. The peak years of 1935, 1943, and 1964 are evident. In the period since 1960, the peak number of cases occurred in 1964, with 488,796 reported. At the time that vaccine was introduced in 1969, some 50,000 cases were reported annually. By 1974, the number had dropped to approximately 12,000; from 1976 to 1978, it ranged between 16,000 and 20,000, but fell to 4,000 in 1980.

Congenital rubella became reportable in the United States in 1966, when nationwide reporting of rubella was instituted. To encourage better notification of congenital cases, a National Registry for the Congenital Rubella Syndrome was established by the CDC in 1969. The results of retrospective and ongoing surveillance reveal some decline in the congenital disease since 1969; however, delays in diagnosis are common and result in underestimates for the most recent years (Fig. 2).

The risk of congenital rubella depends primarily on the month of pregnancy in which infection is acquired. Overall, approximately 16% of infants have major defects at birth following maternal rubella in the first 3 months of pregnancy.[76,77,100,103] If children are followed through childhood for the late appearance of abnormalities, this rises to approximately 30–35%.[57] On the basis of review of 15 prospective studies, Lundstrom[76] in 1962 estimated the risk of fetal damage to be 33% when maternal infection occurs in the first month of pregnancy, 25% if in the second month, 9% in the third month, and 4% in the fourth month.

Prevalence studies of rubella antibody in healthy populations have been carried out in many countries of the world. In an extensive collaborative survey in 1967 sponsored by the World Health Organization,[93] some 80–87% of women 17–22 years old in the mainland areas of Europe, Britain, Japan, and Australia were found to possess antibodies against rubella. A second collaborative study in 1968 of Caribbean and Middle and South American populations[17] again revealed an 80% antibody prevalence in women of childbearing age. A much lower rate was encountered in certain island groups in these and other surveys, and this is discussed in more detail in Section 5.3.

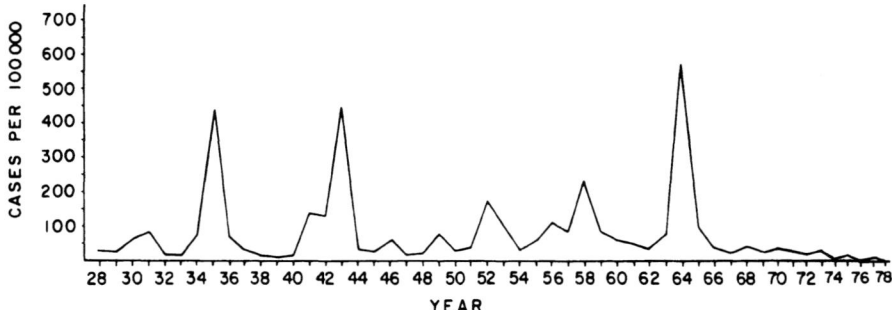

Fig. 1. Incidence of rubella, 1928–1978, in ten selected United States areas. From the CDC[11]

5.2. Epidemic Behavior

In the United States, before the introduction of vaccines, sizable epidemics occurred approximately every 6–9 years, with major ones at intervals up to 30 years (see Fig. 1).[118] Like the United States, European countries and Australia have endemic rubella, with the regular occurrence of cases each year and periodic epidemics. This behavior resulted in an approximate 85% immunity level as determined by serological surveys.[21,71,102,108]

A puzzling epidemiological feature was the sudden eruption of extensive outbreaks after long intervals of time in countries such as the United States. In the intervening periods, the disease ran its usual epidemic cycle of 6–9 years. This pattern succeeded in immunizing approximately 85% of the population by 15–19 years of age. Why, then, did a particular epidemic suddenly gather force and result in such an extraordinary onslaught as characterized the one in 1964? No significant antigenic differences among strains have been documented, yet conceivably viruses with altered biological characteristics and an enhanced capacity to spread may account for such behavior. Host factors may also be involved: there is evidence that infected persons differ in their ca-

Fig. 2. Reported cases of rubella (by year of report) and of congenital rubella (by year of birth), United States, 1966–1978. **Provisional. †Reporting incomplete due to delays in diagnosis. From the CDC.[11a]

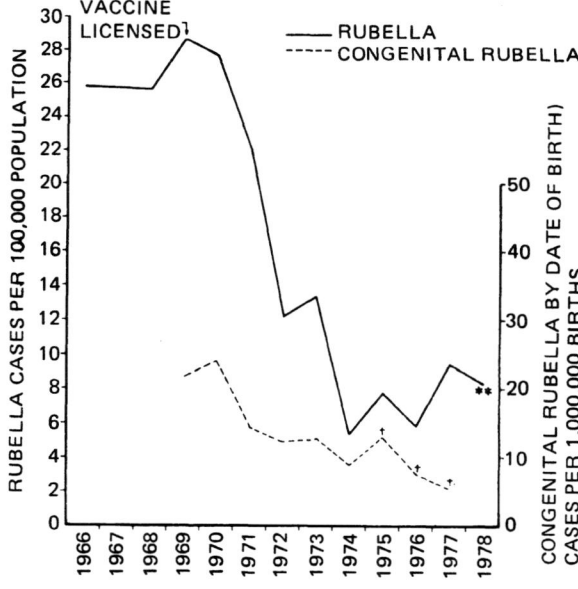

pacity to transmit rubella, and "spreaders" and "nonspreaders" have been identified in an epidemiological study of an outbreak of the disease in Hawaii.[41a] It seems that there must be something—an x factor that we don't know about—that affects the dissemination of rubella virus.

5.3. Geographic Distribution

Although serological surveys have documented the worldwide distribution of rubella infection, there are a number of puzzling features that characterize the behavior of the disease in certain island populations. Some of these are illustrated by the history of the disease on Taiwan,[30,31] which is a semitropical island with a dense population and extensive communication with the rest of the world. Large epidemics of rubella occurred there in 1944, 1957–1958, and 1968–1969. In both 1957–1958 and 1968–1969 outbreaks, the disease began in the north, where attack rates were highest, and moved toward the south, where the rates were considerably lower and the occurrence of cases ceased although significant numbers of susceptibles remained. A serological survey conducted before the 1968–1969 outbreak began indicated that none of the children born in the 10 years since the previous epidemic had acquired antibodies—evidence that the virus had not been circulating since that time. Similarly, serological tests in 1971 showed no change in antibody patterns of schoolchildren since the 1968–1969 epidemic, confirming the results of disease surveillance that documented absence of cases since the outbreak. Thus, by 1971, for unexplained reasons, rubella had not succeeded in becoming endemic on the island of Taiwan. The situation was not unique, for similar results were found in 1972 in Barbados, where no one born there during the previous 10 years had rubella antibodies despite the likelihood of introduction of the agent associated with a tourist influx of some 250,000 persons yearly.[23] Factors such as population size and density and climate do not seem to provide the answers to this puzzling behavior, for on the much smaller and more isolated island of Quemoy near Taiwan, a survey indicated that rubella was endemic there, since 97% of persons aged 6–50 years possessed rubella antibody.[31] No information was available about previous epidemics on Quemoy, but at the time of the survey, no cases

were seen and none had been known to occur in recent months.

The epidemiology of rubella on islands is clearly different from its behavior on the mainland, but no common pattern seems to emerge. Thus, Iceland, a small island that is sparsely populated, has had endemic rubella for many years, and the disease has been reportable since 1888.[104] The conditions for establishing endemicity would seem to be far less suitable than on Taiwan or Barbados, yet rubella long ago gained a foothold in Iceland and has maintained it ever since.

5.4. Temporal Distribution

Epidemics of rubella occur in the continental United States about every 6–9 years (see Fig. 1). The largest number of cases regularly appear in the months of March, April, and May, whether the year is one of low, moderate, or high incidence. The reason for this consistent seasonal pattern is unknown.

5.5. Age and Sex

In the prevaccine era, rubella in the United States was primarily a disease of school-aged children, with a peak incidence in the 5–9 year age group; the disease was uncommon in preschool children, but cases occurred in adolescents and young adults[118]; as vaccination rates among prepubertal children have increased, the peak incidence of the disease has shifted to the 15–24 year age group.[11] In other parts of the world, marked differences in the age at which rubella infection occurs have been revealed by seroepidemiological surveys. Figure 3 compares five countries with the United States. In three South American countries were the incidence of the disease is unknown (since it is not reported) and where congenital rubella does not seem to occur, infection is acquired at an early age; by 5–9 years, as high as 90% may be immune, as in Chile (Fig. 3).[17] In contrast, among island populations such as those of Hawaii[38] and Trinidad and Jamaica,[17] slow acquisition of antibodies has been documented, only 30–40% being immune in the age groups over 20 years. No appreciable differences are apparent in age-specific attack rates by sex in children, but more cases are reported in women than in men.

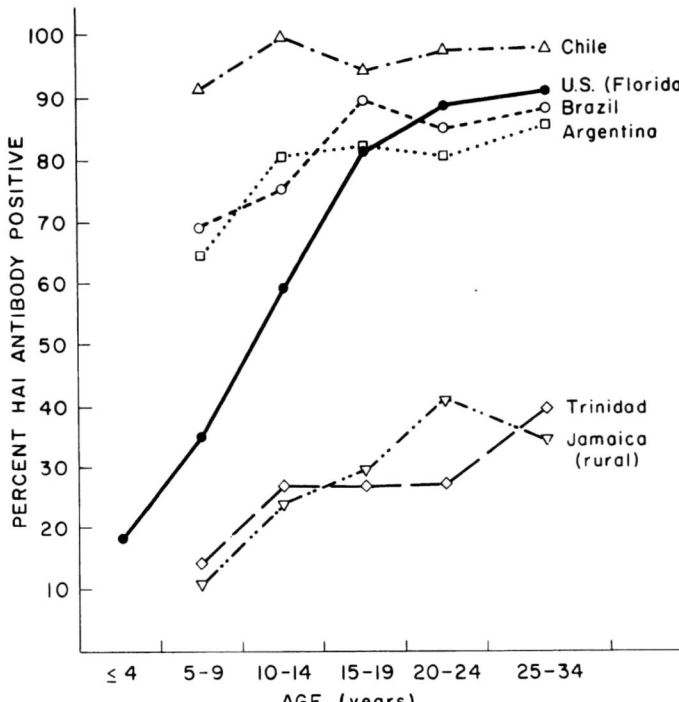

Fig. 3. Age-specific rubella HI antibody patterns in different population groups. Reprinted from Paul and White.[87a]

The significant proportion of adults who remain susceptible reflects the lower communicability of rubella as compared to measles.

5.6. Other Factors

No ethnic differences in incidence have been clearly shown, although the characteristic rash is more difficult to diagnose in persons with dark skin. A lower incidence of congenital rubella was found in outbreaks in Japan,[61] but it seems more likely that this was due to the relative avirulence of the strain rather than to ethnic differences.[6] There is a trend toward higher rates in lower than in upper socioeconomic groups; this may be due to increased exposure in crowded homes.

6. Mechanisms and Routes of Transmission

As with many infections, the exact mode of transmission is not clear, but close person-to-person contact seems to be necessary. The virus is present in the oropharyngeal secretions, and spread is probably via the respiratory route. The period of communicability is estimated to be from 5–7 days before to 3–5 days after the appearance of clinical signs, but is greatest just before and on the day of onset. Infants with the congenital infection shed relatively large amounts of virus from the throat and are effective sources of contagion for susceptible contacts.[14,48] Persistence of virus in the throat may continue for many months in these infants.[14,91] In women, the agent can be recovered from the genital tract[99]; the significance of the presence of virus in this site in terms of transmission is unknown.

7. Pathogenesis and Immunity

Following implantation of the virus on the mucosa of the upper respiratory tract, primary multiplication is thought to occur in the respiratory epithelium or local lymph nodes or both. This is followed by viremia and virus shedding from the throat. Rubella virus has been detected in pharyngeal secretions and in the blood as long as a week before the appearance of rash.[32,53] During the few days before onset, the agent has also been recovered from leukocytes, conjunctival swabs, and synovial fluid.[43]

Viremia apparently results in wide distribution of the virus, including dissemination in the respiratory tract, as suggested by the coryza, cough, and conjunctivitis that sometimes occur. The virus has been recovered from skin lesions within 24 hr of appearance of rash[42]; despite this, the rash is probably a manifestation of an antigen–antibody reaction, rather than a result of direct viral damage.

In the *fetal infection*, transmission is by hematogenous spread during maternal viremia; the recent demonstration of the presence of the agent in the female genital tract raises the possibility of involvement by the ascending route as well. During the course of maternal viremia, the placenta is seeded with virus, followed by development of inflammatory foci in the chorionic villi, granulomatous changes, and necrosis.[18] Infected chorionic cells may break off and act as emboli to target organs.[109]

The mechanisms by which rubella virus induces pathological changes in fetal organs and tissues are not clearly understood. Small size is a striking feature of infants infected *in utero*; this has been shown by Naeye and Blanc[83] to be due to an actual diminution in the total number of cells. One hypothesis is that the reduction in size of infants with the congenital disease results from the dropping out of infected clones of cells, which are known to have a shortened life-span.[105]

There is a high mortality in congenital rubella, especially in the first few months of life.[14,48] At autopsy, lesions have been demonstrated at one time or another in virtually every organ and tissue.[22,109] Inflammatory infiltrates occur in the heart, lungs, middle ear, and choroid plexus. Other lesions include giant-cell hepatitis, nephritis, vasculitis with intimal proliferation and epithelial necrosis, iridocyclitis, and meningitis.

Immunity following natural postnatal infection, as measured both serologically[108] and by tests for cell-mediated immunity,[93a] is in general long-lasting. However, inapparent reinfection has been shown to occur in approximately 4% of persons with naturally acquired immunity who are exposed during epidemics,[24,52] and frank clinical rubella has been documented in subjects with natural as well as vaccine-induced immunity.[20a,27,27a,117] Inapparent

reinfection occurs far more commonly in vaccinees, following certain vaccine preparations.[12,52] There is close correlation between antibody levels and resistance: reinfection occurs primarily in those with low HI and N antibody levels. In addition, there appear to be qualitative as well as quantitative differences between the resistance acquired through experience with wild virus and that acquired by vaccination with some attenuated vaccine strains, since reinfection rates 10 times higher have been observed in vaccinees compared to natural immunes with comparably low HI titers.[52]

A high level of antibody prevalence, and resultant *herd immunity*, was originally thought to deter the occurrence of epidemic rubella. This has not proved to be necessarily the case. In prospective studies, prior antibody-prevalence rates of 75% in college students[24] and the rates of 85–95% or higher in military recruits[52,70] have not prevented the occurrence of rubella outbreaks in which 64–100% of the remaining susceptibles are infected.

Immune responses in congenital rubella are different from those induced by postnatal infection.[106,106a] In some infants, there are immune-system defects that result in failure of antibody production.[106a] Among others with normal serological responses early in life, approximately 20% may lose detectable HI levels by the time they are 5 years old.[13,41] Hardy[39] has reported that a seronegative child with congenital rubella developed the clinical disease on exposure at school when aged 5 years. Similarly, apparent[16] and inapparent reinfections[58] in adults who were diagnosed as having congenital rubella in infancy have also been noted, and Menser et al.[78] have described a woman with the syndrome who was apparently reinfected during her own pregnancy and gave birth to an infant with congenital rubella. The reasons for the more rapid decline in antibody levels and the loss of immunity in persons with congenital rubella are not understood. In addition to unusual humoral antibody patterns, there is evidence that cellular immunity is impaired in congenital rubella[28]; this defect may explain the long persistence of virus excretion in infected infants.

8. Patterns of Host Response

In postnatally acquired rubella, the ratio of inapparent to apparent infections has been estimated to be from 1:1 to as high as 6:1[7,10,24,29,52,53] Age probably plays some role in conditioning the clinical expression of infection, although the relationship is not as clear as in diseases such as poliomyelitis and hepatitis. The observations of Brody[9] during an epidemic on the Pribiloff Islands led him to conclude that there were two groups of adults involved in the outbreak, one whose members had lost detectable antibody and experienced reinfection, largely inapparent, and another group who had their first experiences with the virus and exhibited a high clinical attack rate. In two prospective studies of young adult Hawaiian military recruits at Fort Ord, California, there was a 1.9:1 ratio of inapparent infections to apparent cases in one epidemic in which the men were screened intensely for clinical signs[52] and a 3.7:1 ratio in a subsequent outbreak during which clinical surveillance was less assiduous. The spectrum of the host response is shown in Table 1.

Table 1. Patterns of Host Response to Rubella

I. Acquired rubella
  A. Inapparent infection
  B. Rubella without rash
  C. Rubella with rash
  D. Complications
      1. Joint involvement (arthralgia, arthritis)
      2. Encephalitis
      3. Thrombocytopenic purpura
II. Congenital rubella
  A. Inapparent infection
  B. Congenital rubella syndrome with single or multiple organ involvement
      1. Cardiovascular lesions (patent ductus arteriosus, ventricular septal defect, coarctation of aortic isthmus, pulmonary stenosis)
      2. Eye defects (cataracts, retinopathy, microphthalmia, glaucoma)
      3. Hearing impairment (deafness)
      4. Growth retardation
      5. Thrombocytopenic purpura
      6. Hepatosplenomegaly
      7. Jaundice (regurgitative)
      8. Hepatitis
      9. Central nervous system involvement (psychomotor retardation, encephalitis, microcephaly, asceptic meningitis)
      10. Bone lesions (long bone radiolucencies, bone malformations)
      11. Genitourinary tract (undescended testicle, renal lesions).

8.1. Clinical Manifestations

8.1.1. Acquired Infection.
In the postnatally acquired infection, rash is the most prominent clinical feature and the first evidence of the disease in 95% of affected children. Adults frequently experience a prodrome lasting several days, with malaise, low-grade fever, and tender, swollen postauricular and posterior cervical lymph nodes. Mild sore throat, corzya, cough, and conjunctivitis may be present in the more severe cases. The rash begins on the face, spreads rapidly to the chest and abdomen, and within a day or two extends to the extremities; it is pink, maculopapular, and not distinctive in appearance. The lesions are at first discrete, but later tend to coalesce, particularly on the face. A helpful diagnostic point is that the rash is *always* present on the face.

The most characteristic clinical feature of rubella is the involvement of specific lymph nodes, i.e., postauricular, suboccipital, and posterior cervical, which are often enlarged and tender, sometimes as long as a week before onset. Arthralgia and arthritis are common complications in young adults, particularly women, their frequency increasing with age. The disease is usually a mild one lasting no more than a few days, but in rare instances, complications such as encephalitis, thrombocytopenic purpura, and neuritis may occur.

8.1.2. Congenital Infection.
Like postnatally acquired rubella, the congenital infection may be inapparent, but much more commonly one or more of the characteristic features are present. The risk to the fetus is greatest early in pregnancy, particularly in the first month, and in the second month, which is the period of organogenesis, but fetal involvement can also occur in the second trimester.[40] Maternal rubella in the first trimester is associated with congenital anomalies recognizable at birth in approximately 15–20% of infants. Late manifestations, particularly deafness, raise the proportion of those affected to 30–50%.[57] The rate of virus isolation from placenta or fetus or both obtained at abortion is considerably higher than this, supporting the probability that inapparent infection *in utero* is more common than previously suspected.[2,48,91,92]

In affected infants, the chief abnormalities are heart lesions (most frequently patent ductus arteriosus), cataracts or other ocular lesions (retinopathy, microphthalmia, glaucoma), purpuric and petechial skin lesions associated with thrombocytopenia, hepatosplenomegaly, meningoencephalitis, and lesions of the long bones.[18,22] Hearing loss and psychomotor retardation become apparent later. Multiple system involvement is frequent, especially when infection occurs in the second month of fetal life, when organs are developing. The prognosis in severely involved infants is poor, the mortality being particularly high in the first year of life.[14,48]

8.2. Serological Responses

The time course of appearance of antibodies is shown in Fig. 4. In addition to HI, CF, N, and other antibodies, local secretory IgA antibody has been demonstrated in the nasopharyngeal secretions.[85] PA antibodies are strikingly high in patients with postrubella thrombocytopenia.[112] HI antibodies are usually present on the day of onset and rise rapidly; it may therefore not be possible to show a significant increase in titer unless the first serum specimen is obtained early. CF antibodies appear considerably later—often not until a week or more after onset—so that 4-fold or greater rises in titer between paired specimens can be detected when the first specimen has been collected too late in the course to do so by HI test. The presence of rubella-specific IgM antibody in convalescent sera is also a useful market of recent infection.[21,62a] IgM antibody disappears after 4–8 weeks, leaving only IgG antibody.

The immune response to intrauterine rubella infection differs from that of the postnatal infection.[1,2,5,19,106] It is evident that the fetus can make specific IgM after the 16th week.[2] At birth, rubella IgM is present and continues to rise in titer for approximately 6 months; it commonly persists through the first year of life. Maternal IgG, detectable at 12–16 weeks of fetal life, declines over the first few months after birth as the infant's own rubella IgG rises.

9. Control

9.1. Vaccine Development

As soon as the virus was isolated in tissue culture in 1962, efforts to develop a vaccine were under way. At first, a killed virus vaccine was considered to be the only safe approach, but it soon became apparent that inactivation of the agent by various

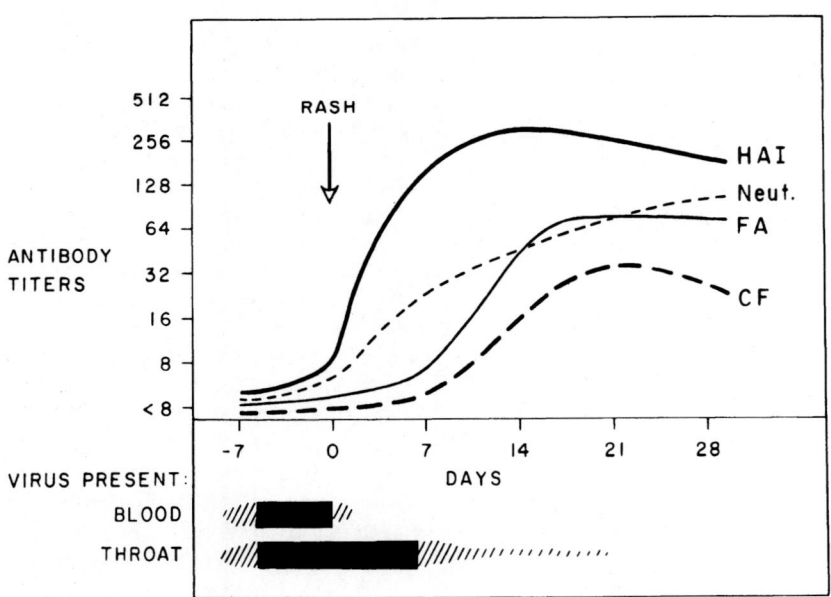

Fig. 4. Antibody responses to primary infection with rubella virus. (HAI) Hemagglutination-inhibition antibodies; (Neut.) neutralizing antibodies; (FA) fluorescent antibodies; (CF) complement-fixing antibodies. Reprinted from Paul and White.[87a]

means inevitably led to loss of antigenicity. Attention was therefore turned to attenuation of the virus by serial passage in tissue culture, and by 1966, Meyer et al.[80] had successfully developed an experimental live virus vaccine. The attenuated strain that they used, "high-passage virus$_{77}$" (HPV$_{77}$), represented the 77th passage of the agent in primary GMK cells. A further 5 passages in duck-embryo (DE) tissue culture resulted in the HPV$_{77}$DE$_5$ vaccine that was licensed in the United States in 1969, after extensive field trials proved its safety and immunogenicity. Shortly afterward, another vaccine strain, Cendehill, developed by Huygelen et al.,[56] was also licensed. This strain was isolated in GMK and passaged 51 times in primary rabbit-kidney cells. A third vaccine, the RA 27/3 of Plotkin[89] recovered and passaged 25 times in human diploid W138 cells, became available in the United States in 1979. The three vaccines are similar in that they induce seroconversion in approximately 95% of susceptibles. The RA 27/3 vaccine has advantages over the others in that it retains the ability to infect by a natural route, viz., intranasally. Furthermore, it induces a broader range of antibody responses than does either HPV$_{77}$DE$_5$ or Cendehill, including the regular appearance of precipitating antibodies,[68] and local secretory IgA in the oropharynx.[85] In addition, RA 27/3 provides greater resistance to reinfection.[25a,33a] A Japanese vaccine, TO 336, has also been described; there is suggestive evidence that it may be less transmissible to the fetus than are other vaccine strains.[6]

At present, only the RA27/3 strain is distributed in the United States. Two preparations are available: one containing only rubella vaccine (Mervuvax II®), and the other containing rubella vaccine combined with measles and mumps vaccine (MMR II®).

9.2. Responses to Rubella Vaccines

9.2.1. Clinical Reactions.

Some reaction occurs in approximately 10–15% of vaccinees, depending on age and sex. By and large, the symptoms and signs are those of mild rubella: low-grade fever, lymphadenopathy, and occasionally rash appearing after 10–20 days. As in the natural disease, transient arthritis and arthralgia lasting up to a week may occur, particularly in women over 20 years old. Joint involvement is uncommon in children, its frequency and severity increasing with increasing age; in

women in the 26–41 year age group, it may reach close to 60%.[115a] Fingers, wrists, and knees are most commonly involved; joint effusions may develop, as in infection with wild virus. Recurrent pain and swelling of the joints over a period of months have been reported, and in at least three cases, the virus has been recovered from knee-joint fluid 4–5 months after vaccination.[11,84] An HPV$_{77}$ strain grown in dog kidney (HPV$_{77}$DK$_{12}$) that was responsible for most of the cases of recurrent arthritis as well as the late neuropathies involving wrists and hands or legs ("catcher's crouch")[59] was withdrawn from distribution in March 1973. The HPV$_{77}$DE$_5$, Cendehill, and RA 27/3 vaccines do not appear to differ significantly in terms of clinical reactions, although there have been few large-scale comparative studies.

9.2.2. Shedding of Virus.

Virus excretion from the throat occurs briefly and in relatively small amounts in most vaccinees.[15] Nevertheless, contact spread is so rare as to be a negligible hazard[37] even for susceptible pregnant women exposed to their vaccinated children.[97] Viremia has rarely been documented in vaccinees, but that it occurs is substantiated by transmission of infection to the fetus in susceptible pregnant women who have inadvertently been given rubella vaccine.[72,81a] Another site from which vaccine virus can be recovered transiently is the genital tract in females.[111]

9.2.3. Serological Responses.

Following vaccine administration, antibody develops in approximately 95% of susceptibles. The responses are similar to those that follow natural infection, but HI and N antibody titers are considerably lower[81] and CF antibodies appear only in those who have brisk HI responses.[49] Local IgA and precipitin antibodies (anti-θ, anti-i) comparable to those that result from wild virus infection occur only with the RA 27/3 vaccine.[47,68,85]

9.3. Vaccination of Children: Impact on Rubella Incidence

In the United States, the decision was made to focus primarily on prepubertal children as the main target for vaccination. An alternate method was adopted in England, where the immunization program is directed toward 13-year-old girls with the view of permitting natural infection in childhood to provide some protection. Recent large outbreaks of rubella in the United Kingdom have raised questions about the wisdom of this approach. The goal in the United States, as set forth by the U.S. Public Health Service Advisory Committee on Immunization Practices, was based on the concept that congenital rubella could be prevented indirectly by inducing a high degree of herd immunity, thus blocking the circulation of virus in the segment of the population in which most infections occur, i.e. young children, who may act as sources of infection for pregnant women. The vaccine is available for use either alone or combined with measles and mumps virus vaccines. The recommendation of the Academy of Pediatrics Committee on Infections is that all children between the ages of 1 year and puberty be immunized against rubella.

In the 12 years since introduction of vaccines, approximately 100 million doses of live rubella virus vaccine have been distributed in the United States. This has resulted in a substantial decrease in the incidence of the disease,[11,44b,63] and as Fig. 1 indicates, the usual cyclic pattern of major epidemics has been interrupted. The number of cases of congenital rubella has also apparently declined, but since there is often a delay of several years in making the diagnosis, recent figures are considered provisional[11,11a] (see Fig. 2).

Localized outbreaks of rubella have nevertheless continued to occur every year throughout the United States. It is thus evident that the concept of controlling the epidemic disease by providing a high degree of herd immunity in the childhood population has not been entirely successful. Outbreaks have been recorded in areas where 83–95% of schoolchildren have been vaccinated.[11b,60] Apparently, close to 100% immunity rates are necessary to prevent the introduction and spread of the virus.[52,70]

A striking change that has occurred in the epidemiology of rubella in the vaccine era has been a shift in the age distribution of cases (Fig. 5). Recent epidemics have been centered largely in unvaccinated high school and university students.[11,60] As a result, instead of being a disease of 5- to 9-year olds, the largest number of cases now occurs in those 15–24 years of age. Hospital associated outbreaks have also caused problems,[89a] especially when they have involved obstetric units.[10b] As immunization rates of the childhood population increase, a higher percentage of those moving into the older age groups should be protected, with a resultant decline in incidence in adolescents and young adults.

9.4. Vaccination of Women of Childbearing Age

Recent recommendations for vaccine use have placed increasing emphasis on immunization of adolescents and young women.[11c,50] However, since the vaccine contains live virus that is capable of infecting the placenta and the fetus, caution is necessary in giving it to postpubertal females because of the possibility that they may be pregnant. The optimum procedure is first to determine by sero-

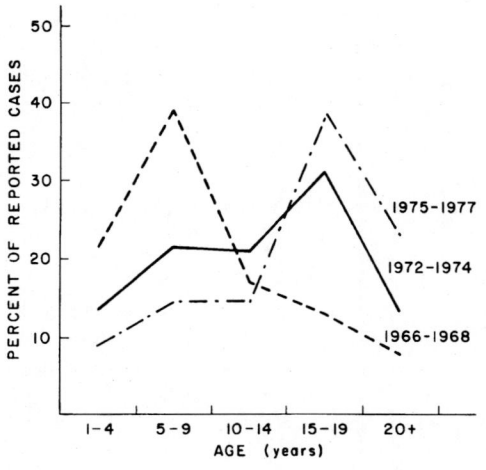

Fig. 5. Shift in age distribution of cases reported to the Center for Disease Control, United States. From the CDC.[11]

logical test whether the woman lacks antibody and is therefore susceptible. Before the vaccine is given, the presence of pregnancy should be excluded and the necessity for suitable birth control measures for the next 3 months should be emphasized.

Despite all warnings, inadvertent vaccination in pregnancy has occured with some frequency.[72,81a,120] In a 1974 review, Levine et al.[72] noted that among the reported instances, the immune status of most of the 471 women given rubella vaccine within 91 days of conception was unknown, and only 81 (17%) had been shown to lack rubella antibodies. Of the 33 known susceptible women given $HPV_{77}De_5$ vaccine strains, the placenta or decidua obtained at abortion yielded virus in 8 cases, and in 1 case the fetus was virus-positive. Fleet et al.[25] recovered rubella virus from fetal eye 20 weeks after maternal immunization; the histopathology was typical of the lesion induced by wild virus.[25] There is less information concerning the effects of other vaccine strains, but virus has been recovered from fetal tissues in 1 of 12 abortuses from susceptibles given Cendehill vaccine; no isolations were made from abortion material from 15 susceptible women who had received RA27/3 vaccine during pregnancy.[11c]

Like wild virus, the $HPV_{77}DE_5$ attenuated strain can induce chronic infection and has been recovered from decidua as long as 20 weeks after vaccine administration.[66] The teratogenic potential of the several attenuated strains is unknown, but it is apparently considerably less than is the case with wild virus.[81a] Up to October, 1980, 101 susceptible women vaccinated within 3 months before and 3 months after conception have been followed to term.[11c] HPV_{77} or Cendehill vaccines had been given to 93, and 8 had received RA27/3 vaccine. All women delivered infants who appeared normal at birth, but evidence of inapparent infection was documented in 3 of 30 tested for the presence of rubella specific IgM.[41b] Based on available evidence, the theoretical risk of congenital malformations attributable to infection with rubella vaccine strains in utero was estimated to be 0–4%.[11c] Although the risk is thus minimal, it cannot be ignored, and inadvertent immunization during pregnancy still constitutes reason for considering termination.

While vaccination is contraindicated during pregnancy, the screening of women for antibodies to rubella should be a routine part of prenatal care. An optimum time to immunize the susceptibles identified by this means is during the first few days postpartum, before they leave the hospital.[51] This takes advantage of the very low risk of pregnancy in the ensuing weeks; nevertheless, depending on the patient, some contraceptive measure may be desirable.[3]

9.5. Management of the Rubella Problem in Pregnancy

The situation that arises most frequently involves a woman in early pregnancy who gives a history of possible exposure to rubella. Under these circumstances, a serum sample should be obtained as soon as possible to determine serologically whether or not she is susceptible. A past history of the disease is unreliable because a number of other viruses induce "rubelliform" rashes. If an HI test reveals the presence of antibody and the blood sample was collected within a few days of exposure, the patient can be reassured that she is immune and therefore not at risk. If a titer of less than 1:8 is obtained, the patient is susceptible and should be followed to determine whether or not she has been infected. A second blood specimen should be obtained approximately 3 weeks after exposure and retested *along with the first specimen*. If infection has occurred, antibodies will be detected in the second serum, and appropriate action can then be discussed with the patient.

Difficulty in interpreting HI results may be encountered when there has been a delay of several weeks in obtaining the first postexposure serum sample. If HI antibodies are present, the question arises of whether they represent a recent or current infection or one that was experienced years before. This can often be answered by determining the immunoglobulin class to which the antibodies belong. As in other viral infections, the first antibody response in a primary infection is IgM, which persists for 4–8 weeks along with a rising level of IgG, which eventually represents virtually all the detectable antibody. Several methods other than separation by density-gradient centrifugation for measurement of IgM are available. They include a fluorescence test,[35] removal of IgG by absorption with *Staphylococcus aureus* protein A,[2a] and an ELISA test.[62a]

Another serological method that may be used to establish the current nature of the infection is the

CF test. Because CF antibodies appear later in the course of the infection (7–10 days after onset of rash), it is often possible to show a rise in CF titer when the serum has been obtained too late in the course to detect a significant increase in HI levels (see Fig. 4).

9.6. Use of Immune Serum Globulin

In the case of the pregnant woman who has been exposed to rubella, immune serum globulin (ISG) has frequently been given in the hope of preventing infection should the patient be susceptible. The results have been disappointing. That ISG, given in adequate dosage *immediately* after exposure, has a modifying effect has been shown by Green *et al.*,[32] who demonstrated in volunteers that under these circumstances it may prevent the *disease* but not the *infection*. There was some suggestion in the data and in those of others[16] that the duration of viremia was shortened, but the numbers were small and no firm conclusions could be drawn. In any event, there are well-documented examples both of rubella with rash and of inapparent infection in women given ISG in optimum doses soon after exposure. The effectiveness of this form of prophylaxis is thus unreliable and unpredictable. The only circumstance in which its use might be considered is in the case of a woman who, because of religious or other reasons, would not consent to termination of the pregnancy should infection—clinical or inapparent—occur in the first trimester of pregnancy.

10. Unresolved Problems

The unpredictable behavior of rubella and the peculiarities of the virus mandate a note of caution to any forecast of the ultimate impact of vaccination on the epidemiological behavior of the disease. Despite favorable trends evidenced by a decline in reported cases of rubella and the rubella syndrome, certain problems still remain. The 1977 immunization survey indicates that in the United States, only 64% of children 10–14 years old have received rubella vaccine—a figure far short of the one necessary to prevent epidemics. While the total number of cases remains low, some estimate of the true number of infections that occur has been suggested by

Sabin,[93c] who points out that if the low rate of reporting (approximately 1 in 10 cases) and the high inapparent infection rate are taken into account, the actual incidence of infection must be many times the rate suggested by the number of reported cases. The continued circulation of wild virus may reinforce the immunity of vaccinees and provide infection and resistance to those who have not been vaccinated, but unfortunately it also carries the hazard of potential exposure of susceptible women. This possibility is emphasized by the continued occurrence of cases in those over the age of 15 (Figs. 5 and 6), a pattern that is in line with other evidence that immunizaton programs have had scant impact on immunity rates among young adults. Age-specific attack rates in this group have shown little change, and serological surveys of women aged 15–40 indicate that some 15% are still susceptible, as was the case before vaccines were introduced.[11,50] Since wild rubella virus continues to circulate, the risk of fetal infection therefore remains.

There have also been problems related to the limited persistence of immunity in some vaccinees and their greater susceptibility to reinfection than is the case after natural infection.[12,52] Neither HPV$_{77}$DE$_5$ nor Cendehill vaccine induces local IgA antibody in the oropharynx, the first line of defense,[85] and this may be a major factor in the higher reinfection rates associated with immunization with these strains. Prospective serological surveillance has shown that vaccine-induced antibodies persist in the majority of persons over a period of 7–10 years.[11,54,114] However, a close correlation has been observed between the original serological response and subsequent maintenance of antibody levels: if this response was brisk, the titers persist well over the 7–9 years that they have been followed, but if the response to vaccination was feeble (HI 1:8–16) approximately 25% may be seronegative by 3–5 years.[49] Of particular concern with respect to poor responders is the observation that 3–5 years after immunization, N antibodies, considered to be the protective ones, are low or absent in 46% of such persons.[54] Absence of N in the presence of HI antibodies has been observed in a small percentage of persons who have experienced natural infection, and recently it has been reported that pregnant women with this antibody profile may be vulnerable to reinfection leading to fetal involvement.[20a,27a] Consequently, it is of concern that the HI-positive, N-negative profile

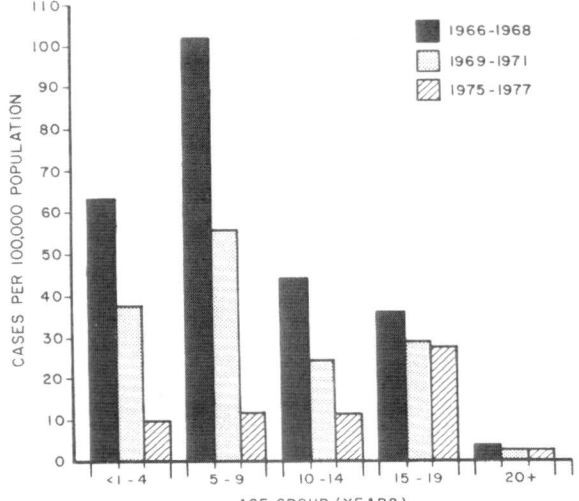

Fig. 6. Reported rubella incidence rates in Massachusetts, New York City, and Illinois, by age group, 1966–1977. From the CDC.[11]

has been found to occur with some frequency in vaccinees. In contrast to those given $HPV_{77}DE_5$ or Cendehill vaccines, however, recipients of RA 27/3 vaccine promptly acquire high levels of N antibody, comparable to those following natural rubella, and most maintain relatively high titers for long periods.[11,44a,97a,114a]

Little information is available on the development and persistence of cell-mediated immunity (CMI) following vaccination, but Rossier *et al.*[93a] have shown that 5 years after immunization, only 24% of $HPV_{77}DE_5$ vaccinees were CMI-positive, in contrast to 88% of young adults who had experienced natural infection some time in the past.

Much also remains to be learned about the epidemiology of rubella, including its enigmatic behavior in certain island populations, and the importance of "super-virus shedders" in influencing the transmission of infection and the course of epidemics. Progressive rubella panencephalitis has been described as a rare late complication of both the acquired and the congenital form of the disease[115]; whether it occurs after vaccine-induced infection is unknown. The possible association of rubella with chronic diseases such as arthritis and diabetes also deserves ongoing attention.

Future success in improving the immune status of the population and thus achieving better control of the rubella problem will require increased efforts

to vaccinate not only children but also young adults. Requirement by many states of proof of immunization on entering school should increase the childhood vaccination rate above the current 65% level, and the recent emphasis on reaching those in their teens or older should also provide an enhanced barrier to circulation of wild rubella virus. In addition, widespread use of the more immunogenic RA 27/3 vaccine promises a sturdier and more durable immunity and a population better protected against rubella. Nevertheless, long-term clinical and serological surveillance of vaccinated populations is necessary in order to monitor immunity levels and to assess the possible need for revaccination of those immunized in infancy.

11. References

1. ALFORD, C. A., Studies on antibody in congenital rubella infections, *Am. J. Dis. Child.* **110**:455–463 (1965).
2. ALFORD, C. A., NEVA, F. A., AND WELLER, T. H., Virologic and serologic studies on human products of conception after maternal rubella, *N. Engl. J. Med.* **271**:1275–1281 (1964).
2a. ANKERST, J., CHRISTENSEN, P., KJELLEN, L., AND KRONVALL, G., A routine diagnostic test for IgA and IgM antibodies to rubella virus: Absorption of IgG with *Staphylococcus aureus*, *J. Infect. Dis.* **130**:268–273 (1974).

3. BALDWIN, J. A., AND FREESTONE, D. S., Risk of early post-partum pregnancy in context of post-partum vaccination against rubella, *Lancet* **2:**366–367 (1971).

4. BANATVALA, J. E. POTTER, J. E., AND BEST, J. M., Interferon response to Sendai and rubella viruses in human foetal cultures, leukocytes and placental cultures, *J. Gen. Virol.* **13:**193–201 (1971).

5. BELLANTI, J. A., ARTENSTEIN, M. S., OLSON, L. C., BUESCHER, E. L., LUHRS, C. E., AND MILSTEAD, K. L., Congenital rubella, *Am. J. Dis. Child.* **110:**464–472 (1965).

6. BEST, J. M., BANATVALA, J. E., AND BOWEN, J. M., New Japanese rubella vaccine: Comparative trials, *Br. Med. J.* **3:**221–224 (1974).

7. BISNO, A. L., SPENCE, L. P., STEWART, J. A., AND CASEY, H. L., Rubella in Trinidad, sero-epidemiologic studies of an institutional outbreak, *Am. J. Epidemiol.* **89:**74–81 (1969).

8. BROWN, G. C., MAASSAB, H. F., VERONELLI, J. A., AND FRANCIS, T., JR., Rubella antibodies in human serum: Detection by the indirect fluorescent-antibody technic, *Science* **145:**943–945 (1964).

9. BRODY, J. A., The infectiousness of rubella and the possibility of reinfection, *Am. J. Public Health* **56:**1082–1087 (1966).

9a. BYRNE, E. B., EVANS, A. S., FONTS, D. W., AND ISRAEL, H. L., A seroepidemiologic study of Epstein–Barr virus and other antigens in sarcoidosis, *Am. J. Epidemiol.* **97:**355–363 (1973).

10. BUESCHER, E. L., Behavior of rubella virus in adult populations, *Arch. Gesamte Virusforsch.* **16:**470–476 (1965).

10a. CAPPEL, R., SCHLUEDERBERG, A., AND HORSTMANN, D. M., Large-scale production of rubella precipitinogens and their use in the diagnostic laboratory, *J. Clin. Microbiol.* **1:**201–205 (1975).

10b. CARNE, S., DEWHURST, C. J., AND HURLEY, R., Rubella epidemic in a maternity unit, *Br. Med. J.,* **1:**444–446 (1973).

11. CENTER FOR DISEASE CONTROL, *Rubella Surveillance, January 1976–December 1978,* pp. 1–26 (issued May, 1980).

11a. CENTER FOR DISEASE CONTROL, Rubella and congenital rubella, United States, 1977–1978, *Morbid. Mortal. Weekly Rep.* **27:**495–497 (1978).

11b. CENTER FOR DISEASE CONTROL, Rubella—Hawaii, *Morbid. Mortal. Weekly Rep.* **26:**272–247 (1977).

11c. CENTER FOR DISEASE CONTROL, Rubella prevention, *Morbidity and Mortality Weekly Report* **30:**37–47 (1981).

11d. CENTER FOR DISEASE CONTROL, *Morbidity and Mortality Weekly Report* **27:**532 (1979).

12. CHANG, T.-W., DESROSIERS, S., AND WEINSTEIN, L., Clinical and serologic studies of an outbreak of rubella in a vaccinated population, *N. Engl. J. Med.* **283:**246–248 (1970).

13. COOPER, L. Z., FLORMAN, A. L., ZIRING, P. R., AND KRUGMAN, S., Loss of rubella hemagglutination inhibition antibody in congenital rubella, *Am. J. Dis. Child.* **122:**397–403 (1971).

14. COOPER, L. Z., ZIRING, P. R., OCKERSE, A. B., FEDUN, B. A., KIELY, B., AND KRUGMAN, S., Rubella: Clinical manifestations and management, *Am. J. Dis. Child.* **118:**18–29 (1969).

15. DAVIS, W. J., LARSON, H. E., SIMSARIAN, J. P., PARKMAN, P. D., AND MEYER, H. M., JR., A study of rubella immunity and resistance to infection, *J. Am. Med. Assoc.* **215:**600–608 (1971).

16. DOEGE, T. C., AND KIM, K. S. W., Studies of rubella and its prevention with immune globulin, *J. Am. Med. Assoc.* **200:**584–590 (1967).

17. DOWDLE, W. R., FERREIRA, W., DE SALLES GOMES, L. F., KING, D., KOURANY, M., MADALENGOITIA, J., PEARSON, E., SWANSTON, W. H., TOSI, H. C., AND VILCHES, A. M., WHO collaborative study on the sero-epidemiology of rubella in Caribbean and Middle and South American populations in 1968, *Bull. WHO* **42:**419–422 (1970).

18. DRISCOLL, S. G., Histopathology of gestational rubella, *Am. J. Dis. Child.* **118:**49–53 (1969).

19. DUDGEON, J. A., Congenital rubella: Pathogenesis and immunology, *Am. J. Dis. Child.* **118:**35–44 (1969).

20. Editorial, Rubella and congenital malformations, *Lancet* **1:**316 (1944).

20a. EILARD, T., AND STRANNEGÅRD, O., Rubella reinfection in pregnancy followed by transmission to the fetus, *J. Infect. Dis.* **129:**594–596 (1974).

21. ENDERS-RUCKLE, G., Seroepidemiology of rubella and reinfection, *Am. J. Dis. Child.* **118:**139–142 (1969).

22. ESTERLY, J. R., AND OPPENHEIMER, E. H., Pathological lesions due to congenital rubella, *Arch. Pathol.* **87:**380–388 (1969).

23. EVANS, A. S., COX, F., NANKERVIS, G., OPTON, E. M., SHOPE, R. E., WELLS, A. V., AND WEST, B., A health and seroepidemiological survey of a community in Barbados, *Int. J. Epidemiol.* **3:**167–175 (1974).

24. EVANS, A. S., NIEDERMAN, J. C., AND SAWYER, R. N., Prospective studies of Yale University freshmen. II. Occurrence of acute respiratory infections and rubella, *J. Infect. Dis.* **123:**271–278 (1971).

25. FLEET, W. J., JR., BENZ, E. W., JR., KARZON, D. T., LEFKOWITZ, L. B., AND HERRMANN, K. L., Fetal consequences of maternal rubella immunization, *J. Am. Med. Assoc.* **227:**621–627 (1974).

25a. FOGEL, A., GERICHTER, C. B., BARNEA, R., HANDSHER, R., AND HEEGER, F., Response to experimental challenge in persons immunized with different rubella vaccines, *J. Pediatr.* **92:**26–29 (1978).

26. FORBES, J. A., Rubella, historical aspects, *Am. J. Dis. Child.* **118:**5–11 (1969).

27. FORREST, J. M., MENSER, M. A., AND HONEYMAN, M. C., Clinical rubella eleven months after vaccination, *Lancet* **2:**399–400 (1972).

27a. Forsgren, M., Carlström, G., and Strangert, K., Case of congenital rubella after maternal reinfection, *Scand. J. Infect. Dis.* **11**:81–83 (1979).

28. Fuccillo, D. A., Steele, R. W., Hensen, S. A., Vincent, M. M., Hardy, J. B., and Bellanti, J. A., Impaired cellular immunity to rubella virus in congenital rubella, *Infect. Immun.* **9**:81–84 (1974).

29. Gale, J. L., Detels, R., Kim, K. S. W., Beasley, R. P., Chen, K. P., and Grayston, J. T., The epidemiology of rubella on Taiwan. III. Family studies in cities of high and low attack rates, *Int. J. Epidemiol.* **1**:261–265 (1972).

30. Gale, J. L., Grayston, J. T., Beasley, R. P., Detels, R., and Kim, K. S. W., The epidemiology of rubella on Taiwan. II. 1968–1969 epidemic, *Int. J. Epidemiol.* **1**:253–260 (1972).

30a. Grandien, M., Espmark, A., and Norrby, E. Evaluation of an immunodiffusion test for screening of rubella immunity, *Acta Pathol. Microbiol. Scand. Sect. C* **84**:153–160 (1976).

31. Grayston, J. T., Gale, J. L., and Watten, R. H., The epidemiology of rubella on Taiwan. I. Introduction and description of the 1957–1958 epidemic, *Int. J. Epidemiol.* **1**:245–252 (1972).

32. Green, R. H., Balsamo, M. R., Giles, J. P., Krugman, S., and Mirick, G. S., Studies on the natural history and prevention of rubella, *Am. J. Dis. Child.* **110**:348–365 (1965).

33. Gregg, N. M., Congenital cataract following German measles in the mother, *Trans. Ophthalmol. Soc. Aust.* **3**:35–46 (1941).

33a. Grillner, L., Immunity to intranasal challenge with rubella virus two years after vaccination: A comparison between three rubella vaccines, *J. Infect. Dis.* **133**:637–641 (1976).

34. Habel, K., Transmission of rubella to *Macacus mulatta* monkeys, *Public Health Rep.* **57**:1126–1139 (1942).

35. Haire, M., and Hadden, D. S. M., Immunoglobulin responses in rubella and its complications, *Br. Med. J.* **3**:130–132 (1970).

36. Halonen, P. E., Ryan, J. M., and Stewart, J. A., Rubella hemagglutinin prepared with alkaline extraction of virus grown in suspension culture of BHK-21 cells, *Proc. Soc. Exp. Biol. Med.* **125**:162–167 (1967).

37. Halstead, S. B., and Diwan, A. R., Failure to transmit rubella virus vaccine: A close-contact study in adults, *J. Am. Med. Assoc.* **215**:634–636 (1971).

38. Halstead, S. B., Diwan, A. R., and Oda, A. I., Susceptibility to rubella among adolescents and adults in Hawaii, *J. Am. Med. Assoc.* **210**:1881–1883 (1969).

39. Hardy, J. B., In discussion of Florman, A. L., Cooper, L. Z., Ziring, P. R., and Krugman, S., Response to rubella vaccination among seronegative children with congenital rubella, *Pediatr. Res.* **4**:513–514 (1970).

40. Hardy, J. B., McCracken, G. H., Gilkeson, M. R., and Sever, J. L., Adverse fetal outcome following maternal rubella after the first trimester of pregnancy, *J. Am. Med. Assoc.* **207**:2414–2420 (1969).

41. Hardy, J. B., Sever, J. L., and Gilkeson, M. R., Declining antibody titers in children with congenital rubella, *J. Pediatr.* **75**:213–220 (1969).

41a. Hattis, R. P., Halstead, S. B., Herrmann, K. L., and Witte, J. J., Rubella in an immunized island population, *J. Am. Med. Assoc.* **223**:1019–1021 (1973).

41b. Hayden, G. F., Herrmann, K. L., Buimovici-Klein, E., Weiss, K. E., Nieberg, P. I., and Mitchell, J. E., Subclinical congenital rubella infection associated with rubella vaccination in early pregnancy, *J. Pediat.* **96**:869–872 (1980).

42. Heggie, A. D., Pathogenesis of the rubella exanthem: Isolation of rubella virus from the skin, *N. Engl. J. Med.* **285**:664–666 (1971).

43. Heggie, A. D., and Robbins, F. C., Natural rubella acquired after birth, clinical features and complications, *Am. J. Dis. Child.* **118**:12–17 (1969).

44. Hess, A. F., German measles (rubella): An experimental study, *Arch. Intern. Med.* **13**:913–916 (1914).

44a. Hillary, I. B., and Freestone, D. S., Persistence of antibody induced by rubella vaccine (Wistar RA 27/3 strain) after six years, *J. Hyg. Camb.* **75**:407–411 (1975).

44b. Hinman, A. R., Preblud, S. R., and Brandling-Bennett, A. D., Rubella: The U.S. experience, in: *Developments in Biological Standardization*, Vol. 43, *Immunization: Benefits versus Risk Factors* (W. Hennessen and C. Huygelen, acting eds.), Proceedings of the 36th Symposium, International Association Biologic for Standardization pp. 315–326, S. Karger, Basel, 1979.

45. Hiro, Y., and Tasaka, S., Die Röteln sind eine Viruskrankheit, *Monatsschr. Kinderheilkd.* **76**:328–332 (1938).

46. Holmes, I. H., Wark, M. C., and Warburton, M. F., Is rubella an arbovirus? II. Ultrastructural morphology and development, *Virology* **37**:15–25 (1969).

47. Horstmann, D. M., Rubella: The challenge of its control, *J. Infect. Dis.* **123**:640–654 (1971).

48. Horstmann, D. M., Banatvala, J. E., Riordan, J. T., Payne, M. C., Whittemore, R., Opton, E. M., and Florey, C. DuVe, Maternal rubella and the rubella syndrome in infants, *Am. J. Dis. Child.* **110**:408–415 (1965).

49. Horstmann, D. M., Controlling rubella: Problems and perspectives, *Ann. Intern. Med.* **83**:412–417 (1975).

50. Horstmann, D. M., Viral vaccines and their ways, *Rev. Infect. Dis.* **1**:502–516 (1979).

51. HORSTMANN, D. M., LIEBHABER, H., AND KOHORN, E. I., Post-partum vaccination of rubella-susceptible women, *Lancet* **2:**1003–1006 (1970).

52. HORSTMANN, D. M., LIEBHABER, H., LeBOUVIER, G. L., ROSENBERG, D. A., AND HALSTEAD, S. B., Rubella: Reinfection of vaccinated and naturally immune persons exposed in an epidemic, *N. Engl. J. Med.* **283:**771–778 (1970).

53. HORSTMANN, D. M., RIORDAN, J. T., OHTAWARA, M., AND NIEDERMAN, J. C., A natural epidemic of rubella in a closed population, *Arch. Gesamte Virusforsch.* **16:**483–487 (1965).

54. HORSTMANN, D. M., AND SCHLUEDERBERG, A., Long term surveillance of rubella vaccinees, *Acta Pathol.*, Supplement No. 275 (in press) (1981).

55. HOVI, T., AND VAHERI, A., Infectivity and some physicochemical characteristics of rubella virus ribonucleic acid, *Virology* **42:**1–8 (1970).

56. HUYGELEN, C., PEETERMANS, J., AND PRINZIE, A., An attenuated rubella virus vaccine (Cendehill 51 strain) grown in primary rabbit kidney cells, *Prog. Med. Virol.* **11:**107–125 (1969).

57. JACKSON, A. D. M., Deafness following maternal rubella: Results of a prospective investigation, *Lancet* **2:**1241–1244 (1958).

58. KENRICK, K. G., SLINN, R. F., DORMANN, D. C., AND MENSER, M. A., Immunoglobulins and rubella-virus antibodies in adults with congenital rubella, *Lancet* **1:**548–551 (1968).

59. KILROY, A. W., SCHAFFNER, W., FLEET, W. F., JR., LEFKOWITZ, L. B., JR., KARZON, D. T., AND FENICHEL, G. M., Two syndromes following rubella immunization: Clinical observations and epidemiological studies, *J. Am. Med. Assoc.* **214:**2287–2292 (1970).

60. KLOCK, L. E., AND RACHELEFSKY, G. S., Failure of rubella herd immunity during an epidemic, *N. Engl. J. Med.* **288:**69–72 (1973).

61. KONO, R., Rubella epidemiology in Japan, in: *International Symposium on Rubella Vaccines*, pp. 37–42, S. Karger, Basel, 1969.

62. KONO, R., HIBI, M., HAYAKAWA, Y., AND ISHII, K., Experimental vertical transmission of rubella virus in rabbits, *Lancet* **1:**343–347 (1969).

62a. KRECH, U., AND WILHELM, J. A., A solid-phase immunosorbent technique for the rapid detection of rubella IgM by hemagglutination inhibition *J. Gen. Virol.* **44:**281–286 (1979).

63. KRUGMAN, S., Present status of measles and rubella immunization in the United States: A medical progress report, *J. Pediatr.* **90:**1–12 (1977).

64. KRUGMAN, S., AND WARD, R., Rubella: Demonstration of neutralizing antibody in gamma globulin and re-evaluation of the rubella problem, *N. Engl. J. Med.* **259:**16–19 (1958).

65. KRUGMAN, S., WARD, R., JACOBS, K. G., AND LAZAR, M., Studies on rubella immunization. I. Demonstration of rubella without rash, *J. Am. Med. Assoc.* **151:**285–288 (1953).

66. LARSON, H. E., PARKMAN, P. D., DAVIS, W. J., HOPPS, H. E., AND MEYER, H. M., JR., Inadvertent rubella virus vaccination during pregnancy, *N. Engl. J. Med.* **284:**870–873 (1971).

67. LE BOUVIER, G. L., Rubella precipitins, in: *International Symposium on Rubella Vaccines, London, 1968: Symposium Series Immunobiological Standardization*, Vol. 11, pp. 133–138, S. Karger, Basel, 1969.

68. LE BOUVIER, G. L., AND PLOTKIN, S., Precipitin responses to rubella vaccine RA 27/3, *J. Infect. Dis.* **123:**220–223 (1971).

69. LEERHØY, J., Neutralization of rubella virus in a rabbit cornea cell line (SIRC), *Acta Pathol. Microbiol. Scand.* **67:**158–159 (1966).

70. LEHANE, D. E., NEWBERG, N. R., AND BEAM, W. E., JR., Evaluation of rubella herd immunity during an epidemic, *J. Am. Med. Assoc.* **213:**2236–2239 (1970).

71. LEHMANN, N. I., FERRIS, A. A., BENNETT, N. M., AND NEWMAN, J. W., Rubella: Results of serological survey of pregnant patients in Melbourne during 1968, *Med. J. Aust.* **1:**1282–1283 (1969).

72. LEVINE, M. M., EDSALL, G., AND BRUCE-CHWATT, L. J., Live-virus vaccines in pregnancy-risks and recommendations, *Lancet* **2:**34–38 (1974).

73. LIEBHABER, H., Measurement of rubella antibody by hemagglutination inhibition. I. Variables affecting rubella hemagglutination, *J. Immunol.* **104:**818–825 (1970).

74. LIEBHABER, H., Measurement of rubella antibody by hemagglutination inhibition. II. Characteristics of an improved HAI test employing a new method for the removal of non-immunoglobulin HA inhibitors from serum, *J. Immunol.* **104:**826–834 (1970).

75. LIEBHABER, H., AND GROSS, P. A., The structural proteins of rubella virus, *Virology* **47:**684–693 (1972).

76. LUNDSTRÖM, R., Rubella during pregnancy: A follow-up study of children born after an epidemic of rubella in Sweden, 1951, with additional investigations on prophylaxis and treatment of maternal rubella, *Acta. Paediatr. Scand.* **51:**1–88, Suppl. 133 (1962).

77. MANSON, M. M., LOGAN, P. D., AND LOY, R. M., Rubella and other virus infections during pregnancy, in: *Report on Public Health and Medical Subjects*, No. 101, Her Majesty's Stationery Office, London, 1960.

78. MENSER, M. A., SLINN, R. F., DODS, L., HERTZBERG, R., AND HARLEY, J. D., Congenital rubella in a mother and son, *Aust. Paediatr. J.* **4:**200–202 (1968).

79. METTLER, N. E., PETRELLI, R. I., AND CASALS, J., Absence of cross-reactions between rubella virus and arbovirus, *Virology* **36:**503–504 (1968).

80. MEYER, H. M., PARKMAN, P. D., AND PANOS, T. C.,

Attenuated rubella virus: Production of an experimental live virus vaccine and clinical trial, *N. Engl. J. Med.* **275**:575–580 (1966).

81. MEYER, H. M., PARKMAN, P. D., HOBBINS, T. E., LARSON, H. E., DAVIS, W. J., SIMSARIAN, J. P., AND HOPPS, H. E., Attenuated rubella viruses: Laboratory and clinical characteristics, *Am. J. Dis. Child.* **118**:155–165 (1969).

81a. MODLIN, J. F., HERRMANN, K. L., BRANDLING-BENNETT, A. D., EDDINS, D. L., AND HAYDEN, G. F., Risk of congenital abnormality after inadvertent rubella vaccination of pregnant women, *N. Engl. J. Med.* **294**:972–974 (1976).

82. MURPHY, F. A., HALONEN, P. A., AND HARRISON, A. K., Electron microscopy of the development of rubella virus in BHK-21 cells, *J. Virol.* **2**:1223–1227 (1968).

83. NAEYE, R. L., AND BLANC, W., Pathogenesis of congenital rubella, *J. Am. Med. Assoc.* **194**:1277–1283 (1965).

83a. NELSON, D. B., QUIRIN, E. P., AND INHORN, S. L., Compatibility of trypsin-modified human erythrocytes in the rubella hemagglutination-inhibition test employing three serum treatment procedures, *Appl. Microbiol.* **27**:767–770 (1974).

84. OGRA, P. L., AND HERD, J. K., Arthritis associated with induced rubella infection, *J. Immunol.* **107**:810–813 (1971).

85. OGRA, P. L., KERR-GRANT, D., UMANA, G., DZIERBA, J., AND WEINTRAUB, D., Antibody response in serum and nasopharynx after infections with rubella virus, *N. Engl. J. Med.* **285**:1333–1339 (1971).

86. PARKMAN, P. D., BUESCHER, E. L., AND ARTENSTEIN, M. S., Recovery of rubella virus from army recruits, *Proc. Soc. Exp. Biol. Med.* **11**:225–230 (1962).

87. PARKMAN, P. D., MUNDON, F. K., MCCOWN, J. M., AND BUESCHER, E. L., Studies of rubella. II. Neutralization of the virus, *J. Immunol.* **93**:608–617 (1964).

87a. PAUL, J. R., AND WHITE, C. (eds.), *Serological Epidemiology*, Academic Press, New York, 1973.

88. PERLINO, C. A., AND ISACSON, P., Direct hemadsorption by cell cultures infected with rubella virus, *Am. J. Dis. Child.* **118**:83–88 (1969).

89. PLOTKIN, S. A., Attenuation of RA 27/3 rubella virus in WI-38 human diploid cells, *Am. J. Dis. Child.* **118**:178–185 (1969).

89a. POLK, B. F., WHITE, J. A., DEGIROLAMI, P. C., AND MODLIN, J. F., An outbreak of rubella among hospital personnel, *N. Engl. J. Med.* **303**:541–545 (1980).

90. PRINZIE, A., HUYGELEN, C., GOLD, J., FARQUHAR, J., AND MCKEE, J., Experimental live attenuated rubella virus vaccine: Clinical evaluation of Cendehill strain, *Am. J. Dis. Child.* **118**:172–177 (1969).

91. RAWLS, W. E., Congenital rubella: The significance of virus persistence, *Prog. Med. Virol.* **10**:238–285 (1968).

92. RAWLS, W. E., DESMYTER, J., AND MELNICK, J. L., Serologic diagnosis and fetal involvement in maternal rubella, criteria for abortion, *J. Am. Med. Assoc.* **203**:627–631 (1968).

93. RAWLS, W. E., MELNICK, J. L., BRADSTREET, C. M. P., BAILEY, M., FERRIS, A. A., TIEHMANN, N., NAGLER, F. P., FURESZ, J., KONO, R., OHTAWARA, M., HALONEN, P., STEWART, J., RYAN, J. M., STRAUSS, J., ZDRAZILEK, J., LEERHØY, J., VON MAGNUS, H., SOHIER, R., AND FERRIERA, W., WHO Collaborative study on the sero-epidemiology of rubella, *Bull. WHO* **37**:79–88, (1967).

93a. ROSSIER, E., PHIPPS, P. H., POLLEY, J. R., AND WEBB, T., Absence of cell-mediated immunity to rubella virus 5 years after rubella vaccination, *Can. Med. Assoc. J.* **116**:481–485 (1977).

93b. ROTHFIELD, N. F., EVANS, A. S., AND NIEDERMAN, J. C., Clinical and laboratory aspects of raised antibody titers in systemic lupus erythematosus, *Ann. Rheum. Dis.* **32**:238–246 (1973).

93c. SABIN, A. B., Overview and horizons in prevention of some human infectious diseases by vaccination, *Am. J. Clin. Pathol. Suppl.* **70**:114–127 (1978).

94. SCHMIDT, N. J., AND LENNETTE, E. H., Rubella complement-fixing antigens derived from the fluid and cellular phases of infected BHK-21 cells: Extraction of cell-associated antigen with alkaline buffers, *J. Immunol.* **94**:815–821 (1966).

95. SCHMIDT, N. J., AND LENNETTE, E. H., Antigens of rubella virus, *Am. J. Dis. Child.* **118**:89–93 (1969).

96. SCHMIDT, N. J., AND STYK, B., Immunodiffusion reactions with rubella antigens, *J. Immunol.* **101**:210–216 (1968).

97. SCOTT, H. D., AND BYRNE, E. B., A serologic study of susceptible pregnant women exposed to a statewide rubella (HPV-77 DE 5) immunization campaign, *J. Am. Med. Assoc.* **215**:609–612 (1971).

97a. SCHLUEDERBERG, A., HORSTMANN, D. M., ANDIMAN, W. A., AND RANDOLPH, M. F., Neutralizing and hemagglutination-inhibiting antibodies to rubella virus as indicators of protective immunity in vaccinees and naturally immune individuals, *J. Infect. Dis.* **138**:877–883 (1978).

98. SEDWICK, W. D., AND SOKOL, F., Nucleic acid of rubella virus and its replication in hamster kidney cells, *J. Virol.* **5**:478–489 (1970).

99. SEPPÄLÄ, M., AND VAHERI, A., Natural rubella infection of the female genital tract, *Lancet* **1**:46–47 (1974).

100. SEVER, J. L., HARDY, J. B., NELSON, K. B., AND GILKESON, M. R., Rubella in the collaborative perinatal research study. II. Clinical and laboratory findings in children through 3 years of age, *Am. J. Dis. Child.* **118**:123–132 (1969).

101. SEVER, J. L., HUEBNER, R. J., CASTELLANO, G. A., SARMA, P. S., FABIYI, A., SCHIFF, G. M., AND CUSUMANO, C. L., Rubella complement fixation test, *Science* **148**:385–387 (1965).

102. SEVER, J. L., SCHIFF, G. M., BELL, J. A., KAPIKIAN, A. Z., HUEBNER, R. J., AND TRAUB, R. G., Rubella: Frequency of antibody among children and adults, *Pediatrics* **35**:996–998 (1965).

103. SIEGEL, M., AND GREENBERG, M., Fetal death, malformation and prematurity after maternal rubella: Results of prospective study, 1949–1958, *N. Engl. J. Med.* **262**:389–393 (1960).

104. SIGURJONSSON, J., Rubella and congenital deafness, *Am. J. Med. Sci.* **240**:712–720 (1961).

105. SIMONS, M. J., Congenital rubella: An immunological paradox?, *Lancet* **2**:1275–1278 (1968).

106. SOOTHILL, J. F., HAYES, K., AND DUDGEON, J. D., The immunoglobulins in congenital rubella, *Lancet* **1**:1385–1388 (1966).

106a. SOUTH, M. A., MONTGOMERY, J. R., AND RAWLS, W. D., Immune deficiency in rubella and other viral infections, *Birth Defects: Orig. Artic. Ser.* **11**:234–238 (1975).

106b. STRANNEGÅRD, Ö., GRILLNER, L., AND LINDBERG, I.-M., Hemolysis-in-gel test for the demonstration of antibodies to rubella virus, *J. Clin. Microbiol.* **1**:491–494 (1975).

107. STEWART, G. L., PARKMAN, P. D., HOPPS, H. E., DOUGLAS, R. D., HAMILTON, J. P., AND MEYER, H. M., Rubella virus hemagglutination-inhibition test, *N. Engl. J. Med.* **276**:554–557 (1967).

107a. SUGISHITA, C., O'SHEA, S., BEST, J. M., AND BANATVALA, J. E., Rubella serology by solid-phase radioimmunoassay: Its potential for screening programs, *Clin. Exp. Immunol.* **31**:50–54 (1978).

108. SVEDMYR, A., LUNDSTRÖM, R., AND THOREN, C., Rubella immunity as correlated to age and history of overt disease, *Arch. Gesamte Virusforsch.* **22**:48–54 (1967).

109. TONDÜRY, G., AND SMITH, D. W., Fetal rubella pathology, *J. Pediatr.* **68**:867–879 (1966).

109a. TRIGER, D. R., KURTZ, J. B., MCCALLUM, F. O., AND WRIGHT, R., Raised antibody titres to measles and rubella viruses in chronic active hepatitis, *Lancet* **1**:665–667 (1972).

110. VAHERI, A., AND HOVI, T., Structural proteins and subunits of rubella virus, *J. Virol.* **9**:10–16 (1972).

111. VAHERI, A., VESIKARI, T., OKER-BLOM, N., SEPPÄLÄ, M., PARKMAN, P. D., VERONELLI, J., AND ROBBINS, F. C., Isolation of attenuated rubella vaccine virus from human products of conception and uterine cervix, *N. Engl. J. Med.* **286**:1071–1074 (1972).

112. VAHERI, A., VESIKARI, T., PENTTINEN, K., AND MYLLYLÄ, G., Soluble rubella antigens, platelet aggregation and postrubella thrombocytopenia, *Inter-national Symposium on Rubella Vaccines, London, 1968: Symposium Series Immunobiological Standardization,* Vol. 11, pp. 107–108, S. Karger, Basel and New York, 1969.

113. VEALE, H., History of an epidemic of Rötheln, with observations on its pathology, *Edinburgh Med. J.* **12**:404–414 (1866).

113a. VOLLER, A., AND BIDWELL, D. E., A simple method for detecting antibodies to rubella, *Br. J. Exp. Pathol.* **56**:338–339 (1975).

114. WEIBEL, R. E., BUYNAK, E. B., MCLEAN, A. A., ROEHM, R. R., AND HILLEMAN, M. R., Persistence of antibody in human subjects for 7 to 10 years following combined live attenuated measles, mumps and rubella vaccines, *Proc. Soc. Exp. Biol. Med.* **165**:260–263 (1980).

114a. WEIBEL, R. E., VILLAREJOO, V. M., KLEIN, E. B., BUYNAK, E. B., MCLEAN, A. A., AND HILLEMAN, M. R., Clinical and laboratory studies of live attenuated RA 27/3 and HPV$_{77}$-DE rubella virus vaccines, *Proc. Soc. Exp. Biol. Med.* **165**:44–49 (1980).

115. WOLINSKY, J. S., BERG, B. O., AND MAITLAND, C. J., Progressive rubella panencephalitis, *Arch. Neurol.* **33**:722–723 (1976).

115a. WEIBEL, R. E., STOKES, J., JR., BUYNAK, E. B., AND HILLEMAN, M. R., Influence of age on clinical responses to HPV$_{77}$ duck rubella vaccine, *J. Am. Med. Assoc.* **222**:805–807 (1972).

116. WELLER, T. H., AND NEVA, F. A., Propagation in tissue culture of cytopathic agents from patients with rubella-like illness, *Proc. Soc. Exp. Biol. Med.* **111**:215–225 (1962).

117. WILKINS, J., LEEDOM, J. M., SALVATORE, M. A., AND PORTNOY, B., Clinical rubella with arthritis resulting from reinfection, *Ann. Intern. Med.* **77**:930–932 (1972).

118. WITTE, J. J., KARCHMER, A. W., CASE, G., HERRMANN, K. L., KASSANOFF, I., AND NEILL, J. S., Epidemiology of rubella, *Am. J. Dis. Child.* **118**:107–111 (1969).

119. WOODS, W. A., JOHNSON, R., HOSTETLER, D. D., LEPOW, M., AND ROBBINS, F., Immunofluorescent studies on rubella infected tissue cultures and human tissues, *J. Immunol.* **96**:253–260 (1966).

120. WYLL, S. A., AND HERRMANN, K. L., Inadvertent rubella vaccination of pregnant women: Fetal risk in 215 cases, *J. Am. Med. Assoc.* **225**:1472–1476 (1973).

12. Suggested Reading

ALFORD, C. A., Rubella, in: *Infectious Diseases of the Fetus and Newborn Infant* (J. S. REMINGTON AND J. O. KLEIN, eds.), pp. 71–106, W. B. Saunders, Philadelphia, 1976.

BRODY, J. A., SEVER, J. L., MCALISTER, R., SCHIFF, G. M., AND CUTTING, R., Rubella epidemic on St. Paul Island in the Pribilofs, 1963. I. Epidemiologic, clinical, and serologic findings, *J. Am. Med. Assoc.* **191:**83–87 (1965).

GREGG, N. M., Congenital cataract following German measles in the mother, *Trans. Ophthalmol. Soc. Aust.* **3:**35–46 (1941).

HORSTMANN, D. M., Problems in measles and rubella, *Dis.-Mon.* **14:**28–52 (1978).

HORSTMANN, D. M., Rubella: The challenge of its control, *J. Infect. Dis.* **123:**640–654 (1971).

CHAPTER 22

Smallpox

Abram S. Benenson

1. Introduction

The story of smallpox is a dramatic tale of a disease with such potential epidemic violence that it has shaped the history of the past, certainly of the New World. Now the disease has been eradicated from the face of the earth. This was done by discovering and developing an effective preventive method and defining the epidemiology of the disease. In an unprecedented exercise of international cooperation, the preventive measures were applied to the critical population groups to achieve the planned goal, the eradication of a disease for the first time in history.

The last case of smallpox occurred October 1977. On October 13, 1977, Ali Maow Maalin was employed as a cook in the hospital in the small town of Merka, Somalia. A vehicle carrying a 6-year-old girl with severe smallpox and a 2-year-old boy in the papular stage of the rash stopped at the hospital, asking directions to the smallpox isolation camp in the area. Ali Maow Maalin traveled with them to the home of the local smallpox surveillance team leader, a distance of less than 1 km. On October 22, he developed a fever and went home; on October 25, he was admitted to the medical ward of the hospital with a diagnosis of malaria, for which he was treated. The following evening, October, 26, he developed a rash; on October 27, he was discharged

home with a diagnosis of chickenpox. He continued to feel very ill, but, suspecting the correct diagnosis, remained silent. However, on October 30, a male nurse from the hospital reported the case to the health authorities. On October 31, the diagnosis of smallpox was made with a rash at the pustular stage and maximal lesions on the extremities, including palms and soles. Ali was isolated in his house with a 24-hour guard, but 2 days later he was moved to a smallpox isolation camp. The clinical course was one of moderately severe smallpox with a discrete rash. By November 15, the rash had reached the scab stage. He was discharged from the isolation center at the end of November. The clinical diagnosis was confirmed by the WHO Collaborating Centre, Centers for Disease Control (CDC), Atlanta, Georgia, by electron microscopy, by isolation of the virus on the chorioallantoic membrane of chick embryos, and by precipitation in gel.

During his illness, Ali had exposed 161 persons, 91 of them face to face. None of these contacts developed smallpox. No subsequent cases of naturally acquired smallpox has been discovered on the face of the earth despite intense surveillance. It is to be hoped that the case of Ali Maow Maalin closes the book for all time on the formerly dread disease of smallpox.

Smallpox remains among the diseases presented in this volume as an example of a class of diseases, as a historical document of an important disease, and because, even though the disease has been eradicated, the virus of smallpox still persists, and it is conceivable that cases may occur following unnatural exposure.

Abram S. Benenson · Gorgas Memorial Laboratory, Panama, Republic of Panama. Present address: School of Graduate Studies and Public Health, San Diego State University, San Diego, California.

2. Historical Background

There are reasons to believe that smallpox has existed since earliest times; for example, the lesions on the mummified face of Rameses V, dated 1160 B.C., suggest that he died of smallpox.[14] While smallpox has apparently existed in China and India for thousands of years, the disease is not mentioned by the early Greek writers. A Syrian epidemic was described in A.D. 302, and during the next several hundred years, reports of epidemics that could have been smallpox became more frequent. The term *variola* was used by Bishop Marius of Avenches in 570 to describe an epidemic in Italy and France, but the disease was not clearly described until about A.D. 900 by the Persian physician Rhazes.[42] Smallpox was spread through Europe by the invasion of the Continent by the Saracens and then by returning Crusaders.[16] The Spaniards brought smallpox with them to the West Indies in 1507 and to Mexico in 1520, resulting in devastating epidemics that decimated the Indians. The phenomenal success of a few conquistadores in subjugating the Aztec and Inca kingdoms may well have been abetted by an advancing pandemic of smallpox that is estimated to have caused the death of $3\frac{1}{2}$ million people within a few years.[85] While on the whole this occurred naturally, in certain instances, there is documentation that hostile Indians were deliberately exposed to smallpox with the intent of generating an epidemic.[86]

In the 17th and 18th centuries, smallpox was the most devastating disease in the Western world.[32] Queen Mary died of the disease in 1694; the Duke of Gloucester, son of Anne, died in 1700. In 1711, Emperor Joseph also succumbed to smallpox. In 1707, 18,000 of the population of 50,000 in Iceland, or 36% of the total population, died from smallpox in a single year. In the New World, Boston experienced eight epidemics during the 18th century with attack rates as high as 52% of the population.[16]

Inoculation of smallpox has been practiced as a protective measure in Asia and apparently in Africa for some time. Reverend Cotton Mather in Boston learned of the practice from his slave,[93] and when the *Philosophical Transactions of the Royal Society of London* published in 1714 the letter by Timoni in which were described inoculations against smallpox in Turkey, Mather resolved to introduce the practice should smallpox "again enter into or City."[49] When

a major epidemic occurred in 1721, which ultimately afflicted half the population of Boston, with a fatality rate of approximately 15%, Cotton Mather induced Dr. Zabdiel Boylston to try the technique. On June 26, 1721, Boylston inoculated his 6-year-old son and two slaves without mishap, and not long afterward a 13-year-old son and seven other persons. Despite professional, clinical, and public opposition, Boylston persisted and vaccinated at least 247 people, with a fatality rate of 2% in comparison to the 15% fatality among those who acquired smallpox naturally. Despite the continued opposition of Boylston's medical colleagues, the public began to recognize and seek the beneficial effects of variolation. Concurrently, Lady Mary Wortley Montagu, who had lived in Turkey as the wife of the British ambassador and had had her son inoculated in 1717, introduced the practice to the British Court.

The acceptance of variolation as a protective measure was marred by the fact that although fatalities among the inoculated were relatively few, the virus in use was fully pathogenic and could and did initiate epidemics of typical and fatal disease among uninoculated contacts. Self-styled, untrained inoculators went into business, and their activities resulted in not only epidemics but also sepsis. As a consequence, many communities outlawed variolation.[7]

Smallpox exerted so strong an influence on operations during the American Revolution[85] that in 1977, Washington ordered the inoculation of all Continental troops who had not had the disease.[25] The practice became so well accepted that when smallpox hit Boston in 1792, 97% of the population had been inoculated![16]

The truly great advance in the smallpox story was the experiment carried out by Edward Jenner in testing the old wives' tale that those who had had cowpox were not susceptible to smallpox. After confirming that those who had a history of cowpox were insusceptible to variolation, on May 14, 1796 he vaccinated 8-year-old James Phipps with material obtained from a pustule on the hand of a milkmaid; 6 weeks later he challenged Phipps with pus from a patient who had smallpox, with no take. After 12 or more successful other vaccinations, his submitted report was rejected, and he had to publish his work privately.[41]

As with the news of variolation, the Atlantic Ocean posed no barrier to the news of vaccination[8,60]; by 1799, vaccine had been received and vaccinations carried out in the New World. However, Dr. Benjamin Waterhouse of Boston is acknowledged to be the Jenner of America. He received vaccine and in 1800 vaccinated four of his children, a 12-year-old servant boy, and two adults. To assure protection against smallpox, they were admitted to the smallpox hospital and variolated; this resulted in a lesion that was gone after 2 days, and smallpox was not acquired from exposure to the highly contaminated environment.[92] Demand for vaccination was immediate, but unfortunately, many vaccinations were performed with material obtained from pyogenic reactions, so that the next exposure to smallpox resulted in disease, or the "vaccines" were contaminated with smallpox virus, resulting in outbreaks of this disease. The problem of spurious vaccine was complicated by a proliferation of spurious vaccinators, "such as stage-drivers, peddlers, and in one instance the sexton of a church."[61] Strong opposition to vaccination and questions of its effectiveness developed. Water-

house organized a conclusive public test of the efficacy of vaccination[92,93] and involved Jefferson in spreading vaccine and vaccine use through much of the country.[38,61] To avoid the mischance of contaminated or spurious vaccine, central sources were established such as the Vaccine Institute set up in Baltimore in 1802 by James Smith.[50]

Despite the availability of vaccine, smallpox continued to be endemic within the United States into the 1940s, its incidence varying with the level of vaccination. The decline of smallpox has been correlated by Leake[48] with improved vaccine potency as electric refrigeration came into use. Military personnel returning from the Far East in 1946 produced outbreaks in Seattle and in San Francisco.[70] In 1947, a traveler from Mexico created a small outbreak in New York City, with 12 cases and 2 deaths.[91] In 1949, 8 cases occurred in the lower Rio Grande Valley in Texas[39]; since that time, no smallpox has occurred within the United States. Smallpox vaccination programs that reached all segments of the population removed smallpox from country after

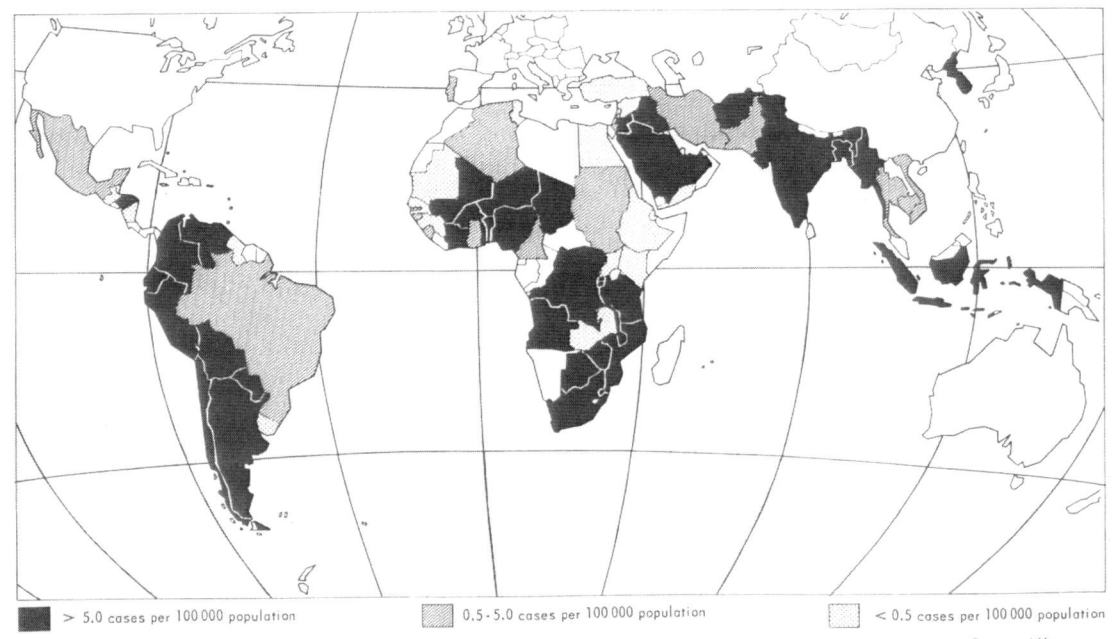

> 5.0 cases per 100 000 population   0.5 - 5.0 cases per 100 000 population   < 0.5 cases per 100 000 population

No reports received from China (mainland), Kuwait, Liberia, Morocco, Muscat & Oman, Nepal, Panama, Quatar, South-West Africa, Trucial Oman and Yemen

Fig. 1. Smallpox incidence in endemic countries, 1950 (cases per 100,000). From the World Health Organization.[96]

country. The world situation in 1950 is presented in Fig. 1.

In 1966, the World Health Organization (WHO) embarked on a program of eradication, and today no known focus of smallpox exists on the face of the earth.

3. Methodology Involved in Epidemiological Analysis

3.1. Sources of Mortality Data

Smallpox is one of the internationally quarantinable diseases, so that the occurrence of any cases of or deaths from smallpox is to be reported by any member nation to the WHO. Since approximately 90% of smallpox patients had skin lesions characteristic of the disease and recognized as such by the general public, with a good disease-reporting system, mortality data on smallpox could be more accurate than those for any other disease. However, in many parts of the world, cases were hidden by families to avoid the removal of their relatives to truly deplorable isolation hospitals, and on occasion communities or countries deliberately concealed the presence of disease for political–economic reasons. Deaths were generally more accurately reported than the number of cases.

3.2. Sources of Morbidity Data

As noted above, as a quarantinable disease, smallpox must be reported to the WHO from all member nations. While the barriers to reporting of deaths were even more applicable to the reporting of cases, among vaccinated persons there could be cases for which the differentiation from chickenpox, if the two diseases were occurring simultaneously, could be established with certainty only by laboratory studies.

The reliability of reporting could be deduced from the reported death/case ratios; a case-fatality rate over 15–20% was indicative of underreporting. Where a poor reporting system exists, gross underreporting is to be expected. Thomas et al.[87] established by inquiry in July 1967 that 119 cases of smallpox with 29 deaths had occurred within a circumscribed population in East Pakistan (Bangladesh) during the preceding year; only 13 cases of

smallpox had been reported to the government from only five of the 23 affected villages. In these five villages, there had in fact been a total of 54 cases. In West Pakistan during a period when 121 outbreaks occurred with a total of 1040 smallpox cases, only 23 (19%) of these outbreaks and 14% of the cases had been officially reported.[88] It is evident that routine reporting methods must often be supplemented by more aggressive epidemiological explorations if accurate data are required, even with a disease for which the diagnosis is evident in the vast majority of cases.

3.3. Surveys

3.3.1. Serological Surveys. Serological surveys to assess the immunity of a community against smallpox were relatively unsatisfactory. While the neutralizing antibody level correlates best with immunity of the individual and thus the population, its performance is cumbersome, so that large numbers of tests can be carried out only with difficulty. Hemagglutination-inhibiting (HI) antibodies are more easily measured in large numbers, but the correlation with immunity is poor. Complement-fixation (CF) and precipitating antibodies persist only for relatively short intervals. Their presence is indicative of recent infection with either variola or vaccinia virus; history of vaccination is essential for analysis. Variola usually evokes a much higher antibody level than uncomplicated vaccinia.

3.3.2. Scar Surveys. A unique feature of smallpox is that both the disease and its preventive measure, Jennerian vaccination, leave a dermal record of their occurrence. This makes it possible to survey a population for its past experience with the disease or with its preventive measure by doing a scar survey. By cluster-sampling techniques, acitivity of the disease and of the vaccinators is detailed by recording the ages of those with or without scars. The survey may be carried out on the whole population or on a segment such as the 0–4 or 0–14 year age group.[35]

a. Vaccination-Scar Survey. The vaccination scar provides an immediate indication of those on whom this preventive procedure was carried out; those without vaccination or smallpox scars constitute the susceptible population. Unfortunately, the presence of the scar at the site used for vaccination does not necessarily indicate that the person is at present immune to smallpox. The immunity might have been present but have waned if many years have passed since the last vaccination, or the scar may be the consequence of a pyogenic infection that had been induced, rather than the desired vaccinial infection. THe typical vaccinial scar is foveated, i.e., pitted and depressed.

b. Smallpox-Scar Survey. The smallpox-scar survey is facilitated by the centrifugal distribution of the pocks, so that residual scars are present on the face. A person is considered positive if at least five characteristic round, depressed facial scars, 1 mm or more in diameter, are present. The oldest cohort of children with unscarred faces indicates the period since smallpox was last present in this population group.

It is more difficult to estimate what the incidence of smallpox had been from a scar survey. An approximation, at best, is possible if one corrects for those how did not survive the disease, and for those who survived disease and were spared pockmarks.[55] Rao[74] reported that 30% of smallpox survivors in Madras lost their scars within 5 years; Foster obtained a comparable figure in Nigeria. The outcome was age-related: of cases in the 0–4 year age group, only 30% retained scars; in the 5–9 year age group, 43% were scarred; of those aged 10 years and over, 89% retained scars.[101] In Pakistan, Mack et al.[55] found pockmarks on 65.9% of smallpox survivors examined after 1 year; only 46% of the 63 survivors under 5 years old were scarred as against 76.5% among the 119 who were 5 years old or older.

3.4. Laboratory Methods

3.4.1. Virus or Antigen Identification. Virus or antigen identification may be accomplished from the skin lesions at any stage and from the blood usually during the prodromal state; when viremia persists, the prognosis is very poor.[18] Blood is collected with sterile anticoagulant. From the skin lesions in the maculopapular stage, five or six lesions should be scraped with a scalpel or a Hagedorn needle to obtain blood-free serous and cellular material from the lower epithelial layers of the skin. This is spread thinly on several clean glass slides, and the slides are dried in the air without heat or preservative. From cases with vesicles or pustules, fluid from several lesions is aspirated into capillary glass tubes or a tuberculin syringe; the floor of these lesions is

scraped gently to obtain cellular (but not bloody) material that is spread on slides. If the disease is at the scabbing stage, at least six scabs are collected in a screw-cap bottle. The virus is stable and can be shipped (with due regard for postal regulations) without refrigeration.[17,97]

Electron-microscopic examination of the smears, if available, provides the most rapid answer. Visualization of the characteristic brick-shaped virus particles identifies the lesion as due to a member of the variola–vaccinia group; the presence of the smaller and spherical herpes-type elementary body is consistent with chickenpox or herpes disease.[51] Thin smears may be examined under the light microscope for the presence of the elementary bodies that have been stained by appropriate methods; this cannot be done with material from the pustular stage.[17]

Fluorescent-antibody techniques may also give a rapid answer, but false-positive results may occur.[65] Diffusion of vesicular or pustular fluid or of a crust extract in agar gel against a specific antiserum and with a positive control may show a line of precipitation within 2 hr, fusing with the lines from the positive control to indicate antigenic identity with the known vaccinal antigen within 6–8 hr.[65,97] The CF procedure may also be used to detect the presence of antigen in the lesion, but this requires 18–24 hr before the test can be read.[65]

In all cases, virus should be isolated, preferably on the chorioallantoic membranes (CAM) of embryonated hen's eggs or on appropriate tissue culture. In 2 or 3 days, CAM lesions distinguish between variola and vaccinia virus, or the differentiation is made by subculturing at 35.25, 38.25, and 39–40°C. The virus of variola minor, or alastrim, will grow only at the lowest temperature; only vaccinia virus will grow at a temperature of 39°C or above.[2,67] Varicella virus will not grow on the CAM.

In support of the WHO eradication program, Nakano and Bingham[65] report that at the CDC, Atlanta, Georgia, electron microscopy, CAM culturing, and agar-gel precipitation detected 95.6, 89.1, and 78.8%, respectively, of the 367 positive specimens. Nakano[64] would add tissue culture to these three tests to assure complete confidence in a negative report. Of course, the validity of any laboratory testing depends on the quality of the material submitted to the laboratory.

3.4.2. Serological Tests. The usual serological tests now available cannot differentiate the antivariola from antivaccinial antibodies, so that recent vaccination must be considered when a titer rise is observed. In general, titers following variola are much higher than those seen after vaccination. Serological tests have their greatest value for detecting subclinical infections or variola sine eruptione.

The agar–gel precipitation (or immunodiffusion) test is positive after the 8th day of illness from smallpox and not infrequently after recent vaccination; within several months, this antibody is no longer detectable. In the CF test, a titer as high as 1:320 appears by the 10th to the 12th day; after vaccination or revaccination, antibodies appear at a much lower titer. CF antibodies are rarely detectable 12 months after infection. HI-antibody titers in the convalescent smallpox patient are much higher than those seen after vaccination; they tend to drop or disappear after a year or more.[19,62] With high-titered sera, it is possible to differentiate antivaccinial from antivariolar antibody by an indirect radioimmunoassay after absorption with CAM antigens.[38a]

4. Biological Characteristics of the Virus

Smallpox is caused by a member of the genus *Orthopoxvirus*, which also includes the viruses of cowpox, monkeypox, ectromelia, buffalopox, camelpox, Turkmenia rodent-pox, "whitepox," as well as variola (including alastrim) and vaccinia viruses.[22a] All these viruses are morphologically indistinguishable; they are large double-stranded DNA viruses, brick-shaped and ranging in size from 250–300 nm by 200–250 nm wide; this places them just within the visibility of the light microscope. Electron microscopy reveals the presence of a central denser area with certain characteristics of a nucleus. While the elementary bodies (Paschen bodies) are indistinguishable and share common antigens and cross-immunity, the members of the group do vary in their biological attributes; for example, the variola viruses can be differentiated into variola major, variola minor, and an intermediate type based on differential growth temperatures and chick lethality.[2] The variola viruses produce disease in man and monkeys; they multiply but do not produce disease in suckling mice. Cowpox and vaccinia viruses, on the other hand, have a wide host range. The purported derivation of present vaccine strains from virus taken from smallpox patients and modified by passage through rabbits and calves was tested by Herrlich *et al.*[36] Despite as many as 100 passages, it was impossible to change the host range of either variola or alastrim strains. These workers concluded that "modification" was due to the presence in the original material of vaccinia virus, which has the broadest host spectrum. Gispen and Brand-Saathof[27] showed by agar-gel precipitation the presence of specific antigens by which one could differentiate the variola and monkeypox viruses from each other and from the other members of the group; vaccinia, rabbitpox, buffalopox, and camelpox could not be differentiated from each other by this technique.

The smallpox virus is stable in the dried condition. It has survived at room temperatures in crusts for over a year and, when dried on slides, for nearly 3 months in the dark and for over a month in the light.[15] Viability is greater at lower levels of relative humidity. When moist, the virus is killed by heating at 60°C for 10 min; when dry, it may withstand 100°C for 5–10 min. It is sensitive to ultraviolet light (sunlight); vaccinia virus (used as the laboratory model) is inactivated by oxidizing disinfectants such as hypochlorites or potassium permanganate; formaldehyde at a concentration of 0.2% destroys infectivity in 24 hr at room temperature. The virus is resistant to 1% phenol for weeks at 4°C, but is inactivated within 24 hr when the temperature is raised to 37°C; it is resistant to 1:10,000 brilliant green.[15]

The range of severity of illness and varying case-fatality rates observed in different outbreaks raise the question of the relative virulence of different strains. In outbreaks due to variola minor virus, mild cases predominate, but hemorrhagic cases occur and the fatality rate is approximately 1%; deaths are more frequent in outbreaks due to the intermediate strains. But even in outbreaks caused by variola major virus, there are variations in the severity of disease among the unvaccinated from place to place and year to year. Sarkar and Mitra,[81] using lethality for chick embryos and for mice, histological changes produced on the CAM, and the viral count in the liver of the chick embryos, tested 25 strains isolated from discrete rash cases. All four tests were positive with 48% of the strains from hemorrhagic cases and 9 and 0% of strains from confluent and discrete cases, respectively. While this indicates a relationship between severity and strain characteristics, it must be noted that 8 (32%) of the strains isolated from hemorrhagic cases were negative in all four tests.

5. Descriptive Epidemiology

5.1. Incidence and Prevalence Data

From a situation in which the disease was once so prevalent that recovery from smallpox was considered essential for survival in large areas of the earth, we have progressed to the point that no case has been discovered since October 1977. The incidence in various countries had varied markedly from year to year depending on the intensity and conscientiousness with which vaccination programs were carried out and with which cases were sought out and reported. In 1962, 14 African countries reported to the WHO smallpox incidence rates over 10 per 100,000 population, ranging from 10 to 144; the rate in Brazil was 4; in Asia, three countries—India, Indonesia, and Pakistan—reported rates of 10, 1, and 4 per 100,000 population, respectively.[94] By 1971, only two countries, Ethiopia and Sudan, had rates over 5 per 100,000, i.e., 10.1 and 6.9, respectively.[98] In 1974, disease was endemic in only four countries: Ethiopia in Africa, with a rate of 16 per 100,000, and Pakistan, Bangladesh, and India in Asia, with rates of 12, 20, and 32 per 100,000 population, respectively. During 1974, five countries reported cases introduced from these endemic countries.[104] By July 1975, smallpox transmisson persisted in only two countries on the globe—Ethiopia in Africa and Bangladesh in Asia; between October 1975 and October 1977, smallpox occurred only in Ethiopia, Kenya, and Somalia.[105]

The total number of reported cases and continents from which these cases were reported are shown in Table 1, which is derived from WHO reports. The increase in Africa in 1971 was accounted for by the epidemic in Ethiopia; that in Asia in 1973–1974 occurred in Bangladesh and India following the social and natural catastrophes of war and flood. Of greater import than the number of reported cases is the reduction in the number of countries reporting cases, and especially of those in which smallpox is still endemic. Where intensive studies were carried out in restricted areas, higher rates were found; in their Bangladesh study area in 1966–1967, Thomas

et al.[87] found an incidence of 106 per 100,000; in West Pakistan during 1967–1968, Mack et al.[56] found 100 per 100,000 in their study area. On the basis of scar surveys, only 19 and 12% of the study populations, respectively, had not previously been vaccinated or had smallpox.[87]

The study carried out in West Africa after indigenous smallpox had been eradicated from the area found that 17.6% of the population was still susceptible to smallpox. Vaccination scars were present in 82.4%, and 12.8% also had smallpox scars.[35] While the overall susceptibility based on scars was comparable to that found in Bengal and Punjab, where disease was still endemic, the West African vaccination scars resulted from the recent WHO vaccination program and were associated with a high level of immunity.

5.2. Epidemic Behavior

By reputation, smallpox has been considered the most highly contagious of infectious diseases, so that when it appeared in a community an explosive outbreak was expected among all susceptibles even remotely exposed to the case. In the big cities of Europe during the 17th and 18th centuries, disease was constantly present, with epidemics occurring periodically in rural areas. In less densely populated America, severe epidemics followed the arrival of infected ships; then the disease would disappear until reintroduced.

Careful epidemiological studies carried out during the smallpox eradication program in West Africa changed this picture of high infectivity to one of a slowly moving disease with as many as 80 days elapsing between the onset of symptoms in the first and last cases among 15 susceptible persons living within a single compound and a secondary attack rate of 26–44% in three different areas.[24] In Madras, only 36.9% of unvaccinated family contacts developed smallpox.[75] In East Pakistan (Bangladesh), 42.9% of unvaccinated family contacts developed disease; the risk of infection among susceptibles varied with the characteristics of the source of infection. When the introducer had no scar of prior vaccination or had died from the disease (presumptive evidence of no prior vaccination), 50% of susceptible family members were infected, but only 8.3% were infected when the introducer had previously been vaccinated.[87] Rao et al.[75] found that

Table 1. World Incidence

Year	Africa		Americas		Asia	
	Number of countries	Number of cases	Number of countries	Number of cases	Number of countries	Number of cases
1959	34	16,916	6	6,974	19	72,354
1960	30	18,027	6	9,075	13	39,989
1961	32	27,516	5	9,045	14	53,962
1962	37	25,030	6	10,032	15	63,558
1963	33	17,580	6	7,385	11	108,406
1964	30	13,583	8	3,712	8	58,903
1965	32	17,049	6	3,632	9	91,598
1966	30	14,759	5	3,670	10	74,303
1967	29	15,529	2	4,544	12	111,619
1968	25	11,069	2	4,375	9	64,578
1969	21	3,584	1	7,410	8	43,208
1970	12	3,220	2	1,795	8	28,669
1971	9	27,679	1	19	7	25,108
1972	6	18,999	—	—	11	45,978
1973	4	5,462	—	—	7	130,392
1974	4	4,467	—	—	6	213,900
1975	2	3,949	—	—	3	15,329
1976	2	954	—	—	—	—
1977	2	3,234	—	—	—	—
1978	—	—	—	—	—	—
1979	—	—	—	—	—	—
1980	—	—	—	—	—	—

[a] Data based on WHO summary: "World: number of smallpox cases reported by year, 1920–1979," submitted to the 33rd World Health Assembly as part of the Report of the Global Commission for the Certification of Smallpox Eradication.
[b] The number in parentheses is the number of countries with endemic disease at the end of the year.
[c] Laboratory acquired cases.

66% of unvaccinated family contacts developed smallpox when the member with the primary case died, in contrast to 32% when he survived.

The pattern of the disease between July 1, 1966, and June 30, 1967, was studied in a rural area of East Pakistan.[89] While there were 132 villages in the study area, 30 outbreaks of smallpox occurred in only 27 villages. The origin of 22 outbreaks was established; 21 of these were introduced from outside the area, and only once did smallpox spread from one village to another within the area. Over two thirds of the outbreaks were brought from large cities, the introducers being adult males from landless families of the villages who had gone to the big city seeking employment and returned to their homes, usually when they became ill. The risk of introduction into a village did not relate to accessibility or any other factor except increased risk with larger village populations.

The situation with regard to transmission differed in the Punjab area of West Pakistan. In 1967–1968, Mack et al.[56] found a 96% attack rate among unvaccinated compound (household) contacts; virtually all secondary compound cases occurred within one generation of the index case. Greater spread occurred within the village to other compounds when the index case was one of severe smallpox. Like the situation in Bangladesh, introductions were principally from large population centers outside the study area, and the unimmunized were much more likely to become introducers. At no time in this period of relatively high smallpox incidence (100 per 100,000 in this area) did the disease occur simultaneously in more than about 50 of the 1717 communities in the study area; during the study period, disease occurred in only 99 different communities. In the same area, in studies carried out over the next 2 years, Heiner et al.[31] found an in-

of Smallpox, 1959–1980[a]

Europe		Oceania		Total	
Number of countries	Number of cases	Number of countries	Number of cases	Number of countries	Number of cases[b]
4	26	—	—	63	96,270
3	54	1	1	55	67,146
6	32	—	—	57	90,555
5	137	—	—	64	98,757
5	133			55	133,504
—	—			46	76,198
1	1			48	112,280
1	72			46	92,804
3	5			46	131,697
2	2			39	80,024
—	—			31	54,202
3	22			25	33,706
—	—			17	52,806
2	176			19	65,153 (6)
1	5			12	135,859 (4)
—	—			10	218,367 (3)
—	—			5	19,278 (1)
—	—			2	954 (1)
—	—			2	3,234 (0)
—	(2)[c]			(1)[c]	(2)[c] (0)
—	—			—	— (0)
—	—			—	— (0)

cidence of 76.8% amoung unvaccinated contacts, again a much higher rate than had been reported in other endemic areas.

The effect of vaccination on epidemic behavior was clearly brought out in Mack's study in West Pakistan.[56] In sharp contrast to a 96% attack rate in the unvaccinated, smallpox occurred in only 4% of those who had been vaccinated within 10 years and in 12% of those vaccinated over 10 years before. In Bangladesh, 15% of cases occurred among vaccinated persons; 8.4% of cases were among those vaccinated 20 years or more previously.[89]

In western Europe, the epidemic behavior varied with the time of the year, with very little transmission after introductions during the warm months of the year (three subsequent cases after eight introductions) but a significant number of secondary cases during the dry seasons.[90] More intimate contact would seem to be essential in West Africa and India for infection to occur. Under certain circumstances, minimal contacts could lead to major outbreaks. In the Seattle outbreak in 1946,[70] 51 cases and 16 deaths came from the illness of a woman convalescent from diphtheria who was housed diagonally across the hall from a smallpox patient; she had never been in his room, but had wandered up and down the hall. An orderly who attended the smallpox patient had contact with this patient, but purportedly carried out usual isolation techniques. Three generations of disease occurred in the community after the epidemic was recognized. In the 1972 experience in Yugoslavia, 173 cases followed the arrival of a pilgrim from Mecca who had a mild or subclinical illness. His contact with several persons was minimal; one of greatest importance was a man who developed a fever for which he was given penicillin. A rash appeared that was interpreted to be allergic, and he was hospitalized and transferred to Belgrade, where he died of a hemorrhagic diathesis; he was the source of infection for 37 secondary cases and 8 tertiary cases.[100] In both outbreaks, the hospital environment was involved; this is considered further in Section 5.9.

The reported risk of acquiring infection varied in different studies. These differences are best interpreted as the varying likelihood of appropriate contact between the index case and the susceptibles; incidence is obviously greatly influenced by the vaccination history of the people, by their social habits, and by environmental factors. The extent and character of the lesions, partly dependent on virus strain, determine the amount of virus shedding.

5.3. Geographic Distribution

The geographic distribution of smallpox 100 years ago was essentially the distribution of man; it became a reflection of the organized activities directed toward its eradication. While 25 years ago the disease existed on every continent except Australia (Fig. 1), national control programs constricted this appreciably.[96] When the WHO Global Eradication Program was initiated in 1967, South America, Africa, and Asia were important foci; today endemic disease no longer exists anywhere.

5.4. Temporal Distribution

No characteristic periodicity had been described for smallpox; outbreaks had followed viral introduction into susceptible groups. It had a seasonal disease,[13,74,84] but no direct correlation with any specific meteorological condition had been defined. In Bangladesh, the seasonality was so marked that the Bengali word for the spring of the year, *bashunto*, was the word for smallpox. While the virus is more stable under lower humidities and lower temperature, the spring of the year (late dry season) in East Bengal is both hot and humid.

In the Punjab, there was a distinct winter peak (November-February), with very few cases between June and September. Mack *et al.*[57] found that the high (96%) infection rate within the compound of the index cases remained high throughout the year; there were differences in the attack rates in other compounds. During the periods of increasing incidence, the mean intergeneration interval from index case to first-generation cases appearing in different compounds was lengthened (17.6 vs. 20.6 days), but not within the same compound (13.6 vs. 13.9 days). This was taken to indicate longer viral survival under conditions of lower relative humidity, consistent with the hypothesis that infection might have been occurring within the compound of the source case—in essence, a model of "hospital" spread.

Data covering the 27 introductions of smallpox into Europe between 1961 and 1973[32] are relevant: 20 in the period from December to May were followed by 483 subsequent cases, for an average of 24.2 and a median of 4.5 subsequent cases per introduction; 7 introductions during the June–November period produced 11 subsequent cases, for an average of 1.6 and a median of 1 case per importation.

5.5. Age

The age distribution of smallpox is related to the immune status and to the relative mobility at different ages. In most endemic areas, the overall incidence was highest among the age group 0–4 years simply because this was the group most likely to be unvaccinated. However, when age-specific rates among the unvaccinated are considered, disease often occurred most frequently among males in the 5–14 year age group, a period of greatest mobility, and the incidence was lowest in those under 1 year of age, thanks to passive maternal immunity. Age also affected the case-fatality rate: among the unvaccinated, the highest case fatality rates were found in those in the youngest age group and again in the oldest; those in the 5–14 year group less frequently developed the highly fatal forms of disease (Table 2), and Sarkar *et al.*[83] found a greater frequency of inapparent infections in this age group.

5.6. Sex

Differences in sex incidence are related to cultural patterns that may have influenced the likelihood of exposure to an infectious case. In Bangladesh in 1966–1967, the incidence rate per 100,000 for males was 122 and for females, 89. The excess was probably related to the fact that the disease was introduced into the communities by males who had gone to the cities to work.[89] In the Punjab, attack rates of village-acquired disease in 1967–1968 among the unvaccinated were comparable for boys and girls

Table 2. Frequency and Case-Fatality Rates of Clinical Types of Smallpox by Age and Vaccination Status, Madras, 1961–1972[a]

Vaccination status	Age	Number of cases	Distribution by age (%)	Incidence of clinical types (%)				Case-fatality rates (%)
				Hemorrhagic	Flat	Ordinary	Modified	
Vaccinated	0–4	9	2.6	1.1	3.3	57.8	37.8	15.6
	5–14	390	11.5	1.8	0.5	57.7	37.4	3.3
	15–24	1159	34.1	2.7	0.6	68.3	28.4	4.1
	25–34	1192	35.1	4.4	1.5	72.5	21.6	7.0
	35–44	356	10.5	4.8	2.8	74.7	17.7	9.3
	45+	211	6.2	3.3	2.4	79.6	14.7	10.4
	TOTALS:	3398	100	3.4	1.3	70.0	25.3	
			Case-fatality rates:	93.9	66.7	3.2	0.0	6.3
Unvaccinated	0–4	2091	59.0	1.1	8.1	87.9	2.9	41.2
	5–14	862	24.3	1.0	4.2	94.0	0.8	20.3
	15–24	304	8.6	8.2	3.9	86.2	1.6	31.6
	25–34	157	4.4	8.3	6.4	84.7	0.6	36.9
	35–44	65	1.8	4.6	1.5	92.3	1.5	43.1
	45+	65	1.8	16.9	12.3	69.2	1.5	63.1
	TOTALS:	3544	100	2.4	6.7	88.8	2.1	
			Case-fatality rates:	98.8	94.1	30.3	0.0	35.8

[a] From Tables 17.1 and 17.2 in Rao.[74]

until puberty; then the incidence for boys residing in infected villages reached a peak of approximately 20%, while that for girls flattened at approximately 10%; after age 20–30 years, there was no difference.[56] This difference is attributable to the restrictions placed on young Moslem women. Pregnancy has an adverse effect on the outcome[76]; this is discussed in Section 8.

5.7. Race

There is no known racial resistance or susceptibility. Such reports have ignored socioeconomic factors, especially the vaccination status of various population groups. However, Dixon[14] suggests that the mortality was lower in populations among whom the disease had been endemic for three or four generations, since those who were genetically most susceptible would have been removed.

5.8. Occupation

As was noted above, in Bangladesh the disease predominated among the unskilled and semiskilled who had gone afield to find employment[89]; in Pun-

jab, the incidence was highest among the unskilled and lowest among landowners.[56]

5.9. Occurrence in Different Settings

In Europe, the hospital was a major focus for infection; those at greatest risk were those who were in contact with a patient on the ward and those who handled the laundry. In the 1970 outbreak in Meschede, Germany, 13 of the 17 secondary cases occurred among patients, 3 among nurses, and 1 in a hospital visitor.[90] In the 1972 outbreak in Yugoslavia, 48% of the 173 cases were acquired in hospitals, and 42 of the 48 cases that occurred in Belgrade involved hospital transmission.[100] The two fatal cases in England in 1973 occurred in visitors to a patient hospitalized for arthritis.[28]

About one half the indigenous cases occurring in Europe between 1950 and 1973 were hospital-acquired[32,54]: about 20% among hospital staff and 30% among patients and visitors.[54]

It would seem somehow inevitable that the last case of smallpox, in Africa, should have been a hospital employee.

5.10. Socioeconomic Status

Disease has been most common among the lower socioeconomic classes, particularly in the floating population, which has been most difficult to vaccinate. With overcrowding, transmission is more likely.

5.11. Other Factors

Important factors in the epidemiology of smallpox lie in the cultural patterns of the population. Those population segments or religious groups who refused or resisted vaccination were at greatest risk of acquiring and harboring smallpox. Social groups among whom illness in a family member is a signal for all family members to gather at the bedside experience increased transmission. The persistence of smallpox for more than 175 years after vaccination was introduced is evidence of continued resistance and refusal to accept vaccination; active and effective antivaccination movements have existed from the days of Jenner and Waterhouse.

6. Mechanisms and Routes of Transmission

6.1. Period of Communicability

When the exanthem appears, virus is present in high concentration in the deeper layers of the skin, but does not penetrate through the epithelium. Concurrent with the exanthem, there is an enanthem in the mouth and throat from which virus has ready access to the saliva, which then becomes the medium for disseminating the infection. Downie et al.[20] recovered virus most frequently from the mouth washings of smallpox patients from the 6th to the 9th day of disease, with the last positive isolation on the 14th day; virus was not isolated during the first 2 days of the febrile illness. The appearance of the rash, usually on the 3rd or 4th day after the fever, thus coincided with the period of greatest infectivity. The blood of patients with hemorrhagic smallpox remained highly infectious until death.[18] From throat swabs, Sarkar et al.[82] recovered 10^5 pock-forming units (PFU) of virus per milliliter of swab-washed fluid from hemorrhagic and severely

ill nonhemorrhagic patients between the 2nd and the 5th day of illness; throat-swab fluids from patients with a discrete rash had a maximal virus titer of 10^3 PFU. Urine and conjunctival swabs from these patients had comparable virus titers. Virus was recovered from patients with fatal, severe nonhemorrhagic cases as late as the 14th day and from no survivors after the 13th day. The authors noted that the hemorrhagic patients were indeed highly infectious, but since they died early (all in this series by the 7th day), they had less opportunity to spread infection. On an epidemiological basis, Rao et al.[75] concluded that transmission occurred predominantly during the first 7 days of illness, especially between the 4th and 7th days, and no contact became infected after the 13th day of disease in the primary case. Virus remained viable in crusts for a prolonged period of time, but there was no evidence that scabs were involved in the transmission of the disease.

6.2. Contact Spread

In some areas, transmission occurred principally by direct person-to-person contact through droplet spread of the saliva and respiratory secretions. The secondary infection rates on the order of 30% reported from West Africa, India, and Bangladesh are consistent with direct contact or droplet spread, as are the observed intervals of up to 80 days for disease to be transmitted within a family group, representing four or five generations of disease.[24]

6.3. Airborne Spread

Traditionally, smallpox has been assumed to be a highly infectious disease, consistent with airborne spread. Many reports, usually anecdotal, indicate transmission at distances or with very minimal contact, such as the episode when a man with smallpox walked into a barber shop: two customers fled and both came down with the disease; the barber, whose flight took him to the doctor's office for vaccination, remained well.[37] The episode in the hospital in Meschede, Germany, in 1970 was more carefully documented, and direct face-to-face or personal contact with the subsequent patients was clearly excluded. By use of a smoke generator a few months later under similar meteorological conditions, it was observed that the central stairwell served as a chimney and that smoke flowed out of the window of the patient's room and entered rooms at the higher floors where secondary infection had been acquired. The authors refer to an outbreak in 1961 in Monshau in which one 9-year-old girl infected ten persons with whom face-to-face contact was excluded. Both she and the Meschede patient had clinical illnesses associated with a considerable amount of coughing, which could effectively aerosolize the pathogen.[90]

Heiner et al.,[31] studying family contacts of smallpox cases in West Pakistan during the period 1968–1970, found a secondary attack rate of 76.8% among unvaccinated persons; DeQuadros et al.[12] reported a secondary attack rate of 69.1% among previously unvaccinated persons in their analysis of 27 rural outbreaks of variola minor in Brazil. These rates are generally comparable to the secondary attack rate of about 80% for measles, which is accepted to be airborne.

6.4. Spread by Fomites

The smallpox patient saturates his pillowcase and bedding copiously with mouth secretions and sometimes abraded vesicle fluid, both heavily laden with virus. As a consequence, laundry workers and hotel chambermaids have experienced disproportionately high incidences of smallpox. Rao[74] could isolate variola virus as long as 66 days from clothing that had been placed in a wooden box; when clothing was spread out on a bed and exposed to indirect light, virus was not recovered after 7 days. MacCallum and McDonald[53] wrapped crusts and material from smallpox patients in raw cotton and held these at 30°C under various humidities; they were unable to recover infectivity from pus or vesicle fluid 3 months later; however, virus survived in the crusts for over 6 months at a relative humidity of 58%. In the room-temperature (20–24°C) controls, in which crusts were held in screw-cap bottles in diffuse light, virus was still recoverable 18 months after the study was begun. Wolff and Croon[92a] recovered viable alastrim virus from crusts that had been held for 13 years in unsealed envelopes at the room temperature of a Dutch laboratory. Thus, smallpox virus could be moved internationally by inanimate objects. While methods for processing raw cotton could break up crusts and could effectively disperse

the contained virus into an aerosol, it is not proven that this has occurred.[14]

6.5. Vectors

The density of houseflies hovering about smallpox patients and on their lesions was often indeed remarkable, creating a potential for mechanical transmission; however, flies have not been unequivocally implicated in any outbreaks. Even though Sarkar et al.[80] found that Culex pipiens and Aedes aegypti retained viable smallpox virus for up to 4 days after feeding on viremic suckling mice and that indeed the virus could be recovered from the proboscides, they felt that, while possible, mosquito transmission "is much less likely than transmission by direct contact with the patients."

6.6. Animal Reservoirs

After the control of smallpox in West Africa had been achieved, cases of pox disease appeared in man in 1970 in the absence of any known smallpox disease. From these, the isolated virus was identified as monkeypox virus.[58] To April 1979, 36 cases of human monkeypox had been recognized, and 6 patients (17%) had died. Secondary infections occurred in 2 of 56 susceptible household contacts, a transmission rate of 4% compared to the 30–45% rate that had applied for smallpox in this geographic area.[102] Of these cases, 27 occurred in Zaire, 4 in Liberia, 3 in Nigeria, and 1 each in Sierra Leone and the Ivory Coast; 28 of known monkeypox cases had occurred among children 9 years of age or younger.[110]

Intensive studies have been carried out seeking an animal reservoir for monkeypox virus. No poxvirus antibody was found in sera from monkeys in Malaysia or in other Asiatic and various African countries.[1a] However, among West African wild monkeys, Breman et al.[8a] found poxvirus antibodies among Cercopithecus (C. aethiops, C. mona, C. petaurista, and C. nictitans) and Colobus (C. badius and C. polykomos) monkeys. The antibodies detectable by immunofluorescent testing in the sera of three monkeys were completely absorbed by monkeypox antigen; antibodies against monkeypox virus persisted after absorption with vaccinia.[27a] In a serological study of the wild-animal population carried out in the Ivory Coast 1½ years after a child in the area had developed monkeypox (4 years after the last case of smallpox in the country), neutralizing poxvirus antibodies were found in three rodent species, three monkey species, and two bird groups. Hemagglutinating antibodies were found only in the African giant squirrel (*Protexuris strangeri*).[8b] No monkeypox virus was recovered from any of the primates or rodents; the virus was isolated from anteaters with a vesicular disease in the Rotterdam Zoo. Laboratory studies by Marennikova and Seluhina[59a] have shown the susceptibility of which mice and rabbits to oral and nasal exposure, as well as contact transmission in young animals.

Of greater concern, however, is the repeated isolation of virus strains that are indistinguishable from variola virus. Two strains of "whitepox" virus, as these variolalike strains are called, were isolated in 1964 from routine monkey-kidney cultures from Malaysian cynomolgus monkeys in Utrecht, Holland.[26] In the search for the reservoir of monkeypox virus, a strain of a similar virus was isolated from a chimpanzee caught in 1970 in the region of Zaire where the first human monkeypox case had been recognized 4 months before.[59] This strain is identified as "chimp-9." In 1973, a whitepox strain was isolated from the kidney of a "sala" monkey that had been captured in the area in Zaire where two cases of monkeypox had occurred. Whitepox strains were recovered in September 1974 from the kidneys of the rodent *Mastomys natalensis* and in March 1975 from the kidneys of another rodent species (*Helios-ciurus rufobrachium*) captured in the region of Zaire in which a monkeypox case had occurred in August 1974.[1a] In 1968, a poxvirus was isolated from a healthy wild gerbil (*Tatera kempii*) caught in Benin while human smallpox was occurring. In laboratory studies, it resembled variola minor virus.[51a]

Whitepox virus is indistinguishable from variola virus in the laboratory; while monkeypox has a characteristic antigen *mo*, variola *va*, and vaccinia *vc* and *va*, whitepox has only *va*.[27] Heberling *et al.*[29a] serially passed vaccinia, variola, monkeypox, and chimp-9 through baboons and found that the patterns of disease produced by chimp-9 and variola were similar and that the lesions produced by monkeypox virus resembled those caused by vaccinia. Fenner[22a] indicates that the only known difference between whitepox and variola viruses lies in the unanswerable question of the former's infectivity for man.

The infectivity of variola virus for monkeys has been shown,[29,68] and while it has been suggested, no human variola case could be traced to monkey disease.[1,34] In the laboratory, the virus died out after several monkey-to-monkey aerosol passages.[68] These isolates, obtained in the wild in the absence of human smallpox disease, raise the question whether a reservoir may exist among rodents as well as in primates[2a] and indicate the need for continued close surveillance of potential animal reservoirs and especially of all human cases with poxlike lesions in possible contact with suspect reservoirs after the human-to-human disease has been globally eradicated.

7. Pathogenesis and Immunity

7.1. Pathogenesis

The classic studies by Fenner on mousepox (infectious ectromelia) have provided the clearest concept of the pathogenesis of smallpox. Normally, as outlined by Downie,[16] the virus of variola enters the body through the respiratory tract, and while some multiplication in mucosal cells of the lower respiratory tract cannot be excluded, the virus probably passes through the mucosa without producing lesions and is taken up by phagocytes and carried to neighboring lymph nodes. Here, the virus multiplies; an early nondetectable viremia probably occurs, with virus entering reticuloendothelial cells in the liver, lymph nodes, spleen, bone marrow, and probably lungs and multiplying during the incubation period of approximately 12 days during which the subject is noninfectious. Roberts,[78] working with ectromelia, and Hahon and Wilson,[29] working with monkey variola, showed that considerable local multiplication of virus took place in the lungs after aerosol exposure.

At the end of the incubation period, the virus spills out of these reticuloendothelial cells to create a viremia that is of short duration in mild cases, usually persisting no more than 2 days. A high viral titer or a viremia persisting after the first 2 days of fever indicates a poor prognosis. The fever of 39.5–40.5°C appears at the time of this massive viral release and is probably due to pyrogens released from the damaged cells in which virus had been multiplying.

The circulating virus localizes mainly in the skin and mucous membranes of the mouth and upper respiratory tract, resulting in dilatation of the capillaries in the dermal papillae, swelling of the endothelial cells, and a perivascular mononuclear-cell accumulation. Virus spreading to the overlying epithelium produces the initial rash. Macules and papules appear after virus has proliferated in the cytoplasm of the epithelial cells of the Malpighian layer with the formation of acidophilic inclusions (Guarnieri bodies). The cells undergo ballooning degeneration, fluid accumulates, and vesicles are formed that have a roof of keratinized cells and a floor either of degenerating epithelial cells or of the dermis; remaining strands of cell walls give the vesicle an umbilicated appearance and a loculated structure. Polymorphonuclear cells accumulate in response to the epithelial-cell necrosis, converting the lesion into a pustule, and then the contents dry, producing the thick crust under which reepithelization occurs. The same initial events occur in the lesions in the mouth and pharnyx, but since there is no keratinized layer, these rapidly become shallow ulcers from which virus is discharged, so that the patient is now highly infectious. Lesions are relatively sparse in the internal organs, a finding that may be related to the fact that variola virus does not produce lesions on chorioallantoic membranes at a temperature over 38.5°C; in the febrile smallpox patient, only the skin surfaces, and particularly the exposed skin surfaces, are below this temperature.

In hemorrhagic smallpox, the viremia at the onset of clinical disease is much more intense and presumably reflects a great multiplication of virus in the internal organs during the incubation period. Enormous amounts of virus are present in the skin even in the absence of microscopically visible lesions; the basic pathological changes are similar, with the added hemorrhagic factor. Death, which has been attributed to a shock syndrome induced by toxic damage to the vascular endothelium, terminates further development of the lesions. At autopsy, the same hemorrhagic phenomena present in the skin may be found in all the viscera.

Scarring is caused by destruction of sebaceous glands, and since these are more numerous on the face, this is the site of most marked scarring. Should secondary bacterial infection supervene, there is involvement of deeper levels of the dermis with resultant permanent scarring. Conjunctival disease with no sequelae is not uncommon; keratitis with residual corneal opacities and iritis and panophthalmitis with blinding can occur.

7.2. Immunity

Susceptibility to smallpox is considered to be universal, but in each outbreak there is a spectrum of severity with some very mild cases, while others have a fatal fulminating course. Recovery requires the development of specific immunity. While the individual skin lesion may be limited in its local extension by the production of interferon, recovery from the disease is related to development of circulating antibody, presumably the neutralizing antibody produced by B lymphocytes, and of cell-mediated immunity dependent on T lymphocytes. Virus neutralizing antibodies appear at about the time vesiculation occurs, about the 4th or 5th day; their appearance is usually associated with clinical improvement, but the lesions continue through their course. In fatal hemorrhagic cases, the antibodies appear later and at a lower level than in the nonhemorrhagic cases.[79]

Rao[74] reported that second attacks of smallpox might occur in 1 in 1000 cases after recovery from clinical smallpox. Such attacks were more frequent among women, and the average interval between the two attacks was 15–20 years; a major reaction to smallpox vaccination could be obtained within 1–2 years after clinical smallpox, indicating that resistance to variola was greater than that to percutaneously inoculated vaccinia. In his experience, second attacks were never fatal.

Passive immunity, induced by the injection of vaccinia-immune γ-globulin, was shown by Kempe et al.[43] to produce a 70% reduction in the incidence of smallpox among contacts. Given in the incubation period, it had the effect on circulating virus of preventing or modifying the disease; it was ineffective against intracellular virus.

Jennerian vaccination provided the tool for smallpox eradication; vaccinia, an immunologically related virus, multiplies at the site of inoculation without disseminating and evokes immunity that is even more effective against variola than against itself. The duration of this protection is difficult to establish, because there is always uncertainty whether the last vaccination did in fact elicit an immunizing vaccinial infection. In general, a high level of immunity against smallpox exists for the first 4 or 5 years, diminishing thereafter. Against variola minor, Dixon[14] expected complete protection for 5 years, and almost complete for 10 years. Revaccination results in an earlier recall of antibodies, and attainment of higher levels, which implies a longer duration of protection.[62,69] Heiner et al.[31] found secondary attack rates of 78.5% among unvaccinated contacts, 8.1% among those who had only primary vaccination, and 3.1% among those who had also been revaccinated.

Smallpox in a vaccinated person is usually milder than that in the unvaccinated, although deaths do occur (Table 2), especially among pregnant women.[73] Vaccination will normally protect against death from smallpox for at least 20 years. Of the cases acquired in Europe between 1950 and 1971, the case-fatality rate among the 149 unvaccinated patients was 40%, compared to 9% among the 412 previously vaccinated; the case-fatality rate was only 11.1% among the 297 patients whose last vaccination had been over 20 years before.[54]

Immunity develops by about the 8th day after primary vaccination, so that vaccination within the first 24–48 hr after contact with a smallpox case will usually prevent an attack; successful revaccination as late as 7 days after exposure may afford complete protection.[33]

8. Patterns of Host Response

The clinical picture of smallpox is superbly described by Christie.[9] Various classifications of variations in this picture have been used. Dixon[14] describes nine types; others[55,87] use lesion density; the classification of Rao,[74] which is essentially that of Christie,[9] is used here.

In the typical case of smallpox, the incubation period (usually 12 or 13 days but ranging from 8 to 17 days) is followed by an acute preeruptive illness lasting 2–4 days, with fever, headache, back pain, and prostration. This is easily confused with influenza, meningitis, or pneumonia; patients have been admitted to hospitals with such diagnoses as acute surgical abdomen and lumbosacral strain. The initial rash appears as maculopapules, first on the face or hands and forearms, then on the trunk and lower limbs. The distribution is centrifugal, with lesions maximal in the distal areas, including the palms and soles. In each region of the body, the lesions are in a similar stage. When the rash appears, the temperature falls and toxemia lessens, so that about the 2nd or 3rd day of the rash, the fever may be gone. The maculopapular lesions become vesicular within 24–48 hr. These may be umbilicated, and become turbid and pustular within a day or so more. The number of lesions can vary markedly, and there is a relationship between prognosis and the density of lesions.[56] The pustules dry and scabbing begins from the 8th to the 10th day of the eruption, and some crusts begin to separate about the 12th or 13th day. A secondary fever may recur during the pustular stage; this is not the consequence of secondary pyogenic infection but part of the disease itself. There is marked facial edema, particularly when the lesions are confluent. The concurrent lesions on the mucous membrane of the mouth and throat can produce marked discomfort and inability to swallow. This form, the *ordinary* type, constitutes the vast majority of cases and had a case-fatality rate in Madras between 1961 and 1972 of 3.2% among the vaccinated and 30.3% among the unvaccinated (Table 2).[74]

More serious cases are those characterized as the *flat* type. The focal lesions project little, if any, above the surrounding skin and are soft and velvety to the touch, rather than hard and pearly. This type is relatively rare, having occurred in Madras in 1.3 and 6.7% of vaccinated and unvaccinated cases with fatality rates of 66.7 and 94.1%, respectively (Table 2).[74]

Most serious is the *hemorrhagic* type, which, during the preeruptive illness, may involve a dusky flush of the skin, hemorrhagic manifestations (petechial or more of a purpura) with subconjunctival bleeding, bleeding from mouth and gums, epistaxis, hematuria, and vaginal bleeding; death sometimes occurs before a diagnostic focal rash appears. In late hemorrhagic disease, death occurs on the 8th to 10th day after hemorrhages have appeared in and between the focal lesions, which are of the flat type. The disease occurred in Madras in 3.4 and 2.4% of the vaccinated and unvaccinated, with fatality rates of 93.9 and 98.8%, respectively (Table 2).[74]

The *modified* type of smallpox occurs principally in vaccinated persons. While the preeruptive illness may be severe, few lesions develop, and these are completely crusted within 10 days. The lesions are superficial and evolve quickly. All patients survive. This type occurred in 25.3% of the vaccinated and 2.1% of those who denied vaccination or prior smallpox (Table 2). *Variola sine eruptione* is a febrile illness with constitutional symptoms not followed by a rash, which represents the clinical manifestations seen in well-vaccinated persons, usually recognized only in doctors and nurses.

The distribution of clinical types and case-fatality rates seen in Madras over the period 1961–1972, as influenced by vaccination status, is presented in Table 3.

Subclinical infections had been considered to be rare but Heiner *et al.*[30] reported that in West Pakistan, 54.5% of 143 previously vaccinated household contacts of smallpox patients developed CF titers equal to or over 1:40 with no reported illnesses, compared to 6.5% among village controls with no household contact. On the basis of positive agar-gel precipitation tests with variola antigen, Rao[74] in Madras reported 34 cases of subclinical infection among 109 family contacts, 5 of whom were unvaccinated. Throat washings were obtained from 37 of these contacts, and virus was isolated from 5 of these; all 5 also had serological positivity. Dekking *et al.*[11] noted conjunctivitis in smallpox patients during the clinical disease and isolated virus from the conjunctivae of 3 of 4 patients. They "were struck by the fact that several mothers whose children died of smallpox had red eyes for many more days than could be explained by their grief alone"; therefore, they prepared cultures from the eyes of 7 patients and recovered virus from all. Six had no other symptoms; one did have 1 day of fever. Of the 7, 5 had not previously been vaccinated.

Sarkar *et al.*[83] recovered virus at a titer of 10^2 to $10^{3.95}$ from the throats of 34 contacts of smallpox patients after 4–8 days of contact; only 4 developed clinical smallpox 5–6 days later. No serological studies were done; the fact that virus was recovered from 6.7% of the 269 vaccinated contacts vs. 27.1% (16) of the 59 unvaccinated contacts suggests that at least some of these represented inapparent infections rather than mechanical carriage.

Inapparent infections, then, must not be considered unusual. They may have been important in maintaining immunity where the incidence of smallpox was high. When the incidence of disease became very low, they seemed to have no epidemiological importance, especially since there was no suggestion that these cases might have been involved in disease transmission. However, Sarkar and co-workers suggest that these cases might have explained apparent discrepancies from the usually accepted incubation period.

Rao[73,76] brought attention to the frequency with which the pregnant woman develops hemorrhagic smallpox. He noted that 50% of hemorrhagic smallpox cases in his hospital had occurred among pregnant women and that prior vaccination afforded poor protection against this severe form should a pregnant woman develop smallpox. Rao *et al.*[77] duplicated the phenomenon in monkeys. Normal animals showed little more than a mild rash and a slight fever appearing the 5th day; however, when a pregnant monkey was infected, she died in 12 days with hemorrhagic disease. Of 14 nonpregnant monkeys given cortisone before and after intradermal infection with variola, 11 died; all 14 non-cortisone-treated controls survived. Viremia was detected in 2 of 10 controls tested before the onset of symptoms; after the fever had appeared, only 1 blood culture was positive of the 16 tested from control monkeys, while 11 of the 26 blood cultures from the steroid-treated animals were positive.

Variola minor (alastrim) and intermediate strains produce the same clinical types of smallpox, but the spectrum is heavily shifted toward the "modified" type, with discrete lesions and rapid recovery. Variola minor (alastrim) does have a case-fatality rate of 1–1.5%. The intermediate type of virus was isolated from patients in Tanganyika, where the case fatality rates varied from 2.8 to 10.9%, averaging 5.6% over the period 1954–1963.[2] The case-fatality rate in Ethiopia in 1971 was 2.1%; if all deaths occurred only among the unvaccinated, the rate would be 2.3%, with a maximal age-specific rate of 12.5% in those under 1 year of age.[99]

9. Control and Prevention Based on Epidemiological Data

9.1. Control Program

Control of smallpox was based on vaccination's breaking the chain of transmission by eliminating

Table 3. Distribution of Clinical Varieties and
1961–

Clinical type	Unvaccinated and unsuccessfully vaccinated			Primary vaccination only after exposure		
	Number	Frequency (%)	CFR (%)	Number	Frequency (%)	CFR (%)
Hemorrhagic	81	2.7	97.5	4	0.8	100
Flat	208	6.8	98.1	28	5.6	96.4
Ordinary	2721	89.5	31.8	426	84.8	20.6
Modified	31	1.0	0.0	44	8.8	0.0
Totals:	3041	100	37.8	502	100	23.6

a From Tables 5.1 and 17.3 in Rao.[74] (CFR) Case-fatality rate.

susceptible hosts. The WHO Smallpox Eradication Program, which was set in motion in 1967, was based on the facts that smallpox is transmitted from man to man, that infection is manifest and carriers do not exist, and that the incubation period is almost 2 weeks, allowing time for appropriate intervention. Happily, it was found that the disease spread relatively slowly through the population in the endemic areas, with several generations of disease within a single family.

The obvious first approach in an area with very high endemicity was to start an effective mass vaccination program. However, the success of the global eradication program shows the great value of the earliest possible institution of "selective epidemiological control," in which vaccination is concentrated on case contacts and places where cases are occurring.[23]

9.1.1. Preparatory Phase. Before an active eradication operation was initiated, time was allowed for an appropriate epidemiological assessment of the distribution of smallpox and of immunity, for personnel to be recruited and trained and supplies and transport to be arranged, and for the population to be educated for cooperation, including not only health education of the public to assure acceptance of vaccination but also recruitment of agencies, voluntary or governmental, that could be suborned into becoming active participants in the control program.

9.1.2. Attack Phase. The active program was divided into three phases.[95] During the *attack phase* (while the incidence of smallpox was 5 or more cases per 100,000 population per year and less than 80% of the population had vaccination scars), a system-

atic mass vaccination campaign was initiated, supported by a concurrent but separate assessment program to assure adequate and effective vaccination coverage. The ultimate success of the program depended heavily on surveillance, i.e., locating and following up all cases of possible smallpox, with localized intensive vaccination in the communities where the cases occurred. As the program proceeded, an active surveillance network was established, enlisting the cooperation of the existing health facilities and all other sources for rapid reporting of possible cases.

Foege *et al.*[23] found that at the beginning of the program in West and central Africa, 95% of smallpox cases coming to attention between January and July 1968 did so through the official health-reporting system. However, 58% of the cases were discovered through the nonofficial reporting system by January 1969. When emphasis was placed on immediate and effective response to each of these reported cases, a very sharp drop took place in the number of cases, and smallpox was eradicated at least a year earlier than had been expected.

9.1.3. Consolidation Phase. The *consolidation phase* was reached when the incidence was below 5 cases per 100,000 and over 80% of all segments of the population showed scars of primary vaccination. A "maintenance vaccination program" provided primary vaccination to immigrants, newborns, and those who had been missed initially. Revaccination was performed on a 3- to 5-year cycle. The surveillance network became of greater importance, and now each report of possible smallpox must result in an epidemiological investigation, laboratory study,

Case-Fatality Rates of Smallpox Patients, Madras, 1972[a]

Primary vaccination scar only			Primary vaccination and revaccination scars			Total	
Number	Frequency (%)	CFR (%)	Number	Frequency (%)	CFR (%)	Number	CFR (%)
111	3.4	94.0	4	3.0	100	200	95.7
45	1.4	66.7	8	—	—	281	92.9
2302	70.5	3.3	75	56.8	0.0	5524	18.6
808	24.7	0.0	53	40.2	0.0	936	0.0
3266	100	6.5	132	100	3.0	6941	21.3

vaccination and observation of case contacts, and containment of infection by isolation of cases and appropriate disinfection.

9.1.4. Maintenance Phase. The *maintenance phase* existed when there had been no endemic smallpox for more than 2 years and the disease persisted on the continent. Maintenance vaccination was continued, particularly of the new members of the population, and intense surveillance was maintained (see Section 9.4.3). Each report of a suspected case was treated as an emergency. From each case or outbreak, specimens were submitted for laboratory confirmation.

9.1.5. Program Execution. The program was carried out essentially as planned. In the programs of many countries, there was a blending of phases, with early implementation of the program of surveillance and case detection, isolation of patients, and localized intensive vaccination in the community, which resulted in cessation of disease before mass vaccination programs had in fact been completed. Surveillance and case-reporting became more effective when cases became few enough that a financial award could be given to anyone who first reported a case of smallpox to the smallpox-eradication teams.

9.2. Immunization Concepts and Practice

9.2.1. Vaccination Problems. The long interval between the introduction of smallpox vaccination and the achievement of global eradication can be explained by the complexities involved in the simple procedure of infecting a susceptible person with vaccinia virus by introducing viable elementary bodies into the stratum germinativum and the upper layers of dermis. These complexities warrant consideration.

Early in the history of vaccination, contaminated vaccines resulted in "spurious takes" with dermal reactions and scars of pyogenic infections, which conferred no immunity to smallpox. The usual vaccines were of low potency to begin with and rapidly lost potency during storage unless kept at below-freezing temperatures. To compensate for the low concentration of vaccinial virus, various instruments and techniques were developed that introduced vaccine into such a large area of skin surface that many takes, when the vaccine was still relatively potent, resulted in a morbidity so severe that the populace fled from the vaccinator. Less traumatic techniques—such as the multiple pressure and scratch methods—involved individual skill, with considerable variation in take rates in the hands of different vaccinators.[5] Furthermore, to assure that the vaccination did result in a good vaccinial infection, strains were selected that were most "potent." These were selected by their greater take rate and were often associated with a more intense, systemic illness after primary vaccination.[72]

9.2.2. Vaccination Reactions

a. Primary Vaccination. A papule appears at the vaccination site about 3 days after vaccination; within 2–3 more days, this vesiculates to constitute the umbilicated and multilocular "Jennerian vesicle." The contents become turbid, and erythema and induration surround this central lesion. The area of erythema reaches its maximal diameter between the

8th and the 12th day, most usually on the 9th or 10th day. At this time, axillary lymph nodes are enlarged and tender, and about 50% of patients have a fever over 37.8°C. The pustule dries from the center out, becoming the dry brown or black scab that falls off in about 3 weeks, leaving the typical foveated pockmark.

b. *Revaccination.* Successful primary vaccination creates not only humoral immunity but also a longer lasting cell-mediated immunity.[3,16] Humoral immunity can wane, but the persisting dermal hypersensitivity to vaccinial protein will result in a reaction maximal in 24–48 hr after revaccination, which is elicited equally well by noninfectious vaccine. This is an "allergic" reaction. It confers no immunity but is associated with increased resistance to vaccination, even in susceptible persons.[21] It is the reaction of the fully immune person to potent vaccine properly applied; this was recognized and described by Jenner.[41] With impotent vaccine or poor technique, infection fails and immunity is incorrectly assumed.[3]

In those who have lost some immunity, a successful revaccination initially produces the "allergic" reaction, which is followed by an enlarging area of skin erythema that becomes maximal earlier than a primary take. The area of erythema surrounding the central lesion becomes maximal later in time as immunity decreases until it occurs 8–10 days after revaccination, the same time course as that of primary vaccination. An allergic reaction can be associated with an increase in circulating antibodies in those nearly fully immune, but the reaction is indistinguishable from the nonprotective reaction elicited by noninfectious vaccine; therefore, this has been termed an *equivocal reaction.* In contrast, when there is still evidence after 1 week of an active inflammatory reaction, in contrast to the simple scab that often follows an equivocal reaction, an immunizing *major reaction* is manifested.[94]

9.2.3. Complications of Smallpox Vaccination

a. *Progressive Vaccinia.* Infection by a live virus, even an attenuated one, involves multiplication of the organism within the host's body until immune processes terminate the infection. When vaccine is applied to a person whose cell-mediated immunity is impaired because of thymic dysplasia or leukemia or similar malignant disease, or because of immunosuppression (chemical or by irradiation), the virus continues to multiply and spreads cell to cell to constitute *progressive vaccinia* (vaccinia necrosum). While this occurs in the United States in one or fewer per million vaccinations,[46] when it does occur it is a dramatic event. Treatment with methisazone as a direct antiviral agent, coupled with vaccinia immune globulin, resulted in the survival in 1968 of 7 of 11 patients whose overall survival prognosis was grave, even without this vaccination complication.

b. *Postvaccinial Encephalitis.* Postvaccinial encephalitis, a puzzling complication, consists of "postvaccinial central nervous system involvement, including separately or in combination the following symptoms: meningeal signs, ataxia, muscular weakness, paralysis, lethargy, coma or convulsions."[45] It has been reported to occur as frequently as 1 in every 4000 primary vaccinations in Holland,[71] and yet in the United States it occurs in 2.9 per million primary vaccinations,[46] a rate similar to the background rate of "nonspecific" encephalitis in the United States.[4] In Austria[6] and in Holland,[71] the incidence fell dramatically with change from the Bern and Copenhagen vaccinal strains, respectively, to the Lister strain. This can be a very serious complication, with reported case-fatality rates ranging from 50+% in Holland[71] to 3–17% in Sweden[22]; in the 1968 United States survey, 25% died.[46] Severe permanent neurological deficiencies remain in some who survive.

c. *Eczema Vaccinatum.* Eczema vaccinatum constitutes more of a threat to eczematous contacts than to the vaccinated person, since vaccination is usually deferred when active weeping lesions are present. When a large area of raw skin surface is exposed to and infected with vaccinia, the pathological event is not too different from that of smallpox. This was reported to occur in the United States 38 times per million primary vaccinations in 1968; an equal number of cases with one death occurred in an unknown number of unvaccinated contacts.[46]

d. *Other Reactions.* In addition to these potentially serious complications of smallpox vaccination, a large number of reactions occur that have no adverse prognostic significance. These include *generalized vaccinia,* frequent *exanthematous reactions,* and *accidental infections* in which virus is transferred to other places. These conditions are rarely of consequence, and while they are often of great concern to physicians and parents, they have little adverse effect on the prognosis or well-being of the vaccinee.

About 20 cases of *congenital vaccinia* of the fetus have been reported since 1932; however, a comparative study disclosed no evidence of an increased frequency of congenital malformations among approximately 8000 infants whose mothers were vaccinated during pregnancy when compared to a similar number whose mothers were not vaccinated.[44]

e. Importance of Vaccination Complications. These complications assume real importance where smallpox does not exist, so that it can truly be said that the preventive measure is costing more lives than the disease itself. Unfortunately, emphasis in the Western world on these complications results in fear of vaccination and overresponse when the unimportant reactions are seen.

9.2.4. Resolution of Some Vaccination Problems. Success of the eradication program depended on solution of many of these problems.[5] Inadequate potency or excessive bacterial contamination of the vaccines was resolved by the use of a stable freeze-dried vaccine and establishment of WHO International Reference Centres for Smallpox Vaccine to assure that high-quality vaccines would be used for the eradication program. Need for skilled individual vaccinators was avoided by the development of the mechanical jet injector, which introduces approximately 0.1 ml intradermally of a potent vaccine containing $10^{6.5}$ PFU/ml and free of detectable bacteria.[63] This was the method of vaccination used in the West and Central African and in the Brazilian campaigns.

The bifurcated needle made available a much cheaper instrument, also very conserving of vaccine. When it is used in the multiple-puncture method[101] with vaccine meeting WHO standards (a virus titer of 10^8 PFU/ml after incubation at 37°C for 4 weeks), infection is reliably produced in susceptibles and is the method used in Asia and Ethiopia. The vaccines to be used were restricted to the Lister or Elstree strain, the EM-63 strain prepared in Moscow, and the New York Board of Health strains used in the United States[101]; in comparative studies, these had been shown to be the preferable strains because they caused fewer systemic symptoms.

9.3. Success of the Program

The global eradication program defined eradication as "the elimination of clinical illness caused by variola virus. . . . Recent experience indicates that, in all countries with a reasonably effective surveillance programme, residual foci can be detected within 12 months of apparent interruption. Thus, in countries with active surveillance programmes, at least 2 years should have elapsed after the last known case . . . before it is considered probable that smallpox transmission has been interrupted."[101] By these criteria, smallpox has been eradicated; no natural transmission of the disease has occurred since October 1977.[113]

The last case in the western hemisphere was detected in suburban Rio de Janeiro, Brazil, in April 1971; the last known case in West Africa occurred in May 1970; the last case in South Africa was reported in January 1971; and the last case in Indonesia was found in January 1972. The last case in Pakistan had its onset on October 12, 1974; in Nepal, on April 6, 1975; in India, on May 24, 1975; and in Bangladesh, on October 16, 1975. The last focus of smallpox has been in Africa, with the last case detected in Ethiopia, with onset on August 9, 1976; in Kenya, on February 5, 1977; and the final case of Ali Maow Maalin in Somalia, on October 26, 1977.

International Commissions had been appointed by WHO after regions had been free of reported disease for at least 2 years to confirm the reports of freedom from disease and to assure that an adequate system existed to recognize any resurgence of disease. They reviewed the activities of the programs in these areas and carried out field visits for on-the-spot verification. Such a commission declared South America free of disease in August 1973; another declared Indonesia clear in April 1974, western Africa in April 1976, and Afghanistan and Pakistan in November and December 1976. During 1977, International Commissions visited and cleared Nepal, Bhutan, and India; nine countries in Central and West Africa; and Bangladesh and Burma.

In October 1977, an Informal Consultation on Worldwide Certification of Smallpox Eradiction met. This group identified those countries in which smallpox had recently been endemic or where there was a high risk that importation might lead to an endemic focus.[108] After careful review of all data, on December 9, 1979, the Global Commission for the Certification of Smallpox Eradication certified that smallpox had been eradicated from the world.

Finally, on May 8, 1980, the Thirty-third World Health Assembly adopted a resolution that "declares solemnly that the world and all its people have won freedom from smallpox, which was a most devastating disease sweeping in epidemic form through many countries since earliest times, leaving death, blindness and disfigurement in its wake and which only a decade ago was rampant in Africa, Asia and South America. . . ."[114]

9.4. Plans for the Future

9.4.1. Vaccination Program. While there has been dispute on the need for routine vaccination in the past,[4,47] the issue has been resolved by the eradication of smallpox. In September 1980, the U.S. Public Health Service Advisory Committee on Immunization Practices stated that smallpox vaccination in civilians is now indicated *only* for laboratory workers directly involved with smallpox or closely related orthopox viruses (e.g., monkeypox, vaccinia, and others). With regard to international travel, as of January, 1982 only Chad continued to require an up-to-date certification of smallpox vaccination as a condition of entry. Since WHO International Health Regulations provide for waiver of vaccination when this is contraindicated for health reasons, it is suggested that the small risk of serious complications in the absence of known smallpox justifies giving waiver letters to travelers to these countries.[10]

9.4.2. Smallpox Laboratories. Laboratories holding variola stock virus will constitute the only known source of disease when eradication is complete. The last two outbreaks of smallpox in Europe arose from the laboratory handling of the virus. In March 1973, a medical laboratory technician was infected in London; two secondary cases were both fatal.[28] In August 1978, a medical photographer working in a room directly over the smallpox laboratory in Birmingham, England, presumably exposed through a ventilation duct, developed fatal smallpox.[106] The photographer's mother developed mild disease[107]; the virologist took his own life. To minimize this hazard, laboratories have been requested to destroy their stocks or justify their retention. As of February 1981, variola virus is known to be held in only five laboratories, all of which are able to meet stringent WHO Safety Requirements,[115] in contrast to 76 laboratories that held variola virus in 1976.[109]

9.4.3. Surveillance. The surveillance system for possible smallpox cases must continue at a high level of efficiency to ensure that no case of smallpox can occur without early recognition and prompt containment.[14] The appearance of a single case will constitute a major medical emergency and will call for concerted international cooperation. The area for most intensive surveillance must be the region of West Africa from Zaire to Sierra Leone, where monkeypox cases have occurred and whitepox isolations were made. In 1978, 4577 specimens were submitted to two WHO Collaborating Centres through the Smallpox Eradication Unit, WHO, coming from 35 countries in Africa and Asia. All were negative for variola virus.[112] The testing of specimens should continue even after certification of smallpox eradication, so that competent and safe laboratory support will be able to rule out smallpox in cases in which smallpox cannot be excluded on clinical or epidemiological grounds, and to identify suspected cases of animal poxviruses affecting man. Continuing surveillance of animal populations for poxviruses will be essential, as will careful study of poxvirus isolates using techniques of DNA analysis and the possibility of viral mutations.

9.4.4. Vaccine Reserves. Should poxvirus disease break out now that eradication has been certified, there will be immediate need for vaccine with which to vaccinate all contacts. For emergency purposes only, the Global Commission has recommended that the WHO store 300,000,000 doses of vaccine in Geneva, New Delhi, and Toronto, stored at −20°C and monitored regularly for potency.[111]

There will continue to be a requirement for vaccination of persons potentially exposed to smallpox (including military personnel, since smallpox will become an increasing attractive bacteriological warfare agent[22a]); thus, there will continue to be a requirement for vaccine.

This will involve primary vaccination of adults. It is argued by some[13] that childhood vaccination affords no protection against complications of revaccination in later life and that it is therefore more logical to withold primary vaccination until required; others argue that early vaccination is associated with fewer complications and protects against complications after revaccination. The experience in Holland reported by Polak,[71] summarized in Table 4, indicates that despite a significant reduction in

Table 4. Central Nervous System Complications Following Primary Vaccination of Infants and Adults with Different Strains of Vaccinia Virus in Different Time Periods, Netherlands[a]

	Vaccinial strain Copenhagen		Vaccinial strain Elstree	
	Infants 1959–1962	Adults 1959–1963	Infants 1963–1970	Adults 1964–1970
Vaccinations	821,000	15,000	1,708,000	21,000
CNS disease (deaths)	31 (16)	4 (1)	19 (11)	1
Rate/million	38	267	11	48

[a] From Polak et al.[72]

incidence related to the change to the Elstree strain, the risk of postvaccinial encephalitis remains significantly higher among adults; the single adult case in the later time period occurred in a person who had been given vaccinia-immune globulin at the time of vaccination, the usual Dutch prophylaxis against CNS complications.[66] Thus, if we are to cope with introduction of smallpox into a nonimmune population with present immunization practices, we must anticipate an increase in the frequency of adverse reactions as well as the probability of relatively wide spread among an unvaccinated population before the infection is recognized.

The vaccines used in the United States, derived from the New York City Board of Health vaccine, were compared with the Elstree vaccine and with the attenuated CV-1 vaccine for effectiveness and reactogenicity in a study carried out at four medical centers. The Elstree and United States vaccines were generally comparable; the CV-1 vaccine was less effective (and produced fewer adverse reactions), and even 28 days after revaccination with reference-standard freeze-dried vaccine, neutralizing antibodies were present in significantly fewer vaccinees and at a lower mean titer.[10c,62a]

10. Unresolved Problems

The meticulous prosecution of the eradication program with the extensive educational component that produced general familiarity with and concern over the disease and enlisted wide popular support, together with the care involved in the certification process, make it most unlikely that foci of disease can persist in the human population.

But might infection arise from the animal kingdom? Monkeypox virus has proven not to have epidemic potential with its very low secondary attack rate of 4% among susceptible family members. Whitepox virus may or may not be infective for man; there has been no smallpox in the human population when these viruses were isolated; this may be because whitepox virus is noninfectious for man or because appropriate contact has not been made between the reservoir animal and man. The possibility that a noninfectious virus might mutate to acquire infectivity for man must be considered. The Global Commission recommended that "research on orthopoxviruses employing the recently developed technique of DNA analysis should continue, to ensure the permanent status of eradication after certification has been completed."[109]

Is all variola virus on earth now present in the five listed laboratories and will it be maintained in the future only in those that establish the stringent WHO safety requirements? Can we destroy all known variola virus and leave no reference material for study when new techniques or new problems arise? Can we be sure that every laboratory that had virus on hand did in fact report it and destroy it? Are there misplaced vials of virus in other laboratories that had believed they had destroyed all their stocks of variola virus?[10a] Is the world secure from malicious dissemination of virus from illicit stocks by misguided fanatics?

How will we maintain an alertness among members of the medical profession so that they will recognize the reemergence of a supposedly nonexistent disease before the second or third generation of cases?

We have achieved the objective foreseen when Jenner introduced smallpox vaccine.[40] "The condition upon which God hath given liberty to man is eternal vigilance" (J. P. Curran, 1790); this applies as much to liberty from smallpox as it does to political liberty. This was foreseen by James Bryce[8c] when he wrote in 1802, four years after Jenner published his report:

> Dr. Jenner has thus acted his part; it remains for the other members of society to act theirs; he has shown how important advantages may be obtained; it is theirs to carry this plan into execution by co-operating, both by example and by precept, to render general the practice of inoculation for the cowpox: the reward being no less than the exterminating one of the most loathsome and fatal diseases to which mankind are liable—The smallpox. I must here, however, observe, that it is not the prevention of smallpox in a country for a few years, or perhaps a century, that ought to be regarded sufficient . . . if it should then unfortunately so happen, that the advantages resulting from vaccination are forgotten, or undervalued . . . then the smallpox may again be imported from some remote corner where the influence of cowpox was unknown, or it may originate *de novo*, . . . and hold a course among mankind nearly as terrific as that described by authors who relate the ravages of this dreadful disease. . . .

11. References

1. ARITA, I., AND HENDERSON, D. A., Smallpox and monkeypox in non-human primates, *Bull. WHO* **39**:277–283 (1968).

1a. ARITA, I., AND HENDERSON, D. A., Monkeypox and whitepox viruses in West and Central Africa, *Bull. WHO* **53**:347–353 (1976).

2. BEDSON, H. S., DUMBELL, K. R., AND THOMAS, W. R. G., Variola in Tanganyika, *Lancet* **2**:1085–1088 (1963).

2a. BAXBY, D., Poxvirus hosts and reservoirs, *Arch. Virol.* **55**:169–179 (1977).

3. BENENSON, A. S., Immediate (so-called "immune") reaction to smallpox vaccination, *J. Am. Med. Assoc.* **143**:1238–1240 (1950).

4. BENENSON, A. S., Routine vaccination for all is still indicated, in: *Controversy in Internal Medicine II* (F. J. INGELFINGER, R. V. EBERT, M. FINLAND, AND A. J. RELMAN, eds.), pp. 371–381, W. B. Saunders, Philadelphia, 1974.

5. BENENSON, A. S., Vaccination factors critical for eradication of smallpox, in: *International Symposium on Smallpox Vaccine* (R. REGAMEY AND H. COHEN, eds.), pp. 17–22, S. Karger, Basel, 1973.

6. BERGER, K., AND HEINRICH, W., Decrease of post-vaccinal deaths in Austria after introducing a less pathogenic virus strain, in: *International Symposium on Smallpox Vaccine* (R. REGAMEY AND H. COHEN, eds.), pp. 199–203, S. Karger, Basel, 1973.

7. BERNSTEIN, S. S., Smallpox and variolation: Their historical significance in the American colonies, *J. Mt. Sinai Hosp.* **18**:229–244 (1951).

8. BLAKE, J. B., *Benjamin Waterhouse and the Introduction of Vaccination*, p. 61, University of Pennsylvania Press, Philadelphia, 1957.

8a. BREMAN, J. G., BERNADOU, J., AND NAKANO, J. H., Poxvirus in West African nonhuman primates: Serological survey results, *Bull. WHO* **55**:605–612 (1977).

8b. BREMAN, J. G., NAKANO, J. H., COFFI, E., GODFREY, H., AND GAUTUN, J. C., Human poxvirus disease after smallpox eradication, *Am. J. Trop. Med. Hyg.* **26**:273–281 (1977).

8c. BRYCE, J., *Practical Observations on the Inoculation of Cowpox, Pointing Out a Test of a Constitutional Affection in Those Cases in which the Local Inflammation is Slight, and in which no Fever is Perceptible*, William Couch, Edinburg, Scotland, 1802.

9. CHRISTIE, A. B., *Infectious Diseases: Epidemiology and Clinical Practice*, pp. 185–237, E. & S. Livingstone, Edinburgh, 1969.

10. CENTER FOR DISEASE CONTROL, Recommendation of the Immunization Practices Advisory Committee, Smallpox Vaccine, *Morbid. Mortal. Weekly Rep.* **29**:417 (1980).

10a. CENTER FOR DISEASE CONTROL, Destruction of variola virus stock—California, *Morbid. Mortal. Weekly Rep.* **28**:172 (1979).

10b. CENTER FOR DISEASE CONTROL, Laboratory-associated smallpox—England, *Morbid. Mortal. Weekly Rep.* **27**:319–320 (1978).

10c. CHERRY, J. D., MCINTOSH, K., CONNOR, J. D., BENENSON, A. S., ALLING, D. W., ROLFE, U. T., TODD, W. A., SCHANBERGER, J. E., AND MATTHEIS, M. J., A clinical and serologic study of four smallpox vaccines comparing variations of dose and route of administration: Primary percutaneous vaccination, *J. Infect. Dis.* **135**:145–154 (1977).

11. DEKKING, F., RAO, A. R., ST. VINCENT, L., AND KEMPE, C. H., The weeping mother, an unusual source of variola virus, *Arch. Gesamte Virusforsch.* **22**:215–218 (1967).

12. DEQUADROS, C. C. A., MORRIS, L., DACOSTA, E. A., ARNT, N., AND TIGRE, C. H., Epidemiology of variola minor in Brazil based on a study of 33 outbreaks, *Bull. WHO* **46**:165–171 (1972).

13. Dick, G., Smallpox: A reconsideration of public health policies, *Prog. Med. Virol.* **8**:1–29 (1966).

14. Dixon, C. W., *Smallpox*, J. & A. Churchill, London, 1962.

15. Downie, A. W., Smallpox (variola major and variola minor), in: *Virus and Rickettsial Disease of Man*, 4th ed. (S. Bedson, A. W. Downie, F. O. MacCallum, and C. H. Stuart-Harris), pp. 84–111, Edward Arnold, London, 1967.

16. Downie, A. W., Smallpox, in: *Infectious Agents and Host Reactions* (S. Mudd, ed.), pp. 487–518, W. B. Saunders, Philadelphia, 1970.

17. Downie, A. W., and Kempe, C. H., Variola and other pox virus infections, in: *Diagnostic Procedures for Viral and Rickettsial Disease*, 4th ed. (E. H. Lennette and N. J. Schmidt, eds.), pp. 281–320, American Public Health Association, New York, 1969.

18. Downie, A. W., McCarthy, K., MacDonald, A., MacCallum, F. O., and Macrae, A. D., Virus and virus antigen in the blood of smallpox patients: Their significance in early diagnosis and prognosis, *Lancet* **2**:164–166 (1953).

19. Downie, A. W., and McCarthy, K., The antibody response in man following infection with viruses of the pox group. III. Antibody response in smallpox, *J. Hyg.* **56**:479–487 (1958).

20. Downie, A. W., St. Vincent, L., Meiklejohn, G., Ratnakannan, N. R, Rao, A. R., Krishnan, G. N. V., and Kempe, C. H., Studies on the virus content of mouth washings in the acute phase of smallpox, *Bull. WHO* **25**:49–53 (1961).

21. Espmark, J. A., Smallpox vaccination studies with serial dilutions vaccine. 1. Primary vaccination and revaccination in human adults, *Acta Pathol. Microbiol. Scand.* **63**:97–115 (1965).

22. Espmark, J. A., Rabo, E., and Heller, L., Smallpox vaccination before the age of three months: Evaluation of safety, in: *International Symposium on Smallpox Vaccine* (R. H. Regamey and H. Cohen, eds.), pp. 243–248, S. Karger, Basel, 1973.

22a. Fenner, F., The eradication of smallpox, *Prog. Med. Virol.* **23**:1–21 (1977).

23. Foege, W. H., Millar, J. D., and Lane, J. M., Selective epidemiologic control in smallpox eradication, *Am. J. Epidemiol.* **94**:311–315 (1971).

24. Foege, W. H., Millar, J. D., and Henderson, D. A., Smallpox eradication in West and Central Africa, *Bull. WHO* **52**:209–222 (1975).

25. Gibson, J. E., *Dr. Bodo Otto and the Medical Background of the American Revolution*, pp. 88–103 and 131–135, Thomas, Baltimore, 1937.

26. Gispen, R., and Brand-Saathof, B., White poxvirus strains from monkeys, *Bull. WHO* **46**:585–592 (1972).

27. Gispen, R., and Brand-Saathof, B., Three specific antigens produced in vaccinia, variola, and monkey-pox infection, *J. Infect. Dis.* **129**:289–295 (1974).

27a. Gispen, R., Brand-Saathof, B., and Hekker, A. C., Monkey-pox-specific antibodies in human and simian sera from the Ivory Coast and Nigeria, *Bull. WHO* **53**:355–360 (1976).

28. Great Britain Report of the Committee of Inquiry into the Smallpox Outbreak in London in March and April, 1973, Report, Her Majesty's Printing Office, London, 1974.

29. Hahon, N., and Wilson, B. J., Pathogenesis of variola in *Macaca irus* monkeys, *Am. J. Hyg.* **71**:69–80 (1959).

29a. Heberling, R. L., Kalter, S. S., and Rodriguez, A. R., Poxvirus infection of the baboon (*Papio cynocephalus*), *Bull. WHO* **54**:285–294 (1976).

30. Heiner, G. G., Fatima, N., Daniel, R. W., Cole, J. L., Anthony, R. L., and McCrumb, F. R., Jr., A study of inapparent infection in smallpox, *Am. J. Epidemiol.* **94**:252 (1971).

31. Heiner, G. G., Fatima, N., and McCrumb, F. R., Jr., A study of intrafamilial transmission of smallpox, *Am. J. Epidemiol.* **94**:316–326 (1971).

32. Henderson, D. A., Importations of smallpox into Europe, *WHO Chron.* **28**:428–430 (1974).

33. Henderson, D. A., Smallpox, in: *Preventive Medicine and Public Health by Maxcy–Rosenau*, 10th ed. (P. E. Sartwell, ed.), pp. 104–116, Appleton-Century-Crofts, New York, 1973.

34. Henderson, D. A., and Arita, I., Monkeypox and its relevance to smallpox eradication, *WHO Chron.* **27**:145–148 (1973).

35. Henderson, R. H., Davis, H., Eddins, D. L., and Foege, W. H., Assessment of vaccination coverage, vaccination scar rates, and smallpox scarring in five areas of West Africa, *Bull. WHO* **48**:183–194 (1973).

36. Herrlich, A., Mayr, A., Mahnel, H., and Munz, E., Experimental studies on transformation of the variola virus into the vaccinia virus, *Arch. Gesamte Virusforsch.* **12**:479–599 (1963).

37. Hull, E., Smallpox contagiousness, *J. Am. Med. Assoc.* **219**:750, 755 (1972).

38. Hunt, J. H., Dr. Benjamin Waterhouse and the introduction of vaccination into the United States, *Brooklyn Med. J.* **10**:391–395 (1896).

38a. Hutchinson, H. D., Ziegler, D. W., Wells, D. E., and Nakano, J. H., Differentiation of variola, monkeypox, and vaccinia antisera by radioimmunoassay, *Bull. WHO* **55**:613–623 (1977).

39. Irons, J. V., Sullivan, T. D., Cook, E. B. M., Cox, G. W., and Hale, R. A., Outbreak of smallpox in the lower Rio Grande Valley of Texas in 1949, *Am. J. Public Health* **43**:25–29 (1953).

40. Jefferson, T., Letter from Thomas Jefferson to Dr.

Jenner (quoted in Hunt[38]), *Brooklyn Med. J.* **10**:395 (1896).

41. Jenner, E., *An Inquiry into the Causes and Effects of the Variolae Vacciniae, a Disease Discovered in Some of the Western Counties of England, Particularly Gloucestershire, and Known by the Name of Cowpox,* Sampson Low, London, 1798.

42. Kahn, C., History of smallpox and its prevention, *Am. J. Dis. Child.* **106**:597–609 (1963).

43. Kempe, C. H., Berge, T. O., and England, B., Hyperimmune vaccinal gamma globulin: Source, evaluation and use in prophylaxis and therapy, *Pediatrics* **18**:177–188 (1956).

44. Koplan, J. P., Goldstein, J., and Foster, S. O., Congenital vaccinia: Some doubts, *Pediatrics* **50**:971–972 (1972).

45. Lane, J. M., Complications following smallpox vaccination, in: *International Symposium on Smallpox Vaccine* (R. H. Regamey and H. Cohen, eds.), pp. 217–226, S. Karger, Basel, 1973.

46. Lane, J. M., Ruben, F. L., Neff, J. M., and Millar, J. D., Complications of smallpox vaccination, 1968, *N. Engl. J. Med.* **281**:1201–1208 (1969).

47. Langmuir, A. D., Vaccination should be abolished in the United States except for selected populations, in: *Controversy in Internal Medicine II* (F. J. Ingelfinger, R. V. Ebert, M. Finland, and A. J. Relman, eds.), pp. 363–370, W. B. Saunders, Philadelphia, 1974.

48. Leake, J. P., Smallpox or variola, *Med. Clin. North Am.* **27**:603–616 (1943).

49. Leikind, M. C., Variolation in Europe and America, *Ciba Symp.* **3**:1090–1101 (1942).

50. Leikind, M. C., The introduction of vaccination into the United States, *Ciba Symp.* **3**:1114–1124 (1942).

51. Long, G. W., Noble, J., Murphy, F. A., Herrmann, K. L., and Lourie, B., Experience with electron microscopy in the differential diagnosis of smallpox, *Appl. Microbiol.* **20**:497–504 (1970).

51a. Lourie, B., Nakano, J. H., Kemp, G. E., and Setzer, H. W., Isolation of poxvirus from an African Rodent, *J. Infect. Dis.* **132**:677–681 (1975).

52. Macaulay, T. B., *The History of England from the Accession of James the Second,* Vol. 4, p. 369, E. H. Butler, Philadelphia, 1856.

53. MacCallum, F. O., and McDonald, J. R., Survival of variola virus in raw cotton, *Bull. WHO* **16**:247–254 (1957).

54. Mack, T. M., Smallpox in Europe, 1950–1971, *J. Infect. Dis.* **125**:161–169 (1972).

55. Mack, T. M., Thomas, D. B., and Khan, M. M., Variola major in West Pakistan, *J. Infect. Dis.* **122**:479–488 (1970).

56. Mack, T. M., Thomas, D. B., Ali, A., and Khan, M. M., Epidemiology of smallpox in West Pakistan. I.

57. Mack, T. M., Thomas, D. B., and Khan, M. M., Epidemiology of smallpox in West Pakistan. II. Determinants of intravillage spread other than acquired immunity, *Am. J. Epidemiol.* **95**:169–177 (1972).

58. Marennikova, S. S., Seluhina, E. M., Mal'ceva, N. N., Cimiskjan, K. L., and Macevic, G. R., Isolation and properties of the causal agent of a new variola-like disease (monkeypox) in man, *Bull. WHO* **46**:599–611 (1972).

59. Marennikova, S. S., Seluhina, E. M., Mal'ceva, N. N., and Ladnyj, I. D., Poxviruses isolated from clinically ill and asymptomatically infected monkeys and a chimpanzee, *Bull. WHO* **46**:613–620 (1972).

59a. Marennikova, S. A., and Seluhina, E. M., Susceptibility of some rodent species to monkeypox virus, and course of the infection, *Bull. WHO* **53**:13–20 (1976).

60. Marshall, M. S., The first smallpox vaccine in the Americas, *Am. Soc. Microbiol. News* **40**:443–445 (1974).

61. Martin, H. A., Jefferson as a vaccinator, *N. C. Med. J.* **7**:1–35 (1881).

62. McCarthy, K., and Downie, A. W., The antibody response in man following infection with viruses of the pox group. II. Antibody response following vaccination, *J. Hyg.* **56**:466–478 (1958).

62a. McIntosh, K., Cherry, J. D., Benenson, A. S., Connor, J. D., Alling, D. W., Rolfe, U. T., Todd, W. A., Schanberger, J. E., and Mattheis, M. J., A clinical and serologic study of four smallpox vaccines comparing variations of dose and route of administration: Primary percutaneous vaccination: Standard percutaneous revaccination of children who received primary percutaneous vaccination, *J. Infect. Dis.* **135**:155–166 (1977).

63. Millar, J. D., Roberto, R. R., Wulff, H., Wenner, H. A., and Henderson, D. A., Smallpox vaccination by intradermal jet injection. I. Introduction, background and results of pilot studies, *Bull. WHO* **41**:749–760 (1969).

64. Nakano, J. H., Evaluation of virological laboratory methods for smallpox diagnosis, *Bull. WHO* **48**:529–534 (1973).

65. Nakano, J. H., and Bingham, P. G., Smallpox, vaccinia, and human infections with monkeypox viruses, in: *Manual of Clinical Microbiology,* 2nd ed. (E. H. Lennette, E. H. Spaulding, and J. P. Truant, eds.), pp. 782–794, American Society for Microbiology, Washington, D.C., 1974.

66. Nanning, W., Prophylactic effect of antivaccinia gamma-globulin against post-vaccinal encephalitis, *Bull. WHO* **27**:317–324 (1962).

67. Nizamuddin, M. D., and Dumbell, K. R., A simple

laboratory test to distinguish the virus of smallpox from that of alastrim, *Lancet* **1**:68–69 (1961).

68. Noble, J., Jr., and Rich, J. A., Transmission of smallpox by contact and by aerosol routes in *Macaca irus*, *Bull. WHO* **40**:279–286 (1969).

69. Nyerges, G., Erdos, L., and Melly, E., Smallpox vaccination immunity in relation to number of insertions, *Bull. WHO* **48**:397–400 (1973).

70. Palmquist, E. E., The 1946 smallpox experience in Seattle, *Can. J. Public Health* **38**:213–218 (1947).

71. Polak, M. F., Complications of smallpox vaccination in the Netherlands, 1959–1970, in: *International Symposium on Smallpox Vaccine* (R. H. Regamey and H. Cohen, eds.), pp. 235–242, S. Karger, Basel, 1973.

72. Polak, M. F., Beunders, J. J. W., Van Der Werff, A. R., Sanders, E. W., Van Klaveren, J. N., and Brans, L. M., A comparative study of clinical reaction observed after application of several smallpox vaccines in primary vaccination of young adults, *Bull. WHO* **29**:311–322 (1963).

73. Rao, A. R., Haemorrhagic smallpox, a study of 240 cases, *J. Indian Med. Assoc.* **43**:224–229 (1964).

74. Rao, A. R., *Smallpox*, The Kothari Book Depot, Bombay 12, 1972.

75. Rao, A. R., Jacob, E. S., Kamalakshi, S., Appaswamy, S., and Bradbury, Epidemiological studies in smallpox: A study of intrafamilial transmission in a series of 254 infected families, *Indian J. Med. Res.* **56**:1826–1854 (1968).

76. Rao, A. R., Prahlad, I., Swaminathan, M., and Lakshmi, A., Pregnancy and smallpox, *J. Indian Med. Assoc.* **40**:353–363 (1963).

77. Rao, A. R., Sukumar, M. S., Kamalakshi, S., Paramasivam, T. V., Parasuraman, T. A. R., and Shantha, M., Experimental variola in monkeys. Part 1. Studies on disease enhancing property of cortisone in smallpox: A preliminary report, *Indian J. Med. Res.* **56**:1855–1865 (1968).

78. Roberts, J. A., Histopathogenesis of mousepox. I. Respiratory infection, *Br. J. Exp. Pathol.* **43**:451–461 (1962).

79. Sarkar, J. K., Chatterjee, S. N., Mitra, A. C., and Mondal, A., Antibody response in haemorrhagic smallpox, *Indian J. Med. Res.* **55**:1143–1149 (1967).

80. Sarkar, J. K., Hati, A. K., and Mitra, A. C., Role of mosquitoes in the spread of smallpox, *J. Infect. Dis.* **128**:781–783 (1973).

81. Sarkar, J. K., and Mitra, A. C., Virulence of variola virus isolated from smallpox cases of varying severity, *Indian J. Med. Res.* **55**:13–20 (1967).

82. Sarkar, J. K., Mitra, A. C., Muhkerjee, M. K., De, S. K., and Mazumdar, D. G., Virus excretion in smallpox. 1. Excretion in the throat, urine, and conjunctiva of patients, *Bull. WHO* **38**:517–522 (1973).

83. Sarkar, J. K., Mitra, A. C., Mukherjee, M. K., and De, S. K., Virus excretion in smallpox. 2. Excretion in the throats of household contacts, *Bull. WHO* **48**:523–527 (1973).

84. Sarkar, J. K., Ray, S., and Manji, P., Epidemiological and virological studies on the off-season smallpox cases in Calcutta, *Indian J. Med. Res.* **58**:829–839 (1970).

85. Simpson, H. N., The impact of disease on American history, *N. Engl. J. Med.* **250**:679–682 (1954).

86. Stearn, E. W., and Stearn, A. E., *The Effect of Smallpox on the Destiny of the Amerindian*, pp. 44–45, Bruce Humphries, Boston, 1945.

87. Thomas, D. B., Arita, I., McCormack, W. M., Khan, M. M., Islam, S., and Mack, T. M., Endemic smallpox in rural Pakistan. II. Intravillage transmission and infectiousness, *Am. J. Epidemiol.* **93**:373–383 (1971).

88. Thomas, D. B., Mack, T. M., Ali, A., and Khan, M. M., Epidemiology of smallpox in West Pakistan. III. Outbreak detection and interlocality transmission, *Am. J. Epidemiol.* **95**:178–189 (1972).

89. Thomas, D. B., McCormack, W. M., Arita, I., Khan, M. M., Islam, M. S., and Mack, T. M., Endemic smallpox in rural East Pakistan. II. Methodology, clinical and epidemiological characteristics of cases, and intervillage transmission, *Am. J. Epidemiol.* **93**:361–372 (1971).

90. Wehrle, P. F., Posch, J., Richter, K. H., and Henderson, D. A., An airborne outbreak of smallpox in a German hospital and its significance with respect to other recent outbreaks in Europe, *Bull. WHO* **43**:669–679 (1970).

91. Weinstein, I., An outbreak of smallpox in New York City, *Am. J. Public Health* **37**:1376–1384 (1947).

92. Winslow, O. E., *A Destroying Angel: The Conquest of Smallpox in Colonial Boston*, Houghton Mifflin, Boston, 1974.

92a. Wolff, H. L., and Croon, J. J. A. B., The survival of smallpox virus (variola minor) in natural circumstances, *Bull. WHO* **38**:492–493 (1968).

93. Woodward, S. B., The story of smallpox in Massachusetts, *N. Engl. J. Med.* **206**:1182–1191 (1932).

94. World Health Organization, WHO Expert Committee on Smallpox, First Report, *WHO Tech. Rep. Ser.*, No. 283 (1964).

95. World Health Organization, WHO Scientific Group, Smallpox Eradication, *WHO Tech. Rep. Ser.*, No. 393 (1968).

96. World Health Organization, A decade of smallpox, *WHO Chron.* **22**:134–141 (1968).

97. World Health Organization, *Guide to the Laboratory Diagnosis of Smallpox for Smallpox Eradication Programmes*, WHO, Geneva, 1969.

98. WORLD HEALTH ORGANIZATION, Smallpox surveillance, *Weekly Epidemiol. Rec.* **47:**18 (1972).

99. WORLD HEALTH ORGANIZATION, Smallpox surveillance, *Weekly Epidemiol. Rec.* **47:**144 (1972).

100. WORLD HEALTH ORGANIZATION, Smallpox, *Weekly Epidemiol. Rec.* **47:**161–162 (1972).

101. WORLD HEALTH ORGANIZATION, WHO Expert Committee on Smallpox Eradication, Second Report, *WHO Tech. Rep. Ser.*, NO. 493 (1972).

102. WORLD HEALTH ORGANIZATION, Smallpox surveillance, *Weekly Epidemiol. Rec.* **49:**9–17 (1974).

103. WORLD HEALTH ORGANIZATION, Progress in smallpox eradication, *WHO Chron.* **28:**361 (1974).

104. WORLD HEALTH ORGANIZATION, Smallpox surveillance, *Weekly Epidemiol. Rec.* **50:**13–28 (1975).

105. WORLD HEALTH ORGANIZATION, Smallpox surveillance, *Weekly Epidemiol. Rec.* **53:**9–15 (1978).

106. WORLD HEALTH ORGANIZATION, Smallpox surveillance, *Weekly Epidemiol. Rec.* **53:**265–266 (1978).

107. WORLD HEALTH ORGANIZATION, Smallpox surveillance, *Weekly Epidemiol. Rec.* **53:**279 (1978).

108. WORLD HEALTH ORGANIZATION, Smallpox surveillance, *Weekly Epidemiol. Rec.* **48:**349 (1978).

109. WORLD HEALTH ORGANIZATION, Smallpox surveillance, *Weekly Epidemiol. Rec.* **54:**1–8 (1979).

110. WORLD HEALTH ORGANIZATION, Human monkeypox in West Africa, *Weekly Epidemiol. Rec.* **54:**12–13 (1979).

111. WORLD HEALTH ORGANIZATION, Smallpox eradication, *Weekly epidemiol. Rec.* **54:**36–37 (1979).

112. WORLD HEALTH ORGANIZATION, Smallpox surveillance, *Weekly Epidemiol. Rec.* **54:**85 (1979).

113. WORLD HEALTH ORGANIZATION, No more smallpox, *Weekly Epidemiol. Rec.* **54:**391 (1979).

114. WORLD HEALTH ORGANIZATION, Declaration of global eradication of smallpox, *Weekly Epidemiol. Rec.* **55:**148 (1980).

115. WORLD HEALTH ORGANIZATION, Smallpox eradication, *Weekly Epidemiol. Rec.* **56:**56 (1981).

12. Suggested Reading

CHRISTIE, A. B., *Infectious Diseases: Epidemiology and Clinical Practice*, pp. 185–237, E. & S. Livingstone, Edinburgh, 1969.

DICK, G., Smallpox: A reconsideration of public health policies, *Prog. Med. Virol.* **8:**1–29 (1966).

DIXON, C. W., *Smallpox*, J. & A. Churchill, London, 1962.

DOWNIE, A. W., Smallpox, in: *Infectious Agents and Host Reactions* (S. MUDD, ed.), pp. 487–518, W. B. Saunders, Philadelphia, 1970.

FENNER, F., The eradication of smallpox, *Prog. Med. Virol.* **23:**1–21 (1977).

FENNER, F., Portraits of viruses: The poxviruses, *Intervirology* **11:**137–157 (1979).

CHAPTER 23

Varicella–Herpes Zoster Virus

Thomas H. Weller

1. Introduction

1.1. Definition

Varicella–zoster virus (*Herpesvirus varicellae*), commonly abbreviated to "V-Z virus" or "VZV," is the etiological agent of two diseases of man, varicella and herpes zoster. Varicella (chickenpox) is a ubiquitous, contagious, generalized exanthematous disease of seasonally epidemic propensities that follows primary exposure of a susceptible person, most often a child. Herpes zoster (shingles) is an endemic sporadic disease, most frequent in elderly people, characterized by the appearance of a unilateral, painful, vesicular eruption localized to the dermatome innervated by a specific dorsal root or extramedullary cranial ganglion. In contrast to varicella, which follows primary exogenous contact with the causative virus, zoster reflects endogenous activation of a VZV infection that has survived in latent form following an attack of varicella. The two clinical entities are not as distinct as is customarily assumed. The patient with zoster frequently develops a disseminated varicelliform eruption; rarely, the person with varicella may exhibit a zosteriform concentration of lesions.

Thomas H. Weller · Department of Tropical Public Health, Center for Prevention of Infectious Diseases, Harvard School of Public Health, Boston, Massachusetts.

1.2. Social Significance

Varicella remains on the ever-shortening list of ubiquitous infectious diseases of childhood for which no vaccine is available in the United States. The social significance of chickenpox supports the need for prophylactic measures; some 4 million cases occur per year in the United States.[111] Usually relatively benign, the disease may be fatal in immunocompromised children. Although rare, a congenital varicella syndrome occurs. The prevalence of its delayed manifestation, herpes zoster, is now increasing in the developed world in proportion to the relative number of older people in the population. Additionally, iatrogenic herpes zoster is more common with the widespread usage of immunosuppressive and cytotoxic drugs that adversely influence host defense mechanisms.

2. Historical Background

2.1. Clinical Recognition

Herpes zoster was described in premedieval times. Varicella, however, was not differenitated from smallpox (variola) until the end of the 19th century. It is of interest that Osler [97] in 1892 deemed it necessary to emphasize that "there can be no question that varicella is an affection quite distinct from variola and without at present any relation whatever to it." However, to this day, the mild or atypical case of smallpox may pose a problem in differential diagnosis vis-à-vis varicella, resolvable only with the aid of virological investigations.

The infectious nature of varicella was demonstrated in 1875 by Steiner,[123] who induced the disease in volunteers by inoculating them with vesicular fluid from patients with chickenpox. Herpes zoster was experimentally transmitted in similar fashion by Kundratitz[75] in 1925, with the production of varicelliform cutaneous lesions.

2.2. Association of Varicella with Herpes Zoster

Interest in the relationship between varicella and herpes zoster dates from the clinical observations of von Bokay[15] in 1888 that susceptible children acquired varicella after contact with persons with herpes zoster. (Subsequently, this association was repeatedly observed; the report of the School Epidemics Committe of Great Britain[117] in 1938, for example, linked 18 outbreaks of varicella to an exposure to zoster.) Additional evidence in support of the monistic etiological concept of the two clinical entities slowly accrued. Tyzzer,[136] in 1906 described superbly the histopathology of the cutaneous lesion in varicella, with its characteristic intranuclear inclusion-containing multinucleate giant cells. An identical histopathological picture for the skin lesion of zoster was recorded by Lipschütz[79] in 1921. Technically difficult studies in the 1930s by several workers who employed vesicular-fluid material as antigen suggested an immunological relationship. In the early 1940s, Zinsser[160] and Sabin[110] alluded to the probable close relationship of the two etiological agents; emphasis at that period focused on the theoretical existence of strains of virus that possessed differing dermatropic or neurotropic affinities. Garland[42] suggested in 1943 that zoster reflected activation of a latent varicella virus, a mechanism similar to that obtaining with the virus of herpes simplex, and he should be credited with first expressing this now generally accepted thesis.

2.3. Isolation and Propagation of the Etiological Agent of Varicella–Zoster

Substantiation of the view that varicella and herpes zoster have a common etiology followed the isolation and propagation *in vitro* by us of the etiological virus.[140,144] By 1958, we[143,145,146] had completed various investigations on agents recovered from patients with varicella and with herpes zoster. These studies revealed no differences in the biological or immunological attributes of viruses isolated from patients with the two clinical entities. We therefore referred to the agent as *varicella-zoster (V-Z) virus* and concluded that "the accumulation of epidemiologic and laboratory evidence in support of the hypothesis that a single etiologic agent is responsible for varicella and herpes zoster appears so impressive that the burden of proof must now logically shift to those who desire to refute the monistic concept."[145]

Since the isolation of VZV the concept that cases of herpes zoster reflect activation of a preexisting latent VZV has been generally accepted. Interest has shifted from the hypothesis that dermatropic and neurotropic strains of VZV exist to the study of the as yet ill-defined mechanisms of host resistance that, when depressed, permit activation of a previously latent VZV.

Parenthetically, confusion with herpes simplex virus (HSV) is to be avoided; while VZV and HSV are both members of the herpes group of viruses, the relationship is distant and the agents are distinct.

3. Methodology Involved in Epidemiological Analysis

3.1. Sources of Mortality Data

In the United States, deaths attributable to chickenpox and to herpes zoster are coded separately and are recorded annually in *Vital Statistics of the United States*, National Center for Health Statistics. Deaths from varicella, most often due to a specific pneumonia or a diffuse hemorrhagic process, have a high probability of accurate attribution; however, those resulting from a postinfectious varicella encephalitis are subject to errors of diagnosis.

Reported deaths[25] from herpes zoster (averaging 108 per year from 1972 to 1976) have slowly increased and now approach those ascribed to varicella (average 111 per year from 1972 to 1976). Some of the deaths attributed to zoster might be more accurately attributed to the inciting disease process, but severe zoster is increasing with the expanded use of immunodepressant therapy.

3.2. Sources of Morbidity Data

3.2.1. Reporting of Cases

a. Requirement for Notification in the United States. Varicella, prior to 1972, was not reportable nationally in the United States. While in certain states chickenpox has been notifiable for many years—for example, since 1910 in Massachusetts—in four states, the disease remained unnotifiable as of 1977. Herpes zoster is generally not reportable.

b. Inadequacies of Notification. Only a fraction of the cases of varicella occurring in the United States are reported. In 1936, 200,000 families in 28 cities in the United States were surveyed to establish the occurrence of communicable diseases; the notification rate of chickenpox cases was estimated to be 20–40% of the actual number.[27] In 1947, Feemster, as cited by Gordon,[56] concluded that only 25% of the cases in Massachusetts were reported. This comparatively high rate probably has not been maintained as interest in infectious diseases has waned. It is currently estimated that the level of reporting in New York City is of the order of 8–10%.[80] A report from the national Center for Disease Control[67] suggests an average figure of 10% for the country. That the level of reporting is totally inadequate and extremely variable from state to state is shown by the fact that three states in which the disease is notifiable reported fewer than 100 cases of varicella in 1977.[25]

c. Occurrence of Inapparent Infections. In contrast to an infection such as mumps, most cases of varicella are clinically apparent. However, in a fraction of infected persons, probably less than 5%, the exanthem is so sparse and transient that its occurrence, especially in the dark-skinned patient, may be missed by the qualified observer. From an analysis of secondary and tertiary attack rates after home exposure, Ross[105] concluded that no more than 4% of cases are unrecognized. The visibility of the disease is indicated by the study by Ross of the number of pocks per child as established by a single home visit on the 6th day to the 9th day of illness. In four groups, mean counts of pocks per child varied from 207 to 510, with a range of 10–1968. Herpes zoster also may exhibit minimal cutaneous lesions. Cases have been described of zosterlike pain in the absence of an overt segmental eruption, with a concurrent rise in specific antibody.

3.2.2. Clinical Observation and Retrospective Histories.
Data on the communicability of varicella derive primarily from the careful study of exposed susceptible children in households, in schools, or on hospital wards. The accuracy of a negative history of varicella depends on the informant and on the time span since the period of maximum risk. The parent of the young child is a better informant than is the subject at an older age. However, in a large-scale retrospective study on the occurrence of chickenpox in the United States,[27] it was concluded that the "forgetting factor" became important for subjects as young as 9 years of age, a period when the parent would be the major informant. Inability to remember past events certainly accounts for the low exposure attack rate of 12% observed by Hope-Simpson[61] in intimately exposed "susceptibles" aged 15 years or more. Ross[105] reported an attack rate of 5% in "susceptible" parents in contrast to a rate of 87% in "susceptible" children. Conversely, the attack rate in children with "positive" histories was 7%. In a serological investigation of children with "negative" histories, one-third of those tested were reactive with a VZV antigen.[49]

The defective memory of the older person with herpes zoster, when questioned regarding the previous occurrence of varicella, has led to confusion. Indeed, the "forgetting factor" played a significant role in the slow acceptance of the monistic view of the etiology of VZV. Contrast, for example, the study in Great Britain of herpes zoster in schoolchildren,[117] wherein a history of varicella could be obtained for 71% of 66 boys with the disease, with the observations of the astute country practitioner of epidemiology, W. N. Pickles,[100] who observed 56 cases of herpes zoster in older people. Pickles specifically queried of his patients with shingles regarding prior chickenpox; only one gave a postive response, leading to the erroneous conclusion that "in view of the suffering caused by herpes zoster in adults it would seem a great misfortune not to acquire chickenpox in early life."

3.3. Serological Surveys

3.3.1. Methodology.
New or improved methods for detection of VZV antibody are being introduced, and serodiagnosis is in a state of evolution. Addi-

tionally, a skin test,[10,70] in the preliminary phase of investigation, may provide a convenient means of rapid assessment of the cellular immune state. These developments have been stimulated by the need to establish quickly the state of susceptibility or lack of susceptibility of the high-risk varicella-exposed subject as justification for institution of specific preventive measures. Criteria for selection of a procedure therefore include availability and rapidity of performance as well as those of specificity and sensitivity.

Of the classic tests, complement fixation (CF)[142,145] has been widely used, and antigen is available from commercial sources; the limitations of the test are discussed below. The neutralization (N) test as performed by plaque reduction is definitive, but time-consuming, and requires cell-free live virus. The problem of obtaining cell-free virus is being resolved, but precludes widespread use of the N test.[9] Labeling of plaques by the direct immunoperoxidase technique shortens the time of performance.[43]

The indirect fluorescent antibody (IFA) test,[116] which utilizes intracytoplasmic and nuclear VZV antigen in acetone-fixed infected cells, can be used as a rapid indicator of the immune state of an exposed person.[57] A modification of the IFA test based on visualization of a viral-induced specific antigen on the membrane of infected cells,[49] referred to as FAMA, is a sensitive indicator of past infection.[47] The FAMA procedure now can be carried out with glutaraldehyde-fixed infected target cells,[159] thus eliminating the constraints and danger inherent in the use of living infected cells.

Two types of hemagglutination procedure have been applied. An indirect hemagglutination (IHA) reaction,[41,83,135] employing fixed red cells as the carrier for culture-derived antigen, is relatively simple to use. The immune adherence hemagglutination (IAHA) test[46] is technically more involved in that antigen–antibody complexes with complement, resulting in activation of the C3 component, which in turn reacts with receptor sites on the red cells to cause agglutination. The sensitivity of the IAHA test approaches that of FAMA[53,69,155]; however, IAHA is slightly less sensitive for the detection of reactive persons, especially those over age 40.[38,69]

While the procedure of radioimmunoassay can be used to detect VZV antibody,[39] it is probable that the highly sensitive enzyme-linked immunosorbent assay (ELISA), recently adapted to studies of VZV antibody,[38] will, because of ease of performance, rapidly come into general use.

3.3.2. Limitations of the Seroepidemiological Approach. Two problems, sensitivity and specificity, deserve consideration in the interpretation of seroepidemiological data. Of the commonly used tests, CF is the least sensitive. Within months after a primary attack of VZV, titers of antibody detectable by CF begin to fall and may reach subdetectable levels. In surveys using CF in the United States[148] and in England,[134] a peak reactivity of around 70% was demonstrable in the 10–20 year age group; in the Seattle study, the rate had fallen to 35% by age 45–49. Parenthetically, in comparison to the persistent antibody responses that follow use of the experimental Japanese VZV vaccine, the CF response after vaccination is labile and of short duration.[8]

The problem of specificity relates to nonspecific rises in titer of VZV antibodies that occur in the person infected with herpes simplex virus (HSV), and vice versa.[71,107,129] However, heterologous responses, as for example a rise in VZV titer in a patient infected with HSV, occur only when the subject has previously been infected with the heterologous agent[113,115]; in each instance, the rise in titer to the current agent greatly exceeds that to the heterologous virus. In general, the more sensitive the serological test, the greater the probability of the detection of low-order heterotypic rises.[38,53,155] While VZV–HSV cross-reactions pose diagnostic problems, the problems are not important in seroepidemiological surveys. Application of one of the new sensitive techniques will eliminate the false negatives commonly observed when the VZV CF reaction is applied to older persons.

3.4. Laboratory Methods

3.4.1. Isolation of Virus. The definitive diagnosis of varicella or herpes zoster is based on the isolation of the etiological agent.[142] Since common laboratory animals are not susceptible, cultures of susceptible cells must be used. While VZV exhibits a lesser degree of host specificity *in vitro* than *in vivo*, cultures of human cells are the most sensitive indicators of VZV; a further consideration is that confluent, transparent, well-organized sheets of cells provide optimal conditions for microscopic detection of the focal lesions induced by VZV. These criteria are satisfied by actively growing cultures of fibroblasts, kidney cells, or amnion cells, all of human origin. One of these culture systems is usually employed for the isolation of VZV.

VZV can be recovered with ease by inoculation of cultures of human cells with the aspirated contents of vesicular lesions. Selection of the young "dewdrop" lesion containing clear fluid is important. Chances of recovery of virus decrease as the lesion becomes pustular, and VZV, in contrast to variola virus, cannot be isolated from crusts or scabs. VZV can be readily isolated during the first 3 days of the exanthem in varicella; isolation of virus thereafter is rare unless the disease is atypical, as in the immunologically compromised host.[54,133,146] Virus can be recovered from the cutaneous lesions of patients with zoster for a longer period of time, i.e., at times to the 7th day or later after the appearance of the segmental vesiculopustular process.

The focal cytopathic process produced by VZV in cultures of susceptible cells has to be differentiated from the transiently focal lesions of the virus of herpes simplex (HSV) or the more persistent focal lesions induced by the human cytomegaloviruses (CMVs). The VZV focal lesion in a sheet of susceptible cells may be apparent as early as 2 days after inoculation—or as late as 3–4 weeks. Microplaques develop, observable under $100\times$ magnification as consisting of a few small, refractile cells. Each microplaque enlarges slowly by involvement of contiguous cells, with progressive degeneration of the older central portion. Very little infectious virus is released from the infected cells, and the number of foci increases slowly. However, peripheral extension of the process continues, with eventual involvement of most of the cell sheet. Stained preparations reveal intranuclear inclusions in involved cells, particularly at the marginal plaque interface. Confirmation of identity of the isolate, and in particular differentiation from CMV, can be accomplished immunologically by use of specific VZV antisera in direct fluorescent antibody (FA) tests or by performance of CF or other serological tests in which the antigen derives from the infected culture. For technical details, the reader is referred to a standard reference on diagnostic procedures.[142]

3.4.2. Rapid Diagnostic Approaches in Urgent Clinical Situations. The diagnosis of the patient presenting with a vesiculopustular eruption re-

quires that varicella and varicelliform eruptions due to HSV be differentiated from those caused by variola–vaccinia viruses. Unless smallpox can be ruled out with certainty, specimens from the patient should be considered as highly infectious and dangerous and should be handled accordingly. Standard procedures should be followed.[29,142] Usually, this will involve transmittal of specimens to a reference laboratory.

In the interim, however, simple procedures can be applied to differentiate the two groups of etiological agents. Examination of stained smears from the base of a fresh lesion, or of a biopsy thereof, will, if the patient is infected with VZV or HSV, reveal multinucleate giant cells and other cells with intranuclear inclusions as originally described by Tyzzer[136]; neither giant cells nor intranuclear inclusions are present in the lesions of variola and vaccinia. Microgel precipitin diagnostic techniques are also useful. As applied to varicella,[137] the procedure has two advantages: A definitive answer can be obtained in 12–24 hr. Also, antigenically reactive material can be demonstrated in extracts of crusts of involuting lesions; positive tests have been obtained from materials collected as late as 14 days after onset of varicella and 23 days after onset of herpes zoster.

If appropriately absorbed antisera and FA facilities are available, application of the IFA test to biopsy material from a cutaneous lesion will rapidly differentiate VZV and HSV lesions.[96]

4. Biological Characteristics of the Virus That Affect the Epidemiological Pattern

4.1. Latency in the Human Host: Primary Infection, Latency, and Reactivation

VZV shares with other herpesviruses the capacity to persist in the body after the primary infection. Decades later, the virus may again become manifest with renewed replication and the production of the clinical syndrome of herpes zoster. Immunologically inexperienced persons in intimate contact with the patient with herpes zoster can contact varicella. Thus, VZV is epidemiologically unique in that it can persist for years in a mobile human incubator, roam globally, and when host defense mechanisms decay again, replicate and initiate an outbreak of the primary disease.

4.2. Failure of Varicella–Zoster Virus to Persist in Scabs or Fomites: Limited Period of Communicability

In contrast to the variola–vaccinia viruses, which survive for long periods in scabs, VZV cannot be recovered from crusts or from the involuting lesions. The period of communicability is therefore discrete and coincident with the duration of vesicular lesions. Room dust is not infectious and terminal disinfection is not indicated.

5. Descriptive Epidemiology

5.1. Incidence and Prevalence Data

5.1.1. General Comments on Varicella. In modern industrialized societies in the temperate areas of the world, almost all persons contract varicella, usually during childhood. Reported annual incidence rates of 85.7 and 87.1 per 100,000 population in the United States for the years 1976 and 1977 are misleading[25]; application of a corrective factor of 10- to 20-fold would probably yield data closer to the actual situation. Figure 1A summarizes the reported cases of chickenpox per 100,000 population in Massachusetts from 1910 through 1977; these data reflect an unknown degree of underreporting.

Varicella is a benign disease in the immunologically uncompromised child in the United States; the few deaths that do occur usually reflect illness in the infant or the adult. However, as physicians increasingly employ immunosuppressant agents in the therapy of conditions such as nephrosis in children, and as the mean life expectancy of children with malignancies, especially leukemia, is prolonged by medical means, fatalities due to a complicating varicella infection can be expected to increase. Thus, the downtrend in mortality associated with varicella as reflected in Table 1, which summarizes mortality data for Massachusetts by decade, can be expected to reverse. The benign nature of varicella in England has been emphasized[76]; in a population of approximately 1 million, only 12 cases that required hospitalization occurred in 10 years. In 1965, about 20 deaths a year were reported from

England and Wales. In Australia, there were only 9 deaths among 1612 patients with varicella admitted to one hospital between 1943 and 1959.[16]

In tropical regions and the less developed regions of the world, the situation with respect to varicella is less clear. Morbidity and mortality statistics are essentially nonexistent. However, as noted below, fragmentary evidence suggests that climatic factors combine to inhibit transmission and to extend susceptibility into the older age groups as compared with industrialized societies.

5.1.2. General Comments on Herpes Zoster. Herpes zoster is a sporadic endemic disease reflecting reactivation of a latent host-contained infection with VZV, with incidence determined by factors influencing the host–parasite relationship. The primary determinant of prevalence is the age composition of the population, with particular reference to time elapsed since acquisition of the primary VZV infection. In a panel practice of some 3500 persons in England observed over a period of 16 years by Hope-Simpson[62] herpes zoster occurred at an annual rate of 3.4 per 1000 persons. Under similar circumstances in a panel practice in Scotland, McGregor[88] recorded an annual rate of 4.8 per 1000.

5.1.3. Risk of Infection in Susceptible Persons. Although varicella has a justifiable reputation as a highly contagious disease, intimate rather than casual contact is required for a high transmission rate. In an analysis based on reported cases of varicella in New York City, the infectivity of chickenpox in households and in society as expressed as annual exposures divided by average number of susceptibles was 0.61 and 0.12, respectively.[156] In comparison with measles (rubeola), which was arbitrarily assigned an infectivity potential of 100%, chickenpox was 80% as infectious in households and 46% as infectious in society.

The most accurate data on the infectivity of varicella derive from experimental studies on attempts to modify varicella in which carefully observed control populations of susceptible children were at risk. In such a study, Ross[105] observed a secondary attack rate of 87% in susceptible siblings in households following the introduction of the primary case of varicella; a tertiary attack rate of 71% was observed among those siblings (i.e., 13% of the original group) who had escaped infection on exposure to the primary household contact.

Hope-Simpson[61] summarized data on the infec-

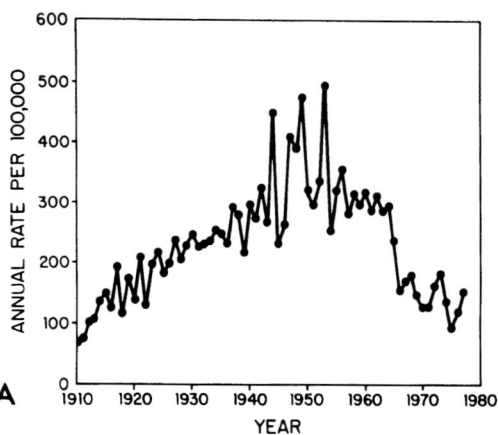

Fig. 1. Reported cases of chickenpox per 100,000 population per year in Massachusetts from 1910 through 1977 (A) and in the United States from 1972 through 1977 (B). Sources: Massachusetts Department of Public Health, Division of Communicable Diseases, Dr. Nicholas J. Fiumara, Director, and the Center for Disease Control, Atlanta, Georgia.

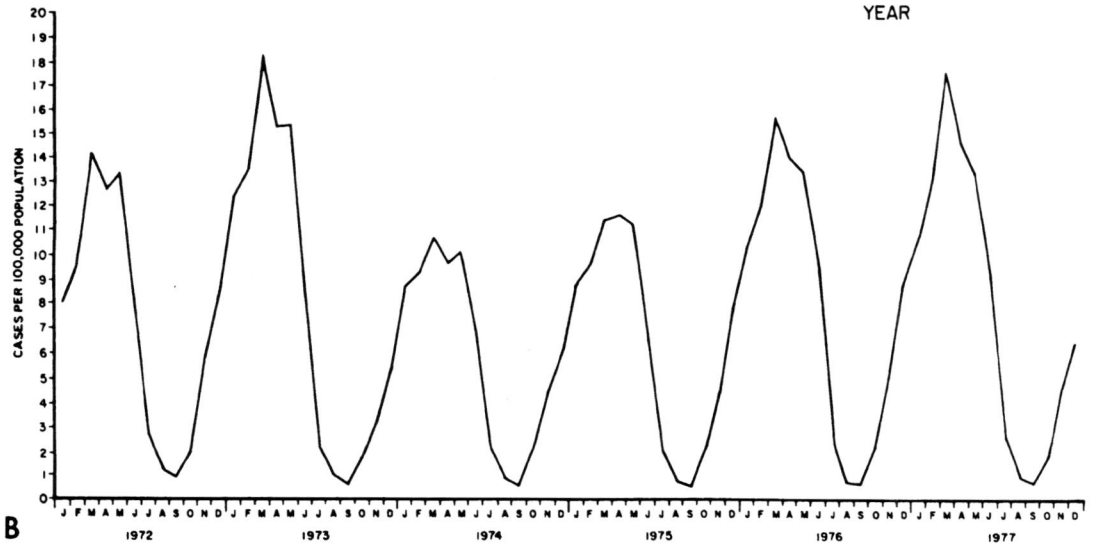

Table 1. Deaths from Chickenpox and Mean Annual Death Rate per 100,000 Population, by Decades, Massachusetts, 1910–1969[a]

Years	Mid-decade population	Deaths	Mean annual death rate
1910–1919	3,701,000	48	0.13
1920–1929	4,158,000	83	0.20
1930–1939	4,361,000	69	0.16
1940–1949	4,511,000	39	0.08
1950–1959	4,853,000	30	0.06
1960–1969	5,343,255	22	0.04

[a] Source: Massachusetts Department of Public Health, Division of Communicable Diseases, Dr. Nicholas J. Fiumara, Director.

tiousness of varicella in a semirural area in Gloucestershire, England; the exposure attack rate among susceptibles, aged 0–15 years, in homes was 61%. In a hospital environment, Gordon[56] cites an experience with a dozen outbreaks of varicella on the wards in which the attack rate among 81 susceptibles was 68%.

The patient with herpes zoster is also infectious. Anecdotal evidence suggests that the patient with zoster poses less of a risk than does the patient with varicella. It has been postulated that the zoster patient is less infectious because the lesions are circumscribed and often covered by clothing. The validity of this thesis is mitigated by the fact that approximately one third of patients with zoster exhibit disseminated cutaneous lesions, indicating the occurrence of a viremia.[95] Perhaps of more import is the fact that patients with zoster often possess significant titers of specific antibody at the time the exanthem is fully developed[145]; therefore, partial neutralization of free infectious virus in the evolving lesion may occur *in vivo* before it is released into the environment.

5.2. Epidemic Behavior

5.2.1. Varicella. In industrialized societies in temperate regions, varicella is endemic in the total population, but epidemic in susceptible clustered subgroups, and exhibits a characteristic seasonal fluctuation in incidence. Data from Massachusetts reveal a pattern of low levels of endemicity at the beginning of the 60-year period that started in 1910 (Fig. 1A and Table 2). Gordon,[56] who examined the data from Massachusetts in 1962, concluded that the pattern to that time was one of mildly fluctuating increasing endemicity, with superimposed recurring epidemics about equally divided between outbreaks at intervals of 2 years and 3 years; two had an interval of 4 years. The increase in annual rates from 1910 to the 1940s was attributed by Gordon to a gradual improvement in reporting.

With data since 1962 now available, in retrospect it would appear that the peak rates of over 400/100,000 in 1944, 1947, 1949, and 1953 in Massachusetts, with intervening extreme fluctuations, reflect the dislocations of the population in the war years,

followed by postwar spurts in the birth rate. A similar but less marked period of fluctuation in annual incidence is reflected by the data for the period of World War I and immediately thereafter. Thus, except for the war periods, reported rates reflect a relatively smooth increase in annual incidence between 1910 and 1940, little influenced by epidemics, with a tendency to plateau at a level of 300/100,000 between 1940 and 1964. Between 1964 and 1966, rates in Massachusetts fell abruptly to the current level of under 200/100,000 per year. Thus, varicella in Massachusetts is at its lowest ebb in half a century, a phenomenon not unique to this state, for data from New York City reveal a parallel decrease in annual incidence.[156]

The apparent 50-year rise and fall in the level of endemicity of varicella in Massachusetts and in New York is of interest. Much of the decline in prevalence observed during the past decade is probably artifactual due to deterioration of the reporting process. This explanation is supported by authorities in New York City.[86] However, as noted below, current low levels of prevalence are paralleled by an altered pattern of seasonal incidence and, to a lesser extent, of age-specific attack rates; therefore, the cyclical phenomenon is not solely an artifact of reporting. It is likely that the recent decrease in prevalence also reflects a declining birth rate and a decrease in the relative number of susceptible children. Other hypotheses deserve examination. Has, for example, some subtle shift in the host–parasite relationship occurred? Is the disease now associated with fewer pocks and thus more often overlooked, perhaps because the average child is better nourished or is less likely to experience another concurrent infectious process? Has the virus become attenuated in nature? These questions are unanswerable. Time will reveal whether current low levels of prevalence will persist or whether rates will again gradually rise and then fall, indicating the existence of long-term cyclic fluctuations in the prevalence of varicella heretofore unrecognized.

In contrast to the endemic nature of varicella in the population at large, epidemics follow introduction of varicella into intimately associated subgroups or clusters of susceptibles. Typical is the school situation described by Wells and Holla[147]; of 67 susceptible children in grades 0–4, 61 contracted the disease in an explosive outbreak. Within elements of larger population groups, as in different boroughs

Table 2. Reported Cases of Chickenpox and Mean Annual Case Rate per 100,000, by Decades, Massachusetts, 1910–1969[a]

Decade	Cases per decade	Mean annual rate per 100,000 (based on mid-decade population)
1910–1919	45,689	123.4
1920–1929	79,765	191.8
1930–1939	106,979	245.3
1940–1949	151,163	335.1
1950–1959	158,084	311.5
1960–1969	125,598	235.1

[a] Source: Massachusetts Department of Public Health, Division of Communicable Diseases, Dr. Nicholas J. Fiumara, Director.

in New York City, levels of endemicity vary annually, reflecting the varying summation of epidemic outbreaks in clusters of susceptibles[156] within each borough.

5.2.2. Herpes Zoster. Herpes zoster is an endemic disease that shows no seasonal pattern and appears in "epidemic proportions" only when induced iatrogenically in specialized groups of patients such as those under chemotherapy because of malignancy. In this instance, the situation reflects chance concurrent reactivation of a latent agent in each patient and not person-to-person transmission.

5.3. Geographic Distribution

5.3.1. Varicella. Varicella and herpes zoster occur throughout the world. There is evidence that in tropical regions, as contrasted to temperate regions, varicella is seen more often in adults. Annual rates for varicella in the U.S. Army in World War II in the Latin American area, where a large number of soldiers from Puerto Rico were stationed, were 1.41 and 2.27 per 1000, respectively, in 1944 and 1945; the comparable figures for the continental United States were 0.71 and 0.61 for the same years.[127] Brunell[18] notes that a majority of pregnant women with varicella observed in New York are of Caribbean origin; of a group studied by Siegel[119] 52% were Puerto Ricans. In Ceylon, varicella was observed to be at least as common in adults as in children.[85] In an Indian village observed over a period of 5 years, 63% of cases of varicella occurred in persons over the age of 15 years.[121] Investigation of cases of varicella in 1976 in the State of Kerala, India, carried out in the terminal phase of the smallpox eradication program, revealed that 50% of cases occurred in those 15 years of age or older.[149]

Three hypotheses have been proposed to explain the relative prevalence of varicella at older ages in the tropics. Transmission may be slowed by the relative isolation of familial clusters in rural areas.[149] It has been suggested that there may be "epidemiological interference" with other prevalent viruses, especially HSV.[121] Probably of equal or greater import is a decreased transmission potential due to ambient temperatues that enhance the relatively labile nature of VZV outside the human host.

As emphasized by Black et al.,[13] VZV can persist because of its latent capacity (i.e., zoster) on introduction into a geographically isolated, small human population; a single isolated Indian tribe in the Amazon, when surveyed serologically, was found to have levels of reactivity comparable to those in the United States.

5.3.2. Herpes Zoster. Available data do not suggest geographic differences in the distribution of herpes zoster. If, however, varicella is acquired at a mean older age in tropical areas, herpes zoster should also occur at a relatively older age. In Kerala, India, herpes zoster is said to be almost unknown.[149]

5.4. Temporal Distribution

5.4.1. Varicella. In the United States, varicella regularly shows a striking seasonal distribution. At the national level for the years 1975 and 1976, annual lows occurred in September (about 2000 cases), rose to peaks of 23,000 and 30,000 cases in March and April, remained relatively high through May, and then abruptly fell to typical summertime lows.[25] [In evaluating data on temporal distribution in terms of date of transmission, corrective factors for the duration of the incubation period (10–21 days) and for the lag in reporting must be considered.]

A somewhat similar seasonal distribution of cases reported in Massachusetts for the 5-year period ending in 1973 is depicted in Fig. 2. The peak incidence, however, is in May, as contrasted to the peak in March at the national level. Gordon[56] analyzed data for the 5 years between September 1956 and August 1961 (a period of relatively high prevalence, when 78,000 cases of varicella were reported, as contrasted to the 1968–1973 period, when 42,000 cases were reported); a bell-shaped monthly distribution was obtained, with peak mean numbers of cases in March and with slowly decreasing numbers through April, May and June. Comparison of the data for 1956–1961 with those for 1968–1973 (presented in Fig. 2) suggests that transmission differs seasonally in years of high prevalence as contrasted to periods of low prevalence. In years of high prevalence, a greater percentage of the pool of susceptibles is infected earlier in the transmission season. During periods of low prevalence, there is a temporal lag in progression of varicella through a community with extension of the seasonal epidemic into the late spring. A similar conclusion was reached by Yorke and London,[156] who calculated that in New York City, the mean monthly contact rates for 14 years

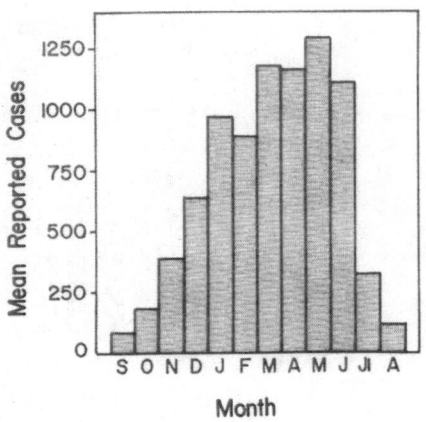

Fig. 2. Reported cases of chickenpox, mean numbers by month, state of Massachusetts, for the 5-year period September 1968 through August 1973. Source: Massachusetts Department of Public Health, Division of Communicable Diseases, Dr. Nicholas J. Fiumara, Director.

of high prevalence are about 5% higher in September and October ($p < 0.01$) and about 4% lower in May and June ($p < 0.05$) than the mean monthly contact rates for 16 years of low prevalence. Using the seasonal data on varicella in New York City, we have summarized the mean monthly cases reported for two 5-year periods, one of high and one of low prevalence (see Fig. 3). For the periods of low prevalence in New York City, the seasonal pattern of gradually increasing rates that peak in the late spring is even more striking than in Massachusetts.

Varicella in the United States is primarily a disease

of winter and spring. The customary explanation of the seasonal pattern relates to aggregation of susceptible children in schools in the fall, the introduction of the agent, and its subsequent dissemination to contacts in the classroom and to susceptible siblings in the home. This epidemiological pattern is dominant in the United States. It is questionable whether physical clustering of susceptibles should be considered the sole factor influencing transmission. Do similar patterns obtain when exposed susceptibles cluster under climatic conditions that are less favorable to the survival of VZV in the envi-

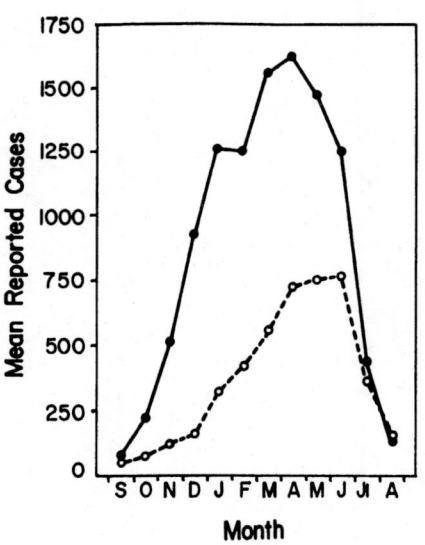

Fig. 3. Reported cases of chickenpox, mean numbers by month, New York City, for two 5-year periods, one of high prevalence, i.e., September 1937 to August 1942 (●) and one of low prevalence, i.e., September 1966 to August 1971 (○). Prepared from tabular data appended by Yorke and London.[156]

ronment, as for example in summer schools and camps?

5.4.2. Herpes Zoster. Herpes zoster has no temporal proclivities, appearing sporadically throughout the year and independently of the prevalence of varicella.[62]

5.5. Age

5.5.1. Varicella. Varicella, in industrialized societies in temperate climates, is primarily a disease of childhood. In Massachusetts, 60–65% of reported cases are in the 5–9 year age group and 20–25% of cases occur in children under 5 years of age (see Fig. 4). In the United States, varicella can be considered as an occupational hazard of nursery and primary-school attendance that few children escape. Figure 4 summarizes data for Massachusetts indicating that varicella tends to be acquired at a younger age during periods of high prevalence than during periods of low prevalence. This trend, while not pronounced, is also apparent on examination of age-specific attack rates for 2 years of high and 2 years of low prevalence (Table 3).

Varicella may occur in the neonatal period as a consequence of infection acquired either *in utero* or at birth if the mother is in the acute phase of the disease shortly prior to or during labor.[91] Brunell[17] demonstrated that VZV antibody crosses the placental barrier, With a sensitive serological indicator (FAMA), the antibody titer of the infant at birth has

been shown to parallel that of the mother; the level then falls, and 50% of positive infants have no demonstrable titer by 5½ months of age.[48] The occurrence and nature of varicella in the near postnatal period mirrors the passively acquired immune state. In the absence of such immunity, infantile varicella may be severe and even fatal. With such protection, infants may experience a modified illness with few pocks or appear to escape completely. The observed failure of varicella to spread in a newborn nursery following introduction of a case has been attributed to the passively protected state of susceptible contacts.[87]

The age distribution of varicella in rural, underdeveloped, upland, populated areas may differ from that in industrialized countries and from that in the lowland tropics. In the course of an epidemic in a rural mountain village in Guatemala, 85% of cases were in children under 6 years of age, and varicella was common in children under 2 years of age.[112] Mention has previously been made of the frequency of varicella in adults in the lowland tropics.

5.5.2. Herpes Zoster. Herpes zoster may occur at any age in the subject who has had a prior attack of varicella, but is age-related, with risk increasing sharply in the later decades of life. McGregor[88] and Hope-Simpson[62] reviewed data on age distribution based on observations in their panel practices in Scotland and in England. McGregor recorded 81 cases of zoster over a 7-year period in a practice of 2400 patients; 61 (75%) of these were in patients

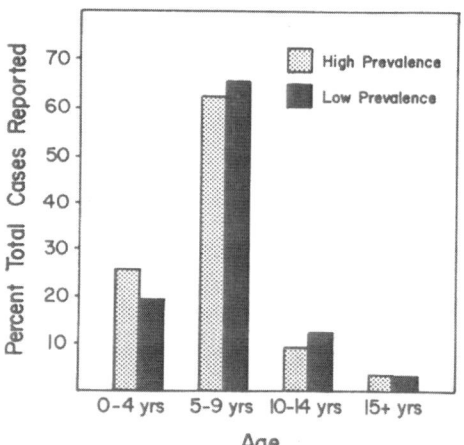

Fig. 4. Distribution of reported cases of chickenpox by age in Massachusetts during a 4-year period of relatively high prevalence (1962–1965; mean annual rate 281.9/100,000; total cases 59,652) and during a 4-year period of relatively low prevalence (1969–1972; mean annual rate 138.9/100,000; total cases 31,164). Source: Massachusetts Department of Public Health, Division of Communicable Diseases, Dr. Nicholas J. Fiumara, Director.

Table 3. Age-Specific Rates per 1000 for Reported Cases of Chickenpox in Massachusetts for 2 Years of High Prevalence and for 2 Years of Low Prevalence[a]

Year	Rate by age group					Total	
	<5 yr	5–9 yr	10–14 yr	15–19 yr	>20 yr	Cases	Rate
High prevalence							
1960	7.8	20.9	2.8	0.5	0.1	16,352	3.2
1962	8.0	20.4	2.6	0.4	0.1	16,359	3.1
Low prevalence							
1970	2.5	9.2	1.6	0.2	0.03	7,115	1.3
1971	3.0	8.2	1.5	0.2	0.1	6,996	1.2

[a] Source: Massachusetts Department of Public Health, Division of Communicable Diseases, Dr. Nicholas J. Fiumara, Director.

over 45 years of age. Hope-Simpson tabulated data on 192 cases observed over a 16-year period in a population of 3534 persons (Table 4). Incidence rose gradually to age 29, tended to plateau through the ages of 30–49, and thereafter again increased.

The amply documented occurrence of cases of herpes zoster in young children with a past history of varicella continues to be the subject of case reports in the literature. With the application of specific virological and serological techniques, unusual cases of zoster are now being recognized in children in whom the possibility of prior undetected intrauterine infection with VZV or an inapparent postnatal infection must be considered.[74,78]

5.6. Sex

No convincing data suggesting differences in susceptibility by sex have been recorded for either varicella or herpes zoster. The prevalence of zoster in women over 70 years of age as observed in a clinical setting is a reflection of the longer life expectancy of the female.

5.7. Race

There is no indication of differing racial susceptibilities to VZV. The previously noted occurrence of varicella pneumonia in adult black or Puerto Rican immigrants to the continental United States is explainable on the basis of diminished opportunities for infection during childhood in their countries of origin.

5.8. Occupation

Since varicella is predominantly a disease of childhood in this country, no specific occupational associations have been described. For the susceptible adult in the United States, in decreasing order parenthood, primary school teaching, and patient-associated medical professions could be considered as occupations of high risk. In Ceylon, where varicella in adults is common, many cases occur in hospital personnel.[85] Trauma has repeatedly been described as a precipitating factor in herpes zoster. If trauma does play a causal role, then physically hazardous occupations may involve an increased risk of precipitating this disease.

5.9. Occurrence of Varicella in Different Settings

5.9.1. In the Home and in Schools. As previously emphasized, varicella is highly infectious on intimate contact. Introduction of VZV into the home or into a primary school with a large percentage of susceptible children characteristically results in an epidemic, usually with exhaustion of the susceptible population by the second or third cycle of transmission.

5.9.2. In the Military. In contrast to the situation in primary-school populations, varicella is of little consequence in the military of the United States with its predominantly immune population. In World War I, there were only 1757 hospital admissions with varicella for the entire U.S. Army.[127] In terms of man-days lost from duty, 31,534 in all, varicella was a relatively insignificant cause; the noneffective rate for measles was 62 times higher and for mumps 129 times higher than that recorded for chickenpox. Similarly, in World War II, varicella posed no problem[55]; between 1942 and 1945, 10,664 cases were reported in the U.S. Army, an annual incidence rate of 0.42. per 1000 average strength. No deaths from varicella occurred in the army during the same period.

5.10. Socioeconomic Status

Little information has been published on the epidemiological role of socioeconomic factors. Ström[128] carried out a retrospective analysis in Sweden of 2000 children born in 1939 and of 2000 born in 1949 in which the children were divided into three social classes. In contrast to pertussis, scarlet fever, and measles, which were less frequent in the 1949 group, varicella had occurred in the 1939 and 1949 groups with equal frequency (67 and 69% by history) by age 12, peaking at 5–6 years of age. No differences in attack rates were noted in the three social classes.

However, on *a priori* grounds, the risk of acquisition of varicella early in childhood would appear directly related to family size and to density of housing and of classroom populations.

5.11. Other Factors

5.11.1 Nutrition. While there is no evidence that malnutrition influences susceptibility to varicella, concurrence enhances the severity of both pathological conditions. In studies on six children in the recovery phase of kwashiorkor, the onset of varicella reduced intake of food and diminished nitrogen retention.[152] In a rural Guatemalan village, varicella was commonly accompanied by diarrhea. In children under 5 years of age with varicella, diarrhea was observed 3 times more frequently than in an uninfected control group.[112] While only 12.5% of well-nourished children with varicella developed diarrhea, this symptom developed in 75% of those who were moderately malnourished. Five of 50 children with varicella-associated diarrhea developed kwashiorkor; one subsequently died.

5.11.2. Genetic Factors. Hook *et al.*[60] described an unusual situation wherein five children in a family contracted severe varicella within a 2-week interval; three developed pneumonia and two died. McKusick,[89] referring to this episode, called attention to his observation that varicella may be severe and even fatal in persons with cartilage–hair hypoplasia (CHH), a recessively inherited skeletal dysplasia. Lux *et al.*[82] studied two patients with CHH, both of whom had severe varicella; one had successive crops of vesicles over a 9-day period, and the other for 14 days. Immunological studies revealed normal humoral responses. A cellular immune defect residing in the small lymphocytes was reflected by chronic neutropenia, lymphopenia, diminished delayed skin hypersensitivity, diminished responsiveness of lymphocytes *in vitro* to phy-

Table 4. Distribution by Age of 192 Cases of Herpes Zoster Observed over a 16-Year Period in a Population of 3534 People in England[a]

Age (yr)	Population	Number of cases	Rate per 1000	Annual incidence per 1000
0–9	510	6	11.8	0.74
10–19	455	10	22.0	1.38
20–29	412	17	41.3	2.58
30–39	491	18	36.6	2.29
40–49	492	23	46.7	2.92
50–59	454	37	81.5	5.09
60–69	350	38	108.6	6.79
70–79	263	27	102.7	6.42
80–89	99	16	161.6	10.10
90–99	8	0	—	—
Total or mean:	3534	192	54.3	3.39

[a] After Hope-Simpson.[62] By personal communication, Hope-Simpson states that the population in each age group represents the mean obtained from 6 of the annual censuses taken during the 16-year period.

tohemagglutinin and to allogeneic cells, and delayed rejection of a skin allograft. These findings have been confirmed in studies on 28 persons with CHH.[138]

As cited by Lux et al.[82] varicella is also severe in patients with another hereditary immunological disease, Nezelof's syndrome, in which there is an autosomal recessive lymphopenia.

5.11.3. Iatrogenic Factors

a. Varicella. Varicella may be life-threatening in children with leukemia and other malignant diseases[26]; with advances in therapy now prolonging the life of the leukemic child, severe infections are a relatively common complication. Corticosteroid,[26,45] immunosuppressive, and cytotoxic therapy may convert a benign illness into a fulminating disease.[58] In 60 children who developed varicella while on anticancer therapy, 32% had visceral involvement and 7% died.[35]

b. Herpes Zoster. Immunosuppressive or antimetabolite therapy may disturb the delicate balance that maintains VZV in a latent state. Rifkind[104] studied 73 patients for 21–37 months after renal transplantation; 6 (8%) aged 12–40 years developed herpes zoster. In other series of renal-transplant patients, zoster developed in 7%[92] and 13%.[73] That the VZV–host relationship is unstable in the immunosuppressed transplant recipient, and to a lesser degree in normal persons, is suggested by results of a longitudinal serological study. Significant fluctuations in antibody titers occurred in asymptomatic subjects, as well as in those developing overt zoster.[81]

Certain types of malignancy, especially Hodgkin's disease and lymphatic leukemia, are recognized as inducers of attacks of herpes zoster, a relationship enhanced by chemotherapy. Analysis of a group of 1132 hospitalized children with cancer revealed that 9% developed herpes zoster; the attack rate was highest in Hodgkin's disease, occurring in 22% of 97 cases[37] The literature on this relationship has been summarized recently.[28,103]

6. Mechanisms and Routes of Transmission

6.1. Varicella

6.1.1. Congenital Infections. While extremely rare, a distinctive congenital varicella syndrome is gradually being defined. Associated with maternal infection in the first or second trimester, the afflicted infant has prominent cicatricial skin scarring often associated with hypoplastic limbs and eye lesions; recently, the diagnosis in one long-term survivor has been confirmed immunologically.[40] The condition is so rare that two large-scale prospective studies involving a total of 433 varicella-complicated pregnancies failed to establish an association.[84,120] A subsequent cohort study in New York City, involving a 5-year follow-up of children born after maternal varicella, revealed no associated malformations.[119]

Onset of varicella in an infant within 10 days of birth is arbitrarily considered as indicating congenital transmission. Perinatal infection occurs less frequently than would be expected. Meyers[91] collected data on 43 cases of congenital varicella; the case-fatality rate was 10%. Reports were available on 46 women with varicella in the last 17 days of pregnancy who were delivered of live infants at term; only 11 (24%) infants had overt varicella. It has been suggested that VZV may not regularly cross the placenta.[40]

6.1.2. Postnatal Transmission. The typical case of varicella is probably infectious for 1–2 days prior to the appearance of the generalized eruption and for 4–5 days therafter, i.e., until the last crop of vesicles has evolved to the purulent and crusted state. The period of infectivity is prolonged in the immunoincompetent host who exhibits successive crops of cutaneous lesions over a period of 1 week or more. Airborne-droplet infection has been emphasized in the past as an important mode of transmission. Evidence on the role of intimate association suggests that infections are also spread by direct contact, and less frequently by indirect contact. The duration of infectivity of droplets containing labile virus must be relatively limited.

The mechanism whereby virus is shed is ill defined. A viremia occurs in the prodromal stage as indicated by disseminated cutaneous lesions and by the observation by Tyzzer[136] that specific histological changes in the evolving cutaneous lesion first appear in the capillary endothelium. Lesions are not confined to the skin, but also occur in the respiratory, urinary, and gastrointestinal tracts; thus, theoretically, various routes exist for dissemination of virus. However, virus has been recovered with regularity only from the cutaneous lesions. Gold[54] could not recover virus from respiratory-tract secretions that were obtained daily from three children, beginning in the latter part of the incubation period and continuing to after appearance of the rash. From an additional case, a single isolate was made from pharyngeal secretions collected 1 day after the exanthem developed. In another study[93] of 29 children, VZV could not be isolated from oropharyngeal swabbings collected before or after appearance of the rash; most of the specimens, however, were frozen before examination. Interpretation of the significance of failures to isolate VZV *in vitro* is an uncertain endeavor. There is no reason to assume that the sensitivity of a culture of human cells as an indicator of VZV equals that of the susceptible human host.

6.1.3. Vectors and Animal Reservoirs. There is no indication that arthropod vectors play a role in the transmission of VZV. Animal reservoirs are unknown and unlikely to exist. VZV is highly host-specific, and rodents are not susceptible. Old World monkeys do not develop generalized disease on inoculation with VZV although a varicellalike disease, produced by a virus closely related to but distinct from VZV, has been described in macaques.[14] While monkeys have not been shown to be susceptible, anthropoid apes apparently can contract varicella if in contact with a human case.[150] Thus, theoretically, the higher apes could maintain VZV in nature.

6.2. Herpes Zoster

The individual with herpes zoster is infectious and can initiate an outbreak of varicella in susceptibles. The mechanism of transmission is even less well defined than in varicella, although probably it is basically similar. Not sufficiently appreciated is the fact that in herpes zoster, a chickenpoxlike dissemination of cutaneous lesions, apparently reflecting a transient viremia, is a common occurrence. In a prospective study in Sweden of 100 consecutive hospitalized patients with herpes zoster, Oberg and Svedmyr[95] observed the appearance of disseminated cutaneous lesions—usually several days after development of the segmental process—in 33% of their patients.

7. Pathogenesis and Immunity

7.1. Varicella

7.1.1. Pathogenesis. Circumstantial rather than factual evidence and analogies to experimental

models of other virus–host interactions provide the basis for hypotheses bearing on the sequence of events following infection of the human host. Entry of the virus is probably via the mucosa of the oropharynx, the upper respiratory tract, the conjunctiva, or, less likely, the skin. Viral replication occurs intracellularly at the site of lodgement, with subsequent cycles of replication involving contiguous cells and leading to dissemination via the blood and lymphatics. Data on growth curves of VZV *in vitro* suggest that multiple cycles of focal replication (perhaps in reticuloendothelial cells) occur during the relatively prolonged incubation period. Early in this stage, nonspecific host immune responses as well as a developing specific immunity partially contain the virus. After 7 days or more, these responses are overwhelmed, the viremia increases quantitatively, and prodromal symptoms develop, followed by cutaneous lesions. Successive crops of vesicles probably reflect a cyclic viremia. In the immunologically competent subject, specific humoral and cellular immune responses thereafter rapidly terminate the viremic phase, although direct cell-to-cell extension with enlargement of established focal lesions continues briefly. Documentation of this sequence of events is incomplete. Gold[54] first established the presence of viremia by a single isolation of virus. However, viremia can be demonstrated frequently and over a period of days in the leukemic child with varicella.[34]

Information on the nature of the immune mechanisms that contain the infectious process is accruing. Rises in titer of immunoglobulin classes IgG, IgM, and IgA are demonstrable by the FAMA method within 5 days of onset.[21] Suspensions of lymphocytes and monocytes from VZV-immune donors have an enhanced capacity to inactivate VZV when examined *in vitro* by a plaque-reduction technique.[50] Mononuclear cells from immune donors exposed to VZV antigen exhibit a blastogenic response[66] that is specific and not elicited by antigens derived from other numbers of the herpesvirus group.[157] VZV induces production of interferon *in vitro* and is inhibited by it[2]; the amount of interferon required for inhibition is directly related to the multiplicity of infection.[102] Interferon can be demonstrated in varicella and zoster vesicular fluids[1]; the appearance and amount correlate directly with the development of the cellular infiltrate in the lesion.[124]

As previously mentioned, the natural history of

varicella is influenced by various host factors. Additionally, physical factors that injure the skin, including trauma and ultraviolet light,[52] may produce focal concentrations of lesions. Thus, while the well-cared-for baby shows no concentration of lesions in the diaper area, in infants with a constantly wet excoriated anogenital skin surface, as high as 68% of the total-body pocks count may be concentrated in that region.[105]

7.1.2. Incubation Period. The average incubation period of varicella is 14 or 15 days. In the carefully studied series of Ross,[105] the range was 10–23 days, with 99% of cases falling between 11 and 20 days.

7.1.3. Immunity. An attack of varicella confers a lasting immunity. While second attacks have been reported, these rare sporadic episodes lack virological or serological confirmation.

7.2. Herpes Zoster

7.2.1. Pathogenesis

a. General. Knowledge of the pathogenesis of herpes zoster is incomplete, and currently, assumption dominates fact. In the great majority of cases, if not all, VZV must be present in the body during the years that intervene between the attack of varicella and the appearance of herpes zoster. It is not known whether in the interim the infection is *persistent*, i.e., one in which at least a few virions are constantly being elaborated, or is *latent*, i.e., one in which the viral genome persists but without viral replication. In either case, the onset of herpes zoster reflects an episode of renewed replication of VZV in a host sensitized and partially immune as the consequence of a prior attack of varicella. The clear-cut evidence, repeatedly recorded, that cases occur sporadically with no temporal or spatial relationship to varicella in epidemic form documents endogenous reactivation as the usual source of virus. Whether herpes zoster exceptionally may follow exogenous reinfection of the partially immune host is not clear. Most reports of cases attributed to exogenous infection[12] may also be interpreted as reflecting the accidental concurrence of two relatively common diseases. Statistically impressive aggregations of cases of herpes zoster—disregarding clusters iatrogenically induced—have not been reported.

The site wherein VZV persits in the quiescent intervening period is not known. Hope-Simpson[62] theorizes that most sensory ganglia harbor latent VZV following varicella. He further suggests that when the defense mechanisms deteriorate below the threshold of viral containment, VZV replicates selectively in a sensory ganglion. Virions are then transported antidromically down the sensory nerve and released around sensory nerve endings in the skin, producing characteristic clusters of zoster vesicles; virus thereafter can be shed into the environment. That this is not the complete picture is apparent from the previously cited data on the common appearance of disseminated cutaneous lesions within a few days of appearance of the segmental eruption; a viremia must often occur. Indeed, in four of eight patients studied recently, virus could be isolated from leukocyte-rich plasma immediately before, or coincident with, the onset of cutaneous dissemination.[33]

There is no evidence indicating that VZV does in fact persist in the dorsal root ganglia following recovery from varicella; unpublished efforts in our laboratory and by others[101] to recover virus from ganglia obtained randomly at autopsy from varicella-immune adults have been unsuccessful. In contrast, during an acute attack of zoster, virus can be recovered from affected ganglia[118] and its presence *in situ* demonstrated by ultrastructural[32,51] and immunofluorescent procedures.[32].

b. Intrinsic Factors. Zoster develops when the host defense mechanisms decay below the containment level. Evidence that the level of cellular immune activity is an important factor is increasing. The person who develops zoster has significant levels of humoral antibody at onset; in some, a further increase in titer beyond an initial high level may not be demonstrable on examination of paired sera. The antibody response, being secondary in nature, might be expected to lack a significant IgM macroglobulin component. However, employing immunofluorescence methods, Ross and McDaid[106] demonstrated IgM VZV antibody in 20 of 40 sera from convalescent zoster patients, and Brunell et al.[21] concluded that localized zoster was accompanied by synthesis of IgM. These reports contrast with the observations of Leonard et al.[77] and Schmidt and Lennette,[114] who could not demonstrate rises in IgM in neutralizing antibody in zoster. Leonard et al.[77] established that the IgG humoral responses differ in varicella and in zoster; sera from zoster cases contained a rapidly migrating IgG subclass with VZV-neutralizing activity that was not present in varicella sera. Differences in the nature of the antibody response were also observed by Palosuo,[99] who could demonstrate platelet-aggregating antibody only in sera from cases of zoster. In patients with disseminated lesions, as contrasted to those with the nondisseminated form, the antibody response as assessed by CF may be delayed.[126]

An impaired cellular immunity is probably an important factor in the pathogenesis of herpes zoster, as reflected by the association with iatrogenic immunosuppression and with malignancies associated with depressed cellular immunity. There is increasing evidence that a transient state of cellular hyporesponsiveness occurs in the acute phase of herpes zoster. White cells harvested from two acute-phase patients inactivated VZV poorly, [50] and Russell et al.[109] found that lymphocytes obtained from patients in the acute phase of herpes zoster, as assessed by transformation on exposure to VZV antigens, exhibited an impaired response. The defect is apparently repaired rapidly, for Jordan and Merigan[66] found that lymphocytes collected from zoster patients 2–11 weeks convalescent responded on stimulation, as did those from varicella-immune children.

Recent studies demonstrate that the untreated patient with lymphoma who is "varicella-immune" has an impaired cellular capacity to respond to VZV antigen.[5,108] Arvin et al.[5] observed that while antibody levels in persons with lymphoma were equivalent to those of control subjects, the capacity of their lymphocytes to transform and to produce interferon on exposure to VZV antigen was depressed. Studies of disseminated zoster in children under treatment for cancer revealed a suggestive, but not definitive, correlation between lymphocyte responsiveness and the appearance of new lesions.[59]

Epidemiological data clearly establish "elapsed time," i.e., time since the attack of varicella, as an important determinant in the pathogenesis of zoster. Regardless of extrinsic factors that may impinge, it is the ill-defined gradual decay with advancing age of the constraining immune processes that allows reactivation of latent VZV. Herpes zoster is a benchmark of immunological senility.

c. *Extrinsic Factors.* Iatrogenic herpes zoster is not a new entity. An association with administration of metallic drugs, especially lead and arsenic, has long been established. Only recently, however, has depression of immunological activity become a desirable therapeutic objective in medicine; whether achieved by physical, biological, or chemotherapeutic means, the result entails an enhanced risk that zoster will appear if the subject has had a prior attack of varicella.

The role of trauma as a precipitant of zoster is controversial. Hope-Simpson[62] established an association in only 2 of 192 cases and considered that these episodes might have been coincidental.

7.2.2. Incubation Period. There is no information on the interval between endogenous reactivation and the appearance of symptoms. Exceptionally, pain in the dermatome subsequently involved may develop 10–14 days prior to the appearance of the eruption; usually the interval is 2–4 days.

7.2.3. Immunity. In contrast to varicella, there are numerous reports in the literature of the occurrence of second and rarely of third attacks of herpes zoster. Hope-Simpson[62] summarized data on age incidence and concluded that if a cohort of 1000 people were to live to be 85 years old, half would have experienced one attack of herpes zoster, 10 would have had two attacks, and possibly 1 would had a third attack.

8. Patterns of Host Response

8.1. Clinical Patterns

8.1.1. Varicella

a. *Prodromal Symptoms.* Adults may have 1 or 2 days of fever and malaise prior to appearance of the rash. In children, premonitory symptoms are usually mild, and appearance of the exanthem is often the first evidence of illness.

b. *Exanthem.* There are three aspects of the vesicular eruption that are of diagnostic significance: the nature and evolution of individual lesions, the concurrent presence of lesions at different stages of development, and the distribution of the process over the body. Individual lesions develop as small, irregular, rose-colored macules in the center of which appears a delicate 1- to 4-mm "dewdroplike" vesicle containing clear fluid. This may rupture; if not, within a few hours the contents become purulent and then dry and crusted. Successive crops of new lesions appear over a period of 2–4 days so that characteristically at the peak of the illness, there are in any one area cutaneous lesions at all stages of evolution and of resolution. Lesions appear first on the scalp and then on the trunk. The distribution of the lesions is centripetal. The greatest concentration is on the trunk, and the distal extremities are the least involved. It is misleading to assume that lesions are confined to the skin; similar involvement of the mucosa of the oropharynx and vagina can be seen, and it is probable that lesions comparable to those in the skin develop to a varying degree in each patient in the respiratory and the gastrointestinal tracts.

c. Course. In the immunocompetent child, the illness is typically benign, accompanied by mild malaise, and reflected by pruritus and fever (100–102°F) for 2–3 days. In the adult, systemic symptoms are more marked, and varicella pneumonia that may be life-threatening is a common complication. In one series of 114 consecutive cases in a military population (average age 25 years), lung involvement was demonstrable roentgenographically in 16%.[139] Secondary bacterial infection of the cutaneous lesions occurs frequently. Reference should be made to a text on infectious diseases for information on rarer complications such as encephalitis.

In the immunologically compromised subject, all clinicopathological manifestations may be enhanced. Focal pocklike lesions may occur throughout the gastrointestinal and respiratory tracts and in the liver and spleen; there may be widespread vascular damage with prominent hemorrhagic lesions.[26]

d. Inapparent Infections. Inapparent infections obviously occur, although, as noted earlier, observational studies suggest a frequency of less than 5% in susceptible children.

8.1.2. Herpes Zoster.

a. Exanthem. The varicelliform eruption in zoster is characteristically unilateral and initially sharply limited in a band or patchlike distribution to the dermatome (or, rarely, associated dermatomes) supplied by a specific dorsal root or extramedullary cranial nerve ganglion. Within the segmental area of localization, lesions may be scattered and few or may be so numerous as to form an almost confluent large plaque. Hope-Simpson[62] noted that the dermatomes most frequently involved in herpes zoster—i.e., the region supplied by the fifth cranial

nerve, and the trunk supplied by ganglia extending from the third dorsal to the second lumbar segments—are those areas wherein the lesions of varicella are also most prominent. The lesions of zoster rarely involve the extremities.

b. Course. Prior to the appearance of the eruption, there may be pain and extreme paresthesia in the involved segment. The lesions appear in crops and, while often larger in comparison, evolve and resolve as in varicella, but at a slower pace, so that virus may be recovered from vesicles for as long as a week after appearance of the eruption. Scabs, as in varicella, are noninfectious but may persist for 2 weeks or more. A regional lymphadenopathy is a characteristic feature if the segmental process is extensive. Severe postherpetic neuralgia that is refractory to treatment is a distressing complication.

It is to be noted that evidence of central nervous system involvement with a spinal fluid pleocytosis is common and that motor involvement with weakness or paralysis may occur, but that a fatal outcome attributable to zoster *per se* is extremely rare. Reference should be made elsewhere for a discussion of other complications.

c. Inapparent Infections. The term "zoster sine herpete" has been applied to situations wherein unilateral focal zosterlike premonitory pain is experienced but vesicles fail subsequently to develop over the involved area.[68] Such transitory imbalances in the host–virus relationship would be epidemiologically unimportant unless accompanied by patterns of viral dissemination now unrecognized.

8.2. Diagnosis

When presented with a patient with a vesiculopustular rash of unknown etiology, the immediate priority is to exclude variola. The atypical modified case of smallpox may closely simulate varicella, and the case of severe hemorrhagic varicella may resemble variola. Such distinctions cannot be made clinically with certainty, and the assistance of the laboratory (Section 3.4) must be immediately sought. Typical cases can be differentiated on clinical grounds by the experienced observer; the criteria are summarized in textbooks on infectious disease, to which reference may be made. However, smallpox has now retreated beyond the experience of most physicians; if the slightest doubt exists, confirmatory evidence from the laboratory should be obtained.

Infections caused by VZV therefore should first be distinguished from variola and other pox viral infections, such as generalized vaccinia or circumscribed inoculation vaccinia. Infections due to herpes simplex virus (HSV) that present as a generalized vesiculopustular eruption (eczema herpeticum) or as a circumscribed zosterlike process are more difficult to differentiate from clinically similar eruptions produced by VZV. Lesions caused by either VZV or HSV will morphologically manifest intrauclear inclusions and multinucleate giant cells. Reliance on the demonstration of a rise in titer of CF antibody against VZV, contrary to statements in some texts, cannot be considered as diagnostic unless tests for HSV CF antibodies fail to show a concurrent increase in titer; this is due, as earlier noted, to the heterologous anamnestic response induced by either agent in immunologically experienced subjects. Other serological approaches such as FA or attempts at isolation of the responsible agent must be undertaken.

The eruption of varicella should also be distinguished from that of rickettsial pox, of infections caused by certain coxsackieviruses, of secondary syphilis in some forms, and from dermatitis herpetiformis. The focal process of zoster, most frequently simulated by herpes simplex, may also be confused with impetigo contagiosa.

9. Control and Prevention

9.1. General Concepts

New approaches to the treatment, control, and prevention of varicella are evolving. Since herpes zoster is endogeneous in origin, prevention of varicella *a priori* should prevent zoster; this may or may not be the case if varicella is prevented through use of a live viral vaccine. The evaluation of the safety of the new varicella vaccine (see Section 9.3.4) developed in Japan, and of similar products, will require observational epidemiological studies over a period of decades. In the interim, improved antiviral compounds, and modification of the virus–host relationship by use of interferon and of transfer factor, will have an increasing role in treatment and prevention of varicella.

9.2. Interruption of Transmisson

9.2.1. Isolation and Quarantine in Homes and Schools. Neither isolation nor quarantine is effective in interrupting the spread of the disease in groups of susceptible children; therefore, both practices generally have been abandoned. Indeed, since practically all persons will eventually acquire the disease, there is merit in the acquisition of varicella in childhood, for the illness then will be less severe and less socially disruptive than if experienced in adulthood. For the same reason, the movement of adults with herpes zoster is not usually constrained.

9.2.2. Protection of Groups at Special Risk. Varicella is a potentially fatal disease in susceptible children who are undergoing immunosuppressive therapy or who concurrently have malignant diseases such as leukemia or Hodgkin's disease. Therefore, efforts should be made to minimize infectious contacts with such high-risk persons by protective isolation procedures. Contact with adults with herpes zoster and with nonimmune children who might be incubating varicella should be precluded if possible. However, the appearance of a case among patients on a ward poses problems, even with the strictest of precautions. Sporadic cases may mysteriously appear for several generations, reflecting either unrecognized breaks in isolation technique or airborne spread. The customary solution is to remove all known susceptibles for a 3-week period. Children at high risk with a known exposure should be given zoster-immune globulin (see Section 9.3.1).

9.3. Modification or Prevention of Varicella

9.3.1. Administration of Specific Antibody. Ross[105] demonstrated in 1962 that administration to susceptible children exposed to varicella of γ-globulin obtained from adults at large did not prevent disease but modified the illness as indicated by fewer pocks and a diminished febrile response. Since patients with zoster develop high titers of specific antibody, a logical extension of this observation was to utilize zoster-immune globulin (ZIG) prepared from blood collected from zoster convalescent patients with high VZV CF titers[22]; a 2-ml dose given within 3 days of exposure prevented varicella in exposed susceptible children. Collaborative studies followed, to evaluate ZIG as a preventive measure in children at high risk, specifically those with leukemia or lymphoma, with immunodeficiency syndromes, or under treatment with immunosuppressive medications.[20,67]

A review of the results of administration of ZIG to 358 exposed persons at high risk revealed an overall attack rate of 22%.[24] Gershon et al.[49] found that use of ZIG in 15 exposed immunocompromised children, known to be susceptible by the FAMA test, resulted in subclinical infection in 5, attenuated overt disease in 9, and severe illness in 1. The period between exposure and administration is critical; a Norwegian study records a 97% protection rate if the period is 3 days or less and a 50% protection rate if the delay is 5 days or more.[153] ZIG is in short supply and its use is restricted to high-risk children meeting defined criteria; currently, the material can be obtained in the United States through American Red Cross regional blood donor centers. The selective use of units of outdated plasma that have significant VZV antibody titers should improve the supply of ZIG.[158] Zoster-immune plasma (ZIP) is useful if ZIG is not available.[11]

9.3.2. Use of Interferon and of Transfer Factor. Merigan and co-workers at Stanford University, in a series of studies, gradually accumulated evidence that interferon is involved in the host defense mechanism against VZV[1,124–126] and could be administered safely to patients with zoster.[65] The usefulness of human leukocyte interferon for the treatment of zoster in patients with cancer has now been established in three controlled, randomized double-blind trials involving 90 patients.[90] No dissemination of the cutaneous process occurred in patients receiving the highest dosage (5.1×10^5 u/ kg per day). Decreases were observed in the number of days of new-vesicle formation, in the amount of acute pain, in the severity of postherpetic neuralgia, and in the frequency of visceral complications. These results are in accord with those achieved with zoster in earlier less well controlled experiments.[31] A trial of relatively low dosages of human interferon in the treatment of varicella in children with cancer yielded suggestive beneficial results.[4]. The topical application of an interferon inducer to the localized lesions of zoster in children with cancer had earlier been shown to be ineffective.[36] Of interest is the beneficial effect of the systemic use of human interferon in the experimental treatment of a simian-

varicella-virus infection in immunosuppressed monkeys.[94]

The interesting results with interferon in the treatment of infections with VZV focus attention on brief reports that the transfusion of white cells from an immune donor[122] and the injection of transfer factor[30] are dramatically beneficial. Winsnes et al.[154] treated 15 patients suffering from lymphoproliferative disease or sarcoid complicated by VZV infection with transfer factor; the results were assessed as favorable, and an increase in serum interferon was observed in several of those treated. These developments provide a promising new approach in the handling of VZV infections in persons at high risk.

9.3.3. Antiviral Chemotherapy. Three compounds that interfere with the synthesis of viral DNA—namely, *Idoxuridine* [(IUdR) 5-iodo-2-deoxyuridine], cytosine arabinoside [(ARA-C) 1-β-D-arabinofuranosylcytosine], and adenine arabinoside [(ARA-A) *Vidarabine*, 9-β-D-arabinofuranosyladenine]—have been used for the treatment of VZV infections. Of these, only ARA-A, a purine nucleoside, is currently promising; IUdR is toxic on systemic administration, and ARA-C potentiates viral dissemination by depressing defense mechanisms of the host.[125]

The potential usefulness of ARA-A for the therapy of herpes zoster in the immunosuppressed has been established by a multi-institutional collaborative study.[151] A randomized crossover study wherein ARA-A was given intravenously for 5 days (10 mg/ kg per day) followed by a placebo for 5 days—or vice versa—was carried out. Because of rapid healing, only data covering the first 5-day period could be analyzed. In the treated group, acute pain disappeared more rapidly, as did virus from the vesicles, the vesicles pustulated sooner, and there were fewer new vesicles. However, information on the therapeutic indications and usefulness of ARA-A is far from complete. In studies carried out *in vitro*, strains of VZV exhibited 20-fold differences in sensitivity to ARA-A.[64] This finding may reflect the variable deamination by adenosine deaminase (ADA) of ARA-A to ARA-Hx (hypoxanthine arabinoside) in the culture system, ARA-Hx being much less active[23]; the role of ADA *in vivo* is unknown. Nevertheless, ARA-A provides a new therapeutic approach. In an unusual patient, who had developed new cutaneous lesions continuously over an 8-

month period, ARA-A therapy yielded dramatic results,[3] with cessation of the process by the 4th day of treatment.

9.3.4. Vaccine Prospects. A live varicella virus vaccine developed by Takahashi et al.[131,132] in Japan in 1974 is under study in that country. The vaccine, derived by serial cultivation of VZV in human and in guinea pig embryonic cells, when given subcutaneously, induces a high degree of immunity in the absence of acute reactions. Asano and Takahashi[8] provide data on 179 children followed for 2 years postvaccination; 50 of 51 children had persistent neutralizing antibodies. Of 80 vaccinated children subsequently exposed to varicella, only 1 developed clinical evidence of infection. Herpes zoster was not observed in the vaccinees. A group of 18 vaccinated children hospitalized with nephrosis or nephritis, including 12 on steroid therapy, remained varicella-free in the presence of four outbreaks of varicella or zoster on the ward.[6] Some of the exposed children exhibited striking rises in titers of VZV neutralizing antibody, suggesting that an inapparent infection had occurred in the absence of clinical disease.

The vaccine also confers protection if administered at the time of exposure or shortly thereafter.[7] A total of 26 children exposed to a familial index case who were vaccinated within 5 days of exposure failed to develop varicella, whereas the attack rate in 19 comparable unvaccinated children was 100%. However, in the studies of Baba et al.,[10] a proportion of vaccinees subsequently developed mild varicella; of 33 infants receiving a small dose of vaccine, i.e., 80 plaque-forming units (PFU), 8 developed an exanthem, and one of 17 older children given 500 PFU developed varicella. These investigators also demonstrated that the varicella skin test introduced by Kamiya et al.[70] was a rapid and useful index of the immune state of an exposed child.

In view of the dangerous potential of varicella in children under therapy for leukemia or other malignant disease, the response of such patients to live varicella vaccine is of particular interest. Vaccine was given to 17 such children with the precaution that anticancer medication was suspended from 1 week before to 1 week after vaccination; a "minute" rash in 3 patients was the only complication.[63] Too few leukemic children have received vaccine without suspension of antitumor therapy to permit appraisal of the procedure.[98,130]

The promising results with a live VZV vaccine in Japan are currently the subject of discussion. The propensity for latency of VZV is a major deterrent to the investigation of comparable vaccines in the United States, for vaccine-induced zoster in a mild form—or even in an exaggerated bizarre form—might develop decades later.[141] Other potential problems have been summarized.[19] The long-term hazards of use of a live virus vaccine are of serious concern, but currently remain hypothetical. In contrast, evidence continues to accrue documenting short-term benefits. Trials of live varicella vaccine are now underway on a limited basis in the United States on the assumption that benefits will outweigh hypothetical risks.[44,72,111]

10. Unresolved Problems

10.1. Prevention

Varicella is second only to gonorrhea in incidence among reportable diseases in the United States. Spontaneous and iatrogenic herpes zoster increase in proportion to the relative number of older people in the population and to those requiring immunosuppressive therapy. An effective varicella vaccine that will prevent the primary attack without inducing a persistent infection is a primary objective.

10.2. Pathogenesis

The deficiencies in the host defense mechanism that permit a latent VZV infection to become active remain unknown, and the site where VZV persists after the primary attack, has not been defined. It is likely that current investigative emphasis on the role of cellular, as contrasted to humoral, immunity in VZV infections will assist in elucidation of these questions.

Other problems require resolution. How does VZV enter the susceptible host? What are the primary or secondary sites of replication that precede or intervene in the viremic phase? If latent VZV does persist in sensory ganglia, was this anatomical site infected by centripetal movement along nerves or was there selective anatomical invasion following a viremic phase?

10.3. Epidemiological Unknowns

The manner in which VZV is disseminated by the infected host has not been defined. Does failure to demonstrate virus in oropharyngeal secretions indeed indicate that the primary source of infectious material is the cutaneous lesion? If so, what is the relative infective potential of the person with herpes zoster? How do varying environmental conditions, particularly temperature and humidity, influence transmission? What is the relative importance of airborne dissemination of VZV as contrasted to direct or indirect contact?

ACKNOWLEDGMENTS

The continuing support of the National Institute of Allergy and Infectious Diseases of the National Institutes of Health (Grants AI-01023 and AI-16154) for studies on varicella–zoster virus is acknowledged.

11. References

1. ARMSTRONG, R. W., GURWITH, M. J., WADDELL, D., AND MERIGAN, T. C., Cutaneous interferon production in patients with Hodgkin's disease and other cancers infected with varicella or vaccinia, *N. Engl. J. Med.* **283**:1182–1187 (1970).
2. ARMSTRONG, R. W., AND MERIGAN, T. C., Varicella-zoster virus: interferon production and comparative interferon sensitivity in human cell cultures, *J. Gen. Virol.* **12**:53–54 (1971).
3. ARONSON, M. D., PHILLIPS, C. F., GUMP, D. W., ALBERTINI, R. J., AND PHILLIPS, C. A., Vidarabine therapy for severe herpesvirus infections: An unusual syndrome of chronic varicella and transient immunologic deficiency, *J. Am. Med. Assoc.* **235**:1339–1342 (1976).
4. ARVIN, A. M., FELDMAN, S., AND MERIGAN, T. C., Human leukocyte interferon in the treatment of varicella in children with cancer: A preliminary controlled trial, *Antimicrob. Agents Chemother.* **13**:605–607 (1978).
5. ARVIN, A. M., POLLARD, R. B., RASMUSSEN, L. E., AND MERIGAN, T. C., Selective impairment of lymphocyte reactivity to varicella zoster virus antigen among untreated patients with lymphoma, *J. Infect. Dis.* **137**:531–540 (1978).
6. ASANO, Y., NAKAYAMA, H., YAZAKI, T., ITO, S., ISOMURA, S., AND TAKAHASHI, M., Protective efficacy of vaccination in children in four episodes of natural varicella and zoster in the ward, *Pediatrics* **59**:8–12 (1977).
7. ASANO, Y., NAKAYAMA, H., YAZAKI, T., KATO, R., HIROSE, S., TSUZUKI, K., ITO, S., ISOMURA, S., AND

TAKAHASHI, M., Protection against varicella in family contacts by immediate inoculation with live varicella vaccine, *Pediatrics* **59**:3–7 (1977).
8. ASANO, Y., AND TAKAHASHI, M., Clinical and serologic testing of a live varicella vaccine and two year followup for immunity of the vaccinated children, *Pediatrics* **60**:810–814 (1977).
9. ASANO, Y., AND TAKAHASHI, M., Studies on neutralization of varicella-zoster virus and serological followup of cases of varicella and zoster, *Biken J.* **21**:15 (1978).
10. BABA, K., YABUUCHI, H., OKUNI, H., AND TAKAHASHI, M., Studies with live varicella vaccine and inactivated skin test antigen: Protective effect of vaccine and clinical application of the skin test, *Pediatrics* **61**:550–555 (1978).
11. BALFOUR, H. H., JR., GROTH, K. E., McCULLOUGH, J., KALIS, J. M., MARKER, S. C., NESBIT, M. E., SIMMONS, R. L., AND NAJARAN, J. S., Prevention or modification of varicella using zoster immune plasma, *Am. J. Dis. Child.* **131**:693–696 (1977).
12. BERLIN, B. S., AND CAMPBELL, T., Hospital acquired herpes zoster following exposure to chickenpox, *J. Am. Med. Assoc.* **211**:1831–1833 (1970).
13. BLACK, F. L., HIERHOLZER, W. J., PINHEIRO, F. DEP., EVANS, A. S., WOODALL, J. P., OPTON, E. M., EMMONS, J. E., WEST, B. S., EDSALL, G., DOWNS, W. G., AND WALLACE, G. D., Evidence for persistence of infectious agents in isolated human populations, *Am. J. Epidemiol.* **100**:230–250 (1974).
14. BLAKELY, G. A., LOURIE, B., MORTON, W. G., EVANS, H. H., AND KAUFMANN, A. F., A varicella-like disease in macaque monkeys, *J. Infect. Dis.* **127**:617–623 (1973).
15. VON BOKAY, J., Über den aetiologischen Zussammenhang der Varicellen mit gewissen Fällen von Herpes zoster, *Wien. Klin. Wochenschr.* **22**:1323–1326 (1909).
16. BOUGHTON, C. R., Varicella-zoster in Sydney. I. Varicella and its complications, *Med. J. Aust.* **2**:392–397 (1966).
17. BRUNELL, P. A. Placental transfer of varicella-zoster antibody, *Pediatrics* **38**:1034–1038 (1966).
18. BRUNELL, P. A., Varicella-zoster infections in pregnancy, *J. Am. Med. Assoc.* **199**:315–317 (1967).
19. BRUNELL, P. A., Protection against varicella, *Pediatrics* **59**:1–2 (1977).
20. BRUNELL, P. A., GERSHON, A. A., HUGHES, W. T., RILEY, H. D., JR., AND SMITH, J., Prevention of varicella in high risk children: A collaborative study, *Pediatrics* **50**:718–722 (1972).
21. BRUNELL, P. S., GERSHON, A. A., UDUMAN, S. A., AND STEINBERG, S., Varicella-zoster immunoglobulins during varicella, latency, and zoster, *J. Infect. Dis.* **132**:49–54 (1975).
22. BRUNELL, P. A., ROSS, A., MILLER, L. H., AND KUO,

B., Prevention of varicella by zoster immune globulin, *N. Engl. J. Med.* **280:**1191–1194 (1969).

23. BRYSON, Y. J., AND CONNOR, J. D., *In vitro* suscepti-bility of varicella zoster virus to adenine arabinoside and hypoxanthine arabinoside, *Antimicrob. Agents Chemother.* **9:**540–543 (1976).

24. CENTER FOR DISEASE CONTROL, Zoster immune glob-ulin, *Morbid. Mortal. Weekly Rep.* **25:**211–212 (1976).

25. CENTER FOR DISEASE CONTROL, Reported morbidity and mortality in the United States, *Morbid. Mortal. Weekly Rep.* **26**(53):1–80 (1978).

26. CHEATHAM, W. J., WELLER, T. H., DOLAN, T. F., JR., AND DOWER, J. C., Varicella: Report of two fatal cases with necropsy, virus isolation, and serologic studies, *Am. J. Pathol.* **32:**1015–1035 (1956).

27. COLLINS, S. D., WHEELER, R. E., AND SHANNON, R. D., *The Occurrence of Whooping Cough, Chickenpox, Mumps, Measles, and German Measles in 200,000 Surveyed Fam-ilies in 28 Large Cities,* Special Study Series, No. 1, Division of Public Health Methods, NIH, USPHS, Washington, D.C., 1942.

28. DOLIN, R., REICHMAN, R. C., MAZUR, M. H., AND WHITLEY, R. J., Herpes zoster-varicella infections in immunosuppressed patients, *Ann. Intern. Med.* **89:**375–388 (1978).

29. NAKANA, J. H., Poxviruses, in: *Diagnostic Procedures for Viral, Rickettsial, and Chlamydial Infections* 5th ed. (E. H. LENNETTE AND N. J. SCHMIDT, eds.), pp. 257–308, American Public Health Association, Wash-ington, 1979.

30. DREW, W. L., BLUME, M. R., MINER, R., SILVERBERG, I., AND ROSENBAUM, E. H., Herpes zoster: Transfer factor therapy, *Ann. Intern. Med.* **79:**747–748 (1973).

31. EMÖDI, G., RUFLI, T., JUST, M., AND HERNANDEZ, R., Human interferon therapy for herpes zoster in adults, *Scand. J. Infect. Dis.* **7:**1–5 (1975).

32. ESIRI, M. M., AND TOMLINSON, A. H., Herpes zoster: Demonstration of virus in trigeminal nerve and gan-glion by immunofluorescence and electron micros-copy, *J. Neurol. Sci.* **15:**35–48 (1972).

33. FELDMAN, S., CHAUDARY, S., OSSI, M., AND EPP, E., A viremic phase for herpes zoster in children with cancer, *J. Pediatr.* **91:**597–600 (1977).

34. FELDMAN, S., AND EPP, E., Isolation of varicella-zoster virus from blood, *J. Pediatr.* **88:**265–267 (1976).

35. FELDMAN, S., HUGHES, W. T., AND DANIEL, C. B., Var-icella in children with cancer: Seventy-seven cases, *Pediatrics* **56:**388–397 (1975).

36. FELDMAN, S., HUGHES, W. T., DARLINGTON, R. W., AND KIM, H. K., Evaluation of topical polyinosinic acid–polycytidylic acid in treatment of localized herpes zoster in children with cancer: A randomized, double-blind controlled study, *Antimicrob. Agents Chemother.* **8:**289–294 (1975).

37. FELDMAN, S., HUGHES, W. T., AND KIM. H. Y., Herpes

zoster in children with cancer, *Am. J. Dis. Child.* **126:**178–184 (1973).

38. FORGHANI, B., SCHMIDT, N. J., AND DENNIS, J., Anti-body assays for varicella-zoster virus: Comparison of enzyme immunoassay with neutralization, immune adherence hemagglutination and complement fixa-tion, *J. Clin. Microbiol.* **8:**545–552 (1978).

39. FORGHANI, B., SCHMIDT, N. J., AND LENNETTE, E. H., Sensitivity of a radioimmunoassay method for detec-tion of certain viral antibodies in sera and cerebro-spinal fluids, *J. Clin. Microbiol.* **4:**470–478 (1976).

40. FREY, H. M., BIALKIN, G., AND GERSHON, A. A., Con-genital varicella: Case report of a serologically proved long-term survivor, *Pediatrics* **59:**110–112 (1977).

41. FURUKAWA, T., AND PLOTKIN, S. A., Indirect hemag-glutination test for varicella-zoster infection, *Infect. Immun.* **5:**835–839 (1972).

42. GARLAND, J., Varicella following exposure to herpes zoster, *N. Engl. J. Med.* **228:**336–337 (1943).

43. GERNA, G., ACHILLI, G., AND CHAMBERS, R. W., De-termination of neutralizing antibody and IgG anti-body to varicella-zoster virus and of IgG antibody to membrane antigens by the immunoperoxidase tech-nique, *J. Infect. Dis.* **135:**975–979 (1977).

44. GERSHON, A. A., Varicella-zoster virus: Prospects for active immunization, *Am. J. Clin. Pathol.* **70:**170–174 (1978).

45. GERSHON, A. A., BRUNELL, P. A., DOYLE, E. F., AND CLAPS, A. A., Steroid therapy and varicella, *J. Pediatr.* **81:**1034 (1972).

46. GERSHON, A. A., KALTER, Z. G., AND STEINBERG, S., Detection of antibody to varicella-zoster virus by im-mune adherence hemagglutination, *Proc. Soc. Exp. Biol. Med.* **151:**762–765 (1976).

47. GERSHON, A. A., AND KRUGMAN, S., Seroepidemio-logic survey of varicella: Value of specific fluorescent antibody test, *Pediatrics* **56:**1005–1008 (1975).

48. GERSHON, A. A., RAKER, R., STEINBERG, S., TOPF-OL-STEIN, B., AND DRUSIN, L. M., Antibody to varicella-zoster virus in parturient women and their offspring during the first year of life, *Pediatrics* **58:**692–696 (1976).

49. GERSHON, A., STEINBERG, S., AND BRUNELL, P. A., Zos-ter immune globulin: A further assessment, *N. Engl. J. Med.* **290:**243–245 (1974).

50. GERSHON, A. A., STEINBERG, S., AND SMITH, M., Cell-mediated immunity to varicella-zoster virus demon-strated by viral inactivation with human leucocytes, *Infect. Immun.* **13:**1549–1553 (1976).

51. GHATAK, N. R., AND ZIMMERMAN, H. M., Spinal gan-glion in herpes zoster: A light and electron micro-scopic study, *Arch. Pathol.* **95:**411–455 (1973).

52. GILCHREST, B., AND BADEN, H. P., Photodistribution of viral exanthems, *Pediatrics* **54:**136–138 (1974).

53. GILLANI, A., AND SPENCE, L., Immune adherence hem-

agglutination test applied to the study of herpes simplex and varicella-zoster virus infections, *J. Clin. Microbiol.* **7:**114–117 (1978).

54. GOLD, E., Serologic and virus-isolation studies of patients with varicella or herpes-zoster infection, *N. Engl. J. Med.* **274:**181–185 (1966).

55. GORDON, J. E., General considerations of modes of transmission, in: *Preventive Medicine in World War II,* Vol. IV, *Communicable Diseases,* p. 27, Department of the Army, Washington, D.C., 1958.

56. GORDON, J. E., Chickenpox: An epidemiological review, *Am. J. Med. Sci.* **244:**362–389 (1962).

57. GRANDIEN, M., APPELGREN, P., ESPMARK, A., AND HANNGREN, K., Determination of varicella immunity by the indirect immunofluorescence test in urgent clinical situations, *Scand. J. Infect. Dis.* **8:**65–69 (1976).

58. HAGGERTY, R. J., AND ELEY, R. C., Varicella and cortisone, *Pediatrics* **18:**160–162 (1956).

59. HAYES, F. A., AND FELDMAN, S., Cell mediated immunity to varicella zoster virus in children being treated for cancer, *Cancer* **42:**159–163 (1978).

60. HOOK, E. B., ORANDI, M., TEN BENSEL, R. W., SCHAMBER, W. F., AND ST. GEME, J. W., JR., Familial fatal varicella, *J. Am. Med. Assoc.* **206:**305–311 (1968).

61. HOPE-SIMPSON, R. E., Infectiousness of communicable diseases in the household (measles, chickenpox, and mumps), *Lancet* **2:**549–554 (1952).

62. HOPE-SIMPSON, R. E., The nature of herpes zoster: A long-term study and a new hypothesis, *Proc. R. Soc. Med.* **58:**9–20 (1965).

63. IZAWA, T., IHARA, T., HATTORI, A., ISAWA, T., KAMIYA, H., SAKURAI, M., AND TAKAHASI, M., Application of a live varicella vaccine in children with acute leukemia or other malignant diseases, *Pediatrics* **60:**805–809 (1977).

64. JOHNSON, M. T., LUBY, J. P., BUCHANAN, R. A., AND MIKULEC, D., Treatment of varicella-zoster virus infections with adenine arabinoside, *J. Infect. Dis.* **131:**225–229 (1975).

65. JORDAN, G. W., FRIED, R. P., AND MERIGAN, T. C., Administration of human leukocyte interferon in herpes zoster. I. Safety, circulating antiviral activity, and host responses to infection, *J. Infect. Dis.* **130:**56–62 (1974).

66. JORDAN, G. W., AND MERIGAN, T. C., Cell-mediated immunity to varicella-zoster virus: *In vitro* lymphocyte responses, *J. Infect. Dis.* **130:**495–501 (1974).

67. JUDELSOHN, R. G., Prevention and control of varicella-zoster infections, *J. Infect. Dis.* **125:**82–84 (1972).

68. JUEL-JENSEN, B. E., A new look at infectious diseases: Herpes simplex and zoster, *Br. Med. J.* **1:**406–410 (1973).

69. KALTER, Z. G., STEINBERG, S., AND GERSHON, A. A., Immune adherence hemagglutination: Further observations on demonstration of antibody to varicella-zoster virus, *J. Infect. Dis.* **135:**1010–1013 (1977).

70. KAMIYA, H., IHARA, T., HATTORI, A., IWASA, T., SAKURAI, M., IZAWA, T., YAMADA, A., AND TAKAHASHI, M., Diagnostic skin test reactions with varicella virus antigen and clinical application of the test, *J. Infect. Dis.* **136:**784–788 (1977).

71. KAPSENBERG, J. G., Possible antigenic relationships between varicella/zoster virus and herpes simplex virus, *Arch. Gesamte Virusforsch.* **15:**67–73 (1964).

72. KEMPE, C. H., AND GERSHON, A. A., Varicella vaccine at the crossroads, *Pediatrics* **60:**930–931 (1977).

73. KORANDA, F. C., DEHMEL, E. M., KAHN, G., AND PENN, I., Cutaneous complications in immunosuppressed renal homograft recipients, *J. Am. Med. Assoc.* **229:**419–424 (1974).

74. KOUVALAINEN, K., SALMI, A., AND SALMI, T. T., Infantile herpes zoster, *Scand. J. Infect. Dis.* **4:**91–96 (1972).

75. KUNDRATITZ, K., Experimentelle Übertragung von Herpes zoster auf den Menschen und die Beziehungen von Herpes zoster zu Varicellen, *Monatsschr. Kinderheilkd.* **29:**516–522 (1925).

76. Leading article, Fatal chickenpox, *Br. Med. J.* **2:**954–955 (1965).

77. LEONARD, L. L., SCHMIDT, N. J., AND LENNETTE, E. H., Demonstration of viral antibody activity in two immunoglobulin G subclasses in patients with varicella-zoster infection, *J. Immunol.* **104:**23–27 (1970).

78. LEWKONIA, I. K., AND JACKSON, A. A., Infantile herpes zoster after intrauterine exposure to varicella, *Br. Med. J.* **3:**149 (1973).

79. LIPSCHÜTZ, B., Untersuchungen über die Ätiologie der Krankheiten der Herpesgruppe (Herpes zoster, Herpes genitalis, Herpes febrilis), *Arch. Dermatol. Syph. Orig.* **136:**428–482 (1921).

80. LONDON, W. P., AND YORKE, J. A., Recurrent outbreaks of measles, chickenpox, and mumps. I. Seasonal variations in contact rates, *Am. J. Epidemiol.* **98:**453–468 (1973).

81. LUBY, J. P., RAMIREZ-RONDA, C., RINNER, S., HULL, A., AND VERGNE-MARINI, P., A longitudinal study of varicella-zoster virus infections in renal transplant recipients, *J. Infect. Dis.* **135:**659–663 (1977).

82. LUX, S. E., JOHNSTON, R. B., JR., AUGUST, C. S., SAY, B., PENCHASZADEH, V. B., ROSEN, F. S., AND McKUSICK, V. A., Chronic neutropenia and abnormal cellular immunity in cartilage–hair hypoplasia, *N. Engl. J. Med.* **282:**231–236 (1970).

83. MANKIKAR, S. D., PETRIC, M., AND MIDDLETON, P. J., Indirect microhemagglutination test for varicella-zoster antibody determination, *Can. J. Microbiol.* **22:**1245–1251 (1976).

84. MANSON, M. M., LOGAN, W. P. D., AND LOY, R. M., Rubella and Other Virus Infections During Preg-

nancy, Report 101, pp. 1–101, Ministry of Health, Her Majesty's Stationery Office, London, 1960.

85. MARETIC, A., AND COORAY, M. P. M., Comparisons between chickenpox in a tropical and a European country, *J. Trop. Med. Hyg.* **66**:311–315 (1963).

86. MARR, J. S. (Director, Bureau of Infectious Disease Control, New York City Department of Health), Personal communication, 1974.

87. MATSEOANE, S. L., AND ABLER, C., Occurrence of neonatal varicella in a hospital nursery, *Am. J. Obstet. Gynecol.* **92**:575–576 (1965).

88. MCGREGOR, R. M., Herpes zoster, chickenpox and cancer in general practice, *Br. Med. J.* **1**:84–87 (1957).

89. MCKUSICK, V. A., Fatal varicella (letter to the editor), *J. Am. Med. Assoc.* **207**:370 (1969).

90. MERIGAN, T. C., RAND, K. H., POLLARD, R. B., ABDALLAH, P. S., JORDAN, G. W., AND FRIED, R. P., Human leukocyte interferon for the treatment of herpes zoster in patients with cancer, *N. Engl. J. Med.* **298**:981–987 (1978).

91. MEYERS, J. D., Congenital varicella in term infants: Risk reconsidered, *J. Infect. Dis.* **129**:215–217 (1974).

92. NARAQUI, S., JACKSON, G. G., JONASSON, O., AND YAMASHIROYA, H. M., Prospective study of prevalence, incidence, and source of herpes virus infections in patients with renal allografts, *J. Infect. Dis.* **136**:531–540 (1977).

93. NELSON, A. N., AND ST. GEME, M. W., JR., On the respiratory spread of varicella-zoster virus, *Pediatrics* **37**:1007–1009 (1966).

94. NEUMANN-HAEFELIN, D., SHRESTHA, B., AND MANTHEY, K. F., Effective antiviral prophylaxis and therapy by systemic application of human interferon in immunosuppressed monkeys, *J. Infect. Dis.* **133**(Suppl. A):211–216 (1976).

95. OBERG, G., AND SVEDMYR, A., Varicelliform eruptions in herpes zoster—Some clinical and serological observations, *Scand. J. Infect. Dis.* **1**:47–49 (1969).

96. OLDING-STENKVIST, E., AND GRANDIEN, M., Early diagnosis of virus-caused vesicular rashes by immunofluorescence on skin biopsies. I. Varicella, zoster, and herpes simplex, *Scand. J. Infect. Dis.* **8**:27–35 (1976).

97. OSLER, W., *The Principles and Practice of Medicine*, p. 65, D. Appleton, New York, 1892.

98. OZAKI, T., NAGAYOSHI, S., MORISHIMA, T., ISOMURA, S., SUSUKI, S., ASANO, Y., AND TAKAHASHI, M., Use of a live varicella vaccine for acute leukemic children shortly after exposure in a children's ward, *Biken J.* **21**:69–72 (1978).

99. PALOSUO, T., Varicella and herpes zoster: Differences in antibody response revealed by the platelet aggregation technique, *Scand. J. Infect. Dis.* **4**:83–89 (1972).

100. PICKLES, W. N., *Epidemiology in Country Practice*, pp. 46–47, Williams and Wilkins, Baltimore, 1939.

101. PLOTKIN, G. A., STEIN, S., SNYDER, M., AND IMMESOETE, P., Attempts to recover varicella virus from ganglia, *Ann. Neurol.* **2**:249 (1977).

102. RASMUSSEN, L., HOLMES, A. R., HOFMEISTER, R., AND MERIGAN, T. C., Multiplicity-dependent replication of varicella-zoster virus in interferon treated cells, *J. Gen. Virol.* **35**:361–368 (1977).

103. REBOUL, F., DONALDSON, S. S., AND KAPLAN, H. S., Herpes zoster and varicella infections in children with Hodgkin's disease: An analysis of contributing factors, *Cancer* **41**:95–99 (1978).

104. RIFKIND, D., The activation of varicella-zoster virus infections by immunosuppressive therapy, *J. Lab. Clin. Med.* **68**:463–474 (1966).

105. ROSS, A. H., Modification of chickenpox in family contacts by administration of gamma globulin, *N. Engl. J. Med.* **267**:369–376 (1962).

106. ROSS, C. A. C., AND MCDAID, R., Specific IgM antibody in serum of patients with herpes zoster infections, *Br. Med. J.* **4**:522–523 (1972).

107. ROSS, C. A. C., SUBAK SHARPE, J. H., AND FERRY, P., Antigenic relationship of varicella-zoster and herpes simplex, *Lancet* **2**:708–711 (1965).

108. RUCKDESCHEL, J. C., SCHIMPFF, S. C., SMYTH, A. C., AND MARDINEY, M. R., JR., Herpes zoster and impaired cell-associated immunity to the varicella-zoster virus in patients with Hodgkin's disease, *Am. J. Med.* **62**:77–85 (1977).

109. RUSSELL, A. S., MAINI, R. A., BAILEY, M., AND DUMONDE, D. C., Cell mediated immunity to varicella-zoster antigen in herpes zoster (shingles), *Clin. Exp. Immunol.* **14**:181–185 (1973).

110. SABIN, A. B., Neurotropic virus diseases of man, *J. Pediatr.* **19**:445–451 (1941).

111. SABIN, A. B., Varicella-zoster vaccine: Commentary, *J. Am. Med. Assoc.* **238**:1731–1733 (1977).

112. SALOMON, J. B., GORDON, J. E., AND SCRIMSHAW, N. S., Studies of diarrheal disease in Central America. X. Associated chickenpox, diarrhea and kwashiorkor in a highland Guatemalan village, *Am. J. Trop. Med.* **15**:997–1002 (1966).

113. SCHAAP, G. J. P., AND HUISMAN, J., Simultaneous rise in complement fixing antibodies against herpesvirus hominis and varicella-zoster virus, *Arch. Gesamte Virusforsch.* **17**:495–503 (1968).

114. SCHMIDT, N. J., AND LENNETTE, E. H., Neutralizing antibody responses to varicella-zoster virus, *Infect. Immun.* **12**:606–613 (1975).

115. SCHMIDT, N. J., LENNETTE, E. H., AND MAGOFFIN, R. L., Immunologic relationship between herpes simplex and varicella-zoster viruses demonstrated by

complement-fixation, neutralization, and fluorescent antibody tests, *J. Gen. Virol.* **4**:321–328 (1969).

116. SCHMIDT, N. J., LENNETTE, E. H., WOODIE, J. D., AND Ho, H. H., Immunofluorescent staining in the laboratory diagnosis of varicella-zoster virus infections, *J. Lab. Clin. Med.* **66**:403–412 (1965).

117. SCHOOL EPIDEMICS COMMITTEE OF GREAT BRITAIN, Epidemics in Schools, Medical Research Council, Special Report Series No. 227, London, His Majesty's Stationery Office, 1938.

118. SHIBUTA, H., ISHIKAWA, T., HONDO, R., AOYAMA, Y., KURATA, K., AND MATUMOTO, M., Varicella virus isolation from spinal ganglion, *Arch. Gesamte Virusforsch.* **45**:382–385 (1974).

119. SIEGEL, M., Congenital malformations following chickenpox, measles, mumps, and hepatitis: Results of a cohort study, *J. Am. Med. Assoc.* **226**:1521–1524 (1973).

120. SIEGEL, M., AND FUERST, H. T., Low birth weight and maternal virus disease: A prospective study of rubella, measles, mumps, chickenpox, and hepatitis, *J. Am. Med. Assoc.* **197**:680–684 (1966).

121. SINHA, D. P., Chickenpox—a disease predominantly affecting adults in West Bengal, India, *Int. J. Epidemiol.* **5**:367–374 (1976).

122. SPIRER, Z., Prevention and treatment of varicella during steroid therapy, *Lancet* **1**:635 (1975).

123. STEINER, Zur Inokulation der Varicellen, *Wien. Med. Wochenschr.* **25**:306 (1875).

124. STEVENS, D. A., FERRINGTON, R. A., JORDAN, G. W., AND MERIGAN, T. C., Cellular events in zoster vesicles: Relation to clinical course and immune parameters, *J. Infect. Dis.* **131**:509–515 (1975).

125. STEVENS, D. A., JORDAN, G. W., WADDELL, T. F., AND MERIGAN, T. C., Adverse effect of cytosine arabinoside on disseminated zoster in a controlled trial, *N. Engl. J. Med.* **289**:873–878 (1973).

126. STEVENS, D. A., AND MERIGAN, T. C., Interferon, antibody, and other host factors in herpes zoster, *J. Clin. Invest.* **51**:1170–1178 (1972).

127. STOKES, J., JR., Chickenpox, in: *Preventive Medicine in World War II*, Vol. IV, *Communicable Diseases, Transmitted Chiefly Through Respiratory and Alimentary Tracts*, pp. 55–56, Department of Army, Washington, D.C., 1958.

128. STRÖM, J., Social development and declining incidence of some common epidemic diseases in children: A study of the incidence in different age groups in Stockholm, *Acta Paediatr. Scand.* **56**:159–163 (1967).

129. SVEDMYR, A., Varicella virus in HeLa cells, *Arch. Gesamte Virusforsch.* **17**:495–503 (1965).

130. TAKAHASHI, M., Some risk to varicella vaccine use (letter to the editor), *Pediatrics* **61**:504 (1978).

131. TAKAHASHI, M., OTSUKA, T., OKUNO, Y., ASANO, Y., YAZAKI, T., AND ISOMURA, S., Live vaccine used to prevent the spread of varicella in children in hospital, *Lancet* **2**:1288–1290 (1974).

132. TAKAHASHI, M., OKUNO, Y., OTSUKA, T., OSAME, J., TAKAMIZAWA, A., SASADA, T., AND KUBO, T., Development of a live attenuated varicella vaccine, *Biken J.* **18**:25–33 (1975).

133. TAYLOR-ROBINSON, D., Chickenpox and herpes zoster. III. Tissue culture studies, *Br. J. Exp. Pathol.* **40**:521–532 (1959).

134. TOMLINSON, A. H., AND MACCALLUM, F. O., The incidence of complement-fixing antibody to varicella-zoster virus in hospital patients and blood donors, *J. Hyg.* **68**:411–416 (1970).

135. TRLIFAJOVA, J., RYBA, M., AND JELINEK, J., Indirect hemagglutination reaction (IH)—the method of choice for the detection of anamnestic antibodies to varicella-zoster (VZ) virus, *J. Hyg. Epidemiol. Microbiol. Immunol. (Prague)* **20**:101–106 (1976).

136. TYZZER, E. E., The histology of the skin lesions in varicella, *Philipp. J. Sci.* **1**:349–372 (1906).

137. UDUMAN, S. A., GERSHON, A. A., AND BRUNELL, P. A., Rapid diagnosis of varicella-zoster by agar-gel diffusion, *J. Infect. Dis.* **126**:193–195 (1972).

138. VIROLAINEN, M., SAVILAHTI, E., KATILA, I., AND PERHENTUPA, J., Cellular and humoral immunity in cartilage-cell hypoplasia, *Pediatr. Res.* **12**:961–966 (1978).

139. WEBER, D. M., AND PELLECCHIA, J. A., Varicella pneumonia: Study of prevalence in adult men, *J. Am. Med. Assoc.* **192**:572–573 (1965).

140. WELLER, T. H., The propagation *in vitro* of agents producing inclusion bodies derived from varicella and herpes zoster, *Proc. Soc. Exp. Biol. Med.* **83**:340–346 (1953).

141. WELLER, T. H., Prospects for immunization against varicella and cytomegalovirus infections, in: *First International Conference on Vaccines Against Viral and Rickettsial Diseases of Man*, pp. 276–282, Scientific Publication 147, Pan American Health Organization, Washington, D.C., 1967.

142. WELLER, T. H., Varicella-zoster virus, in: *Diagnostic Procedures for Viral, Rickettsial, and Chlamydial Infections*, 5th ed. (E. H. LENNETTE AND N. J. SCHMIDT, eds.), pp. 375–398, American Public Health Association, Washington, 1979.

143. WELLER, T. H., AND COONS, A. H., Fluorescent antibody studies with agents of varicella and herpes zoster propagated *in vitro*, *Proc. Soc. Exp. Biol. Med.* **86**:789–794 (1954).

144. WELLER, T. H., AND STODDARD, M. B., Intranuclear inclusion bodies in cultures of human tissue inoculated with varicella vesicle fluid, *J. Immunol.* **68**:311–319 (1952).

145. WELLER, T. H., AND WITTON, H. M., The etiologic agents of varicella and herpes zoster: Serologic stud-

ies with the viruses as propagated *in vitro, J. Exp. Med.* **108**:869–890 (1958).

146. Weller, T. H., Witton, H. M., and Bell, E. J., The etiologic agents of varicella and herpes zoster: Isolation, propagation, and cultural characteristics *in vitro, J. Exp. Med.* **108**:843–868 (1958).

147. Wells, M. W., and Holla, W. A., Ventilation in the flow of measles and chickenpox through a community, *J. Am. Med. Assoc.* **142**:1337–1344 (1950).

148. Wentworth, B. B., and Alexander, E. R., Seroepidemiology of infections due to members of herpesvirus group, *Am. J. Epidemiol.* **94**:496–507 (1971).

149. White, E., Chickenpox in Kerala, *Indian J. Public Health* **22**:141–151 (1978).

150. White, R. J., Simmons, l., and Wilson, R. B., Chickenpox in young anthropoid apes: Clinical and laboratory findings, *J. Am. Vet. Med. Assoc.* **161**:690–692 (1972).

151. Whitley, R. J., Ch'ien, L. T., Dolin, R., Galasso, G. J., and Alford, C. A., Jr. (eds.), and the Collaborative Study Group, Adenine arabinoside therapy of herpes zoster in the immunosuppressed, NIAID Collaborative Antiviral Study, *N. Engl. J. Med.* **294**:1193–1199 (1976).

152. Wilson, D., Bressani, R., and Scrimshaw, N. S., Infection and nutritional status. I. Effect of chickenpox on nitrogen metabolism in children, *Am. J. Clin. Nutr.* **9**:154–158 (1961).

153. Winsnes, R., Efficacy of zoster immunoglobulin in prophylaxis of varicella in high-risk patients, *Acta Paediatr. Scand.* **67**:77–82 (1978).

154. Winsnes, R., Froland, S. S., and Degre, M. I., Effect of transfer factor and zoster immunoglobulin in patients with varicella-zoster infection and malignancy, *Scand. J. Infect. Dis.* **10**:21–27 (1978).

155. Wong, C. L., Castriciano, S., Chernesky, M. A., and Rawls, W. E., Quantitation of antibodies to varicella-zoster virus by immune adherence hemagglutination, *J. Clin. Microbiol.* **7**:6–11 (1978).

156. Yorke, J. A., and London, W. P., Recurrent outbreaks of measles, chickenpox, and mumps. II. Systematic differences in contact rates and stochastic effects, *Am. J. Epidemiol.* **98**:469–482 (1973).

157. Zaia, J. A., Leary, P. L., and Levin, M. J., Specificity of the blastogenic response of human mononuclear cells to herpesvirus antigens, *Infect. Immun.* **20**:646–651 (1978).

158. Zaia, J. A., Levin, M. J., Wright, G. G., and Grady, G. F., A practical method for preparation of varicella-zoster immune globulin, *J. Infect. Dis.* **137**:601–604 (1978).

159. Zaia, J. A., and Oxman, M. N., Antibody to varicella-zoster virus-induced membrane antigen: Immunofluorescence assay using monodisperse glutaraldehyde-fixed target cells, *J. Infect. Dis.* **136**:519–530 (1977).

160. Zinsser, H., Immunology of infections by filterable virus agents, in: *Virus and Rickettsial Diseases*, p. 106, Harvard University Press, Cambridge, 1940.

12. Suggested Reading

12.1. Monographic Summaries of Information on Varicella and on Herpes Zoster

Juel-Jensen, B. E., and MacCallum, F. O., *Herpes Simplex, Varicella and Zoster*, Lippincott, Philadelphia, 1972, 194 pp.

Taylor-Robinson, d., and Caunt, A. E., *Varicella Virus*, Virology Monograph No. 12, Springer-Verlag, New York, 1972, 88 pp.

12.2. Comprehensive Review of the Epidemiology of Varicella, with 257 References Covering the Literature through 1961

Gordon, J. E., Chickenpox: An epidemiological review, *Am. J. Med. Sci.* **244**:362–389 (1962).

12.3. Summary of Procedures for Isolation and Study of Varicella–Zoster Virus in the Laboratory

Weller, T. H., Varicella-zoster virus, in: *Diagnostic Procedures for Viral and Rickettsial Infections*, 5th ed. (E. H. Lennette and N. J. Schmidt, eds.), pp. 375–398, American Public Health Association, Washington, 1979.

12.4. Clinical Descriptions of Varicella and of Zoster, Including Complications and Differential Diagnosis

Brunell, P. A., Chickenpox, in: *Communicable and Infectious Diseases*, 8th ed. (F. H. Top, Sr., and P. R. Wehrle, eds.), pp. 165–173, C. V. Mosby, St. Louis, 1976.

Krugman, S., Ward, R., and Katz, S. L., Varicella and zoster infections, in: *Infectious Diseases of Children*, 6th ed., pp. 451–471, C. V. Mosby, St. Louis, 1977.

Marcy, S. M., and Kibrick, S., Varicella and herpes zoster, in: *Infectious Diseases*, 2nd ed. (P. D. Hoeprich, ed.), pp. 744–758, Harper and Row, Hagerstown, Md., 1977.

12.5. An Encyclopedic, Multiauthored Summary of Knowledge of the Herpesviruses of Man and of Animals

Kaplan, A. S., (ed.), with 26 co-authors, *The Herpesviruses*, Academic Press, New York, 1973, 739 pp.

PART III

Malignant and Chronic Neurological Diseases Associated with Viruses

CHAPTER 24

Burkitt Lymphoma

George Miller

1. Introduction

Burkitt lymphoma (BL) is a malignant lymphoma of children occurring with highest frequency in certain parts of Africa and New Guinea where malaria is hyperendemic. It is found in low frequency throughout the world and in nonmalarious areas.

The epidemiology of the disease is highly characteristic and provoked Burkitt's hypothesis that the causal agent might be vectored virus. It is a disease of children and is rare before the age of 2 years and after the age of 20 years. The median age of patients in endemic areas is approximately 8 years.[4] Burkitt tumor is the most common childhood tumor in Africa, and its incidence in the two major endemic areas, equatorial Africa and Papua New Guinea, may reach as high as 10/100,000 in children living in certain districts. The tumor is found primarily in the hot, wet, lowlands of Africa and New Guinea, although sporadic cases have been described throughout the world.[1,120]

Given the state of our knowledge at this time, it would seem justified to make an association with the Epstein–Barr virus (EBV) part of the definition of the disease as it occurs in the endemic areas. The tumor itself contains, in nearly all instances, the EBV genome[92,128] and certain EBV antigens,[77] and EBV-producing cell lines can be derived from the tumors, as initially shown by Epstein and co-workers.[37,38] Patients with BL have elevated antibody

George Miller · Department of Pediatrics and Department of Epidemiology and Public Health, Yale University School of Medicine, New Haven, Connecticut.

titers to EBV[57] and certain unique EBV-related antibodies.[60] The etiological association of EBV with BL is strengthened by experimental observations that EBV is capable of providing immortality *in vitro* to normal lymphocytes of humans and certain primates[58,82,100] and that EBV induces a lymphoma on inoculation into certain species of New World nonhuman primates.[40,85,110]

The majority of BLs in America and Europe do not contain detectable EBV DNA, and a rare case of BL in the endemic region is also free of EBV DNA.[72,125] This suggests that the tumor may have multiple etiologies.

2. Historical Background

The clinical syndrome described in detail by Burkitt[13] in 1958 during his tour as a surgeon in East Africa had been, in retrospect, known to clinicians and pathologists since the beginning of the 20th century.[25,30] However, through Burkitt's efforts, the disease was unified into a clearly delineated entity with characteristic clinical, pathological, and epidemiological features.[13,15,18,19]

The concept that this lymphoma might be due to a virus was suggested by Burkitt[14] in 1962, but the initial search for an agent was unsuccessful. In 1964, Epstein and Barr[37] and Pulvertaft[102] simultaneously reported in the same issue of *The Lancet* the successful growth of tumor cells from BL tissue in the laboratory; this was rapidly followed by the observation of herpeslike particles in these cultured cells under the electron microscope.[39] The agent was found to be distinct from other known herpesviruses of man, and it was designated as *Epstein–Barr virus*. Attempts to cultivate EBV in other tissue-culture systems were unsuccessful, but the development of an immunofluorescent test for EBV antibody by Henle and Henle[56] in 1966 facilitated epidemiological and diagnostic inquiry. The presence of EBV genome in lymphoma cells was demonstrated by zur Hausen *et al.*[128] in 1970, and the experimental production of lymphomas with EBV in nonhuman primates was reported in 1973 by Shope *et al.*[110] and by Epstein *et al.*[40]

3. Methodology

3.1. Mortality and Morbidity Data

Three methods have been used to estimate the number of children with BL. After Burkitt observed the disease in Uganda, he undertook a series of "tumor safaris," traveling thousands of miles by jeep throughout Africa.[15] Similar informal surveys have been conducted in New Guinea. In areas where the disease is common—for example, in East Africa—tumor registries and records of cancer hospitals have served as a source of case-finding, particularly the Kenyatta National Hospital in Nairobi, Kenya, the Mulogo Hospital in Kampala, Uganda, and the Makerere University College Medical School in Kampala, Uganda. Finally, the epidemiology of BL has been studied intensively by close surveillance of limited geographic areas where there is a high incidence of disease. In particular, the West Nile district of Uganda was intensively studied on a house-to-house basis and was the site of a prospective serological survey in which the protective effects of EBV antibodies were assessed.[34,68,99] In this study, which involved over 40,000 children, it was determined that the sera of BL patients contain elevated titers of antibody to EB viral capsid antigen (VCA) from 7 to 54 months prior to the clinical detection of the tumors.

3.2. Serological Surveys

Studies for the presence of antibody to EBV have been carried out throughout the world using the indirect immunofluorescence test of the Henles for antibody to VCA as the major epidemiological tool. Immunoglobulin M (IgM) antibodies to VCA have served as an indication of recent primary infection.[5,108] Antibody determinations against the diffuse (D) and restricted (R) components of the "early antigen" (EA) complex have been used as indicators of tumor burden and for prognosis of survival.[59] Occasionally, antibodies directed against neoantigens located in the nucleus (EBNA) or on the membrane (MA) of infected cells have been measured in serological surveys.

3.3. Laboratory Diagnosis

The pathological criteria of BL have been well established through conferences under the auspices of the U.S. National Cancer Institute, the International Agency for Cancer Research, and the World Health Organization.[7] The virological features of African lymphomas associated with EBV are (1) presence of antibody to EBV, (2) elevation of VCA antibody titers to 1:160 or higher, and (3) presence of antibodies to early and membrane antigens and, if tissue is available, demonstration of the EBV genome by hybridization[92,128] with EBV nucleic acid and by the EBNA or anticomplement immunofluorescence test.[78]

4. Biology of Epstein–Barr Virus

4.1. Structure and Morphology

To appreciate the nature of the evidence relating EBV to BL, a brief introduction to the biology of this agent is necessary. On the basis of its morphology and the size of its nucleic acid, which is double-stranded DNA, this virus belongs to the herpes group.[109] The mature virus possesses a lipoprotein envelope and inner capsid structure with regular capsimeres, 162 in number, and a nucleoid that contains the nucleic acid. Physical maps prepared with the EcoRI and Sal restriction endonucleases are now available for the DNAs of two transforming strains of EBV, B95-8 (Hawley) from mononucleosis and W91 (Nyevu) from BL.[49] These genomes are greater than 95% homologous and share several features. The ends of the DNA are identical and composed of varying numbers of repeating subunits.[70] This permits circularization of the genome following exonuclease digestion. There is also an internal area within the genome of serial repeats of 2.0×10^6 dalton sequence.[107] One segment of DNA is found in W91 but is absent in B95-8.

There are two biological variants of EBV. One, represented by the unique P3JHR-1 virus, is cytolytic to B lymphocytes, is efficient at superinfection and antigen induction in genome carrier cells, and fails to transform cells *in vitro* or to induce tumors in primates.[62,84] The virus has apparently lost its transforming potential on laboratory passage. All other strains analyzed so far are not cytolytic on their initial interactions and are transforming and tumorigenic. The structural basis for these biological differences is not yet clear, but the DNAs of both biological variants are highly similar. However, based on partial thermal denaturation mapping, the P3JHR-1 virus is heterogeneous and appears to contain two different types of genomes. One genome seems to be a rearrangement of the sequences found in the transforming genome.[32]

The question whether different virus strains are consistently associated with different diseases is not yet resolved, but most available evidence indicates that there are not specific strains for each EBV-associated disease.

4.2. Epstein–Barr Virus Cell-Associated Antigens

The mature EBV has been seen only rarely in BL biopsies.[51] However, if lymphoid tissues from the tumors are cultivated *in vitro*, continuous lymphoid-cell lines are obtained in which mature EBV may be found in a small proportion of the cells.[38,90] Such continuous lymphoid-cell lines have served to define a number of cell-associated EBV-related antigens. Such antigens have served as one basis for search for evidence of the virus in human tumors. A *membrane antigen* (MA) is found on the surface of BL biopsies as well as on the surface of certain continuous lymphoblastoid-cell lines.[71] An intracellular antigen, designated *viral capsid antigen* (VCA), is found in a small percentage of cells of continuous lymphoblastoid-cell lines that are productive of virus.[56] This antigen is not usually detected in biopsies of BL and is present only in those cell lines that are also productive of virus. Some continuous cell lines produce MA but not VCA. A third antigen, called *early antigen* (EA), appears on abortive infection of continuous lymphoblastoid cells by EBV.[60] This antigen is not detected *in vivo* but appears in a subpopulation of cells of productive lymphoblastoid-cell lines. EA can also be induced in nonproductive cell lines by treatment with halogenated pyrimidines.[46,53,54] A *nuclear antigen* (EBNA) is found in all living cells of continuous lymphoblastoid-cell lines that contain the EBV genome.[104] It is also found *in vivo* in BL, in nasopharyngeal carcinoma, and in experimental EBV-induced lymphoma of marmosets.[77,80,105,122] This important antigen is present whether or not the cells are producing mature virus. The EBNA has been purified to homogeneity; it appears to consist of four identical subunits, each with molecular weight of 40,000 daltons. EBNA binds to DNA, but otherwise its biological function is not known.[78]

Antigen complexes have also been detected in cell extracts by complement fixation (CF) and represent at least three distinct components.[117] Some of the CF reactivity of cell lines is no doubt due to the EBNA reactivity. A soluble antigen has been found in continuous lymphoblastoid-cell lines detectable by immunodiffusion.[96]

There are as yet no studies that demonstrate differences between the cell-associated antigens found in BL cells and comparable antigens found in cells derived from patients with infectious mononucleosis or nasopharyngeal cancer or from normal persons. A summary of EBV-related antigens found in BL biopsies and in cell lines derived therefrom is presented in Table 1.

4.3. Cell–Virus Relationships

Only a fraction of cells in continuous lymphoblastoid-cell lines from BL contain viral particles or the VCA; nonetheless, all the cells contain the viral genome. If single cells are plated from a line that contains only 1–5% of cells with virus, all the daughter clones contain virus.[87] This finding demonstrates that the viral genome is present in cells that are not making virus but its expression is somehow inhibited. Furthermore, continuous cell lines completely lacking in signs of mature virus production have been derived from BL. The prototype of such a cell line is called *Raji*.[36] Raji nonetheless contains

Table 1. A Scheme Illustrating Differences in the Expression of the Epstein–Barr
Virus Genome in Burkitt Lymphoma Cells

	Burkitt lymphoma		
Viral function detected	Biopsies	Nonproductive cell lines	Productive cell lines
Viral DNA	+	+	+
Viral-specific RNA	+	+	+
Complement-fixing (CF) antigen	+	+	+
Nuclear antigen (EBNA)	+	+	+
Membrane antigen (MA)	+	−	+
Early antigen (EA)	−	Inducible	+
Viral capsid antigen (VCA)	−	−	+
Nucleocapsids	−	−	+
Enveloped virus	−	−	±

certain viral antigens, particularly EBNA, and contains the viral genome detectable by nucleic acid hybridization.[93,127]

Considerable effort has gone into defining the state of the viral genome in Raji cells. The genome appears to be associated with cellular chromosomes.[93] The number of copies of EBV genes per Raji cell is relatively constant between 40 and 60 per cell as the line is maintained in culture. The number of EBV-genome copies doubles early in the S (DNA synthesis) phase of the cell mitotic cycle.[53] The majority of EBV DNA in Raji cells is not covalently integrated into cellular DNA.[93] These viral genomes exist as circles with superhelical twists.[2] There is also some evidence that a minor population of genomes present in Raji cells is linearly integrated into cellular DNA.[3] Only a small fraction of the genome in Raji is transcribed.[101]

Several lines of evidence indicate that the host cell modulates the expression of the resident viral genome. For example, when a somatic-cell hybrid is produced between a cell line productive of EBV and an epithelioid-cell line, the resulting cell hybrid contains the EBV genome detectable by nucleic acid hybridization but no longer produces virus particles.[50] Furthermore, there is a marked difference in the expression of the viral genome in cells of different species, all containing the same strain of EBV. Human cells derived from umbilical-cord lymphocytes are nonproductive and express only EBNA; by contrast, marmoset lymphocytes containing the same strain of virus are fully productive and release considerable quantities of extracellular virus.[81]

4.4. Cell Transformation and Oncogenicity

When EBV is added *in vitro* to normal human lymphocytes derived from an antibody-negative subject or from umbilical-cord blood, the cells acquire the ability to grow continuously in culture and to grow in semisolid medium.[58,114,123] This process is often referred to as *immortalization*.[79] Morphological changes, consisting of enlargement, clumping, and rapid cell growth, are preceded by the appearance of EBNA and stimulation of cellular DNA synthesis.[47,106] The usual target cell for immortalization by the virus is a small resting lymphocyte derived from bone marrow.[55,64] There is evidence that an intact EBV genome is required to immortalize the cell, and B cells immortalized *in vitro* usually contain the entire viral genome.[113] The efficiency of immortalization by EBV is very high. It has been estimated that 1 in 50 viral genomes produced in tissue culture is capable of immortalization. At least 20–30% of a cell population enriched in B lymphocytes can be immortalized. EBV can also immortalize nonhuman primate B cells,[41,86,118] and the virus produces a lymphoma in nonhuman primates.[40,79,80,85,110] The experimental disease reproduces many of the characteristics of the human infections. There is a spectrum of responses of the inoculated marmosets varying from inapparent infection to transient lymphoid hyperplasia to malignant lymphoma that originates in the germinal follicle and resembles the immunoblastic sarcoma of man.[85] Those tumored animals that live for a long time develop elevated antibody levels to EBV. The virus can be recovered from the abdominal lymph nodes in the form of continuous lymphoblastoid-cell lines, and EBNA appears in imprints made directly from tumor cells. The EBV genome has been detected in several experimental tumors.[121] The incidence of tumors in inoculated marmosets is increased by treatment with immunosuppressive drugs.

4.5. Relationship of Epstein–Barr Virus to Burkitt Lymphoma

4.5.1. Demonstration of EBV in the Tumor.
Biopsies of BL from the endemic areas regularly contain the viral genome detectable by nucleic acid hybridization with radioactive complementary RNA or DNA probes.[92,128] A rare tumor in the endemic area, histologically compatible with BL fails to demonstrate the viral genome. In BL occurring outside the endemic area, EBV DNA is associated with approximately 20% of the tumors, and the remainder are genome-negative.[125] The viral DNA has only rarely been detected in lymph nodes affected with other lymphoproliferative diseases. For example, Lindahl et al.[77] have studied 21 Swedish patients with Hodgkin's disease, lymphocytic lymphoma, or chronic leukemia and have failed to detect the EBV genome by hybridization. Recently, Bornkamm et al.[11] have found EBV DNA in a condition known as immunoblastic lymphadenopathy.

When EBV DNA is present in a BL, there are between 6 and 100 copies of the viral genome per cell. Sugden[113] has found, using the Southern transfer technique, that the tumors contain a large portion of the viral DNA, probably all of it, and not just a fragment of the genome. The viral DNA in BL cells is mainly in the form of superhelically twisted circular molecules; integrated DNA may also be present.[69]

Viral-specific RNA has been found in the BL biopsies by Kieff and co-workers. These transcripts represent about 3–6% of the genome, and they map at various locations on the viral DNA. One transcript appears to come from a portion of the DNA that is present in an EBV strain derived from BL and absent in a strain from mononucleosis.[29]

Cell lines that contain EBV antigens (EBNA and often VCA and EA) and the viral genome can be regularly established from BL. In the initial biopsy from which the cell lines are derived, only EBNA is detectable, and there is usually no evidence for

mature virus or VCA. However, these appear within several days after the cells have been cultivated in vitro. A small number of continuous cell lines have been established from genome-negative tumors; these lines lack EBV antigens or DNA. Both EBV-genome-positive and -genome-negative lymphoblastoid cell lines from BL have the characteristics of B lymphocytes. Most contain intracellular and surface Ig, and they often secrete Ig. They also contain a receptor for the third component of complement.

4.5.2. Seroepidemiological Relationships.
Seroepidemiological surveys of antibodies against the VCA have demonstrated that EBV is worldwide in its distribution and there is no major difference in the incidence of antibodies in patients and control groups from the endemic area.[57,76] However, the relative rate of acquisition of antibodies differs markedly by geographic locale and socioeconomic class. For example, in East Africa, nearly 80% of 2- to 4-year-olds have antibodies to VCA; by contrast, only 40% of sera from 2- to 4-year-olds of American lower socioeconomic classes are positive for antibodies to the same antigen.[57] This result strongly suggests that in the endemic area, infection is acquired at a very early age (see Fig. 1)

A recent study of infants in Ghana by Biggar et al.[9,10] has shown that maternal antibodies against VCA are acquired via the transplacental route by all infants. These disappear by 6 months of age. Between 6 and 18 months of age, 80% of the infants studied developed their own antibodies to EBV without any clinically discernible illness. It was notable that these silent primary EBV infections in infants were accompanied by transient appearance of antibody to the R component of early antigen, whereas primary infection in adults, i.e., mononucleosis, has classically been associated with an anti-D (EA) response. Anti-R (EA) is also seen in infantile EBV infections in America.[45]

As part of the prospective study in the West Nile district of Uganda, the rate at which susceptibles in East Africa become infected has been investigated: 50% of the susceptibles aged 0–5 years acquired antibodies in the 18 months between a first and a second serum sample. The infection was not as readily transmitted in older subjects, for the rate of seroconversion of susceptibles was 37% in the age group 6–10 and nil in the age group 11–15.[68] There does not seem to be any marked difference in incidence of positive antibody titers in BL patients and in a wide variety of control groups including subjects matched for age, sex, and tribe. Siblings and neighbors, subjects from areas of high BL incidence, or subjects from areas of low BL incidence all seem to have approximately the same frequency of antibody to EBV.

Thus, the picture that emerged from initial seroepidemiological study was that infection with EBV was ubiquitous. However, marked differences were encountered in antibody titers between BL patients and control populations.[57] For example, the Henles and their collaborators found that of 139 patients with BL, 81.3% had antibodies with titers of 1:160 or greater, and the geometric mean titer was 275. By contrast, the geometric mean titer of 489 control patients was 1:37, and only 14% of the positive titers were greater than 1:160. Patients with other cancers, including patients with lymphomas, did not have elevated EBV antibodies as a rule, although patients with Hodgkin's disease have slightly higher geometric mean titers than normal.[33,74]

The association of elevated EB VCA antibody titers with Burkitt tumors is most striking in the endemic area. In contrast, studies reported from two laboratories indicate that between one sixth and one third of American patients with a histological diagnosis of BL failed to demonstrate antibodies to EBV, and the levels of such antibodies in sera of American BL patients are in the range found in normal persons.[63,75]

Elevated antibody titers to EBV have been encountered in other diseases such as sarcoidosis.[20] The cause of antibody elevation in patients with BL remains conjectural. Elevated EBV titers are not a feature of malignancy in general.[33]

Few studies have attempted to compare the height of the titers of antibodies to viruses other than EBV. One study has shown that antibody titers to cytomegalovirus (CMV) and varicella–zoster virus were approximately 4-fold higher in BL patients than in matched controls.[61] However, this finding has not been confirmed in other laboratories. In the prospective study in Uganda, there were no differences between BL patients and controls in antibody titers to herpes simplex virus, CMV, or measles virus in sera taken either before or after tumor development[34] (see Section 4.5.3).

4.5.3. Prospective Seroepidemiological Study of BL. Under the auspices of the International Agency for Research on Cancer and under the direction of Dr. G. de-Thé, a prospective study was conducted in the West Nile district of Uganda to determine the relationship of EBV infection to BL.[34] Serum samples were taken from 42,000 children who were then followed for 5 years. In this group, 14 cases of BL developed. This rate, of approximately 7 per 10^5 per year, was lower than expected and was associated with a declining incidence of BL in the study area. All the patients with BL had antibodies to EBV in the initial serum samples obtained between 7 and 54 months before the diagnosis of BL (see Fig. 2). Thus, BL is not associated with primary EBV infection, but is possibly a late sequela. Of the 14 BL patients, 10 had antibody titers to VCA that were 2-fold or more higher than those found in sera of matched controls. Thus, in BL patients, the phenomenon of elevated anti-VCA seems to precede the development of the tumor. Tumor tissue from 5 patients with elevated anti-VCA antibodies was tested for EBV DNA; 4 contained between 40 and

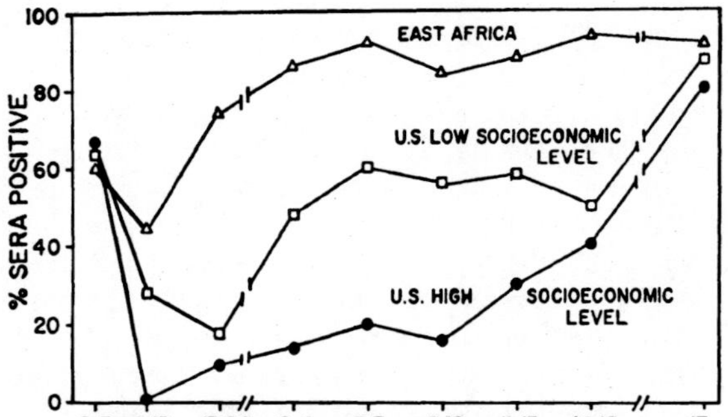

Fig. 1. Age distribution of antibodies to EBV in East Africa and the United States. From Henle et al.[57]

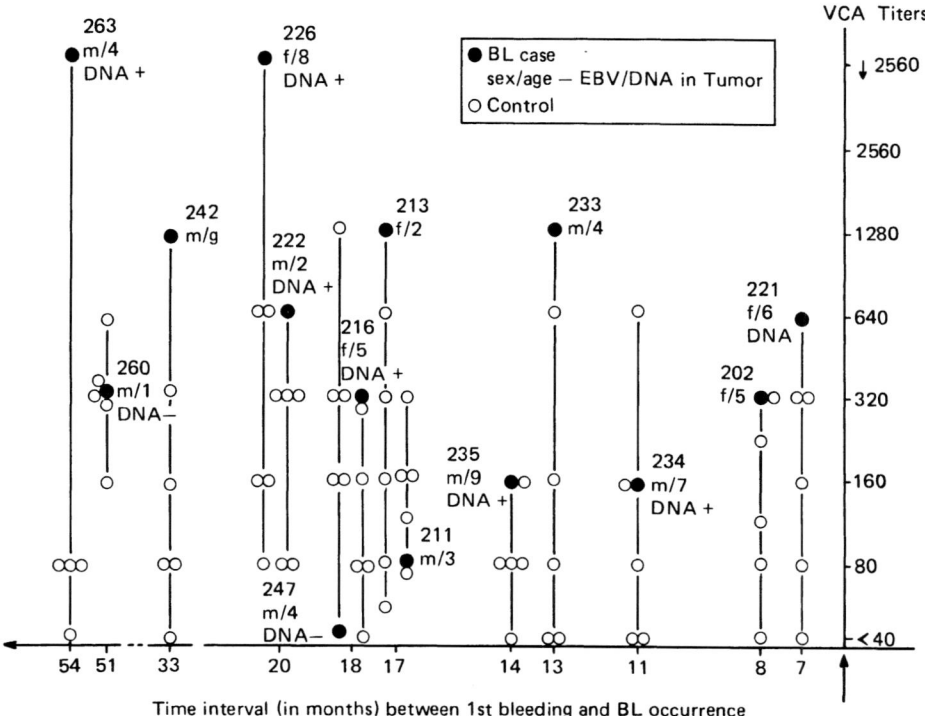

Fig. 2. EBV VCA titers in sera collected from BL cases prior to tumor manifestation and from controls, by length of interval between bleeding and case detection.

116 genomes per cell; the fifth was negative. The tumor of 1 of the 4 patients without elevated anti-VCA did not contain the EBV genome; one tumor from a patient with normal anti-VCA titers was genome-positive; the other tumor was not available for testing. Antibody titers to other EBV-associated antigens such as EA, EBNA, or the soluble CF antigen were not different in the initial bleeding sera of BL patients and controls. However, 10 of the 14 BL patients and none of the controls developed antibody to the EA-R component. In general, the study supports an association between EBV and BL. In the study population, a 2-fold or higher elevation of anti-VCA titer was associated with a 30-fold increased risk for development of BL. It was conjectured that anti-VCA elevation was associated with increased virus burden. Whether this was due to virus strain variation, to increased permissiveness of certain subjects' cells to viral replication, or to

specific deficiencies in anti-EBV control mechanisms is not known.

5. Descriptive Epidemiology

5.1. Incidence

In the endemic areas, BL is the most common childhood cancer and may reach an incidence of as high as 8–10 cases per 100,000 per year in certain circumscribed geographic locales. Within Kenya, for example, as illustrated in Table 2, the incidence of childhood lymphoma varies markedly among tribes in different geographic areas. This variation in incidence is not seen in adult lymphoma or in squamous-cell carcinoma. In Kenya, the highest incidence occurs in the Bantu tribes living along the coast, whereas a low incidence (approximately one

Table 2. Tribal Distribution of Lymphomas and Epitheliomas in Kenya[a]

| Ethnic groups | Tribes | Lymphomas[b] | | | | Squamous-cell carcinoma (adults and children, per 100,000)[b] |
| | | Children | | Adults | | |
		Number	Per 100,000	Number	Per 100,000	
Bantu	Coastal	31	8.2	11	2.9	8.3
Nilotic	Luo	48	6.3	21	2.8	5.7
Bantu	Luhya	30	4.5	13	2.0	6.6
Bantu	Kisii	9	3.5	9	3.5	9.7
Bantu	Kamba	18	3.1	28	4.6	9.2
Bantu	Kikuya	31	2.0	53	3.3	9.5
Nilo-Hamitic	Kalenjin	5	1.2	9	2.2	8.5

[a] From Dalldorf et al.[28]
[b] This is not the annual incidence per 100,000, but the number of tumors identified in the Nairobi Cancer Registry during 1957–1962 inclusive, related to the standardized tribal breakdown of the population in Kenya.

eighth the incidence among the coastal tribes) occurs in tribes living in central highlands.[30] Similar variations in incidence have been described for Uganda districts (see Fig. 3), with high rates in the northern districts and low rates in the southwestern districts.[18]

In certain areas of Uganda—for example, the Mengo districts in central Uganda—there appears to have been a marked decrease in incidence in recent years. In the Mengo districts, the rate was 30/ 1,000,000 per year early in the 1960s and declined to 9/1,000,000 per year by the end of the 1960s, at a time when case-finding efforts were probably increased.[88] By contrast, in other areas of Uganda— for example, the northern region—the incidence remained stable at a rate of 5–10/100,000 per year.

In many areas of the world, a clinical pathological entity resembling BL has been identified. In some countries—for example, Malaysia, Colombia, and Brazil[1,16,22]— the incidence of BL is intermediate between that in the endemic areas of Africa and New Guinea and that in the rest of the world where the disease is only sporadic.

BL occurs in endemic pattern in areas of the world where malaria is either "hyper- or holoendemic." In these areas, malaria infection is universal, occurs very early in life, and is transmitted throughout the year.[17,28,67] Conversely, endemic BL has not been encountered in nonmalarious areas of the world. Of great interest is the low incidence of disease in certain isolated areas—for example, the islands of Zanzibar and Pemba, which are only 20 miles from the

coast of Tanzania, where the tumor is endemic.[17] The low tumor incidence can also be correlated with a very low incidence of malaria resulting from malaria eradication campaigns. Furthermore, the decreasing incidence of disease in Uganda and in Natal, as well as in New Guinea, can be correlated with programs of malaria eradication.

The incidence of childhood lymphoma in the endemic areas of Africa is approximately twice the incidence in the United States of acute lymphoblastic leukemia, the most common malignant disease of childhood. In the United States, lymphoma is third as a cause of childhood cancer and is approximately one eighth as common as leukemia. Thus, Dalldorf[27] suggested that there appeared to be a reciprocal relationship between the incidence of leukemia and that of lymphoma. However, the low incidence of leukemia in Africa may be related to ease of diagnosis rather than to real differences in incidence.[116]

5.2. Geographic Factors

As a general rule, BL occurs in hot, wet, rural lowlands. Exceptions to this generalization have been found,[8] but it appears that this constellation of geographic attributes is characteristic for those areas where the disease is endemic. On the basis of his personal surveys, Burkitt suggested that endemic areas for the tumor are lower than 3000 feet above sea level and have an annual rainfall of more than 40 inches. Figure 4 is one of the early maps showing the distribution of the tumor in a belt across central Africa.

Within the endemic areas, there are some instances of microepidemics that result in marked clustering of cases in space and time.[89,99] For example, Pike et al.[99] noted that in the West Nile district of Uganda five cases in 2 years occurred in one village and that most cases occurred in adjacent counties. Morrow et al.[89] identified seven cases in 27 months in Bwamba County, Uganda. In the West Nile district, new cases are diagnosed twice as often

in the second half of the year as in the first, although cases appear during each month.[119]

Recently, a cluster of four young adults with EBV-associated BL was observed in rural Pennsylvania in one year. The patients lived within 30 miles of one another, and two had shared the same household.[66]

5.3. Age and Sex

The ages of 661 patients recorded in Uganda by Burkitt are given in Fig. 5. The median age of pa-

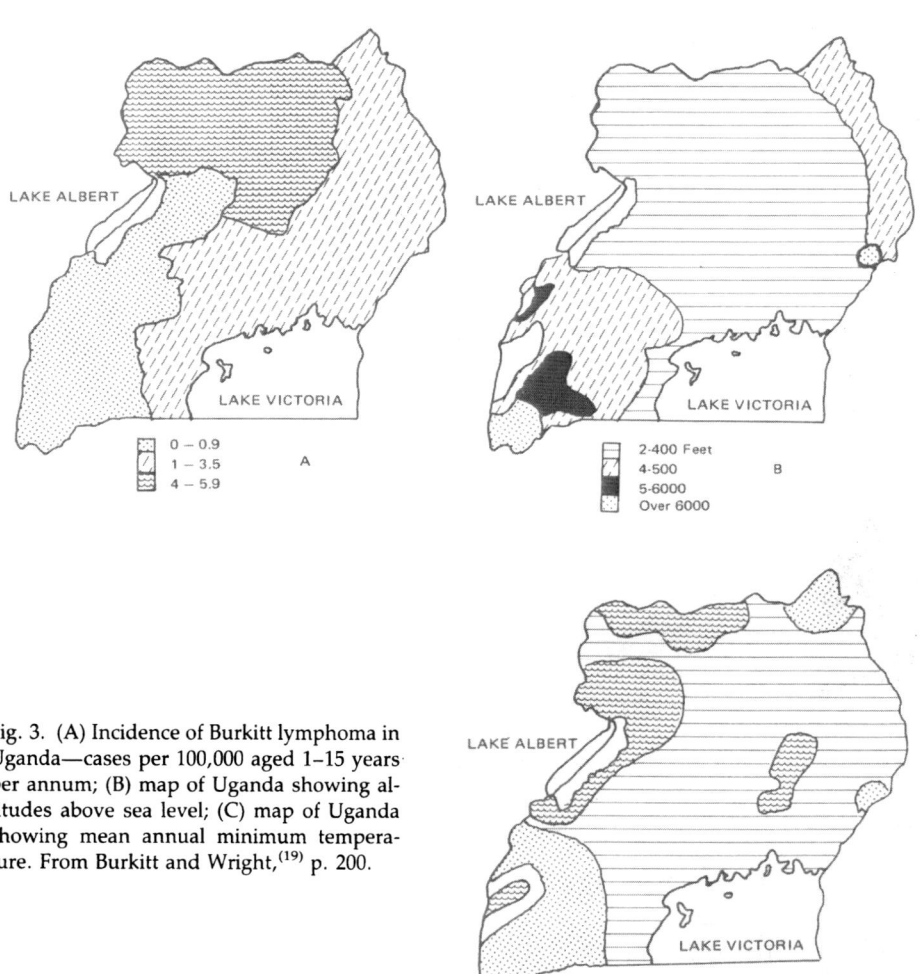

Fig. 3. (A) Incidence of Burkitt lymphoma in Uganda—cases per 100,000 aged 1–15 years per annum; (B) map of Uganda showing altitudes above sea level; (C) map of Uganda showing mean annual minimum temperature. From Burkitt and Wright,[19] p. 200.

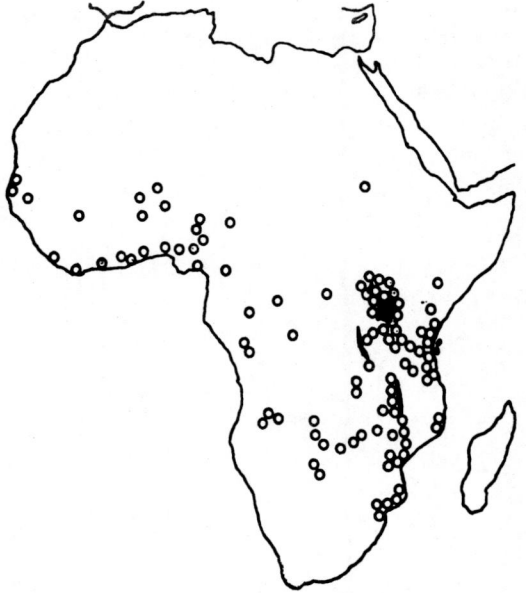

Fig. 4. Known tumor distribution in Africa. From Burkitt.[15]

ample, nearly 50% of patients who are immigrant Banyarwanda and Bakiga tribesmen from Rwanda and Burundi to the southwest, where there is a low incidence of Burkitt lymphoma, are over 15 years old, and 26% are over 30 years old. Furthermore, within Uganda, the age of patients is greater in low-incidence areas than in the high-incidence areas. Outside the endemic area—for example, in America—BL patients are slightly older; the median age of 20 patients was 10.5 years.[125]

The overall sex incidence is 2.3 males to 1 female. This is apparently a real difference, for the sex ratio of cases of Wilm's tumor and retinoblastoma recorded in the Kampala registry is approximately 1.

5.4. Genetic and Other Host Factors

Since BL is endemic in both East Africa and New Guinea, it is unlikely that there is a genetic predisposition limited to a relatively small ethnic or tribal group. However, since the association between malaria and BL appears so strong, some effort has been made to determine whether genetic factors that protect against malaria might influence the epidemiology of BL. For example, Pike et al.[98] studied the frequency of the sickle-cell hemoglobin heterozygous trait in patients with Burkitt tumor as compared with hospitalized and normal control subjects. They found AS hemoglobin in approximately 17% of Burkitt tumor patients compared to 24–29% of controls. Since the sickle-cell trait is associated

tients is remarkably constant from one area to another. For example, in Uganda, Nigeria, Ghana, and New Guinea, the median age ranges from 7.7 to 9.2 years.[4] Burkitt noted that the age of patients with African lymphoma who are immigrant to central Uganda is greater than the age of lymphoma patients who are born in the endemic areas. For ex-

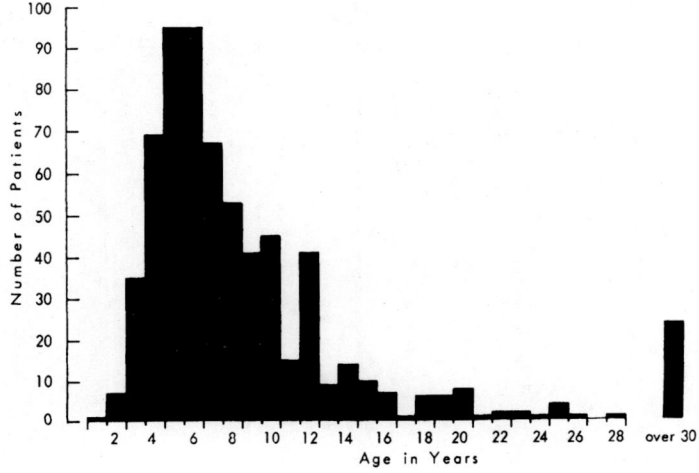

Fig. 5. Age distribution of 661 patients recorded in Uganda. From Burkitt and Wright,[19] p. 7.

Table 3. Hemoglobin Genotype in Nigerian Burkitt Tumor Patients and Controls

Hemoglobin genotype	Ibadan Hospital				Ilora village controls	
	Patients		Controls			
AA	78	(78.0%)	225	(68.0%)	142	(70.3%)
AS	17	(17.0%)	95	(28.7%)	49	(24.3%)
SC,SS,CC,AC	5	(5.0%)	11	(3.3%)	11	(5.4%)
TOTALS:	100	(100.0%)	331	(100.00%)	202	(100.00%)

with protection against malaria, this observation is compatible with the hypothesis that sickle-cell trait may also be somewhat protective against BL (see Table 3).

6. Mechanism and Route of Transmission

The geographic and climatic distribution of BL was found to correspond to the distribution of yellow fever in Africa; this prompted the initial suggestion that the disease was transmitted by an arthropod vector. This route of transmission has not been proved. However, EBV has been demonstrated in the oropharyngeal secretions of patients with infectious mononucleosis and BL and in healthy persons.[23,48,83] Although the exact site of viral replication has not been defined, the virus is preferentially present in saliva, including saliva obtained by cannulation of the parotid duct.[91] It is attractive to speculate that BL begins in the vicinity of the oropharynx, because this is the first site of viral exposure and replication. A form of stomatitis appears to precede or coincide with the onset of BL. The etiology of the stomatitis is not known, but its existence may also help account for the original site of tumor involvement.[31]

7. Pathogenesis

7.1. Cell Transformation

Presumably, during the course of oropharyngeal replication of the virus, some lymphoid cells in the vicinity are transformed by the virus; that is, their growth potential is increased by interaction with the virus. Following this event, there is thought to be an additional event or events that result in the conversion of one of the cells with increased growth potential into a clone of malignant cells. Several types of studies support the concept that Burkitt tumors arise from single cells.[43]

BL biopsy specimens examined for the presence of IgM on their surface fall into two groups: in approximately 84% of the tumors, all the cells demonstrate Ig staining, and in about 16% of the tumors, there is no Ig staining. Thus, the majority of Burkitt tumors are clonal with respect to Ig heavy-chain production.

A proportion of female BL patients are heterozygous for the glucose-6-phosphate dehydrogenase (G-6-PD) enzyme, which is associated with the X chromosome. In females, one or the other of the X chromosomes is inactivated in each cell. Consequently, if the Burkitt tumor had a multicellular origin, then one might anticipate that Burkitt tumors from heterozygous patients would demonstrate both the A and B subtypes of G-6-PD. However, 33 of 34 individual Burkitt tumors from 19 patients had single-enzyme phenotypes. Tumors from different sites in the same patient had the same single-enzyme phenotype.

Recent cytogenetic studies provide further evidence for a clonal origin of the Burkitt tumor cells. Nearly all the tumor cells have a marker chromosome number 14 that contains an extra band on its long arm; hence, the marker is called 14 q +.[124] This is usually derived by a translocation from the long arm of the 8th chromosome. The 14 q + marker is not found in the peripheral blood of BL patients; thus, it presumably arises following cell transformation. This marker is seen in other lymphomas; it is not unique to BL. It is not found in lymphoblastoid-cell lines established either spontaneously or by *in vitro* transformation of the lymphocytes of normal subjects.

These findings suggest that the disease has a clonal origin; that is, it emerges from one cell and then spreads to the other part of the body.

The mode of spread of the transformed cells has not been defined for Burkitt tumor patients, and there are no published studies about the circulation of transformed cells in the peripheral blood. However, in the experimental infection of marmosets, EBV-converted cells can be detected in the peripheral blood from the 2nd to the 4th week after inoculation of the virus.

7.2. Immunological Surveillance

It is assumed but not demonstrated that cell transformation occurs regularly as part of the initial EBV infection in all persons. Presumably, in the majority of persons, transformed cells are eliminated rapidly through an interaction of various immune mechanisms and new antigens that appear on the surface of the transformed cells. The exact nature of the new antigens that call forth the immune response is not known. These antigens may include viral-specified alterations in the cell membrane, which are known to occur with the herpesvirus group, and they also may include cell determinants that are unmasked or rearranged following virus transformation.

Two types of neoantigens present on the surface of EBV-transformed cells have been described. One antigen, the *membrane antigen* (MA), was originally demonstrated on the surface of BL cells and is also present on some lymphoid-cell lines. MA is likely to reflect part of the viral replicative cycle; since MA seems to induce viral neutralizing antibody, it is probable that MA contains glycoproteins also present in the viral envelope.[97] BL patients have antibodies to MA. The other cell-surface antigen is referred to as *lymphocyte-detected membrane antigen* (LYDMA). This antigen is detected by cytotoxic T cells that will kill all EBV-carrying lines but not lymphoid lines that are EBV-negative. The demonstration of LYDMA requires that natural killer cells first be eliminated. The natural killer cells are cytotoxic in a nonspecific fashion for lymphoid and other target cells with or without EBV. Cytotoxic T cells that react with LYDMA are present in the blood of patients with infectious mononucleosis; they disappear in convalescence.[115] They are not detectable

in the blood of BL patients, but can be found in small numbers in tumor tissue of BL patients.[65] LYDMA may also stimulate cytotoxic-T-cell activity during the course of *in vitro* transformation by EBV when mixed leukocytes from adults are used.

The type of effector mechanism that recognizes these neoantigens and eliminates tumor cells *in vivo* is not well understood. The exact role of cytotoxic antibodies, complement, cytotoxic T lymphocytes, nonspecific killer cells, or macrophages in the intact host is not worked out.

Patients with BL exhibit some form of cell-mediated sensitivity to their own tumors, for they develop delayed-type skin reactions when inoculated with extracts of autologous tumor cells.[42]

In general, untreated BL patients appear to be somewhat hyporeactive in their capacity to mount delayed hypersensitivity reactions (see Table 4). For example, only 2 of 10 untreated Burkitt tumor patients could be sensitized to respond to a chemical hapten, dinitrochlorobenzene (DNCB), in comparison to 11 of 15 controls of the same age.[111] With chemotherapy or in remission, the ability to respond to DNCB rose to 13 of 32 and 5 of 7 respectively. Similarly, the response of untreated BL tumor patients' lymphocytes to phytohemagglutinin (PHA) was approximately 60% that of the control group; BL patients under chemotherapy or in remission showed normal responses to PHA.

An important problem to solve is the relationship between malaria and successful immunosurveillance against EBV-transformed cells. There are two theories about the way in which malaria might act as a promoter in BL: (1) Malaria induces a state of reticuloendothelial hyperplasia secondary to reactions involved in disposal of the malaria parasites and of the products of hemolysis. The frequency of transformation by an exogenous virus such as EBV may be markedly greater in the already stimulated reticuloendothelial system of the young child with malaria.[95] (2) Alternatively, malaria may produce a degree of immunological paralysis and allow a small number of virus-transformed cells to multiply beyond the point where they can be eliminated by immune mechanisms. The total dose of tumor cells is a well-known determinant of experimental tumorigenesis by virally transformed cells and may be crucial in determining the outcome of viral transformation *in vivo*.

Finally, the environmental circumstances associ-

Table 4. Delayed Hypersensitivity Reaction against DNCB and PHA Response of Lymphocytes of Burkitt Lymphoma Patients in Relation to the Tumor Burden of the Patients[a]

Tumor burden	Number of DNCB-positive patients over number tested	Reactivity of patients' lymphocytes toward PHA		
		cpm/10^6 cells	Percentage of age controls	Number of patients tested
Untreated with tumor	2/10 (20%)	4500	58	25
Under chemotherapy	13/32 (40%)	7400	96	24
Without tumor	5/7 (71%)	9700	126	11
Controls				
5–12 years old	11/15 (73%)	7700	100	34
20–50 years old	29/31 (97%)	8600	100	30

[a] From Burkitt and Wright,[19] p. 165.

ated with malaria and EBV infection at an early age may permit the operation of still unidentified cocarcinogens to function to bring about a cellular mutation that increases the oncogenicity of EBV.

Several observations support the general hypothesis that EBV-induced lymphomas are highly antigenic and that failure of immune recognition is responsible for their tumorigenicity. The histological appearance of the tumors with extensive histiocytic infiltration suggests a process of cell killing and elimination. The relatively high frequency of long-term remissions following chemotherapy suggests that natural immune mechanisms can eliminate the remainder of the tumor cells once the tumor mass is reduced to a low level. Finally, the fall of membrane-reactive antibodies prior to tumor relapse suggests that these antibodies may be important in maintaining tumor regression. The experimental model provides support for this concept of pathogenesis, since marmosets treated with immunosuppressive drugs develop malignant lymphoma at a higher rate than nontreated animals.

8. Patterns of Host Response

8.1. Clinical and Pathological Features

The disease presents in more than half the children as a unilateral swelling of the jaw. Jaw tumors are characteristically found as the presenting sign in younger children and abdominal masses in older children. However, even in young children, the disease is multifocal at the time of diagnosis, and there are usually additional sites of tumor involvement in abdominal viscera, kidney, liver, and lymphatic tissue of the gastrointestinal tract.[19] Other favored sites for occurrence of the tumor are the endocrine and exocrine glands, particularly thyroid, ovary, and salivary glands. The anatomical distribution of the disease is characteristic not only for the organs involved but also for the organs and sites spared. Characteristically, the lymphoma less frequently involves peripheral lymph nodes, lung, and the lymphatic tissue of Waldeyer's ring in the nasopharynx; it has never been found in the thymus. A summary of anatomical involvement from an autopsy series is shown in Table 5.

In addition to anatomical location of the tumors, a clinical characteristic of the disease is its favorable response to cytoxic chemotherapy. In earlier series, long survival was not usual: approximately 20% of the patients survived more than 2 years.[19] With improvements in chemotherapy, the 2-year survival rate for BL approaches 80% and is markedly better than the survival rate for lymphoblastic or histiocytic lymphomas.[21,126] It is characteristic of the survival curves that additional deaths are rare after the second year (see Figs. 6 and 7).

Although the histopathological definition of the disease was initially somewhat confused, O'Conor et al.[94] classified the tumor as a poorly differentiated, diffuse lymphoma. A group of experts in the pathology of the lymphoreticular system defined the entity as an undifferentiated malignant lymphoma in which the predominant cell type is usually a primitive stem cell and much less frequently either a lymphoblast or a reticulum cell.[7] Interspersed

Table 5. Organ Involvement in Burkitt Lymphoma: Postmortem Series 1953–1967 Inclusive[a]

	Children (65)		Adults (23)		Total (88)	
	Number	%	Number	%	Number	%
Skeleton						
Jaw	37	57	7	30	42	48
Skull vault	6	9	6	26	12	14
Other bones	8	12	7	30	15	17
Central nervous system						
Brain	12	18	3	13	15	17
Spinal cord (paraplegia)	6	9	4	17	10	11
Thoracic cavity						
Pericardium	3	5	1	4	4	5
Heart	21	32	5	22	26	30
Pleura	6	9	3	13	9	10
Lung	11	17	2	9	13	15
Digestive system						
Salivary glands	6	9	3	13	9	10
Peritoneum	8	12	2	9	10	11
Stomach	17	26	3	13	20	23
Small intestine	18	28	6	26	24	27
Large intestine	9	14	3	13	12	14
Liver	24	37	10	43	34	39
Gallbladder	3	5	2	9	5	6
Pancreas	28	43	9	39	37	42
Lymphoreticular system						
Lymph nodes	45	69	16	70	60	68
Spleen	20	31	8	35	28	32
Genitourinary system						
Kidney	50	77	16	70	64	73
Bladder	2	3	2	9	4	5
Prostate[b]	1	2	—	—	1	1
Testes[b]	6	12	1	5	7	10
Ovaries[c]	14	82	3	75	17	81
Breast	1	2	3	13	3	3
Endocrine system						
Pituitary	8	12	3	13	11	12
Thyroid	24	37	8	35	30	34
Adrenals	38	58	11	48	49	56

[a] From Burkitt and Wright,[19] p. 65.
[b] Percentages based on the number of males in the series.
[c] Percentages based on the number of females in the series.

among the tumor are histiocytes or macrophages giving the tumor a starry-sky appearance; this appearance is not seen only in BL. The tumors show large areas of necrosis, presumably because of rapid growth, and cell death is thought to account for the histiocytic infiltration. The tumor is generally thought to arise in the trabecular marrow of the mandible, but this point is not definitely established. Usually, the tumor does not involve the distal bone marrow and leukemia is not a feature of the disease.

8.2. Serological Features

The sera of nearly 100% of African patients with BL contain antibody against the viral capsid antigen (VCA) and approximately 70% antibody directed

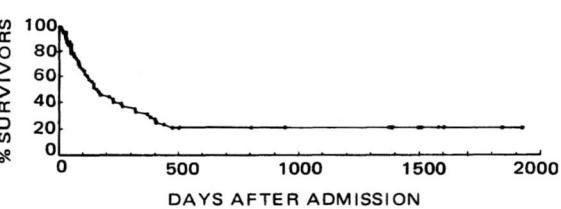

Fig. 6. Survival of patients with childhood malignant lymphoma in Uganda. From Burkitt and Wright,[19] p. 48.

against the EBV early antigen (EA). Antibodies to EA are not usually found in the sera of normal subjects and, if present, are of low titer. The presence of high-titered antibody to EA correlates with a poor prognosis: it is found in 100% of BL patients with a short course between diagnosis and death, but only 43% of patients surviving more than 2 years.[59]

Following therapy with local radiation to the Burkitt tumor, there is a small increase (one 2-fold serum dilution or less) to the EA and VCA. This result might be anticipated if local therapy allowed release of antigen into the circulation.[35] Gunven *et al.*[52] found that in three out of four BL patients studied sequentially, a small decrease in the antibody titer to the membrane antigen (MA) precedes relapse. The interpretation of this finding is that with progressive increase in tumor mass, the circulating antibodies are removed by MA on the tumor cells.

9. Therapy and Control

9.1. Chemotherapy

Chemotherapy, particularly with the alkylating agent cyclophosphamide (cytoxan), is highly effec-

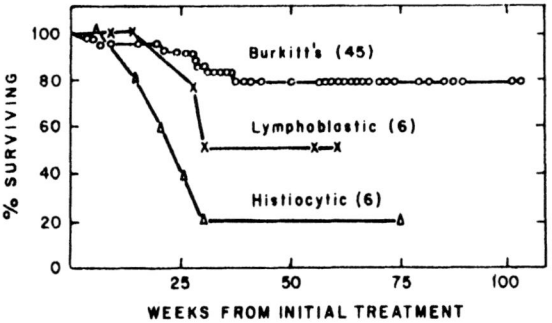

Fig. 7. Comparison of survival of patients with BL, lymphoblastic lymphoma, and histiocytic lymphoma. From Ziegler *et al.*[126]

tive in BL. Long-term survivals of 1 year or more can be obtained in as many as 80% of patients. It would appear that chemotherapy will provide the mainstay of treatment for the foreseeable future.

9.2. Malaria Control

The disease rarely occurs in nonmalarious areas even in the endemic belt, and whatever the mechanisms involved, it would seem that control of malaria in the form of control of its vectors is associated with a decreased incidence of BL. Consequently, the long-range control of BL will be closely linked with success in malaria eradication.

Since malaria has been postulated as a cofactor in BL, a field trial to reduce malaria prevalence in Tanzania through chloroquine prophylaxis is in progress to determine whether the BL incidence also decreases. If this proves to be so, the control of malaria in very early life might be a more practical approach to lowering BL incidence than a vaccine.

9.3. Vaccines

The successful application of live attenuated vaccines in the prevention of Marek's disease, a malignant lymphoma of chickens caused by a herpesvirus, has raised hopes that a similar approach might be tried in man.[24] The major problem envisioned is that the herpes viruses establish long-term residence in their host and can be reactivated by a variety of stimuli. This phenomenon appears to be the case for EBV as well, which is apparently reactivated under conditions of renal transplantation and immunosuppressive therapy.[112] Consequently, it would be very difficult to determine the ultimate safety of a live vaccine against EBV if the vaccine virus could be reactivated in future years and cause disease. Nonetheless, immunization against cell-membrane-associated EBV-determined antigens that are important in surveillance of the transformed cells might ultimately be attempted.

These membrane-antigen vaccines will need to be free of nucleic acid, since it has been shown that the naked DNA of another lymphoma-inducing virus, herpes ateles virus, is oncogenic in animals.[44] The surveillance of vaccine efficacy in a geographic area that is politically unstable and for a disease that seems to be declining in frequency presents a major obstacle.

10. Unresolved Problems

The major unresolved problem is the geographic oncogenesis of a ubiquitous virus. EBV is associated with inapparent infections, with infectious mononucleosis, and with two malignant diseases, BL and nasopharyngeal carcinoma. The malignancies occur in sharply circumscribed geographic locales, yet the virus is worldwide in distribution. One possibility to explain this paradox is that different viral strains or subtypes are involved. This hypothesis seems increasingly unlikely. Extensive cross-reaction has been found in a variety of cell-associated antigens among various EBV strains. Neutralization tests, which might be anticipated to be the most sensitive indicators of subtle antigenic differences, have not shown distinctive serotypes.[26] The EBV DNA fragments generated by the restriction endonuclease EcoRI are very similar in biopsies of Burkitt tumors and in DNA obtained from virions originating from mononucleosis.[113] The EcoRI fragments of viral DNAs obtained from tumors or nonmalignant conditions show some differences, but these variations do not seem to be disease-related. However, it is possible that important biological differences among strains may be attributable to subtle structural variations that have not yet been seen with the techniques employed.

If host factors underlie the different responses of different population groups to the same virus, one would very much like to know how such host factors operate. One hypothesis explored in some detail by Kufe et al.[73] is that BL results from cooperative infection with EBV and an endogenous RNA tumor virus. Although the presence of RNA tumor viruses in BL has not yet been confirmed in other laboratories, the mere presence of the RNA tumor virus does not indicate its causal role. Many other host factors may be operative in the transition from transformation of cell growth properties to oncogenic

conversion. The cells of certain persons may be unstable following transformation and permit further mutations or cytogenetic changes. Certain persons may have target cells that, because of an unusual state of differentiation, are more susceptible to malignant change. Other hosts may lack one or more elements of the immune surveillance apparatus. There are kindreds in which the boys develop fatal lymphoproliferative disease apparently as the result of a failure of specific anti-EBV Ig production, and other children have died with disseminated malignant EBV infection apparently because of lack of cell-mediated immunity.[6,12,103]

Part of the problem of the limited geographic distribution of the EBV-associated lymphoid tumors is the apparent lack of association of EBV with most cases of American BL and certain rare cases of histologically consistent BL in Africa. This leads to the inevitable conclusion that multiple etiological agents may be associated with the same histopathological entity. This, of course, is not an uncommon finding in the epidemiology of infectious diseases. The alternate explanation is that EBV is a passenger virus even in the endemic area and is not etiologically related to the Burkitt tumor. This hypothesis now seems very unlikely, for several reasons. First, EBV is now known to possess oncogenicity on the basis of animal experiments. Second, one fails to understand why, if EBV is a passenger virus, it should be present in every cell of Burkitt tumor in the endemic area and in nearly every Burkitt tumor. Third, if it is a passenger virus, why does it specifically select a particular tumor in a particular geographic locale and not appear regularly in other lymphomas?

ACKNOWLEDGMENTS

This work was supported by grants from the American Cancer Society (VC-107), and the U.S. Public Health Service (CA16038, CA12055).

11. References

1. Collected reports of cases of Burkitt's lymphoma from countries outside the endemic areas, *Int. J. Cancer* **2:**559–609 (1967).
2. ADAMS, A., AND LINDAHL, T., Epstein–Barr virus genomes with properties of circular DNA molecules in carrier cells, *Proc. Natl. Acad. Sci. U.S.A.* **72:**1477–1481 (1975).

3. ADAMS, A., LINDAHL, T., AND KLEIN, G., Linear association between cellular DNA and EBV DNA in a human lymphoblastoid cell line, *Proc. Natl. Acad. Sci. U.S.A.* **70**:2888–2892 (1973).

4. ARMENIAN, H. K., AND LILLIENFELD, A. M., The distribution of incubation periods of neoplastic diseases, *Am. J. Epidemiol.* **99**:92–100 (1974).

5. BANATVALA, J. E., BEST, J. M., AND WALLER, D. K., Epstein–Barr virus-specific IgM in infectious mononucleosis, Burkitt lymphoma, and nasopharyngeal carcinoma, *Lancet* **1**:1205–1208 (1972).

6. BAR, R. S., DELOR, C. J., CLAUSEN, K. P., HURTUBISE, P., HENLE, W., AND HEWETSON, J. F., Fatal infectious mononucleosis in a family, *N. Engl. J. Med.* **290**:363–367 (1974).

7. BEARD, C. W., O'CONOR, G. T., THOMAS, L. B., AND TORLONI, H., Histopathological definition of Burkitt's tumor, *Bull. WHO* **40**:601–607 (1969).

8. BERRY, C. G., Lymphoma syndrome in northern Nigeria, *Br. Med. J.* **2**:668–670 (1964).

9. BIGGAR, R. J., HENLE, W., FLEISHER, G., PRÖCKER, J., LENNETTE, E. T., AND HENLE, G., Primary Epstein–Barr virus infections in African infants. I. Decline of maternal antibodies and time of infection, *Int. J. Cancer*, **22**:239–243 (1978).

10. BIGGAR, R. J., HENLE, G., BOCHER, J., LENNETTE, E. T., FLEISHER, G., AND HENLE, W., Primary Epstein–Barr virus infections in African infants. II. Chemical and serological observations during seroconversion, *Int. J. Cancer* **22**:244–250 (1978).

11. BORNKAMM, G. W., STEIN, H., LENNART, K., RÜGGEBERG, F., BARTELS, H., AND ZUR HAUSEN, H., Attempts to demonstrate virus-specific sequences in human tumors. IV. EB viral DNA in European Burkitt lymphoma and in immunoblastic lymphadenopathy with excessive plasmacytosis, *Int. J. Cancer* **17**:177–181 (1976).

12. BRITTON, S., ANDERSSON-ANVRET, M., GERGELY, P., HENLE, W., JONDAL, M., KLEIN, G., SANDSTEDT, B., AND SVEDMYR, E., Epstein–Barr virus immunity and tissue distribution in a fatal case of infectious mononucleosis, *N. Engl. J. Med.* **298**:89–92 (1978).

13. BURKITT, D. P., A sarcoma involving the jaws in African children, *Br. J. Surg.* **46**:218–223 (1958).

14. BURKITT, D. P., A children's cancer dependent on climatic factors, *Nature (London)* **194**:232–234 (1962).

15. BURKITT, D., Determining the climatic limitations of a children's cancer common in Africa, *Br. Med. J.* **2**:1019–1023 (1962).

16. BURKITT, D., Burkitt's lymphoma outside the known endemic areas of Africa and New Guinea, *Int. J. Cancer* **2**:562–565 (1967).

17. BURKITT, D., Etiology of Burkitt's lymphoma—An alternative hypothesis to a vectored virus, *J. Natl. Cancer Inst.* **42**:19–28 (1969).

18. BURKITT, D., AND WRIGHT, D. H., Geographical and tribal distribution of the African lymphoma in Uganda, *Br. Med. J.* **5487**:569–573 (1966).

19. BURKITT, D. P., AND WRIGHT, D. H. (eds.), *Burkitt's Lymphoma*, Livingstone, Edinburgh, 1970.

20. BYRNE, E. B., EVANS, A. S., FONTS, D. W., AND ISRAEL, H. L., A seroepidemiological study of Epstein–Barr virus and other antigens in sarcoidosis, *Am. J. Epidemiol.* **97**:355–363 (1973).

21. CARBONE, P., BERNARD, C. W., BENNETT, J. M., ZIEGLER, J. L., COHEN, M. H., AND GERBER, P., National Institutes of Health clinical staff conference: Burkitt's tumor, *Ann. Intern. Med.* **70**:817–832 (1969).

22. CARVALHO, R. P. S., EVANS, A. S., FROST, P., DALLDORF, G., CAMARGO, M. F., AND JAMRA, M., EBV infections in Brazil. I. Occurrence in normal persons, in lymphomas and in leukemias, *Int. J. Cancer* **11**:191–201 (1973).

23. CHANG, R. S., LEWIS, J. P., AND ABILDGAARD, C. F., Prevalence of oropharyngeal excreters of leukocyte-transforming agents among a human population, *N. Engl. J. Med.* **289**:1325–1329 (1973).

24. CHURCHILL, A. E., PAYNE, L. N., AND CHUBB, R. C., Immunization against Marek's disease using a live attenuated virus, *Nature (London)* **221**:744–747 (1969).

25. COOK, A. R., *Uganda Memories*, Uganda Society, 1945.

26. COOPE, D., HESTON, L., BRANDSMA, J., AND MILLER, G., Cross neutralization of infectious mononucleosis and Burkitt lymphoma strains of Epstein–Barr virus with hyperimmune rabbit antisera, *J. Immunol.* **123**:232–238 (1979).

27. DALLDORF, G., Lymphomas of African children. *J. Am. Med. Assoc.* **181**:1026–1028 (1962).

28. DALLDORF, G., LINSELL, C. A., BARNHART, F. C., AND MARTYN, R., An epidemiologic approach to the lymphomas of African children and Burkitt's sarcoma of the jaws, *Perspect. Biol. Med.* **7**:435–449 (1964).

29. DAMBAUGH, T., NKRUMAH, F. K., BIGGAR, R. J., AND KIEFF, E., Epstein–Barr virus RNA in Burkitt tumor tissue, *Cell* **16**:313–322 (1979).

30. DAVIES, J. N. P., ELMES, S., HUTT, M. S. R., MTIMAVALYE, L. A. R., OWOR, R., AND SHAPER, L., Cancer in an African community, 1897–1956: An analysis of the records of Mengo Hospital, Kampala, Uganda: Part 2, *Br. Med. J.* **1**:336–341 (1964).

31. DEAN, A. G., WILLIAMS, E. H., ATTOBUA, G., OMEDA, J., GADI, A., AMUTI, A., AND ATIMA, S. B., Clinical events suggesting herpes-simplex infection before onset of Burkitt's lymphoma, *Lancet* **2**:1225–1228 (1973).

32. DELIUS, H., AND BORNKAMM, G. W., Heterogeneity of Epstein–Barr virus. III. Comparison of a transforming and a nontransforming virus by partial denaturation mapping of their DNAs, *J. Virol.* **27**:81–89 (1978).

33. DESCHRYVER, A., KLEIN, G., HENLE, G., HENLE, W.,

CAMERON, H. M., SANTESSON, L., AND CLIFFORD, P., EB-virus associated serology in malignant disease: Antibody levels to viral capsid antigens (VCA), membrane antigens (MA) and early antigens (EA) in patients with various neoplastic conditions, *Int. J. Cancer* **9**:353–364 (1972).

34. DE-THÉ, G., GESER, A., DAY, N. E., TUBEI, P. M., WILLIAMS, E. H., BEIR, D. P., SMITH, P. G., DEAN, A. G., BORNKAMM, G. W., FEORINO, P., AND HENLE, W., Epidemiological evidence for causal relationship between Epstein–Barr virus and Burkitt's lymphoma from Ugandan prospective study, *Nature (London)* **274**:756–761 (1978).

35. EINHORN, N., HENLE, G., HENLE, W., KLEIN, G., AND CLIFFORD, P., Effect of local radiotherapy on the antibody levels against EBV-induced early and capsid antigens (EA and VCA) in patients with certain malignant tumours, *Int. J. Cancer* **9**:182 (1972).

36. EPSTEIN, M. A., ACHONG, B. G., BARR, Y. M., ZAJAC, B., HENLE, G., AND HENLE, W., Morphological and virological investigations on cultured Burkitt tumor lymphoblasts (strain Raji), *J. Natl. Cancer Inst.* **34**:547–559 (1966).

37. EPSTEIN, M. A., AND BARR, Y. M., Cultivation *in vitro* of human lymphoblasts from Burkitt's malignant lymphoma, *Lancet* **1**:252–253 (1964).

38. EPSTEIN, M. A., HENLE, G., ACHONG, B. G., AND BARR, Y. M., Morphological and biological studies on a virus in cultured lymphoblasts from Burkitt's lymphoma, *J. Exp. Med.* **121**:761–770 (1965).

39. EPSTEIN, M. A., ACHONG, B. G., AND BARR, Y. M., Virus particles in cultured lymphoblasts from Burkitt's lymphoma, *Lancet* **1**:702–703 (1964).

40. EPSTEIN, M. A., HUNT, R. D., AND RABIN, H., Pilot experiments with EB virus in owl monkeys (*Aotus trivirgatus*). I. Reticuloproliferative disease in an inoculated animal, *Int. J. Cancer* **12**:309–318 (1973).

41. FALK, L., WOLFE, L., DEINHARDT, F., PACIGA, J., DOMBOS, L., KLEIN, G., HENLE, W., AND HENLE, G., Epstein–Barr virus: Transformation of non-human primate lymphocytes *in vitro*, *Int. J. Cancer* **13**:353–376 (1974).

42. FASS, L., HERBERMAN, R. B., AND ZIEGLER, J., Delayed cutaneous hypersensitivity reactions to autologous extracts of Burkitt-lymphoma cells, *N. Engl. J. Med.* **282**:776–780 (1970).

43. FIALKOW, P. J., KLEIN, E., KLEIN, G., CLIFFORD, P., AND SINGH, S., Immunoglobulin and glucose-6-phosphate dehydrogenase as markers of cellular origin in Burkitt lymphoma, *J. Exp. Med.* **138**:89–101 (1973).

44. FLECKENSTEIN, B., DANIEL, M. D., AND HUNT, R. D., Tumor induction with DNA of oncogenic primate herpesviruses, *Nature (London)* **274**:57–59 (1978).

45. FLEISHER, G., HENLE, W., HENLE, G., LENNETTE, E. T., AND BIGGAR, R. J., Primary infection with Epstein—Barr virus in infants in the the United States: Clinical and serologic observations, *J. Infect. Dis.* **139**:553–558 (1979).

46. GERBER, P., Activation of Epstein–Barr virus by 5-bromodeoxyuridine in virus free human cells, *Proc. Natl. Acad. Sci. U.S.A.* **69**:83–85 (1972).

47. GERBER, P., AND HOYER, B. H., Induction of cellular DNA synthesis in human leucocytes by Epstein–Barr virus, *Nature (London)* **231**:46–47 (1971).

48. GERBER, P., NKRUMAH, F. K., PRITCHETT, R., AND KIEFF, E., Comparative studies of Epstein–Barr virus strains from Ghana and the United States, *Int. J. Cancer* **17**:71–81 (1976).

49. GIVEN, D., AND KIEFF, E., DNA of Epstein–Barr virus. IV. Linkage map of restriction enzyme fragments of the B95-8 and W91 strains of Epstein–Barr virus, *J. Virol.* **28**:524–542 (1978).

50. GLASER, R., AND RAPP, F., Rescue of Epstein–Barr virus from somatic cell hybrids of Burkitt lymphoblastoid cells, *J. Virol.* **10**:288–296 (1972).

51. GRIFFIN, E. R., WRIGHT, D. H., BELL, T. M., AND ROSS, M. G. R., Demonstration of virus particles in biopsy material from cases of Burkitt's tumour, *Eur. J. Cancer* **2**:353–358 (1966).

52. GUNVEN, P., KLEIN, G., CLIFFORD, P., AND SINGH, S., Epstein–Barr virus-associated membrane-reactive antibodies during long term survival after Burkitt's lymphoma, *Proc. Natl. Acad. Sci. U.S.A.* **71**:1422–1426 (1974).

53. HAMPAR, B., DERGE, J. G., MARTOS, L. M., TAGAMETS, M. A., CHANGE, S. Y., AND CHAKRABARTY, M., Identification of a critical period during the S phase for activation of the Epstein–Barr virus by 5-iododeoxyuridine, *Nature (London) New Biol.* **244**:214–217 (1973).

54. HAMPAR, B., DERGE, J. G., MARTOS, L. M., AND WALKER, J. L., Synthesis of Epstein–Barr virus after activation of the viral genome in a virus negative human lymphoblastoid cell (Raji) made resistant to five bromodeoxyuridine, *Proc. Natl. Acad. Sci. U.S.A.* **69**:78–82 (1972).

55. HENDERSON, E., ROBINSON, J., FRANK, A., AND MILLER, G., Epstein–Barr virus: Transformation of lymphocytes separated by size or exposed to bromodeoxyuridine and light, *Virology* **82**:196–205 (1977).

56. HENLE, G., AND HENLE, W., Immunofluorescence in cells derived from Burkitt's lymphoma, *J. Bacteriol.* **91**:1248–1256 (1966).

57. HENLE, G., HENLE, W., CLIFFORD, P., DIEHL, V., KAFUKO, G. W., KIRYA, B. G., KLEIN, G., MORROW, R. H., MUNUBE, G. M., R., PIKE, M. C., TUKEI, P. M., AND ZIEGLER, J. L., Antibodies to Epstein–Barr virus in Burkitt's lymphoma and control groups, *J. Natl. Cancer Inst.* **43**:1147–1157 (1969).

58. HENLE, W., DIEHL, V., KOHN, G., ZUR HAUSEN, H.,

AND HENLE, G., Herpes-type virus and chromosome marker in normal leukocytes after growth with irradiated Burkitt cells, *Science* **157**:1064–1065 (1967).

59. HENLE, W., HENLE, G., GUNVEN, P., KLEIN, G., CLIFFORD, P., AND SINGH, S., Patterns of antibodies to Epstein–Barr virus-induced early antigens in Burkitt's lymphoma: Comparison of dying patients with long term survivors, *J. Natl. Cancer Inst.* **50**:1163–1173 (1973).

60. HENLE, W., HENLE, G., ZAJAC, B. A., PEARSON, G., WAUBKE, R., AND SCRIBA, M., Differential reactivity of human serums with early antigens induced by Epstein–Barr virus, *Science* **169**:188–190 (1970).

61. HILGERS, J., DEAN, A. G., AND DE-THÉ, G. B., Elevated immunofluorescence titers to several herpes viruses in Burkitt's lymphoma patients: Are high titers unique? *J. Natl. Cancer Inst.* **54**:49–51 (1975).

62. HINUMA, Y., KONN, M., YAMAGUCHI, J., WUDARSKI, D. J., BLAKESLEE, J. R., AND GRACE, J. T., JR., Immunofluorescence and herpes-type virus particles in the P₃HR-1 Burkitt lymphoma cell line, *J. Virol.* **1**:1045–1051 (1967).

63. HIRSHAUT, Y., COHEN, M. H., AND STEVENS, D. A., Epstein–Barr virus antibodies in American and African Burkitt's lymphoma, *Lancet* **2**:114–116 (1973).

64. JONDAL, M., AND KLEIN, G., Surface markers on human B and T lymphocytes. II. Presence of Epstein–Barr virus receptors on B lymphocytes, *J. Exp. Med.* **138**:1365–1378 (1973).

65. JONDAL, M., SVEDMYR, E., AND KLEIN, E., Killer T cells in a Burkitt's lymphoma biopsy, *Nature (London)* **255**:405–407 (1975).

66. JUDSON, S. C., HENLE, W., AND HENLE, G., A cluster of Epstein–Barr virus-associated American Burkitt's lymphoma, *N. Engl. J. Med.* **297**:464–468 (1977).

67. KAFUKO, G. W., AND BURKITT, D. P., Burkitt's lymphoma and malaria, *Int. J. Cancer* **6**:1–9 (1970).

68. KAFUKO, G. W., HENDERSON, B. E., KIRYA, B. G., MUNUBE, G. M. R., TUKEI, P. M., DAY, N. E., HENLE, G., HENLE, W., MORROW, R. H., PIKE, M. C., SMITH, P. G., AND WILLIAMS, E. H., Epstein–Barr virus antibody levels in children from the West Nile District of Uganda, *Lancet* **1**:706 (1972).

69. KASCHKA-DIERICH, C., ADAMS, A., LINDAHL, T., BORNKAMM, G., BJURSELL, G., KLEIN, G., GIOVANELLA, B., AND SINGH, S., Intracellular forms of Epstein–Barr virus DNA in human tumor cells *in vivo*, *Nature (London)* **260**:302–306 (1976).

70. KINTER, C. R., AND SUGDEN, B., The structure of the termini of the DNA of Epstein–Barr virus, *Cell* **17**:661–672 (1979).

71. KLEIN, G., CLIFFORD, P., KLEIN, E., AND STJERNSWARD, J., Search for tumor specific immune reactions in Burkitt lymphoma patients by the membrane immunofluorescence reaction, *Proc. Natl. Acad. Sci.*

U.S.A. **55**:1628–1635 (1966).

72. KLEIN, G., LINDAHL, T., JONDAL, M., LEIBOLD, W., MÉNÉZES, J., NILSSON, K., AND SUNDSTRÖM, C., Continuous lymphoid cell lines with B-cell characteristics that lack the Epstein–Barr virus genome, derived from three human lymphomas, *Proc. Natl. Acad. Sci. U.S.A.* **71**:3283–3286 (1974).

73. KUFE, D., HEHLMANN, R., AND SPIEGELMAN, S., RNA related to that of a murine leukemia virus in Burkitt's tumors and nasopharyngeal carcinoma, *Proc. Natl. Acad. Sci. U.S.A.* **70**:5–9 (1973).

74. LEVINE, P. H., ABLASHI, D. V., AND BERARD, C. W., Elevated antibody titers to Epstein–Barr virus in Hodgkin's disease, *Cancer* **27**:416–421 (1971).

75. LEVINE, P. H., O'CONOR, G. T., AND BERARD, C. W., Antibodies to Epstein–Barr virus (EBV) in American patients with Burkitt's lymphoma, *Cancer* **30**:610–615 (1972).

76. LEVY, J. A., AND HENLE, G., Indirect immunofluorescence tests with sera from African children and cultured Burkitt cells, *J. Bacteriol.* **92**:275–276 (1966).

77. LINDAHL, T., KLEIN, G., REEDMAN, B. M., JOHANSON, B., AND SINGH, S., Relationship between Epstein–Barr virus (EBV) DNA and the EBV-determined nuclear antigen (EBNA) in Burkitt lymphoma biopsies and other lymphoproliferative malignancies, *Int. J. Cancer* **13**:764–772 (1974).

78. LUKA, J., LINDAHL, T., AND KLEIN, G., Purification of the Epstein–Barr virus-determined nuclear antigen from Epstein–Barr virus-transformed human lymphoid cell lines, *J. Virol.* **27**:604–611 (1978).

79. MILLER, G., Oncogenicity of Epstein–Barr virus, *J. Infect. Dis.* **130**:187–205 (1974).

80. MILLER, G., AND COOPE, D., Epstein–Barr viral nuclear antigen (EBNA) in tumor cell imprints of experimental lymphoma of marmosets, *Trans. Assoc. Am. Physicians* **87**:205–218 (1974).

81. MILLER, G., AND LIPMAN, M., Comparison of the yield of infectious virus from clones of human and simian lymphoblastoid lines transformed by Epstein–Barr virus, *J. Exp. Med.* **138**:1398–1412 (1973).

82. MILLER, G., LISCO, H., KOHN, H. I., AND STITT, D., Establishment of cell lines from normal adult human blood leukocytes by exposure to Epstein–Barr virus and neutralization by human sera with Epstein–Barr virus antibody, *Proc. Soc. Exp. Biol. Med.* **137**:1459–1465 (1971).

83. MILLER, G., NIEDERMAN, J. C., AND ANDREWS, L., Prolonged oropharyngeal excretion of EB virus following infectious mononucleosis, *N. Engl. J. Med.* **288**:229–232 (1973).

84. MILLER, G., ROBINSON, J., HESTON, L., AND LIPMAN, M., Differences between laboratory strains of Epstein–Barr virus based on immortalization, abortive

infection and interference, *Proc. Natl. Acad. Sci. U.S.A.* **71**:4006–4010 (1974).

85. MILLER, G., SHOPE, T., COOPE, D., WATERS, L., PAGANO, J., BORNKAMM, G. W., AND HENLE, W., Lymphoma in cotton-top marmosets after inoculation with Epstein–Barr virus: Tumor incidence, histologic spectrum, antibody responses, demonstration of viral DNA, and characterization of viruses, *J. Exp. Med.* **145**:948–967 (1977).

86. MILLER, G., SHOPE, T., LISCO, H., STITT, D., AND LIPMAN, M., Epstein–Barr virus: Transformation, cytopathic changes, and viral antigens in squirrel monkey and marmoset leukocytes, *Proc. Natl. Acad. Sci. U.S.A.* **69**:383–387 (1972).

87. MILLER, M. H., STITT, D., AND MILLER, G., Epstein–Barr viral antigen in single cell clones of two human leukocytic lines, *J. Virol.* **6**:699–701 (1970).

88. MORROW, R. H., PIKE, M. C., AND SMITH, P. G. Epidemiology of Burkitt's lymphoma in the Mengo Districts, Uganda, 1957–1968, Presented at the annual meeting of the American Epidemiological Society, April 5–6, 1974.

89. MORROW, R. H., PIKE, M. C., SMITH, P. G., ZIEGLER, J. L., AND KISUULE, A., Burkitt's lymphoma: A time–space cluster of cases in Bwamba County of Uganda, *Br. Med. J.* **2**:491–492 (1971).

90. NADKARNI, J. S., NADKARNI, J. J., KLEIN, G., HENLE, W., HENLE, G., AND CLIFFORD, P., EB viral antigens in Burkitt tumor biopsies and early cultures, *Int. J. Cancer* **6**:10–17 (1970).

91. NIEDERMAN, J., MILLER, G., PEARSON, H., AND PAGANO, J., Patterns of excretion of Epstein–Barr virus in saliva and other oropharyngeal sites during infectious mononucleosis, *N. Engl. J. Med.* **294**:1355–1359 (1976).

92. NONOYAMA, M., HUANG, C. H., PAGANO, J. S., KLEIN, G., AND SINGH, S., DNA of Epstein–Barr virus detected in tissue of Burkitt's lymphoma and nasopharyngeal carcinoma, *Proc. Natl. Acad. Sci. U.S.A.* **70**:3265–3268, (1973).

93. NONOYAMA. M., AND PAGANO, J. S., Separation of Epstein–Barr virus DNA from large chromosomal DNA in non-virus producing cells, *Nature (London) New Biol.* **238**:169 (1972).

94. O'CONOR, G. T., Malignant lymphoma in African children. II. A pathological entity, *Cancer* **14**:270–283 (1961).

95. O'CONOR, G. T., Persistent immunologic stimulation as a factor in oncogenesis, with special reference to Burkitt's tumor, *Am. J. Med.* **48**:279–285 (1970).

96. OLD, L. J., BOYSE, E. A., OETTGEN, H. F., deHARVEN, E., GEERING, G., WILLIAMSON, B., AND CLIFFORD, P., Precipitating antibody in human serum to an antigen present in cultured Burkitt's lymphoma cells, *Proc. Natl. Acad. Sci. U.S.A.* **56**:1669–1704 (1966).

97. PEARSON, G. R., AND QUALTIERE, L. T., Papain solu-

98. PIKE, M. C., MORROW, R. H., KISUULE, A., AND MAFIGIRI, J., Burkitt's lymphoma and sickle cell trait, *Br. J. Prev. Soc. Med.* **24**:39–41 (1970).

99. PIKE, M. C., WILLIAMS, E. H., AND WRIGHT, B., Burkitt's tumour in the West Nile District of Uganda 1961–5, *Br. Med. J.* **2**:395–399 (1967).

100. POPE, J. H., HORNE, M. K., AND SCOTT, W., Identification of the filtrable leukocyte-transforming factor of QIMR-WIL cells as herpes-like virus, *Int. J. Cancer* **4**:255–260 (1969).

101. POWELL, A. L. T., KING, W., AND, KIEFF, E., Epstein–Barr virus-specific RNA. III. Mapping of DNA encoding viral RNA in restringent infection, *J. Virol.* **29**:261–274 (1979).

102. PULVERTAFT, R. J. V., Cytology of Burkitt's tumor (African lymphoma), *Lancet* **1**:238–240 (1964).

103. PURTILO, D. T., DE FLORIO, D., HUTT, L. M., BHAWAN, J., YANG, J. P. S., OTTO, R., AND EDWARDS, W., Variable phenotypic expression of an X-linked recessive lymphoproliferative syndrome, *N. Engl. J. Med.* **297**:1077–1081 (1977).

104. REEDMAN, B. M., AND KLEIN, G., Cellular localization of an Epstein–Barr virus (EBV)-associated complement-fixing antigen in producer and non-producer lymphoblastoid cell lines, *Int. J. Cancer* **11**:499–520 (1973).

105. REEDMAN, B. M., KLEIN, G., POPE, J. H., WALTERS, M. L., HILGERS, J., SINGH, S., AND JOHANSSON, B., Epstein–Barr virus-associated complement-fixing and nuclear antigens in Burkitt lymphoma biopsies, *Int. J. Cancer* **13**:755–763 (1974).

106. ROBINSON, J., AND MILLER, G., Assay for Epstein–Barr virus based on stimulation of DNA synthesis in mixed leukocytes from human umbilical cord blood, *J. Virol.* **15**:1065–1072 (1975).

107. RYMO, L., AND FORSBLOM, S., Cleavage of Epstein–Barr virus DNA by restriction endonucleases EcoRI, Hind III, and Bam I, *Nucleic Acids Res.* **5**:1387–1402 (1978).

108. SCHMITZ, H., AND SCHERER, M., IgM antibodies to Epstein–Barr virus in infectious mononucleosis, *Arch. Gesamte Virusforsch.* **37**:332–339 (1972).

109. SCHULTE-HOLTHAUSEN, H., AND ZUR HAUSEN, H., Partial purification of the Epstein–Barr virus and some properties of its DNA, *Virology* **40**:776–779 (1970).

110. SHOPE, T., DECHAIRO, D., AND MILLER, G., Malignant lymphoma in cotton-top marmosets following inoculation of Epstein–Barr virus, *Proc. Natl. Acad. Sci. U.S.A.* **70**:2487–2491 (1973).

111. STJERNSWARD, J., CLIFFORD, P., AND SVEDMYR, E., General and tumor destructive cellular immunological reactivity, in: *Burkitt's Lymphoma* (D. P. BURKITT AND D. H. WRIGHT, eds.), pp. 164–171, Livingstone, Edinburgh, 1970.

112. STRAUCH, B., SIEGEL, N., ANDREWS, L., AND MILLER,

G., Oropharyngeal excretion of Epstein–Barr virus by renal transplant recipients and other patients treated with immunosuppressive drugs, *Lancet* **1**:234–237 (1974).

113. SUGDEN, B., Comparison of Epstein–Barr viral DNA's in Burkitt lymphoma biopsy cells and in cells clonally transformed *in vitro*, *Proc. Natl. Acad. Sci. U.S.A.* **74**:4651–4655 (1977).

114. SUGDEN, B., AND MARK, W., Clonal transformation of adult human leukocytes by Epstein–Barr virus, *J. Virol.* **23**:503–508 (1978).

115. SVEDMYR, E., AND JONDAL, M., Cytotoxic effector cells specific for B cell lines transformed by Epstein–Barr virus are present in patients with infectious mononucleosis, *Proc. Natl. Acad. Sci. U.S.A.* **72**:1622–1626 (1975).

116. VANIER, T. M., AND PIKE, M. C., Leukemia incidence in tropical Africa, *Lancet* **1**:512–513 (1967).

117. WALTERS, M. K., AND POPE, J. H., Studies of the EB virus-related antigens of human leukocyte cell lines, *Int. J. Cancer* **8**:32–40 (1971).

118. WERNER, J., HENLE, G., PINTO, C. A., HAFF, R. F., AND HENLE, W., Establishment of continuous lymphoblast cultures from leukocytes of gibbons (*Hylobates lar*), *Int. J. Cancer* **10**:557–567 (1972).

119. WILLIAMS, E. H., DAY, N. E., AND GESER, A. G., Seasonal variation in onset of Burkitt's lymphoma in the West Nile District of Uganda, *Lancet* **2**:19–22 (1974).

120. WITKEY, I. S., Malignant lymphoma in Papua, New Guinea: Epidemiologic aspects, *J. Natl. Cancer Inst.* **50**:1703–1711 (1973).

121. WOLF, H., WERNER, J., AND ZUR HAUSEN, H., EBV DNA in nonlymphoid cells of nasopharyngeal carcinomas and in a malignant lymphoma obtained after inoculation of EBV into cottontop marmosets, *Cold Spring Harbor Symp. Quant. Biol.* **39**:791–796

122. WOLF, H., ZUR HAUSEN, H., AND BECKER, V., EB viral genomes in epithelial nasopharyngeal carcinoma cells, *Nature (London) New Biol.* **244**:245–247 (1973).

123. YAMAMOTO, N., AND HINUMA, Y., Clonal transfor-

mation of human leukocytes by Epstein–Barr virus in soft agar, *Int. J. Cancer* **17**:191–196 (1976).

124. ZECH, L., HAGLUND, A., NILSSON, K., AND KLEIN, G., Characteristic chromosomal abnormalities in biopsies and lymphoid-cell lines from patients with Burkitt and non-Burkitt lymphomas, *Int. J. Cancer* **17**:47–56 (1976).

125. ZIEGLER, J. L., ANDERSSON, M., KLEIN, G., AND HENLE, W., Detection of Epstein–Barr virus DNA in American Burkitt's lymphoma, *Int. J. Cancer* **17**:701–706 (1976).

126. ZIEGLER, J. L., MORROW, R. H., JR., TEMPLETON, A., C., TEMPLETON, C., BLUMING, A. Z., FASS, L., AND KYALWAZI, S. K., Clinical features and treatment of childhood malignant lymphoma in Uganda, *Int. J. Cancer* **5**:415–425 (1970).

127. ZUR HAUSEN, H., AND SCHULTE-HOLTHAUSEN, H., Presence of EB virus nucleic acid homology in a "virus-free" line of Burkitt tumor cells, *Nature (London)* **227**:245–248 (1970).

128. ZUR HAUSEN, H., SCHULTE-HOLTHAUSEN, H., KLEIN, G., HENLE, W., HENLE, G., CLIFFORD, P., AND SANTESSON, L., EB-virus DNA in biopsies of Burkitt tumors and anaplastic carcinomas of the nasopharynx, *Nature (London)* **228**:1056–1057 (1970).

12. Suggested Reading

EPSTEIN, M. A., AND ACHONG, B., (eds), *The Epstein–Barr Virus*, Springer-Verlag Berlin, Heidelberg, New York, 1979.

MILLER, G., Biology of EB virus, in: *Viral Oncology* (G. KLEIN, ed.), pp. 713–738, Raven Press, New York, 1980.

DE-THÉ, G., The epidemiology of Burkitt lymphoma, *Epidemiol. Rev.* **1**:32–54, (1979).

HENLE, W., HENLE, G., AND LENNETTE, E. T., The Epstein–Barr virus. *Sci. Am.* **241**:48–59 (1979).

CHAPTER 25

Nasopharyngeal Carcinoma

G. de-Thé, J. H. C. Ho, and C. S. Muir

1. Introduction

Nasopharyngeal carcinoma (NPC) and Burkitt lymphoma (BL) are neoplasms for which there is strong evidence of a viral association. Their study exemplifies the problems inherent in chronic-disease epidemiology and in demonstrating a causal relationship between viruses and cancer in man.[42a]

There are two complementary approaches in exploring the possible oncogenic role of viruses in humans. The first is to investigate, according to the hypothesis of Huebner and Todaro,[98] the fundamental role of vertically transmitted oncornaviruses (oncogenic RNA viruses), which are held to be "activated" by various chemical, physical, or viral agents. This approach has far-reaching implications for humans, for whom only indirect evidence, but not as yet proof, of the existence of oncornalike agents has so far been obtained (see the review by Gallo et al.[55]).

The second avenue is to consider horizontally transmitted viruses as part of the environment. In humans, the geographical distribution of the main types of cancers is such that variations up to 100-fold exist for some sites, suggesting that the environment plays a critical role in their development.[45] If chemicals are generally believed to play the major role, environmental, physical, and microbiological agents should not be overlooked. Carcinogenesis is accepted by most epidemiologists to represent a multistep and multifactorial process,[147] the clinical onset of the tumor being the last and obvious one.

The Epstein–Barr virus (EBV) may act as an initiator in the causation of BL and malaria as a promoter (both are environmental agents)[32,41,141] (see Chapter 24). NPCarcinoma is another example of close association between a virus (the EBV) and a human tumor. The pathogenesis and role of the EBV in NPC are not yet understood, but the level of association is very strong the world over, in contrast to Burkitt-type lymphomas.[42,120,143]

Two conferences have set the stage of knowledge of the etiology of NPC, the first, in 1967, published by the UICC,[102] the second in 1978, published by the IARC.[100]

2. Historical Background

On the basis of the work of Derry,[23] Smith and Dawson,[168] Krogman,[115] and Wells,[183,184] Clifford[21] has stated that the oldest known patholog-

G. de-Thé · CNRS, Faculty of Medicine A. Carrel, Lyon and Cancer Institute—CNRS, Villejuif, France. J. H. C. Ho · Institute of Radiology and Oncology, Queen Elizabeth Hospital, Kowloon, Hong Kong. C. S. Muir · International Agency for Research on Cancer, Lyon, France.

ical specimens of NPC were derived from inhabitants of northeast Africa and the Middle East from the period 3500–3000 B.C. Reviewing the evidence, Ho[82] concluded that only one of the Romano-Egyptian cases described by Smith and Dawson[168] could have been a nasopharyngeal cancer. In Europe, Durand-Fardel[46] is generally credited as giving the first clinical description of a case of NPC, while Michaux[129] reported the first histologically proven case.

In China, NPC has been recognized, at least since the early part of this century, as the "Kwantung (Guangdong) tumor," stressing the high frequency of this neoplasm in Kwantung, the southernmost province. Ho,[82] in his search for a description of the disease in early Chinese medical writings, could find only a fatal disease called *shih ying*, also known as *shih yung*, both meaning literally "loss of nutrition." The description given in the *Encyclopaedia of Chinese Medical Terms*, edited by Wu,[191] of the clinical picture of *shih ying* is consistent with that of the "mainly metastatic type" of NPC[80] (see Section 8.2.1). However, no mention was made in the encyclopedia as to when the disease was first described. The apparent lack of a full description of NPC in early Chinese medical writings may be because the disease is largely confined to the south, whereas practically all the early writings were by physicians in northern and central China.[79]

In parts of Asia, it was some time before it was realized that the malignant deposits in the neck lymph nodes were secondary to a nasopharyngeal primary tumor, and Bonne and others continued to describe such neoplasms as "reticuloendothelioma lymphoglandulae colli lateralis." It was probably Digby et al.[43] who first drew attention to the unusual frequency of NPC among Chinese in Hong Kong and over large parts of China in a remarkably detailed description of the clinical and pathological features in 103 cases in which it was stated categorically that the tumors arose in the epithelium of the nasopharynx.[122]

While pathologists in Europe and North America debated the classification and histogenesis of the neoplasms, notably the so-called lymphoepithelioma and transitional-cell carcinomas, New and Kirch, and later others including Digby et al.[43] concluded that all were variants of squamous-cell carcinoma—a view since upheld by ultrastructural studies.[56,172]

Before 1962, there was no real attempt to study the epidemiology of NPC. The medical profession seemed to be quite satisfied with the hypothesis advanced by Dobson[44] that the high frequency of NPC in Chinese was related to the poorly ventilated houses in which they lived, inhaling the carcinogen-laden domestic smoke. This was later disputed by Ho[82] when he found that the frequency of NPC in Chinese fisherfolk who lived practically all their lives in boats and cooked their food in the open was significantly higher than that in the rest of the Chinese population in Hong Kong, the majority of whom lived in congested dwellings on land.

3. Methodology Involved in Epidemiological and Virological Studies

3.1. Sources of Mortality Data

Mortality data are derived from cause-of-death statements on death certificates. The figures available for nasopharyngeal cancer* for a wide variety of countries have been aggregated by the World Health Organization[188] and age-specific rates, but not age-adjusted rates, provided. In general, the disease is exceedingly rare. Further, national mortality data rarely give figures for racial groups within a country. Although rates for administrative divisions such as provinces are often available on request, these are usually based on small numbers of cases and are subject to considerable statistical fluctuation.

3.2. Sources of Morbidity (Incidence) Data

Morbidity data for nasopharyngeal cancer are obtained from cancer registries, being derived from reports on newly diagnosed cases of cancer occurring in a defined population. Regrettably, such information is generally lacking for much of the United States, for most of South America, Africa,

---

* All rates in this chapter are age-adjusted to the world population distribution[176] and are expressed per 100,000 per annum. In this chapter, *nasopharyngeal cancer* refers not only to the carcinomas (NPC) but also to neoplasms of other cell types, e.g., chordoma, multiple myeloma, and the malignant lymphomas.

Asia, and Oceania, and for large parts of Europe and the U.S.S.R. Even though there are large gaps in geographic coverage,[135] the morbidity from cancer is probably better measured than for any other chronic disease and for many infectious and acute processes. Available morbidity data of good quality are published in the *Cancer Incidence in Five Continents* monographs[99,175,176] and are presented in Fig. 1. It will be observed that for the vast majority of cancer registries, not only are the age-adjusted rates

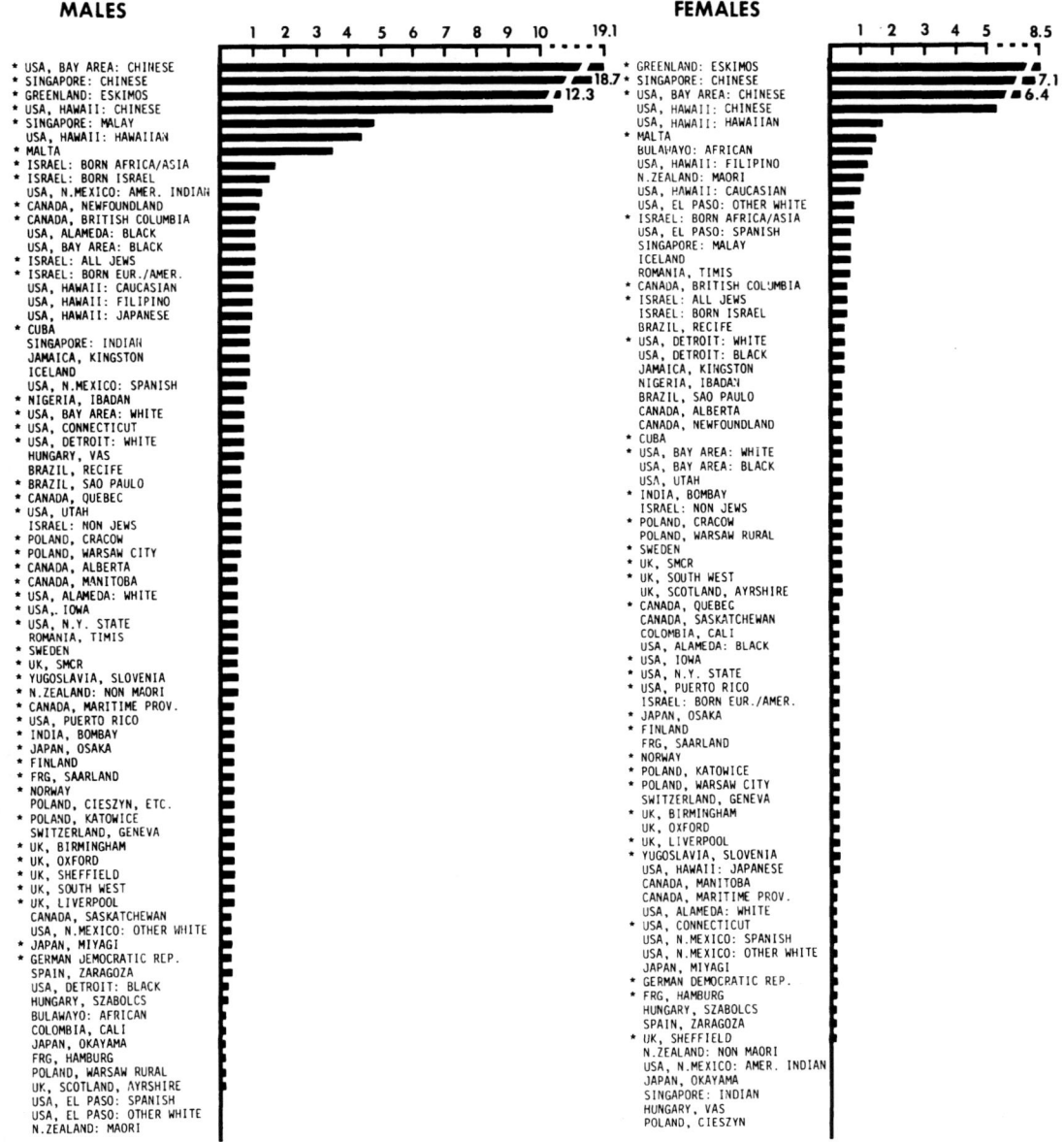

Fig. 1. Age-adjusted mortality rates for NPC by sex. All rates are standardized to the world population distribution. Data were derived mainly from *Cancer Incidence in Five Continents*, 1976.[99] *Rates based on more than 10 cases.

below 1 per 100,000 per annum, but also many rates are based on fewer than 10 cases.

3.3. Sources of Relative-Frequency Data

Relative-frequency data, indicating the proportion of nasopharyngeal cancer observed in a series of patients with all types of cancer, are derived from the files of pathology and radiotherapy departments. The sources of bias in measuring relative frequency as well as in mortality and morbidity data have been analyzed.[77,135]

3.4. Serological Surveys

Two types of serological surveys have been carried out to unravel the relationship between the Epstein–Barr herpesvirus (EBV) and NPC. The first type is represented by case–control studies aimed at evaluating the humoral immune response of the NPC patients compared to that of various controls.[37,40,74] The second type is population-based surveys aimed at establishing the epidemiological characteristics of the virus in populations at different risk for EBV-associated diseases. We have been conducting such a study covering Chinese in Hong Kong, Indians, Chinese and Malays in Singapore, Nilotic tribes in Uganda, and Caucasians in France.[36]

3.4.1. Selection of Groups. In the first type of studies, controls were usually selected among patients of the same age group and sex with tumors other than NPC. Whenever possible, normal subjects such as volunteer blood donors also served as controls. In these seroepidemiological studies, the choice of groups to be bled was a matter of compromise between representativeness and feasibility, and included volunteers in maternity and child clinics, primary and secondary schools, universities, and army and police groups. Soon it was found that such selected groups were not a good representation of the population at large. Successful efforts were then made to obtain representative samples of the general population, and *randomly* selected families were visited and interviewed and the eligible members bled.

3.4.2. Serological Tests. Three techniques are mainly utilized in EBV serology: immunofluorescence, complement-fixation (CF), and immunoprecipitation. Two classes of immunoglobulins, IgG

and IgA, appear to play an important role in the relationships between EBV and NPC.

a. Immunofluorescence Tests. Immunofluorescence (IF) is the main tool of EBV serology as it is used for the detection of four different groups of EBV-determined antigens: viral capsid antigen (VCA), early antigen (EA), membrane antigen (MA), and Epstein–Barr nuclear antigen (EBNA).

VCA Test: As described by Henle and Henle,[67] the VCA test is an indirect IF test, detecting intracellular structural antigens (viral capsid antigens) in EBV-producing cell lines. In routine testing, one detects IgG, and a positive test (i.e., ≥1:10) merely reflects that the person concerned has been infected and has reacted to the infection. The titers of VCA antibodies obtained in various laboratories on the same sera can vary from one to three dilutions; the causes of such variations are multiple, the main ones being the lymphoblastoid-cell line and the proportion of VCA-positive cells at the time of testing.[60] All serological tests carried out within the International Agency for Research on Cancer seroepidemiological survey were done using the Jijoye cell line as the source of antigen. Large antigen batches were prepared to minimize the variation of titers related to the percentage of IF-positive cells. The small variations still observed were evaluated and, if necessary, were corrected during statistical analysis.

EA Test: Also described by Henle and co-workers,[69,71] the EA test detects "early antigens" produced within a few hours after superinfection by EBV of non-virus-producing lymphoblastoid lines such as Raji. EA synthesis does not require DNA replication, and appears to consist of two different antigens: a diffuse (D) antigen and a restricted (R) one.[70] Antibodies against EA reflect an *active infection* of the organism concerned.

MA Test: Developed and extensively used by Klein *et al.*,[107,108] the MA test detects EBV-determined membrane-bound antigens. The test is done on live cells, in contrast to the VCA and EA tests, in which acetone fixation is used. MAs are comprised of at least three different antigenic components.[109] Antibodies against MA seem to be of clinical and prognostic value in BL and NPC patients.[107,109]

EBNA Test: As described by Reedman and Klein,[150] the EBNA test detects the EBV-determined nuclear antigen(s) that appears to be related to the soluble antigen, as detected by the CF test.[37,112,119] This nuclear antigen appears a few hours after EBV infection[7,193] and is present in EBV-transformed lymphoid cells even when they are not virus producers.

EBNA is also detected in BL[151] and NPC[34,95] biopsies, as well as in NPC biopsies transplanted into nude mice.[111]

b. Complement-Fixation Tests. CF is used in EBV serology with either particulate antigen, i.e., semi-purified virus,[57] or soluble antigen, extracted from non-virus-producing cell lines.[170,177] These CF antigens seem to divide into three components: one is sedimentable and heat-resistant, corresponding to a structural antigen, one is heat-labile and sedimentable, and one is heat-stable and soluble, the last two components being nonstructural antigens.[181] Antibodies against particulate antigen(s) parallel those directed against VCA, whereas antibodies directed against soluble antigen from a non-virus-producing line (Raji) appear to parallel those directed against EBNA and seem to reflect a prolonged infection with this virus. The CF soluble (CF/S) antibodies develop only weeks or months after infectious mononucleosis.[169,178]

c. Immunoprecipitation Test. This test for EBV was developed by Old *et al.*[142] using the Ouchterlony immunodiffusion technique. This immunoprecipitation (IP) antigen seems to be closely related, if not identical, to CF/S antigen.[149] This test needs large amounts of antigen, and is not quantitative.

d. Antibodies of the IgA Class. As discussed in Section 3.6.2b, IgA antibodies are becoming increasingly useful in NPC management. Their detection is possible in the VCA, EA, and MA indirect IF tests, simply by using fluorescein-labeled immunoglobulins directed against purified human IgA.

3.5. Sociological Surveys

When no clear lead to the etiology of a neoplasm or a plausible hypothesis to test exists, it is often useful to survey the way of life of groups at high and low risk for the disease to determine whether there are habits or exposures that may be pertinent to disease development. Such surveys are usually best conducted by anthropologists or sociologists. Since the sum total of life style embraces so many factors, it is essential to describe the current etiological hypothesis of carcinogenesis to such investigators so that their studies may have specific areas

of focus. The very detailed analysis of the way of life in the Caspian region of Iran carried out in connection with esophageal cancer in that area typifies the possible scope of such investigations.[114]

Because of the long induction time for cancer, attempts should be made to determine conditions as they were 20–30 years ago as well as those prevailing at the time of the survey.

3.6. Laboratory Diagnosis

3.6.1. Histopathology. Diagnosis depends on the demonstration of the neoplasm in a biopsy of the nasopharynx.[1] Biopsies from many areas and at several times may be needed, since the tumorous process often infiltrates underneath an apparently normal mucosa. The microscopic appearance of the neoplasms was reviewed by Shanmugaratnam and Muir[155] and by Yeh.[195] The World Health Organization (WHO) has now published an illustrated classification of upper respiratory tract neoplasms, including those of the nasopharynx, and listing the appropriate ICD-O codes.[189] Pathologists were urged to use the WHO classification at the NPC conference in Kyoto,[100] and are increasingly doing so. This is essential to be able to compare the disease in different geographical areas. The vast majority of NPCs arise from the nasopharyngeal epithelium and should be considered, irrespective of their appearance on light microscopy, as variants of squamous-cell carcinomas. This statement is based on electron-microscopic studies that have revealed the presence of tonofibrils and other epithelial markers in most of the histological variants.[56,171,172] Any of the histological types of NPC may be infiltrated by varying amounts of lymphocytes: this feature is not restricted to the lymphoepitheliomas and may be pertinent to the association with a lymphotropic virus. For the experienced pathologist working in a high-incidence area, diagnosis rarely poses any problems; however, the Schminke variant composed of single or small loose aggregations of malignant cells set in a dense lymphoid stroma and the rarer spindle-cell and clear-cell variants may cause difficulties for those unfamiliar with the region. While the diagnosis, particularly of the Regaud variant of the neoplasm, can usually be made with confidence from the biopsied secondary deposits in a neck lymph node, this practice is to be deprecated, since it does not indicate unequivocally the site of the primary tumor and nasopharyngeal biopsy is simpler to perform.

The pathologist working in a low-incidence area should ask himself, when confronted by a nasopharyngeal biopsy or a secondary deposit in an upper neck lymph node, "Is this a Schminke variant?" and "What about the nasopharynx?"

3.6.2. Serology   *a. IgG Antibodies.* There is a characteristic EBV antibody pattern associated with NPC. Patients with undifferentiated carcinoma of the nasopharynx, regardless of their ethnic or geographic origin, have high EBV VCA, EA, and EBNA serological reactivities (IgG class) when compared to patients with other tumors (OT) or to normal subjects (NS).[40] As can be seen in Table 1, the EBV reactivity that separates best between NPC and either OT or NS relates to antibodies directed against EA. This regularity in humoral response of NPC patients to EBV EA, regardless of origin,[40] contrasts with the situation of BL patients from Africa, who have high EBV reactivities and high EBV DNA content, whereas patients from the United States have inconsistently elevated EBV reactivities and EBV-genome content in tumor cells.[120,143]

Antibodies against early antigen (EA)[69] are of special interest, since they reflect an active EBV infection. In NPC patients, as in patients with infectious mononucleosis, EA antibodies are mostly directed against the diffuse (D) component of the EA complex, whereas in BL, patients' EA antibodies are directed against the restricted (R) component.[70,113] The EA reactivity in NPC patients is also stage-dependent, and Henle et al.[74] are of the opinion that reactivity to D component probably reflects the degree of lymph-node involvement.

Antibodies against complement-fixation soluble (CF/S) antigen are already very high in Chinese NPC patients in stage I[33] (see Fig. 1), in contrast to BL patients, in whom CF/S antibodies are low at an early stage and increase with clinical deterioration.[169,170] CF antibodies against CF/S antigen increase slightly from stage I to stage V of NPC and in both diseases appear to have a prognostic value and can be used as a useful clinical guide. Antibodies against MA are also regularly high in NPC patients.[25]

As can be seen in Fig. 2, the serological response to VCA, EA, and EBNA antigens increases with the severity of the disease, from stages I to V of Ho,[37,68] the EA reactivity being again the most useful one to follow, possibly associated with lymph-node involvement.[74]

Table 1. Epstein–Barr Virus Serological Reactivities in Nasopharyngeal Carcinoma Patients, Patients with Other Tumors, and Normal Subjects Originating from Three Geographic Areas[a]

Group and EBV reactivities		NPC patients		OT patients		NS	
		GMT	Number of sera	GMT	Number of sera	GMT	Number of sera
Hong Kong	VCA	1316		376		119	
Chinese	**EA**	**182**		**8**		**9**	
	CF	88		18		21	
	EBNA	776		86		ND	
			49		39		45
Tunis	VCA	1677		190		114	
Arabs	**EA**	**119**		**8**		**7**	
	CF	75		ND		24	
	EBNA	593		142		ND	
			65		65		65
Paris	VCA	978		166		91	
Caucasians	**EA**	**194**		**6**		**7**	
	CF	32		10		10	
	EBNA	118		ND		ND	
			18		37		40

[a] From de-Thé et al.[40] Abbreviations here and in Tables 2 and 3: (CF) Complement fixation; (CF/S) CF soluble; (EA) early antigen; (EBNA) Epstein–Barr nuclear antigen; (EBV) Epstein–Barr virus; (GMT) geometric mean titer; (ND) not done; (NPC) nasopharyngeal carcinoma; (NS) normal subjects; (OT) other tumors; (VCA) viral capsid antigen.

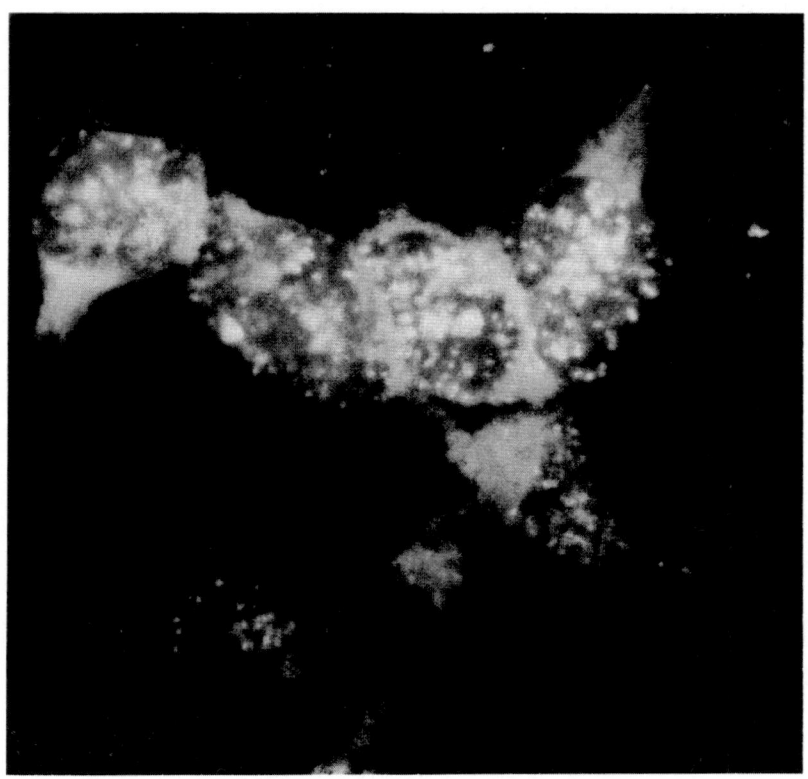

Fig. 6. Touch smear from an NPC biopsy originating from Hong Kong (Reg. No. 74/1173), stained for EBNA by the anticomplement immunofluorescence test (ACIF) using an NPC serum (Tu 125) having no detectable antinuclear factor. Note the coarse, granular aspect of the EBNA. The positive cells here are believed to be epithelial.

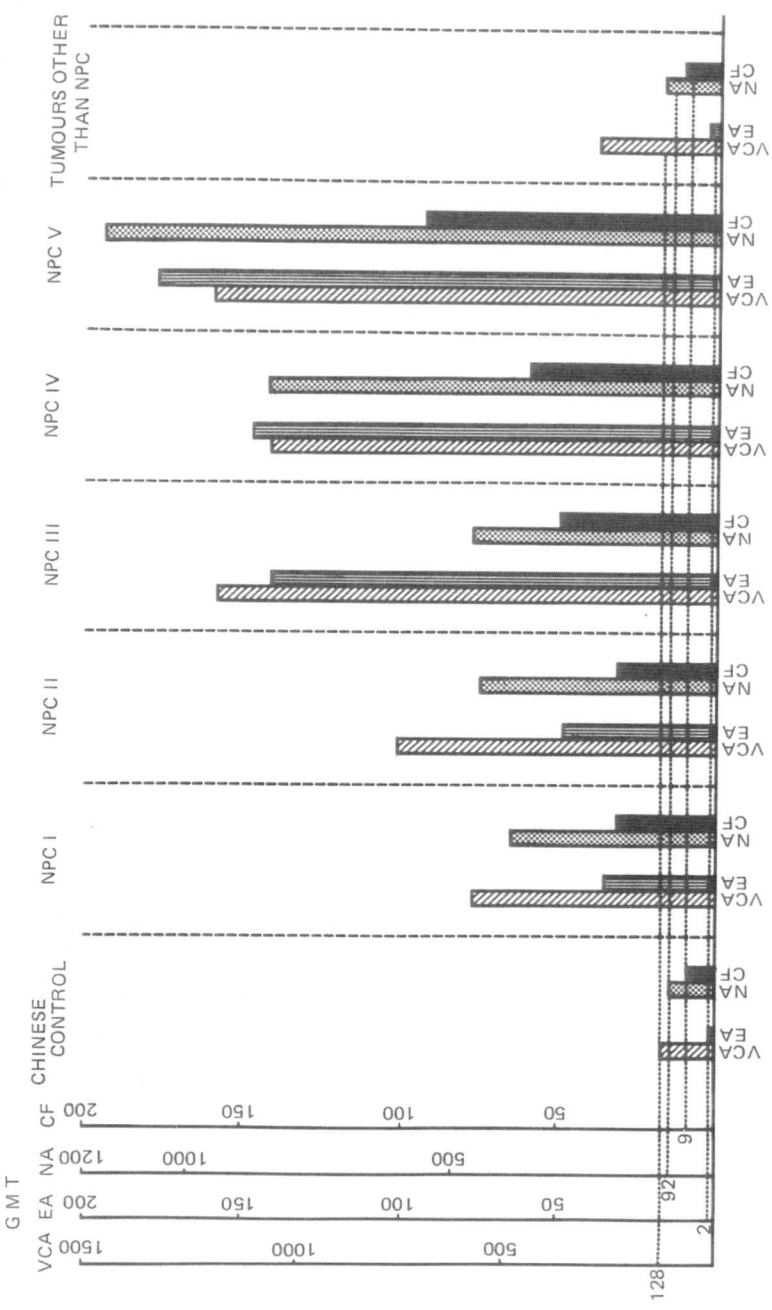

Fig. 2. Histogram giving the various EBV antibody reactivities (IgG class) in Chinese NPC patients at different stages of the disease and, for comparison, the reactivities of normal subjects (Chinese controls) and of Chinese patients with tumors other than NPC. (GMT) Geometric mean titer; (VCA) viral capsid antigen; (EA) early antigen; (NA) nuclear antigen; (CF) complement-fixation (soluble) antigen. From de-Thé et al.[37]

b. IgA Antibodies in Serum and Saliva of NPC Patients. Following the observations of Wara *et al.*[182] that NPC patients had very high levels of IgA antibodies in their sera, Henle and Henle[75] found that such IgA antibodies were directed against EBV-determined antigens (VCA and EA-D). These authors found that among healthy donors or patients with tumors of the ear, nose, and throat (ENT) other than NPC, only 5% had antibodies to VCA and none to EA.[75,101] Ho *et al.*[88] confirmed the importance of IgA antibodies directed to EA in NPC patients, whereas Desgranges *et al.*[27] and Pearson *et al.*[145] extended their observations to non-Chinese NPC patients, namely Tunisian and American cases. This IgA response increases with advancing stages of the disease (see Table 2) and represents systemic (7 S) antibodies restricted to EBV, since IgA antibody titers to herpes simplex virus did not differ between NPC patients and controls. Zeng *et al.*[200] detected Ig A/VCA in NPC patients from 8 provinces and cities in China.

Desgranges *et al.*[27] and Ho *et al.*[89,91] extended these serological studies to the salivas of NPC patients, which were found to contain high levels of secretory IgA (11 S), specific for VCA and EA-D in 75 and 35% of the salivas of NPC patients, respectively. As can be seen in Fig. 3, IgA antibodies to EBV were found confined to the saliva of 50% of NPC patients, but were not detected in saliva from patients with infectious mononucleosis (IM), BL, or other tumors. Further, Desgranges *et al.*[28] found that plasma cells surrounding the epithelial tumor cells contained IgA antibody molecules that were secondarily found to be specific for EBV VCA, whereas epithelial-tumor cells were seen to exhibit the secretory piece at their surface (x, a) (Figs. 4 and

5). These results, confirmed by Ho *et al.*,[91,92] raise the possibility that the EBV IgA present in NPC saliva has its origin in the tumor itself, possibly representing blocking antibodies. The presence of serum and salivary IgA to VCA and EA could have a practical value, not only for the diagnosis of NPC (with a very high sensitivity and specificity), but also as a possible marker for prognosis in the management of the disease.

3.6.3. Viral Markers in NPC Biopsies. There is a regular presence of viral fingerprints in NPC tumor tissue. EBV DNA sequences have been found by DNA/DNA hybridization, DNA/cRNA hybridization, and DNA/DNA reassociation kinetics in most NPC biopsies.[140,144,198] Because EBV is a lymphotropic virus and NPC is an epithelial tumor (see Section 3.6.1), it was believed that the EBV DNA detected was localized in lymphoid cells, which are regularly present in NPC tumors, and not in the epithelial-tumor cells. However, the opposite has now been demonstrated by Wolf *et al.*,[187] showing that EBV DNA sequences were predominantly in epithelial cells, and confirmed by Desgranges *et al.*,[26] who detected EBV DNA in separated epithelial-cell populations from NPC biopsies originating from different geographic areas. It appears that the level of differentiation of tumor cells has a bearing on the viral expression, since only undifferentiated types of NPC regularly show detectable EBV DNA and EBNA.[3,4] In parallel, EBV-specific nuclear antigen (EBNA) was detected by indirect IF in touch smears of NPC biopsies (see Fig. 6).[34,95,201] Klein *et al.*[111] successfully grafted NPC tumor biopsies to nude mice and observed that these grafted tumors contained only epithelial cells and regularly exhibited EBNA. These epithelial characteristics were

Table 2. Epstein–Barr VCA and EA IgG and IgA Geometric Mean Titers in Sera from Chinese NPC Patients in Different Stages of the Disease, in Patients with Other Tumors, and in Controls[a]

Subjects	Number of sera tested	VCA IgA		EA IgA		VCA IgG		EA IgG	
		GMT	S.E.M.	GMT	S.E.M.	GMT	S.E.M.	GMT	S.E.M.
NPC Stage I	38	44.4	0.6	10	0.5	512	0.4	48.5	0.7
NPC Stage II	42	69.6	0.5	12.3	0.6	803.4	0.4	54.9	0.4
NPC Stage III	50	85.7	0.6	23	0.6	1097.5	0.3	97	0.6
NPC Stage IV	50	56.6	0.6	20	0.6	630.4	0.4	84.4	0.7
NPC Stage V	35	52.8	0.9	16.8	0.9	724.1	0.5	101.6	0.5
OT	50	3.3	0.1	2.5	0.0	279.2	0.3	3.3	0.3
NS	50	2.8	0.1	2.5	0.0	92.1	0.3	2.2	0.1

[a] For abbreviations, see Table 1 footnote. (S.E.M.) Standard error of the mean.

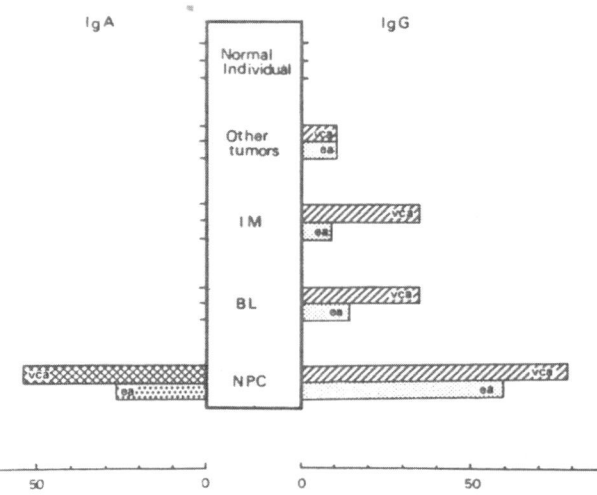

Fig. 3. IgA and IgG in throat-washings from patients with NPC, BL, IM, other tumors, and normal individuals. From Desgranges and de-Thé.[29]

% Ig positive throat washings

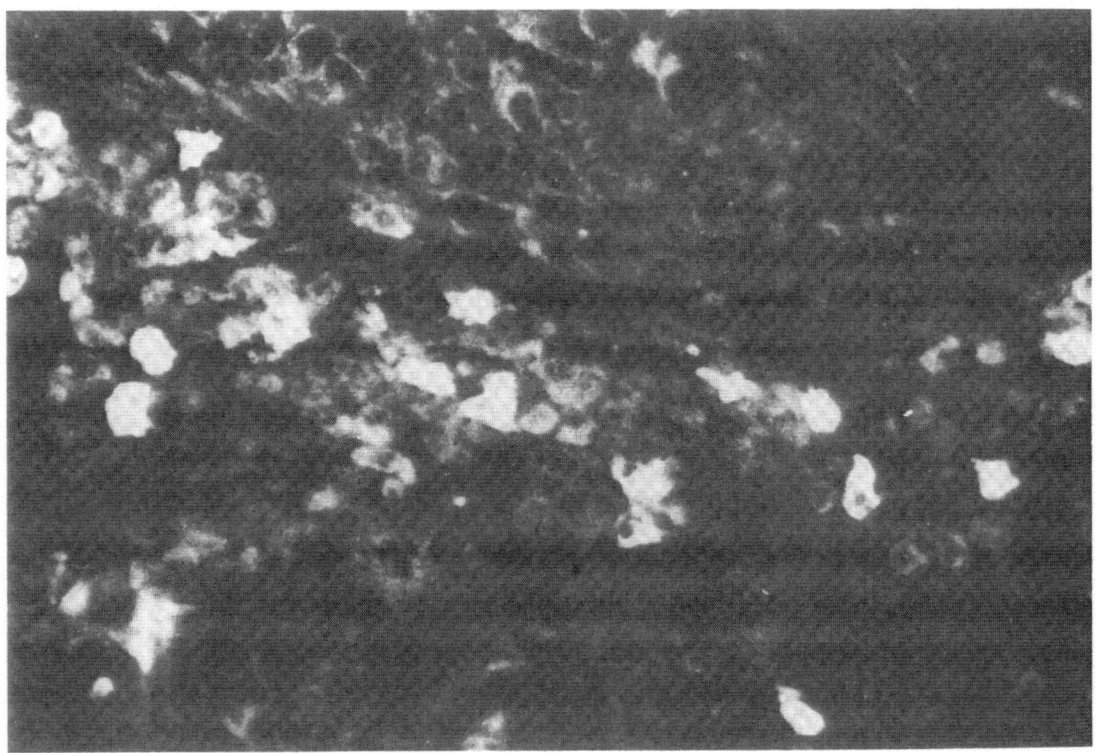

Fig. 4. IgA (α) in plasmocytes surrounding epithelial-tumor cells. ×300. From Desgranges and de-Thé.[29]

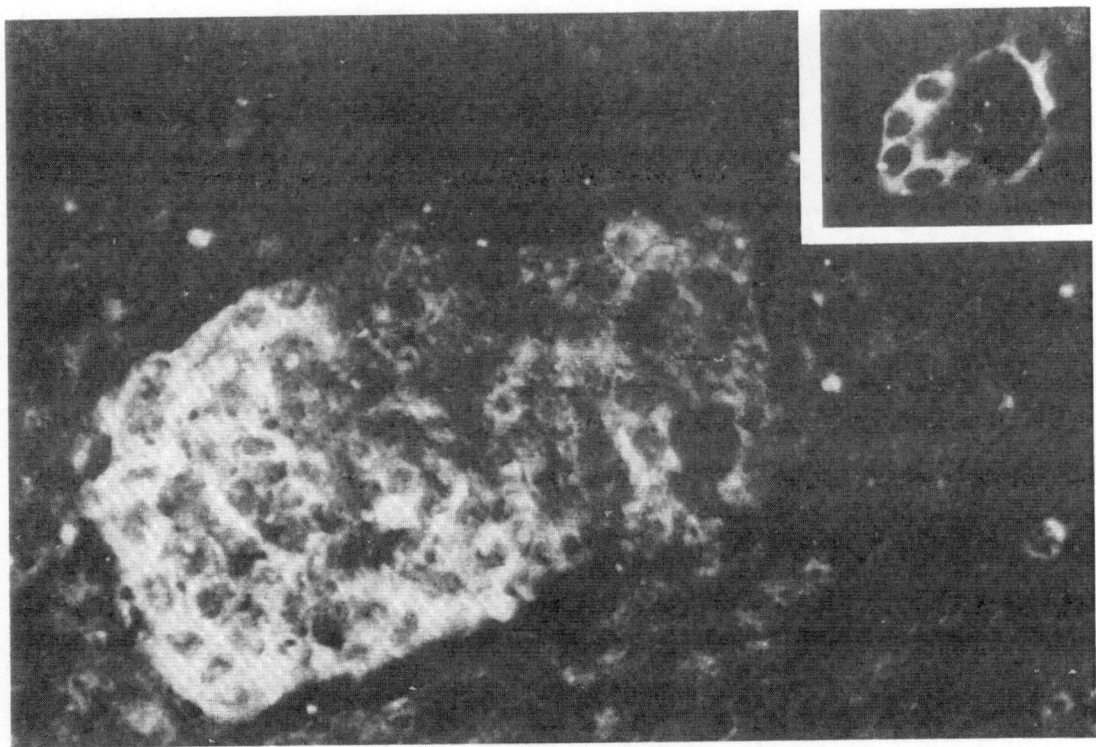

Fig. 5. IgA (SP) in the glandular acini and on the surface of epithelial-tumor cells. ×300. From Desgranges and de-Thé.[29]

confirmed by electron microscopy.[38] After treatment with 5-iodo-2-deoxyuridine [(IUdR) Idoxuridine] or 5-bromodeoxy-uridine (BUdR), or after superinfection with HR1-EBV, epithelial-tumor cells can synthesize EA,[62] suggesting that such epithelial cells have surface receptors for EBV and that, under certain circumstances, the viral genome can be derepressed in tumor cells. Full replication of EBV was observed in epithelial-tumor cells after passage in nude mice, and the virus was isolated.[174]

4. Biological Characteristics of Epstein–Barr Virus in Its Relationship with Nasopharyngeal Carcinoma

The herpesvirus discovered by Epstein *et al.*[47,48] in 1964 in a culture derived from a BL biopsy is a widespread and silent parasite of human B-lymphoid cells. The lack of a permissive cell system allow-

ing *in vitro* virus titration and virus cloning makes virological studies on the EBV rather difficult. *In vivo*, the EBV probably infects B lymphocytes in circulating blood, lymph nodes, spleen, and other sites, where the viral infection becomes latent.

A number of investigators have searched for a reservoir of EBV in the human organism outside the lymphocytes (which represent a semipermissive system), but with no success to date. Only B lymphocytes appear to be permissive for EBV infection: when B- and T-lymphoid populations are separated from the blood of EBV-seropositive subjects, only B-cell populations eventually give rise to permanent lymphoblastoid-cell lines, the best marker for EBV infection.[193] Epithelial cells in the nasopharynx are obvious candidates to replicate the virus under normal conditions. It is regrettable that the interesting claim of Lemon *et al.*[118] that EBV replicates in epithelial cells of the ororhinopharynx during IM could not be confirmed. On the other hand, the lymphoid cells regularly present in the submucosa of the nasopharynx might play a critical role both in the replication of the virus and in tumor development, since the EBV is mainly lymphotropic, and since this tumor arises only in the area of the lymphoepithelium. The B or T nature of the lymphocytes present in the tumor is a matter of controversy: Yata et al.[192,194] found that both B and T cells were present in tumor tissue, but that a relative increase of B cells was observed in the lymphoid-depleted areas as well as in direct contact with epithelial cells. In contrast, Jondal and Klein[103] found that the lymphocytes present in tumor biopsies were mostly of T type. The study of the lymphocytes of the normal nasopharyngeal mucosa and in NPC is therefore of great importance in understanding the pathogenesis of such tumor, as well as the cell-mediated immune response of NPC patients to EBV.[17,121]

Latent infection by EBV is present in every population around the world, but age at primary infection varies greatly among ethnic groups and geographic areas. As is true for other herpesviruses, EBV reinfection might occur, as well as *reactivation of a latent infection* by factors that are unknown at present. One abnormal condition that "turns on" viral replication is the transfer of circulating lymphocytes to *in vitro* culture, leading to the establishment of lymphoblastoid lines. This phenomenon (called "lymphoblastoid transformation"[9]) is of as great interest to oncovirologists as it is to immunologists. Although it is poorly understood (see the review of Klein[110]), there is agreement that such a phenomenon is caused by the presence of EBV-infected lymphocytes.[30,31,139]

Does "lymphoblastoid transformation" occur *in vivo*, and are such transformed cells eliminated by immunosurveillance mechanisms? Expression of viral-determined antigens occurs in BL tumor cells, where the EBNA and MA (see Section 3.4.2a)[107,151] can be detected.

In vitro (i.e., in lymphoblastoid lines), viral replication is also controlled by unknown factors and synthesis of VCA, EA, and other antigens taking place in a changing proportion of cells. Such variation in "viral expression" is line-dependent, and also time-dependent for most lines.[31,58] Early functions include the EBNA, MA, and EA, and those appearing later include structural VCA and probably the IP antigens.

The mode of transmission of EBV is not fully established, but saliva appears to play an important role in horizontal transmission, since infectious and transforming EBV has regularly been found in the saliva of IM patients and of seropositive normal subjects.[49,59,130,137] Sociocultural customs or habits, in which exchange of saliva between adults and young infants takes place, could play a role in EBV infection in early infancy. Breast feeding may play a role in EBV transmission, since milk does contain EBV-infected cells, as demonstrated by the establishment of lymphoblastoid lines from human milk (Feller, personal communication). All data available indicate that EBV infection is not transmitted through placenta,[50,72,146] but there is no reason that under exceptional circumstances (in pregnant women), or under severe malaria infection (known to damage the placenta), congenital EBV infection could not occur.

The full spectrum of host response to EBV in the human organism is still ill defined. This virus causes Paul-Bunnell-positive IM in young adults.[50,72,73] Most primary infections, however, are asymptomatic, and this virus would have been considered as a mild, inoffensive parasite if it had not been associated with two malignancies: BL and NPC. We saw in Section 3.4 that the association between EBV and NPC is based on serological data and on the evidence for the presence of EBV fingerprints (DNA and EBNA) in tumor cells of both BL and NPC.

This characteristic pattern is found in NPC patients originating from various parts of the world (see de-Thé et al.[40] and Table 1), and such consistency is of particular importance, since NPC is a distinctive pathological entity that cannot be readily confused with other conditions. The lack of similar serological reactivities in patients with other carcinomas localized in nearby tissues such as the oro- and hypopharynx (Table 3), and even in patients with tumors of the nasopharynx other than carcinomas,[24] indicates that a peculiar relationship must exist between EBV and NPC.

The nature of the association between EBV and NPC remains to be established. The regular presence of viral fingerprints in tumor cells and the specific immune response to EBV in NPC patients in regions with high, intermediate, or low risk for the disease makes the passenger hypothesis very unlikely.[40] That EBV is the causative agent of most IM is universally accepted (see Chapter 10). Further evidence for the causal nature of the relationship between EBV and BL lies in the results of the prospective seroepidemiological study in Uganda, in-

Table 3. Geometric Mean Titers of Epstein–Barr Virus Reactivities in Different Groups of Chinese Sera[a]

Type of Sera	EBV reactivities				
	VCA Jijoye	EA Raji	EBNA (ACIF) Raji	CF/S Raji	Number of sera
NPC patients	937.3	93.3	605.4	49.9	91
Tumor other than NPC	296.2	3.9	115.2	11.6	37
Normal subjects	128	2.2	92.1	9.0	47

[a] For abbreviations, see Table 1.

dicating that children who are to develop BL have high VCA titers years prior to tumor onset, with an increased relative risk of 30 for children having VCA titers 2 dilutions higher than the mean of the titers of the sex/age/locality-matched normal children[32–41] (see Chapter 24). That early infection by EBV plays the role of an initiating factor in BL development has been hypothesized by one of us.[32,41] The situation for NPC should be entirely different.

5. Descriptive Epidemiology

5.1. Incidence, Frequency, and Geographic Distribution

For the vast majority of population groups, the incidence rates for nasopharyngeal cancer are below 1 per 100,000 per annum. In persons of Chinese descent, much higher rates have been found, and morbidity rates have recently become available for selected Chinese populations. As can be seen in Fig. 7, the largely similar rates for Chinese in Zhongshan (Chungshan) county of Kwantung (Guangdong), Hong Kong, and the Bay Area of California are almost twice those for Chinese in Hawaii. The risk in Singapore Cantonese is significantly higher than for the remainder of the Singapore Chinese.[160] The rates in Shanghai and in Japan are half those observed in Hawaii.

With respect to the principal Chinese-language groups living in Singapore, the rates for both sexes in the Cantonese are twice those of the Teochew (known as Chiu Chau in Hong Kong) and the Hokkien (who come from the province of Fukien, which is to the north of and in continuity with the Chiu Chau district, northeast of Hong Kong). Since the Cantonese have a much lower risk of esophageal

cancer than the Hokkien and Teochew, it is unlikely that these differences could be due to differential reporting among the various groups.[159]

In his studies of Hong Kong Chinese, Ho[78,82] noted that the lowest incidence rate* was found in Chinese originating from the central coastal provinces (4.0) and that a 3–4 times higher incidence was observed in persons originating from Kwantung (Guangdong) Province. The Chiu Chau area of this province, located to the northeast of Hong Kong, showed a rate of 8.0. On further examination of the Hong Kong population,[90] it was noted that nasopharyngeal cancer incidence among the Cantonese "boat people" was higher (age-adjusted rates of 54.7 for males and 18.8 for females) than that among the land-dwellers (18.8 for males and 10.2 for females). The sex-incidence ratio of NPC in the boat group was 2.9 males to 1 female, even higher than for land-dwellers. The boat people are so called because they live on boats with only occasional visits to land. They speak their own distinctive dialects of Cantonese and have been present in the Hong Kong region since time unknown.

Incidence data from China are scanty.[104] Relative-frequency material published in 1959 suggested an increase from north to south.[94] As is apparent in Fig. 7, incidence in the metropolitan area of Shanghai seems to be considerably lower than mortality in the Chungshan (Zhongshan) county of Kwantung (Guangdong) province. While data quality are probably not strictly comparable, nonetheless the data are consistent with lower incidence rates in the north. There are few migrants from North China in Southeast Asia to form a comparison

---

* These rates are not strictly comparable to those in Fig. 1, being adjusted to the 1961 Hong Kong census population.

group. Data from Taiwan show a 2-fold excess of risk for males born in China compared to those born in Taiwan.[125] However, the unusual sex ratio of the incidence rates (M, 11.4; F, 11.7) among the China-born undermines confidence in these findings.

The Malay people of Singapore, who in general use the medical facilities much less than the other groups, have comparatively high rates (see Fig. 1). This group tends to live in the rural districts of the island and has a way of life that varies considerably from that of the Chinese. The incidence rates in the Caucasoid Indian and Pakistani moiety of the Singapore population are very low (see Fig. 1).

Incidence rates for all ethnic groups living on Hawaii are raised, but these are based on very small numbers (see Fig. 1).

High frequencies of NPC have been reported in Greenland Eskimos with some admixture of Caucasian blood[138] (Fig. 1) and in Alaskan natives.[12] Unpublished tabulations from the North West Territories of Canada show that this disease is considerably more common than elsewhere in the country,

probably due to an excess risk in the Eskimo population. Why these Mongoloid groups should have such high rates when northern Chinese and Japanese do not remains to be determined. Are cultural factors rather than racial stock, *per se*, more important in determining NPC risk? In Israel, although the cancer is at a much lower incidence level, there are still interesting differences among Jews coming from various parts of the world. The highest rates are noted in the Jews born in Asia or Africa (M, 1.7; F, 0.7) but rates in Jews born in Israel (M, 1.5; F, 0.5) are almost as high. For those born in America or Europe, rates are low. Many of the Jews from Africa migrated from Morocco, Algeria, and Tunisia, where there is evidence (see below) that NPC is of raised frequency. Minimum incidence rates in Kuwait are also raised (M, 2.2; F, 1.0).

Most of the other information on the distribution of NPC comes from relative-frequency series (Table 4). This has been summarized by Muir.[132,134] NPC is common in many populations of Southeast Asia such as Malays, Thais, Vietnamese, and Javanese in which Chinese admixture and racial intermin-

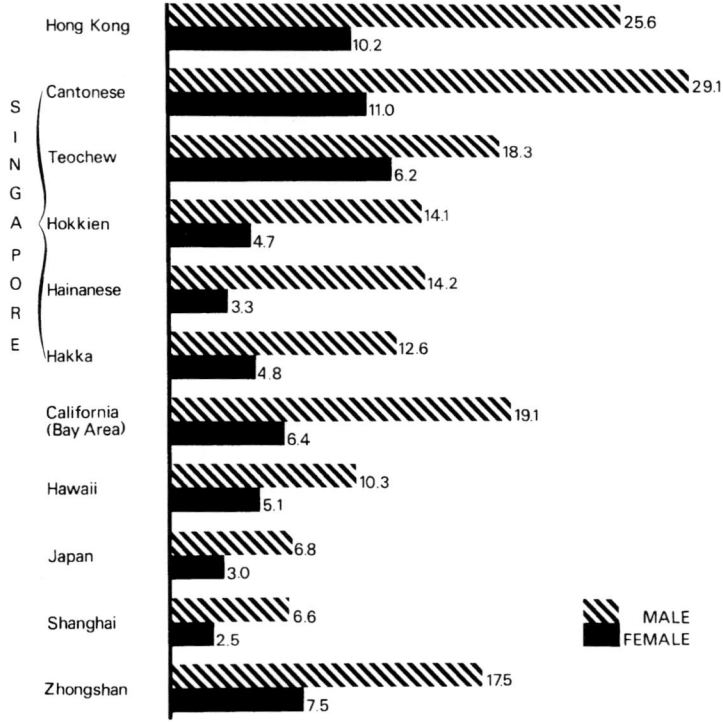

Fig. 7. Age-adjusted morbidity for NPC for selected Chinese populations, by sex (see the text). Figures for Zhongshan (Chungshan) county are mortality.

Table 4. Relative Frequency[a] of Nasopharyngeal Cancer in African and Asian Populations[b]

Population group	Cases M	Cases F	Relative frequency (%) M	Relative frequency (%) F	Population group	Cases M	Cases F	Relative frequency (%) M	Relative frequency (%) F
Malaysia					Vietnamese	105	58		
Chinese	150	77	11.5	6.0		163		3.7	
Malays	54	20	10.6	4.2	Algeria				
Indians	7	2	1.3	0.4	Algerians	364		5.0	
Thailand (Bangkok)					Europeans	83		3.5	
Chinese	27		15.9		Tunisia				
Chinese/Thai	20		10.3		Tunisians			6.7	2.9
Thais	29		4.6		Europeans			2.5	0.8
North Thais	34	19	3.7	2.1	Congo (Brazzaville)	1	0	0.4	0
(Chiang Mai)					Senegal (Dakar)	1	0	0.1	0
Sabah					Ivory Coast (Abidjan)	2	0	0.5	0
Chinese	9	0	8.9	0	Iraq (Baghdad)	73	—	1.3	—
Indigenous	11	3	9.2	3.4	Egypt (Alexandria)	26	—	1.3	—
Sarawak					Morocco	95	46	8.5	3.8
Chinese	6	5	4.8	3.8	Sudan	87	14	7.8	1.2
Malays	1	1	3.2	4.2	Zanzibar				
Dayaks	8	4	8.6	4.9	Negroes	1		0.4	
Java					Arabs	1		1.3	
Chinese	31	3	18.2	1.4	Mozambique	3	0	0.7	0
Javanese	108	44	10.3	2.9	(Lourenço Marques)				
Formosa	1260	446	23.2	5.2	Nigeria (Ibadan)	5	3	0.7	0.4
Filipinos (Philippines)	182		2.9		South Africa (Cape				
Filipinos (Hawaii)	8	0	2.5	0	Province: Coloureds)	4	1	0.5	0.1

[a] Relative frequency is taken here as the percentage of NPC among malignancies observed in the referred populations.
[b] For references, see Muir.[134]

gling cannot be excluded, although it is very rare in Japanese and probably infrequent in the populations of Korea,[195–196] Mongolia, and North China.[94] Ho[78] has clearly shown that the Macaonese in Hong Kong, the descendants of Portuguese settlers in Macao who intermarried with Chinese from Kwantung (Guangdong), have a much higher frequency of NPC than the rest of the non-Chinese population.

Clifford[19,20] has claimed that NPC is of high relative frequency among head and neck malignancies treated in Nairobi. However, Linsell[127] noted a more modest relative frequency of 2.3% in Kenya biopsy material in 1957–1961, this being greatest in the Kalenjin tribe (3.2%) and least in the coastal Bantu (0.2%). Computing crude incidence rates from Clifford's material, Muir[134] noted a maximum rate of 1.3 in male Nandi. This rate is not age-adjusted, and it is likely that there is considerable un-

derdiagnosis. Nevertheless, it is doubtful that the "true" age-adjusted rate would be greater than 5.

In Uganda, Schmauz and Templeton[153] noted a higher minimum age-adjusted incidence rate in Nilotics and para-Nilotics than in the Bantu–Sudanic groups. In general, the north of the country showed a higher incidence than did the south, despite the better hospital and transport systems in the south.

Relative-frequency studies from Algeria, Morocco, and Tunisia suggest a moderately elevated NPC level. In Tunisia, Zaouche[197] noted that in 23 months, 156 nasopharyngeal cancers were diagnosed at the Institut National de Cancérologie (Institut Salah Azaiz) in Tunis. If these cases are related to the entire Tunisian population, the crude minimum rates for males and females are 2.6 and 0.9, respectively. Since the period covered represents when the institute was begun, it is likely that there was gross underreporting.

In summary, the disease is very common in Southern Chinese, Eskimos, and native Greenlanders (an Eskimo population with admixture of Caucasian blood). The Chinese-mixed populations of Southeast Asia have a lower incidence rate. Rare in Japan and infrequent in north China, NPC is of moderate incidence in the Maghreb (Tunisia, Algeria, and Morocco), in Kuwait (Y.T. Omar, personal communication), in Sudan,[133] in northern parts of Kenya and Uganda, and in Israel, in the Israel-born, and in migrants from North Africa. Elsewhere, it is rare.

5.2. Epidemic Behavior

There have not been any reports of clustering in nasopharyngeal cancer. This does not preclude a part-viral etiology because, as with a varying and lengthy latent period, the cases resulting from an infectious process occurring every few years would be unlikely to appear in cyclical fashion.

5.3. Sex and Age

Most series show a male preponderance of around 2-fold.

The curves of age-specific incidence for nasopharyngeal cancer in Chinese populations in Hong Kong and Singapore are very similar in that they show a fairly steep rise from 20–24 years of age to about 50–54, with a fall thereafter.[82] This could be interpreted as representing a cessation of exposure at around 40 years of age, a cohort effect such as has been noted for breast cancer,[11] or the exhaustion of a pool of susceptibles.

The curve for NPC in Swedes is dissimilar in that the rise occurs two decades later and continues until age 70–74.[82] Bailar[8] noted that NPC tends to appear at an earlier age than most other forms of cancer in Caucasian populations. However, comparison of the age distribution of patients in areas where NPC is common and elsewhere is difficult because it is likely that each series contains some systemic malignant lymphomas that first presented in the nasopharyngeal region, and such neoplasms are proportionately much more common in low-incidence populations.[154,155,195]

Green et al.[63] point out that within the United States, nasopharyngeal cancer has three age peaks with racial and epidemiological differences held to reflect different etiologies. Under the age of 20, nasopharyngeal cancer incidence was 7 times higher in blacks than in whites, although these rates are based on small numbers. This trimodal age curve comprised a small peak under age 10 resulting from rhabdomyosarcoma of the nasopharynx in whites; a second mode at 15–24 due to NPC, more pronounced in blacks than in whites; and a third, larger peak in older adults, the rates being higher in blacks than in whites until middle life, and lower thereafter. However, these curves were quite overshadowed after the age of 25 by the rates among the United States Chinese.

It is of interest to note that in Tunisia, Kuwait, and the Sudan, the age curve appears to be bimodal, 20% of cases in the Sudan appearing before the age of 20 years.[16,152] In Constantine, Algeria,[117] the peak frequency was in the age group 15–24 with a 10-fold male excess. Here, 18% of neoplasms were seen below the age of 15.

5.4. Occupation

Analysis of mortality rates in males by occupation in Taiwan[126] revealed excess risks in those engaged in salt production, national defense, public service, and mining. The higher risk in salt workers and miners did not, of course, account for the overall high rate, and the higher rates in the other two groups could be due to the high proportion of mainlanders engaged in these occupations (see Fig. 7). The "boat people" of Hong Kong are largely fishermen, but fishermen elsewhere do not have a high risk of NPC. The bizarre finding of three cases of NPC in Canadian bush pilots could be due to chance.[5]

Henderson and co-workers' case–control study in the United States[65] showed that those occupationally exposed to fumes, smoke, and chemicals were at a higher risk. Within the United States, those areas with a high mortality from NPC were also prone to bladder cancer, a correlation that Fraumeni and Mason[54] hold to be consistent with the finding that British workers in leather and shoe factories are also more likely to have both nasal-cavity and bladder neoplasms.

5.5. Change of Risk on Migration

An environmental theory of causation would be much more convincing if it could be shown that groups not normally at high risk for NPC acquired such a risk after a sojourn in a high-incidence area, or if migrants from a high-incidence area were to lose their risk on moving to a low-incidence area. This is an oversimplification, since migrants often take much of their environment with them in the form of diet and culture.[153a,190]

Buell[13,14] reviewed California death certificates for 1955–1964 and found that 5 of 273 white male decendents with NPC were born in the Philippines or China, areas where the disease is endemic. The expected number, based on death certificates for other cancer deaths, was much less than 1. Analysis of name and birthplace of parents of the decendents showed that all were of Caucasian stock.

Fraumeni and Mason[54] noted that the mortality from NPC was 26-fold in Chinese males and 22-fold in Chinese females when compared to the black and white populations of the United States. During the study period, 1950–1969, there was, however, a diminution in risk. This decline could be due to changed food habits or other environmental factors or to an increase in the proportion of low-risk central and northern Chinese in the United States following 1945. Prior to this period, immigration was largely confined to high-risk southern Chinese. King and Haenszel[105] examined mortality among the foreign and native-born Chinese in the United States. There was an indication of a lower risk for Erdai (the United-States-born Chinese). However, Shanmugaratnam and Tye[157] have suggested that the rate is increased for Singapore-born Chinese, but this question is being reexamined using the most recent Singapore Cancer Registry data. Any rise in incidence among Indians and Pakistanis living in Singapore (see Fig. 1) would be of greatest interest, but this has not been observed.

5.6. Environmental Factors

Polunin[148] reviewed the ways of life of peoples with high risk of nasopharyngeal cancer and was unable to identify any single distinguishing feature. Indeed, Muir and Oakley[131] commented on the large differences in life style among Chinese, Malays, and Dayaks living in Sarawak (Borneo) who had, nevertheless, substantially the same frequency of the disease.

While there has been no lack of speculation and anecdote since the disease was first characterized, Shanmugaratnam and Higginson[156,158] were the first to conduct a retrospective survey on a group of patients with histologically proven primary NPC. This study was essentially negative. A further case–control study involving 379 Singapore Chinese patients with NPC, together with 595 patients with other ENT diseases and 1044 patients with diseases other than cancer or ENT disease, showed that NPC patients differed significantly from both groups of controls, in that they showed stronger associations for both personal and family history of nasal illnesses, the use of traditional Chinese medicines for the nose and throat, and exposure to smoke from antimosquito coils.[161] These latter exposures are not necessarily causal and could be interpreted as reflecting a more traditional household.

Armstrong et al.[6] noted that NPC risk in urban Chinese in Selangor, Malaysia, was elevated in those whose life style was based on a low socioeconomic status, eating few fresh foods, with little variety in meals, and living in old, poor-quality housing.

Ho[80,81,85,87,90,93,97] suggested that salted fish might be an etiological factor, being a traditional food commonly consumed by rich and poor southern Chinese from early childhood, especially those from Kwangtung (Guangdong), whether resident in China or abroad. An unusual dietary item in central and northern China, this salted fish contains appreciable quantities of nitrosodimethylamine.[52,53,96,173] The fact that NPC has been known to be common among southern Chinese for well over 50 years suggests the influence of a traditional rather than a modern environment.[90] Further, the factor is more likely to be ingested than inhaled, since in Hong Kong NPC is twice as common in "boat people" who live in boats and cook in the open than in land-dwellers mostly living in congested apartments.[80,90] The sharp rise in age-specific incidence after the age of 20–24 years suggests the importance in Chinese patients of early childhood.[90]

Since adults will not be able to recall diet in childhood, let alone infancy and weaning, such data have to be obtained by interview of mothers and older relatives of young patients. Thus, Anderson et al.[2] interviewed 24 Hong Kong Chinese NPC patients diagnosed before the age of 25 years. Most interviews took place in the homes where they were born, in the presence of older members of their families. The only foods eaten by all subjects, and worth consideration, were laap cheung (Cantonese pork sausage), salted fish, tau si (a black fermented product made of salted soya beans), and dried squid. Salted fish was the most common item and the only one fed to babies. In childhood, the NPC patients had rarely or never been fed vegetables or fruits. Most, since childhood, were stated to have been sickly, inactive, withdrawn, and choosy about their food. It was suggested that consumption of salted fish and vitamin C deficiency in early childhood could be important environmental factors and that a certain personality type may be associated with an increased risk. Furthermore, the study eliminated household inhalants and aerial contaminants as likely factors.

Geser et al.[61] undertook a case–control study of Chinese NPC patients admitted to the Queen Elizabeth Hospital, Hong Kong, the controls being inpatients with other cancers. Healthy members of the households of cases and controls were also interviewed to obtain information unbiased by the experience of having cancer. Positively associated with NPC were: belonging to the four lowest occupational classes, practicing Buddhism or ancestor worship, having religious altars in the house, and a history of previous illness of the ear or nose after the age of 15 years. Negatively associated factors included eating of bread and tinned food and the use of spices. Weaning habits were compared in the households of NPC patients and those of controls, by asking women who had ever breast fed a child about food supplements given to the baby during and immediately after weaning. Salted fish was given to babies just after weaning more often in households with an NPC case than in control households. Multivariate analysis showed that traditional life style, and the consumption of salted fish during weaning, were independent risk factors. This analysis also demonstrated that two, or three, of the many expressions of a traditional life style included in the study could account for the total increase in NPC risk associated with this way of life, although the authors concluded that it is quite possible that other factors, as yet unidentified, are just as important.

Lin et al.[126] in a case–control study in Taiwan,

noted that there was a significant excess of smokers among patients, the relative risk for persons smoking more than 20 cigarettes a day compared with those who had never smoked being greater than 2-fold. Working under poorly ventilated conditions was found to enhance risk, as did the use of herbal drugs and nasal balms or oils.

Clifford[20] suggested that the smoke and benzpyrene-containing soot so prominent in the huts of Kenyan groups with a raised frequency of the disease could be a causal factor, but the disease was found to be more common in males, who spend much less time in the huts.

Henderson et al.[65] undertook a case–control study on 156 patients and 267 controls in California, finding a highly significant increased relative risk (RR) of 1.8 for a prior history of ENT disease, occupational exposure to fumes (RR 2.0), smoke (RR 3.0), and chemicals (RR 2.4). In this study, over 50% were Chinese and most of the others whites. The white and Chinese patients were analyzed separately, the results being the same. This study is particularly valuable in that a group of patients with cancers elsewhere in the pharynx were also interviewed; unlike those with nasopharynx cancer, these showed clearly the effects of tobacco and alcohol. The history of previous ENT disease was common to both patients with cancer of the nasopharynx and elsewhere in the pharynx and is probably nonspecific. Exposure to fumes was most common in cooks among the Chinese, but studies in Singapore and Hong Kong have not shown such an association; among Chinese patients and controls, there was no significant difference in the current use of salted fish, but frequency of use was significantly greater in patients.[66]

EBV titers were not found to correlate with the risk factors cited above, i.e., prior ENT disease, occupational exposures, or American birthplace for either Chinese or white populations or for their controls. Birth or early childhood in the homeland was an important risk factor, particularly for patients diagnosed before the age of 50.

5.7. Genetic Factors

Descriptive epidemiology has established that persons of southern Chinese descent, no matter where they live, or Southeast Asian populations who have genetic similarities to southern Chinese, e.g., the Malays, are at high risk for this cancer. The disease is less common in north China and rare in the Japanese, who are also of north Mongoloid origin.

Familial aggregation of NPC cases takes place both in high-risk areas, as repeatedly stressed by Ho,[78,82,85,86] and in low-risk areas.[136,186]

Walshe,[180] in a review of the physical anthropology of races with a high incidence of nasopharyngeal cancer, suggested that in the absence of a single physical characteristic common to populations of those countries with a high incidence of the disease, and not found in others, the most profitable approach to the problem would be to concentrate on patients and controls. One approach was to study blood genetic markers (e.g., red cell antigens, red cell enzymes, HLA) to determine whether NPC patients had a characteristic genetic profile.[162]

Red cell blood group analyses were unrewarding,[64] but genetic studies involving 25 red cell enzymes and 5 serum protein systems indicated that NPC tends to concentrate on genetically distinct subpopulations of Chinese in Singapore.[106] More significant differences in human leukocyte antigen (HLA) types were found between Chinese NPC patients and controls. An HLA profile associated with increased risk of NPC consisted of an increase in the frequency of the first-locus antigen (HL-A2) and a deficit in the frequency of antigens detected at the second locus ("blank").[162] This blank was later demonstrated to represent a new HLA antigen named Sin-2,[163,164,165] now named BW46. The haplotype A2-B-Sin-2 was shown to carry an increased RR of 1.96.[166] When attention was directed to newly diagnosed cases, it was found that the haplotype AW 19-BW 17 was more frequently seen in NPC than in controls.[167] Among long-term survivors, BW 17 was found significantly decreased in frequency, as though this marker were associated with poor prognosis.[167]

Betuel *et al.*[10] have obtained evidence suggesting that the second-sublocus deficit is also seen among Tunisian NPC patients, but to a much lesser extent than in Chinese.

The high-risk HLA pattern is not present in all NPC patients, and conversely, such a pattern is present in some persons with no NPC. The most likely interpretation is that the HLA data reveal the existence of NPC-disease-susceptibility gene(s). A reasonable postulate[128] is that the putative disease-susceptibility genes function as immune-response genes.

5.8. Epidemiological Behavior of Epstein–Barr Virus

EBV infection is present in every population around the world, but age at primary infection seems to vary with socioeconomic level. There seems to exist a gradient of prevalence of infection in young children from cold to tropical countries.[51]

From data accumulated in experimental viral oncology, age at infection, dose and route of infection, and genetic susceptibility were known to be critical factors. It was therefore felt essential to have reliable data on the epithemiology of EBV in populations at different risk for EBV-related diseases (IM, BL, NPC). An international collaborative seroepidemiological study on EBV among Chinese (high risk for NPC, nil for IM and BL), Ugandans (high risk for BL, low for NPC, nil for IM), and Europeans (high risk for IM, low to nil for NPC and BL) took place in Hong Kong, Singapore, Uganda, and France.[36] In a first phase, volunteers from various sources were accepted: maternity and child clinics, army and police, university students, and others. Since such groups did not cover all age groups and did not represent the populations at large, randomly selected families were visited, interviewed, and bled.

The age at primary infection by EBV varies markedly among the groups studied. As seen in Fig. 8, in the 2–3 year age group, 97% of Ugandans were EBV-antibody positive, compared with only 20% of Singapore Chinese and 30% of Indians. Such differences tapered off at around 10 years of age, when 100% of Ugandans, 75% of Chinese, 85% of Indians, and 65% of Europeans were found to be EBV-antibody positive. An unexpected finding was that Hong Kong Chinese might have earlier EBV infection than Singapore Chinese (de-Thé *et al.*, unpublished data).

Ugandan children respond to EBV infection early in life by a strong humoral response. The geometric mean titers of VCA antibodies in the 1–5 year age group reached or passed 420 (Fig. 9). After this initial stress, Ugandan children populations show a dramatic fall of detectable EBV antibodies, possibly due to formation of antigen–antibody complexes or to loss of immunity.

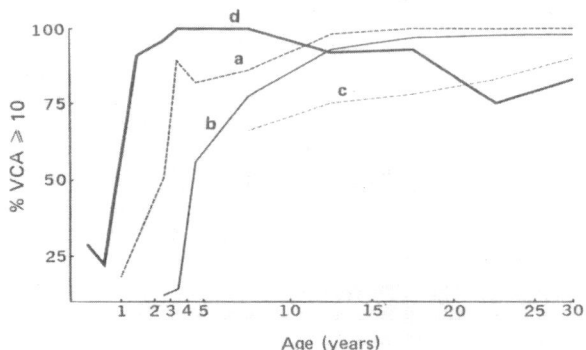

Fig. 8. Age-specific prevalence of antibodies to EBV VCA in Singapore Indians (a), Singapore Chinese (b), Caucasians (c), and Ugandans (d). Note the important difference between 1 and 5 years of age in these groups.

Indians in Singapore, who are at very low risk for NPC, BL, and IM, have the strongest immune response to EBV VCA.

The aforementioned differences in the infection rate and the immune response to EBV among ethnic groups and geographic areas may reflect cultural differences. They may also reflect a genetically dependent immune response to EBV antigens. The latter is an attractive hypothesis, since NPC has a strong genetic component (see above), and since genetics plays an important role in determining the susceptibility of animals to oncogenic viruses in general[123,124] and to herpesviruses in particular (Marek's disease).

6. Mechanism of Transmission

While primary EBV infection is probably transmitted through saliva, current serological and epidemiological evidence suggests that NPC is a con-sequence of reactivation, rather than a primary infection. The history of a higher frequency of upper respiratory infections in NPC patients than in controls, prior to tumor development, raises the possibility that some respiratory virus, occurring in adult life, might either reactivate EBV locally, or make epithelial cells permissive to EBV infection in genetically susceptible persons, or both. At present, EBV is known to infect only B lymphocytes, so some added factor, like a virus, or some environmental chemical, might be critical to permit the entry of EBV into epithelial cells. Future studies will determine whether the epithelial cells of the nasopharynx infected by EBV are normal, precancerous, or tumorous.

7. Pathogenesis

The evidence available thus far does not permit the conclusion that EBV alone is the cause of NPC.

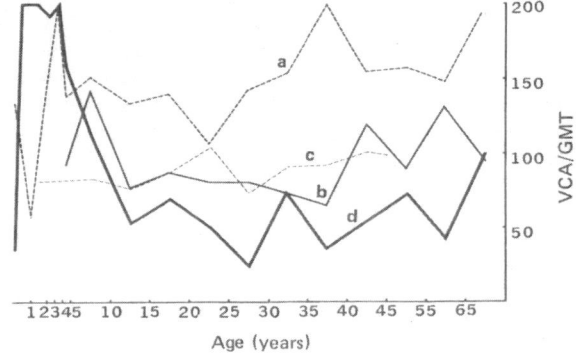

Fig. 9. Geometric mean antibody titers against EBV VCA in the different age and ethnic groups (ad identified in the Fig. 8 caption). Note that the Ugandans, after a very high peak between 1 and 3 years of age, become the lower responders, whereas the Indians exhibit a relatively stable and high humoral response against the virus.

While the various forms of serological reactivity to EBV in NPC patients can be interpreted as either cause or effect, the regular presence of EBV fingerprints in epithelial-tumor cells leaves no doubt that there is a strong link between the two. Evidence of close contacts and cytoplasmic bridges between epithelial and lymphoid cells both in normal nasopharyngeal mucosa and in NPC[56,179] might indicate a mode of intercelular interaction through which EBV might operate.

That chemical factors may play a part in the carcinogenesis has been suggested in the past by Clifford[22] and more recently by Ho.[86,87,90] The former author suspected benzpyrene in soot as a possible etiological agent of NPC among Kenyans, while the latter found carcinogenic nitrosamines in the salted fish fed during the weaning and postweaning periods in the case of southern Chinese. There are both epidemiological and experimental data in support of the latter hypothesis.[90]

8. Patterns of Host Response

8.1. Clinical Course of Nasopharyngeal Carcinoma

The clinical course of NPC varies widely in duration. Without any form of specific therapy or with only palliative or inadequate radiation therapy, the patient may live from a few months to 13 years from the date of diagnosis.[79,84]

The presenting symptoms depend on the location within the nasopharynx of the primary tumor, its tendency to invade neighboring structures, the direction of invasion, and its predilection to metastasize to regional lymph nodes. Thus, the signs and symptoms in order of frequency (see Table 5) are cervical nodal enlargement, nasal symptoms (obstruction, postnasal discharge, epistaxis), aural symptoms due to eustachian tubal obstruction (impairment of hearing of the conductive type, with or without tinnitus and serous otitis media), involvement of cranial nerves (V, especially its maxillary branch, VI, IX, X, XI, XII, and upper cervical sympathetics), persistent headache, and stiffness of the jaw due to lateral spread of the tumor to the pterygoid muscles. About one fifth of cases have more than one presenting symptom; their frequency distribution is shown in Table 5.

Table 5. Order of Frequency of Signs and Symptoms in Nasopharyngeal Carcinoma Patients: All Cases (513)

Presenting symptoms	Frequency	%
Nodal enlargement	288	43.31
Nasal	132	19.85
Aural	133	20.00
Pain	85	12.78
Cranial nerve impairment	20	3.01
Miscellaneous		
Hawking	4	0.60
Trismus	3	0.45
TOTALS:	665	100.00

8.2. Clinical Types of Disease

The biological behavior of the tumor determines the clinical types of the disease, which may be classified as (1) metastatic, (2) invasive, and (3) combined.[79]

8.2.1. Metastatic Type. The metastatic type, constituting about 33% of all cases, is characterized by the appearance of metastases, initially in the cervical lymph nodes (with the upper nodes involved before the lower) and later in distant organs, or, much less commonly, the two may appear about the same time, while the primary tumor apparently does not extend locally, remaining confined to the nasopharynx throughout. Only in exceptional cases, probably less than 0.1% of patients, have distant metastases been observed after a course of radiation therapy without cervical-nodal metastases being detected before the course or afterward. The spread may be confined to the cervical nodes for 1–3 years and in some for as long as 5 years or more.

Survival is longest with this type, and it is also with this variety that occasional patients are encountered in whom the tumor is apparently controlled for long periods, following what is normally considered as inadequate radiation therapy.

The common sites of distant metastases are the skeleton, especially the spine, liver, lung, and skin. The lymph nodes below the clavicles to as low as the femoral and inguinal nodes may be involved. Epidural and meningeal metastases occur, but metastases in the brain have not been encountered, although the brain is susceptible to direct invasion by the upward spread of the primary tumor or by adjacent meningeal metastases. The brain is believed to be devoid of a lymphatic system, but is nevertheless a common site of metastases from carcinomas of bronchus and breast. It is possible that NPC may be peculiar in that blood-borne metastases require the presence of lymphatics for their establishment.

8.2.2. Invasive Type. The invasive type occurs in only about 8% of all cases. There is evidence of direct spread to adjacent muscles, bones, cranial nerves, paranasal sinuses, the orbit, veins, and venous sinuses at the base of the skull. Cervical nodal metastases are either insignificant or not detected, even until the death of the patient. However, in some patients, hematogenous metastases occur, usually after intracranial spread has become evident. Presumably, these metastases are the result of tumor invasion of the basal venous sinuses that communicate with the internal jugular vein and perivertebral plexus of veins.

8.2.3. Combined Type. The combined type, constituting about 59% of all cases, is characterized by a combination of direct spread of the primary tumor and the appearance of cervical nodal metastases. These may occur at about the same time or one after the other, with varying intervals in between. What causes the change in behavior in the latter group is not known.

9. Control and Prevention

The treatment of NPC with localized disease or only regional spread is by megavoltage radiation therapy. Ho[90] has shown that for tumors clinically confined to the nasopharynx (stage I), prophylactic cervical lymph nodal irradiation does not confer improved survival or tumor-control prospects. Cervical irradiation should therefore be withheld until nodal metastasis becomes clinically evident. There may be a place for adjuvant chemotherapy following a course of regional radiation therapy for patients with cervical nodal involvement down to the supraclavicular fossae (stage IV), because over 50% of such patients showed clinical evidence of distant metastases within 18 months of the completion of a course of radiation therapy. Until the immune status (tumor-specific and EBV-specific) of NPC patients is better understood, immunotherapy is not recommended, although research in this direction must be encouraged.

The cumulative proportional actuarial survival and relapse-free survival after commencement of treatment by clinical stage according to Ho's classification[79] for Chinese patients treated by 4.5 MeV photons at Queen Elizabeth Hospital, Hong Kong, during 1969–1971 are shown in Fig. 10.

Prevention of NPC should concentrate on groups suspected from epidemiological studies to be at very high risk. These include first-degree relatives of NPC patients, especially those with more than one member of the family affected,[85,86] and possibly persons with an HLA profile to be characterized further. Apart from education of the general public to discontinue the practice of giving salted fish to babies (which will take a long time), groups at high risk should have their sera tested for EBV reactivities (especially IgA VCA), found to be a useful screening test for NPC.[92] Persons found to have elevated EBV serology should have a thorough clinical examination, including the radiological examination recommended by Ho,[78,83] initially and thereafter at yearly intervals or more frequently when there are suggestive symptoms. However, negative clinical and radiological evidence of a tumor does not exclude NPC. Multiple biopsy of the nasopharynx should be done in the presence of a positive serological EBV IgA VCA test and repeated subsequently when the titer rises.

Education of the public, as well as the medical profession, on the early signals of the disease is essential in high-risk populations. The lack of awareness of these signals has been the cause of unnecessary delay in seeking medical advice on the part of the patient and in early diagnosis by the profession. A painless lump high up in the neck in an adult southern Chinese should be considered as due to NPC until proved otherwise. This is as much an aphorism for NPC as a lump in the breast in a female over 40 years is for breast carcinoma.

If inspection of the lateral pharyngeal recesses (fossa of Rosenmüller) by the use of a Yankauer speculum were routinely employed in examination, fewer tumors would be considered occult. In the mainly submucosal primary tumors, the earliest detectable sign is a hemorrhagic finely granular or velvety patch, which can be missed if only the postnasal mirror is used. Exfoliative cytology, using a saline-soaked swab rubbed against different areas of the mucosa and dropped into a test tube of saline, which is later passed through a Millipore filter membrane for collection of cells that are then fixed and stained *in situ*, has been found by Ho (unpublished

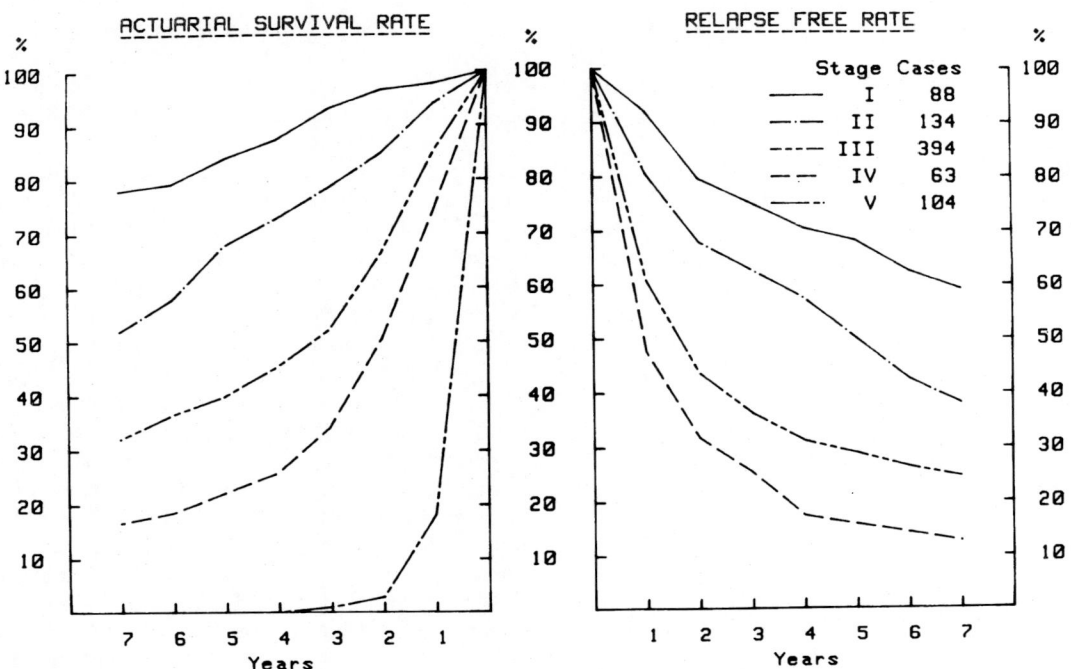

Fig. 10. Actuarial survival rate and relapse-free rate for Chinese NPC patients from Hong Kong by stage according to Ho's classification[79] and year after commencement of treatment.

data) to detect "occult" carcinomatous areas. These were subsequently confirmed by tissue biopsy.

10. Unresolved Problems and Projects for the Future

Three main avenues remain to be followed in the understanding of the etiology of this disease. The first is continued assessment of the role of the virus so closely associated with the tumor. The second is to clarify further the place of the life style and that of chemical and other environmental factors associated with this cancer. The third is to define better the genetic components responsible for susceptibility or resistance to the disease.

10.1. Role of Epstein–Barr Virus in the Management and Control of Nasopharyngeal Carcinoma

There are so many questions that one would like to see answered concerning the role of EBV in NPC pathogenesis that it would be senseless to discuss all of them. Replication of EBV takes place in the ororhinopharynx, as shown by the presence of EBV in saliva, but the nature of the replicating cells at the time of primary infection and in disease process is unclear, even if the epithelial cells of the nasopharynx mucosa are prime candidates. The claim of Lemon et al.[118] that EBV replicates in epithelial cells has not yet been confirmed, and study of the immunovirological events in the ororhinopharynx in normal and diseased subjects is a matter of urgency. The factors that govern the reactivation of the latent EBV infection would be another important theme of research, since such knowledge should help in the development of new therapy and in the prevention of EBV-associated diseases including NPC.

The control of NPC is a major public health problem in south China and in large parts of Southeast Asia.[35] To achieve early detection, our colleagues from the Peoples Republic of China have conducted a mass seroepidemiological survey in the adult population of the autonomous region of the Guang-Si province. In testing 56,000 normal subjects aged 30 years or more for the presence of high IgA antibodies to VCA, they showed that NPC could be detected very early with this technique.[199] Expanding their surveys, they have detected among IgA carriers some lesions of the nasopharynx that they consider as premalignant (Zeng Yi, personal communication). The investigation of these premalignant lesions from the virological and immunological points of view should clarify the role of EBV and open new avenues for prevention.[35]

That high IgA antibodies to VCA could long precede the clinical onset of NPC was suggested by the results of Ho et al.,[92] who observed that 3–5 years prior to tumor onset, three NPC patients already had IgA VCA titers ranging from 20 to 320. It is hoped that the Chinese mass surveys will be used to conduct a prospective study, aimed at assessing the kinetics of IgA immediately preceding NPC. The assessment of EBV serology and especially of IgA antibodies to VCA and EA as a tool for clinical management of NPC (diagnosis and prognosis) is under way.

Can an EBV vaccine be contemplated for NPC?[39a,76] Live vaccine, using turkey herpesvirus, has been found very efficient in preventing Marek's disease.[18] Laufs[116] has demonstrated that a killed vaccine for *Herpesvirus saimiri* (HVS) can prevent HVS-induced lymphomas in cotton-top marmosets. The major problem with EBV and NPC is that it would be most difficult to propose to vaccinate everyone prior to primary infection, i.e., in the first years of life, since one would have to wait for 40–50 years to evaluate the effect. The only practical possibility would be to investigate the immune status (both humoral and cell-mediated immunity) prior to clinical onset. If the reactivation of a latent EBV infection were the precipitating event leading to tumor development, then a specific immunointervention might represent a real possibility of preventing the disease.

Antiviral chemotherapy, a meager possibility at present, might become a developing field in the coming decade and help in the control of NPC.

10.2. Chemical and Environmental Factors in the Causation of Nasopharyngeal Carcinoma

The salted-fish hypothesis needs to be further assessed, by both experimental and epidemiological means. In a recent review, Henderson and Louie,[66] listing the risk factors, concluded that the salted-fish hypothesis was worth pursuing. Comparative investigation of the consumption of salted fish in the young age groups and NPC incidence should be carried out in different populations of Southeast Asia. It is doubtful, however, that the salt-fish-at-weaning hypothesis could be tested by case–control study of NPC patients, since recollection would be very poor.

Further work also needs to be done on the exposure to dust and fumes in terms of presence of carcinogens and nasopharyngeal physiology. It is curious that while several investigators have implicated cigarette smoking, generally in Caucasian populations, Taiwan excepted, this risk factor has not been found in Chinese.

10.3. Genetic Markers and Nasopharyngeal Carcinoma

The specificity of the constitutional type delineated by Anderson et al.[2] needs to be determined together with the possibility for this type of person of having a particular HLA profile.

Future studies will have to identify HLA profiles associated with NPC in geographic areas having intermediate and low risk for the disease. The main goal of immediate interest among Chinese patients will be to identify genotypes related to NPC in the *Ia* and locus *D* regions of chromosome 6, preferably by studying families having multiple cases of NPC.

10.4. Conclusion

NPC is among the very few human tumors in which genetic, environmental, chemical, and viral factors are involved. The understanding of the interplay among these sets of factors should yield fundamental knowledge on cancer causation, pathogenesis, and prevention, the latter being our final goal.

ACKNOWLEDGMENTS

Financial help from the Hong Kong Anti-Cancer Society, the World Health Foundation (Hong Kong), and the Cancer Research Institute Inc. (New York) is acknowledged.

11. References

1. ALI, M. Y., AND SHANMUGARATNAM, K., Cytodiagnosis of nasopharyngeal carcinoma, *Acta Cytol.* **11**:51–60 (1967).
2. ANDERSON, E. N., JR., ANDERSON, M. L., AND HO, J. H. C., A study of the environmental backgrounds of young Chinese nasopharyngeal carcinoma patients, in: *Nasopharyngeal Carcinoma: Etiology and Control* (G. DE-THÉ AND Y. ITO, eds.), pp. 231–239, IARC Scientific Publication No. 20, IARC, Lyon, France, 1978.
3. ANDERSSON-ANVRET, M., FORSBY, N., KLEIN, G., AND HENLE, W., Studies on the occurrence of Epstein–Barr virus DNA in nasopharyngeal carcinomas in comparison with tumors of other head and neck regions, *Int. J. Cancer* **20**:702–707 (1977).
4. ANDERSSON-ANVRET, M., FORSBY, N., KLEIN, G., AND HENLE, W., The association between undifferentiated nasopharyngeal carcinoma and Epstein–Barr virus shown by correlated nucleic acid hybridization and histopathological studies, in: *Nasopharyngeal Carcinoma: Etiology and Control* (G. DE-THÉ AND Y. ITO, eds.), pp. 347–358, IARC Scientific Publication No. 20, IARC, Lyon, France, 1978.
5. ANDREWS, P. A. I., AND MICHAELS, I., Nasopharyngeal carcinoma in Canadian bush pilots, and aviator's cancer, *Lancet* **2**:85, 640 (1968).
6. ARMSTRONG, R. W., KANNAN-KUTTY, M., AND ARMSTRONG, M. J., Self-specific environments associated with nasopharyngeal carcinoma in Selangor, Malaysia, *Soc. Sci. Med.* **12**:149–156 (1978).
7. AYA, T., AND OSATO, T., Early events in transformation of human cord leukocytes by Epstein–Barr virus: Induction of DNA synthesis, mitosis and the virus associated nuclear antigen synthesis, *Int. J. Cancer* **14**:341–347 (1974).
8. BAILAR, J. C., III, Race, environment and family in the epidemiology of cancer of the nasopharynx, in: *Cancer of the Nasopharynx* (C. S. MUIR AND K. SHANMUGARATNAM, eds.), pp. 101–105, UICC Monograph Series, Vol. 1, Munksgaard, Copenhagen, 1967.
9. BENYESH-MELNICK, M., FERNBARCH, D. J., AND LEWIS, R. T., Studies on human leukemia. I. Spontaneous lymphoblastoid transformation of fibroblastic bone marrow cultures derived from leukemic and non-leukemic children, *J. Natl. Cancer Inst.* **31**:1311–1331 (1963).
10. BETUEL, H., CAMMOUN, M., COLOMBANI, J., DAY, N. E., ELLOUZ, R., AND DE-THÉ, G., The relationship between nasopharyngeal carcinoma and the HL-A system among Tunisians, *Int. J. Cancer* **16**:249–254 (1975).
11. BJARNASON, O., DAY, N., SNAEDAL, G., AND TULINIUS, H., The effect of year on the breast cancer age incidence curve in Iceland, *Int. J. Cancer* **13**:689–696 (1974).
12. BLOT, W. J., LANIER, A., AND FRAUMENI, J. F., JR., Cancer mortaliy among Alaskan natives 1960–1969, *J. Natl. Cancer Inst.* **55**:547–554 (1975).
13. BUELL, P., Nasopharyngeal cancer in Chinese of California, *Br. J. Cancer* **19**:459–470 (1965).
14. BUELL, P., Race and place in the etiology of nasopharyngeal cancer: A study based on California death certificates, *Int. J. Cancer* **11**:268–272 (1973).
15. BURKITT, D. P., The trail to a virus, in: *Oncogenesis and Herpesviruses* (P. M. BIGGS, G. DE-THÉ, AND L. N. PAYNE, eds.), pp. 345–348, IARC Scientific Publication No. 2, Lyon, France, 1972.
16. CAMMOUN, M., VOGT-HOERNER, G., ANd MOURALI, N., Les tumeurs du naso-pharynx en Tunisie: Étude anatomo-clinique de 143 observations, *Tunis Med.* **49(3)**:131–141 (1971).
17. CHAN, S. H., CHEW, T. S., GOH, E. H., SIMONS, M. J., AND SHANMUGARATNAM, K., Impaired general cell-mediated immune functions *in vivo* and *in vitro* in patients with nasopharyngeal carcinoma, *Int. J. Cancer* **18(2)**:139–144, (1976).
18. CHURCHILL, A. E., PAYNE, L. N., AND CHUBB, R. C., Immunization against Marek's disease using a live attenuated virus, *Nature (London)* **221**:744–747 (1969).
19. CLIFFORD, P., Carcinoma of the nasopharynx in Kenya, *East Afr. Med. J.* **42**:373–396 (1965).
20. CLIFFORD, P., Malignant diseases of the nasopharynx and paranasal sinuses in Kenya, in: *Cancer of the Nasopharynx* (C. S. MUIR AND K. SHANMUGARATNAM, eds.), pp. 82–94, UICC Monograph Series, Vol. 1, Munksgaard, Copenhagen, 1967.
21. CLIFFORD, P., A review on the epidemiology of nasopharyngeal carcinoma, *Int. J. Cancer* **5**:287–309 (1970).
22. CLIFFORD, P., Carcinogens in the nose and throat: Nasopharyngeal carcinoma in Kenya, *Proc. R. Soc. Med.* **65**:682–686 (1972).
23. DERRY, D. E., Anatomical report (B), in: *Archaeological Survey of Nubia, Cairo, Egyptian Ministry of Finance* (Bulletin No. 3), pp. 40–42, 1909.
24. DE SCHRYVER, A., FRIBERG, S., JR., KLEIN, G., HENLE, W., HENLE, G., DE-THÉ, G., CLIFFORD, P., AND HO, H. C., Epstein–Barr associated antibody patterns in carcinoma of the post-nasal space, *Clin. Exp. Immunol.* **5**:443–459 (1969).
25. DE SCHRYVER, A., KLEIN, G., HENLE, G., HENLE, W., CAMERON, H., SANTESSON, L., AND CLIFFORD, P., Epstein–Barr virus associated serology in malignant disease: Antibody levels to viral capsid antigens (VCA), membrane antigens (MA) and early antigens (EA) in patients with various neoplastic conditions, *Int. J. Cancer* **9**:353–364 (1972).
26. DESGRANGES, C., WOLF, H., DE-THÉ, G., SHANMUGARATNAM, K., ELLOUZ, R., CAMMOUN, N., KLEIN, G., AND ZUR HAUSEN, H., Nasopharyngeal carcinoma X—

Presence of Epstein–Barr genomes in epithelial cells of tumours from high and medium risk areas, *Int. J. Cancer* **16**:7–15 (1975).

27. DESGRANGES, C., DE-THÉ, G., HO, J. H. C., AND EL-LOUZ, R., Neutralizing EBV-specific IgA in throat washings of nasopharyngeal carcinoma (NPC) patients, *Int. J. Cancer* **19**:627–633 (1977).

28. DESGRANGES, C., LI, J. Y., AND DE-THÉ, G., EBV specific secretory IgA in saliva of NPC patients: Presence of secretory piece in epithelial malignant cells, *Int. J. Cancer* **20**:881–886 (1977).

29. DESGRANGES, C., AND DE-THÉ, G., Presence of Epstein–Barr virus specific IgA in saliva of nasopharyngeal carcinoma patients: Their activity, origin, and possible clinical value, in: *Nasopharyngeal Carcinoma: Etiology and Control* (G. DE-THÉ AND Y. ITO, eds.), pp. 459–469, IARC Scientific Publication No. 20, IARC, Lyon, France, 1978.

30. DE-THÉ, G., AMBROSIONI, J. C., HO, H. C., AND KWAN, H. C., Lymphoblastoid transformation and presence of herpes-types viral particles in a Chinese nasopharyngeal tumour cultured *in vitro*, *Nature (London)* **221**:770–771 (1969).

31. DE-THÉ, G., HO, H. C., KWAN, H. C., DESGRANGES, C., AND FAVRE, M. C., Nasopharyngeal carcinoma (NPC). I. Types of cultures derived from tumour biopsies and non-tumorous tissues of Chinese patients with special reference to lymphoblastoid transformation, *Int. J. Cancer* **6**:189–206 (1970).

32. DE-THÉ, G., GESER, A., DAY, N. E., TUKEI, P. M., WILLIAMS, E. H., BERI, D. P., SMITH, P. G., DEAN A. G., BORNKAMM, G. W., FEORINO, R., AND HENLE, W., Epidemiological evidence for causal relationship between Epstein-Barr virus and Burkitt's lymphoma from Ugandan prospective study, *Nature* **274**:756–761 (1978).

33. DE-THÉ, G., SOHIER, R., HO, J. H. C., AND FREUND, R., Nasopharyngeal carcinoma. IV. Evolution of complement fixing antibodies during the course of the disease, *Int. J. Cancer* **12**:368–377 (1973).

34. DE-THÉ, G., ABLASHI, D. V., LIABEUF, A., AND MOURALI, N., Nasopharyngeal carcinoma (NPC). VI. Presence of an EBV nuclear antigen in fresh tumour biopsies: Preliminary results, *Biomedicine* **19**:349–352 (1973).

35. DE-THÉ, G., DESGRANGES, C., ZENG, Y., WANG, P. C., BORNKAMM, G. W., ZHU, J. S. AND SHANG, M., Search for pre-cancerous lesions and EBV markers in the Nasopharynx of IgA positive individuals, in: *Nasopharyngeal Carcinoma*, Cancer Campaign, Vol. 5, (Grundmann, E., Krueger, G. R. F., Ablash, D. V., eds.), pp. 111–117, Gustav Fisher Verlag, Stuttgart, 1981.

36. DE-THÉ, G., DAY, N. E., GESER, A., HO, J. H. C., LAVOUE, M. F., SIMONS, M. J., SOHIER, R., AND TUKEI, P., Epidemiology of the Epstein–Barr virus: Prelimi-

nary analysis of an international study, in: *Oncogenesis and Herpesviruses II* (G. DE-THÉ, M. A. EPSTEIN, AND H. ZUR HAUSEN, eds.), pp. 3–16, IARC Scientific Publication No. 11, Vol. 2, IARC, Lyon, France, 1975.

37. DE-THÉ, G., HO, J. H. C., ABLASHI, D. V., DAY, N. E., MACARIO, A. J. L., MARTIN-BERTHELON, M. C., PEARSON, G., AND SOHIER, R., Nasopharyngeal carcinoma. IX. Antibodies to EBNA and correlation with response to other EBV antigens in Chinese patients, *Int. J. Cancer* **16**:713–721 (1975).

38. DE-THÉ, G., VUILLAUME, M., GIOVANELLA, B. C., AND KLEIN, G., Epithelial characteristics of tumour cells in nasopharyngeal carcinoma (NPC) passaged in nude mice—an ultrastructural study, *J. Natl. Cancer Inst.* **57**:1101–1105 (1976).

39. DE-THÉ, G., Is Burkitt's lymphoma (BL) related to a perinatal infection by Epstein–Barr virus?, *Lancet* **1**:335–338 (1977).

39a. DE-THÉ, G., Epstein–Barr virus: Is it time to discuss a vaccine? *Biomed. Comm.* **28**:15–17 (1978).

40. DE-THÉ, G., LAVOUÉ, M.-F., AND MUENZ, L., Differences in EBV antibody titres of patients with nasopharyngeal carcinoma originating from high, intermediate and low incidence areas, in: *Nasopharyngeal Carcinoma: Etiology and Control* (G. DE-THÉ AND Y. ITO, eds.), pp. 471–481, IARC Scientific Publication No. 20, IARC, Lyon, France, 1978.

41. DE-THÉ, G., The epidemiology of Burkitt's lymphoma: Evidence for a causal association with Epstein–Barr virus—a review, *Am. J. Epidemiol.* **1**:32–57 (1979).

42. DE-THÉ, G., The role of the Epstein–Barr virus in human diseases: Infectious mononucleosis (IM), Burkitt's lymphoma (BL), nasopharyngeal carcinoma (NPC), in: *Viral Oncology* (G. KLEIN, ed.), Raven Press, New York, 1979 (in press).

42a. DE-THÉ, G., Multistep carcinogenesis, Epstein–Barr virus and human malignancies, in: *Viruses in Naturally Occurring Cancers* (M. ESSEX, G. TODARO, H. ZUR HAUSEN, eds.), pp. 11–21, Cold Spring Harbor Conferences on Cell Proliferation, Vol. 7, Cold Spring Harbor Laboratory Publ., Cold Spring Harbor, New York, 1980.

43. DIGBY, K. H., THOMAS, G. H., AND HSIU, S. T., Notes on carcinoma of the nasopharynx, *Caduceus* **9**:45–64 (1930).

44. DOBSON, W. C., Cervical lymphosarcoma (letter to the editor), *Chin. Med. J.* **38**:786 (1924).

45. DOLL, R., Epidemiology of cancer: Current perspectives, *Am. J. Epidemiol.* **104**:396–408 (1976).

46. DURAND-FARDEL, Cancer du pharynx—ossification dans la substance musculaire du coeur, *Bull. Soc. Anat. (Paris)* **12**:73–80 (1837).

47. EPSTEIN, M. A., ACHONG, B. G., AND BARR, Y. M., Virus particles in cultured lymphoblasts from Burkitt's lymphoma, *Lancet* **1**:702–703 (1964).

48. EPSTEIN, M. A., AND ACHONG, B. G., Recent progress in EB virus research, *Annu. Rev. Microbiol.* (1977).

49. EVANS, A. S., AND NIEDERMAN, J. C., Epidemiology of infectious mononucleosis, in: *Oncogenesis and Herpesviruses* (P. M. BIGGS, G. DE-THÉ, AND L. N. PAYNE, eds.), pp. 351–356, IARC Scientific Publications No. 2, Lyon, France, 1972.

50. EVANS, A. S., The history of infectious mononucleosis, *Am. J. Med. Sci.* **267**:189 (1974).

51. EVANS, A. S., New discoveries in infectious mononucleosis, *Mod. Med.* **1**:18–24 (1974).

52. FONG, Y. Y., AND WALSH, E. O., Carcinogenic nitrosamines in Cantonese salt-dried fish, *Lancet* **1**:1032 (1971).

53. FONG, Y. Y., AND CHAN, W. C., Bacterial production of di-methyl nitrosamine in salted fish, *Nature (London)* **243**:421–422 (1973).

54. FRAUMENI, J. F., JR., AND MASON, T. J., Cancer mortality among Chinese Americans, 1950–69, *J. Natl. Cancer Inst.* **52**:659–665 (1974).

55. GALLO, R. C., SAXINGER, W. C., GALLAGHER, R. E., GILLESPIE, D. A., AULAKH, G. S., AND WO NG-STAAL, F., Some ideas on the origin of leukemia in man and recent evidence for the presence of type-C viral related information, in: *Origins of Human Cancer* (H. HIATT, J. D. WATSON, AND J. A. WINSTEN, eds.), pp. 1253–1285, Cold Spring Harbor Conferences on Cell Proliferation, Vol. 4, Book B, Cold Spring Harbor Publ., Cold Spring Harbor, New York, 1977.

56. GAZZOLO, L., DE-THÉ, G., AND VUILLAUME, M., Nasopharyngeal carcinoma. II. Ultrastructure of normal mucosa, tumor biopsies and subsequent epithelial growth *in vitro*, *J. Natl. Cancer Inst.* **48**:73–86 (1972).

57. GERBER, P., AND BIRCH, S., Complement-fixing antibodies in sera of human and non-human primates to viral antigens derived from Burkitt's lymphoma cells, *Proc. Natl. Acad. Sci. U.S.A.* **58**:478–484 (1967).

58. GERBER, P., WHANG-PENG, J., AND MONROE, J., Transformation and chromosome changes induced by Epstein–Barr virus in normal human leukocyte cultures, *Proc. Natl. Acad. Sci. U.S.A.* **63**:740–747 (1969).

59. GERBER, P., NONOYAMA, M., LUCAS, S., PERLIN, E., AND GOLDSTEIN, L., Oral excretion of EBV by healthy subjects and patients with infectious mononucleosis, *Lancet* **2**:988–989 (1972).

60. GESER, A., DAY, N. E., DE-THÉ, G., CHEW, T. S., FREUND, R. J., KWAN, H. C., LAVOUÉ,, M. F., SIMKOVIC, D., AND SOHIER, R., The variability in immunofluorescent viral capsid antigen antibody testing in population surveys of Epstein–Barr virus infection, *Bull WHO* **50**:389–400 (1974).

61. GESER, A., CHARNAY, N., DAY, N. E., DE-THÉ, G., AND HO, H. C., Environmental factors in the etiology of nasopharyngeal carcinoma: Report on a case–control study in Hong Kong, in: *Nasopharyngeal Carcinoma: Etiology and Control* (G. DE-THÉ AND Y. ITO, eds.), pp.

213–229, IARC Scientific Publication No. 20, Lyon, France, 1978.

62. GLASER, R., DE-THÉ, G., LENOIR, G., AND HO, J. H. C., Superinfection of nasopharyngeal carcinoma epithelial tumour cells with Epstein–Barr virus, *Proc. Natl. Acad. Sci. U.S.A.* **73**:960–963 (1976).

63. GREEN, M. H., FRAUMENI, J. F., JR., AND HOOVER, R., Nasopharyngeal cancer among youngs in United States: Racial variations by cell type, *J. Natl. Cancer Inst.* **58**:1267–1270 (1977).

64. HAWKINS, B. R., SIMONS, M. J., GOH, E. H., CHIA, K. B., AND SHANMUGARATNAM, K., Immunogenetic aspects of nasopharyngeal carcinoma. II. Analysis of ABO, Rhesus and MNS's red cell systems, *Int. J. Cancer* **13**:116–121 (1974).

65. HENDERSON, B. E., LOUIE, E., JING, J. S. H., BUELL, P., AND GARDNER, M. B., Risk factors associated with nasopharyngeal carcinoma, *N. Engl. J. Med.* **295**: 1101–1106 (1976).

66. HENDERSON, B. E., AND LOUIE, E., Discussion of risk factors for nasopharyngeal carcinoma, in: *Nasopharyngeal Carcinoma: Etiology and Control* (G. DE-THÉ AND Y. ITO, eds.), pp. 251–260, IARC Scientific Publication No. 20, Lyon, France, 1978.

67. HENLE, G., AND HENLE, W., Immunofluorescence in cells derived from Burkitt's lymphoma, *J. Bacteriol.* **91**:1248–1256 (1966).

68. HENLE, W., HENLE, G., BURTIN, P., CACHIN, Y., CLIFFORD, P., DE SCHRYVER, A., DE-THÉ, G., DIEHL, V., HO, H. C., AND KLEIN, G., Antibodies to Epstein–Barr virus in nasopharyngeal carcinoma, other head and neck neoplasms and control groups, *J. Natl. Cancer Inst.* **44**:225–231 (1970).

69. HENLE, W., HENLE, G., ZAJAC, B. A., PEARSON, G., WAUBKE, R., AND SCRIBA, M., Differential reactivity of human serums with early antigens induced by Epstein–Barr virus, *Science* **169**:188–190 (1970).

70. HENLE, G., HENLE, W., AND KLEIN, G., Demonstration of two distinct components in the early antigen complex of EBV infected cells, *Int. J. Cancer* **8**:272–282 (1971).

71. HENLE, G., Antibodies to EBV-induced early antigens in infectious mononucleosis, Burkitt's lymphoma and nasopharyngeal carcinoma, in: *Recent Advances in Human Tumor Virology and Immunology* (W. NAKAHARA, K. NISHIOKA, T. HIRAYAMA, AND T. ITO, eds.), pp. 343–359, University of Tokyo Press, Tokyo, 1971.

72. HENLE, W., AND HENLE, G., Epstein–Barr virus: The cause of infectious mononucleosis, in: *Oncogenesis and Herpesviruses* (P. M. BIGGS, G. DE-THÉ, AND L. N. PAYNE, eds.), pp. 358–370, IARC Scientific Publication No. 2, Lyon, France, 1972.

73. HENLE, W., AND HENLE, G., Epstein–Barr virus and infectious mononucleosis, *N. Engl. J. Med.* **288**:263–264 (1973).

74. HENLE, W., HO, H. C., AND KWAN, H. C., Antibodies

to Epstein–Barr virus related antigens in nasopharyngeal carcinoma: Comparison of active cases with long term survivors, *J. Natl. Cancer Inst.* **51**:361–369 (1973).

75. HENLE, G., AND HENLE, W. Epstein–Barr virus-specific IgA serum antibodies as an outstanding feature of nasopharyngeal carcinoma, *Int. J. Cancer* **17**:1–7 (1976).

76. HIGGINSON, J., DE-THÉ, G., GESER, A., AND DAY, N. E., An epidemiological analysis of cancer vaccines, *Int. J. Cancer* **7**:565–574 (1971).

77. HIGGINSON, J., AND MACLENNAN, R., The world pattern of cancer incidence, in: *Modern Trends in Oncology—Research Progress* (R. W. RAVEN, ed.), pp. 9–27, Butterworths, London, 1973.

78. HO, H. C., Nasopharyngeal carcinoma in Hong Kong, in: *Cancer of the Nasopharynx* (C. S. MUIR AND K. SHANMUGARATNAM, eds.), pp. 58–63, UICC Monograph Series, Vol. 1, Munksgaard, Copenhagen, 1967.

79. HO, J. H. C., The natural history and treatment of nasopharyngeal carcinoma (NPC), in: *Oncology*, Vol. 4 (Proceedings of the 10th International Cancer Congress) (R. LEE-CLARK, R. W. CUMLEY, J. E. McCAY, AND M. COPELAND, eds.). pp. 1–14, Year Book Medical Publishers, Chicago, 1970.

80. HO, H. C., Incidence of nasopharyngeal cancer in Hong Kong, UICC Bulletin, *Cancer* **9(2)**:5 (1971).

81. HO, J. H. C., Genetic and environmental factors in nasopharyngeal carcinoma, in: *Recent Advances in Human Tumor Virology and Immunology* (Proceedings of the First International Cancer Symposium of the Princess Takamatsu Cancer Research Fund) (W. NAKAHARA, K. NISHIOKA, T. HIRAYAMA, AND Y. ITO, eds.), pp. 275–295, University of Tokyo Press, Tokyo, 1971.

82. HO, J. H. C., Nasopharyngeal carcinoma (NPC), in: *Advances in Cancer Research* (G. KLEIN, S. WEINHOUSE, AND A. HADDOW, eds.), pp. 57–92, Academic Press, New York and London, 1972.

83. HO, H. C., Radiologic diagnosis of nasopharyngeal carcinoma with special reference to its spread through the base of skull, in: *Cancer of the Nasopharynx* (C. S. MUIR AND K. SHANMUGARATNAM, eds.), pp. 238–246, UICC Monograph Series, Vol. 1, Medical Examination Publishing Co., New York, 1972.

84. HO, H. C., Head and neck—Radiologic diagnosis, *J. Am. Med. Assoc.* **220**:396 (1972).

85. HO, H. C., Current knowledge of the epidemiology of nasopharyngeal carcinoma—A review, in: *Oncogenesis and Herpesviruses* (P. M. BIGGS, G. DE-THÉ, AND L. N. PAYNE, eds.), pp. 357–366, IARC Scientific Publication No. 2, Lyon, France, 1972.

86. HO, H. C., Epidemiology of nasopharyngeal carcinoma (NPC), in: *Proceedings of the 1st Asian Cancer Conference*, Shima and Tokyo, September 22–25, 1973.

87. HO, H. C., Epidemiology of nasopharyngeal carcinoma, *J. R. Coll. Surg. Edinburgh* **20**:223–235 (1975).

88. HO, J. H. C., NG, M. H., KWAN, H. C., AND CHAN, J. C. W., Epstein–Barr virus-specific IgA and IgG serum antibodies in nasopharyngeal carcinoma, *Br. J. Cancer* **34**:655–660 (1976).

89. HO, H. C., NG, M. H., AND KWAN, H. C., IgA antibodies to Epstein–Barr viral capsid antigens in saliva of nasopharyngeal carcinoma patients, *Br. J. Cancer* **35**:888–890 (1977).

90. HO, J. H. C., An epidemiologic and clinical study of nasopharyngeal carcinoma, *Int. J. Radiat. Oncol. Biol. Phys.* **4**:181–198 (1978).

91. HO, H. C., KWAN, H. C., AND NG, M. H., Immunohistochemistry of local immunoglobulin production in nasopharyngeal carcinoma, *Br. J. Cancer* **37**:514–519 (1978).

92. HO, H. C., KWAN, H. C., NG, M. H., AND DE-THÉ, G., Serum IgA antibodies to Epstein–Barr virus capsid antigen preceding symptoms of nasopharyngeal carcinoma, *Lancet* **1**:436–437 (1978).

93. HO, J. H. C., HUANG, D. P., AND FONG, Y. Y., Salted fish and nasopharyngeal carcinoma in southern Chinese, Lancet **1**:626 (1978).

94. HU, C. H., AND YANG, C., A decade of progress in morphologic pathology, *Chin. Med. J.* **79**:409–422 (1959).

95. HUANG, D. P., HO, J. H. C., HENLE, W., AND HENLE, G., Demonstration of Epstein–Barr virus-associated nuclear antigen in nasopharyngeal carcinoma cells from fresh biopsies, *Int. J. Cancer* **14**:580–588 (1974).

96. HUANG, D. P., GOUGH, T., AND HO, J. H. C., Analysis for volatile nitrosamines of salt-preserved foodstuffs traditionally consumed by southern Chinese, in: *Nasopharyngeal Carcinoma: Etiology and Control* (G. DE-THÉ AND Y. ITO, eds.), pp. 309–314, IARC Scientific Publication No. 20, IARC, Lyon, France, 1978.

97. HUANG, D. P., SAW, D., TEOH, T. B., AND HO, J. H. C., Carcinomas in rats fed with Cantonese salted marine fish, in: *Nasopharyngeal Carcinoma: Etiology and Control* (G. DE-THÉ AND Y. ITO, eds.), pp. 315–328, IARC Scientific Publication No. 20, IARC, Lyon, France, 1978.

98. HUEBNER, R. J., AND TODARO, G. T., Oncogenesis of RNA tumor viruses as determinants of cancer, *Proc. Natl. Acad. Sci. U.S.A.* **64**:1087–1–94 (1969).

99. INTERNATIONAL AGENCY FOR RESEARCH ON CANCER (IARC), *Cancer Incidence in Five Continents*, Vol. III (J. WATERHOUSE, C. S. MUIR, P. CORREA, AND G. POWELL, eds.), IARC Scientific Publication No. 15, Lyon, France, 1976.

100. INTERNATIONAL AGENCY FOR RESEARCH ON CANCER (IARC), *Nasopharyngeal Carcinoma: Etiology and Control* (G. DE-THÉ AND Y. ITO, eds.), IARC Scientific Publication No. 20, Lyon, France, 1978.

101. INTERNATIONAL AGENCY FOR RESEARCH ON CANCER

(IARC), Annual Report, pp. 75–76, IARC, Lyon, France, 1978.

102. INTERNATIONAL UNION AGAINST CANCER [UNION INTERNATIONAL CONTRE LE CANCER (UICC)], *Cancer of the Nasopharynx*, Monograph Series, Vol. 1 (C. S. MUIR AND K. SHANMUGARATNAM, eds.), Munksgaard, Copenhagen, 1967.

103. JONDAL, M., AND KLEIN, G., Classification of lymphocytes in nasopharyngeal carcinoma (NPC) biopsies, *Biomedicine* **23**:163–165 (1975).

104. JUNG, P. F., AND YU, C., Nasopharyngeal cancer in China, *Postgrad. Med.* **33**:A77–A82 (1963).

105. KING, H., AND HAENSZEL, K., Cancer mortality among foreign and native-born Chinese in the United States, *J. Chron. Dis.* **26**:623–646 (1972).

106. KIRK, R. L., BLAKE, N. M., SERJEANTSON, S., SIMONS, M. J., AND CHAN, S. H., Genetic components in susceptibility to nasopharyngeal carcinoma, in: *Nasopharyngeal Carcinoma: Etiology and Control* (G. DE-THÉ AND Y. ITO, eds.), pp. 283–297, IARC Scientific Publication No. 20, IARC, Lyon, France, 1978.

107. KLEIN, G., CLIFFORD, P., KLEIN, E., AND STJERNSWÄRD, J., Search for tumor-specific immune reactions in Burkitt lymphoma patients by the membrane immunofluorescence reaction, *Proc. Natl. Acad. Sci. U.S.A.* **55**:1628–1635 (1966).

108. KLEIN, G., PEARSON, G., HENLE, G., HENLE, W., DIEHL, V., AND NIEDERMAN, J. C., Relation between Epstein–Barr viral and cell membrane immunofluorescence in Burkitt tumour cells. I. Dependence of cell membrane immunofluorescence on presence of EB virus, *J. Exp. Med.* **128**:1011–1020 (1968).

109. KLEIN, G., EBV associated membrane antigens, in: *Oncogenesis and Herpesviruses* (P. M. BIGGS, G. DE-THÉ, AND L. N. PAYNE, eds.), pp. 295–301, IARC Scientific Publication No. 2, Lyon, France, 1972.

110. KLEIN, G., The Epstein–Barr virus, in: *The Herpesviruses* (A. KAPLAN, ed.), pp. 521–555, Academic Press, New York, 1973.

111. KLEIN, G., GIOVANELLA, B. C., LINDAHL, T., FIALKOW, P. J., SINGH, S., AND STEHLIN, J., Direct evidence for the presence of Epstein–Barr virus DNA and nuclear antigen in malignant epithelial cells from patients with anaplastic carcinoma of the nasopharynx, *Proc. Natl. Acad. Sci. U.S.A.* **71**:4737–4741 (1974).

112. KLEIN, G., AND VONKA, V., Relationship between the Epstein–Barr virus (EBV) determined complement fixing antigen and the nuclear antigen (EBNA) detected by anti-complement fluorescence, *Int. J. Cancer* **53**:1645–1646 (1974).

113. KLEIN, G., *Viral Oncology*, Raven Press, New York, 1979.

114. KMET, J., AND MAHBOUBI, E., Esophageal cancer in the Gaspian littoral of Iran: Initial studies, *Science* **175**:846–853 (1972).

115. KROGMAN, W. M., The skeletal and dental pathology of an early Iranian site, *Bull. Hist. Med.* **8**:28–48 (1940).

116. LAUFS, R., Immunisation of marmoset monkeys with a killed oncogenic herpesvirus, *Nature (London)* **249**:571–572 (1974).

117. LEMAIGRE, G., DIEBOLD, J., TEMMIM, L., ARSENIEV, L., LECHARPENTIER, Y., ALLOUACHE, A., DELAITRE, B., AND ABELANET, R., Carcinome du nasopharynx chez les sujets jeunes—Étude clinique, anatomique et ultrastructurale de 50 cas observés dans l'est algérien, *Nouv. Presse Med.* **6**:3509–3513 (1977).

118. LEMON, S. M., HUTT, L. M., SHAW, J., LI, J. L., AND PAGANO, J., Replication of EBV in epithelial cells during infectious mononucleosis, *Nature (London)* **268**:268–270 (1977).

119. LENOIR, G., MARTIN-BERTHELON, M. C., FAVRE, M. C., AND DE-THÉ, G., Characterization of EBV antigens. I. Biochemical analysis of the complement-fixing soluble antigen and relationship with EBNA, *J. Virol.* **17**:672–674 (1976).

120. LEVINE, P., CHO, B., CONNELLY, R., DE VITA, C., BERARD, C., O'CONOR, G., AND DORHMAN, R., The American Burkitt's lymphoma registry: A progress report, *Ann. Intern. Med.* **83**:82–83 (1975).

121. LEVINE, P. H., DE-THÉ, G., BRUGERE, J., SCHWAAB, G., MOURALI, N., HEBERMAN, R. B., AMBROSIONI, J. C., AND REVOL, P., Immunity to antigens associated with a cell line derived from nasopharyngeal carcinoma (NPC) in non-Chinese NPC patients, *Int. J. Cancer* **17**:155–160 (1976).

122. LIANG, P. C., Studies on nasopharyngeal carcinoma in the Chinese: Statistical and laboratory investigations, *Chin. Med. J.* **83**:373–390 (1964).

123. LILLY, F., The inheritance of susceptibility of the Gross leukemia virus in mice, *Genetics* **53**:529–539 (1966).

124. LILLY, F., Mouse leukemia: A model of a multiplegene disease *J. Natl. Cancer Inst.* **49**:927–934 (1972).

125. LIN, T. M., HSU, M. M., CHENG, K. P., CHIANG, T. C., JUNG, P. F., AND HIRAYAMA, T., Morbidity and mortality of cancer of the nasopharynx in Taiwan, *Gann Monogr.* **10**:137–144 (1971).

126. LIN, T. M., CHEN, K. P., LIN, C. C., HSU, M. M., TU, S. M., CHIANG, T. C., JUNG, P. F., AND HIRAYAMA, T., Retrospective study on nasopharyngeal carcinoma, *J. Natl. Cancer Inst.* **51**:1403–1408 (1975).

127. LINSELL, C. A., Cancer in Kenya, in: *Cancer in Africa* (P. CLIFFORD, C. A. LINSELL, AND G. L. TIMMS, eds.), pp. 7–12, East African Publishing House, Nairobi, 1968.

128. MCDEVITT, H. O., AND BODMER, W. J., HL-A, immune response genes, and disease: Occasional survey, *Lancet* **1**:1269–1275 (1974).

129. MICHAUX, L., Carcinome de base du crâne, Cited by GODTFREDSON, E., Ophthalmologic and neurologic symptoms of malignant nasopharyngeal tumours:

Clinical study comprising 454 cases, with special reference to histo-pathology and possibility of earlier recognition, *Acta Psychiatr. Scand. Suppl.* **34**:1–323 (1944).

130. MILLER, G., NIEDERMAN, J. C., AND STILL, D. A., Infectious mononucleosis: Appearance of neutralizing antibody to Epstein–Barr virus measured by inhibition of formation of lymphoblastoid cell lines, *J. Infect. Dis.* **125**:403–406 (1972).

131. MUIR, C. S., AND OAKLEY, W. F., Nasopharyngeal carcinoma in Sarawak (Borneo), *J. Laryngol.* **81**:197–207 (1967).

132. MUIR, C. S., AND SHANMUGARATNAM, K., The incidence of nasopharyngeal cancer in Singapore, in: *Cancer of the Nasopharynx* (C. S. MUIR AND K. SHANMUGARATNAM, eds.), pp. 47–53, UICC Monograph Series, No. 1, Munksgaard, Copenhagen, 1967.

133. MUIR, C. S., Nasopharyngeal carcinoma in non-Chinese populations with special reference to South East Asia and Africa, *Int. J. Cancer* **8**:351–363 (1971).

134. MUIR, C. S., Nasopharyngeal carcinoma in non-Chinese populations, in: *Oncogenesis and Herpesviruses* (P. M. BIGGS, G. DE-THÉ, AND L. N. PAYNE, eds.), pp. 367–371, IARC Scientific Publication No. 2, Lyon, France, 1972.

135. MUIR, C. S., Geographical differences in cancer patterns, in: *Host Environment Interactions in the Etiology of Cancer in Men* (R. DOLL AND I. VODOPIJA, eds.), pp. 1–13, IARC Scientific Publication No. 7, IARC, Lyon, France, 1973.

136. NEVO, S., MEYER, W., AND ALTMAN, M., Carcinoma of nasopharynx in twins, *Cancer* **28**:807–809 (1971).

137. NIEDERMAN, J. C., AND EVANS, A. S., Infectious mononucleosis, in: *Serological Epidemiology*, pp. 119–132, Academic Press, New York, 1973.

138. NIELSEN, N. H., MIKKELSEN, F., AND HART-HANSEN, J. P., Nasopharyngeal cancer in Greenland: Incidence in an arctic Eskimo population, *Acta Pathol. Microbiol. Scand. Sect. A* **85**:850–858 (1977).

139. NILSSON, K., KLEIN, G., HENLE, G., AND HENLE, W., The role of EBV in the establishment of lymphoblastoid cell lines from adult and foetal lymphoid tissue, in: *Oncogenesis and Herpesviruses* (P. M. BIGGS, G. DE-THÉ, AND L. N. PAYNE, eds.), pp. 285–290, IARC Scientific Publication No. 2, Lyon, France, 1972.

140. NONOYAMA, M., AND PAGANO, J. S., Homology between Epstein–Barr viruses DNA and viral DNA from Burkitt's lymphoma and nasopharyngeal carcinoma determined by DNA–DNA reassociation kinetics, *Nature (London)* **242**:44–47 (1973).

141. O'CONOR, G. T., Persistent immunological stimulation as a factor in oncogenesis with special reference to Burkitt's tumour, *Am. J. Med.* **48**:279–285 (1970).

142. OLD, L. J., BOYSE, E. A., OETTGEN, H. F., DE HARVEN, E., GEERING, G., WILLIAMSON, E., AND CLIFFORD, P., Precipitation antibody in human serum to an antigen present in cultured Burkitt's lymphoma cells, *Proc. Natl. Acad. Sci. U.S.A.* **56**:1699–1704 (1966).

143. PAGANO, J. S., HUANG, C. H., AND LEVINE, P., Absence of Epstein–Barr viral DNA in American Burkitt's lymphoma, *N. Engl. J. Med.* **289**:1395–1399 (1973).

144. PAGANO, J. S., HUANG, C. H., KLEIN, G., DE-THÉ, G., SHANMUGARATNAM, K., SIMONS, M. J., AND YAN, C. S., Homology of Epstein–Barr viral DNA in nasopharyngeal carcinoma from Kenya, Taiwan, Singapore and Tunis, in: *Oncogenesis and Herpesviruses II* (G. DE-THÉ, M. A. EPSTEIN, AND H. ZUR HAUSEN, eds.), pp. 191–193, IARC Scientific Publication No. 11, Vol. 2, IARC, Lyon, France, 1975.

145. PEARSON, G. R., COATES, H. L., NEEDL, H. B., LEVINE, P., ABLASHI, D., AND EASTON, J., Clinical evaluation of EBV serology in American patients with nasopharyngeal carcinoma, in: *Nasopharyngeal Carcinoma: Etiology and Control* (G. DE-THÉ AND Y. ITO, eds.), pp. 439–448, IARC Scientific Publication No. 20, Lyon, France, 1978.

146. PEREIRA, M. S., FIELD, A. M., BLAKE, J. M., RODGERS, F. G., AND BAILEY, L. A., Evidence for oral excretion of EB virus in infectious mononucleosis, *Lancet* **1**:710–711 (1972).

147. PETO, R., Epidemiology, multistage models, and short-term mutagenicity tests, in: *Origins of Human Cancer* (H. HIATT, J. D. WATSON, AND J. A. WINSTEN, eds.), pp. 1403–1428, Cold Spring Harbor Conferences on Cell Proliferation, Vol. 4, Book C, Cold Spring Harbor Laboratory Publ., Cold Spring Harbor, New York, 1977.

148. POLUNIN, I., The ways of life of people with high rates of nasopharyngeal carcinoma, in: *Cancer of the Nasopharynx* (C. S. MUIR AND K. SHANMUGARATNAM, eds.), pp. 106–111, IUCC Monograph Series, Vol. 1, Munksgaard, Copenhagen, 1967.

149. REEDMAN, B. M., POPE, J. H., AND MOSS, D. J., Identity of the soluble EBV associated antigens of human lymphoid cell lines, *Int. J. Cancer* **9**:172–181 (1972).

150. REEDMAN, B. M., AND KLEIN, G., Cellular localization of an Epstein–Barr virus (EBV) associated complement-fixing antigen in producer and nonproducer lymphoblastoid cell lines, *Int. J. Cancer* **11**:499–520 (1973).

151. REEDMAN, B. M., KLEIN, G., POPE, J. H., WALTERS, M. K., HILGERS, J., SMITH, S., AND JOHANSSON, B., Epstein–Barr virus associated complement fixing and nuclear antigens in Burkitt's lymphoma biopsies, *Int. J. Cancer* **13**:755–763 (1974).

152. SAAD, A., Observations on nasopharyngeal carcinoma in the Sudan, in: *Cancer in Africa* (C. A. LINSELL AND G. L. LIMMS, eds.), pp. 281–285, East African Publishing House, Nairobi, 1968.

153. SCHMAUZ, R., AND TEMPLETON, A. C., Nasopharyngeal cancer in Uganda, *Cancer* **29**:610–621 (1972).

153a. SCOTT, G. C., AND ATKINSON, L., Demographic features of the Chinese population in Australia and the relative prevalence of nasopharyngeal cancer among Caucasians and Chinese, in: *Cancer of the Nasopharynx* (C. S. MUIR AND K. SHANMUGARATNAM, eds.), pp. 64–72, UICC Monograph Series, Vol. 1, Munksgaard, Copenhagen, 1967.

154. SHANMUGARATNAM, K., Nasopharyngeal carcinoma in Asia, in: *Racial and Geographical Factors in Tumour Incidence* (A. A. SHIVAS, ed.), pp. 169–188, Pfizer Medical Monograph, Vol. 2, Edinburgh University Press, Edinburgh, 1967.

155. SHANMUGARATNAM, K., AND MUIR, C. S., Nasopharyngeal carcinoma: Origin and structure, in: *Cancer of the Nasopharynx* (C. S. MUIR AND K. SHANMUGARATNAM, eds.), pp. 153–162, UICC Monograph Series, Vol. 1, Munksgaard, Copenhagen, 1967.

156. SHANMUGARATNAM, K., AND HIGGINSON, J., Aetiology of nasopharyngeal carcinoma: Report on a retrospective survey in Singapore, in: *Cancer of the Nasopharynx* (C. S. MUIR AND K. SHANMUGARATNAM, eds.), pp. 130–137, UICC Monograph Series, Vol. 1, Munksgaard, Copenhagen, 1967.

157. SHANMUGARATNAM, K., AND TYE, C. Y., A study of nasopharyngeal cancer among Singapore Chinese with special reference to migrant status and specific community (dialect group), *J. Chron. Dis.* **23**:433–441 (1970).

158. SHANMUGARATNAM, K., Studies on the etiology of nasopharyngeal carcinoma, *Int. Rev. Exp. Pathol.* **10**:361–413 (1971).

159. SHANMUGARATNAM, K., Cancer in Singapore—Ethnic and dialect group variations in cancer incidence, *Singapore Med. J.* **14**:68–81 (1973).

160. SHANMUGARATNAM, K., AND WEE, A., "Dialect group" variations in cancer incidence among Chinese in Singapore, in: *Host Environment Interaction in the Etiology of Cancer in Humans* (R. DOLL AND I. BODOPIJA, eds.), pp. 67–82, IARC Scientific Publication No. 7, Lyon, France, 1973.

161. SHANMUGARATNAM, K., TYE, C. Y., GOH, E. H., AND CHIA, K. B., Etiological factors in nasopharyngeal carcinoma: A hospital-based, retrospective case–control questionnaire study, in: *Nasopharyngeal Carcinoma: Etiology and Control* (G. DE-THÉ AND Y. ITO, eds.), pp. 199–212, IARD Scientific Publication No. 20, Lyon, France, 1978.

162. SIMONS, M. J., WEE, G. B., DAY, N. E., DE-THÉ, G., MORRIS, P. J., AND SHANMUGARATNAM, K., Immunogenetic aspects of nasopharyngeal carcinoma. I. Differences in HL-A antigen profiles between patients and comparison groups, *Int. J. Cancer* **13**:122–134 (1974).

163. SIMONS, M. J., DAY, N. E., WEE, G. B., SHANMUGARATNAM, K., HO, H. C., WONG, S. H., TI, T. K., YONG, N. K., DARMALINGAM, S., AND DE-THÉ, G., Nasopharyngeal carcinoma. V. Immunogenetic studies of South East Asian ethnic groups with high and low risk for the tumor, *Cancer Res.* **34**:1192–1195 (1974).

164. SIMONS, M. J., WEE, G. B., DAY, N. E., CHAN, S. H., SHANMUGARATNAM, K., AND DE-THÉ, G., Immunogenetic aspects of nasopharyngeal carcinoma (NPC). IV. Probable identification of an HL-A second antigen associated with a high risk for NPC, *Lancet* **1**:142–143 (1975).

165. SIMONS, M. J., DAY, N. E., WEE, G. B., CHAN, S. H., SHANMUGARATNAM, K., AND DE-THÉ, G., Immunogenetic aspects of nasopharyngeal carcinoma (NPC). III. HL-A type as a genetic marker of NPC predisposition to test the hypothesis that EBV is an aetiologic factor in NPC, in: *Oncogenesis and Herpesviruses II* (G. DE-THÉ, M. A. EPSTEIN, AND H. ZUR HAUSEN, eds.), pp. 249–258, IARC Scientific Publication No. 11, Vol. 2, IARC, Lyon, France, 1975.

166. SIMONS, M. J., WEE, G. B., GOH, E. H., CHAN, S. H., SHANMUGARATNAM, K., DAY, N. E., AND DE-THÉ, G., Immunogenetic aspects of nasopharyngeal carcinoma. IV. Increased risk in Chinese of nasopharyngeal carcinoma associated with a Chinese-related HLA profile (A2, Singapore 2), *J. Natl. Cancer Inst.* **57**:977–980 (1976).

167. SIMONS, M. J., CHAN, S. H., WEE, G. B., SHANMUGARATNAM, K., GOH, E. H., HO, J. H. C., CHAU, J. C. W., DARMALINGAM, S., PRASAD, U., BETUEL, H., DAY, N. E., AND DE-THÉ, G., Nasopharyngeal carcinoma and histocompatibility antigens, in: *Nasopharyngeal Carcinoma: Etiology and Control* (G. DE-THÉ AND Y. ITO, eds.), pp. 271–282, IARC Scientific Publication No. 20, IARC, Lyon, France, 1978.

168. SMITH, G. E., AND DAWSON, W. R., in: *Egyptian Mummies*, p. 157, Allen and Unwin, London, 1924.

169. SOHIER, R., AND DE-THÉ, G., Fixation du complément avec un antigène soluble: Différences d'activité importantes entre les sérums de lymphoma de Burkitt, de cancer du rhinopharynx et de mononucléose infectieuse, *C. R. Acad. Sci.* **273**:121–124 (1971).

170. SOHIER, R., AND DE-THÉ, G., Evolution of complement-fixing antibody titers with the development of Burkitt's lymphoma, *Int. J. Cancer* **9**:524–528 (1972).

171. SVOBODA, D. J., KIRCHNER, K. R., AND SHANMUGARATNAM, K., Ultrastructure of nasopharyngeal carcinomas in American and Chinese patients: An application of electron microscopy to geographic pathology, *Exp. Mol. Pathol.* **4**:189–204 (1965).

172. SVOBODA, D. J., KIRCHNER, K. R., AND SHANMUGARATNAM, K., The fine structure of nasopharyngeal carcinoma, in: *Cancer of the Nasopharynx* (C. S. MUIR AND K. SHANMUGARATNAM, eds.), pp. 163–171, UICC Mon-

ograph Series, Vol. 1, Munksgaard, Copenhagen, 1967.

173. TERRACINI, B., MAGEE, P. N., AND BARNES, J. M., Hepatic pathology on low dietary levels of dimethylnitrosamine, *Br. J. Cancer* **21**:599–565 (1967).

174. TRUMPER, P. A., EPSTEIN, M. A., GIOVANELLA, G. C., AND FINERTY, S., Isolation of infectious EB virus from epithelial tumor cells of nasopharyngeal carcinoma, *Int. J. Cancer* **20**:655–662 (1977).

175. UNION INTERNATIONAL CONTRE LE CANCER, *Cancer Incidence in Five Continents—Technical Report* (R. DOLL, P. PAYNE, AND J. WATERHOUSE, eds.), UICC, Geneva, 1966.

176. UNION INTERNATIONAL CONTRE LE CANCER, *Cancer Incidence in Five Continents*, Vol. 2 (R. DOLL, C. MUIR, AND J. WATERHOUSE, eds.), UICC, Geneva, 1970.

177. VONKA, V., BENYESH-MELNICK, M., LEWIS, R. T., AND WIMBERLY, I., Some properties of the soluble (S) antigen of cultured lymphoblastoid cell lines, *Arch. Gesamte Virusforsch.* **31**:113–124 (1970).

178. VONKA, V., VLCHOVA, I., ZAVADOVA, H., KOUBA, K., LASOVSKA, J., AND DUBEN, J., Antibodies to EB virus capsid antigen and to soluble antigen of lymphoblastoid cell in infectious mononucleosis patients, *Int. J. Cancer* **9**:529–535 (1972).

179. VUILLAUME, M., AND DE-THÉ, G., Nasopharyngeal carcinoma. III. Ultrastructure of different growths leading to lymphoblastoid transformation *in vitro*, *J. Natl. Cancer Inst.* **51**:67–80 (1973).

180. WALSHE, R. J., The physical anthropology of races with a high incidence of nasopharyngeal cancer, in: *Cancer of the Nasopharynx* (C. S. MUIR AND K. SHANMUGARATNAM, eds.), pp. 112–118, UICC Monograph Series, Vol. 1, Munksgaard, Copenhagen, 1967.

181. WALTERS, M. K., AND POPE, J. H., Studies of the EB virus-related antigens of human leukocyte cell lines, *Int. J. Cancer* **8**:32–40 (1971).

182. WARA, W. M., WARA, D. W., PHILLIPS, T. L., AND AMMAHH, A., Elevated IgA in carcinoma of the nasopharynx, *Cancer* **35**:1313–1315 (1975).

183. WELLS, C., Ancient Egyptian pathology, *J. Laryngol.* **77**:261–265 (1963).

184. WELLS, C., Two mediaeval cases of malignant disease, *Br. Med. J.* **1**:1611–1612 (1964).

185. WILLIAMS, E. H., DAY, N. E., AND GESER, A., Seasonal variation in onset of Burkitt's lymphoma in the West Nile district of Uganda, *Lancet* **2**:19–22 (1974).

186. WILLIAMS, E. H., AND DE-THÉ, G., Familial aggregation in nasopharyngeal carcinoma (letter to the editor), *Lancet* **2**:295 (1974).

187. WOLF, H., ZUR HAUSEN, H., AND BECKER, V., EB viral genomes in epithelial nasopharyngeal carcinoma cells, *Nature (London) New Biol.* **244**:245–257 (1973).

188. WORLD HEALTH ORGANIZATION, *Mortality from Malignant Neoplasms 1955–1965*, Geneva, 1970.

189. WORLD HEALTH ORGANIZATION (WHO), *Histological Typing of Upper Respiratory Tract Tumours: International Classification of Tumours*, No. 19 (K. SHANMUGARATNAM AND L. H. SOBIN, eds.), 1978.

190. WORTH, R. M., AND VALENTINE, R., Nasopharyngeal carcinoma in New South Wales, Australia, in: *Cancer of the Nasopharynx* (C. S. MUIR AND K. SHANMUGARATNAM, eds.), pp. 73–76, UICC Monograph Series, Vol. 1, Munksgaard, Copenhagen, 1967.

191. WU, C. H. (ed.), *The Encyclopaedia of Chinese Medical Terms*, Vol. 1, p. 756, Commercial Press, Shanghai, 1921 (in Chinese).

192. YATA, J., DESGRANGES, C., DE-THÉ, G., AND TACHIBANA, T., Lymphocytes in infectious mononucleosis: Properties of atypical cells and origin of the lymphoblastoid lines, *Biomedicine* **19**:479–483 (1973).

193. YATA, J., DESGRANGES, C., NAKAGAWA, T., FAVRE, M. C., AND DE-THÉ, G., Lymphoblastoid transformation and kinetics in the appearance of Epstein–Barr viral nuclear antigen (EBNA) in cord blood B cells by Epstein–Barr virus infection, *Int. J. Cancer* **15**:377–384 (1975).

194. YATA, J., DESGRANGES, C., DE-THÉ, G., AND TACHIBANA, T., Nasopharyngeal carcinoma. VII. Lymphocyte subpopulations in the blood and tumour tissue, *Biomedicine* **21**:244–250 (1974).

195. YEH, S., Histology of nasopharyngeal cancer, in: *Cancer of the Nasopharynx* (C. S. MUIR AND K. SHANMUGARATNAM, eds.), pp. 147–152, UICC Monograph Series, Vol. 1, Munksgaard, Copenhagen, 1967.

196. YUN, I. S., A statistical study of tumours among Koreans, *Cancer Res.* **9**:370–371 (1949).

197. ZAOUCHE, A., Les tumeurs malignes de la sphère ORL en Tunisie: A propos des 644 tumeurs des voies aerodigestives superieures à l'Institut National de Carcinologie de Tunis due 1.10.67 au 15.8.69, Thesis, Paris, 1970.

198. ZUR HAUSEN, H., SCHULTE-HOLTHAUSEN, H., KLEIN, G., HENLE, W., HENLE, G., CLIFFORD, P., AND SANTESSON, L., EBV DNA in biopsies of Burkitt tumours and anaplastic carcinomas of the nasopharynx, *Nature (London)* **228**:1056–1058 (1970).

199. ZENG Y., LIU Y. X., LIU C. R., CHEN S. W., WEI J. N., ZHU J. N., AND ZAI H. J., Application of immunoenzymatic method and immunoautoradiographic method for the mass survey of nasopharyngeal carcinoma, *Intervirology* **133**:166–168 (1980).

200. ZENG, Y., SHANG, M. AND LIU, C. R., Detection of anti Epstein–Barr virus IgA in NPC patients in 8 provinces and cities in China, *Chinese Oncology* **1–2** (1979).

201. ZENG, Y., SHEN, S., PI, G., MA, J. L., ZHANG, Q., ZHAO, M. G., AND DONG, H. J., Application of anticomplement immunoenzymatic method for the detection of EBNA in carcinoma cells and normal epithelial cells from the nasopharynx, in: *Nasopharyngeal*

Carcinoma, Cancer Campaign, Vol. 5, (GZUNDMAN, E., KZUEGER, G., ZUNDMAN, E., KZUEGER, G. R. F., AND ABLASHI, D. B., eds.), Gustav Fischer Verlag, Stuttgart, 1981.

12. Suggested Reading

DE-THÉ, G., The Chinese epidemiological approach of nasopharyngeal carcinoma research and control, *The Yale J. Biol. Med.* **54**:33–39 (1981).

DE-THÉ, G. Epidemiology of Epstein–Barr virus and associated diseases in man, in: *Herpesviruses, Vol. 1,* (B. ROIZMAN, ed.), Plenum Press, New York, 1982, in press.

DE-THÉ, G. AND YTO, X., eds., *Nasopharyngeal Carcinoma: Etiology and Control.* IARC Scientific Publication No. 20, IARC, Lyon, France, 1978.

GZUNDMAN, E., KZUEGER, G., ZUNDMAN, E., KZUEGER, G. R. F., AND ABLASHI, D. V., eds. *Nasopharyngeal Carcinoma*, Cancer Campaign, Vol. 5, Gustav Fischer Verlag, Stuttgart, 1981.

MUIR, C. S. Nasopharyngeal carcinoma in non Chinese populations with special reference to South East Asia and Africa, *Int. J. Cancer*, **8**:351–363 (1971).

MUIR, C. S., AND SHANMUGARATNAM, K., eds., *Cancer of the Nasopharynx*, UICC Monograph Series, No. 1, Munksgaard, Copenhagen, 1967.

CHAPTER 26

Cervical Cancer

André J. Nahmias, William E. Josey,
and James M. Oleske

1. Introduction

Carcinoma of the uterine cervix is one of the most
common cancers in women in the United States and
throughout the world. Because of its frequency and
accessibility to methods of early detection, cervical
cancer is among the most thoroughly studied of all
human malignant diseases. Its natural history has
been extensively investigated, and the gradation
from intraepithelial neoplastic cervical changes
(dysplasia and carcinoma *in situ*) to invasive carcinoma has been well documented. Although such
progression of the disease does not appear to be an
inevitable process, ample evidence has accumulated
to indicate that when invasive cancer occurs, it is
practically always preceded by a preinvasive phase
in its development.

The intraepithelial and early invasive stages of
cervical cancer are infrequently detected by the traditional methods of history-taking, speculum examination, palpation, and probing. However, their
detection can be accomplished without removal of
tissue by cytological examination of exfoliated cervical cells, by direct magnified observations made
with the colposcope, or by both measures. The mor-

tality associated with cervical cancer has decreased
significantly in most places where these early detection methods are employed.

A small percentage of cervical malignancies are
adenocarcinomas rather than squamous-cell (epidermoid) carcinomas. Such adenocarcinomas may
also occur *in situ*. An even smaller number are ad-
enocanthomas (mixed type), sarcomas, and lymphomas. The discussion herein is concerned primarily with the common squamous-cell type.

A large number of epidemiological studies have
been conducted in various countries to elucidate risk
factors associated with cervical cancer. These investigations, which have shown greatest consistency
for such variables as early onset of coitus and exposure to multiple sexual consorts, strongly support
the concept that one or more sexually transmitted
agents are involved in cervical carcinogenesis. Over
the past 15 years, genital herpes simplex viruses
(HSVs) have received increasing attention as possible etiological agents. Emphasis will be given in
this chapter to studies relating these viruses to cervical cancer.

2. Historical Background

In the 19th century, clinicopathological studies
established that squamous carcinoma of the cervix
was distinct from cancer of the body of the uterus.
In the last part of that century and in the early part
of the 20th century, the microscopic features of in-

André J. Nahmias · Department of Pediatrics
William E. Josey · Department of Gynecology and Ob-
stetrics, Emory University School of Medicine, Atlanta,
Georgia. **James M. Oleske** · Department of
Pediatrics, New Jersey College of Medicine, Newark,
New Jersey.

653

traepithelial carcinoma were described, but the term *carcinoma in situ* was not introduced until 1932, by Broders.[18] In the late 1920s, Schiller introduced the iodine test, which distinguishes glycogen-containing epithelium (positive stain) from epithelium lacking glycogen (no staining). Although this test helped to delineate normal from abnormal epithelium, it did not establish a diagnosis of the abnormal epithelium. In 1925, Hinselmann developed the colposcope to allow direct magnified observation of the cervix. His discovery that the earliest cancer focus originated from atypical epithelium rather than from a nodule was an important initial step toward elucidation of the natural history of the disease. Although exfoliative cytology of the cervix had been described earlier, the systematic 15-year studies of Pananicolaou and Traut,[91] published in 1943, provided great impetus for the use of that technique for the detection of precancer and cancer. In addition to facilitating diagnosis, the application of these various methods, including histopathology, either singly or in combination, contributed significantly to present-day understanding of the biology of cervical carcinoma.

Significant epidemiological observations related to cervical cancer were first reported in 1842 by an Italian physician, Rigoni-Stern.[105] This investigator was the first to point to the rarity of the cancer in nuns and its greater frequency in married than in unmarried women, observations that took another century to be confirmed and extended. The more recent epidemiological studies have led to the concept that early sexual intercourse is the pivotal event in setting up risk, allowing the transmission of some carcinogenic agent from the coital male to the female at risk.[107] Speculations on the nature of the putative carcinogen have included various noninfectious factors such as smegma and spermatozoa, as well as a variety of infectious agents such as *Treponema pallidum* and *Trichomonas vaginalis*.[5] The possible role of genital HSV in cervical carcinogenesis was first suspected from a different line of evidence.

In 1964, studies of an infant with neonatal HSV infection and of his mother's cervical HSV infection led to further investigations by our group at Emory that provided the first suspicion of an association between genital herpes and cervical neoplasia.[81] We observed that women with cytological findings consistent with HSV infection in cervicovaginal smears had an increased frequency of cervical pre-

cancer and cancer. During studies to confirm the specificity of the cytological changes—first in humans, then in mice—it was noted that mice genitally infected with human genital HSV isolates died at a much higher frequency than mice inoculated with nongenital HSV strains. Other biological differences were also found between genital and nongenital strains.[72] Serological testing permitted differentiation of HSV strains according to their most frequent site of origin and mode of transmission into two antigenic types, HSV-1 and HSV-2, described earlier by Schneweis[111] and Plummer[94] (see Chapter 13). The differences in virus types between those most often associated with genital infections (HSV-2) and nongenital infections (HSV-1) thus provided another approach to the study of the genital herpes–cervical cancer association, since serological differentiation of antibodies to the two types then became possible. These early seroepidemiological studies demonstrated a higher frequency of HSV-2 antibodies in women with cervical cancer as compared to controls.[8,73,99] Many other types of approaches, from the molecular to the epidemiological and comparative, have provided further evidence linking genital herpes to cervical cancer. Results of these studies and the problems of establishing a causal relationship are discussed in later sections.

3. Methodology

3.1. Mortality and Morbidity of Cervical Neoplasia

Several factors have contributed to the problem of defining mortality and morbidity data in various geographic regions. First is the fact that until the 1940s, cervical cancer and cancer of the corpus uteri were reported together as cancer of the uterus.[53] Another problem is that it is not always clear whether the number of new cases per year is comprised of both *in situ* and invasive cancer or only the latter. In the United States, for instance, estimates of new cases of cervical cancer that have been obtained from the NCI National Cancer Survey do not include cases of carcinoma *in situ* (CIS). Mortality rates are also available from the SEER Program[113] and vital statistics records of the United States and other countries. The true rates may be compromised by the problem of whether the cancer is listed as the cause of death on the death certificate.[57] Another factor that has greatly influenced mortality rates is the extent to which methods for the detection of cervical cancer in its early stages have been employed in a particular geographic region. Improved methods of therapy in certain areas would also be expected to influence mortality rates. Access to optimum medical care might therefore affect the differences encountered in age-specific rates, particularly mortality rates, since symptoms are not usually apparent until the disease has progressed to a relatively advanced stage.

Prevalence rates of dysplasia, CIS, and invasive cancer have been obtained in several surveys by application of detection methods, chiefly cytological techniques, followed by histological confirmation.[53] Incidence rates have been determined by following over varying periods of years women who had previously negative cytological findings. The incidence rates for women with dysplasia who went on to develop CIS or invasive cancer have also been compared with the rates for those whose initial smears were cytologically negative. Of course, the duration of follow-up studies in a disease with a long latency period affects the results obtained.

The rates obtained in the various studies will depend on the adequacy of the methods and on the interpretations employed.

3.1.1. Cytological Methods. The sensitivity of the cytological methods will depend on how the smears were obtained, the adequacy of the specimen, the number of smears obtained, and the competence of the observer.[121] Variations in interpretation are not uncommon. Also, in case of advanced invasive disease, concomitant inflammation may obscure the cytological diagnosis. Overall, the technique has an 80–95% reliability in detecting cervical-cell abnormalities.

3.1.2. Colposcopic Methods. The competence of the observer is also important when colposcopic methods are used. Such techniques are also about 80–95% reliable in detecting cervical neoplasia.[17] Since some negative results obtained by cytological methods may be positive by colposcopy and vice versa, the combined use of the two techniques increases the accuracy.

3.1.3. Histological Methods. Since the histopathological diagnosis is the most usually accepted finite criterion, albeit occasionally yielding false-negative results,[122] differences in interpretation

would make comparison of results obtained in different areas problematical. Diagnostic variability has been repeatedly demonstrated in studies wherein the same slide sections were submitted to a number of different pathologists, particularly in case of intraepithelial abnormalities.[104] It is also appreciated that diagnostic biopsies may affect the progression of the process by removal of some of the tumor tissue.[103]

3.1.4. Appropriate Controls. In studies attempting to determine specific risk factors in women with cervical neoplasia as compared to those with no evidence of cervical precancer or cancer, there arises the problem of the validity of historical information, e.g., number of sexual partners and contraceptive usage. In reference particularly to whether or not the male contacts were circumcised, the adequacy of historical information has been challenged repeatedly.[107]

3.2. Studies Relating Herpes Simplex Virus to Cervical Cancer

Several of the methods used for diagnosing HSV-1 and/or HSV-2 infections and associated problems have been detailed in Chapter 13. The features related more specifically to studies attempting to link genital HSV infection to cervical cancer are emphasized here.

3.2.1. Epidemiological Studies

a. Prospective studies. Women with active genital herpetic lesions can be identified clinically, but because of occasional confusion with other entities, at least cytological confirmation of the diagnosis is required. Since genital infections can be caused by HSV-1,[72] which is also potentially oncogenic (see Section 4.2), it would be important to obtain virus isolation and typing. Furthermore, to differentiate between the possibility that a primary infection is more or less likely to be followed by cervical neoplasia than is a recurrent genital infection, serological studies on acute and convalescent sera are required. Similarly, although it is also possible to follow prospectively women with subclinical cervical herpetic infections who have been detected cytologically during routine Papanicolaou screening smears for cervical neoplasia,[82] a primary infection could not be differentiated from a recurrent one without such serological tests.

For control purposes, in view of the large number

of subclinical genital HSV infections,[51] it is not possible to rule out infection at any specific time unless virological or cytological tests are applied continuously at weekly intervals, an obviously impractical approach. Therefore, serological techniques demonstrating the absence of HSV-2 antibodies constitute one potential way of identifying control groups. This is predicated on the sensitivity and specificity of the serological assay used to detect HSV-2 type-specific antibodies and again on the premise that there would be only a small number of HSV-1-related cervical neoplasias.

Another approach could be to follow prospectively women with or without antibodies to certain tumor-associated HSV antigens (see Table 1 and Section 7.1). It might also be possible to differentiate cervical dysplastic cells that react with certain HSV antibodies from those that do not by such methods as immunofluorescence and to follow the progression to more severe cervical neoplastic disease. Such approaches are dependent on the characterization and specificity of the neoplasia-related HSV antigens or antibodies to such antigens.

b. Retrospective studies. Such studies have the problems related to the methods of serological testing noted above. In case cell-mediated immunological tests are used, the responses in patients with cervical neoplasia must be carefully compared with those in women with no prior exposure to HSV-1 and/or HSV-2 infection and in those with active primary or recurrent infections. There is also the need of defining accurately the type of cervical neoplasia being studied and whether any form of potential therapy, including biopsies, has been used.

c. Appropriate controls. The problem of appropriate controls for either prospective or retrospective studies is critical. Because of the possibility that genital HSV infection and cervical neoplasia may be codependent, both tending to be found in women whose sexual habits or those of their consorts would enhance the likelihood of occurrence of the two entities, it is particularly important to control for a number of variables related to sexual attributes.

3.2.2. Detection of Virus or Virus Markers in Neoplastic Cells. The induction of virus replication and its isolation in cervical-cancer tissues or cells in culture constitute the most direct approach. However, such isolation does not necessarily establish a causal role for HSV. It might also result from coincidental active HSV infection in a woman with cervical neoplasia or from laboratory contamination of the cell culture by the virus.

Attempts to detect HSV antigens in exfoliated cervical cells or biopsy specimens can be performed by immunofluorescence, immunoperoxidase, or radioimmunoassay techniques. Problems with nonspecific positive reactions can occur, and here again confirmatory work and characterization of the antigens would provide greater reliability to results obtained.

The detection of viral DNA or RNA in cancer cells by molecular hybridization techniques is limited by the sensitivity of these assays. If only a small fraction of the viral genome is present in the cancer, the assay might not be sensitive enough to allow its detection or that of its transcripts. It is also to be emphasized that the cancer tissue being tested should be examined for the proportion of cancer cells and normal cells in the tissue. In case of *in situ* hybridization techniques performed on tissue sections, there is also a problem with nonspecific positive reactions, and controls with viral probes other than those for HSV are mandatory.

4. Biology of the Cancer and the Virus

4.1. Cervical Cancer

Knowledge of the natural history of cervical cancer is of particular importance in delineating the phase at which a potentially oncogenic agent might act. Despite a large amount of past and current (see the summaries in Section 8.1) research in this area, controversial points need to be resolved. For instance, it is still not clear whether dysplasia begins in a single precursor cell or within a larger field of cells, nor is it clear whether it spreads by multiplication of the single abnormal cell or by conversion of neighboring normal epithelium into dysplastic epithelium.[50,104] The various possibilities of the progression from normal cells to invasive cancer include (1) directly, (2) via dysplasia only, (3) via CIS to invasion, or (4) via dysplasia to CIS to invasion. The evidence is strongest for the fourth alternative, although the other pathways cannot be ruled out entirely.[50] This progression is suggested by the peak age distribution of dysplasias, which precedes by several years that for CIS, which in turn precedes by several years that for invasive cancer. Similar progression has also been observed in mouse models in which chemical carcinogens have been applied to the cervix.[26] Of special interest is the finding from these animal studies that the rate of progression depends on genetic features of the host and on the frequency of application of the carcinogen. It is also accepted by most investigators, though not all, that dysplasias can regress in varying frequencies and that not all cases of CIS progress to invasive cancer.[27,39,50]

There is now almost general acceptance of the concept that cervical neoplasia usually begins in the region of the squamocolumnar junction, in accordance with findings from the early studies of Pund and Auerbach.[96] Colposcopic examination of the cervix reveals a transformation zone wherein the columnar epithelium is often replaced by squamous cells (metaplasia). It has not been established whether the metaplastic cells originate from embryonal rests of urogenital sinus epithelium, directly from columnar cells, or from multipotential "reserve" cells in the underlying stroma. The studies of Coppleson and Reid[27] indicate that this normally occurring process of squamous metaplasia, which can be noted in varying frequencies in the cervix of women, occurs with highest frequency in association with the first pregnancy. These authors concluded that dysplasia and CIS do not originate from native squamous epithelium, but rather from metaplastic cells. They further postulated that transformation of metaplastic cells to atypical cells is caused by some oncogenic agent(s).

This concept would explain the peculiar susceptibility of the cervix to neoplastic transformation if it is assumed that the immature metaplastic epithelium is more sensitive to an oncogenic agent like HSV than is mature squamous epithelium. It is also attractive in offering an explanation for the disparity in frequency of cervical cancer and penile cancer, despite the approximately equal frequencies of penile and cervical herpetic infections. Vulvar carcinoma, although sometimes discovered to be associated with cervical carcinoma,[32] also occurs at a much lower frequency. An association between genital herpes and vulvar cancer has very recently been made.[139] Neither penile nor vulvar epithelium demonstrates squamous metaplasia. It is worth noting here that female sexual contacts of males with penile cancer show a higher frequency of cervical cancer than control women whose contacts do not have penile cancer.[59] This suggests that the same oncogenic agents may be involved, even though the incidence of penile cancer is much lower.

4.2. Herpes Simplex Viruses

The biological characteristics of HSVs have already been described in Chapter 13. Of particular relevance to the coherence of a possible role of HSV in cervical carcinogenesis was the need to establish that the cervix is indeed a common site of infection by the virus. Several studies have confirmed this point, which was not well appreciated previously, since cervical herpetic infections are most often subclinical and require laboratory methods for their detection.[51] Histopathological studies have also revealed that the virus commonly infects areas at or near the squamocolumnar junction,[82] the site of origin of most cervical neoplastic lesions.

The oncogenic potential of herpesviruses in general, and of HSV in particular, has been established only relatively recently. Since the 1960s, a large number of herpesviruses have been discovered from species as widely different as fungi and man, and include HSV-2 and the Epstein–Barr virus.[77] Several herpesvirus have been associated with neoplastic disease in animals and humans.[97] The evidence for a causal relationship of the herpesviruses to neoplasia, whether of lymphohematopoeitic or solid organs, varies from weak to strong. The point to stress, however, is that because herpesviruses have been definitely linked causally to cancer in some species, all other herpesviruses are rendered suspect of the same capability.

More specifically in regard to HSVs, it has now been shown that when HSV-1 or HSV-2 is inactivated by any of several methods (ultraviolet or photodynamic inactivation), it can transform hamster or other rodent cells in vitro (reviewed in a number of publications[79,97,98,101]). Transformation can also be accomplished with temperature-sensitive mutants and with fragments of the DNA of the virus.[19,54] The transforming event is apparently infrequent, and some, but not all, of the in-vitro-transformed cells can cause tumors when inoculated into hamsters. Tumor-bearing hamsters have been shown to possess HSV antibodies in their serum, and HSV antigens can be demonstrated in a varying number of the tumor cells. Viral-specific genetic information has been detected in some of the hamster transformed cell lines.[35] As yet, no convincing evidence of *in vitro* transformation by HSV in primate cells, including human cervical epithelium, has been obtained.[136]

Sarcomas have been found at the site of inoculation of about 1% of newborn hamsters inoculated directly with several strains of HSV-2.[75] Viral antigens have been detected in some of the transplanted or cultured tumors.[45] Several mice genitally inoculated with live HSV-2 have developed cervical neoplasia,[68,74] although cervical cancers have also been noted in mice treated only with female hormones.[71] Using formalin-inactivated HSV-2, or ultraviolet-inactivated HSV-1 or HSV-2, a significant number of cervical and endometrial neoplasms were produced in mice.[134,135] In *Cebus* monkeys, genital inoculation of live HSV-2 produced only a few cervical dysplasias.[90]

Important points raised by these *in vitro* and *in vivo* studies, which of course cannot be used as proof of the oncogenic potential of HSV in humans, are possible differences in the oncogenic potential of different strains of HSV and the low frequency of transformation obtained. There is also some suggestion that the HSV genome may no longer be detectable in hamster tumors after many serial passages, pointing to the possibility that the HSV genome may no longer be detectable in human cervical cancers.[117] Technical variations may, however, account for these results obtained by various methods.

The first three investigations to compare the occurrence of antibodies to HSV-2 in women with cervical neoplasia and controls were performed by the Baylor, Emory, and Hopkins groups.[8,73,99] Different neutralization assays (kinetic neutralization, microneutralization potency, and multiplicity analysis) and different HSV-1 and HSV-2 strains were employed. All three studies indicated that the frequency of HSV-2 antibodies is higher in women with invasive cervical cancer than in control groups matched for age and socioeconomic status. Variabilities in results were observed, however. Thus, two of the three studies showed a higher frequency of HSV-2 antibodies in women with intraepithelial neoplasia than that found in the control group, whereas one study did not. Furthermore, the percentage of women positive for HSV-2 antibodies by the use of the multiplicity-analysis test in both the study and control groups was higher than that found with the use of the other two serological tests.

In a later study, comparing the multiplicity-analysis tests with the microneutralization index (HSV-2/HSV-1), the correlation between the two assays was found to be poor.[53]

A large number of other seroepidemiological studies have been conducted since that time in many parts of the world[2,15,48,61,87] and have been reviewed elsewhere.[53,65,66,78,95,100,102] In a limited number of studies, comparisons of titers between cancer and control women have indicated higher mean titers in the cancer group.[1,2] The large majority of studies, however, measured primarily the frequency of antibodies to HSV-2 in women with cervical cancer and controls, most often comparable in age, race, and socioeconomic status. In a few studies in which certain attributes of sexual promiscuity were equalized among cases and controls, significant differences in the frequency of HSV-2 antibodies in the women with cervical cancer were observed.[1,8,78] In some studies, the frequency of HSV-2 antibodies was so high in the controls that no significant excess could be detected in the cancer cases. To circumvent this difficulty, we studied 57 women with CIS who were 21 years of age or younger, since the frequency of HSV-2 antibodies in the control group of 87 young women was only 15%. The 65% frequency of HSV-2 antibodies in the CIS group constituted a significant difference.[78]

Even in studies in which the frequency of HSV-2 antibodies was significantly higher than in controls, the percentage of those with antibodies in the cancer cases has been as low as 30–40%. Together with negative studies in New Zealand, Israel, Colombia, and Taiwan, these findings provide important questions to be resolved as regards the herpes–cancer association. Several explanations for these findings could be given, including: (1) the difficulty of detecting HSV-2 antibodies in subjects with prior HSV-1 infection[78,95,101]; (2) the possible variability in strains of HSV-2[114] or the possibility that HSV-1 may be more involved in cervical neoplasia in some countries in which genital HSV-1 is more common than HSV-2[52]; and (3) different causes of cervical cancer, of which HSV may be only one[102] and in which geographic variabilities in causation may occur. The problem of the serological test used to measure HSV-2 antibodies is exemplified by the results obtained when sera from the Columbia study were reexamined with a more specific and sensitive radioimmunoassay[60]: whereas the frequency of HSV-2 antibodies detected by microneutralization had been 30% in both cervical and control groups, a significant difference was found when the new assay was employed.

Prospective studies of the incidence of cervical cancer in relation to various risk factors could provide a different approach to this problem. Ideal prospective studies, as described in detail elsewhere,[76] would require very specific serological tests and would be extremely expensive as well. They would be particularly warranted if some method of preventing HSV infection (see Section 9) could be incorporated in the overall investigation. Nevertheless, several prospective studies of a less idealized nature have been conducted, or are currently being conducted, by several groups.

We are currently engaged[4,76] in a follow-up study of about 600 women whom we had identified over the years as having evidence of genital herpetic or HSV-2 infection and of about 400 women who had no HSV-2 antibodies by our assay (80–85% sensitivity and specificity). Both groups of women had cytologically negative smears for cervical abnormalities on entry into the study. Evaluations of the two groups for various epidemiological variables have not revealed significant differences between the two groups, particularly as regards sexual and parity variables. A 4-fold higher frequency of severe cervical dysplasia and CIS has so far been detected in the herpes groups as compared to the control group.

Of particular interest was the finding that 6 (21%) of 28 women identified serologically with a primary genital HSV-2 infection went on to develop severe dysplasia or CIS.[4] This is 10 times the rate found in the control group. Although the series is small, it has important implications in terms of the possible causality issue. These preliminary observations also raise the possibility that oral HSV-1 acquired in childhood may protect from cervical neoplasia in the same way perhaps as the turkey herpesvirus administered to young chicks protects them from the neoplasia induced by Marek's disease virus in older chickens. Such a possibility has also been raised by British workers using seroepidemiological methods.[118]

Another approach has been used by Swedish workers who defined a group of women clinically diagnosed to have genital herpes between 1948 and 1958 and a group of control women attending the same clinics over this period in whom this *clinical* diagnosis was not made.[49] The availability of a tumor registry in Sweden permitted these investigators to determine the number of women in the herpes and control groups who developed cervical cancer in later years. A significantly higher frequency of cervical cancer was observed in the herpes group, particularly in patients in whom genital herpes was diagnosed when they were 15–19 years old. Major deficiencies with this approach are the lack of information regarding subclinical genital herpetic infection in either group and the absence of information regarding possibly important epidemiological variables in the two groups.

A third approach is to collect and store sera from large numbers of women and test only those who develop cervical neoplasia at a later time, as well as an appropriate number of controls. For instance, sera of women without evidence of cervical neoplasia had been stored during the NIH Perinatal Viral Disease Study in Boston.[21] Serum was then obtained around the time some of these same women were diagnosed as having CIS. Serial samples from women without cervical cancer were also available for testing. The frequency of serological evidence of HSV-2 infection in women developing CIS was significantly higher than that noted in control women. A similar type of approach is currently being used in much larger numbers of women by Czech and by Danish workers.[84,130]

5. Descriptive Epidemiology

In this section, the epidemiological patterns of cervical neoplasia are presented and compared, wherever possible, with the epidemiological patterns found with HSV-2 infection. Even though the incidence and mortality rates for cervical neoplasia will be listed according to various attributes—e.g., geographic, socioeconomic, ethnic origin—the pivotal points will be tied up in the latter part of the discussion.

5.1. Incidence and Mortality Data

The incidence of cervical cancer has been ascertained from time trends in mortality and by incidence data obtained from national cancer surveys, as well as from a number of cancer registries and special studies, such as the SEER Program,[113] performed in various areas. Most striking are differences in mortality and incidence rates between the United States white and nonwhite population, the rates in nonwhite females being over twice as high as those in white females.[57,113] A reduction in the mortality rates for cervical cancer has been noted over recent years. Thus, the rates for 1950–1955 of 9.6 per 100,000 women for whites and 22.6 per 100,000 for nonwhites declined to 5.8 and 15.8 by 1967–1968[53] and to 4.1 and 11.8, respectively, by 1973–1976.[113]

Kessler[53] has reviewed a number of community-based cytological surveys for cervical neoplasia during the past two decades. These surveys incorporate cases detected at the start of the survey (prevalence) and those identified later (incidence). The rates obtained in these surveys are generally 5–25 times higher than those obtained by incidence statistics from cancer registries or special surveys. The longer the follow-up studies are conducted during such surveys, the closer the results would reflect incidence rates. These cytological studies have demonstrated several points of value: (1) with single cervical cytological screening, up to 1% of women will be found with CIS or invasive cancer; (2) fewer invasive cancers are usually detected on later screenings of the same women; (3) women found to have cervical dysplasia in their initial smears will have a higher likelihood of developing CIS or invasive cancer on later screening than women with initially negative smears.

5.2. Lifetime Risk

It has been estimated that the likelihood, from birth onward, of a woman's developing cervical cancer is around 1–2%.[38,39] On the basis of various serological studies done in the United States, the probability of a woman's developing HSV-2 infection in her lifetime is 10–50%. As will be indicated later, both these probabilities depend on certain attributes of the woman. Nevertheless, these estimates suggest that if HSV-2 is indeed causally related to cervical cancer, the case/cancer rate would be around 1:8–40. Since about one quarter of genital herpetic infections are primary, if the risk of developing cervical cancer is chiefly related to a primary genital herpetic infection, the case/cancer rate would

be closer to 1:2–10. Indeed, in a small number of women with primary genital herpes,[4] the risk of severe dysplasia and CIS was about 1:5.

Rawls and Campione-Piccardo[102] arrived at a risk estimate of the contribution of HSV-2 to cervical cancer in a different fashion. By analyzing all the seroepidemiological reports of the frequency of HSV-2 antibodies in cervical cancer cases, these workers found the data to fit best a model in which HSV-2 is one of two (or more) causes of cervical cancer. They estimated that for each 10% of the population infected with HSV-2, there will be an increase of about 5 cases in the annual incidence of cervical cancer.

5.3. Age

The incidence rate for CIS is highest in the 30–39 year age group, and that for invasive cancer is highest after the age of 40 years. The age-adjusted incidence of cervical cancer has almost doubled in the United States since 1950 and is due primarily to *in situ* cancer.[57] This may reflect the increased use of cytological screening. It could also be that concomitant with the overall increase of gonorrhea during this period, other venereally transmitted agents, such as HSV, may have been on the rise.

5.4. Geographic Distribution

There are significant variations in the mortality and age-specific rates for cervical cancer in different countries. Muñoz[70] has separated countries in those of high risk, intermediate risk, and low risk. Among the high-risk countries are Colombia, Chile, and Poland; in the intermediate-risk group are the Scandinavian countries and the United States; in the low-risk group are Israel and New Zealand. These differences may be due to a large number of factors, including the extent of application of early detection methods, sexual practices in various socioeconomic levels, and other national and cultural variables to be discussed below. Within the United States, a higher mortality rate for cervical cancer has been recorded generally in southern cities as compared to northern cities, the lowest rate being found in the Northeast. Women from urban counties have higher mortality rates than those from suburban counties; women from rural areas have higher rates than either urban or suburban women. These differences may reflect the availability of diagnostic and therapeutic facilities in different settings.

The frequency of HSV-2 antibodies has been determined in a relatively small number of adult women between the ages of 30 and 50 years in various countries.[53,102] It was found to be 10–70% in the United States, 20–50% in several European and Asian countries, and over 50% in some African countries. It should be reemphasized that the methods used in the serological surveys differed greatly and that the composition of the populations serologically tested varied widely.

5.5. Socieconomic Status

Studies in the United States and abroad have indicated that the highest incidence of cervical cancer is in women of the lowest economic groups.[69,137] A decreasing cancer incidence was noted with improved socioeconomic status. A similar relationship exists for HSV-2 infections.[64,102]

5.6. Ethnic or Religious Origin

The lowest frequency of cervical cancer has been noted in Jewish women and in Amish women in the United States, and the highest frequency in black and Puerto Rican women.[57] American Indians also have a higher rate of cervical cancer than whites. In general, migrant women to the United States have a lower mortality from cancer of the cervix compared to native United States whites. However, excess mortality has been recorded in Mexican, Canadian, and Yugoslavian migrants to the United States.

5.7. Other Variables

It was recognized over a century ago that celibate women, such as nuns, are very unlikely to develop cervical cancer.[105] This point has been confirmed more recently.[107] We have found only 1 of 34 nuns to have HSV-2 antibodies; higher rates were found in all other populations studied. Increased rates of cervical cancer have been found in women with syphilis, in prisoners, and in prostitutes.[107] The rate of HSV-2 antibodies in prostitutes is very high, approaching 70%.[30]

Rotkin[107] has reviewed studies that assayed the following variables: early marriage, multiple marriages, broken marriage, early coitus, multiple sexual consorts, coital frequency, unstable sexual relationship, parity, gravidity and abortions, contraception, and circumcision. This worker portrayed the relative strength, consistency, and inconsistency of accumulated trends for specific variables in a simplified table. A remarkable consistency was found for variables associated with early onset of coitus, including early marriage. Variables related to multiple sex partners were also observed to be significantly increased in women with cervical cancer as compared to controls. Obstructive methods of contraception, including condoms and diaphragms, were more widely used in controls than in cancer cases. The hypothesis that noncircumcision of sexual consorts increases the risk of cervical cancer has not been corroborated in the majority of recent studies.

A possible genetic predisposition to the development of cervical cancer is suggested by two studies reporting an increased frequency of HLA B-12 in women with this neoplasm.[55,123] A higher frequency of HSV-2 antibodies was noted in such patients with HLA B-12.[56] There does not appear to be an increased risk of cervical neoplasia in women on steroid contraceptives.[16]

6. Mechanisms and Routes of Transmission

One conclusion to be drawn from all of the studies discussed above is that the most important determinant for cervical carcinogenesis is sexual intercourse. These epidemiological findings strongly support the concept that the oncogenic agent is acquired sexually, often during the period of adolescence. Exposure to many males would increase the likelihood of acquisition of oncogenic agents, although sexual contact with only one partner who had acquired the agent from other sources must also be considered. One study has indicated that second wives of men whose first consort developed cervical cancer had a greater likelihood of developing this neoplasia.[53]

The data noted earlier regarding geographic area, socioeconomic status, and ethnic origin are most likely related to the more critical factors associated with sexual variables. Although the numbers of pregnancies and deliveries do not appear to contribute to an increased risk, little attention has been paid to the age at first pregnancy. This is a more objective criterion than age at first coitus. In addition, it may have significant bearing regarding the possible role of metaplasia in cervical carcinogenesis, because metaplasia occurs with higher frequency in the first pregnancy.[27]

The epidemiological aspects of cervical cancer could thus fit several possible etiological agents, any one of which could be introduced with sexual intercourse. Epidemiological observations make it unlikely that sperm would represent the oncogenic factor, as suggested by Australian and British workers.[27,116] Smegma would also be an unlikely candidate in view of the negative epidemiological data related to circumcision.[107] Alexander[5] reviewed several candidate infectious agents other than HSV, including *Trichomonas vaginalis, Treponema pallidum, Neisseria gonorrhoeae,* mycoplasmas, chlamydiae, and cytomegaloviruses (CMVs). The relative frequency of genital infection with all these agents, except possibly *Trichomonas pallidum,* is higher than that for HSV. The milder forms of cervical dysplasia have been associated with chronic inflammation and infection with such agents as *Trichomonas vaginalis* and chlamydiae.[110,126]

There is little epidemiological or biological information on the oncogenic potential of any of the aforenamed agents with the exception of CMVs.[97] One of three serological studies[37,119,129] noted a higher frequency of CMV antibodies in women with cervical cancer as compared to controls, although the difference was less than that observed for HSV-2 antibodies. The more recent finding that genital wart viruses involve the cervix[63] and the well-appreciated oncogenic potential of this group of papovaviruses make it important to pursue the possible involvement of these viruses in cervical carcinogenesis.

Current knowledge on the epidemiology of genital HSV infection (Chapter 13) fits well the epidemiological pattern of the suspect factor. The virus has been demonstrated to be sexually transmitted. The infection is particularly common in adolescents and young adults, with a peak age of around 20–22 years. From a temporal viewpoint, this peak age is several years earlier than that for cervical dysplasia and cancer. The similarities in the epidemiological patterns for genital HSV infection and cervical cancer, however, provide one of the most difficult problems in establishing causality, since it is well appreciated that a woman who acquires one venereally transmitted agent is likely to be exposed to other agents, either concurrently or at another time.

7. Pathogenesis and Immunity

7.1. Pathogenesis

The pathogenesis of preinvasive cervical neoplasia has been described in Section 4. Progression of the invasive cancer occurs primarily by involvement of contiguous areas and lymphatic channels. This local extension of the tumors and its consequent effects on the ureters, with subsequent urinary-tract obstruction, infection, and uremia, are the principal causes of death in patients with advanced disease. Death often intervenes before the development of metastases to other organs.

The pathogenesis of HSV in primary or recurrent infections has been discussed in Chapter 13. It is amplified here to develop a possible scheme for the events leading to cell transformation. Such a scheme, presented in Fig. 1, is based on a variety of *in vitro* and *in vivo* animal or human observations. It should be appreciated that several of these findings, as noted earlier, require confirmation for validation.

Three types of cell–virus interactions can be considered: (1) a productive infection, which causes cell death and results in a subclinical or clinically apparent infection; (2) a latent infection, with later reactivation of a presumably intact virus genome resulting in a productive infection in mucocutaneous, CNS, or ocular sites; (3) cell transformation, wherein the cell survives and retains the ability to multiply, but may contain an incomplete viral genome having a limited capacity to be expressed.

The presence of defective viral DNA in some HSV strains has been demonstrated *in vitro.*[33] Ultraviolet irradiation and photodynamic inactivation, both of which can cause defects in the viral DNA, have been shown to cause the virus to transform cells.[98] The presence of latent HSV in human sensory and autonomic nervous system ganglia[13,132] has also been demonstrated. As noted earlier, there are as yet only preliminary observations suggesting that primary infections might be more important than genital infections occurring in women with prior HSV-1 infection. Nevertheless, the recurrence of a cervical herpetic infection would explain why, in some

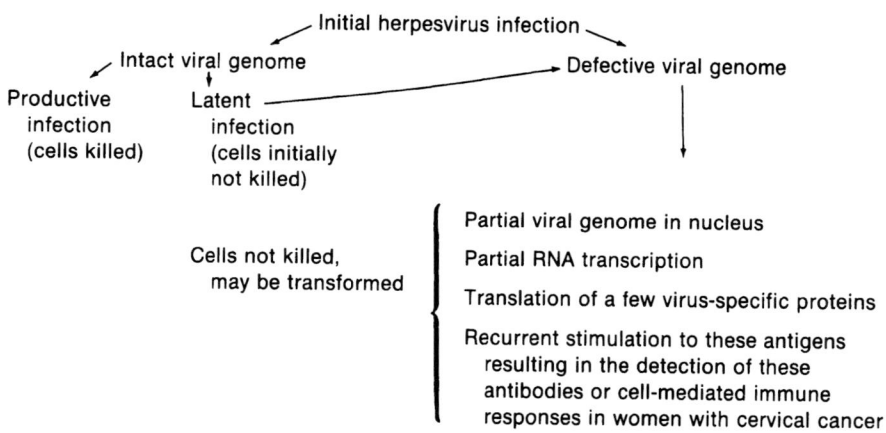

Fig. 1. A tentative scheme of various herpes virus–cell interactions.

cases, HSV has been isolated around, or after, the time of the detection of the cervical neoplasia. Another less likely possibility is that the virus could remain latent in the cancer cell, as suggested by the still unduplicated recovery of HSV from a culture of CIS in one instance.[9]

Molecular hybridization studies in HSV-2-transformed hamster cells have provided evidence for the presence of only a fraction of the virus genome varying from 8 to 32% in one to three copies per cell.[35] Several workers are now attempting to define where on the viral genetic maps the transforming genes are located.[19,20,62,92]

Concurrent with the hamster model, investigators have used similar technology to attempt to detect HSV DNA or RNA in human cervical neoplasias. In one large human invasive cervical cancer in which no infectious virus could be demonstrated, a fraction of the viral DNA was detected.[34] By techniques that may not have been sensitive enough to detect less than one complete viral genome, negative results were obtained by other workers.[138] More recently, several workers have used *in situ* hybridization to attempt to detect HSV RNA transcripts in tissue-sectioned cells of cervical neoplasias. Three groups have recently reported on finding evidence of such transcripts in varying frequency in cervical dysplastic or invasive cancer cells.[31,58,62] These variable results may represent differences in the sensitivity or specificity of the methods employed. If the probes are indeed specific (positive results were, for instance, also obtained with an adenovirus probe

by one group[58]), such observations would provide further evidence for the causal role of HSV in at least some cervical neoplasias.

Current methodology is also being used to define in human cervical neoplasms the localization of genes associated with transformation on the HSV genetic map. If this can be ascertained, it would then be possible to determine which protein antigens are coded by these genes. A search could then be made for these proteins in cervical neoplastic cells or for antibodies or cell-mediated immune responses to these particular proteins in patients with cervical neoplasias or other HSV-associated tumors. Such genetic and molecular information[106] could also provide the most cogent explanation for the disparate results obtained with the tumor-associated HSV antigen studies presented below.

Some evidence for cross-reacting antigen between HSV and cervical cancer has been obtained by immunodiffusion tests.[38,45] Of interest is the recent demonstration that HSV antibodies can be eluted from cervical cancer cells,[115] providing support for corss-reacting antigens.

Immunofluorescence tests, using antisera to unpurified HSV-2 applied to exfoliated cervical cells or biopsies, have yielded conflicting results.[3,88,89,108] Several workers have, however, described various HSV antigens that appear to be associated with either cervical cancer or squamous-cell carcinomas of nongenital sites. As can be noted in Table 1, these antigens appear to be different HSV proteins. They have been used in various ways to determine their

Table 1. Tumor-Associated Herpes Simplex Virus Antigens: Detection of These Antigens in Cervical Neoplasias and for Serological and Cell-Mediated Immune Studies

Antigen	Characteristics	Detection of antigen in cervical neoplasms (Ref. nos.)	Used for detection of antibodies in sera of patients with cancer	Used in cell-mediated assays (Ref. nos.)
HSV-TAA (HSV-1 and 2)	Nonstructural membrane-associated mol. wt. = 40,000–60,000	—	Squamous-cell carcinomas, including cervical cancer—antibody not prognostic[41–44]	42
AG-4 (HSV-2)	Structural membrane-associated mol. wt. = 161,000	9	Cervical neoplasias—antibody prognostic[7,9–11,40,52,86,93]	—
VP 143 (HSV-2)	Nonstructural DNA-binding protein, cytoplasmic and nuclear mol. wt. = 143,000	67	Cervical neoplasias[6]	—
AG-e (HSV-1 and 2)	Structural cytoplasmic and nuclear, two proteins mol. wt. = 130,000 and 140,000	11	Cervical neoplasia—antibody not prognostic[11,93]	14
ICSP 34/35[a] (HSV-2)	Nonstructural DNA-binding protein mol. wt. = 140,000	29		

[a] May be similar to VP143—also found in vulvar cancers.[139]

association with cervical neoplasia or other squamous-cell tumors. In some cases, antibodies to these proteins were used to detect the antigens in cervical cancers or exfoliated cells. In other studies, the frequency of antibodies to these antigens in the sera of patients with cervical neoplasias, squamous-cell cancers, and controls was ascertained. The prognostic value of such antibodies in relation to progression of the cervical cancer has also been investigated. Cell-mediated immune responses were also studied with some of these antigens.

Detailed results of these various studies have been recently reviewed.[80,93] In general, a small to great difference in the frequency of detection of these antigens in cervical neoplastic cells, as compared to those from the normal cervix or other cancers, has been noted. Similarly, a small to great difference in positive reactions using antibody or cell-mediated assays has been reported. One possible explanation for the disparate results is that there is a varying amount of viral genetic information in different neoplastic cells with variable transcription and translation of one or more of these proteins. As noted in the scheme presented in Fig. 1, such HSV anti-gens, expressed in tumor cells, would then be able to stimulate specific immune responses as the transformed cells carrying them multiply. Antibodies to some of these antigens might be less readily stimulated by productive infection, even with multiple recurrences. Thus, women with cervical neoplasias might be found to possess antibodies to these antigens in a higher frequency than that occurring in women with primary or recurrent infections. In the event the cancer or precancer is eliminated by treatment, the stimulus for such antibodies might no longer be present. There is some indication that the antibodies can be of the IgM class, favoring this hypothesis.[112,125]

7.2. Immunity

Immune mechanisms may provide surveillance to remove transformed cells before they multiply. They may thus help in causing a regression of some of the precancerous cervical lesions or in delaying the progress of the tumor or its metastases. If HSV-1 does indeed afford some protection from HSV-2-associated neoplasia, as suggested earlier, the cross-immunity known to exist between HSV-1 and HSV-2 might explain this observation.

The presence of mononuclear and plasma cells in invasive cancer sites has been noted.[27] Some evidence has also been obtained, using *in vitro* assays, that lymphocytes or serum (plus complement) from women with cervical cancer can lyse cervical-cancer target cells.[28,121,131,133] A leukocyte migration-inhibition test using cervical-cancer antigens demonstrated more positive responses in the cervical-neoplasia patients than in controls.[22] The lymphocytes of women with cervical cancer have also been found to differ in their susceptibility to antilymphocyte serum.[109] Results of testing for delayed hypersensitivity with a variety of common skin-test antigens, such as *Candida* antigens, showed that there was no depression of skin reactivity until the women were in late stages of invasive cancer.[83]

8. Patterns of Host Response

8.1. Clinical and Pathological Features

There are no symptoms characteristic of cervical cancer. The most significant manifestation is bleeding, which occurs in some cases when the cancer breaks through the protective epithelium. However, there may be extensive spread of the cancer through the pelvis without any bleeding.

In case of intraepithelial cervical lesions (dysplasia or CIS), physical examination is usually negative. Similarly, many cases of early invasive cancer are clinically inapparent. Invasive cancer may manifest itself as an erosion, an ulcer, and a mass with or without ulceration. The most readily diagnosed cervical cancer is that associated with an exophytic type of growth.

Dysplasia is a disturbance in the normal orderly arrangement of cells in the epithelial lining of the cervix and its glands, and can be further differentiated into mild, moderate, or severe, according to the extent of involvement of the surface epithelium. When cellular alterations are noted through the full thickness of the cervical epithelium, the process is classified as carcinoma *in situ* (intraepithelial carcinoma, stage 0 carcinoma). The diagnosis of invasive cervical carcinoma is made when there is stromal penetration by the abnormal cells. For clinical, therapeutic, and prognostic purposes, invasive carcinoma is classified as stage I (confined to the cervix), stage II (extending beyond the cervix, but not to the pelvic wall or lower vagina), stage III (extending to the pelvic wall or lower third of the vagina), stage IV (with invasion of the bladder or rectum, or with metastases beyond the true pelvis). Subdivisions of stages I and II are also recognized for further refinement in clinical staging of the disease.

It has been very difficult to determine the time required for progression of the cancer from one stage to another in any one woman. Lymph-node involvement occurs with increasing frequency from stage I on—about 15% in stage I, 30% in stage II, and 50% in stage III. The extent of spread of cancer is limited in the majority of cases to involvement of pelvic structures, with perhaps 5% causing death rapidly by metastases.[39] The low frequency of distant spread may be partially a result of death from ureteral obstruction, hemorrhage, infection, or intercurrent disease before metastatic involvement of vital organs. Immune host factors might also be operative in preventing spread to distant body sites. Although metastases are uncommon, they have been encountered with increasing frequency in patients previously treated for advanced cervical carcinoma. They can occur in a large number of tissues, although the majority are found in the lungs and liver.[39] Local extension of the tumor is mainly in a lateral direction, rather than vertically. The ureters are most frequently affected, the bladder is less commonly involved, and intrinsic rectal involvement is unusual.

Squamous-cell carcinomas comprise over 90% of cervical cancers; adenocarcinomas and rare tumors, such as sarcomas, comprise the remainder. The squamous tumors can be differentiated into three histological grades: grade I, keratinizing type; grade II, large-cell nonkeratinizing; grade III, small-cell cancer.[103] These types differ in their frequency in that grade II is more common than grade I, which in turn is more common than grade III. Their location in the cervix and their prognosis may differ, although data on these points are still limited.

8.2. Serological Features

Some evidence has been obtained on the ability to detect circulating cervical-cancer-tumor-associated antigens in the sera of women with invasive cancers, less frequently in precancerous lesions.[22,46]

Since a small percentage of control women were also positive, attempts are currently being made to purify these antigens. With the use of an immunofluorescence test, the sera of women with cervical cancer have also been noted to react with cervical cells in higher titers than controls.[22]

As noted earlier, some correlation has been found between the progression or successful therapy of cervical cancer and antibodies to certain HSV-asociated tumor antigens (Table 1). A correlation with progression of disease has also been noted between increasing HSV-2 neutralizing antibody titers and decreasing complement-antibody and antibody-dependent cell-mediated cytotoxic titers.[23-25,120,124] In addition, progressively increasing lymphocyte transformations, using mitomycin-treated HSV-2-transformed human cells, were noted from normal subjects to those with invasive cancer.[124] Progressively rising plasma levels of carcinoembryonic antigen (CEA) predicted recurrent disease in over 80% of women whose tumors stained positively for CEA.[128]

9. Therapy and Control

The possible approaches to control of cervical cancer include (1) eradication of the causal agent(s); (2) prevention of transmission of the disease, whether the causal agent(s) is known or not; and (3) early detection of the disease and treatment, preferably in its preinvasive form. Of these three approaches, the most desirable in the long run is the first. As regards the second approach, on the basis of the epidemiological evidence, it is likely that sexual abstention could prevent cervical cancer, but that approach is not very acceptable. The use of obstructive forms of contraception, such as condoms, does not appear to be very practical or to be based on sufficient evidence of success at present.

The third approach, which is the one currently employed, is associated with a great number of problems. First, it requires that all women, from adolescence on, have repeat cytological screening at frequent intervals. One of the major problems is that of obtaining Pap smears on those women who are at highest risk of developing cervical cancer. Since such women are the least likely to seek preventive services, this approach requires a great amount of public education and community effort.

A second problem is the enormous cost of routine screening programs, which includes the cost of educating qualified personnel. This cost, in the long run, would probably be less than that associated with the hospitalization and treatment costs for invasive carcinomas and, of course, does not enter into the discussion of the worth of a human life. A third problem is that of the need of adequate follow-up in mobile populations for fear of progression to more serious forms. In this regard, even though cervical conization or cryotherapy may be sufficient to treat severe dysplasia or CIS in most cases, the problems of adequate follow-up have forced many physicians to prefer hysterectomy for these lesions.[36] One suggested scheme for the "detection/follow-up/treatment/follow-up" approach has been described.[85] This scheme emphasizes all the problems at the human level—as regards necessary health personnel and patient education—associated with its satisfactory accomplishment. To obviate the difficulties and cost of yearly Papanicolaou smears, the American Cancer Society has recently proposed that screening can be reduced to every 3 years in women with two previous negative Papanicolaou smears. We believe, however, that on the basis of current evidence, women detected with genital herpes comprise a high-risk group and that annual screening should be continued in such cases. It might also be possible that a fluorescent-activated cell sorter to identify cervical neoplastic cells using HSV antigenic markers could facilitate screening.[12]

The therapy for invasive cancer is still relatively individualized and consists of various forms of surgical and radiological treatment. These methods can be found in standard textbooks. The value of such treatment is borne out by earlier data that indicated that the 5-year survival in untreated cases was 5%, whereas today the overall 5-year survival is around 40–50%.[39] The survival rates are greatly dependent on the stage of the disease at which the diagnosis is first made. Thus, intraepithelial cancer is virtually 100% curable, and the 5-year survival of patients in stage I is around 90%. Survival rates decrease with each stage, to reach 5–10% for stage IV cases. Adjunctive chemotherapy and immunotherapy, including use of interferon, which are under investigation in various centers, is still of undetermined value.[127]

Besides its importance in relation to the overall concept of the possible viral causation of human cancers, the studies on the relationship of HSV to cervical cancer have had as their final goal the possibility that preventing the viral infection could prevent the cancer. Indeed, such a demonstration would provide the best evidence of causality.

As noted in Chapter 13, HSV vaccines are currently under development. We have suggested elsewhere[80] the advantages of a prospective study that could provide valuable information regarding both the possible effectiveness of HSV vaccines and the role of genital herpes in cervical carcinogenesis. Such an investigation should be able to determine: (1) how frequently cervical neoplasia developed in women who do not acquire HSV antibodies compared to those with prior HSV-1 experience and those who acquire a primary genital HSV-2 infection and (2) whether the HSV vaccine protects women from developing significant cervical neoplasia. In addition, the role of the vaccine in preventing or decreasing the severity of the initial or recurrent genital infection can be determined, and the possible role of other suspect candidates could also be evaluated in such a prospective study.

10. Unresolved Problems

10.1. Control of Cervical Cancer with Available Knowledge

Control of cervical cancer requires a very large effort in education of the public and of health professionals, as well as a great outlay of support on a continuous rather than a spotty basis for routine cytological screening. The development of serological tests to define women at particular risk for developing cervical cancer or to determine progression or recurrence of the cancer would be most valuable.

10.2. Establishing a Causal Role of Herpes Simplex Virus in Human Carcinogenesis

Two types of approaches appear necessary to establish that HSV plays a causal role in human carcinogenesis. The most likely to provide the firmest evidence of a causal role of HSV in human carcinogenesis is the vaccine approach mentioned above. Improved knowledge of the molecular and genetic aspects of the viruses could provide better types of vaccines. Improvement of our knowledge of immunological responses to HSV and mechanisms of latency and greater application of animal models would greatly assist such an objective.

The second approach is a continued effort to employ every discipline, from the molecular to the epidemiological, to provide evidence so overwhelming that a causal relationship between HSV and cervical neoplasia becomes as likely as that for cigarette smoking and lung cancer. Confirmation of many of the preliminary findings, as noted in Fig. 1, is badly needed, i.e., the presence of viral genome and viral-specified antigens in the suspect human cancers and not in control tissues and the finding of a high frequency of antibodies or cell-mediated immune responses to special well-characterized HSV antigens in women with cervical neoplasia as compared to a well-controlled group of women without cancer. In addition, the results of prospective studies in humans would provide important support. The delineation of the specific part(s) of the viral genome related to oncogenicity should provide extremely important information needed to resolve these problems.

ACKNOWLEDGMENTS

The research reported herein was supported by grants from the American Cancer Society and the National Institutes of Health.

11. References

1. ADAM, E., KAUFMAN, R. H., MELNICK, J. L., LEVY, A. H., AND RAWLS, W. E., Seroepidemiologic studies of herpesvirus type 2 and carcinoma of the cervix. III. Houston, Texas, *Am. J. Epidemiol.* **96:**427–442 (1972).
2. ADAM, E., RAWLS, W. E., AND MELNICK, J. L., The association of herpesvirus type 2 infection and cervical cancer, *Prev. Med.* **3:**122–141 (1974).
3. ADELUSI, B., OSUNKOYA, B., AND FAGIYI, A., Herpes type 2 virus antigens in human cervical carcinoma, *Obstet. Gynecol.* **47:**545–548 (1976).
4. ADELUSI, B., NAIB, Z., MUTHER, J., AND NAHMIAS, A., Epidemiological studies relating genital herpes simplex virus (HSV) infection with cervical neoplasia—an update, in: *The Human Herpesviruses: An Interdisciplinary Perspective* (A. NAHMIAS, W. DOWDLE, AND R. SCHINAZI, eds.), p. 627, Elsevier/North-Holland, New York, 1981.

5. ALEXANDER, E. R., Possible etiologies of cancer of the cervix other than herpesvirus, *Cancer Res.* **33**:1485–1496 (1973).

6. ANZAI, T., DREESMAN, G. R., COURTNEY, R. J., ADAM, E., RAWLS, W. E., AND BINYESH-MELNICK, M., Antibody to herpes simplex virus type 2-induced nonstructural proteins in women with cervical cancer and in control groups, *J. Natl. Cancer Inst.* **54**:1051–1059 (1975).

7. ARSEKANIS, M., GEORGION, G. M., WELSH, J. K., CAUCHI, M. N., AND MAY, J. T., Ag-4 complement fixing antibodies in cervical cancer and herpes infected patients using local herpes simplex virus type 2, *Int. J. Cancer* **25**:67–71 (1979).

8. AURELIAN, L., ROYSTON, I., AND DAVIS, H. J., Antibody to genital herpes simplex virus: Association with cervical atypia and carcinoma *in situ*, *J. Natl. Cancer Inst.* **45**:455–464 (1970).

9. AURELIAN, L., Virions and antigens of herpes virus type 2 in cervical carcinoma, *Cancer Res.* **33**:1539–1547 (1973).

10. AURELIAN, L., STRANDBERG, J. D., AND MARCUS, R. L., Neutralization, immunofluorescence and complement fixation tests in identification of antibody to a herpesvirus type 2-induced, tumor-specific antigen in sera from squamous cervical carcinoma: Immunology of cancer, *Prog. Exp. Tumor Res.* **19**:165–181 (1974).

11. AURELIAN, L., SMITH, F., AND CORNISH, J. D., IgM antibody to a tumour-associated antigen (Ag-4) induced by herpes simplex virus type 2: Its use in location of the antigen in infected cells, *J. Natl. Cancer Inst.* **56**:471–477 (1976).

12. AURELIAN, L., GRUPTA, P., FROST, J., ROSENSHEIM, N., SMITH, C., TYRER, H., MANTIONE, J., AND ALBRIGHT, C., Fluorescence-activated separation of cervical abnormal cells using herpesvirus antigenic markers, *Anal. Quant. Cytol. J.* **1**:89–102 (1979).

13. BARINGER, J. R., Herpes simplex virus infection of nervous tissue in animals and man, *Prog. Med. Virol.* **20**:1–25 (1975).

14. BELL, R. B., AURELIAN, L., AND COHEN, G. H., Proteins of herpesvirus type 2. IV. Leukocyte inhibition responses to type common antigen(s) in cervix cancer and recurrent herpetic infections, *Cell. Immunol.* **41**:86–102 (1978).

15. BEST, J. M., MENDIS, L. N., VESTERGAARD, B. F., AND BANATVALA, J. E., Geographical study of antibodies to membrane antigens of HSV-2 infected cells, HSV-2 specific antibodies and total immunoglobulin levels in patients with cervical cancer, in: *The Human Herpesviruses: An Interdisciplinary Perspective* (A. NAHMIAS, W. DOWDLE, AND R. SCHINAZI, eds.), pp. 628–629, Elsevier/North-Holland, New York, 1981.

16. BOCK, J. E., Steroid contraception and the risk of neoplasia, *Ugeskr. Laeg.* **140**:2596–2597 (1978).

17. BOLTEN, K. A., Practical colposcopy in early cervical and vaginal cancer, *Clin. Obstet. Gynecol.* **101**(4):808–837 (1967).

18. BRODERS, A. C., Carcinoma *in situ* contrasted with benign penetrating epithelium, *J. Am. Med. Assoc.* **99**:1670–1674 (1932).

19. CAMACHO, A., AND SPEAR, P. G., Transformation of hamster embryo fibroblasts by a specific fragment of the herpes simplex virus genome, *Cell* **15**:993–1002 (1978).

20. CAMERON, I. R., AND MACNAB, C. M., Transformation studies using defined fragments of herpes simplex virus type 2, in: *The Human Herpesviruses: An Interdisciplinary Perspective* (A. NAHMIAS, W. DOWDLE, AND R. SCHINAZI, eds.), p. 634, Elsevier/North-Holland, New York, 1981.

21. CATALANO, L. W., JR., AND JOHNSON, L. D., Herpesvirus antibody and carcinoma *in situ* of the cervix, *J. Am. Med. Assoc.* **217**:447–450 (1971).

22. CHIANG, W. T., WEI, P. Y., AND ALEXANDER, E. R., Circulatory and cellular immune responses to squamous cell carcinoma of the uterine cervix, *Am. J. Obstet. Gynecol.* **126**:116–121 (1976).

23. CHRISTENSON, B., AND ESPMARK, A., Long-term follow-up studies on herpes simplex antibodies in the course of cervical cancer. II. Antibodies to surface antigen of herpes simplex virus infected cells, *Int. J. Cancer* **17**:318–325 (1976).

24. CHRISTENSON, B., Antibody-dependent cell-mediated cytotoxicity to herpes simplex virus type 2 infected target cells in the course of cervical carcinoma, *Am. J. Epidemiol.* **108**:125–135 (1978).

25. CHRISTENSON, B., Anticomplement immunofluorescence (ACIF) tests and mixed haemadsorption (MH) tests on HSV-2 transformed cells and on cervical cancer cells with sera from cervical cancer patients, in: *The Human Herpesviruses: An Interdisciplinary Perspective* (A. NAHMIAS, W. DOWDLE, AND R. SCHINAZI, eds.), p. 632, Elsevier/North-Holland, New York, 1981.

26. CHRISTOPHERSON, W. M., Concepts of genesis and development in early cervical neoplasia, *Obstet. Gynecol. Surv.* **24**(2):842–850 (1969).

27. COPPLESON, M., AND REID, B., *Preclinical Carcinoma of the Cervix Uteri*, Pergamon Press, Oxford, 1967.

28. DISAIA, P. J., SINKOVICS, J. G., RUTLEDGE, F. N., AND SMITH, J. P., Cell-mediated immunity to human malignant cells, *Am. J. Obstet. Gyncol.* **114**:979–989 (1972).

29. DREESMAN, G. R., BUREK, J., ADAM, E., KAUFMAN, R. H., MELNICK, J. L., POWELL, K. L., AND PURIFOY, D. J., Expression of herpesvirus-induced antigens in human cervical cancer, *Nature (London)* **283**:591–593 (1980).

30. DUENAS, A., ADAM, E., MELNICK, J. L., AND RAWLS, W. E., Herpesvirus type 2 in a prostitute population, *Am. J. Epidemiol.* **95**:483–498 (1972).
31. EGLIN, R. P., MACLEAN, A. B., SHARP, F., MACNAB, J. C. M., CLEMENTS, J. B., AND WILKIE, N. M., The detection of herpes virus coded material in neoplastic cervical tissue, in: *The Human Herpesviruses: An Interdisciplinary Perspective* (A. NAHMIAS, W. DOWDLE, AND R. SCHINAZI, eds.), pp. 630–631, Elsevier/North-Holland, New York, 1981.
32. FRANKLIN, E. W., III, AND RUTLEDGE, F. D., Epidemiology of epidermoid carcinoma of the vulva, *Obstet. Gynecol.* **39**:165–172 (1972).
33. FRENKEL, N., Defective interfering herpesviruses, in: *The Human Herpesviruses: An Interdisciplinary Perspective* (A. NAHMIAS, W. DOWDLE, AND R. SCHINAZI, eds.), pp. 91–120, Elsevier/North-Holland, New York, 1981.
34. FRENKEL, N., ROIZMAN, B., CASSAI, E., AND NAHMIAS, A., A DNA fragment of herpes simplex 2 and its transcription in human cervical cancer tissue, *Proc. Natl. Acad. Sci. U.S.A.* **69**:3784–3789 (1972).
35. FRENKEL, N., LOCKER, H., COX, B., ROIZMAN, B., AND RAPP, F., Herpes simplex virus DNA in transformed cells, *J. Virol.* **18**:885–893 (1976).
36. FRICK, H. C., Management of non-invasive carcinoma of the cervix, *Surg. Clin. North Am.* **58**:55–60 (1978).
37. FUCCILLO, D. A., SEVER, J. L., MODER, F. L., CHEN, T. C., CATALANO, L. W., AND JOHNSON, L. D., Cytomegalovirus antibody in patients with carcinoma of the uterine cervix, *Obstet. Gyncol.* **38**:599–601 (1971).
38. GALL, S. A., AND HAINES, H., Cervical carcinoma antigens and the relationship to HSV-2, *Gynecol. Oncol.* **2**:451–459 (1974).
39. GUSBERG, S. B., AND FRICK, H. C., II, *Corscaden's Gynecologic Cancer*, 4th ed., Williams & Wilkins, Baltimore, 1970.
40. HEISE, E. R., KUCERA, L. S., RABEN, M., AND HOMESLEY, H., Serological response patterns to herpes virus type-1 early and late antigens in cervical carcinoma patients, *Cancer Res.* **39**:4022–4026 (1979).
41. HOLLINSHEAD, A. C., AND TARRO, G., Soluble membrane antigens of lip and cervical carcinomas: Reactivity with antibody for herpes-virus nonvirion antigens, *Science* **179**:698–700 (1973).
42. HOLLINSHEAD, A. C., LEE, O., CHRETIEN, P. B., TARPLEY, J. L., RAWLS, W. E., AND ADAM, E., Antibodies to herpesvirus nonvirion antigens in squamous carcinomas, *Science* **182**:713–715 (1973).
43. HOLLINSHEAD, A. C., CHRETIEN, P. B., LEE, O'B., TARPLEY, J. L., KERNEY, S. E., SILVERMAN, N. A., AND ALEXANDER, J. C., *In vivo* and *in vitro* measurements of the relationship of human squamous carcinomas to herpes simplex virus tumor-associated antigens, *Cancer Res.* **36**:821–828 (1976).

44. HOLLINSHEAD, A., TARRO, G., CHRETIEN, P. B., AND RAWLS, W., Herpes simplex associated tumor antigens, in: *Viral Immunodiagnosis* (E. KURSTAK AND R. MORRISETT, eds.), pp. 301–317, Academic Press, New York, 1974.
45. IBRAHIM, A., RAY, M., McGAW, J., BROWN, R., AND NAHMIAS, A. J., Common antigens of herpes simplex virus-associated hamster tumors and human cervical cancer, *Proc. Soc. Exp. Biol. Med.* **152**:343–347 (1976).
46. IBRAHIM, A. N., ROBINSON, R. A., MARR, L., ABDELAL, A., AND NAHMIAS, A., Tumor-associated antigens in cervical cancer tissues and in sera of cervix and head and neck cancer patients, *J. Natl. Cancer Inst.* **63**:319–323 (1979).
47. ITO, H., TSUTSUI, F., KURIHARA, S., AKABAYASHI, T., TOBE, T. AND NISHIMURA, C., Serum antibodies to herpesvirus early antigens in patients with cervical carcinoma determined by anticomplement immunofluorescence technique, *Int. J. Cancer* **18**:557–563 (1976).
48. JANDA, Z., KANDA, J., VONKA, V., AND SVOBODA, B., A study of herpes simplex type 2 antibody status in groups of patients with cervical neoplasia in Czechoslovakia, *Int. J. Cancer* **12**:626–630 (1973).
49. JEANSSON, S., AND MOLIN, L., Prospective study of clinically detected genital herpes in Sweden, Presented at the International Cancer Congress, Florence, Italy, 1974.
50. JOHNSON, L. D., The histopathological approach to early cervical neoplasia, *Obstet. Gynol. Surv.* **24**(2):735–767 (1969).
51. JOSEY, W. E., NAHMIAS, A. J., AND NAIB, Z. M., Genital infection with type 2 herpesvirus hominis: Present knowledge and possible relation to cervical cancer, *Am. J. Obstet. Gynecol.* **101**:718–729 (1968).
52. KAWANA, T., CORNISH, J. D., SMITH, M. F., AND AURELIAN, L., Frequency of antibody to a virus-induced, tumor-associated antigen (Ag-4) in Japanese sera from patients with cervical cancer and controls, *Cancer Res.* **36**:1910–1914 (1976).
53. KESSLER, I. I., Perspectives on the epidemiology of cervical cancer with special reference to the herpesvirus hypothesis, *Cancer Res.* **34**:1091–1110 (1974).
54. KIMURA, S., FLANNERY, V. L., LEVY, B., AND SCHAFFER, P. A., Oncogenic transformation of primary hamster cells by herpes simplex virus type 2 (HSV-2) and HSV-2 temperature sensitive mutant, *Int. J. Cancer* **15**:786–798 (1975).
55. KOENIG, U. D., AND MULLER, N., Cervical carcinoma and HLA-antigens, First International Symposium on HLA and Diseases, INSERM, Paris 228 (1976).
56. KOENIG, U. D., MULLER, N., AND SCHNEWEIS, K. E., Herpes-simplex type-2 antibodies and HLA-B12 in cervical cancer, *Lancet* **2**:857 (1976).
57. LILLIENFELD, A. M., LEVINE, M. L., AND KESSLER, I. I.,

Cancer in the United States, Harvard University Press, Cambridge, 1972.

58. MAITLAND, N. J. BUSUTTIL, A., LUDGATE, S. M., SMART, G., AND JONES, K. W., *In situ* hybridizations using herpes simplex virus type 2 DNA to probe for virus-specific RNA in tissue biopsies from patients with abnormal cervical cytology, in: *The Human Herpesviruses: An Interdisciplinary Perspective* (A. NAHMIAS, W. DOWDLE, AND R. SCHINAZI, eds.), p. 631, Elsevier/North-Holland, New York, 1981.

59. MARTINEZ, I., Relationship of squamous cell carcinoma of the cervix uteri to squamous cell carcinoma of the penis, *Cancer* **24**:777–780 (1969).

60. MATSON, D. O., ADAM, E., MELNICK, J. L., AND DREESMAN, G. R., Prevalence of antibodies to herpes simplex virus (HSV) measured with a type-specific radioimmunoassay in cervical neoplasia-case control studies, in: *The Human Herpesviruses: An Interdisciplinary Perspective* (A. NAHMIAS, W. DOWDLE, AND R. SCHINAZI), p. 628, Elsevier/North-Holland, New York, 1981.

61. MCDONALD, A. D., WILLIAMS, M. C., MANFREDA, J., AND WEST, R., Neutralizing antibodies to herpesvirus types 1 and 2 in carcinoma of the cervix, carcinoma *in situ* and cervical dysplasia, *Am. J. Epidemiol.* **100**:130–135 (1974).

62. MCDOUGALL, J. K., AND GALLOWAY, D. A., Detection of viral nucleic acid sequences using *in situ* hybridization, in: *Persistent Viruses* (J. G. STEVENS, ed.), Symposia on Molecular and Cellular Biology. Academic Press, New York, 1978.

63. MEISELS, A., FORTIN, R., AND ROY, M., Condylomatous lesions of the cervix. II. Cytologic, colposcopic and histopathologic study, *Acta Cytol* **21**:379–390 (1977).

64. MELNICK, J. L., AND RAWLS, W. E., Herpesvirus type 2 and cervical carcinoma, *Am. J. Epidemiol.* **100**:130–135 (1974).

65. MELNICK, J. L., ADAM, E., AND RAWLS, W. E., The causative role of herpesvirus type 2 in cervical cancer, *Cancer* **34**:1375–1385 (1974).

66. MELNICK, J. L., AND ADAM, E., Epidemiological approaches to determining whether herpesvirus is the etiological agent of cervical cancer, *Prog. Exp. Tumor Res.* **21**:49–69 (1978).

67. MELNICK, J. L., ADAM, E., LEWIS, R., AND KAUFMAN, R. H., Cervical cancer cell lines containing herpesvirus markers, *Intervirology* **12**:111–114 (1979).

68. MINHU, C., YU, S., QIDA, Z., AND YOUSIN, C. Experimental studies on induction of cervical carcinoma in mice by genital herpes simplex virus, in: *The Human Herpesviruses: An Interdisciplinary Perspective* (A. NAHMIAS, W. DOWDLE, AND R. SCHINAZI, eds.), p. 633, Elsevier/North-Holland, New York, 1981.

69. MORTON, W. E., HORTON, H. B., AND BAKER, H. W., Effects of socioeconomic status on incidences of three sexually-transmitted diseases, *Sex. Transm. Dis.* **6**:206–210 (1979).

70. MUÑOZ, N., Discussion on general aspects of cervical cancer, *Cancer Res.* **33**:1382–1384 (1973).

71. MUÑOZ, N., Effect of herpesvirus type 2 and hormonal imbalance on the uterine cervix of the mouse, *Cancer Res.* **33**:1504–1508 (1973).

72. NAHMIAS, A. J., AND DOWDLE, W. R., Antigenic and biologic differences in herpesvirus hominis, *Prog. Med. Virol.* **10**:110–159 (1968).

73. NAHMIAS, A. J., JOSEY, W. E., NAIB, Z. M., LUCE, C. F., AND GUEST, B. A., Antibodies to herpesvirus hominis types 1 and 2 in humans. II. Women with cervical cancer, *Am. J. Epidemiol.* **91**:547–552 (1970).

74. NAHMIAS, A. J., NAIB, Z. M., AND JOSEY, W. E., Herpesvirus hominis type 2 infection—association with cervical cancer and perinatal disease, *Perspect. Virol.* **7**:73–89 (1970).

75. NAHMIAS, A. J., NAIB, Z. M., JOSEY, W. E., MURPHY, F. A., AND LUCE, C. F., Sarcomas after inoculation of newborn hamsters with herpesvirus hominis type 2 strains, *Proc. Soc. Exp. Biol. Med.* **134**:1065–1069 (1970).

76. NAHMIAS, A. J., NAIB, Z. M., JOSEY, W. E., FRANKLIN, E., AND JENKINS, R., Prospective studies of the association of genital herpes simplex infection and cervical anaplasia, *Cancer Res.* **33**:1491–1497 (1973).

77. NAHMIAS, A. J., The evolution (evovirology) of herpesviruses, in: *Viruses, Evolution and Cancer* (E. KURSTAK AND K. MARAMOROSCH, eds.), pp. 605–624, Academic Press, New York, 1974.

78. NAHMIAS, A. J., NAIB, Z. M., AND JOSEY, W. E., Epidemiological studies relating genital herpetic infection to cervical carcinoma, *Cancer Res.* **34**:1111–1117 (1974).

79. NAHMIAS, A., AND SAWANABORI, S., The genital herpes–cervical cancer hypothesis—10 years later, *Prog. Exp. Tumor Res.* **21**:117–139 (1978).

80. NAHMIAS, A., AND NORRILD, B., The oncogenic potential of herpes simplex viruses and their association with cervical neoplasia, in: *Herpesviruses and Cancer* (F. RAPP, ed.), pp. 25–46, CRC Press, Boca Raton, Florida, 1980.

81. NAIB, Z. M., NAHMIAS, A. J., AND JOSEY, W. E., Cytology and histopathology of cervical herpes simplex infection, *Cancer* **19**:1026–1031 (1966).

82. NAIB, Z. M., NAHMIAS, A. J., JOSEY, W. E., AND ZAKI, S. A., Relation of cytohistopathology of genital herpesvirus infection to cervical anaplasia, *Cancer Res.* **33**:1452–1463 (1973).

83. NALICK, R. H., DISAIA, P. J., REA, T. H., AND MORROW, M. H., Immunological response in gynecologic malignancy as demonstrated by the delayed hypersensitivity reaction: Clinical correlations, *Am. J. Obstet. Gynecol.* **118**:393–405 (1974).

84. NATIONAL CANCER INSTITUTE, International Cancer Research Data, Bank, Special Listing 322, Current Cancer Research on Gynecological Cancer, Feb. 22, 1980.

85. NELSON, J. H., JR., AND HALL, J. E., Detection, diagnostic evaluation, and treatment of dysplasia and early carcinoma of the cervix, *Ca.* 20:150–163 (1970).

86. NOTTER, M. F. D., AND DOCHERTY, J. J., Comparative diagnostic aspects of herpes simplex tumor-associated antigens, *J. Natl. Cancer Inst.* 57:483–488 (1976).

87. ORY, H., CONGER, B., RICHART, R., AND BARRON, B., Relation of type 2 herpesvirus antibodies to cervical neoplasia in Barbados, West Indies, 1971, *Obstet. Gynecol.* 43:901–904 (1974).

88. PACSA, A. S., KUMMERLANDER, L., PEJTSIK, B., AND DORSITS, G., Herpesvirus antibodies and antigens in patients with cervical anaplasia and in controls, *J. Natl. Cancer Inst.* 55:775–781 (1975).

89. PACSA, A. S., KUMMERLANDER, L., PEJTSIK, B., KRIMMER, K., AND PALI, K., Herpes simplex virus-specific antigens in exfoliated cervical cells from women with and without cervical anaplasia, *Cancer Res.* 36:2130–2138 (1976).

90. PALMER, A. E., LONDON, W. T., NAHMIAS, A. J., NAIB, Z. M., TUNCA, J., FUCCILLO, D. A., ELLENBERG, J. H., AND SEVER, J. L., A preliminary report on investigation of oncogenic potential of herpes simplex virus type 2 in *Cebus* monkeys, *Cancer Res.* 36:807–809 (1976).

91. PAPANICOLAOU, G. N., AND TRAUT, H. F., *Diagnosis of Uterine Cancer by the Vaginal Smear*, Commonwealth Fund, New York, 1943.

92. PARK, M., LONSDALE, C. M., TIMBURG, M. C., SUBAK-SHARPE, J. H., AND MACNAB, J. C. M., Genetic retrieval of information from herpes simplex virus transformed rat cells by recombination with superinfecting temperature sensitive mutants, in: *The Human Herpesviruses: An Interdisciplinary Perspective* (A. NAHMIAS, W. DOWDLE, AND R. SCHINAZI, eds.), p. 635, Elsevier/North-Holland, New York, 1981.

93. PEARSON, G. R., AND AURELIAN, L., Immunology of herpesvirus-associated cancers, in: *The Human Herpesviruses: An Interdisciplinary Perspective* (A. NAHMIAS, W. DOWDLE, AND R. SCHINAZI, eds.), pp. 297–308, Elsevier/North-Holland, New York, 1981.

94. PLUMMER, G., Serological comparison of the herpesviruses, *Br. J. Exp. Pathol.* 45:135–141 (1964).

95. PLUMMER, G., A review of the identification and titration of antibodies to herpes simplex viruses type 1 and type 2 in human sera, *Cancer Res.* 33:1469–1476 (1973).

96. PUND, E. R., AND AUERBACH, S. H., Preinvasive carcinoma of the cervix uteri, *J. Am. Med. Assoc.* 131:960–963 (1946).

97. RAPP, F. (ed.), *Oncogenic Herpesviruses*, CRC Press, Boca Raton, Florida, 1980.

98. RAPP, F., AND REED, C., Experimental evidence for the oncogenic potential of herpes simplex virus, *Cancer Res.* 36:800–806 (1976).

99. RAWLS, W. E., TOMPKINS, W. A. F., AND MELNICK, J. L., The association of herpesvirus type 2 and carcinoma of the uterine cervix, *Am. J. Epidemiol.* 89:547–554 (1969).

100. RAWLS, W. E., ADAM, E., AND MELNICK, J. L., An analysis of seroepidemiological studies of herpesvirus type 2 and carcinoma of the cervix, *Cancer Res.* 33:1477–1482 (1973).

101. RAWLS, W. E., BACCHETTI, S., AND GRAHAM, F. L., Relation of herpes simplex viruses to human malignancies, in: *Current Topics in Microbiology and Immunology*, Vol. 77 (W. A. BASLE, W. HENLE, P. H. HOFSCHNEIDER, et al., eds.), pp. 71–85, Springer-Verlag, Berlin, 1977.

102. RAWLS, W. R., AND CAMPIONE-PICCARDO, J., Epidemiology of herpes simplex virus type 1 and type 2, in: *The Human Herpesviruses: An Interdisciplinary Perspective* (A. NAHMIAS, W. DOWDLE, AND R. SCHINAZI, eds.), pp. 137–152, Elsevier/North-Holland, New York, 1981.

103. REAGAN, J. W., AND WENTZ, W. B., Genesis of carcinoma of the uterine cervix, *Clin. Obstet. Gynecol.* 10(4):883–921 (1967).

104. RICHART, R. M., Natural history of cervical intraepithelial neoplasia, *Clin. Obstet. Gynecol.* 10(4):748–784 (1967).

105. RIGONI-STERN, D., Fatti statistici relativi alle malattie cancrose che servirono di base alle poche cose dette dal Dott. G. Servire, *Prog. Pathol. Ter. Ser.* 2:507–517 (1842).

106. ROIZMAN, B. R., The structure and isomerization of herpes simplex virus genomes, *Cell* 16:481–494 (1979).

107. ROTKIN, I. D., A comparison review of key epidemiological studies in cervical cancer related to current searches for transmissible agents, *Cancer Res.* 33:1353–1367 (1973).

108. ROYSTON, I., AND AURELIAN, L., The association of genital herpesvirus with cervical atypia and carcinoma *in situ*, *Am. J. Epidemiol.* 91:531–538 (1970).

109. SAWANABORI, S., ASHMAN, R. B., NAHMIAS, A. J., BENIGNO, B. B., AND LA VIA, M. F., Rosette formation and inhibition in cervical dysplasia and carcinoma *in situ*, *Cancer Res.* 37:4332–4335 (1977).

110. SCHACHTER, J., HILL, E. C., KING, E. B., COLEMAN, V. R., JONES, P., AND MEYERS, K. F., Chlamydial infection in women with cervical dysplasia, *Am. J. Obstet. Gynecol.* 123:753–757 (1975).

111. SCHNEWEIS, K. E., Serolgische Untersuchungen zur Typendifferenzierung des *Herpesvirus hominis*, *Z. Immunitaetsforsch.* 124:24–48 (1962).

112. SCHNEWEIS, K. E., HAAG, A., LEHMKOSTER, A., AND KAENIG, V., Seroimmunological investigations in patients with cervical cancer: Higher rates of HSV-2 an-

tibodies than in syphilis patients and evidence of IgM antibodies to an early HSV-2 antigen, in: *Oncogenesis and Herpesvirus*, Vol. 2 (G. DE-THÉ, M. A. EPSTEIN, AND H. ZUR HAUSEN, eds.), pp. 208–210, International Agency for Research on Cancer, Lyon, France, 1975.

113. SEER, Cancer Incidence and Mortality in the United States (1973–1976), DHEW Publ. No. (NIH) 78-1837, 1979.

114. SETH, P., RAWLS, W. E., DUFF, R., RAPP, F., ADAM, E., AND MELNICK, J. L., Antigenic differences between isolates of herpesvirus type 2, *Intervirology* **3**:1–14 (1974).

115. SETH, P., AND BALACHANDRAN, A., Elution of herpes simplex virus-specific antibodies from squamous cell carcinoma of uterine cervix, in: *The Human Herpesviruses: An Interdisciplinary Perspective* (A. NAHMIAS, W. DOWDLE, AND R. SCHINAZI, eds.), pp. 629–630, Elsevier/North-Holland, New York, 1981.

116. SINGER, A., REID, B. L., AND COPPLESON, M., A hypothesis: The role of a high-risk male in the etiology of cervical carcinoma, *Am. J. Obstet. Gynecol.* **126**:110–115 (1976).

117. SKINNER, G. R., Transformation of primary hamster embryo fibroblasts by type 2 herpes simplex virus: Evidence for a "hit and run" mechanism, *Br. J. Exp. Pathol.* **57**(4):361–376 (1976).

118. SKINNER, G. R. B., WHITNEY, J. E., AND HARTLEY, C., Prevalence of type-specific antibody against type 1 and type 2 herpes simplex virus in women with abnormal cervical cytology: Evidence towards pre-pubertal vaccination of sero-negative female subjects, *Arch. Virol.* **54**:211–221 (1977).

119. SPRECHER-GOLDBERGER, S., THIRY, L., LEFEBVRE, N., DEKEGEL, D., AND DEHALLEUX, F., Complement-fixation antibodies to adenovirus-associated viruses, adenoviruses, cytomegaloviruses and herpes simplex viruses in patients with tumors and in control individuals, *Am. J. Epidemiol.* **94**:351–358 (1971).

120. SPRECHER-GOLDBERGER, S., THIRY, L., GOULD, I., FASSIN, Y., AND GOMPEL, C., Increasing antibody titers to herpes simplex virus type 2 during follow-up of women with cervical dysplasia, *Am. J. Epidemiol.* **97**:103–110 (1973).

121. SPJUT, H. J., AND FECHNER, R. E., Cytologic diagnosis of cervical dysplasia and carcinoma *in situ*, *Clin. Obstet. Gynecol.* **10**(4):785–807 (1967).

122. STAFL, A., FRIEDRICH, E. G., AND MATTINGLY, R. F., Detection of cervical neoplasia: Reducing the risk of error, *Ca* **24**(1):22–30 (1974).

123. TAKASUGI, M., TERASAKI, P. L., HENDERSON, B., MICKEY, M. R., MENCK, H., AND THOMPSON, R. W., HLA antigens in solid tumors, *Cancer Res.* **33**:648–649 (1973).

124. THIRY, L., SPRECHER-GOLDBERGER, S., FASSIN, Y., GOULD, I., GOMPEL, C., PESTIAU, J., AND DEHALLEUX, F., Variations of cytotoxic antibodies to cells with herpes

simplex virus antigens in women with progesssing or regressing cancerous lesions of the cervix, *Am. J. Epidemiol.* **100**:251–261 (1974).

125. THIRY, L., SPRECHER-GOLDBERGER, S., HANNECART-POLORNI, E., GOULD, I., AND BOSSENS, M., Specific non-IgG antibodies and cell-mediated responses to herpes simplex virus antigens in women with cervical carcinoma, *Cancer Res.* **37**(5):1301–1306 (1977).

126. THOMAS, D. B., AND RAWLS, W. E., Relationship of herpes simplex virus type-2 antibodies and squamous dysplasia to cervical carcinoma *in situ*, *Cancer* **42**:2716–2725 (1978).

127. VAN NAGELL, J. R., DONALDSON, E. S., AND GAY, E. C., Evaluation and treatment of patients with invasive cervical cancer, *Surg. Clin. North Am.* **58**:67–85 (1978).

128. VAN NAGELL, J. R., DONALDSON, E. S., GAY, E. C., HUDSON, S., SHARKEY, R. M., PRIMUS, F. J., POWELL, D. F., AND GOLDENBERG, D. M., Carcinoembryonic antigen in carcinoma of the uterine cervix, *Cancer* **44**:944–948 (1979).

129. VESTERGAARD, B. F., HORNSLETH, A., AND PEDERSEN, S. M., Occurrence of herpes and adenovirus antibodies in patients with carcinoma of the cervix uteri, *Cancer* **30**:68–74 (1972).

130. VONKA, V., KANKA, J., JELINEK, J., SUCHANEK, A., HAVRANKOVA, A., AND DOMORAZKOVA, E., Prospective study of the cervical carcinoma: Progress report, in: *The Human Herpesviruses: An Interdisciplinary Perspective* (A. NAHMIAS, W. DOWDLE, AND R. SCHINAZI, eds.), pp. 627–628, Elsevier/North-Holland, New York, 1981.

131. VOX, G., HAMMOND, M., VOS, D., GRABBELAAR, B., AUSLANDER, B., AUSLANDER, H., AND MARESCOTTI, G., An evaluation of humoral antibody responses in patients with carcinoma of the cervix, *J. Obstet. Gynecol. Br. Commonw.* **79**:1040–1046 (1972).

132. WARREN, K. G., BROWN, S. M., WROBLEWSKA, Z., GILDEN, D., KOPROWSKI, H., AND SUBAK-SHARPE, J., Isolation of latent herpes simplex virus from the superior cervical and vagus ganglions of human beings, *N. Engl. J. Med.* **298**:1068–1069 (1978).

133. WEINTRAUB, I., KLISAK, I., LAGASSE, L. D., AND BYFIELD, J. E., Evidence for specific tumor cytotoxic antibodies in serum of cervical cancer patients, *Am. J. Obstet. Gynecol.* **116**:985–992 (1973).

134. WENTZ, W. B., REAGAN, J. W., AND HEGGIE, A. D., Cervical carcinogenesis with herpes simplex virus type 2, *Obstet. Gynecol.* **46**:117–121 (1975).

135. WENTZ, W., REAGAN, J., HEGGIE, A., ANTHONY, D., AND FU, Y., Carcinogenesis of the uterine cervix with inactivated herpesvirus, in: *The Human Herpesviruses: An Interdisciplinary Perspective* (A. NAHMIAS, W. DOWDLE, AND R. SCHINAZI, eds.), p. 633, Elsevier/North-Holland, New York, 1981.

136. WILBANKS, G., TSURUMOTO, D., MARCZYNSKA, B., McPHERON, L., AND DEINHARDT, F., Attempts to transform primate cells *in vitro* by herpes simplex virus, in: *The Human Herpesviruses: An Interdisciplinary Perspective* (A. NAHHMIAS, W. DOWDLE, AND R. SCHINAZI, eds.), pp. 636–637, Elsevier/North-Holland, New York, 1981.

137. WYNDER, E. L., Epidemiology of carcinoma *in situ* of the cervix, *Obstet. Gynecol. Surv.* **24**(2):697–711 (1969).

138. ZUR HAUSEN, J., SCHULTE-HOLTHAUSEN, H., WOLF, H., DORRIES, K., AND EGGER, H., Attempts to detect virus-specific DNA in human tumors. II. Nucleic acid hybridizations with complementary RNA of human herpes group viruses, *Int. J. Cancer* **13**:657–664 (1974).

139. KAUFMAN, R. H., DREESMAN, G. R., BUREK, J., et al., Herpesvirus-induced antigens in squamous-cell carcinoma in situ of the vulva, *N. Engl. J. Med.* **305**:483–488 (1981).

12. Suggested Reading

Conference on early cervical neoplasia, *Obstet. Gynecol. Survey* **24**(2):675–1048 (1969).

COPPLESON, M., AND REID, B., *Preclinical Carcinoma of the Cervix Uteri*, Pergamon Press, Oxford, 1967.

Clinical Obstetrics and Gynecology **10**(4):741–1049 (1967).

LEVINE, P. H., GAYLORD, C. E., AND BURTON, G. J. (eds.), International Symposium on Human Tumors Associated with herpesviruses, *Cancer Res.* **34**:1083–1244 (1974).

Symposium on herpesvirus and cervical cancer, *Cancer Res.* **33**:1345–1563 (1973).

NAHMIAS, A., DOWDLE, W., AND SCHINAZI, R. (eds.), *The Human Herpesviruses: An Interdisciplinary Perspective*, Elsevier/North-Holland, New York, 721 pp., 1981.

RAPP, F. (ed.), *The Oncogenic Herpesviruses*, Vols. 1 and 2, CRC Press, Boca Raton, Florida, 1980.

CHAPTER 27

Chronic Neurological Diseases

Subacute Sclerosing Panencephalitis, Progressive Multifocal Leukoencephalopathy, Kuru, Creutzfeldt–Jakob Disease

Jacob A. Brody and Clarence Joseph Gibbs, Jr.

1. Introduction

Most subacute and chronic progressive degenerative diseases of the central nervous system of man have been classified as disorders of unknown etiology. Few if any are curable, and although some are genetically determined, most are sporadic in occurrence, and there appears not to be a history of the disease in close relatives. That any one or more of these chronic idiopathic disorders might have infection as their etiology was not recognized until the subacute progressive degenerative heredofamilial disease kuru was transmitted to chimpanzees and was subsequently shown to be serially transmissible in experimental animals inoculated with bacteria-free filtrates of brain tissues from animals dying with the disease. Kuru thus became the first subacute fatal central nervous system disease of man to have a virus-induced "slow infection" established as its etiology.

Even though the possibility of a virus etiology for kuru was postulated early in the discovery of the disease, the lack of febrile response or acute inflammatory lesions and the failure to detect abnormal

Jacob A. Brody · Epidemiology, Demography, Biometry, National Institute on Aging, National Institutes of Health, Bethesda, Maryland. Clarence Joseph Gibbs, Jr. · Laboratory of Central Nervous System Studies, National Institute of Neurological and Communicative Disorders and Stroke, National Institutes of Health, Bethesda, Maryland.

Table 1. Slow Infections Caused by Unconventional Viruses

Man	Animals
Kuru	Scrapie
Creutzfeldt–Jakob disease	Mink encephalopathy

clinical, chemical, or hematological values at any stage of the disease in man did not support this hypothesis. Nevertheless, it was the elucidation of the viral etiology of kuru that led to the discovery that both the familial and the sporadic type of Creutzfeldt–Jakob disease (CJD) were caused by a virus that is transmissible to subhuman primates. CJD thus became the first presenile dementia of man to have an established viral etiology.

The transmissible agents of kuru and CJD share biological, physical, and chemical properties with those of scrapie and transmissible mink encephalopathy and have been classified as prototype viruses of the subacute spongiform virus encephalopathies (Table 1). Because of their unusual properties, they have been referred to as "unconventional viruses." They are unconventional in that they do not induce inflammatory lesions, are thermostable, have not yet been shown to induce an immune response, are resistant to ultraviolet light, and have not yet been associated with a nucleic acid type.

There are, however, other slow infections of the human brain that, subsequent to work on kuru and CJD, have been shown to have a virus etiology. These are slow infections caused by "conventional" viruses—viruses that can be visualized by electron microscopy, induce specific antigen–antibody reactions, and have either an RNA or a DNA type of nucleic acid. In Table 2 are listed a number of "slow infections" of man that are caused by conventional viruses.

It has been known since the dawn of classic virology that conventional viruses can and do cause diseases associated with long incubation periods, chronic diseases, persistent infections, and diseases with varied pathological reactions. What is new is the establishment of an unconventional-type virus etiology for heredofamilial and presenile dementias of man as well as the isolation of conventional viruses from the brains of patients with chronic neurological disorders months to years after initial contact with the invading virus.

In this chapter, we present information on two diseases of the central nervous system caused by "conventional viruses," subacute sclerosing panencephalitis (SSPE), caused by defective measles virus, and progressive multifocal leukoencephalopathy (PML), caused by papovaviruses, and two diseases of the central nervous system of man caused by "unconventional viruses," kuru and CJD.

2. Subacute Sclerosing Panencephalitis

2.1. Introduction

SSPE is a progressive, fatal disease of the central nervous system that affects children and young adults. The virus is etiologically related to the measles virus, and as such is easier to work with using conventional laboratory methods than the viruses that cause the other three diseases discussed in this chapter. This has resulted in voluminous literature on SSPE, and in attempting to present the epide-

Table 2. Slow Infections Caused by Conventional Viruses

Disease	Virus
Subacute sclerosing panencephalitis (SSPE)	Measles
Subacute postmeasles leukoencephalopathy	Measles
Multiple sclerosis	(Measles?)
Progressive multifocal leukoencephalopathy (PML)	Papovaviruses (JC and SV40-related)
Progressive congenital rubella	Rubella
Cytomegalovirus brain infection	Cytomegalovirus
Subacute encephalitis	Herpes simplex adenovirus type 32 Echovirus
Homologous serum jaundice	Hepatitis B
Infectious hepatitis	Hepatitis A

miological picture, the authors were forced to be selective in both the data presented and the references cited.

2.2. Historical Background

SSPE was first described by Dawson in 1933 and then again by von Bogaert in 1945. In 1965, paramyxovirus was observed in brain tissue of SSPE patients by electron microscopy, and in 1967, a very high measles-antibody titer was demonstrated in the cerebrospinal fluid (CSF) and in serum. The published proceedings of an international conference on SSPE[68] reviewed the state of knowledge through 1967. Subsequently, the virus was isolated from brain tissue by various groups, and numerous surveys and clinical and laboratory studies have been conducted.

2.3. Methodology

The largest single source of epidemiological data is a registry started by Jabbour *et al.*[44] in 1969. Its chief shortcoming is that it is dependent on voluntary submission of data from medical centers throughout the United States. Various forms of registries have been initiated in other countries. The Israeli data, although limited numerically, are particularly valuable because of relatively complete ascertainment and inclusion of diverse groups of migrants.[73a] Other sources of data are found in numerous case reports and series from clinical centers since 1933. Case–control studies have been published, but they still encompass limited numbers of patients.[17,36c]

2.4. Biological Characteristics of the Virus

There is still dispute as to whether the SSPE virus is classical measles virus or a variant. If it is a variant, this could of course affect the epidemiological pattern. SSPE virus differs biochemically from classic measles virus, but not in a consistent manner.[36b,66a] It seems probable that it results from any of various mutations in measles virus, but it is not clear whether these mutations occur before infection, in the infected person, or even in the prolonged culture period usually needed for isolation in the laboratory. Difficulty encountered in isolating virus from SSPE

specimens suggests that it is defective in the patient.[48a] The absence of antibody against the virus membrane (M) protein suggests that this protein may be the key site of expression of the defect.[36b,79a]

2.5. Descriptive Epidemiology

SSPE is a rare disease with fewer than 50 new patients reported per year in the United States. Accepting the limitations of diagnosis and reporting, the published rates have varied from section to section and from country to country from 0.4 to 2.6 per million.[73a] The rate is higher in the southeastern part of the United States than in other regions of the country.[57a] The disease appears to be worldwide in distribution.

Almost all authors have observed a nonurban preponderance of cases.[17] While some series have not revealed a striking difference, the observation merits increased credence, since the diagnosis of SSPE is made only in urban centers. In the United States, there was not only a higher rural than urban incidence, but also a higher farm than nonfarm incidence and a lower central-city than other urban incidence.[36c] In virtually all series, males have outnumbered females in a ratio of 2:3 or greater.[57a] The mean age at onset is generally about 7 years, with a range of 2–21 years. The great majority of cases occur between ages 4 and 12. SSPE has been reported in all ethnic groups studied; in the United States, the rate in whites was 4 times that in blacks,[57a] but in Cape Province, South Africa, all of 15 reported cases were in blacks.[57]

There are several reports that SSPE occurs more frequently in families of lower socioeconomic level, although there are many exceptions to this observation. Cases tend to occur in large sibships. In a study of 43 patients, median birth order was fourth, and for their controls it was third.[17] There are several reports of SSPE developing in children following exposure to sick animals, primarily dogs, swine, and fowl.[12,13,17,36c,70] The association of SSPE with exposure to birds was very strong ($p < 0.001$) in the largest case–control study yet reported.[36c] Detels *et al.*[17] have also reported a cluster of three patients within a ten-block area near St. Louis in 1968, immediately following a distemper epidemic in the same region. Baguley and Glasgow[4] suggested that the administration of Salk vaccine in New Zealand in 1956 was related to the appearance of SSPE in the community. These various associations with SSPE make it clear that some extrinsic factor often present in the rural environment, and distinct from measles virus, is important in the pathogenesis.

Multiple cases of SSPE have been reported, but are rare in related persons. There is also a report of SSPE occurring in only one of a set of identical twins.[82] Measles-antibody titers among siblings of patients are within the normal range.[8,45] These observations argue against the playing of an important role by genetic factors.

Since 1973, there has been in the Unites States a sharp decline in the incidence of SSPE.[57a,b] The time of this decline coincides with the time at which a majority of measles-vaccine-protected children reached the age of the peak SSPE attack rate. The study of Modlin et al.[57b] found an SSPE attack rate in children with a history of measles that was approximately 10 times that observed in children who had been vaccinated and not had measles. The evidence was not clear as to whether vaccinated children with SSPE had all been infected with measles, sometimes unrecognized, or whether vaccine was associated with a very low rate of SSPE independently of wild measles virus.

2.6. Pathogenesis and Immunity

Clinically and pathologically, the disease is primarily a sclerosing encephalitis. In some instances, the rapidly progressive phase of the disease with paralysis, myoclonus and dementia is preceded by a variable period of unusual behavior or deterioration of learning ability at school.[63a] The diagnosis is frequently made clinically and is readily confirmed by finding very high measles-antibody titer in the serum and the presence of measles-specific antibody in CSF. The virus can be seen by electron microscopy[68] and with special techniques has been isolated from all portions of the brain[43,63] and on two occasions early in the course of the disease from biopsies of lymph nodes.[42] In addition, immune complexes containing measles antigen, complement, and immunoglobulin G (IgG) have been found in organs throughout the body.[16] The virus apparently multiplies in the presence of extraordinarily high amounts of measles antibody in the CSF and serum. IgM as well as IgG is present in these fluids.[15]

SSPE virus, but not measles virus, has produced a subacute encephalitis in dogs,[42,60] calves, and lambs[74] in the absence of a detectable serological response. There appears to be an encephalitogenic factor for ferrets[49,75] and hamsters, and in rats, an encephalitis was produced by inoculation at a critical age.[11]

Adult female hamsters were immunized with measles virus and subsequently bred. At 48–72 hr after birth, the offspring were challenged with measles virus, and most survived. The challenge apparently produced a latent infection in the hamsters. After 1 month, the animals were given an immunosuppressive drug and rapidly developed fatal measles encephalitis.[79]

2.7. Patterns of Host Response

While laboratory data are considerable, some of the observations are unconfirmed, and in a sense, the implications of various reports are contradictory. Epidemiological observations may prove of considerable importance in elucidating the pathogenesis of SSPE and possibly in clarifying the implications of the available laboratory data. We have already alluded to the observation that it is a disease of childhood with a considerable male excess and for the most part confined to nonmetropolitan areas. A key finding was that in a large proportion of SSPE patients, measles occurred very early in life.[7] This finding was subsequently confirmed by the observation that in the United States, 55% of 198 patients with SSPE had measles under age 2 years.[44] In Finland, 12 of 14 patients had measles between 6 and 24 months of age.[18] In a case–control study of 52 patients, the mean age at measles infection was 2.4 years among SSPE patients and 4.0 years in controls.[36b] In this latter series, 11 patients had no history of measles and 12 had measles under age 1 year. Those with no history of measles had known household exposure, and measles-antibody titer was present in the same range as in other SSPE patients. Presumably, some of these had measles so early in life that there was sufficient passively acquired maternal antibody to modify the clinical manifestations of the disease. Thus, early onset of measles, perhaps in the presence of maternal antibody, which interfered with the normal complete host response, may have permitted the measles virus to establish itself as a chronic infection. In this context, it was reassuring to find that measles vaccine virus, which is usually given at an early age, was associated with a reduced, not an increased, SSPE incidence.[57a] Since early age of measles was not observed in about half the SSPE patients, other factors attendant on the measles infection may exist that permit the virus to become established as a chronic infection.

The observation that an aberrant immunological host response to measles is etiologically involved is supported by the finding in one large series that the interval between measles and SSPE is nonrandom and fairly close to 6 years.[67] The absence of or low titer of antibody to the M protein of measles virus in SSPE patients also supports this finding.[36b] The failure of Machamer *et al.*[52b] and of Wechsler[79a] to find anti-M antibody in a Protein-A-absorbed fraction from sera of long-term immune persons suggests that the normal response to this protein does not include globulins of the IgM^1 or IgM^2 class. Depressed skin reactivity to test antigens and reduced IgA levels have been reported.[31]

The observation that SSPE occurs primarily in nonurban males[12,13,17,44] has prompted several workers to suggest that a sequence of an unusual triggering event and measles infection initiates the process of cellular destruction in the central nervous system. It is probable that early onset of measles and events such as chickenpox preceding measles infection occur more frequently in urban inner-city populations, which seem to be relatively immune to SSPE. An equally compelling argument is that the group at highest risk, the nonurban males, are exposed to higher doses of numerous environmental factors including zoonotic infections.[8] Support for this latter thesis is (1) more frequent contact with sick fowl and dogs; (2) the observation of a second virus in the central nervous system in an SSPE patient; and (3) the observation that an immunosuppressive drug precipitated a latent measles infection into a fatal measles encephalitis in hamsters.

2.8. Control and Prevention

As noted above, measles vaccine appears to be capable of greatly reducing the incidence of SSPE. Clearly, general early use of this vaccine is the best defense and an effective one against this disease. In this respect, the control of SSPE is further advanced than control of the other chronic neurological diseases except possibly kuru. However, current

scientific information cannot rule out the possibility that measles vaccine virus also causes a small number of SSPE cases or triggers latent disease. Nor is it known whether vaccination at one age is safer than at another age, except that it must presumably precede natural measles infection. Too little is known of the other environmental, i.e., nonurban, factor in measles pathogenesis to permit definition of procedures to reduce its impact.

2.9. Unresolved Problems

While far more is known about SSPE than about other slow virus diseases of man, the basic questions of etiology and pathogenesis are not yet solved. While it seems probable that mutation in the virus leads to establishment of the chronic infection, there is no consensus as to whether this is the initial event or is due to selection of virus capable of growing in neurological tissues of an immunologically sensitized host. Neither do we have any knowledge of how or when the second environmental factor associated with rural life exerts its effect.

3. Progressive Multifocal Leukoencephalopathy

3.1. Introduction and Historical Background

PML is a rare and unusual demyelinating disease first described in 1958. It almost invariably occurs in patients with other severe diseases, usually those that affect the reticuloendothelial system. Thus far, approximately 200–250 cases have been described. Early authors postulated a viral etiology,[64] and papovalike virions were seen by electron microscopy first in 1969[83] and subsequently by many other neuropathologists. Isolation of papovaviruses from brain material was reported in the early 1970s.[62,80]

3.2. Methodology

The only available sources for morbidity and mortality data are case reports and reviews of the literature. Three extensive studies are those by Zu Rhein,[83] Brun *et al.*[10] and Walker.[77a] There have been several serological surveys in patients and in the general population for papovaviruses.[29,61,69] The viruses have been recovered from human brain material either by inoculating homogenated brain tissue into monolayers of human fetal brain cells[62,51] or by using dispersion cultures of brain cells fused to African green monkey kidney cells.[80] These isolation procedures are cumbersome, and rapid identification of the virus in brain cells has been achieved by preparing specific sera to the virus strains and using fluorescent-antibody or electron-microscopic agglutination.[81] In sections of PML brain tissue, common polyomavirus antigen has been demonstrated by the peroxidase–antiperoxidase technique.[30a]

3.3. Biological Characteristics of the Virus

In recent years, viruses have been identified in 53 PML patients.[77b] Two have been indistinguishable from SV40, a simian papovavirus, while the remaining 51 have been the JC virus isolated from a patient in Wisconsin.[62] Another human papovavirus, the BK virus isolated in England[30] from the urine of an immunosuppressed renal-transplant patient, has not been encountered in PML. Serological surveys have indicated that infections with JC and BK viruses are very common, with the majority of adults having antibody.[9a,12a,29,61] SV40 antibody has been observed in a small percentage of humans who received poliomyelitis vaccine contaminated with this virus and also in about 3% of humans who were not vaccinated against poliomyelitis.[69] PML patients in whom virus has been identified do not invariably possess antibody at a detectable level.[58] This may be a result of their generally depressed immunological status or immune-complex formation. Thus, it is difficult to determine from serological data how and when the infection occurred or who is at risk. The JC strain has been found capable of inducing brain tumors in hamsters[78] and in monkeys.[52a] In a very few human brains, PML has been found together with gliomatous or lymphomatous tumors.[39a]

3.4. Descriptive Epidemiology

Limited epidemiological information is available from the 200 or so documented cases. Apparently, occasional cases go undiagnosed, but extensive retrospective reviews of brains of patients who died in large clinical centers of leukemia or lymphoma detected only a handful of previously undiagnosed PML cases.[83] Patients have thus far been reported in the United States, Canada, most European countries, Israel, Australia, and Japan. The disease is very rare under age 30; such a case was reported by Castaigne *et al.*[14] in an 18-year-old male who was diagnosed as having PML and multiple astrocytic tumor nodules in the white matter of the brain. PML has been diagnosed in two children with combined immunodeficiency. They were 5 years old and 11 years old[85] at the time of death. The oldest known patient was 84. The great majority of cases occur from the 5th to the 7th decades of life. There appears to be a slight excess of cases among males of about 1.5:1. Occupation was recorded for about 30 patients. Since this was a highly selected group seen ultimately by a neuropathologist, the information is of limited value. While most of the patients were white-collar workers—some at the executive level—farmers and people engaged in outdoor occupations were also represented.[83]

3.5. Pathogenesis and Immunity

Papovavirus infections without known illness are very common, as shown by antibody surveys, but PML is rare. More than half the known patients have had malignant lymphoproliferative diseases, including lymphosarcoma. Nonlymphoproliferative diseases such as chronic and acute myelogenous leukemia and carcinomatosis and benign disease of the reticuloendothelial system, especially tuberculosis and sarcoidosis, make up the bulk of the residual cases. There are reports of PML developing up to 30 years after pulmonary anthracosilicosis, chronic bronchitis and asthma, idiopathic thrombocytopenic purpura, and lupus erythematosus. Recently, there have been several reports of PML following renal transplants.[52,53,84] There are three cases in which the only prior pathology was senility or severe arteriosclerosis.[83] There are reports of at least three cases of PML occurring in the absence of any associated systemic disease.[21,72]

Because of the background conditions in most patients who develop PML, they have received X-radiation, cytotoxic agents, and steroids, either alone or in combination, prior to onset of the central nervous system disease. These immunosuppressants may be etiologically related to PML, although there are well-documented instances of patients who never received such therapy.[83]

3.6. Patterns of Host Response

The nature and frequency of the background diseases strongly suggest that the papovaviruses become destructive in the central nervous system as a result of a hyporeactive immune system in the host. Whether the virus has been latent for a long period prior to onset of PML or is acquired once the host defenses are weakened cannot be determined.

Neurological signs appear insidiously but progress rapidly, with death occurring in an average of 4 months. There are occasional patients who have survived more than a year, and there is one report of a patient who developed PML, had a remission, and died 5 years later of an apparently unrelated pneumonia.[37]

3.7. Unresolved Problems

PML is an extremely rare disease. It is of great interest, however, because it is caused by apparently widespread viruses that become pathogenic in an apparent hypoactive immune state in the host. Conditions that compromise the host defense mechanisms are common, and a fairly wide range of diseases have been implicated with PML. This suggests that (1) many diseases share a very rare but specific immunosuppressing factor; (2) the host has a very rare immune deficit that permits these background diseases to precipitate PML; or (3) an as yet unknown rare precipitating event is involved. Clarification of this problem could have far-reaching implications in the understanding of diseases that develop in hyporeactive immune states.

4. Kuru

4.1. Introduction

Kuru was the first slow virus disease to be demonstrated in man. Pertinent information through 1964 was presented in a symposium[28] and more recently in review by Gajdusek[22a] and others[73d] and in a book.[63b] Because of the properties of the

kuru virus and the neuropathological appearance of the brain, it has been classified as a subacute spongiform virus encephalopathy along with CJD of man, scrapie of sheep, and mink encephalopathy.[32] The disease is a heredofamilial subacute degeneration of the central nervous system, confined essentially to people of the Eastern Highlands region of Papua New Guinea.

4.2. Historical Background

The great majority of patients belong to the Fore linguistic group, who until recently lived a Stone Age existence. Since 1950, there has been increasing Westernization. Known environmental and cultural changes in the kuru region have been described by Alpers.[2] It appears that kuru was not recognized until the first or second decade of the 20th century. Rates slowly increased and reached "epidemic" proportions during the 1950s.[2]

Intensive study of kuru began in 1956. Initially, while a simple genetic hypothesis was entertained, extensive attempts using classic techniques were employed to detect infectious agents. Subsequently, when no evidence of a sufficient compensatory reproductive advantage with increased fertility in kuru patients was found that would account for the survival of the genes, other explanations were sought.[22] In 1959, Hadlow[36] pointed out the similarity of the neuropathology of scrapie and kuru. This led to renewed attempts to transmit kuru to laboratory animals including primates. In 1965, after 20 months of incubation, chimpanzees inoculated intracerebrally with suspensions of human brain from kuru patients developed the disease.[26]

4.3. Methodology

Since 1956, census information has been available through the Australian administrative offices and patrols in the region and through the efforts of the research group under Dr. Gajdusek, who conduct total population surveys at 6-month intervals. It is believed that case-finding is complete.[22] Appropriate serological and pathological materials have been collected through the years. With the establishment of the Laboratory of Slow, Latent, and Temperate Viruses at the National Institute of Neurological and Communicative Disorders and Stroke in 1962, concentrated efforts using conventional laboratory techniques, plus a wide program of primate inoculation, have been utilized to transmit, identify, and characterize the kuru virus.[32]

4.4. Biological Characteristics of the Virus

To date, no virus has been visualized by electron microscopy, and there are no serological tests that detect antibody or neutralize infectious material. For these reasons, plus the high stability of the infectious particle to many physical and chemical agents and several other unusual properties, some investigators have chosen to refer to the transmitting property of kuru and the other subacute virus encephalopathies as an "agent" rather than a virus. The present authors favor the designation "virus." The virus is filterable through membranes of 100-nm minimum pore diameter and reaches titers of over 10^7 LD_{50} per gram in brain tissue of primates. It is transmissible by peripheral or intracerebral inoculation thus far into chimpanzees and eight species of monkeys in from 10 months to over 8 years on primary inoculation; transmission by the oral route to one squirrel monkey has been reported with an incubation period of 36 months.[31a] The virus is stable for many years at $-70°C$ or on lyophilization and is not totally unactivated by a temperature of $85°C$ for 30 min. There is firm evidence that the virus can be maintained *in vitro* in tissue cultures for many months without losing its virulence for the chimpanzee.[22]

4.5. Descriptive Epidemiology

Kuru is confined to a number of adjacent valleys in the mountainous interior of the Eastern Highlands of New Guinea, which include 160 villages with a total population of 35,000. Approximately 80% of all known cases occur in members of the Fore linguistic group and the remainder from nine other linguistic groups. There have been wide variations in rates in individual villages with considerable change over time.

Since 1956, some 2500 cases have been documented and critically analyzed by age and sex over time.[3,22] In the early years of study, approximately 200 deaths per year occurred from kuru, which at that time approached 1% per annum of the total population. Deaths have been declining steadily

and now number about 30 per year; in 1978, there were 22 deaths and 28 living cases of kuru.[3a] During the years when rates were high, the disease was found to affect all ages beyond infants and toddlers. Among preadolescents, the sex ratio was approximately equal, while among adults, there was a marked female excess, giving an overall rate of almost 3 females to 1 male. During the past decade, the rates among males have been generally stable, while the female rate has declined notably. The female/male ratio at age of death showed a bimodal distribution in the period 1957–1973: for ages 8–9 years, it was 1.5; for ages 10–14 years, 1.0; for ages 15–19 years, 0.9; and for ages 20–29 years, 3.5.[3a] In addition, preadolescent cases are no longer seen, and no child under 10 years old has developed kuru since 1967.[22]

Kuru has been observed among people born in the endemic area many years after they migrated away. There have been no secondary cases among persons in close contact with these migrants. Furthermore, there has been considerable immigration into the endemic area, and despite many thousands of man-years of close contact with the flora, fauna, food, and people of the region, no case of kuru has occurred among these new settlers.

The culture of the kuru region resembles that of the surrounding kuru-free highland people. Women and small children share the women's houses, while adult men, the group least affected by kuru, live separately. Diets, however, are similar for males and females and not distinguishable from those of neighboring kuru-free groups.[22]

4.6. Mechanisms and Routes of Transmission

Ritual cannibalism, the practice of consumption of dead kinsmen as a rite of mourning, was apparently introduced into the kuru region about 1920.[2] There are compelling reasons to believe this practice to have been involved in the transmission of the disease. Women for the most part conducted the butchery of the dead, which was carried out barehanded. Brain tissue was squeezed to a pulp and packed into bamboo cylinders, in which it was steamed. In the mountainous highland area, water boils at 90–95°C. It is likely that the extremely heat-stable virus, which is present at concentrations as high as 10^7, would not be completely inactivated under these conditions.[22] Adult men rarely participated in this ceremony and seldom ate the flesh of dead kuru victims. As mentioned, women lived with small children of both sexes, but young boys went to live with men as they approached adolescence. Thus, in the early days, the rates of kuru among preadolescents were the same for males and females, but the adult rates were higher for females, which coincides with the degree of exposure to kuru brains. Since the virus is infectious by the peripheral route, Gajdusek[22] suggests that the most likely route of infection from contaminated brain was percutaneous, through cuts or sores in the hands or other parts of the body or by being rubbed by unwashed hands into the nose or eyes. The recent experimental transmission to a monkey by the oral route[31a] suggests that this may also occur in nature and have a longer incubation period than by parenteral incubation.

Perhaps the most convincing argument relating cannibalism with kuru is the steady decline in rates since the abandonment of the practice of cannibalism between 1957 and 1962 and the striking observation that no child under 10 years old has developed kuru since 1967.

Contagion can virtually be ruled out as a means of transmission. There were no secondary cases among contacts of kuru victims who had migrated from the kuru region and no cases in immigrants to the endemic area.

4.7. Pathogenesis and Immunity

There is no detectable immunity to kuru. Apparently, the virus accumulates gradually in the central nervous system and destroys enough cells to produce the clinical picture. The incubation period is variable. Children as young as 3 years of age have developed the disease, which would be a minimal estimate of the incubation period. The study has been in progress since 1956. Since there are still living cases in 1981, the maximum incubation period is at least 25 years and may be over 30 years.

4.8. Patterns of Host Response

The symptomatology of kuru is remarkably uniform, leading to total incapacitation and death usually in 3–9 months. The disease is characterized by a cerebellar ataxia and a shiverlike tremor that pro-

gresses to complete motor incapacity.[41] The word *kuru* means "shivering" or "trembling" in the Fore language.

4.9. Control and Prevention

Although impossible to prove, it appears that the kuru virus was introduced into the Eastern Highlands some time after the turn of the century from an unidentified source, perhaps a human or animal with a spongiform encephalopathy. It was allowed to spread because of the ritual of cannibalism and by 1950 had reached astonishing rates in a general familial pattern. Since the disease is disappearing with the cessation of cannibalism, it appears that prevention is achieved by avoiding exposure to infectious brain material.

4.10. Unresolved Problems

The major unresolved problem is to determine the nature of the virus that causes kuru and to determine the relationship between the virus of kuru and the other spongiform virus encephalopathies of man and animals. While the phenomenon in the New Guinea highlands is unique and related to the disappearing practice of cannibalism, humans are exposed to brains from many sources. It is not inconceivable that these exposures present a constant hazard to man. To clarify this matter, it is essential that kuru and related viruses be characterized. Cheaper, less cumbersome, and less time-consuming laboratory methods would greatly facilitate this. The development of serological tests, if possible, would make the overall understanding of the spongiform encephalopathies far easier and more complete.

5. Creutzfeldt–Jakob Disease

5.1. Introduction

Since 1968, convincing evidence has emerged that CJD is one of four classic slow virus infections that involve spongiform degeneration of the central nervous system. Others thus far identified are kuru in man, scrapie in sheep, and transmissible mink encephalopathy.

5.2. Historical Background

CJD, first delineated in the early 1920s by Creutz-feldt and Jakob, occurs throughout the world. It is uncommon, but not rare. The disease was the subject of a neurological symposium,[1] a complete survey of the literature,[56] and an extensive monograph.[50] Gibbs *et al.*[35] provided critical insight into the nature of this disease in 1968 by successfully transmitting it from human brain biopsy material to chimpanzees. Recent data were brought together in a book in 1979.[63b]

Primarily because of the variety of clinical features of CJD and the fact that no person has seen more than a few patients, there are at least 20 synonyms for it in the literature.[50,71] While there is still not complete agreement, there is increasing acceptance of the unity of this disease entity as a destructive process of the gray matter of the central nervous system usually presenting as a variable period of vague psychic disturbance progressing in a few weeks or months to frank dementia complicated by cerebellar, extrapyramidal, or pyramidal symptoms and finally to mutism, rigidity, and death. Various subclassifications have been attempted. A useful though probably not definitive classification of CJD was developed by Bobowick *et al.*[5] (Table 3) and by Roos *et al.*[65] In this scheme, three major types are recognized and presented in order of diminishing severity. The table includes the clinical characteristics and other terms in the literature assigned to these three general types.

5.3. Methodology

Mortality and morbidity data for CJD are limited. Until 1965, the only sources of information were reviews of published clinical series.[50,56] Recently, area-wide surveys were carried out in Israel,[48] France,[8a] Iceland, and Czechoslovakia, and its worldwide occurrence was reviewed[53d]; a case–control study was conducted in the United States, where the source of cases was patients from selected medical centers and patients from whom central nervous system material was sent to Drs. Gajdusek and Gibbs at the National Institutes of Health (NIH) for virus transmission studies. There is also a report on the characteristics of 12 CJD patients whose brain material was used in an unsuccessful attempt to transmit the disease to chimpanzees,[65] as well as one serological study of 13 such patients and of 10 chimpanzees that were inoculated with CJD material.[9] By far the largest series of patients available at present (approximately 824) is represented by those from whom materials have been sent to the NIH for transmission studies.[34,53d]

5.4. Biological Characteristics of the Virus

As with the other spongiform encephalopathies, the disease has been transmitted to a variety of animals inoculated intracerebrally or by multiple peripheral routes. Oral transmission to monkeys has recently been reported.[31a] The causative agent has not been identified by electron-microscopic study, and no serological tests are yet available. On primary transmission from man, the incubation period in parenterally inoculated apes has ranged from 10 to 71 months and in monkeys from 11 to 68 months, and in the domestic cat, it has been 30 months. It was 23 and 27 months in two monkeys by the oral route.[31a] In guinea pigs in primary transmission, the incubation period is approximately 14–17

Table 3. Creutzfeldt–Jakob Disease: Classification System with Equivalent Terms from the Literature and Essential Characteristics

Type I. Names:	Subacute spongiform encephalopathy, Heidenhain, amaurotic, spongy, myoclonic, cortical
Characteristics:	Visual disturbances, dementia, aphasia, myoclonus, "burst suppression" EEG, acute course of 1 to several months
Type II. Names:	Transitional, diffuse cerebral, thalamic, niger, cerebellar, corticostriatal
Characteristics:	Rigidity, dementia, ataxia, tremors, subacute course of less than 9 months
Type III. Names:	Classic, Jakob, spastic pseudosclerosis, amyotrophic, corticostriatospinal, corticospinal
Characteristics:	Parkinsonian features, and/or amyotrophic lateral sclerosis syndrome (ALS) which may or may not have associated parkinsonian features, all features of types I and II, especially terminally, chronic course of 1–2 years

months.[52f] *In vitro* cultures of human tissues and tissues from animals with natural and experimentally induced disease remain infectious for subhuman primates for more than a year. Tissue-culture cells from the brain of one CJD patient spontaneously transformed, and a virus particle akin to oncogenic RNA viruses was present in the transformed cells, but has been shown to have no relationship to CJD.[40] Two types of viruslike particles were observed by electron microscopy in brain-biopsy specimens of two additional patients.[77] The significance of these observations and their etiological relationship to CJD remain obscure, since preparations of purified virus do not reveal classic virions or nucleocapsids. The virus can be transmitted to subhuman primates by inoculation of human liver, kidney, spleen, and lymphoid tissues from patients dying with the disease.[24,25] The consistency with which subhuman primates are affected after inoculation with brain and visceral tissues from patients with CJD, the clinical and neuropathological similarity between the disease in humans and that in apes and monkeys, the ability to transmit the disease with bacteria-free filtrates, and the ability of the agent to self-replicate *in vitro* are all strong evidence that the causative agent is a virus. At present, however, with the exception that brain and visceral tissues are known to contain the transmissible agent in at least some cases, virological studies are not useful in determining the epidemiological pattern of CJD.[32,33,34] The recent reproduction of a scrapielike encephalopathy in goats inoculated with brain suspension from two patients with CJD suggests a close relationship between the two viruses.[36a]

5.5. Descriptive Epidemiology

Exact incidence data are not available, but a reasonable estimate is 1–2 cases per million per year.[53a] Since the average duration is about a year, this would also reflect the prevalence rate. The death rate in the United States in the period 1973–1977 was estimated to be 0.26 per million, varying by state from 0 to 0.6.[52c,53a,d] In France, a systematic search identified 170 fatal cases from 1968 to 1977, a death rate of 0.32 per million.[8a,8b] Other estimated death rates per million are 0.40 in Iceland, 1.2 in Fukuoka province in Japan, and 0.43 for the Boston area in the United States. Information on prevalence comes from an Israeli report[35a,48] wherein a rate of 1 per million was encountered. In this study, there was a marked disparity among immigrants from different countries, with a much higher rate (31 per million) encountered among migrants from Libya. Siedler and Malamud,[71] in a series of autopsied patients from California, found 15 cases of CJD, which made it one fifth as frequent as Alzheimer's disease and one half as frequent as Pick's disease. There is no convincing evidence of contagion among humans or animals for CJD. The only strongly suggestive evidence so far in regard to possible contact transmission comes from the report of Jellinger *et al.*[46] in which they describe CJD in a husband and wife. No maternal transmission has been reported in man or experimentally in guinea pigs[52g] or nonhuman primates.[53b] A total of 73 families with two or more members affected with CJD have been identified.[53c] In these families, there were 286 affected members yielding a proportion of 15% familial occurrence of CJD. From 13 cases in 12 families, brain material has transmitted the disease to nonhuman primates.[20,34,53c] In light of the rarity of these combinations, it is probable that common exposure to an infectious agent, to an extrinsic factor that activated the agent already latent, or to an unidentified toxin was involved, with a possible genetic component in some instances. Indeed, the disease occurs in a pattern consistent with autosomal dominant transmission and is therefore the unique example in man of a virus-induced disease apparently determined by a single gene mechanism.[53c]

Epidemiological patterns on a worldwide basis have been derived from 1435 patients analyzed by Masters *et al.*[53d] The geographic distribution of cases appears to be worldwide. The bulk of reports have come from Europe and North America,[5] while there are reports of CJD in South America, Israel, Japan, India, Africa, and Australia.[5,35a,47,48,54,55] In France, the mortality rate per million was 0.3, but in the most densely populated parts of Paris, it reached 1.33; a significant correlation existed between population density and CJD mortality in the Paris urban agglomeration.[8a] However, no urban–rural differences existed in the rest of France or have been seen in the United States.[5]

There is little information on temporal trends. Tabulations of May[56] and Kirschbaum[50] of case reports from the world literature list about 70 cases

Table 4. Comparison of Certain Features

Disease	Virus	Geographic distribution	Age	M/F ratio	Ethnic group	Other
		Descriptive epidemiology				
SSPE	Defective measles	Worldwide	5–7	3:1	All	Rural, exposure to fowl and dogs
PML	Polyomavirus genus	Many countries	50–70	1.5:1	?	Hodgkin's disease, leukemia, and others
Kuru	Subacute spongiform encephalopathy	Eastern Highlands of Papua New Guinea	All ages	1:3	Fore people only	Ritualistic cannibalism resulting in self-inoculation; heredofamilial
CJD	Subacute spongiform encephalopathy	Worldwide	40–69	About equal	All	Organ/tissue transplantation; head trauma, ?neurosurgical/ neuropathological accidents; sporadic, familial, and conjugal

for the period 1920–1960, and from 1960 to 1968, approximately 150 cases are listed. Following transmission experiments and attendant heightened interest in CJD, another 150 cases have been observed in the past 5 years.[20] In a review of patients from designated neurological centers in the United States from 1966 to 1971, no temporal trend was observed,[5,65] but reports from other countries indicate that clustering does occur.[53d]

Approximately 90% of cases occur in the 40–69 year age group. The mean age at death is about age 60 for types I and II, while for type III disease, it is 48 years,[5,71] (see Table 4). The mean survivorship for type I disease is 5 months after onset, with a range of 2–10 months; for type II disease, the mean is 8 months, with a range of 3–15 months; and for type 3 disease, the mean is 30 months, with a range of 10–72 months. In many instances, there is a rapid progressive evolution over a period of weeks to months, reducing the patient to a vegetative state for a more prolonged period.

Males and females were equally affected in most reports, although in two series[5] there was a slight preponderance of males, primarily of type II patients, and in the first 12 cases transmitted by Roos et al.[65], the ratio was 10 males to 2 females. The Israeli study[48] also had a slight male excess. Present information indicates that all races are susceptible,

although comparative rates are not available. In a case–control study,[5] 38 confirmed patients were compared with their spouse or nearest surviving relative and a designated lifelong friend of the same age and sex. Broad categories of information were ascertained at interview regarding recent health prior to illness, immunological history, previous hospitalization and illnesses, family history, residential history and foreign travel, occupational history, education, smoking habits, vacations, food habits, and animal-exposure history. In this series, approximately half the patients were classified as type I, while 30% were type II and 20% were type III. It is probable that there was an overrepresentation of type I CJD, the most acute form of the disease, since these are the patients who are most likely to be referred for diagnostic and virological studies. We did not detect any patterns or practices that distinguished among the three types of disease, with the exception mentioned above that type III patients die approximately 10 years earlier than the others. Comparison for the numerous parameters referred to above did not yield discernible differences among the patients. In all groups, a wide range of occupations, residencies both urban and rural, degree of education, history of familial illness, and life styles were equally represented. There was a slight excess among patients for severe upper res-

of Slow Virus Infections of Man

Incubation period	Pathogenesis		Animal transmission
	High antibody titer	Depressed immune response	
6 years	+ +	+	+ Dogs, hamsters, calves, lambs
Unknown	±	Usually	— ? Spontaneous occurrence in *M. rhesus*
Years?	No antibody demonstrable	Unknown	+ Chimpanzees, Old World monkeys, New World monkeys, mink goats
4–18 months	No antibody demonstrable	Unknown	+ Chimpanzees, domestic cat, New World monkeys, Old World monkeys, guinea pigs, hamsters, mice, rats, goats

piratory infection during the 6-month interval prior to onset than during the same time period for controls, particularly for patients with type II disease. This observation must be viewed with caution because of the obvious differences in recall among patients with catastrophic illness. There was also a tendency for more mental illness in the families of patients and in the patients themselves than among controls. Antecedent mental illness has been commented on by Roos et al.[65] and by Ferber et al.[20] Evidence of prior hepatic disease was not encountered, although Kirschbaum[50] and Roos et al.[65] have noted abnormal liver-function tests and histological changes in the liver in CJD patients. In their series of cases, Traub et al.[76] have four patients who had experienced traumatic injuries immediately prior to the onset of CJD.

An intriguing observation in the study by Bobowick et al.[5] was that one third of patients and one third of controls gave a history of eating animal brains. Of these, 10 of 14 patients and 3 of 12 controls specifically stated a preference for hog brains. There are no data available on the frequency of brain consumption in the general population or the animal source of the brains eaten.

Interest in genetic factors in CJD has increased greatly.[24] In addition to the 13 cases in the 12 families referred to above from which successful trans-

mission to chimpanzees was accomplished, another 6 families with multiple cases have been documented.[20,24,25] Of 1902 cases recently reviewed, 15% were familial,[53c] and analysis of family cases suggested an incubation period up to 30 years. In some of these families (including one with successful transmission), cases have appeared in multiple generations in an autosomal dominant pattern. This leads to speculation that some families have a genetic defect determining the susceptibility to a latent virus. On the other hand, there might be vertical transmission of the agent within some families, with long incubation periods.[24] Another interpretation would be that shared environment in the absence of any genetic determinants caused these familial patterns.

5.6. Mechanisms and Routes of Transmission

Little is known concerning the mode of acquisition of CJD in humans except for three presumably iatrogenically transmitted infections that have been reported, one via a corneal transplant from a CJD patient[19] and two after use of stereotactic EEG electrodes previously used on a CJD patient.[4a] Human brain material from CJD patients has been successfully transmitted to a wide variety of animals, including the chimpanzee, five species of New World monkeys (spider, squirrel, capuchin, woolly, and marmoset), and six species of Old World monkeys (bushbaby, mangabey, African green, rhesus, cynomolgus, and stumptail), and the domestic cat. Many other species are still under observation.[25,33] CJD has been successfully transmitted to guinea pigs, hamsters, mice, rats, and goats.[32,33,34,36a,52a, d,f,g,h,55a,73b,c] The possible influence of a genetic factor has already been mentioned. All known spongiform encephalopathies can be transmitted by inoculation of infected brain and visceral tissues into susceptible host material. Scrapie and mink encephalopathy have been transmitted from animal to animal by contact and by ingestion of infected tissues. Thus, the aforementioned observation of a high rate of consumption of animal brains by CJD patients, while not different from that of controls except in preference for hog brains, provides a possible tenuous clue. The Israeli data, with high rates in migrants from Libya, a Moslem country where pigs are not eaten, would indicate that consumption of hog brains is not etiologically involved or that other animals, if the brains are ingested, may be capable of transmitting the virus[35a] Herzberg et al.[38] recently suggested that the dietary habit of eating sheep eyeballs, a gastronomic delicacy among Bedouin and Moroccan Arabs and also Libyans, may be associated with the high incidence of CJD in this population, since the tissues could be infected with scrapie, a subacute spongiform virus encephalopathy of sheep. Although an increasing range of animal hosts susceptible to the CJD virus is developing, it must be reemphasized that there are no firm data that ingested animal brains are the source of CJD infection in humans.

5.7. Pathogenesis and Immunity

Little is known about the pathogenesis of CJD in humans. From animal-inoculation data, it may be inferred that a lengthy incubation period precedes onset of clinical manifestations. In general, once symptoms appear, the disease is rapidly progressive. There are suggestions in some patients that mental disturbances many years prior to documented clinical onset may in fact be an early sign of the disease.[65,76] There is also the observation that in some instances the disease appears during severe upper respiratory illness, which is compatible with the hypothesis that a debilitating disease

could cause the release of a latent virus infection. In one series quoted above,[5] the respiratory illness was most frequently encountered in type II (ataxic) CJD. Preliminary information from another report of 22 patients with the ataxic form of CJD has not revealed similar occurrences in hospital records of about half these patients.[39]

CJD has been transmitted from human to human via a cornea transplant[19] and following stereotactic electroencephalographic exploration with the use of silver electrodes that had been previously implanted on a patient with proven CJD.[4a] Since the donor's eye was enucleated prior to removal of the cornea, the cornea was almost certainly contaminated with optic nerve. However, inoculation into the anterior chamber of the eye of cornea removed from infected guinea pigs without enucleation of the eye caused in healthy recipient guinea pigs a spongiform encephalopathy.[52d] In addition, the neurosurgical cases of Nevin et al.[59] suggest that CJD may be transmissible to man by direct inoculation. Inoculation of brain from a neurosurgeon who died of papulosis atrophicans maligna (Köhlmeier-Degos) with associated neuropathological features of CJD has produced experimental spongiform encephalopathy in subhuman primates.[27] It is not known whether this patient developed the disease because of contact with a CJD brain during his neurosurgical practice; however, this must be considered a possibility. These cases, together with the known transmissibility to primates of at least some CJD and the presence of the CJD virus in visceral tissue, have important practical implications. It is unwise to transplant tissues, including skin, kidney, and cornea, from any patient with presenile dementia.[28a] Additionally, exclusion of patients with presenile dementias as blood donors is suggested, since the presence of the virus in the buffy coat of the blood of infected guinea pigs and mice has been demonstrated.[51a,52e] Further, because of the presumed stability of CJD virus by analogy with scrapie virus, tissues from presenile dementia patients may pose a hazard to neurosurgeons, pathologists, and others who come in contact with them.

Transmissibility to the domestic cat raises the possibility of an animal reservoir, although there has been no report of natural disease in cats resembling experimental feline CJD.

Immune mechanisms have not been demonstrated in CJD, and specific antibodies to infected brain material or high antibody titers to a large series of known viruses have not been demonstrated.[9] However, it has recently been demonstrated that greater than 50% of patients with CJD have in their serum heterogeneic autoantibodies directed specifically against neurofilament protein in the axonal process of mature neurons of the central nervous system grown *in vitro*.[72a]

5.8. Patterns of Host Response

The range of clinical manifestations is outlined in Table 3. As mentioned above, with the exception of earlier onset in type III CJD and the questionable data on hepatic involvement or upper respiratory disease prior to onset, there are no detectable patterns of prior host response. As a result, there is little in the way of control and prevention available through epidemiological data other than the suggestion that heightened interest be directed toward the consumption of animal brains as a factor.

There have been reports of three CJD patients treated with amantadine in whom rapid improvement over varying periods of time was observed.[66] In at least one of these, autopsy confirmation of the diagnosis is available. Along with its many other effects, amantadine is an antiviral agent. Another independent action is in the dopaminergic pathways of the central nervous system. Whether either of these actions caused the improvement or whether other CJD patients will improve after treatment with amantadine remains to be determined.

5.9. Control and Prevention

Until the source and mechanism of naturally occurring CJD in humans are established, there is no epidemiological basis for prevention. However, iatrogenic transmissions may be preventable, and a series of precautions for caring for patients with CJD and in handling their tissues have been published[28a] and amended.[28b] Special isolation wards for patients seem unwarranted. Gloves are recommended in handling infected tissues, but not in routine care of patients. Patients should not be used as a donor source of blood or any other tissue (especially cornea). Needles and needle electrodes should be autoclaved (121°C and 15 lb/cm^2 for 1 hr), incinerated, or discarded. The virus resists simple boiling in water, 10% formalin, 70% alcohol, β-propiolac-

tone, and both ionizing and ultraviolet irradiation. Glutaraldehyde data are not available, and tests of ethylene oxide are in progress. Adequate disinfection is achieved with 5% hypochlorite, 0.03% permanganate, phenolics, and iodine solutions.

5.10. Unresolved Problems

It is obvious from the foregoing discussion that CJD is a fascinating human disease that is transmissible to a variety of animal species. Aside from this, most aspects of acquisition, prevention, and control are still to be resolved. While the disease is rare, 1435 cases have been assembled; 824 were reported to the NIH since 1966 and 611 cited from the world literature from 1910 through 1977.[53d] Of these, 111 were experimentally transmissible, 588 were regarded as definite or probable CJD, and 736 were grouped as possible cases.

Since a dominant feature of the disease is dementia, attention has been directed to other human dementias with the thought that there may be possible overlap with CJD or that perhaps they are caused by other slow viruses.[23] In this connection, it is worth mentioning the occurrence of CJD and Alzheimer's disease in members of the same family.[53c] Indeed, the transmission of CJD to subhuman primates has made it possible to define a subgroup of CJD patients whose disease is transmissible and to determine whether some cases diagnosed as CJD may represent a distinct nontransmissible neurological illness. It has further permitted an inquiry into the possibility that there are cases of transmissible virus dementias that are being given clinical or pathological diagnosis other than CJD. These diagnoses may include such syndromes as Alzheimer's or Pick's disease, parkinsonism with dementia, and "cortical atrophy" or "dementia of unknown etiology."[63c]

6. Summary and Comparison

It is a well-established fact that kuru, a rare and disappearing transmissible heredofamilial disease of man in the Eastern Highlands of Papua New Guinea, and scrapie, a subacute progressive degenerative central nervous system disease of sheep that has been recognized for more than 200 years in Europe, have largely been responsible for our knowledge that viruses cause chronic, slowly evolving, relentlessly progressive, fatal diseases of the central nervous system. It was the study of these two diseases that led to the demonstration that Creutzfeldt–Jakob disease, an uncommon but not rare presenile dementia of man, is also caused by a virus closely related or identical to the viruses of kuru and scrapie. Because of their unique physical, biological, and biochemical properties, they are classified as the subacute spongiform virus encephalopathies.

These advances during the past decade led to the elucidation of "conventional" virus etiologies for other chronic neurological diseases such as subacute sclerosing panencephalitis, caused by defective measles virus, and progressive multifocal leukoencephalopathy, caused by papovaviruses. It thus became apparent that a wide diversity of clinical courses and pathological lesions could be produced by viral invasions of the central nervous system.

The studies of "slow infections" of the central nervous system have necessitated new concepts concerning the spectrum of neurological diseases that might be related to viruses. A viral etiology must now be considered in neurological diseases that are manifested by chronic, subacute, progressive, or relapsing degenerative courses with or without associated dementia and in which noninflammatory pathological lesions are observed.

7. Unresolved Problems

A major unresolved problem associated with chronic subacute progressive degenerative diseases of the central nervous system of viral etiology continues to be our lack of knowledge of the definitive nature of the subacute spongiform virus encephalopathies. In the case where more conventional viruses produce chronic infections, the problem is our lack of knowledge of the mechanisms of virus–host cell relationships that permit these viruses to enter the central nervous system and establish progressive and ultimately fatal diseases. New methods will certainly be required to determine whether infection is involved in the etiology of other chronic neurological diseases such as multiple sclerosis, amyotrophic lateral sclerosis, and Parkinson's disease, and perhaps even diseases that appear to follow a genetic pattern.[58a] We must concern ourselves with classic virological knowledge of latency, masking,

persistence, temperateness, existence of proviruses, and defectiveness; we must take into account the problems of host-range specificity and the need for helper viruses. Finally, we must also recognize that viruses will prove to be responsible for only a limited number of chronic neurological diseases.

Acknowledgments

The editor is indebted to Dr. Francis L. Black, Professor of Epidemiology (Microbiology), and Dr. Elias Manuelidis, Professor of Neuropathology and Neurology, Yale University School of Medicine, and to Dr. Gabriele Zu Rhein, Professor of Pathology, and Dr. D. L. Walker, Professor of Microbiology, University of Wisconsin School of Medicine, for their help in updating this chapter.

8. References

1. ALEMA, G., Transmissible and genetic late dementiae, in: *Proceedings of the Tenth International Congress of Neurology*, Abstract No. 29 (A. SUBIRANA AND J. M. BURROWS, eds.), p. 13, Barcelona, September 9–14, 1973, *Int. Congr. Ser.*, No. 319, Excerpta Medica, Amsterdam, 1973.
2. ALPERS, M., Epidemiological changes in kuru, 1957 to 1963, in: *Slow, Latent and Tempurate Virus Infections*, NINDB Monogr. No. 2 (D. C. GAJDUSEK, C. J. GIBBS, JR., AND M. ALPERS, eds.), pp. 65–82, National Institutes of Health, PNS Publ. No. 1378, Department of Health, Education, and Welfare, Government Printing Office, Washington, D.C., 1965.
3. ALPERS, M. P., Kuru: Implications of its transmissibility for the interpretation of its changing epidemiologic pattern, in: *The Central Nervous System* Some Experimental Models of Neurological Diseases, (O. T. BAILEY AND D. E. SMITH, eds.), pp. 234–251, Proceedings of the Fifty-sixth Annual Meeting of the International Academy of Pathology, Washington, D. C., March 12–15, 1967, International Academy of Pathology Monograph No. 9, Williams and Wilkins, Baltimore, 1968.
3a. ALPERS, M. P., Epidemiology and ecology of kuru, in: *Slow Transmissible Diseases of the Nervous System*, Vol. I, *Clinical, Epidemiological, Genetic, and Pathological Aspects of the Spongiform Encephalopathies* (S. B. PRUSINER AND W. J. HADLOW, eds.), pp. 67–90, Academic Press, New York, 1979.
4. BAGULEY, D. M., AND GLASGOW, G. L., Subacute sclerosing panencephalitis and Salk vaccine, *Lancet* 2:763–765 (1973).
4a. BERNOULLI, C., SIEGFRIED, J., BAUMGARTNER, C., REGLI, F., RABINOWICZ, T., GAJDUSEK, D. C., AND GIBBS, C. J., JR., Danger of accidental person-to-person trans-

mission of Creutzfeldt–Jakob disease by surgery, *Lancet* **1**:478–479 (1979).

5. BOBOWICK, A. R., BRODY, J. A., MATTHEWS, M. R., ROOS, R., AND GAJDUSEK, D. C., Creutzfeldt–Jakob disease: A case control study, *Am. J. Epidemiol.* **98**:381–394 (1973).

6. BOLTON, C. F., AND ROZDILSKY, B., Primary progressive multifocal leukoencephalopathy, *Neurology* **21**:72–77 (1971).

7. BRODY, J. A., AND DETELS, R., Subacute sclerosing panencephalitis: A zoonosis following aberrant measles: Hypothesis, *Lancet* **2**:500–501 (1970).

8. BRODY, J. A., DETELS, R., AND SEVER, J. L., Measles-antibody titers in sibships of patients with subacute sclerosing panencephalitis and controls, *Lancet* **1**:177–178 (1972).

8a. BROWN, F., AND CATHALA, F., Creutzfeldt–Jakob disease in France, in: *Slow Transmissible Diseases of the Nervous System*, Vol. I, *Clinical, Epidemiological, Genetic, and Pathological Aspects of the Spongiform Encephalopathies* (S. B. PRUSINER AND W. J. HADLOW, eds.), pp. 213–227, Academic Press, New York, 1979.

8b. BROWN, P., CATHALA, F., AND GAJDUSEK, D. C., Cruetzfeldt–Jakob disease in France. III. Epidemiological study of 170 patients dying during the decade 1968–1977, *Ann. Neurol.* **6**:438–446 (1979).

9. BROWN, P., HOOKS, J., ROOS, R., GAJDUSEK, D. C., AND GIBBS, C. J. JR., Attempt to identify the agent of Creutzfeldt–Jakob disease by antibody relationship to known viruses, *Nature (London) New Biol.* **235**:149–152 (1972).

9a. BROWN, P., TSAI, T., AND GAJDUSEK, C., Seroepidemiology of human papovaviruses, *Am. J. Epidemiol.* **102**:331–340 (1975).

10. BRUN, A., NORDENFELDT, E., AND KJELLEN, L., Aspects on the variability of progressive multifocal leukoencephalopathy, *Acta Neuropathol.* **24**:232–243 (1973).

11. BYINGTON, D. P., AND BURNSTEIN, T., Measles encephalitis produced in suckling rats, *Exp. Mol. Pathol.* **19**:36–43 (1973).

12. CANAL, N., AND TORCK, P., An epidemiological study of subacute sclerosing leucoencephalitis in Belgium, *J. Neurol. Sci.* **1**:380–389 (1964).

12a. CANDEIAS, J. A. N., BARUZZI, R. G., PRIPES, S., AND IUNES, M., Prevalence of antibodies to the BK and JC papovaviruses in isolated populations, *Rev. Saude Publica* **11**:510–514 (1977).

13. CANELAS, H. M., JULIAO, O. F., LEFEVRE, A. B., LAMARTINE de ASSIS, TOGNOLA, W. A., dE JORGE, F. B., FONSECA, L. C., AND XAVIER-LIMA, A., Subacute sclerosing panencephalitis: epidemiological, clinical and biochemical study of 31 cases, *Arch. Neuro-Psychiatr.* (*São Paulo*) **25**:255–268 (1967).

14. CASTAIGNE, P., RONDOT, P., ESCOURELLE, R., RIDADEAU, D., LUMAS, J. L., CATHALA, F., AND HAUW, J., Leucoencephalopathe multifocale progressive et "gliomes" multiples, *Rev. Neurol.* **130**:379–393 (1974).

15. CONNOLLY, J. H., HAIRE, M., AND HADDEN, D. S. M., Measles immunoglobulins in subacute sclerosing panencephalitis, *Br. Med. J.* **1**:23–25 (1971).

16. DAYAN, A. D., AND STOKES, M. I., Immune complexes and visceral deposits of measles antigens in subacute sclerosing panencephalitis, *Br. Med. J.* **2**:374–376 (1972).

17. DETELS, R., BRODY, J. A., McNEW, J., AND EDGAR, A. H., Further epidemiologic studies of subacute sclerosing panencephalitis, *Lancet* **2**:11–14 (1973).

18. DONNER, M., HALONEN, H., AND HALTIA, M., Subakuutti sklerosoiva panenkefaliitti, *Duodecim* **85**:541–553 (1969).

19. DUFFY, P., WOLF, J., COLLINS, G., DEVOE, A. G., STREETEN, B., AND COWEN, D., Person-to-person transmission of Creutzfeldt–Jakob disease, *N. Engl. J. Med.* **299**:692–693 (1974).

20. FERBER, R. A., WIESENFELD, S. L., ROOS, R. P., BOBOWICK, A. R., GIBBS, C. J., JR., AND GAJDUSEK, D. C., Familial Creutzfeldt–Jakob disease: Transmission of the familial disease to primates, in: *Neurology* (A. SUBRIANA AND J. E. BURROWS, eds.), pp. 358–380, Proceedings of the Tenth International Congress of Neurology, Barcelona, September 8–15, 1973, *Int. Congr. Ser.*, No. 319, Excerpta Medica, Amsterdam, 1973.

21. FERMAGLICH, J., HARDMAN, J. M., AND EARLE, K. M., Spontaneous progressive multifocal leukoencephalopathy, *Neurology* **20**:479–484 (1970).

22. GAJDUSEK, D. C., Kuru in the New Guinea highlands, in: *Tropical Neurology*, Vol. 29 (J. D. SPILLANE, ed.), pp. 376–383, Oxford University Press, London, 1973.

22a. GAJDUSEK, D. C., Slow infections with unconventional viruses, *Harvey Lect.* **72**:283–353 (1978).

23. GAJDUSEK, D. C., AND GIBBS, C. J., JR., Kuru and the virus dementias, in: Conference on Biohazards in Cancer Research, Pacific Grove, California, January 22–24, 1973, *Biohazards in Biological Research* (A. HELLMEN, M. N. OXMAN, AND R. POLLACK, eds.), pp. 288–299, Cold Spring Harbor Press, Cold Spring Harbor, New York, 1973.

24. GAJDUSEK, D. C., AND GIBBS, C. J., JR., Subacute and chronic diseases caused by atypical infections with unconventional viruses in aberrant hosts, in: *Persistent Virus Infections*, Vol. VIII, *Perspectives in Virology* M. POLLARD, ed.), pp. 279–311, Academic Press, New York, 1973.

25. GAJDUSEK, D. C., AND GIBBS, C. J., JR., Familial and sporadic chronic neurologic degenerative disorders transmitted from man to primates, in: *Advances in Neurology*, Vol. 10, *Primate Models of Neurological Disorders* (B. S. MELDRUM AND C. D. MARSDEN, eds.), pp. 291–375, Raven Press, New York, 1975.

26. GAJDUSEK, D. C., GIBBS, C. J., JR., AND ALPERS, M., Experimental transmission of a kuru-like syndrome to chimpanzees, *Nature (London)* **209**:794–796 (1966).

27. GAJDUSEK, D. C., GIBBS, C. J., JR., EARLE, K., DAMMIN, G. J., SCHOENE, W. C., AND TYLER, H. R., Transmission of subacute spongiform encephalopathy to the chimpanzee and squirrel monkey from a patient with papulosis atrophicans maligna of Köhlmeier-Degos, in: *Proceedings of the Tenth International Congress on Neurology* (A. SUBIRANA AND J. BURROWS, eds.), pp. 390–392, *Int. Cong. Ser.*, No. 319, Excerpta Medica, Amsterdam, 1973.

28. GAJDUSEK, D. C., GIBBS, C. J., JR., AND ALPERS, M. (eds.), *Slow, Latent and Temperate Virus Infections*, NINDB Monogr. No. 2, National Institutes of Health, PNS Publ. No. 1378, Department of Health, Education, and Welfare, Government Printing Office, Washington, D.C., 1965.

28a. GAJDUSEK, D. C., GIBBS, C. J., JR., ASHER, D. M., BROWN, P., DUVAN, A., HOFFMAN, P., NEMO, G., ROHWER, R., AND WHITE, L., Precautions in medical care of, and in handling materials from, patients with transmitted virus dementia (Creutzfeldt–Jakob disease), *N. Engl. J. Med.* **297**:1253–1258 (1977).

28b. GAJDUSEK, D. C., GIBBS, C. J., JR., AND ASHER, D. M., Letter to the editor, *N. Engl. J. Med.* **298**:976 (1978).

29. GARDNER, S. D., Prevalence in England of antibody to human polyomavirus (B.K.), *Br. Med. J.* **1**:77–78 (1973).

30. GARDNER, S. D., FIELD, A., COLEMAN, D., AND HULME, B., New human papovavirus (B.K.) isolated from urine after renal transplantation, *Lancet* **1**:1253–1257 (1971).

30a. GERBER, M. A., SHAH, K. V., THUNG, S. N., AND ZU RHEIN, G. M., Immunohistochemical demonstration of common antigen of polyomaviruses in routine histologic tissue sections of animals and man, *Amer. J. Clin. Pathol.* **73**:794–797 (1980).

31. GERSON, K. L., AND HASLAM, R. H. A., Subtle immunologic abnormalities in SSPE, *N. Engl. J. Med.* **285**:78–82 (1971).

31a. GIBBS, C. J., JR., AMYX, H. L., BACOTE, A., MASTERS, C. L., AND GAJDUSEK, D. C., Oral transmission of kuru, Creutzfeldt–Jakob disease, and scrapie to nonhuman primates, *J. Infect. Dis.* **142**:205–208 (1980).

32. GIBBS, C. J., JR., AND GAJDUSEK, D. C., Transmission and characterization of the agents of spongiform virus encephalopathies, kuru, Creutzfeldt–Jakob disease, scrapie and mink encephalopathy, in: *Immunological Disorders of the Nervous System*, Vol. XLIX (L. P. ROWLAND, ed.), Res. Publ. A.R.N.M.D., pp. 383–410, Williams and Wilkins, Baltimore, 1971.

33. GIBBS, C. J., JR., AND GAJDUSEK, D. C., Experimental subacute spongiform virus encephalopathies in primates and other laboratory animals, *Science* **182**:67–68 (1973).

34. GIBBS, C. J., JR., AND GAJDUSEK, D. C., Biology of kuru and Creutzfeldt–Jakob disease, in: *Slow Virus Diseases* (W. ZEMAN AND E. H. LENNETTE, eds.), pp. 39–48, Williams and Wilkins, Baltimore, 1973.

35. GIBBS, C. J., JR., GAJDUSEK, D. C., ASHER, D. M., ALPERS, M. P., BECK, E., DANIEL, P. M., AND MATTHEWS, W. B., Creutzfeldt–Jakob disease (subacute spongiform encephalopathy): Transmission to the chimpanzee, *Science* **161**:388–389 (1968).

35a. GOLDBERG, H., ALTER, M., AND KAHANA, E., The Lybian Jewish focus of Creutzfeldt–Jakob disease: A search for the mode of natural transmission, in: *Slow Transmissible Diseases of the Nervous System*, Vol. I, *Clinical, Epidemiological, Genetic, and Pathological Aspects of the Spongiform Encephalopathies* (S. B. PRUSINER AND W. J. HADLOW, eds.), pp. 195–211, Academic Press, New York, 1979.

36. HADLOW, W. J., Scrapie and kuru, *Lancet* **2**:289–290 (1959).

36a. HADLOW, W. J., PRUSINER, S. B., KENNEDY, R. C., AND RACE, R. E., Brain tissue from persons with Creutzfeldt–Jakob disease causes scrapie-like encephalopathy in goats, *Ann. Neurol.* **8**:628–631 (1980).

36b. HALL, W. W., LAMB, R. A., AND CHOPPIN, P. W., Measles and subacute sclerosing panencephalitis virus proteins: Lack of antibodies to the M protein in patients with subacute sclerosing panencephalitis, *Proc. Natl. Acad. Sci. U.S.A.* **76**:2047–2051 (1979).

36c. HALSEY, N. A., MODLIN, J. F., JABBOUR, J. T., DUBEY, L., EDDENS, D. L., AND LUDWIG, D. D., Risk factors in SSPE: A case–control study, *Am. J. Epidemiol.* **111**:415–431 (1980).

37. HEDLEY-WHYTE, E. T., SMITH, B. P., TYLER, H. R., AND PETERSON, W. P., Multifocal leukoncephalopathy with remission and five year survival, *J. Neuropathol. Exp. Neurol* **25**:107–116 (1966).

38. HERZBERG, L., HERZBERG, B. W., GIBBS, C. J., JR., SULLIVAN, W., AMYX, H., AND GAJDUSEK, D. C., Creutzfeldt–Jakob disease: Hypothesis for high incidence in Libyan Jews in Israel, *Science* **186**:848 (1974).

39. HIRANO, A., Personal communication, 1974.

39a. HO, K., GARANCIS, J. C., PAEGLE, R. D., GERBER, M. A., AND BORKOWSKI, W. J., Progressive multifocal leukoncephalopathy and malignant lymphoma of the brain in a patient with immunosuppressive therapy, *Acta Neuropathol. (Berlin)* **52**:81–83 (1980).

40. HOOKS, J. J., GIBBS, C. J., JR., CHOPRA, H., LEWIS, M., AND GAJDUSEK, D. C., Spontaneous transformation of human brain cells grown *in vitro* and characterization of associated virus particles, *Science* **176**:1420–1422 (1972).

41. HORNABROOK, R. W., Kuru—A subacute cerebellar degeneration: The natural history and clinical features, *Brain* **91**:53–74 (1968).

42. HORTA-BARBOSA, L., Subacute sclerosing panencephalitis: Isolation of suppressed measles virus from

lymph node biopsies, *Science* **173**:840–841 (1971).

43. HORTA-BARBOSA, L., FUCCILLO, D. A., LONDON, W. T., JABBOUR, J. T., ZEMAN, W., AND SEVER, J. L., Isolation of measles virus from brain cell cultures of two patients with subacute sclerosing panencephalitis, *Proc. Soc. Exp. Biol. Med.* **132**:272–277 (1969).

44. JABBOUR, J. T., DUENAS, D. A., SEVER, J. L., KREBS, H. M., AND HORTA-BARBOSA, L., Epidemiology of subacute sclerosing panencephalitis (SSPE), *J. Am. Med. Assoc.* **220**:959–962 (1972).

45. JABBOUR, J. T., AND SEVER, J. L., Serum measles antibody titers in patients with subacute sclerosing panencephalitis, compared with parents and siblings, *J. Pediatr.* **73**:905–907 (1968).

46. JELLINGER, V. K., SEITELBERGER, F., HEISS, W. D., AND HOLCZABEK, W., Konjugale Form der subakutem spongiosen Enzephalopathie (Jakob–Creutzfeldt-Erkrankung), *Wien. Klin. Wochenschr.* **84**:245–249 (1972).

47. JOASOO, A., AND WOLFENDEN, W. H., Subacute spongiform encephalopathy, *Med. J. Aust.* **1**:354–356 (1968).

48. KAHANA, E., ALTER, M., BRAHAM, J., AND SOFER, D., Creutzfeldt–Jakob disease: A focus among Libyan Jews in Israel, *Science* **183**:90–91 (1974).

48a. KATZ, M., AND KOPROWSKI, H., The significance of failure to isolate infectious viruses in cases of subacute sclerosing panencephalitis, *Arch. Gesamte Virusforsch.* **41**:390–393 (1973).

49. KATZ, M., RORKE, L. B., MASLAND, W. S., BRODANO, G. B., AND KOPROWSKI, H., Subacute sclerosing panencephalitis: Isolation of a virus encephalitogenic for ferrets, *J. Infect. Dis.* **121**:188–195 (1970).

50. KIRSCHBAUM, W. R., *Jakob–Creutzfeldt Disease*, American Elsevier, New York, 1968, 251 pp.

51. KOPROWSKI, H., Interaction between papova-like virus and paramyxovirus in human brain cells: A hypothesis, *Nature (London)* **225**:1045–1047 (1970).

51a. KURODA, Y., GIBBS, C. J., JR., AMYX, H. L., AND GAJDUSEK, D. C., The pathogenesis of Creutzfeldt–Jakob disease in the mouse, *Infect. Immun.* (in press) (1981).

52. LEGRAIN, M., *et al.*, Leuco-encepholie multifocal progressive après transplantation renale, *J. Neurol. Sci.* **23**:49–62 (1974).

52a. LONDON, W. T., HOUFF, S. A., MADDEN, D. L., FUCILLO, D. A., GRAVELL, M., WALLEN., W. C., PALMER., A. E., SEVER, J. L., PADGETT, B. L., WALKER, D. L., ZU RHEIN, G. M., AND OHASHI, T., Brain tumors in owl monkeys inoculated with a human polyomavirus (JC virus), *Science* **201**:1246–1249 (1978).

52b. MACHAMER, C. E., HAYES, E. C., GOLLOBIN, S. D., WESTFALL, L. K., AND ZWEERINK, H. J., Antibodies against the measles matrix polypeptide after clinical infection and vaccination, *Infect. Immun.* **27**:817–825 (1980).

52c. MALMGREN, R., KURLAND, L., MOKRI, B., AND KURTZKE, J., The epidemiology of Creutzfeldt–Jakob disease, in: *Slow Transmissible Diseases of the Nervous System,*

Vol. I, *Clinical, Epidemiological, Genetic, and Pathological Aspects of the Spongiform Encephalopathies,* (S. B. PRUSINER AND W. J. HADLOW, eds.), pp. 93–112, Academic Press, New York, 1979.

52d. MANUELIDIS, E. E., ANGELO, J. N., GORGACZ, E. J., KIM, J. H., AND MANUELIDIS, L., Experimental Creutzfeldt–Jakob disease transmitted via the eye with infected cornea, *N. Engl. J. Med.* **296**:1334–1336 (1977).

52e. MANUELIDIS, E. E., GORGACZ, E. J., AND MANUELIDIS, L., Interspecies transmission of Creutzfeldt–Jakob disease to the Syrian hamster with reference to clinical syndromes and strains of agent, *Proc. Natl. Acad. Sci. U.S.A.* **75**:3432–3436 (1978).

52f. MANUELIDIS, E. E., KIM, J., ANGELO, J. N., AND MANEULIDIS, L., Serial propagation of Creutzfeldt–Jakob disease in guinea pigs, *Proc. Natl. Acad. Sci. U.S.A.* **73**:223–227 (1976).

52g. MANUELIDIS, E. E., AND MANUELIDIS, L., Experiments on maternal transmission of Creutzfeldt–Jakob disease in guinea pigs, *Proc. Soc. Exp. Biol. Med.* **160**:233–236 (1979).

52h. MANEULIDIS, E. E., MANUELIDIS, L., PINCUS, J. H., AND COLLINS, W. F., Transmission, from man to the hamster, of Creutzfeldt–Jakob disease with clinical recovery, *Lancet* **2**:40–42 (1978).

53. MANZ, H. J., DINSDALE, H. B. AND MOVRIN, P. A. F., Progressive multifocal encephalopathy after renal transplantation, *Ann. Intern. Med.* **75**:77–81 (1971).

53a. MASTERS, C. L., GAJDUSEK, D. C., GIBBS, C. J., JR., BERNOULLI, C., AND ASHER, D. M., Familial Creutzfeldt–Jakob disease and other familial dementias: An inquiry into possible modes of transmission of virus-induced familial disease, in: *Slow Transmissible Diseases of the Nervous System,* Vol. I, *Clinical, Epidemiological, Genetic, and Pathological Aspects of the Spongiform Encephalopathies* (S. B. PRUSINER AND W. J. HADLOW, eds.), pp. 143–194, Academic Press, New York, 1979.

53b. AMYX, H. L., GIBBS, C. J., JR., GAJDUSEK, D. C., AND GREER, W. E., Absence of vertical transmission of subacute spongiform viral encephalopathies in experimental primates, *Proc. Soc. Exp. Biol. Med.* **166(14)**:469–471 (1981).

53c. MASTERS, C. L., GAJDUSEK, D. C., AND GIBBS, C. J., JR., The familial occurrence of Creutzfeldt–Jakob disease and Alzheimer's disease, *Brain* (in press) (1981).

53d. MASTERS, C. L., HARRIS, J. O., AND GAJDUSEK, D. C., Creutzfeldt–Jakob disease: Patterns of worldwide occurrence, in: *Slow Transmissible Diseases of the Nervous System,* Vol. I, *Clinical Epidemiological, Genetic and Pathological Aspects of the Spongiform Encephalopathies* (S. B. PRUSINER AND W. J. HADLOW, eds.), pp. 113–142, Academic Press, New York, (1979).

54. MATHUR, W. V. AND KARANI, H. J., Jakob–Creutzfeldt syndrome, *J. Indian Med. Assoc.* **49(3)**:142–143 (1967).

55. MATSUOKA, T., HAMANAKA, T., TAIL, S., TATEBAYASHI, Y., KIJIMA, S., AND NISHIKAWA, T., Subacute spongi-

form encephalopathy as a subtype of Creutzfeldt–Jakob disease—A report of two cases, *Psychiatr. Neurol. Jpn.* **72:**669–690 (1970).

55a. MATTHEWS, W. B., TOMLINSON, A. H., AND HUGHES, J. T., Transmission of Creutzfeldt–Jakob disease to guinea pigs, *Lancet* **2:**752 (1979).

56. MAY, W. W., Creutzfeldt–Jakob disease. I. Survey of the literature and clinical diagnosis, *Acta Neurol. Scand.* **44:**1–32 (1968).

57. MCDONALD, R., KIPPS, A., AND LEARY, P. M., Subacute sclerosing panencephalitis in the Cape Province, *S. Afr. Med. J.* **48:**7–9 (1974).

57a. MODLIN, J. F., HALSEY, N. A., EDDINS, D. L., CONRAD, J. L., JABBOUR, J. T., CHIEN, L., AND ROBINSON, H., Subacute sclerosing panencephalitis: A report of the national registry, *J. Pediatr.* **94:**231–236 (1979).

57b. MODLIN, J. F., JABBOUR, J. T., WITTE, J. J., AND HALSEY, N. A., Epidemiologic studies of measles, measles vaccine, and subacute sclerosing panencephalitis, *Pediatrics* **59:**505–512 (1977).

58. NARAYAN, O., PENNEY, J. B., JOHNSON, R. T., HERNDON, R. M., AND WEINER, L. P., Etiology of progressive multifocal leukoencephalopathy: Identification of papovavirus, *N. Engl. J. Med.* **289**(24):1278–1282 (1973).

58a. NATHANSON, N., Slow viruses and chronic disease: The contribution of epidemiology, *Public Health Rep.* **95:**436–443 (1980).

59. NEVIN, S., MCMENEMEY, W. H., BEHRMAN, S., AND JONES, D. P., Subacute spongiform encephalopathy—A subacute form of encephalopathy attributable to vascular dysfunction (spongiform cerebral atrophy), *Brain* **83:**519–564 (1960).

60. NOTERMANS, S. L. H., TIJL, W. F. J., WILLENS, F. T. C., AND SLOOFF, J. L., Experimentally induced subacute sclerosing panencephalitis in young dogs, *Neurology* **23:**543–553 (1973).

61. PADGETT, B. L., AND WALKER, D. L., Prevalence of antibodies in human sera against JC virus, an isolate from a case of progressive multifocal leukoencephalopathy, *J. Infect. Dis.* **127:**467–470 (1973).

62. PADGETT, B. L., ZU RHEIN, G. M., WALKER, D. L., ECKROADE, R. J., AND DESSEL, B. H., Cultivation of papova-like virus from human brain with progressive multifocal leukoencephalopathy, *Lancet* **1:**1257–1260 (1971).

63. PAYNE, F. E., BAUBLIS, J. V., AND ITABASHI, H. H., Isolation of measles virus from cell cultures of brain from a patient with subacute sclerosing panencephalitis, *N. Engl. J. Med.* **281:**585–589 (1969).

63a. PETTAY, O., DONNER, M., HALONEN, H., PALOSUO, T., AND ALMI, A., Subacute sclerosing panencephalitis: Preceding intellectual deterioration and deviant measles serology, *J. Infect. Dis.* **124:**439–444 (1971).

63b. PRUSINER, S. B., AND HADLOW, W. J. (eds.), *Slow Transmissible Diseases of the Nervous System*, Vol. I, *Clinical, Epidemiological, Genetic, and Pathological Aspects of the*

Spongiform Encephalopathies, Academic Press, New York, 1979, 472 pp.

63c. REWCASTLE, N. B., GIBBS, C. J., JR., AND GAJDUSEK, D. C., Transmission of familial Alzheimer's disease to primates, *J. Neuropathol. Exp. Neurol.* **37:**679 (1978).

64. RICHARDSON, E. P., Progressive multifocal leukoencephalopathy, in: *The Remote Effects of Cancer of the Nervous System* (L. BRAIN AND F. H. NORRIS, JR., eds.), pp. 6–16, Grune and Stratton, New York, 1965.

65. ROOS, R., GAJDUSEK, D. C., AND GIBBS, C. J., JR., The clinical characteristics of transmissible Creutzfeldt–Jakob disease, *Brain* **96:**1–20 (1973).

66. SANDERS, D., AND POSKANZER, D. C., Personal communication, 1973.

66a. SCHLUEDERBERG, A. E., CHAVANICH, S., LIPMAN, M. B., AND CARTER, C., Comparative molecular weight estimates of measles and subacute sclerosing panencephalitis virus structural polypeptides by simultaneous electrophoresis in acrylamide slab gels, *Biochem. Biophysics Res. Commun.* **58:**547–551 (1974).

67. SEVER, J. L., JABBOUR, J. T., BEADLE, E., AND KREBS, H., Constant incubation period for subacute sclerosing panencephalitis (abstract), *Proc. Soc. Exp. Biol. Med.* (April 1974).

68. SEVER, J. L., AND ZEMAN, W. (eds.), Conference on Measles Virus and Subacute Sclerosing Panencephalitis, Bethesda, Maryland, September 13, 1967, *Neurology* **19**(Part 2):30–51 (1968).

69. SHAH, K. V., DANIEL, R. W., AND WARSZAWSKI, R. M., High prevalence of antibodies to BK virus, and SV-40 related papovavirus, in residents of Maryland, *J. Infect. Dis.* **128:**784–787 (1973).

70. SHAW, C. M., BUCHAN, G. C., AND CARLSON, C. B., Myxovirus as a possible etiologic agent in subacute inclusion-body encephalitis, *N. Engl. J. Med.* **277:**511–515 (1967).

71. SIEDLER, H., AND MALAMUD, N., Creutzfeldt–Jakob disease: Clinicopathologic report of 15 cases and review of the literature (with special reference to a related disorder designated as subacute spongiform encephalopathy), *J. Neuropathol. Exp. Neurol.* **22:**381–402 (1963).

72. SILVERMAN, L., AND RUBINSTEIN, L. G., Electron microscopic observations on a case of progressive multifocal leukoencephalopathy, *Acta Neuropathol.* **5:**215–224 (1965).

72a. SOTELO, J., GIBBS, C. J., JR., AND GAJDUSEK, D. C., Autoantibodies against axonal neurofilaments in patients with kuru and Creutzfeldt–Jakob disease, *Science* **210:**190–193 (1981).

73a. SUTTON, R. N. P., Slow viruses and chronic disease of the central nervous system, *Postgrad. Med. J.* **55:**143–149 (1979).

73b. TATEISHI, J., OHTA, M., KOGA, M., SATO, Y., AND KUROIWA, Y., Transmission of chronic spongiform encephalopathy with kuru plaques from humans to small rodents, *Ann. Neurol.* **5**:581–584 (1979).

73c. TATEISHI, J., SATO, Y., KOGA, M., DOI, H., AND OHTA, M., Experimental transmission of human subacute spongiform encephalopathy to small rodents. 1. Clinical and histological observations, *Acta Neuropathol.* **51**:127–134 (1980).

73d. TER MEULEN, V., AND HALL, W. W., Slow virus infections of the nervous system: Virological, immunological and pathogenetic considerations, *J. Gen. Virol.* **41**:1–25 (1978).

74. THEIN, P., MAYR, A., TER MEULEN, V., KOPROWSKI, H., KACKELL, M. Y., MULLER, D., AND MEYERMANN, R., Subacute sclerosing panencephalitis: Transmission of the virus to calves and lambs, *Arch. Neurol.* **27**:540–548 (1972).

75. THORMAR, H., JERVIS, G. A., KARL, S. C., AND BROWN, H. R., Passage in ferrets of encephalitogenic cell-associated measles virus isolated from brain of a patient with subacute sclerosing panencephalitis, *J. Infect. Dis.* **127**:678–685 (1973).

76. TRAUB, R. D., GAJDUSEK, D. C., AND GIBBS, C. J., JR., Transmissible virus dementia: The relation of transmissible spongiform encephalopathy to Creutzfeldt–Jakob disease, in: *Aging, Dementia and Cerebral Function* (M. KINSBOURNE AND L. SMITH, eds.), pp. 91–146, Spectrum, New York, 1977.

77. VERNON, M. L., HORTA-BARBOSA, L., FUCCILLO, D. A., SEVER, J. L., BARINGER, J. R., AND BIRNBAUM, G., Virus-like particles and nucleoprotein-type filaments in brain tissue from two patients with Creutzfeldt–Jakob disease, *Lancet* **1**:964–967 (1970).

77a. WALKER, D. L., Progressive multifocal leukoencephalopathy: An opportunistic viral infection of the central nervous system, in: *Handbook of Clinical Neurology*, Vol. 34, *Infections of the Nervous System* (P. J. VINKEN AND G. W. BRUYN, eds.), pp. 307–329, Elsevier/North-Holland, New York, 1978.

77b. WALKER, D. L., Personal communication, 1981.

78. WALKER, D. L., PADGETT, B. L., ZU RHEIN, G. M., ALBERT, A. E., AND MARSH, R. F., Human papovavirus (JC): Induction of brain tumors in hamsters, *Science* **181**:674–676 (1973).

79. WEAR, D., AND RAPP, F., Latent measles virus infection of the hamster central nervous system, *J. Immunol.* **107**:1593–1598 (1971).

79a. WECHSLER, S. L., WEINER, H. L., AND FIELDS, B. N., Immune response in subacute sclerosing panencephalitis: Reduced antibody response to the matrix protein of measles virus, *J. Immunol.* **123**:884–889 (1979).

80. WEINER, L. P., HERNDON, R. M., NARAYAN, O., JOHNSON, R. T., SHAH, K., RUBINSTEIN, L. J., PREZIOSI, T. J., AND CONLEY, F. K., Isolation of virus related to SV-40 from patients with progressive multifocal leukoencephalopathy, *N. Engl. J. Med.* **286**:385–390 (1972).

81. WEINER, L. P., NARAYAN, O., PENNEY, J. B., JR., HERN-DON, R. M., FERINGA, E. R., TOURTELLOTTE, W. W., AND JOHNSON, R. T., Papovavirus of JC type in progressive multifocal leukoencephalopathy, *Arch. Neurol.* **29**:1–3 (1973).

82. WHITAKER, J. N., SEVER, J. L., AND ENGEL, W. K., Subacute sclerosing panencephalitis in only one of identical twins, *N. Engl. J. Med.* **287**:864–866 (1972).

83. ZU RHEIN, G. M., Association of papova-virions with a human demyelinating disease (progressive multifocal leukoencephalopathy), *Prog. Med. Virol.* **11**:185–247 (1969).

84. ZU RHEIN, G., AND VARAKIS, J., Progressive multifocal leucoencephalopathy in a renal allograft regiment, *N. Engl. J. Med.* **291**:798 (1974).

85. ZU RHEIN, G. M., PADGETT, B. L., WALKER, D. L., CHUN, R. W. M., HOROWITZ, S. D., AND HONG, R., Letter to the editor: Progressive multifocal leukoencephalopathy in a child with severe combined immunodeficiency, *N. Engl. J. Med.* **299**:256–257 (1978).

9. Suggested Reading

GAJDUSEK, D. C., Kuru and Creutzfeldt–Jakob disease: Experimental models of non-inflammatory degenerative slow virus disease of the central nervous system, *Ann. Clin. Res.* **5**:254–261 (1973).

GAJDUSEK, D. C., Kuru in the New Guinea highlands, in: *Tropical Neurology*, Vol. 29 (J. D. SPILLANE, ed.), pp. 376–383, Oxford University Press, London, 1973.

GAJDUSEK, D. C., Unconventional viruses and the origin and disappearance of kuru, *Science* **197**:943–960 (1977).

GAJDUSEK, D. C., Slow infections with unconventional viruses, *Harvey Lect.* **72**:283–353 (1978).

GAJDUSEK, D. C., AND GIBBS, C. J., JR., Familial and sporadic chronic neurological degenerative disorders transmitted from man to primates, in: *Advances in Neurology*, Vol. 10, *Primate Models of Neurological Disorders* (B. S. MELDRUM AND C. D. MARSDEN, eds.), pp. 291–375, Raven Press, New York, 1975.

GIBBS, C. J., JR., AND GAJDUSEK, D. C., Transmission and characterization of the agents of spongiform virus encephalopathies, kuru, Creutzfeldt–Jakob disease, scrapie and mink encephalopathy, in: *Immunological Disorders of the Nervous System*, Vol. XLIX (L. P. ROWLAND, ed.), Res. Publ. A.R.N.M.D., pp. 383–410, Williams and Wilkins, Baltimore, 1971.

GIBBS, C. J., JR., AND GAJDUSEK, D. C., Atypical viruses as the cause of sporadic, epidemic, and familial chronic diseases in man, in: *Slow Viruses and Human Diseases*, Vol. 10, *Perspectives in Virology* (M. POLLARD, ed.), pp. 161–198, Raven Press, New York, 1978.

GIBBS, C. J., JR., GAJDUSEK, D. C., AND AMYX, H. L., Strain variation in the viruses of Creutzfeldt–Jakob disease and kuru, in: *Slow Transmissible Diseases of the Nervous System*, Vol. 2 (S. B. PRUSINER AND W. J. HADLOW, eds.), pp. 87–110, Academic Press, New York, 1979.

MASTERS, C. L., HARRIS, J. O., GAJDUSEK, D. C., GIBBS, C. J., JR., BERNOULLI, C., AND ASHER, D. M., Creutzfeldt–Jakob disease: Patterns of worldwide occurrence and the significance of familial and sporadic clustering, *Ann. Neurol.* **5:**177–188 (1979).

NARAYAN, O., PENNY, J. B., JOHNSON, R. T., HERNDON, R. M., AND WEINER, L. P., Etiology of progressive multifocal leucoencephalopathy: Identification of papovavirus, *N. Engl. J. Med.* **289(14):**1278–1282 (1973).

PRUSINER, S. B., AND HADLOW, W. J. (eds.), *Slow Transmissible Diseases of the Nervous System*, Vol. 1, *Clinical, Epidemiological, Genetic, and Pathological Aspects of the Spongiform Encephalopathies*, Academic Press, New York, 1979, 472 pp.

WALKER, D. L., Progressive multifocal leukoencephalopathy: An opportunistic viral infection of the central nervous system, in: *Handbook of Clinical Neurology*, Vol. 34, *Infections of the Nervous System* (P. J. VINKEN AND G. W. BRUYN, eds.), pp. 307–329, Elsevier/North-Holland, New York, 1978.

WEINER, L. P., JOHNSON, R. T., AND HERDON, R. M., Viral infections and demyelinating diseases, *N. Engl. J. Med.* **288:**1103–1110 (1973).

ZU RHEIN, G. M., Association of papova-virions with a human demyelinating disease (progressive multifocal leucoencephalopathy), *Prog. Med. Virol.* **11:**185–247 (1969).

Index

Printed by Books on Demand, Germany